ACSM's Advanced Exercise Physiology

Second Edition

Wolters Kluwer | Lippincott Williams & Wilkins
Health

Philadelphia · Baltimore · New York · London
Buenos Aires · Hong Kong · Sydney · Tokyo

AMERICAN COLLEGE
of SPORTS MEDICINE
w w w . a c s m . o r g

Acquisitions Editor: Emily Lupash
Product Manager: Andrea Klingler
Marketing Manager: Christen Murphy
Designer: Doug Smock
Compositor: Absolute Service, Inc.

Second Edition

Copyright © 2012 American College of Sports Medicine

351 West Camden Street   Two Commerce Square
Baltimore, MD 21201   2001 Market Street
                                Philadelphia, PA 19103

Printed in China

9 8 7 6 5 4 3 2 1

Library of Congress Cataloging-in-Publication Data

ACSM's advanced exercise physiology. — 2nd ed.
   p. ; cm.
 Advanced exercise physiology / editors, Peter A. Farrell, Michael Joyner, Vincent Caiozzo.
 Includes bibliographical references and index.
 ISBN 978-0-7817-9780-1 (alk. paper)
 1. Exercise—Physiological aspects. I. Farrell, Peter A. II. Joyner, Michael J. III. Caiozzo, Vincent. IV. American College of Sports Medicine. V. Title: Advanced exercise physiology / editors, Peter A. Farrell, Michael Joyner, Vincent Caiozzo.
 [DNLM: 1. Exercise—physiology. WE 103]
 QP309.A83 2012
 612'.044—dc23

2011023733

DISCLAIMER

Care has been taken to confirm the accuracy of the information present and to describe generally accepted practices. However, the authors, editors, and publisher are not responsible for errors or omissions or for any consequences from application of the information in this book and make no warranty, expressed or implied, with respect to the currency, completeness, or accuracy of the contents of the publication. Application of this information in a particular situation remains the professional responsibility of the practitioner; the clinical treatments described and recommended may not be considered absolute and universal recommendations.

The authors, editors, and publisher have exerted every effort to ensure that drug selection and dosage set forth in this text are in accordance with the current recommendations and practice at the time of publication. However, in view of ongoing research, changes in government regulations, and the constant flow of information relating to drug therapy and drug reactions, the reader is urged to check the package insert for each drug for any change in indications and dosage and for added warnings and precautions. This is particularly important when the recommended agent is a new or infrequently employed drug.

Some drugs and medical devices presented in this publication have Food and Drug Administration (FDA) clearance for limited use in restricted research settings. It is the responsibility of the health care providers to ascertain the FDA status of each drug or device planned for use in their clinical practice.

To purchase additional copies of this book, call our customer service department at (800) 638-3030 or fax orders to (301) 223-2320. International customers should call (301) 223-2300.

Visit Lippincott Williams & Wilkins on the Internet: http://www.lww.com. Lippincott Williams & Wilkins customer service representatives are available from 8:30 AM to 6:00 PM, EST.

CCS0811

EDITORS

Peter A. Farrell, PhD, FACSM
Department of Kinesiology
East Carolina University
Greenville, NC

Michael J. Joyner, MD, FACSM
Department of Anesthesiology
Mayo Clinic
Rochester, MN

Vincent J. Caiozzo, PhD, FACSM
Departments of Orthopaedic Surgery and
    Physiology and Biophysics
College of Medicine
University of California
Irvine, CA

PREFACE

Exercise physiology is similar to other disciplines that have matured not only through an exponential expansion of the literature but also in the need for researchers to specialize in particular systems or functions. This need to specialize, however, poses a fundamental challenge in the education of the next generation of exercise physiologists: there remains a need for an advanced understanding of all systems because of the simple fact that each of the body systems interacts with and, in many cases, regulates other systems. It seems quite unlikely that even talented younger students could read a journal article about specifics of frequency modulation of motor units and come away with a satisfying understanding of data being presented in a primary literature paper.

The American College of Sports Medicine's (ACSM's) *Advanced Exercise Physiology, Second Edition*, bridges the gap between that basic understanding of physiology during exercise (knowledge gained in an introductory course on exercise physiology) and information presented through the primary literature in high-quality journals. The chapters are written by authorities in most of the major areas of investigation in exercise physiology, and the content in this edition has been updated to include the latest facts and concepts available to authorities in the field. Each chapter presents a detailed summary of facts and solidifying concepts necessary for students to embrace before they can understand the specifics in the primary literature.

The chapters provide an in-depth summary of how each system functions and is regulated during the physiological stress of exercise. Our goal in this second edition was to take advantage of the fact that all of the authors are the scientists that a graduate student should seek out when they have a need for detailed information and understanding in the various areas. We have anticipated those needs and have reorganized the chapters so that the major points have been highlighted and presented in terms that a typical graduate/upper-level undergraduate student in exercise physiology could comprehend.

Organization

Students normally seek graduate programs whose faculty has expertise in specific areas of exercise physiology. Unfortunately, most graduate programs do not have sufficient breadth of faculty expertise to teach all the areas included in this textbook. Information in all chapters is at a level that, once understood, will assure that students possess up-to-date, coherent, and accurate information at an advanced level.

This second edition of *Advanced Exercise Physiology* has been reorganized so that each chapter is presented in a similar manner, which makes the information flow more comprehensibly for students. Though the chapters continue to center on specific topics, the second edition cross-references points made that involve concepts/facts pertinent to more than one chapter. This approach emphasizes the fundamental appreciation that no physiological system functions in isolation especially during exercise.

ACSM's Advanced Exercise Physiology, Second Edition, begins with an introductory chapter on the history of exercise physiology that provides excellent insights into how the science of exercise physiology developed through a combination of medicine and, at first, preparation for war or fighting and then physical performance in the Olympics and international competitions. Subsequent chapters discuss specific systems such as nervous system control of movement, muscle architecture, force generation, and, when these processes fail, the fatigue process. Perhaps the most extensive single chapter is Chapter 8, "The Respiratory System," which presents a detailed description of respiratory function and the known causes for increased ventilation during exercise, as well as other aspects of lung function. Extensive coverage of the cardiovascular system is provided in three chapters (Chapters 9–11) that discuss the structure of the cardiovascular system, heart function, and circulatory control at the level of the microcirculation.

An extensive section on metabolism begins with a review of how the gastrointestinal system functions to deliver nutrients before, during, and after exercise and its role in maintaining acid–base, electrolyte, and water balance during exercise (Chapter 12). Because of the importance of providing fuels during exercise, six chapters (Chapters 13–18) are devoted to carbohydrate, fat, and protein metabolism during exercise and in response to regular exercise training. Chapter 19, "The Endocrine System: Integrated Influences on Metabolism, Growth, and Reproduction," provides coverage of many hormonal regulators that control several systems described in other chapters, as well as exercise metabolism. An additional strength of this chapter is the coverage of endocrine changes that alter reproductive function, with a primary, but not exclusive, emphasis on women. The chapter on immunology provides the latest information on how the immune system responds to exercise and equally important how the immune system interacts with exercise metabolism. This chapter also reviews literature supporting the concept of muscle being an endocrine organ. This section of the book culminates with a discussion on body fluid control mechanisms during exercise and includes the renal system (Chapters 20–22).

The final section of the book centers on how environmental factors influence many of the regulatory mechanisms discussed in the previous chapters. Separate chapters discuss heat, cold, hypoxia, hyperbaria, and exercise in space. Chapter 27 is quite futuristic in nature; it covers exercise genomics and proteomics from the perspective of how modern techniques can be used to better understand how exercise alters gene expression and more.

Features

New additions to the chapters include **Key Points**, which highlight the most important concepts or facts, and section **Summaries**, which provide brief synopses of key sections. We also include **Test Yourself** questions, which appear throughout the chapters and will require students to use critical thinking skills to discuss hypotheses and how the information they have learned relates to practical applications. We are hopeful these questions also will help to stimulate class or group discussions.

Additional Resources

ACSM's Advanced Exercise Physiology, Second Edition, includes additional resources for both instructors and students that are available on the book's companion website at http://thepoint.lww.com/ACSMAdvExPhys2e.

Instructors

- Image bank
- PowerPoint lecture outlines
- WebCT/Blackboard/Angel LMS cartridge

Students

- Full text online
- Interactive quiz bank
- Animations

In addition, purchasers of the text can access the searchable full text through the book's website. See the front inside cover of this text for more details and include the passcode to gain access to the website.

Peter Farrell
Mike Joyner
Vince Caiozzo

CONTRIBUTORS

Charles Tipton, PhD
Department of Physiology
University of Arizona
Tucson, AZ
Chapter 1

V. Reggie Edgerton, PhD
Department of Integrative Biology and Physiology
Department of Neurobiology
Brain Research Institute
University of California, Los Angeles
Los Angeles, CA
Chapter 2

Roland R. Roy, PhD, FACSM
Department of Integrative Biology and Physiology
Brain Research Institute
University of California, Los Angeles
Los Angeles, CA
Chapter 2

Ronald F. Zernicke, PhD, DSc, FACSM
School of Kinesiology
Departments of Orthopaedic Surgery and Biomedical
   Engineering
University of Michigan
Ann Arbor, MI
Chapter 3

Gregory R. Wohl, PhD, PEng
Department of Mechanical Engineering
McMaster University
Hamilton, Ontario, Canada
Chapter 3

Jeremy M. LaMothe, MD, PhD
Department of Surgery
University of Calgary
Calgary, Alberta, Canada
Chapter 3

Vincent J. Caiozzo, PhD
Departments of Orthopaedic Surgery and Physiology
   and Biophysics
College of Medicine
University of California
Irvine, CA
Chapter 4

Richard Tsika, PhD
Department of Biomedical Sciences
University of Missouri
Columbia, MO
Chapter 5

Robert H. Fitts, PhD
Department of Biological Sciences
Marquette University
Milwaukee, WI
Chapter 6

Douglas R. Seals, PhD
Department of Integrative Physiology
University of Colorado at Boulder
Boulder, CO
Chapter 7

Lee M. Romer, PhD, FACSM
Reader (Human and Applied Physiology)
Centre for Sports Medicine and Human Performance
Brunel University
Uxbridge Middlesex, UK
Chapter 8

A. William Sheel, PhD
School of Human Kinetics
University of British Columbia
Vancouver, British Columbia, Canada
Chapter 8

Craig A. Harms, PhD, FACSM
Department of Kinesiology
Kansas State University
Manhattan, KS
Chapter 8

Donal S. O'Leary, PhD
Department of Physiology
Wayne State University
School of Medicine
Detroit, MI
Chapter 9

Patrick J. Mueller, PhD
Department of Physiology
Wayne State University School of Medicine
Detroit, MI
Chapter 9

Javier A. Sala-Mercado, MD, PhD
Department of Physiology
Cardiovascular Research Institute
Wayne State University, School of Medicine
Detroit, MI
Chapter 9

Russell L. Moore, PhD
Department of Integrative Physiology
University of Colorado at Boulder
Boulder, CO
Chapter 10

David A. Brown, PhD
Department of Physiology
East Carolina University
Greenville, NC
Chapter 10

Steven S. Segal, PhD, FACSM
Department of Medical Pharmacology and Physiology
University of Missouri–Columbia
Columbia, MO
Chapter 11

Shawn E. Bearden, PhD, FAHA
Department of Biological Sciences
Biomedical Research Institute
Idaho State University
Pocatello, ID
Chapter 11

G. Patrick Lambert, PhD
Department of Exercise Science
Creighton University
Omaha, NE
Chapter 12

Xiaocai Shi, PhD, FACSM
Gatorade Sports Science Institute
Barrington, IL
Chapter 12

Robert Murray, PhD, FACSM
Sports Science Insights, LLC
Crystal Lake, IL
Chapter 12

Ronald A. Meyer, PhD
Departments of Physiology and Radiology
Michigan State University
East Lansing, MI
Chapter 13

Robert W. Wiseman, PhD
Departments of Physiology and Radiology
Michigan State University
East Lansing, MI
Chapter 13

Mark Hargreaves, PhD
Department of Physiology
University of Melbourne
Melbourne, Australia
Chapter 14

Lawrence L. Spriet, PhD
Department of Human Health and Nutritional Sciences
University of Guelph
Guelph, Ontario, Canada
Chapters 15 and 16

Graham P. Holloway, PhD
Department of Human Health and Nutritional Sciences
University of Guelph
Guelph, Ontario, Canada
Chapter 16

Anton J. M. Wagenmakers, PhD
School of Sport and Exercise Sciences
University of Birmingham
Birmingham, United Kingdom
Chapter 17

David A. Hood, PhD
School of Kinesiology and Health Science
Muscle Health Research Centre
York University
Toronto, Ontario, Canada
Chapter 18

Michael F. N. O'Leary, PhD
School of Kinesiology and Health Science
Muscle Health Research Centre
York University
Toronto, Ontario, Canada
Chapter 18

Giulia Uguccioni, PhD
School of Kinesiology and Health Science
Muscle Health Research Centre
York University
Toronto, Ontario, Canada
Chapter 18

Isabella Irrcher, PhD
Department of Ophthalmology
Queen's University
Kingston, Ontario, Canada
Chapter 18

Anne B. Loucks, PhD
Department of Biological Sciences
Ohio University
Athens, OH
Chapter 19

Laurie Hoffman-Goetz, PhD, MPH, FACSM
Department of Health Studies and Gerontology
University of Waterloo
Waterloo, Ontario, Canada
Chapter 20

Bente Klarlund Pedersen, MD, DrSc
The Centre of Inflammation and Metabolism
Faculty of Health Sciences
University of Copenhagen
Rigshospitalet
Copenhagen, Denmark
Chapter 20

Gary W. Mack, PhD
Department of Exercise Sciences
Brigham Young University
Provo, UT
Chapter 21

Edward J. Zambraski, PhD
Military Performance Division
U.S. Army Research Institute of Environmental Medicine
Natick, MA
Chapter 22

Michael N. Sawka, PhD
Thermal and Mountain Medicine Division
U.S. Army Research Institute of Environmental Medicine
Natick, MA
Chapter 23

John W. Castellani, PhD
Thermal & Mountain Medicine Division
U.S. Army Research Institute of Environmental Medicine
Natick, MA
Chapter 23

Samuel N. Cheuvront, PhD, RD
Thermal and Mountain Medicine Division
U.S. Army Research Institute of Environmental Medicine
Natick, MA
Chapter 23

Andrew J. Young, PhD
Military Nutrition Division
U.S. Army Research Institute of Environmental Medicine
Natick, MA
Chapter 23

Carsten Lundby, PhD
The Copenhagen Muscle Research Center
Rigshospitalet
Copenhagen, Denmark
Chapter 24

John R. Claybaugh, PhD
Department of Clinical Investigation
Tripler Army Medical Center
Tripler AMC, HI
Chapter 25

Keizo Shiraki, MD, PhD
Department of Physiology
University of Occupational and Environmental Health
Kitakyushu, Japan
Chapter 25

Robert Elsner, PhD
Institute of Marine Science
University of Alaska
Fairbanks, AK
Chapter 25

Yu-Chong Lin, PhD
Department of Physiology
John A. Burns School of Medicine
University of Hawaii
Honolulu, HI
Chapter 25

Suzanne M. Schneider, PhD
Department of Exercise Science
University of New Mexico
Albuquerque, NM
Chapter 26

Victor A. Convertino, PhD
U.S. Army Institute for Surgical Research
Fort Sam Houston, TX
Chapter 26

Frank W. Booth, PhD
Department of Physiology
School of Medicine
University of Missouri
Columbia, MO
Chapter 27

P. Darrell Neufer, PhD
Departments of Exercise and Sport Science and
  Physiology
East Carolina Diabetes and Obesity Institute
East Carolina University
Greenville, NC
Chapter 27

REVIEWERS

Kenneth Beck, PhD
KC Beck Physiological Consulting, LLC
Saint Paul, MN

Sue Beckham, PhD, FACSM
Cooper Institute for Aerobic Research
Dallas, TX

Phillip A. Bishop, EdD
Department of Kinesiology
University of Alabama
Tuscaloosa, AL

Marvin Boluyt, PhD
Washtenaw Community College
Ann Arbor, MI

Randy W. Bryner, EdD
Department of Human Performance/Exercise Physiology
West Virginia University
Morgantown, WV

J. Richard Coast, PhD, FACSM
Department of Biological Sciences
Northern Arizona University
Flagstaff, AZ

Carol Ewing Garber, PhD, FAHA, FACSM
Department of Biobehavioral Sciences (Program in
    Movement Sciences)
Teachers College, Columbia University
New York, NY

Bill Farquhar, PhD
Department of Kinesiology and Applied Physiology
University of Delaware
Newark, DE

Marty Gibala, PhD
Department of Biological Sciences
McMaster University
Hamilton, Ontario, Canada

Ellen Glickman, PhD, FACSM
Exercise Science Laboratory
Kent State University
Kent, OH

Allan Goldfarb, PhD, FACSM
Department of Kinesiology
University of North Carolina
Greensboro, NC

Jose Gonzalez-Alonso, PhD
Center for Sports Medicine and Human Performance
Brunel University
Uxbridge, Middlesex, United Kingdom

Lisa Griffin, PhD
The University of Texas at Austin
Austin, Texas

John Hawley, PhD
School of Medical Sciences
RMIT University
Victoria, Australia

Vineet B. Johnson, BPT, PGDip(PT), MSc, PhD(c)
Department of Human Kinetics
Capilano University
North Vancouver, British Columbia, Canada

Jill Kanaley, PhD, FACSM
Department of Nutrition and Exercise Physiology
University of Missouri
Columbia, MO

David Leehey, MD
Oak Park, IL

Raymond W. Leung, PhD
Department of Physical Education and Exercise Science
Brooklyn College of the City University of New York
Brooklyn, NY

Mark Loftin, PhD, FACSM
Department of Health, Exercise Science, and Recreation
    Management
University of Mississippi
University, MS

Kevin McCully, PhD, FACSM
Department of Kinesiology
University of Georgia
Athens, GA

Sheri A. Melton, PhD, Fulbright-Nehru Scholar
Department of Kinesiology
West Chester University of Pennsylvania
West Chester, PA

Joel Mitchell, PhD
Department of Kinesiology
Texas Christian University
Fort Worth, TX

David Nieman, DrPH, FACSM
Appalachian State University
Weaverville, NC

François Péronnet, PhD, FACSM
Department of Kinesiology
University of Montreal
Montreal, Canada

Stuart Phillips, PhD, FACSM
Department of Kinesiology
McMaster University
Hamilton, Ontario, Canada

Christian K. Roberts, PhD
School of Nursing
University of California, Los Angeles
Los Angeles, CA

R. Andrew Shanely, PhD
Appalachian State University
Kannapolis, NC

Michael Smith, PhD, FACSM
Department of Integrative Physiology
University of North Texas Health Science Center
Fort Worth, TX

Joseph Starnes, PhD, FACSM
University of North Carolina at Greensboro
Department of Kinesiology
Greensboro, NC

Trent Stellingwerff, PhD
Department of Nutrition and Health
Nestlé Research Centre
Lausanne, Switzerland

Hirofumi Tanaka, PhD, FACSM
Department of Kinesiology
University of Texas at Austin
Austin, TX

Stuart Warden, PhD, FACSM
Department of Physical Therapy
Indiana University
Indianapolis, IN

Jason B. Winchester, PhD, CSCS, USAW
Department of Kinesiology, Leisure, and Sports Sciences
East Tennessee State University
Johnson City, TN

ACKNOWLEDGMENTS

We would like to thank and acknowledge the editors of the first edition of this book: Dr. Charles Tipton, senior editor; and Drs. Michael Sawka, Charlotte Tate, and Ronald Terjung, section editors. The previous edition provided a wonderful foundation for students in all of the major areas of exercise physiology. We gratefully acknowledge the individual authors who gave graciously of their time for one purpose: providing an excellent resource to our next generation of exercise physiologists.

CONTENTS

CHAPTER 1

Historical Perspective: Origin to Recognition

Charles M. Tipton

INTRODUCTION

In prehistoric times, exercise was a way of life and essential for existence. However, this role changed when humans became "civilized" and began to develop the various cultures within different geographical regions of the world. Regardless of the culture involved, two important reasons for a "role change" were the incidence of diseases and an evolving concept of health.

In 1542, the French physician and astronomer Jean Fernel (1497–1558) introduced the term *physiology* to explain bodily function (1) and, more than 300 years later, the words *physiology* and *exercise* were first included in a scientific publication by William H. Byford (2). Readers should realize that the word physiology is derived from the Greek term *physis*, which means nature, and is used by both Hippocrates and Galen as meaning a natural state or the functioning of an organism as a whole (3). Implicit with its use by the Greek philosophers and physicians was the concept that a living organism, under natural conditions, acted primarily as an intact unit, whereas the actions of its parts were subordinate to a supreme function. Hence, the more an organism functioned as a whole, the healthier it became. However, the more the parts of the organism began to function independently of a supreme function, the more unhealthy the organism became (3). Thus, an important linkage of physiology with antiquity (the time period that ended with the death of Galen) was the belief that health existed when disease was absent (4). This ancient view persisted until the beginning of the twentieth century. The intriguing feature of antiquity is how the physiologic effects of exercise became regarded and accepted as being conducive to health.

The purposes of this chapter are to provide a historical background for the idea that exercise is important for one's health status and to identify the beliefs, observations, and findings of ancient and early investigators on the acute and chronic effects of exercise that evolved into physiologic concepts that were occurring with the emergence and subsequent recognition of exercise physiology as a scientific discipline. Keep in mind that, for a discipline to be recognized, a critical body of knowledge and subject matter must be available and sufficiently well organized to be presented as a formal course of learning in an educational environment (5). In addition, an acknowledged reference text must be available such as the one by Brainbridge (6).

Contribution from the River Civilizations

Overview

Ancient humans migrated, via exercise, from Central Africa to the banks of the Tigris, Euphrates, Nile, Indus, and Yellow rivers where the earliest civilizations were established (4). Although all made significant and distinctive contributions to the emergence of culture and its customs including sporting activities, only those settlements near the Indus and Yellow rivers made contributions to exercise physiology (4).

The Indus River Civilization of India

Archeologic excavations in the Indus Valley during the 1920s revealed the existence of an ancient Indus civilization that authorities believe existed earlier than a carbon dated value of 3300 BC and were contemporaries with the civilizations in Mesopotamia, Egypt, and China (4,7). The excavations indicated a culture that was focused on personal hygiene, public health, and sanitation while experiencing myriad diseases that included arteriosclerosis,

1

osteomyelitis, cancer, metal poisoning, and so forth. The excavations also discovered statues with positions that suggested yoga movements were being performed.

Several millennia later, or during 1500 BC, the interest in health and sanitation prevailed as demonstrated within the oldest literature in the world; namely, the 1028 hymns of the Rgveda (Rig-Veda) (8). However, when disease occurred, it was the result of evil spirits that originated from the anger or disposition of gods and goddesses or from a "spell" from a living or deceased enemy. Moreover, when health was mentioned, it was at the pleasure of the gods and had little relevance to the recovery process (9).

Between 1500 and 800 BC, unidentified philosophers and physicians formulated the Tridosa (also listed as the Tridhatu) doctrine (10), which helped to explain the relationships between disease and health or life and death (10,11). The doctrine indicated the elements of water, fire, earth, and ether were responsible for the formation of the human body. These elements interacted with three nutrient substances (derivatives of the wind, sun, and moon), which subsequently became transformed into dosas (humors) of air, bile, and phlegm, which were called vayu, pitta, and kapha, respectively (11). Later, blood was added as the fourth dosa (11). Physiologically, vayu was responsible for movement, activation or response systems (sympathetic nervous system), maintenance of the vital breath, enhancement of digestion, movement of chyle and blood throughout the body, and to sustain life. Pitta promoted the formation of colored pigments from the liver and spleen, enhanced metabolism, increased heat production, and aided fluid movement to and from the heart (10,11), whereas kapha promoted growth, transported body fluids throughout the body, bathed sense organs with fluids, and improved strength, endurance, and the "*healthy functioning of the body*" (8, Vol. I, p. 12).

TEST YOURSELF

What were the contributions to exercise physiology from the Indus River civilization?

As a note to the historical argument between Indian and Greek scholars as to the origin of the humoral theory, the Rgveda contains a hymn that directs the Aswins (twin gods of medicine) to "*preserve the well being of the three humors*" (8, Vol. I, p. 95).

Intrinsic to the Tridosa doctrine were the concepts that (a) vayu, pitta, and kapha dosas controlled and regulated all functions of the body; (b) dosas did not increase or decrease spontaneously—rather, they had to be displaced or deranged; and (c) that disease occurred when they were displaced and health prevailed when they were in equilibrium (10–12). Besides disease, conditions that could modify the equilibrium between the various dosas were climate, food, poisons, mental disturbances, sedentary living, fatigue, and exercise (11,12).

TEST YOURSELF

Why are the Tridosa doctrine and the humoral theory of importance to the history of exercise physiology?

The Legacy of Susruta (Sushruta)

Although Susruta's existence and era have elements of mythology and controversy, he (Fig. 1.1) is regarded as an authentic Indian physician who taught surgery and medicine at the university in Benares during 600 BC (13). Not only is he revered for his contributions to the establishment of medicine and surgery and for his samhitas on medicine in India (12,14,15), he is acclaimed for his contributions to ophthalmology (16) and urology (17).

Susruta accepted the ancient concept of the elements and was a strong advocate of the Tridosa doctrine. He was convinced a sedentary lifestyle of inactivity coupled with protracted periods of sleeping and excessive food and fluid consumption would elevate the kapha dosa to the extent that it would disrupt the equilibrium among the dosas and result in a disease state. Consequently, he recommended exercise in his recommendations to prevent the occurrence of kapha diseases (12–14). He also recommended exercise for conditions of obesity because it was caused by an increase in the vayu dosa associated with lymph chyle. On the other hand, he noted vayu could be "deranged by hard work, carrying heavy loads, and by violent movements" (11). Seldom mentioned in the diabetic literature is the fact that Susruta was the first physician to recommend exercise for

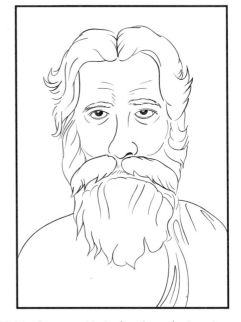

FIGURE 1.1   Susruta of India (ca. 600 BC) who advocated exercise to establish an equilibrium between the dosas. (With permission from Sharma PV. *Ayurveda*. Varansai: Chaukhambha Orientalia; 1975:41.)

individuals with diabetes, which was classified as a disease of the urinary tract (12). Not to be ignored is his belief that excessive exercise could result in coughing, fever, and vomiting and lead to diseases as consumption, tuberculosis, asthma, and potentially death (12).

Exercise was defined as a "sense of weariness from bodily labour and it should be taken every day" (12, p. 485) and included walking, running, jumping, swimming, diving, or riding an elephant as well as participating in activities such as archery, wrestling, and javelin throwing (12). He was the first physician to prescribe exercise and felt it should be moderate in intensity, or to the extent that would elicit labored breathing, but never excessive because it could lead to death. Before exercise was prescribed, the age, strength, physique, and diet had to be considered as did the season and the terrain (12).

Susruta also promoted moderate exercise because it promoted the growth of limbs; enhanced muscle mass (stoutness), strength, endurance, tautness (tone), and resistance against fatigue; reduced corpulence; improved digestion; elevated body temperature and thirst; improved appearances; and promoted mental alertness, memory, and "keen intelligence" (12).

The Legacy of Caraka (Charaka)

Equally renowned in India for his ancient writings and contributions to medicine is Caraka (Fig. 1.2), whose accomplishments in medicine are well accepted although uncertainty prevails concerning his era. Using the research employed to

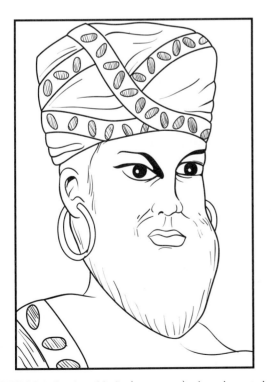

FIGURE 1.2 Caraka of India (ca. 200 BC) who advocated exercise to cure diabetes. (With permission from Bahita SL. *A History of Medicine with Special Reference to the Orient.* New Delhi: Office of the Medical Council of India; 1977:17.)

discern the period of Susruta, his era has been determined to be associated with 200 BC (13).

Careful examination of his Samhita (18, p. 39) indicates views similar to Susruta specifically, "*the disturbance of the equilibrium of tissue elements is the disease while the maintenance of equilibrium is health.*" In addition, he advocated moderate exercise, recommended activity to alleviate dosas, "especially kapha" (18, p. 152), and felt exercise would cure diabetes (19). He cautioned that excessive exercise could result in dyspnea, heart, and gastrointestinal diseases, and bleeding organs. Lastly, he wrote that chronic exercise would inhibit the heart, increase work capacity, result in leanness, and minimize discomfort while enhancing digestion, perspiration, and respiration (18).

The Yellow River Civilization of China

According to the medical historian Bhatia (9), between the Shang Empire (ca. 1800–1000 BC) and the installation of emperors (221 BC), the health of the ancient Chinese was essentially determined by a culture of gods, demons, devils, and spirits. Disease was the result of demons and devils that possessed the body and their removal required incantations, charms, and offerings. When cures or recovery occurred, they were attributed to the presence of supernatural forces.

Within the Shang empire, disease was attributed to a curse from an ancestor or with punishment for a sin previously committed which required prayers, incantations, divination, and herb therapy. For select diseases, rhythmical breathing exercises with arm movements were advocated with cures expected in several months (20,21). However, there are no records of exercise being promoted for other diseases or disorders. The Chou dynasty (1050–256 BC) followed the demise of the Shang empire and is associated with the doctrine of the five elements, the religion of Taoism, and the Yin-Yang doctrine.

In contrasts to the views of the inhabitants of the Indus River Valley, ancient Chinese believed the human body consisted of ratios between the elements of metal, wood, water, fire, and earth, whose union produced life whereas their separation meant death (9). When the ratios were in equilibrium, an individual was regarded as healthy but, if they were "deranged," he or she was at risk of acquiring a disease (9).

To achieve immortality and to live a longer life, ancient Chinese who followed "the way of Tao" were instructed to perform deep breathing exercise in order to eliminate the "bad air" from the body. There is no record of other exercises being advocated for this purpose. As noted, the Yin-Yang doctrine emerged during the Chou dynasty. Accordingly, the universe was not created by divine action but by a self-generated process of nature that operated on the dualistic principles of yin and yang which meant "*the principle of Yin and Yang is the basis of the entire universe. It is the principle of everything in creation. It brings about the transformation to parenthood; it is the root and source of life and death*" (22). Consequently, all animate and inanimate objects plus circumstances and phenomena were a combination of these principles with the human body consisting of three parts of yin and three parts of yang. Yang was associated with health and life, whereas yin was identified with disease and death (22).

The Legacy of Hua T'o (Hua Tuo)

During the Eastern Han dynasty (25–220 AD) and at the time of Galen's death, Hua T'o's surgical skills earned him the distinction of being China's first surgeon (Fig. 1.3). He promoted exercise for its yang effect and reportedly told his disciples: *"The body needs exercise, only it must not to the point of exhaustion for exercise expels the bad air in the system, promotes the free circulation of the blood, and prevents sickness"* (23, p. 54). Besides health, he promoted exercise to strengthen legs, provide a lightness to the body, enhance digestion, and to decrease old age. Like his counterparts in India, he was against performing excessive exercise because of its harmful effects. To achieve the effects of exercise, he advocated performing movements (frolics) that were similar to those performed by deers, tigers, bears, monkeys, and birds.

The "frolic movements" attributed to Hua T'o have similarities to the descriptions of the Daoyin Tu movements and drawings from the Mawangdui medical manuscripts

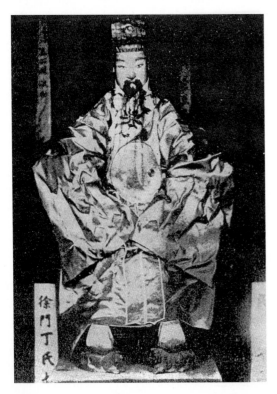

FIGURE 1.3 Hua T'o of China (ca. 25–220 AD) who advocated exercise to promote health and to prevent sickness.

of the Hunan province associated with the era of circa 200 BC (24). Harper translations included terms as "bird stretch, chicken stretch, gibbon jumping, crane listening, bear climbing, and hawk prey" to describe the movements but indicated they were being performed for therapeutic purposes to minimize pains in the ribs, inguinal swelling, abdominal bloating, nape pain, and internal hotness (24).

Contributions from Greece

Overview

Ancient Greece is associated with the Minoan civilization (3000–1100 BC), the Mycenaean civilization (1550–1050 BC), and a Classical period (490–323 BC) (25). The inhabitants were collectively known as the Hellenes and representative of tribes with different dialects, customs, and social organizations who colonized the region by migration and invasions between 1300 and 1100 BC. The Dorians established the city-state of Sparta and the Ionians accomplished the same with Athens.

Like distant cultures, the Hellenic priests and physicians associated disease and illness with punishments from one or more deities while seeking protection, healing, and health from others. To Hellenes, Zeus was the supreme god; Athena was the daughter of Zeus with assorted healing powers; and Apollo was the son of Zeus who could inflict illness and cause natural death to males, whereas his sister Artemis had similar powers with females. When Asclepius became a deity, he was regarded as the physician god of healing and the son of Apollo. His daughters, Hygeia and Panacea, became goddesses of health and treatment, respectively (20).

Readers should realize that competitive athletic games were scheduled at Olympia between 1370 and 1140 BC, as well as during 776 BC (26). However, there is no meaningful information to indicate that advice on how to improve performance was available or given to any competitor. Homer (ca. 750 BC) provides considerable detail about the nature of the funeral games for Patroclus during the Trojan War (ca. 1250 BC); however, there are no passages devoted to training or methods of training (27).

The City-state of Sparta and Its Practices

The Dorians, who established Sparta, wanted an oligarchic form of government with a constitution and educational system with the primary purpose *"to maintain an army of experts who were ready and able at any moment to suppress sedition within the state or repel invasion from without"* (28, p. 165). In essence, the Spartan was to be a professional soldier with his education being directed toward achieving physical fitness and obeying authority. Like all Hellenes, they expected their gods to protect them from death and disease. Health was defined as being physically fit for the state and babies judged to be "unfit" were left to die at a site listed as Apothetae. Men were expected to be healthy warriors with women becoming mothers of healthy warriors. Participation in fitness activities and competitive athletics were expected of both genders and only in Sparta and Chios were women expected to compete against males in wrestling (29).

After the age of seven, children left their homes to live in barracks with others of their age group where they remained until adulthood and marriage. Although their education included arts, music, and gymnastics, the primary focus was on becoming a warrior state. The same is true for their emphasis in sports and competitive games. Although Olympic records indicated Spartans were frequent participants and victors, it is unknown how they prepared for competition. However, it is safe to assume frequency was high, intensity was heavy, and the duration was long (28,30). Other than their focus and dedication to fitness, the Spartans made little contributions to the substance and emergence of exercise physiology.

TEST YOURSELF

Contrast the contribution to exercise physiology from the city-states of Sparta and Athens.

The Emergence of Greek Physiologic Concepts

Thales (639–544 BC) founded a school at Miletus and taught water as the basic element in plant and animal life while also being the source for earth and air (31). Anaximander (611–547 BC) felt that all living creatures, including man, had their beginnings in water (32). Anaxagoras (500–428 BC) also believed that life arose from "the moist" but felt disease originated from bile before entering the blood vessels, lungs, and pleura (32). On the other hand, Anaximenes (610–545 BC) felt that air was divine and responsible for substance, motion, and life (32). Pythagoras (570–490 BC) established a school, laid the foundation for the element and quality components of the humoral theory, refused to accept the idea that gods were responsible for all evil and disease, and promoted the concepts that (a) all disease and bodily functions arose from dissolute behavior and (b) good health was a state of harmony (equilibrium) between the opposing elements, qualities, or tendencies. Moreover, he advocated long walks and participation in events such as running, wrestling, discus throwing, and boxing to achieve this harmony (33).

Alcmaeon (ca. 500 BC), a graduate of the Pythagorean school, proposed that health denoted a harmonious equilibrium between the qualities of wet, hot, dry, sweet, bitter, and so forth, with disease occurring with the dominance of any single quality. Furthermore, he felt diseases occurred with excesses or deficiencies of food and drink, increases in either heat or cold, phlegm from the head, both yellow and black bile from the blood, substances from the marrow, and personal hardship. He also believed that physical fatigue could result in disease (20).

Empedocles (504–443 BC), also a disciple of Pythagoras, championed the concept that the elements of fire, water, earth, and air (aether) were necessary for the formation of the human body and that transformation occurred between elements and qualities without origination or destruction (34).

With time, these transformations between elements and qualities became fluids known as humors with hot + wet = blood, hot + dry = yellow bile, cold + wet = phlegm, and cold + dry = black bile (34,35, p. 77). Around 440 BC, Philolaus proposed that changes in blood, bile, and phlegm were the causes for disease (36).

Gymnasiums, Panhellenic Games, and Trainers

Gymnasiums were dedicated to Apollo, existed before 600 BC in Sparta and Athens and were most prominent during the eras of Hippocrates and Plato (37). It was a public institution; contained stadiums; and provided instruction in music, grammar, and gymnastics (running, wrestling, boxing, throwing the javelin and discus, jumping) for affluent students up to 16 years of age (37). Gymnasiums also served as a discussion site for adults and sage elders and as a training site for gymnastic events (37). Physicians served as the director (gymnasiarch), subdirector (gymnast), and as iatroliptes whose duties were to prepare prescriptions, perform venesections, provide massages, reduce dislocations, and to advise trainers on the performance of gymnastic exercises in order to achieve a healthy body (38). Collectively, the gymnasium physicians were known to favor exercise over medical treatment to restore health (39). This was true for Herodicus of Selymbria (ca. 480 BC), who was the father of therapeutic gymnastics (40), prescribed complex exercises that required an understanding of geometry to perform them, and advised Hippocrates on prescribing exercise—he was criticized by Hippocrates and especially by Plato for advocating strenuous and dangerous exercises (41).

Professional trainers were available at the Panhellenic Games held in the Olympia Valley, with the fifth century games being their zenith. Many competitors trained in the stadiums associated with the gymnasiums. Although Hippocrates, Plato, and Galen had little respect for their advice because of the questionable knowledge they were imparting, trainers did advise athletes to use repetition, to incorporate overload to increase strength (bend rods of wrought iron, pull wagons with yoked animals, lift heavier boxes, stones, or animals), use halters with jumping events, chase animals to improve speed, throw heavier javelins, and to run in the sand and for long distances to improve endurance (42–44).

By the time of Galen, trainers were promoting a 4-day tetrad system which featured preparation, concentration, relaxation, and perfection. The first day the athlete was to perform numerous brief but intense exercise sessions that were to "prime" him for the next day's activities. The second day was to be devoted to maximum efforts, which would exhaust the athlete. On the third day, the athlete was to relax and enjoy a day of recreation, whereas on the fourth day, the intensity level was to be moderate while perfecting skill levels. It is of interest that, after Galen's death, this method of training was harshly criticized by Philostratus (170–247 AD) for its lack of flexibility and individuality (44).

The Legacy of Hippocrates

There are 76 books on Greek medicine that were written between 460–370 BC that have been collectively labeled as the Corpus Hippocraticum. All have been attributed to Hippocrates of Cos, although not all of them have been authenticated (Fig. 1.4) (45). Hence, readers should not become overly annoyed by the contradictions, redundancy, and confusion associated with his texts. However, there is no confusion about his being responsible for separating medicine from philosophy, religion, and magic, or the introduction of rational medicine, or being considered the father of scientific medicine (45–47).

He endorsed the concept that the human body represented the interaction of the elements and their qualities but felt that fire and water were the responsible ones (36). He wrote extensively on diseases, classified them into categories (acute, chronic, endemic, epidemic), and indicated how air, climate, seasons, water, sanitation, food and fluids, and excessive exercise impacted them (36,48). His articulation of humors and the necessity of achieving a "*balance*" (equilibrium) among them in order for health to be present and disease to be absent are likely the reasons he is credited as being the originator of the humoral theory

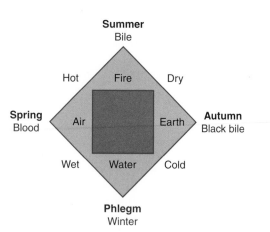

FIGURE 1.5   The components of the humoral theory attributed to Hippocrates. (With permission from Conrad LI, Neve M, Nutton V, Wear A. *The Western Medical Tradition*. Cambridge: Cambridge University Press; 1995:25.)

(Fig. 1.5) (48). Inherent with the discussion on humors is that Hippocrates believed that nature (*physis*) would heal disease and that acquiring an equilibrium was essential to achieve that state (health). It is of interest that Hippocrates advocated exercise so that the "*collected humor may grow warm, become thin, and purge itself away*" (48, p. 363). Thus, when consumption was diagnosed because of the single or collective actions of phlegm, blood, or bile, exercise was prescribed and included within the treatment regimen (49). In fact, Hippocrates should be acknowledged as the first physician to provide a detailed exercise prescription for his patients. He is also extensively acknowledged for his statements concerning disease. In the *Nature of Man* he states: "*Those due to exercise are cured by rest and those due to idleness are cured by exercise*" (36, p. 25).

When Hippocrates referred to exercise, he was relating to walking, running, wrestling, swinging the arms, push-ups, shadow boxing, and ball punching (50). When prescribed, the intensity was usually light or moderate, but seldom heavy or excessive as disease was expected to ensue. He believed air was essential for life, required the process of inspiration and expiration, and that breathing was increased with exercise. Moreover, the rapid breathing of exercise was one method to cool the "innate heat" within the heart. He advocated warming up and believed that running would cause the flesh to heat, concoct, and dissolve while enhancing digestion. Running would eliminate the "moisture of the body" and if "cloaked," would also make the skin "more moist." However, he never addressed the issue as to whether exercise would increase the innate heat of the body. Although the fatigue pains of acute exercise were acknowledged, he felt they could be alleviated by training (36,48,51). Hippocrates knew that muscles would atrophy after fractures and that exercise (walking) minimized the amount of tissue being lost (52). He attributed training for enhanced bone development, increased stature, improved muscle mass and tone (hardness), and improved athletic performance. He had a low opinion of athletes and, as noted earlier, little or no respect for trainers (36).

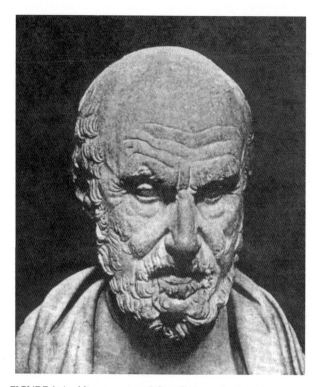

FIGURE 1.4   Hippocrates of Cos. Father of scientific medicine and regarded as the author of the humoral theory for which exercise was advocated to maintain its homeostatic balance. (From Singer S. *Greek Biology and Greek Medicine*. Oxford, UK: Oxford University Press; 1922:91.)

Other Contributors from the Hippocratic and Post-Hippocratic Era

Plato of Athens (427–347 BC), a brilliant philosopher and founder of the Academy, was a younger colleague of Hippocrates who believed it was necessary for the elements of the body to be in a definite order for health to exist. If they were in reverse order or deranged, disease would occur. In fact, if anything was judged to be unhealthy, it could lead to a disease state (53,54). He introduced the concept of a soul that existed in tripartite form—existing in the brain (reason = rational soul), within the heart (spirit = irrational soul), and the liver (desire = irrational soul). He also believed the body could affect the soul and emphasized the necessity of maintaining "due proportion" between the mind (soul) and body to promote health and prevent disease. To achieve this proportion, motion was required that included gymnastic activities (dancing, wrestling, walking, running, racing, track and field events, plus sailing). On this relationship he wrote, *"We should not move the body without the soul or the soul without the body, and, thus, they will be on guard against each other, and be healthy and well balanced"* (53, p. 511).

Like Hippocrates, he was not impressed with athletes and felt they were susceptible to disease if they deviated from their regimens. His best student was Aristotle (384–322 BC), who also supported the concept that the soul was responsible for movement. He promoted gymnastics for its beauty, believed Sparta that physical activities were too harsh, advocated light exercises before puberty to enhance growth and was convinced that strenuous (heavy) exercise should be avoided throughout life (53).

While Erasistratus of Chios in Sicily (310–250 BC) has been considered by select historians as the "father of physiology," he made few contributions to the emergence of exercise physiology. He did endorse the element concepts advanced by Alcmaeon and felt that health was present when balance had occurred among them. Moreover, he included moderate exercise (walking) in his therapeutic regimen (dieting, gymnastic activities, bathing, minimal drugs) for diseases not caused by ascites or pleurisy (38,55).

Contributions from the Roman Empire

An Overview

Archeologic evidence indicates that ancient tribes settled the hills of Rome around 950 BC. Settlers believed spirits existed in animate and inanimate objects, which became the subject of their worship. Later, they directed their efforts to gods and goddesses and enacted rituals and prayers to seek protection against diseases that occurred because of divine displeasure (56). Although the Etruscans occupied the region and already had gods and goddesses, the Romans accepted and renamed the Greek god of medicine (Asclepius to Aesculapius) and the goddess of health (Hygeia to Salus) (37).

Besides their gods and goddesses, the Romans were influenced by the Greek views on health and medical practices. One Greek physician who moved to Rome and prescribed exercise (walking and running) for his patients (with dropsy) was Asclepiades (128–56 BC). Besides not accepting the humoral theory of Hippocrates, he was regarded by Galen as being "either mad or entirely unacquainted with the practice of medicine" (20, p. 633).

The Roman Army, Gladiators, and Training

The effectiveness of the Roman army was a major factor in the transformation of the Roman Republic of 510 BC into the Roman empire that existed between 161–181 AD with Emperor Marcus Aurelius. Individuals recruited into the army were required to be healthy and followed a lifestyle of "reasonable exercise," adequate daily sleep, and a well-regulated diet (57). Once in the army, they were expected to be able to march 32 km in 5 hours with the military step while carrying a 20-kg pack or 38.4 km in 4 hours with the full step and no pack (58,59). In 1998, Whipp and associates (59) simulated marching conditions associated with legionaries and found the full step was associated with a mean VO_2 of $1.43 \text{ L} \cdot \text{min}^{-1}$, whereas the military step mean was $1.42 \text{ L} \cdot \text{min}^{-1}$.

Longer marches were scheduled to experience fatigue, improve endurance, and to "wear out the stragglers." They conducted drills and physical activities (running and charging, broad and long jumping) at the intensity level required for combat while using twofold heavier wooden swords and wickerwork shields to strengthen the arms. The same rationale was followed with the shafts of the practice spear (javelin) and, by the time of Scipio and his battles with Spain (ca. 210 AD), the army was using a 4-day tetrad training schedule that followed the same principles employed by athletes (56).

Gladiatorial contests began between 370 and 340 BC with a small number of paired combatants. By the time of Augustus (27 BC–14 AD), 10,000 pairs had been reported (60). Preparatory schools became the responsibility of the state and all had physicians and trainers on their staff—Claudius Galenus was the most notable (39). Like the army, they performed and repeated running, charging, and jumping activities at high intensity levels while using heavier weapons in their combat drills. Unlike the army, they used warming up exercises (61).

TEST YOURSELF

What were the contributions to exercise physiology from the gladiators and soldiers of the Roman army?

The Legacy of Claudius Galenus

Claudius Galenus, or Galen, was from Pergamon in Asia Minor and studied medicine at Alexandria, settled in Rome in 162 AD, and, 7 years later, became the personal

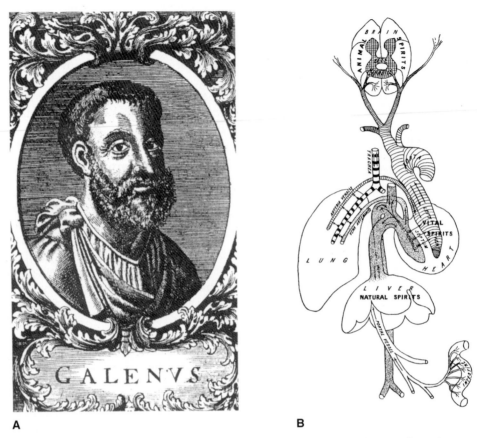

A **B**

FIGURE 1.6 **A.** Claudius Galenus, or Galen of Pergamon. Considered by many historians as the most important figure in medicine and physiology since Hippocrates, Galen was the only individual known to directly influence physiologic thinking and practices for more than 1200 years. **B.** Galen's view of physiology. (From West JB. *Respiratory Physiology: People and Ideas.* New York: Oxford University Press; 2003:76, 141. Courtesy of the American Physiological Society.)

physician to the emperor Marcus Aurelius (Fig. 1.6). He believed in the power of the gods, was a follower of Asclepius and had been an "attendant" at a local temple that revered him. He accepted the concept that living matter was a mixture (crasia) of the elements, their qualities, and the four humors whose proportions affected physiologic functions while determining the uniqueness and temperance of individuals (62). He promoted Plato's idea of a tripartite soul with distinctive souls being represented in the brain, heart, and liver (63). An admirer of Hippocrates, he incorporated many Hippocratic concepts within his own texts. Because of his personality, knowledge, and productivity (434 titles attributed to him of which 350 have been authenticated), his beliefs have impacted universal medical and health practices for more than a millennium (64).

Galen and Exercise

According to Galen, movement had to be vigorous, with increased respiration, to be called exercise. Work and exercise appeared to be equivalent terms, but he was receptive to different organizational approaches if others wished to pursue the point. In fact, activities such as shadow boxing,

leaping, discus throwing, small-or-large ball activities, and climbing ropes were regarded as exercise, whereas digging, rowing, plowing, reaping, riding, fighting, walking, hunting, and so forth, were considered to be work or exercise. Exercises were classified as either being swift or slow, vigorous or atony, violent or gentle. Running and ball exercises were examples of swift exercises; lifting a heavy weight, climbing a slope, and digging were cited for vigorous exercise; whereas discus throwing and continuous jumping were regarded as violent exercises (65). (After the various translations of the writings of Hippocrates and Galen, the terms violent and excessive exercise have been interpreted to be the equivalent of very heavy or maximal exercise.)

Galen and His Physiologic Concepts

Galen believed blood was produced in the liver, carried by the vena cava into the right heart, and distributed through the lungs and interventricular septum into the left ventricle, where it was ejected (pulsations), containing air and heat, into the periphery. However, the blood was propelled not only by the contraction of the ventricle but by the contraction of the arteries as well. Thus, the pulse rate changes recorded by previous cultures were a result of an active dilation of the arteries that was initiated by cardiac contraction. Moreover, Galen appears to be the first to record that pulse rate is increased with exercise (but without providing data). In *The Pulse for Beginners* (66), he notes that moderate exercise "renders the pulse vigorous, large, quick, and frequent." Also mentioned was that, if vigorous movement did not cause an increase in respiration, it should not be labeled as exercise.

Other statements associate exercise with "accelerated movements of respiration" (65). These statements must be placed in this physiologic context: Galen considered air or pneuma to be essential for life, absorbed by the lungs, carried by the left heart to all organs, and the object of respiration—but not the principle responsible for specific respiratory movements (47). He commented that an increase in inspiration would nourish the "vital spirit" and the "vaporization of the humors" that originated in the heart and arteries (44). His views were similar but not identical to those of Aristotle—Galen thought the increased respiration would cool the heart and elevate body temperature. Unlike Aristotle, he believed the increased respiration would increase combustion within the left ventricle (47).

TEST YOURSELF

Alan Ryan, a late sports medicine historian, declared that Galen was the "father of exercise physiology." Do you agree? Provide a rationale for or against his declaration.

Acute and Chronic Exercise

In his description of the uses and values of exercise, he referred to a "readier metabolism" (65). One physiologic interpretation of this observation is that Galen was referring to the combustion of substrates that occurred essentially in the left ventricle and led to the liberation of heat (47). As noted earlier, this process would also elevate body temperature. Acute exercise also increased the digestive process, which involved the heat of digestion, transforming the substrate (food) into lymph and then into humors. Subsequently, the humors would provide the materials for the tissues of the body. In Book I of Galen's *Hygiene* (*De Sanitate Tuenda*), it is evident that the increased evacuation of excrement was considered to be an acute effect of exercise. Moreover, if the excrement was retarded with problems of constituency, one possible cause was the "insufficiency of warmth" (heat for dissolving purposes), which occurred because of the lack of exercise (65). He also proclaimed that some of the fluid consumed would become urine, with components being passed "off as sweat or insensible perspiration," with sweating occurring with the "violence of exercise." However, when exercise was excessive and an overproduction of heat had occurred (immoderation of the heat), fever would result (65). In most circumstances, Galen regarded fever as a disease and usually treated it with an application of cold to the body.

Acute exercise was also associated with fatigue. He stated in Book II, "the art of exercise is no small part of hygienic science, and avoiding fatigue is no small part of the art of exercise" (65, p. 143), while noting that fatigue without exercise is a symptom of disease (he identified several types of fatigue). Exercise physiologists who relate the fatigue of muscular exercise to the presence of lactic acid should realize that Galen wrote in Book II that excessive exercise with faulty secretions would result in "an acidity of the thin and warm fluids, which erode and prick and sting the body" (65, pp. 145–146). Besides the sensations of pain, fatigue was associated with reduced strength, a disinclination to movement, arrhythmias of the pulse, and an impaired power of the mind.

Views Concerning Athletes

Galen considered trained individuals to possess the "peak" condition of health while exhibiting elevated muscle tone (hardness of the organ), accelerated respiration, increased muscle strength, "readier metabolism," an elevated "intrinsic warmth," better nutrition, and diffusion of all substances with enhanced elimination of excrements (65). Despite his responsibilities for the welfare of gladiators, he had a low regard for athletes, especially wrestlers, and the individuals who trained them. Similar to Hippocrates, Galen viewed athletes as "the extremes of good conditions" and, as such, were in a "dangerous state." On the other hand, if they were in good condition, the humors were in equilibrium, and the blood would be well-distributed throughout the body. As for wrestlers, he felt they were overfed and overtrained, which produced an unhealthy body type (unequal distribution of fat and muscle) and humoral imbalance. However, Galen recognized that the energy demands of boxers and wrestlers in training required a diet of pork and "special" breads because the traditional diet of vegetables and "ordinary" bread would be disastrous for the athlete (65).

Philostratus and Training

Despite Hippocrates' and Galen's negative opinions of athletes, athletes and their training were an integral component of the Greek and Roman cultures. Insights on their practices were provided by Flavios Philostratus (170–244 AD), a teacher of rhetoric, philosophy, and fine living, who traveled between Athens and Rome and wrote *Concerning Gymnastics* (44). He extensively commented on Galen's view that trainers were inadequately prepared for their responsibilities or were unable to provide meaningful advice on how to train. He also argued against the rigid tetrad system of training that was being implemented in select gymnasiums because the "whole of gymnastics has been ruined" (44). With this 4-day training schedule, the first day was devoted to preparing the athlete, the second was scheduled so the athlete was "intensively engaged," the third was allocated for recreation, and on the fourth day, the athlete was "moderately exerted." Philostratus felt the system made no allowances for individualized training programs ("they deprived their science of intelligent understanding in respect to the condition of the athlete to be trained"). In addition, athletes must better integrate exercise and diet in their training programs. However, he did note that distance runners (light exercise) were running 8 to 10 laps in their training programs, sprint runners (stade-race = furlong) had trained by running against hares and horses, and the athletes in the heavy exercise category (wrestlers and boxers) were lifting and carrying heavy burdens, bending or straightening out thick iron plates, pulling yokes with oxen, or even wrestling (actually fighting) with bulls and lions! Although his observations contained limited physiologic insights or explanations, he reported that moderately hard exercise by individuals who consumed too much wine would produce secretions of sweat that would be harmful to the blood. Hence, he recommended mild exercise and massage that would keep open the pores and drain off the sweat (44).

Summary of Ancient Exercise Physiology

The history of exercise physiology is inextricably linked to ancient humans' acceptance of supernatural forces, the evolvement of physiology to explain the existence of life and the consequences of disease, and to the emergence of rational medicine. Exercise was a way of life and responsible for the migration from Central Africa to the river civilizations of which India and China were of key importance. Both cultures, and later the Greeks, endorsed the concept that select elements were responsible for the formation of the human body but only the inhabitants of the Indus River and Greece referenced the complex transformations necessary for the formation of dosas (humors), which were first mentioned in the 1500 BC hymns of the Rgveda and integrated into the Indian Tridosa doctrine around 1000 BC. Inherent in the Tridosa doctrine was that disease and illnesses occurred when the three dosas were not in equilibrium and that health prevailed when they were. Around 600 BC, the Indian surgeon Susruta proposed moderate exercise to decrease the diseases associated with the elevation of the kapha humor which could occur with inactivity, excessive consumption of food and fluid, and prolonged sleeping. He also recommended exercise for patients with obesity and diabetes and felt the dosa vayu was displaced by heavy work, and that excessive or heavy exercise could be lethal. Several centuries later, his perspective was championed by the renowned physician Caraka who maintained that diabetes could be cured by exercise.

Although inhabitants of the Yellow River civilization incorporated features of the elemental theory into their concept of the human body, they either ignored or were oblivious of the Tridosa doctrine. They did endorse features of Taoism and the Yin-Yang doctrine in that yang was the principle associated with life and health whereas yin was the principle identified with death and disease. Like the Tridosa doctrine, the principles had to be in equilibrium (balance) before harmony or health was present. Over the centuries, Chinese physicians or philosophers advocated deep breathing exercises to remove the "bad air" and animal movements to minimize body pains and ailments. However, it was not until late in the Han dynasty that exercise was advocated by the Chinese surgeon Hua T'o for its yang effect on health and for its effect on strength, circulation, appetite, and the prevention of old age.

At the time of Homer, the gods and goddesses of Greece reigned supreme on matters of health and disease, with athletic games and competition being an integral component of their culture. The city-state of Sparta was established with the intent of being a warrior state where health was focused on fitness for combat and education was directed toward the use of art, music, and gymnastics for warrior purposes. Although not documented, we can assume that Sparta demonstrated the effectiveness of elevated frequencies, higher intensity levels, and increased durations in the improvement of physical fitness.

In other regions of Greece, philosophers and physicians were advocating concepts that became templates for education and governance, the humoral theory, and the beginning of rational medicine—of which the latter two have generally been attributed to Hippocrates. He felt that disease could occur because of external and internal factors that would alter the balance between the four humors and, like the Hindus, proclaimed health was present when they are in equilibrium. As diet modification and the purging effect of exercise could alter the balance between the humors, they were key regimen components in achieving a healthy status.

Hippocrates advocated moderate exercise for its beneficial effects on the human body and was the first to provide a detailed exercise prescription for diseased individuals. Like other physicians from India, China, and Greece, he was against excessive exercise for its harmful effects.

Prior to the emergence of Hippocrates, trainers were present to provide information to students attending gymnasiums and to athletes competing in games. Although Hippocrates, Plato, and Galen had little respect for their knowledge level, they were advocating practices associated with specificity, overload, endurances, and training schedules. This was also true for trainers or instructors responsible for the combat training of gladiators or legionnaires.

The Romans' greatest contribution was Claudius Galenus because his concepts on vital, animal, and natural spirits; innate heat; and structure existing for the purpose of function dominated physiologic thinking and medical practice until the sixteenth century. Health was regarded as unimpaired capacity for function and occurred when the elements and their qualities were in proportion while disease emerged when they were not. Moderate exercise, especially with the small ball, was advocated because of its beneficial effects on heart rate, breathing, body temperature, digestion, excretion, distribution of spirits, the concentration of humors, and for its training effects. As with Hippocrates, he prescribed exercise for select diseases.

Emergence of Christianity, the Medieval Period, and the Renaissance

Overview

This time period encompassed the Eastern barbarian invasion of the West that started with the Christian era, the anti-Hellenist practices of the Christian church toward Greek and Roman writings, and the establishment of Islam in the seventh century in Arabia and its spread to Greece, Africa, Spain, and some regions of France. It was an era when new medical schools in Italy, France, England, and the Netherlands were formed, and an era whose closing was associated with Vesalius (1514–1564) dismissing Galen's views on anatomy and physiology, and the Swiss chemist Theophrastus Bombastus von Hohenheim, or Paracelsus (1493–1541), "revolting" against Galen and his physiologic concepts (67).

The Legacy of Avicenna

As emphasized by Berryman (64), the Hippocratic and Galenic concepts pertaining to medical practice were dominating influences during most of this period. Their influence was first demonstrated in the Islamic world and later in the Christian sphere because of the Arabic and Latin translations of their texts. When exercise was discussed, it was generally within the context of the nonnaturals advocated by Galen and explained by his complex system of physiology, which included the humors, elements, qualities, members, facilities, operations, and spirits. Within the Arabic world and much of Europe, the prevailing influence was the writings of Abu Ali Sina Balkhi, or Avicenna (980–1037), a Persian physician and author of more than 100 books, of which his most renowned was the *Canon of Medicine* (Fig. 1.7) (68,69). Osler considered this book to be the most famous medical textbook ever written (70), and the text was described by Rothschuh as a "thorough systemization of all the medical knowledge available since antiquity" (47). Avicenna incorporated the galenic concepts of humors, elements, qualities, members, facilities, operations, and spirits into a complex system of principal members (heart, brain, liver), with each member having a controlling influence on the functions of other organs. Inherent in each separate system were virtues (actions), operations (functions), and faculties (selected characteristics of organs). There were three virtues (vital, animal, natural) associated with "*spiritus*" for distribution throughout the body. The most relevant was the vital virtue, the source of innate heat. It was found in the heart and blood, was responsible for heart rate and respiration, contained the "*spiritus*" (vital spirit) that Hippocrates labeled as pneuma and was distributed by the arteries (68).

Avicenna promoted the exercise concepts of Galen and reinforced the idea that moderate exercise was beneficial (a necessary factor with rest) for living because it "*balances the body by expelling residues and impurities and are factors of good nutrition for adults and of happy growth for the young*" (69, p. 24). He also noted that moderate exercise (walking) "*would repel the*

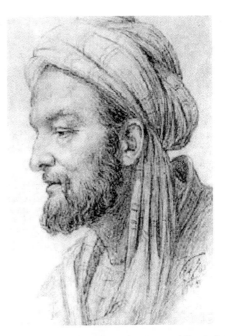

FIGURE 1.7 Abu Ali Sina Balkhi or Avicenna of Persia (980–1037) who promoted the exercise views of Galen and the concept of heat balance. Regarded by some authorities as the father of modern medicine. (From Avicenna—The free encyclopedia.)

bad humors." He indicated that exercise effects were dependent on the degree (intensity), amount (frequency and duration), and rest taken, cautioning his readers that excessive exercise could adversely affect the innate heat and lead to a state "*akin to death*" (69). Avicenna's focal point was the production and consequences of innate heat, which he considered responsible for the large and strong pulse with exercise. In addition, he emphasized that exercise was associated with elevated body temperatures (would make the body "very hot"), that perspiration occurred with physical exhaustion, and that exercise should cease when sweating stops because an abundant sweat was "*a symptom of moist illnesses.*" Although seldom mentioned in the history of thermal regulation, Avicenna was the first to list in tabular form within the *Cannon of Medicine* (68), the factors responsible for heat gain and heat loss.

He recommended chronic exercise for weak and undeveloped limbs, and he was among the first to acquaint Western culture with the ancient Hindu practice of breathing exercises for individuals with respiratory weakness (69). For individuals in geographical areas that were not receptive to or influenced by the writings of Avicenna, the nonnatural concepts of Galen were followed on matters that pertained to exercise and its effects.

In 1553, a Spanish physician, Cristobal Mendez (1500–1561), published in Latin the *Book of Bodily Exercise* (71). In translation, the text consisted of 82 pages containing 40 distinctive chapters that were organized in accordance with four treatises:

1. Exercise and its benefits
2. The division of exercise
3. Common exercises and which ones are the best
4. The time convenient for exercise and its value

The contents were essentially Greek and Roman concepts concerning exercise with an emphasis on its importance to health. To be beneficial, moderate exercise must be frequent, enjoyable, continuous (intermittent exercise will fail to consume and dissipate the humor, causing it to leave by the pores opened by the heat of movement), and associated with shortness of breath (caused by the increased heat within the heart and the need for more air via elevated ventilation). Besides extolling the health virtues of exercise and the need to avoid over exercising, he devoted several chapters to the heat produced by exercise and its consequences. While noting that movement per se will increase body heat, he mentions that with movement caused by exercise, the *"blood rubs very much with the parts as do the spirits and bile, causing subtlety and lightness, and showing heat in them"* (71, p. 19). Although the text has historical significance, it had a limited circulation and a minimal impact on the medical profession.

TEST YOURSELF

Who was Avicenna and what contributions, if any, did he make to exercise physiology?

Summary of This Time Period

Because of the influence of Avicenna, Galen's system of physiology and his views on exercise and its physiology extended into the Islamic world and the regions of Spain and France by the availability of his *Cannon of Medicine.* Although seldom cited, his views on temperature and its effects on the body were far advanced for his era. In contrast, the printing of the Mendez text on the bodily effects of exercise, which essentially consisted of Galen's views, had little impact despite being authored by a physician. Although Galen's views on anatomy and physiology were either rejected or minimized during the closing of this period, this was not the case for exercise and its selective effects on the body.

The Seventeenth Century

Overview

The seventeenth century has been characterized in the history of science as the Age of the Scientific Revolution because it was a time when the emphasis was on how (not why) things happen, speculation changed to experimentation, interpretation became mechanistic, mathematics entered into the language of science, and measurements began in medicine. Moreover, it was when the philosophies of René Descartes (1596–1650) and Sir Francis Bacon significantly contributed to these transitions, and when Jan Baptista van Helmont of Belgium (1577–1644) reported

that disease did not have to originate within the body, that the body contained "ferments" (enzymes) which aided digestion, and that fever had no relationship to the putrefaction of the humors (67). The German Franz de le Boë (1614–1672), or Franciscus Sylvius, ignored the humoral theory and related health to the interactions between bodily acids, bases, and their neutralization. However, for exercise physiology, it was a time of reformulation of ideas and association because the prevailing concepts of Galen were rejected and the ones based on physiologic investigations were evolving as they were discovered.

Circulatory, Respiratory, and Neuromuscular Investigations

The single most important scientific event during this time (67) was the discovery in 1628 of the continuous circulation of the blood by William Harvey (1578–1657) in England (72). His discovery was "completed" in 1661 by Marcello Malpighi (1628–1649), who identified the existence of capillaries in the lung (47). Harvey's epic investigation established that cardiac output and its distribution to the periphery had the capacity to increase, was dependent on the *"strength of the pulse,"* and indicated that *"the heart makes more than a thousand beats in a half hour in some two, three, or even four thousand"* (72). While at Oxford University, Richard Lower (1631–1693) championed the findings of Harvey and declared in his 1669 publication (73), the heart to be a muscle (as had Harvey, Stensen, and Leonardo da Vinci). He noted in Chapter 1 of his publication that the heart is *"more carefully fashioned than all other muscles of the body. For its work is more necessary and continuous than that of all other muscles, and hence it was particularly appropriate that it should also far surpass them in the elegance of its structure"* (73).

According to Lower, the heart was not the source of heat production by the body—the movement of the heart was dependent on the inflow of spirits through the nerves. Moreover, with violent exercise (likely maximal in intensity), the movement of the heart was accelerated in proportion to the blood that was *"driven and poured into its ventricles in great abundance as a result of the movement of muscles"* (73, p. 122). He also has been reported as indicating that exercise would enhance blood flow to the brain and that exercise and movements of the body were an aid to health (74). As for the effects of training, Harvey appears to be the first to indicate that a history of physical activity by animals, and likely humans, would be associated with cardiac enlargement (*"have a more thick, powerful, and muscular heart"* [72]).

During the time of Harvey, van Helmont reported that air was composed of different gases and Robert Boyle (1627–1691) in Oxford proved air was necessary for life and formulated the gas laws that bear his name (75). Sir Michael Foster, a famous English physiologist, described these experiments of Boyle as being the most fundamental in the physiology of respiration (76). Later, Giovanni Borelli

(1608–1679), an ardent Italian physicist and iatrophysicist, began and reported on his studies on the mechanics of respiration (76). Robert Hooke, who was associated with the Oxford physiologists, knew that air and breathing were essential for life but felt that neither lung movements nor blood flow were the most important aspect of breathing; rather, it was the air in the lungs that caused the color change within the venous blood (74). John Mayow (1643–1679), an Oxford contemporary of both Boyle and Hooke, published a text in 1674 entitled *Medico-Physical Works* (77) in which he clarified the findings of Borelli on the mechanics of breathing and emphasized that the lungs passively followed the movements of the thorax. Furthermore, respiration had no relationship to the cooling of the blood or to the promotion of blood flow. But the inspiration of air was essential for the transfer of some elastic nitrous particles, the *spiritus nitroaereus,* from the air into the blood. To Mayow, breathing facilitated the contact between air and blood, enabling the transfer of the niter particles to the blood, which subsequently reacted with sulfurous and combustible particles, resulting in elevated body and blood temperatures and a change in the color of the blood. He was also of the opinion that violent exercise would increase the frequency of breathing and create an intense heat within the body because of the greater effervescence caused by the increased number and presence of nitro-aerial particles (47,74,77).

As noted earlier, during the early decades of the seventeenth century, a prevailing concept was that nerves conveyed "spirits" to muscles, which initiated contraction. Thomas Willis (1621–1675) of Oxford, teacher of Robert Hooke, John Locke, and Richard Lower (78), was a major proponent of the idea that animal spirits from the brain traveled down nerve fibers to muscles, where they met nitrous and sulfurous particles, which caused an "explosion," resulting in inflated muscles when they contracted (78). Giovanni Borelli (1608–1679) of Pisa, Italy, stated that a spirituous juice (*succus nerveus*) was carried by nerves to the brain to cause sensations or to the muscles which interacted with the blood to produce an effervescence (reaction between fermentation and ebullition) causing inflation and contraction of muscles, which resulted in limb movements (47,71). Later, a Cambridge physician, Francis Glisson (1597–1677), challenged the concept that nerves conveyed a "spirit" to muscles which inflated them during contraction. He proved his point by demonstrating that no water displacement took place when a forceful underwater contractile effort was made. In addition, he reported that muscle fibers had the property of irritability, which was later "rediscovered" and made famous by Albrecht Haller (47). A Danish physician, Niels Stensen (1638–1686), noted that skeletal muscle fibers contract in a geometric manner, which decreased their length while increasing their width (47). In 1694, the Swiss mathematician Johann Bernoulli (1667–1748) published a dissertation entitled *On the Mechanics and Movement of the Muscles* (79) in which he described muscles as small machines, used differential calculus to explain their functions, and described the contraction process as follows:

> When the mind wishes that a limb of the body moves, some agitation of animal spirits occurs in the brain so that, by twitching the origin of some nerve, they shake the spirituous juice contained inside over its whole length and, because of the irritation of the origin of the nerve, the last droplet of nervous juice is driven out by the slight vibration at the other orifice (79, p. 139).

According to Bernoulli, muscular strength was related to the availability of the spirituous juice being released, whereas muscular fatigue (tiredness) was dependent on the quantity of consumed spirits. In fact, he states, "*I also assume that carrying same weight at the same height during the same time consumes the same quantity of spirits*" (79, p. 135).

According to William Croone, an English physician (1633–1684), violent exercise was associated with painful and stiff muscles caused by a combination of an inadequate blood flow, sweating, and the removal of "spirits." In addition, he was of the opinion that the presence of sweat on muscles was associated with the swelling and contraction of skeletal muscles (80).

Metabolic and Thermal Investigations

Beginning in the sixteenth century and continuing through the early eighteenth century, contemporary scholars made a concerted effort to use mathematical and physical principles to address medical and biologic questions. One prominent individual in this movement was an Italian physician and professor at Venice and later Padua, Santorio Santorio (1561–1636), who developed accurate instruments to measure changes in heart rate, body temperature, and body weight (balance chair). These instruments were used to measure changes with sitting, sleeping, after exercise, meal consumption, excretion, and so forth, which became the forerunner of metabolic balance studies (47,81). Santorio also conducted studies pertaining to changes in sensible and insensible perspiration (81). His aphorisms indicated (#19, this indicates the 19th aphorism described by Santorio) that violent exercise of both mind and body would result in a lighter body weight while hastening old age and the threat of untimely and early death. To maintain a youthful face, individuals should avoid sweating or perspiring too much in the heat (#36). Another aphorism pertaining to temperature regulation stated that the fluid evacuated by violent exercise was sweat that originated from unconcocted (unheated) juices (#1) and that, if sound bodies did not perspire, this condition could be corrected by exercise (#34).

It is apparent that few seventeenth century scientists advocated strenuous or violent exercise because they, like Hippocrates and Galen, continued to believe it was unhealthy. This belief was prevalent with iatrophysicists and iatromechanicists. The extreme was to relate a specific organ to a machine (67). These individuals felt that heavy or maximal activity (*e.g.*, running, dancing) and especially singing, which markedly increased lung movements, could lead to disorders including asthma, hemoptysis (blood-stained sputum), and phthisis (tuberculosis of the lung) (82).

Summary of the Century

The Age of the Scientific Revolution began with the momentous discovery of the circulation by Harvey. He knew the heart and its circulation had the capacity to increase, as with exercise, and was the first to comment that a history of physical activity was associated with a larger and stronger heart. Lower of Oxford was a leading exponent of muscle contractions being responsible for an increased blood flow to the periphery and to the brain and for the heart not being the source of heat produced by the body. Oxford physiologists championed the concept that air and breathing were essential for life, and Mayow indicated it was air that was responsible for the color change in blood. Willis promoted the idea that animal spirits from the brain traveled to the muscles where an explosion occurred causing inflated muscles when they contracted. Borelli refined the spirits concept into "spirituous juices" that caused limb movements, whereas Bernoulli related muscular strength to the availability of the "juices" being released. Santorio perfected the thermometer and developed a weighing chair in which he measured weight and temperature changes with food consumption, exercise, and sleep, thus conducting the first known balance study. Despite the limited number of exercise studies being conducted, investigators continued to believe that excessive exercise was unhealthy.

The Eighteenth Century

Overview

The eighteenth century has been labeled by both Berryman (64) and Rothschuh (47) as the Age of Enlightenment because it was a time of emergence and implementation of several new and important philosophies. John Locke (1632–1704) of England argued that all knowledge had to be based on experience. Jean le Rond d'Alembert (1717–1783) and Denis Diderot (1713–1784) of France advocated replacing the era of theology and faith with science. Gottfried W. Leibniz (1646–1716) of Germany strove to reconcile existing and opposing views on matter and spirit, mechanism and teleology, experience and knowledge, freedom and necessity, religion and philosophy. Finally, the German Immanuel Kant (1724–1804) advocated that individuals use their intelligence without being guided by another person (47,67). Interestingly, there were few physiologic investigations or discoveries during the first half of the eighteenth century.

Respiratory, Metabolic, and Circulatory Investigations

Near the end of the eighteenth century, Karl W. Scheele (1742–1786) of Sweden discovered oxygen ("fiery air"), and Joseph Priestley of England (1733–1804) proclaimed the existence of "dephlogisticated air." About the same time, the brilliant French chemist Antoine L. Lavoisier (1743–1794) conducted experiments that destroyed the phlogiston theory of Stahl and established the chemical foundations for respiration, metabolism, and animal heat (47). Of the systematists mentioned during this time, all promoted exercise for health reasons, as did other physicians whose texts were not concerned with physiologic thinking or advancement. In such instances, exercise was usually discussed in the Galenic context of the nonnaturals (64,83). However, the most significant respiratory and metabolic studies of the century were conducted by Lavoisier and the French chemist Armand Seguin (1776–1835). They measured the oxygen consumption (of Seguin) that occurred with resting, fasting, digestion, and when performing work (foot moving a treadle) (84). (The work is detailed later in this chapter, in the Milestone of Discovery section.) From prior studies that included animals, they knew the carbon within the body underwent "combustion" to produce heat, water, and carbonic acid (carbon dioxide reacting with water). However, he thought the heat was generated by combustion in the lungs of a substance found in blood.

During this century insights into the circulation came early, from the extensive studies of the English physician John Floyer (1649–1734). Floyer developed an accurate pulse watch in 1707 and used its readings to classify people into different humoral states and identify certain disorders and diseases (85). For example, a pulse of 75 to 80 was listed as being hot in the first degree, associated with a choleric disposition and caused by hot seasons, hot air, exercise, passions, cards, study, hot medicines, hot baths, hot diet, and retained excrements. A rate between 65 and 60 was cold in the second degree and identified with melancholic individuals, occurring in the spleen, and caused by hydropic tumors and cachexias. The normal value was 70 to 75 beats per minute and a value of 140 beats per minute could be associated with death! It was Floyer's belief that changes in blood temperature, spirits, and humoral rarefaction caused by exercise were responsible for the changes in pulse rate. Moreover, if the rate was higher than 140 beats per minute and if death did not occur, it was difficult to count. When serving as the subject, he reported that 30 minutes of moderate walking caused his pulse to increase to 112 beats per minute; also, his pulse was 76 before he rode on a horse and 90 beats per minute after an hour's ride. He also measured respiratory frequency and related it to the pulse rate, but there was no evidence that he measured both during exercise. He did regard respiration as an aid to circulation in the movement of blood (74).

Several decades later, an Irish physician and researcher named Bryan Robinson (1680–1754) published an important but frequently overlooked text, *A Treatise of the Animal Oeconomy* (86). He wrote that an individual in the recumbent position had a pulse rate of 64 beats per minute, which would change to 68 beats per minute when sitting, to 78 beats per minute with standing, to 100 beats per minute after walking 4 miles in 1 hour, and to 140 to 150 beats per minute after running as hard as possible (86). At this time, Seguin and Lavoisier had recognized that the amount of oxygen consumed was related to the frequency of heart rate multiplied by the number of inspirations, and Stephen Hales had noted that exercise was associated with a brisk circulation; an increased number of systoles; and an improved blood flow to dilated and agitated lungs, the stomach, and the gut (intestines) (87). Lastly, Robinson observed that muscle blood flow was related to the force created by the contracting muscles.

Neuromuscular, Digestion, and Thermal Investigations

Robinson also felt the forces that caused limb movements were controlled by the will, which acted on nerves. To him, nerves were *"the principal instruments of sensation and motion"* (86, p. 91). He advocated moderate exercise to increase muscle strength and size and acknowledged that laboring (trained) individuals had larger and stronger muscles than inactive sedentary individuals. During this time, James Keill (1673–1719), an English physician, made the observation that muscle strength was related to the number of fibers present (88). Around 1760, John Theophilus Desaguliers (1683–1744), an English priest, curator, and admirer of strongmen, helped to develop a dynamometer that could accurately measure muscular strength (89,90). In a text pertaining to the benefits of therapeutic exercise, the Paris physician Joseph-Clement Tissot (1747–1826) indicated that motion (exercise) would increase muscle size and strength (91).

The idea that exercise would enhance digestion was repeated by both Hales and Tissot, as was the concept that it would aid the descent and evacuation of bowel contents. Tissot stated that exercise would increase sweating while removing the "sour salts" and "heterogeneous parts" from the blood, which would avoid the possibility of "spoiling" the blood (91). Robinson indicated that exercise should give a "glowing warmth" to the skin as long as it caused a "fever." He also described experiments in which individuals traveled 2 miles in 30 minutes, producing 8 and 9 ounces of sweat, or eight times the amount they produced when not exercising in the summer heat (86). Robinson examined the relationship between sweating and urine production during exercise and observed that both processes were about equal at the beginning of exercise but, as the exercise continued, urine production decreased until it became less than recorded at the start. When expressed on a ratio basis, it changed from 6:1 to 16:1 when the skin exhibited

a "glowing warmth" (86). Before Lavoisier reported that an essential function of insensible perspiration was to control the magnitude of the body heat (*e.g.*, temperature regulation), Black determined the latent heat of the evaporation of water, and Blagden reported a cooling effect from the evaporation of sweat (92). However, there are no reports that Lavoisier conducted exercise experiments with Seguin on this subject.

The Text of Tissot

Tissot's text was published in French in 1780 but was not translated into English until 1964 (91). Because it was associated with therapeutic exercise, these two aspects discouraged citation of it in many of the early publications. This was unfortunate because numerous pages were devoted to the effects of motion on nondiseased individuals and to the principles of the exercise prescription. The most notable was his third rule of gymnastics, which pertained to the intensity and duration of exercise according to the season and the age, sex, and temperament of the patient. He described moderate exercise as the condition that "just leads to perspiration, or lassitude or fatigue." His position on strenuous or violent exercise is unclear, but he does state that *"whether the motion is moderate or violent, as long as its duration is in the proper ratio to the strength of person exercising and conforms to the therapeutic indication for which it was proposed"*; namely, *"it always produces most of the good effects of which we have spoken"* (91, p. 20).

Summary of the Century

For exercise physiology, the discovery of oxygen by Joseph Priestly, Carl Scheele, and Antoine Lavoisier and the measurement of Seguin's oxygen consumption during treadle exercise by Lavoisier were the most significant achievements of the century. Lavoisier made measurements during rest, with and without food, and at different intensity levels; thus, he conducted the first human experiment on energy transformations (see Milestones section). John Floyer and Bryan Robinson were able to record heart rates during exercise with Floyer being concerned when the heart rate was in excess of 140 beats · min^{-1}. Robinson also measured sweat production and urine formation during exercise and found an inverse relationship between the two as the exercise progressed. Robinson wrote that nerves initiated motion and that active individuals had stronger and larger muscles than inactive ones. James Keill projected that muscle strength was related to the number of muscle fibers while John Desaguliers constructed a dynamometer capable of its measurement. Joseph-Clement Tissot published a French text in 1780 with an orientation for therapeutic exercise that contained similar views of Robinson while maintaining the exercise prescription should consider the age, season, sex, and temperament of the subject before intensity and duration should be considered. Unfortunately for North America and Britain, it was not translated into English until 1964.

The Nineteenth Century

Overview

The first decades of the nineteenth century were a continuation of the era of Enlightenment, or an "analysis of the laws of nature, history, and religion with the help of reason . . . leading to the development of liberalism, individualism, and democracy at the social level." The natural sciences, notably physiology and chemistry, "marched from discovery to discovery . . . and established a series of general laws" while providing the foundations of knowledge on which most twentieth-century technologic achievements were based (67). Medical historians Lyons and Pertrucelli (67) have described the nineteenth century as "the beginning of modern medicine"; Rothschuh, the physiology historian (47), labeled this era as "the beginning"; and, to Berryman, an exercise historian (64), it was a time when "exercise was receiving more attention from physicians because of its traditionally important role in the maintenance of health."

Relevant Publications

The nineteenth century was also a time when a large number of publications occurred on subject matter that was intrinsic to exercise physiology.

The Text of Sinclair

Few physiologists in England had an interest in exercise but there was a heightened interest in sports. In 1807, the Earl of Caithness, John Sinclair, published texts that addressed aspects of training for humans and animals (93). An interesting aspect of his views was that they were formulated from observations reported by Herodicus, Asclepiades, Celsus, Galen, Sir Francis Bacon, and Bryan Robinson plus opinions of respected trainers from those eras. The composite conclusion was that training would reduce extraneous fat, increase muscle mass, make bones harder and less likely to be injured, increase perspiration, improve the wind (lungs), prolong breath-holding time, and reduce recovery time. With animals, trained horses exhibited less fatigue and would not wear out sooner than their untrained counterparts. Considering the times and the educational background of the trainers, it is no surprise that Sinclair did not propose to change the "core of all training regimens," namely purging, puking, sweating, diet, and exercise (94).

The Text of Beaumont

In 1833, William Beaumont (1785–1853) attracted the attention of physiologists outside of the United States with his observations of Alexis St. Martin of Canada, who survived a gunshot wound resulting in a gastric fistula. Beaumont described more than 70 experiments, including exercise, with the interior of St. Martin's stomach (95). He concluded that moderate exercise was conducive to rapid and healthy digestion, whereas severe and fatiguing exercise would retard the process. In addition, he stated that:

Exercise, sufficient to produce moderate perspiration, increases the secretions from the gastric cavity and produces an accumulation of a limpid fluid, within the stomach, slightly acid, and possessing the solvent properties of the gastric juice in an inferior degree. This is probably a mixed fluid, a small proportion of which is gastric juice (95, p. 94).

The Text of Combe

Beginning in 1834, an Edinburgh physician named Andrew Combe (1787–1847) wrote a textbook on physiology applied to health and physical and mental education that contained nine chapters and had 16 printings in the United States by 1854 (96). In his text, exercise was advocated for its health benefits because of the effects of movement on bones, muscles, heart, lungs, the digestive system, and the central nervous system. Although moderate and progressive exercise was prescribed, the need for rest intervals was noted. Moreover, lack of exercise was associated with muscle weakness and, in the case of the lungs, the potential for diseases. Concerning muscles, he indicated that exercise increased their blood flow; that they were proportional in size and structure to the effort required of them; that, when used frequently, muscles would increase in thickness and possibly with greater force; and that increased power was associated with increased activity of the nervous system (96).

The Text of Dunglison

Although Beaumont ignored his advice concerning functioning of the digestive system, Robley Dunglison's (1798–1869) views on medicine and physiology, published in 1835, were highly regarded because he had authored prominent textbooks on both subjects. While a faculty member of the hygiene department at the University of Maryland, his text (97) was the first book on preventive medicine for medical students (64). The book contained an 18-page chapter devoted to exercise. Dunglison emphasized that exercise was important for one's health, and that "*inglorious inactivity*" would cause an individual to "suffer" because of a loss of function of the nervous, muscular, circulatory, digestive, secretory, and excretory systems, and that the loss could lead to "*hypochondriasis, hysteria, and the whole train of nervous diseases*," and for many grave "*bodily ailments*" (97, p. 442). He classified exercise as active or passive and emphasized the importance of traveling exercises, which meant covering long distances in unfamiliar outdoor environments for improved digestive and mental functions.

Exercise in moderation was advocated for its beneficial and tonic influences on the body, whereas violent exercises, such as running, dancing, and wrestling, were discouraged because they caused air to contain less oxygen and more carbon dioxide and led to respiratory turmoil leading to suffocation, cardiac dilations, aneurysms of large vessels, hemorrhages from the lungs and nose, body shocks, hernias, dislocations, and more muscle sprains and lacerations. Besides the physiologic effect of enhancing digestion, moderate exercise increased the action of the heart and the connected respiratory movements; promoted blood flow to the capillaries and its functions (nutrition and secretion); increased muscle firmness, elasticity, and bulk; and promoted loss of fat around the muscles (97).

The Publication of Byford

The first time a publication included the words and addressed the subject of the physiology of exercise was in 1855 (2). The author was William H. Byford, a physician and professor at Rush Medical College in Chicago, who had a history of conducting exercise experiments with animals and humans pertaining to heat, circulation, breathing, and secretion. Byford was aware of the health benefits of exercise and was concerned that the medical profession appeared indifferent to the subject. Hence, his article was an attempt to inform and to educate others on its importance while encouraging them to initiate related research. Byford defined exercise as "voluntary discharge of any or all the animal functions, as intellect, sensation, locomotion, and voice" and described the phenomena of exercise as "*vascular excitement, increased heat, redness of the surface, and augmented secretion and excretion*" (2, p. 33). However, he neglected to mention the types or intensity levels being advocated. Because blood was the foundation from which all organs received their nutrients to discharge their functions, it was essential that the supply of blood increase in proportion to the elevated demands of the organ, which was, in turn, dependent on increased muscle activity. As nutritive material was removed from blood and the effete matter it contained, the exchange within the capillaries was also enhanced by muscle contractions. He described the exchange process as the capillary force of the circulation and noted that when the muscles were contracting quickly and frequently, they would attract a large amount of blood from the capillaries and pass it on to the veins and to the heart. Moreover, it was an exchange that was accomplished by the mechanical action of muscles upon the veins. He acknowledged that this explanation was incomplete because it ignored cerebral influences and the important role of capillary circulation. Besides involving circulatory and muscular systems, the excitement of exercise included emotions and possible atomic or molecular changes occurring in nervous centers, as well as organic functions associated with perspiration and urinary excretions. When vascular excitement was specifically mentioned, it referred to the distribution of blood and its nutrients to all of the vital organs and tissues. This role gave importance to exercise because it enhanced organ development and functions of which muscles were deemed the most important. He noted that blood contained high levels of albuminous or protein compounds that provided the structure for other organs and served the exclusive functions of muscle (he thought more than half of the albumin found in blood would likely be consumed by the muscles) (2). Byford then proceeded to discuss the role of albumin in disease states and the value of physical activity in the process. Exercise was important for increasing the warmth of the body and the temperature of the blood because this change enhanced nutrient disintegration. In addition, the digestive process was facilitated. He stated:

It is this beautiful mutual dependence and reciprocal stimulation, by affording the material ready prepared as it were to each other, both in a physiologic and physical sense, that the health, efficiency, and even integrity of the animal and organic are preserved in their proper condition for the support of the whole system (2, p. 40).

Secretions from the skin, kidney, and liver were also facilitated by exercise. However, physiologic consequences arose when organs associated with these secretions were unable to perform their functions, in part, because of a lack of muscular activity.

The Publications of Austin Flint Jr.

Although Byford introduced the terms exercise physiology and described its physiologic foundations, it was Austin Flint Jr. (1853–1914), a physician whose publications promoted and enhanced its scientific entrance (Fig. 1.8). Frequently, Flint failed to identify his junior status as his father was an accomplished physician and author (1812–1886), so his publications have authorship problems. After graduation, he studied with Bernard in France, served as a professor at the medical school in Buffalo, and became renowned while serving on the physiology faculty at Bellevue Hospital Medical College in New York. The 1875 publication of *A Textbook of Human Physiology,* which had four editions, was likely his most influential text because it was extensively used in the medical schools that were educating many of the physicians that assumed teaching and administrative responsibilities in the institutions that were offering exercise physiology courses in physical education departments (98). In this edition, Flint discussed the effect of exercise on the heart and cited the data of Bryan Robinson. He emphasized the changes in blood pressure, mentioned the blood flow data of Chauveau and noted that muscular contractions enhanced venous return. When discussing metabolism, he included the exercise results of Seguin and Lavoisier (see Milestone of Discovery) concerning oxygen consumption changes, the ventilatory increases noted by Vierordt, and the carbon dioxide results of Edward Smith.

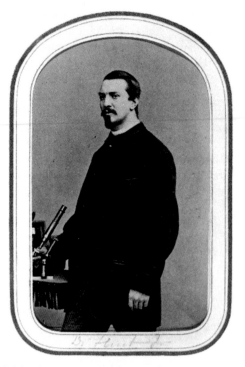

FIGURE 1.8 Austin Flint Jr. (1853–1914). A physician whose investigations and textbook promoted the acceptance of exercise physiology being a scientific discipline. (From McArdle WA, Katch FI, Katch VL. *Exercise Physiology,* 7th ed. Philadelphia: Lippincott Williams & Wilkins; 2010:34.)

Furthermore, he mentioned that with conditions of great fatigue and exhaustion, the carbon dioxide content of the expired air was decreased (hyperventilation). At the time of the first edition, Flint was engaged in a controversy as to whether nitrogen was excreted with muscular exercise (argument was associated with the issue of whether proteins were the prime substrate for muscle function). In 1870, Flint carefully studied the urinary nitrogen excretion of an individual who walked about 318 miles in 5 days and found that for every 100 parts of nitrogen ingested, 154 parts of nitrogen were excreted. Thus, he felt that "violent" exercise would cause tissue breakdown that would be reflected with an increased loss of body proteins (99). In the textbook, muscle action or effort was generally discussed with regard to the responses of frog muscles to electrical stimulation. He wrote that muscles increased in size and power with frequent exercise. In addition, he felt that repeated exercise would increase the size but not the number of the fasciculi. Although muscle fluid (or juice) was slightly alkaline at rest, moderate exercise would cause it to become more neutral but, with strenuous exercise, it would become acidic because of the presence of lactic acid.

The effect of exercise on body temperature was emphasized and an upper limit of 104°F (40°C) was listed with "violent, muscular exercise," which in turn would increase sweating. The fact that muscle activity could increase muscle temperature was verified by inserting a thermoelectric needle into the biceps of an individual sawing wood and observing a rise of 2°F. Lastly, Flint felt that exercise would enhance

the development of bones and suggested that it would prolong life (98).

In 1878, Flint published *On the Source of Muscular Power* in which he detailed the experiments of Liebig, Lehmann, Fick and Wislicenus, Parkes, Pavy, and those he conducted with Weston (100). Not surprisingly, the topic was the effect of exercise on nitrogen balance. Significant conclusions were as follows:

V. Experiments show that excessive and prolonged muscular exercise may increase the waste or wear of certain of the constituents of the body to such a degree that this wear is not repaired by food. Under these conditions, there is an increased discharge of nitrogen, particularly in the urine. . . .

VII. By systemic exercise of the general muscular system or of particular muscles, with proper intervals of repose for repair and growth, muscles may be developed in size, hardness, power, and endurance. The only reasonable theory that can be offered in explanation of the process is the following: While exercise increase the activity of dissimulation of the muscular substance, a necessary accompaniment of this is an increased activity in the circulation of the muscles, for the purpose of removing the products of their physiologic wear. This increased activity of circulation is attended with an increased activity of the nutritive processes, provided the supply of nutriment be sufficient, and provided also that the exercise be succeeded by proper periods of rest. It is in this way only that we can comprehend the process of development of muscles by training; the conditions in training being exercise, rest following the exercise, and appropriate alimentation, the food furnishing nitrogenized matter to supply the waste of the nitrogenized parts of the tissues.

VIII. All that is known with regard to the nutrition and disassimilation of muscles during ordinary or extraordinary work teaches that such work is always attended with destruction of muscular substance, which may not be completely repaired by food, according to the amount of work performed and the quantity and kind of alimentation (100, pp. 94–96).

The Publications of Hartwell

In 1886, Edward M. Hartwell, PhD, MD, of The Johns Hopkins University, addressed a convention of the American Association for the Advancement of Physical Education.

The title of his presentation was *On the Physiology of Exercise*. The speech was subsequently published in two parts in the *Boston Medical and Surgical Journal* (101,102). He spoke on this topic because "the fundamental and essential characteristics of exercise are generally misstated and its proper effects so frequently overlooked, that I have chosen the physiology of exercise as my theme" (101, p. 297). After using du Bois-Reymond's definition of exercise ("*the frequent repetition of a more or less complicated action of the body with the cooperation of the mind, or an action of the mind alone, for the purpose of being able to perform it better*"), he discussed the anatomical and contractile characteristics of muscle tissue and its response to neural stimuli before it "begins working." The importance of an increased blood flow to working skeletal muscles was emphasized. He mentioned that the blood entering muscle was bright red, rich in oxygen, and low in carbonic acid, whereas it was dark blue, had a higher temperature, and contained waste products and "poorer" oxygen when it left to return to the heart. If these conditions could not be reversed, muscle irritability became less and a stronger stimulus was required. He proposed that if muscles received adequate food, oxygen, and rest, they would increase in size and weight because fibers number and sizes would increase. Repeated exercise would make the muscles larger, harder, and stronger. He noted that muscles were "more perfect power-machines" than are steam engines and rifled cannons because of the energy transformations within the tissue ("*the potential energy of organized material is transformed into the work, which we see manifested in motion, animal heat, and the chemical actions involved in nutritive, secretory, and excretory processes*" [101, p. 301]). Exercise was important for achieving a healthy state, and failure to exercise could be associated with incomplete oxidation of food, the accumulation of effete products, disordered digestion, an enfeebled nervous system, flabby muscles, impaired secretions, an onset of ill health, and the occurrence of diseases (101, p. 301). He concluded that to achieve a healthy state, an average individual should walk 8 or 9 miles daily.

Hartwell also focused on the growth and development of individuals from various segments of English society. It was apparent to Hartwell that young individuals from "well-to-do parents" and environments had stature and weight measures that were superior to those from working parents. He inferred that this difference was due, in part, to inadequate play activity and the failure to receive sufficient exercise. In the final segments of his presentation, he addressed the effect of exercise on the nervous system with an emphasis on the brain. After mentioning the effect of use and disuse on the muscular system, he indicated that use and disuse had "similar effects in the case of nerve cells and fibres, both sensory and motor." Hartwell compared the nervous system of a blacksmith with that of a 5-year-old male and attributed the size, branching, and connections of the motor nerves and the cells within the motor area to be larger and more numerous in the motor area in the blacksmith, in part, because of the effect of chronic exercise during the critical phase of growth and development. He then discussed aspects of human inheritance and stated that

> *muscular exercise deserves more attention than is usually given it, and that, when properly chosen, regulated and guided, it not only does a man good, but makes him better; at least, it may make him a better man, in many respects, than his father was, and enable him to transmit to his progeny a veritable aptitude for better thoughts and actions* (102, p. 324).

However, he provided no evidence to support his statements.

The Text of Kolb

In 1893, the accomplished German sportsman and physician George Kolb had his book *The Physiology of Sport*, translated and published in English (103). The text contains results and opinions from his case studies with the members of the "Berliner-Ruder-Club," with a focus on the maximal exertion and training of sportsmen (predominately, rowers). He began his text with a discussion of the fatigue with maximum exertion that is first experienced by the skeletal muscles but is related to the insufficiencies of the circulation of the blood, the respiratory system, the nervous system, and possibly to the fact that the athlete is overtrained. Besides indicating that skeletal muscles were important for sporting activities and associated with "sportsman fatigue," they must be strengthened in "every way." For rowers, this meant daily practice (3 minutes) for the arms and legs with dumbbells weighing 4 to 5 pounds each and deep knee bends for the extensors of the upper thigh. Several chapters were devoted to the responses of the cardiovascular system, with many pages devoted to pulse wave tracings recorded with a sphygmograph (103, p. 33). He reported that maximal effort in rowers was associated with heart rates of 230 to 350 beats per minute and radial artery pressures around 185 mm Hg. After several months of training, heart rates would be reduced by 16 beats per minute, and blood pressure was lowered by 20 mm Hg.

From his analysis of the sphygmographic results, he concluded that maximal exertion would increase the rate and work of the heart, alter cardiac dilation, elevate the velocity of blood flow, and cause muscle and cardiac hypertrophy. The term "cardiac dullness" was invoked to describe dilation or enlargement of the heart. He indicated that there were pathologic conditions in which cardiac dullness was increased, but this condition was not a characteristic in trained rowers. Kolb elaborated on the respiratory changes of rowers and reported that respiratory rates could increase from 12 to 60 per minute and be maintained with heavy exertion. Actually, he reported frequency values as high as 140 before muscle failure occurred (103). Vital capacity values were decreased after rowing events, presumably because of the increased volume of blood within the lungs. Using himself as a subject in rowing races that lasted 1 to 9 minutes, he found the percentage of carbon dioxide in expired air to increase from 4.3% to 6% and to 9.0% once the event had ended. He calculated that in an 8-minute race, he had a gaseous exchange of 600 L of air in the lungs, of which approximately 39 L was carbon dioxide. He felt that dyspnea occurred because of the combined influence of an oxygen lack and an increase in carbon dioxide acting on the respiratory center. In addition, he attributed the fatigue of rowers to the respiratory system because muscles were unable to counteract the increased "*development of carbonic acid.*" Trained rowers were characterized as having lower resting and exercise respiratory frequencies while possessing stronger and hypertrophied respiratory muscles (assumed from force measurements). Kolb felt it was necessary to "exercise the lungs" and recommended a daily short and fast run of 3 minutes.

He reported that rowing frequently increased rectal temperatures to 104°F with no apparent harm to the individual, although cold water douching after practice or competition was a routine procedure with most clubs. Although the energy cost of rowing was calculated to be 33,000 kg · m^{-1} per second, he acknowledged that it was more an approximation than factual. The textbook contains a chapter on urinalysis in which the importance of being hydrated is emphasized, whereas minimal concern is shown about the increases in urea and albumin with exercise. In the chapter on nervous insufficiency, he attempted to explain how it could be a cause of muscular fatigue and used sphygmographic tracings to support his assumptions and position. In essence, he described it as a depressed state associated with overtraining whose cause was related to "*the increased outflow from the arterial system depending on the chronic dilation of the capillaries in the muscles chronically hypertrophied*" (103, p. 163).

The Text of LaGrange

In 1890, the French textbook of the physician Fernand LaGrange, *Physiology of Bodily Exercise,* was translated into English and made available to instructors of exercise physiology (104). It contained 395 pages in 38 chapters containing six parts that listed titles such as muscular work, fatigue, habituation to work, different exercises, results of exercise, office of the brain in exercise, and 20 citations. Since its publication, the book has been surrounded with controversy, initially by George Fitz, for its incomplete and unscholarly presentation and its limited comprehension of the subject matter (105), and recently by McArdle, Katch, and Katch, who challenged Berryman's designation that it was the first textbook in exercise physiology (105). Tipton agrees with Fitz's assessment, disagrees with his distinguished colleagues because a poorly written text with inadequate documentation and incomplete explanations doesn't change its intent, presentation, or date of publication, but suggests that Bryan Robinson's 1734 text (86) has sufficient substance and detail to warrant consideration. However, to claim the distinction of being the first scientific text to merit discipline status and

recognition, the 1919 edition of *The Physiology of Muscular Activity* by F. A. Bainbridge, published by Longmans, Green & Company (6), has been selected for this purpose.

The Nineteenth Century and Establishment of Formal Courses in Exercise Physiology

Overview

Recall that for an academic discipline to be recognized, formal courses within designated programs were expected to be operational. Although Byford's article in 1855 brought focus and attention for exercise physiology, it virtually had no impact on physiologists or departments of physiology in establishing programs or courses on this subject matter.

The Lawrence Scientific School

After the Civil War, there was a heightened interest by the American public in personal and public health, gymnastics, calisthenics, physical training, physical education, outdoor recreation, and competitive athletics (94). Moreover, this interest remained intense well into the twentieth century. Two results were the establishment of secondary school and college physical education programs and professional organizations. Included within their objectives were the promotion of hygiene or bodily health and educational development. Intrinsic to the hygienic goal was the dissemination of information related to the physiology of the circulatory, respiratory, muscular, digestive, and excretory systems (107). One example of a program designed to prepare their graduates for positions in schools, athletic clubs, agencies such as the YMCA, gymnasiums, and the like was the Lawrence Scientific School and its Department of Anatomy, Physiology, and Physical Training at Harvard University in Massachusetts (107). Although the Lawrence Scientific School was established in 1847, it was not until 1892 that a 4-year scientific program in anatomy, physiology, and physical training was initiated to prepare individuals to be responsible for gymnasiums or to enter the second year of medical school. Physiology of exercise was taught in the fourth year as a theory class by George Wells Fitz, MD. This course required a laboratory experience that was the first of its kind in the United States. The program had nine graduates and ended in 1899 because of financial, philosophical, leadership, and political reasons. It remains unknown whether a text was required or what topics were discussed or taught (107). Before the turn of the century, other institutions had established degree programs that required formal instruction in exercise physiology. Observe that all had physicians in leadership positions with select examples being Oberlin College in Ohio (Delphine Hanna, MD), International Young Men's Christian College (currently known as Springfield College) in Massachusetts (Luther Halsey Gulik, MD, and later

James H. McCurdy, MD), Stanford University in California (Thomas Denison Wood, MD), and the one at Harvard University that involved Fitz. The significance of these course offerings was they highlighted an important requirement of an emerging scientific discipline.

Details of the emergence of exercise physiology from the classrooms of physical education departments to the 1996 APS publication of the first *Handbook of Physiology* devoted to exercise physiology can be found in the chapter by Buskirk and Tipton (108).

Nineteenth and Early Twentieth Century Investigations that Enhanced the Recognition of Exercise Physiology

Central, Peripheral, and Autonomic Nervous Systems

In 1888, when German physiology was dominating Europe and, in Berlin, Nathan Zuntz (1847–1920) was achieving recognition for his exercise studies, it was accepted that activation of the nervous system would result in locomotion. During this year, Geppert and Zuntz conducted a hyperpnea experiment that advanced the ideas that neural and autonomic systems were involved, exercise caused the release of a substance into the blood that acted directly on the respiratory center within the brain, and neural receptors within exercising muscle would directly elicit increased respiratory responses (109). Several years later in Stockholm, Jons Erik Johansson showed that passive leg exercise with a rabbit resulted in an increase in heart rate that appeared to be related to activation of neural centers in the brain (110).

After the turn of the century, August Krogh (1862–1949, Nobel laureate in 1920) and Johannes Lindhard (1870–1947) of Denmark (Fig. 1.9) investigated the cardiorespiratory effects of light and heavy exercise and observed that various responses that were likely due to a "neural mechanism" occurred in "less than a second" (111). They associated their results with an "irradiation of impulses from the motor cortex rather than a reflex from the muscles" (111, p. 122). Little did they realize that their observations would become the foundation for the concept of a central command with exercise!

To assess autonomic influences, measurements of heart rate changes were made. In 1895, Heinrich Ewald Herring (1866–1948) of Prague exercised rabbits and explained the increase via an elevation in accelerator nerve activity and a decrease in vagal (parasympathetic) influences (112). Using exercising subjects at the University of Michigan in 1904, Wilbur Bowen measured the latency periods after the initial heart rate cycle and indicated that the increase could be from a decrease in the restraining influence of the inhibitory center (vagal activity) because of the motor cortex and/or nerve endings of muscles (113, p. 243). Ten years later, Herbert Gasser and Walter Meek at the University of Wisconsin studied exercising dogs that had been subjected to a muscarinic receptor blocker (atropine), vagal sectioning, and adrenalectomy.

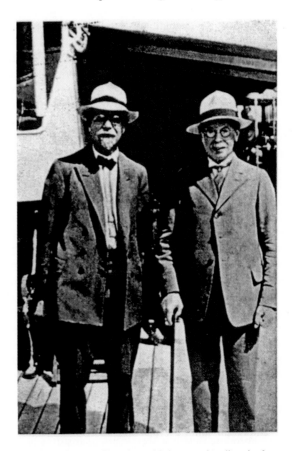

FIGURE 1.9 August Krogh and Johannes Lindhard of Copenhagen. These distinguished investigators conducted seminal exercise studies in respiration, circulation, and metabolism that helped gain recognition for the discipline of exercise physiology. Krogh was awarded the Nobel Prize in Physiology and Medicine in 1920. (From McArdle WA, Katch FI, Katch VL. *Exercise Physiology*. 5th ed. Philadelphia: Lippincott Williams & Wilkins; 2001:xlvii.)

They concluded that inhibition of vagal impulses (vagal withdrawal) was the "most economical means" by which an increase in heart rate could occur (114).

The idea that the sympathetic nervous system would be active during exercise can be attributed to Walter B. Cannon (1871–1945) of Harvard University, who became interested in an extract from the adrenal gland whose physiologic effects were similar to those of the substance released by the adrenal gland with stimulation of the splanchnic nerve. During these times, Cannon regarded epinephrine more as an endocrine product than as a neurotransmitter and considered its actions in raising glucose concentrations useful for the muscle power and redistribution of blood flow needed to fight or to run (115). In a subsequent chapter, details will be provided on the roles of the sympathetic and parasympathetic systems during an exercise response.

The Muscular System

With the development and perfection of dynamometers after the middle of the nineteenth century, the assessment and attainment of strength acquired a new importance that extended for many decades. The subject was of sufficient importance to the Union Army during the 1860s that strength data were collected on soldiers before the practice was extended to student populations at Amherst College or the YMCA International College in Massachusetts (106). Since the time of Milo of Croton or even before, it had been accepted that for an increase in strength to occur, the load or resistance had to be increased. Improvements in coordination and an increase in mass were the most frequent explanation to explain the changes. Park describes the years between 1870 and 1914 as a time when physiologists, physicians, and physical educators in many countries sought to extend scientific understanding of the severe effects of muscle exertion on the body (116). By 1892, Angelo Mosso (1846–1910) at the University of Turin in Italy had developed the first ergograph and was recording work performance and quantifying the process of muscular fatigue (117). Because fatigued muscles would respond to external electrical stimulation, Mosso was a proponent of "central fatigue," an idea attributed to August Waller (1816–1870) in London (118). Although not frequently acknowledged, Mosso had evidence for "peripheral fatigue," which, in voluntary exercise, includes the events of neuromuscular transmission (transmission fatigue) and the process of muscular contraction (contraction fatigue) (118). Using an ergograph to assess fatigue, Theodore Hough at Massachusetts Institute of Technology, after the turn of century, reported the presence of muscle soreness and attributed its existence to diffusible waste products and to possible tissue ruptures (119). In a related investigation concerned with neuromuscular fatigue, he concluded that nerve cells fatigued more rapidly than muscle fibers (120). The association between muscle fatigue and lactic acid levels in humans was increased when Ryffel in 1910 found running 12 laps in 2 minutes and 45 seconds increased blood levels to 71 mg · 100 mL^{-1} and urine levels to 2.3 g · mL^{-1} (121). However, isolated muscle preparations had to be developed and experiments conducted before it was possible to investigate muscle mechanics in exercising humans. Although Heidenhaim and Fick preceded him, A. V. Hill by 1913 had carefully developed and effectively perfected an in vitro muscle preparation that enabled him to quantify work performed and the mechanical efficiency of the responses. In fact, he reported for frog muscle that it could be as high as 50%, although it was usually between 25% and 30% (122). Later, he measured the heat being produced and used the preparation to experimentally develop the essential relationships for the force-velocity equation emphasized in a subsequent chapter.

Morpurgo in 1897 at the University of Siena in Italy reported that the histologic changes in the sartorius muscles of two dogs before and after a 2-month period of wheel running resulted in a 54% increase in cross-sectional areas because of increases in fiber diameter without changes in numbers of fibers or nuclei. Although he was uncertain of the role of spindles, which were measured, their numbers did not increase as well. He concluded that the hypertrophy was due to an increase in sarcoplasm (123). Using the Johansson ergograph to determine the effects of training, Hedvall reported in 1915 that forearm training increased muscular endurance by 819% (124).

TEST YOURSELF

Discuss the progression of physiologic knowledge from 1510 to 1910 of acute and chronic exercise pertaining to the responses of the nervous, cardiovascular, respiratory, skeletal musculature, oxygen transport, metabolic, and the thermoregulatory systems.

The Cardiovascular System

From the time of John Floyer (~1707) to the era of Wilbur Bowen (~1904), heart rates were recorded by palpations of the pulse, palpations of the heart, auscultation of heart sounds, or by graphic records of the pulse. The most accurate and reliable for exercise purposes was the placement of a tambour without button or membrane over the carotid artery, which allowed the pulsations of the artery to be transmitted to a recording drum. In 1904, using this approach, Bowen reported rates while subjects rode a stationary bicycle for various durations. The highest heart rate achieved was 150 beats per minute (113). Several years later, Lowsley reported heart rates of individuals who participated in a 100-yard dash at about 140 beats per minute or a 20-mile run at about 125–100 beats per minute (125). Besides vagal withdrawal, nervous impulses stimulating the accelerator center, elevated blood temperature, waste products within the heart, and increased muscle metabolites were the explanations for the higher values.

Stephen Hales used the horse to make the first measurement of blood pressure and, during 1863, Etienne Marey (1830–1904) in France used the same animal to record the pressure response with exercise. In England during 1898, while using a Hill-Barnard sphygmomanometer, Leonard Hill (1866–1952) had a subject run 400 yards before recording an arterial pressure of 130 mm Hg (126). He was likely the first to report that postexercise blood pressures were lower than normal resting values after "severe muscular work." While at the International YMCA College in Massachusetts, McCurdy was among the first to record blood pressure from humans during exercise. In 1901, he recorded blood pressures (with a Hill and Riva-Rocci sphygmomanometer) of students performing maximum back and leg lifts and noted that the average values increased from 111 to 180 mm Hg (highest was 210 mm Hg). He attributed the increase to an elevation in intrapulmonary and intra-abdominal pressures, which were also measured (127). Several years later, Bowen measured blood pressure of subjects performing light exercise on a bicycle (~400 kg · m · min^{-1}) and felt the elevations (60–70 mm Hg) were a result of the increase in the output of the heart plus the augmented intrapulmonary and intra-abdominal pressures (113). In the subsequent Lowsley study, subjects who trained for a marathon ran 5 to 9 miles and exhibited increases in systolic pressure of 32.5 mm Hg and diastolic pressure of 20.6 mm Hg. As with Hill's findings, there was a decrease in the average after-exercise pressures (125). In 1911, Hooker measured the effect of "violent" cycling exercise on the venous blood pressures of six subjects and observed mean increases of 9.5 cm of water, which were due in part to local vasodilation and the vasoconstriction of the splanchnic bed (128).

Once Harvey explained the existence of circulation, several centuries passed before the theory and methodology of its measurement occurred. The theory was the conservation of mass (*e.g.*, oxygen leaving and entering the lungs), and the methodology was either the direct or indirect Fick (direct Fick measures mixed venous blood from the pulmonary artery and arterial blood from a systemic artery, whereas the indirect Fick measures the dilution effect of rebreathing foreign gases using dyes or isotope clearance procedures) (129). In 1898, Zuntz and Hagerman used the direct Fick method with horses exercising on a treadmill and found the expected increases (130). Using the nitrous oxide rebreathing procedure with humans exercising on a bicycle, in 1915, Johannes Lindhard of Copenhagen found that cardiac output could increase from 4.9 to 28.6 L · min^{-1}, with heart rates changing from 70 to 166 beats per minute (131). Lindhard's data suggested that stroke volume would be increased with exercise and enhanced by training. Since Peterson, Piper, and Ernest H. Starling (1886–1927) of England conducted the research (nonexercise design) in 1914 leading to Starling's "law of the heart," Bainbridge was the first to offer an explanation, which over the years continues to create discussions among physiologists. He stated that "the powerful heart of the athlete, while obeying the law of the heart, is able to respond to a moderate increase of venous inflow by a much larger output per beat" (6, p. 54).

The effect of exercise on the size of the heart has intrigued men of science since the time of Harvey. Soon after the discovery of x-rays in 1895 by the German Wilhelm C. Röntgen (1845–1923), Nobel laureate in 1901, numerous individuals have measured heart size before and after exercise. In a 1915 study by C. S. Williamson that carefully considered the phase of respiration when the photographs (teleroentgens) were taken immediately after the cessation of "severe exercise" (running up and down stairs), 88% of the subjects exhibited decreases (132). Although increased cardiac contractility was mentioned, the results were appropriately criticized because they were not obtained during exercise. Many decades passed before methodology would be available for accurate measurement during exercise. These aspects will be covered in subsequent chapters.

Not unexpectedly, the first insights on changes in blood flow with movement came from the horse. In France during 1887, J. B. Auguste Chauveau (1837–1917) and Kaufman found chewing caused a fivefold increase in flow to the levator labii superioris (levator muscle of upper lip) (133). In studies on capillaries that culminated in a Nobel Prize for physiology and medicine in 1920, Krogh found

that simulated work (electrical stimulation of muscles in guinea pigs and frogs) resulted in marked increases, from 10- to 30-fold in the number of capillaries per millimeter of cross-sectional area being observed (134).

Because of the popularity of rowing and uncertainty as to its healthful effects, the Harvard University athletic committee in 1899 had Eugene Darling conduct physiologic tests on the eight- and four-man varsity crew members during the strenuous component of the competitive season (135). The cardiovascular investigations were concerned with the size of the heart (determined by percussion, the occurrence of abnormal sounds, and the character of the pulse). Cardiac hypertrophy was considered to be a sign of strength and power, whereas cardiac dilation was evidence of cardiac fatigue. The measurements indicated that cardiac enlargement did occur, but Darling could not differentiate the hypertrophy from the dilation. He was unable to demonstrate that the heart was "overtrained" but felt some of the changes were "unpleasantly near to pathologic conditions" and advocated constant supervision and observations when crew members were in training. None of the heart sound results had significance, but the pulse results showed they were "invariably of high tension after unusual effort." Two years later, Darling reported on the effects of training and its aftereffects as they pertained to members of the crew and football team (136). Cardiac hypertrophy was a consistent finding for both groups, but it was not considered to be pathologic. He summarized his findings by noting "that no ill effects, which could reasonably be attributed to training, were to be discovered 9 months after stopping the training" (136, p. 559).

The Respiratory System

During the time of Byford, the English penal system was using scheduled walking on massive treadwheels for punishment and ostensibly for health reasons. In London, from 1856 to 1859, a physician and social activist with an interest in respiration, Edward Smith (1818–1874) (Fig 1.10), conducted systematic respiratory studies on the effects of exercise that included himself and prisoners (137).

Using a mask, a gasometer for inspiratory volumes, an absorption chamber with potassium hydrate, and a dehumidifier chamber, he reported mean values for liters of inspired volumes, respiratory rates, and heart rates with activities, including swimming, rowing, walking 4 mph, walking 3 mph while carrying 50.9 kg, and walking on the treadwheel, which had 43 steps and covered 8.73 meters per minute. The inspired volumes ranged from 23.1 to 39.1 L per minute; the respiratory rates from 20 to 30 breaths per minute, and the heart rates from 114 to 189 beats per minute (138). When he measured the amount of carbonic acid formed during exercise, he found walking at 2 mph expired about 18 grains, or 1.15 g; 3 mph yielded 26 grains, or 1.66 g; treadwheel walking resulted in 48 grains, or 3.07 g (139). Although it is uncertain whether his results significantly changed penal procedures or laws, they provided a foundation for

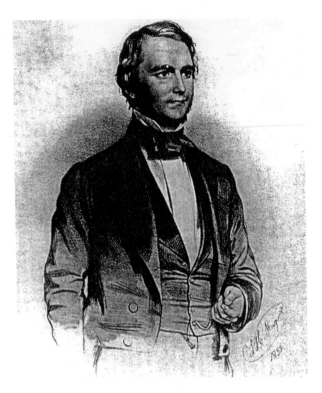

FIGURE 1.10 Edward Smith of Coldbath Fields Prison fame in England. He has been described by Carleton Chapman as a physiologist, ecologist, and reformer. His seminal investigations on the respiratory responses during exercise have become a foundation for the recognition of exercise physiology. (From McArdle WA, Katch FI, Katch VL. *Exercise Physiology*. 5th ed. Philadelphia: Lippincott Williams & Wilkins; 2001:xxxiii.)

subsequent respiratory and metabolic research in the late 19th and early 20th centuries while demonstrating that the production of carbon dioxide was linearly related to the intensity of exercise (137).

Recall that it was hyperpnea experiments by Geppert and Zuntz during 1888 that led to the idea that an exercise stimulus from the brain or from metabolites affecting muscle would activate the respiratory center (109). The rapid pulmonary ventilatory responses observed by Krogh and Lindhard in 1913 conclusively demonstrated that the onset of exercise increased the excitability of the center (111). They also suggested that hydrogen was primarily responsible for the rapid increase in ventilation, and this concept has stimulated much research and will be discussed in the chapter pertaining to the respiratory system. The linear relationships between work performed (0– ~1500 kg · M^{-1}), oxygen consumption (~0.4–3.3 L · min^{-1}), and pulmonary ventilation (~15–65 L · min^{-1}) was best demonstrated by the 1915 investigation of Lindhard in Denmark (131). C. Gordon Douglas (1822–1963) and John S. Haldane (1860–1936) in England found that intense exertion elevated alveolar carbon dioxide pressure by about 10 mm Hg before it decreased (140). This research was followed by Hough, who noted that running at 4 mph increased both oxygen and carbon dioxide tension

but, as the intensity increased and if the run was "hard," carbon dioxide could fall 11 mm Hg, while oxygen values could rise to 112 to 125 mm Hg (141). He attributed these changes to overventilation of the lungs and to the entrance into the blood of a "muscular katabolite."

Douglas and Haldane demonstrated that respiratory dead space increased approximately threefold with exercise (142) during the time of the Copenhagen debate between Christian Bohr (1855–1911) and Krogh concerning whether oxygen reached the blood by secretion or diffusion. Krogh showed that diffusion was the responsible mechanism, while his wife, Marie, reported in 1915 that oxygen diffusion with moderate to heavy exercise was associated with increases ranging from 31% to 66% (143).

The Oxygen Transport System and Maximal Oxygen Consumption

After the Smith experiments with prisoners during the 1850s (137), new apparatus and methods became available for the collection and analysis of expiratory gases. Around the turn of the twentieth century, Zuntz (Fig. 1.11) developed a treadmill that was used mainly for animals. He also had access to the portable Zuntz-Geppert "breathing machine" for metabolic studies with laboratory, sporting, hiking, and high-altitude activities (47).

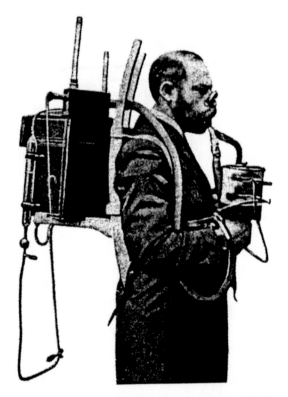

FIGURE 1.11 Nathan Zuntz of Germany. A distinguished investigator, whose metabolic and hemopoietic studies gave a foundation for the establishment of exercise physiology. (From McArdle WA, Katch FI, Katch VL. *Exercise Physiology*. 5th ed. Philadelphia: Lippincott Williams & Wilkins; 2001:lii.)

During the early decades of the twentieth century, Frances G. Benedict (1870–1957) of Wesleyan University in Connecticut, who had been associated with "metabolic leaders" such as Voit and Wilbur O. Atwater (1844–1907), conducted careful and comprehensible metabolic studies with exercising subjects and noted systematic elevations as intensity progressively increased, with 3.06 L · min^{-1} being the highest value recorded (144). In the bicycle ergometer study conducted by Lindhard (131), when cardiac output (28.6 L · min^{-1}) was measured by an improved nitrous oxide method, the oxygen consumption value was 2.8 L · min^{-1}. However, more than three decades would elapse before careful measurements of systemic arteriovenous oxygen differences were used to assess maximal oxygen uptake.

The number of circulating erythrocytes, the concentration of hemoglobin, and the magnitude of the blood volume are important factors for obtaining a maximal response, and select aspects will be mentioned in the discussion on the hemopoietic system. As noted previously, by 1915, Marie Krogh had measured the diffusion of oxygen from the alveolus to the blood during dynamic exercise; this value later was estimated to be 4.0 to 6.0 L · min^{-1} (143).

Metabolic Systems and Their Substrates

Between the Seguin and Lavoisier experiments in the 1790s and the research activities of Edward Smith during the 1850s, the principle leading to the law of the conservation energy was independently proposed by J. Mayer and Hermann von Helmholtz (1821–1894) of Germany (confirmed in 1894 by an energy balance study by Max Rubner). Early investigators after Smith, like Max von Pettenkofer and Carl von Voit, used carbon dioxide production, measured the work performed (foot lathe) with and without fasting, and calculated the oxygen being consumed. With Nathan Zuntz leading the entry into the twentieth century, accurate treadmills for energy transformation studies with animals and humans were constructed (bicycles as well); spirometers, calorimeters, and a portable (Zuntz-Geppert) apparatus were developed; and the 1888 Geppert-Zuntz equation for the determination of "true oxygen" was in use (109). According to Benedict and Cathcart (144), the first metabolic studies concerned with muscular work using either the treadmill or the bicycle were performed in the Zuntz laboratory. However, the most comprehensive and careful were the ones they reported in 1913 pertaining to the metabolic transformations (oxygen consumption, work performed, heat produced, mechanical efficiency) that occurred with subjects walking and running while fasting or consuming diets high and low in carbohydrates (144).

During these formative times, von Pettenkofer and von Voit indicated that Liebig was wrong concerning whether proteins were the substrate of choice for muscular activity. In 1891, George Katzenstein in Zuntz's laboratory reported respiratory exchange ratio (RER) values (but as respiratory quotients [RQ]) that were 0.80 at rest, 0.80 while walking, and 0.80 while climbing (145). Five years later, Chauveau of France cited RQ results of 0.75 at rest and 0.84, 0.87, 0.97, and 0.87 with 70 minutes of stair climbing that became 0.84 after 60 minutes of rest (146). He interpreted the increases with exercise as indicating that carbohydrates were being used and the declines as representing conversions of fats into carbohydrates before oxidation occurred. Immediately, Zuntz and Chauveau became involved in a controversy concerning which substrates were being preferentially used during exercise. It was Zuntz's view that muscles, whether resting or active, would use fat and carbohydrates in the proportion they were presented to the tissues.

In 1913, Benedict and Cathcart observed that muscular activity caused a small increase in the RQ regardless of whether the diet was high or low in carbohydrates (144). When a high-carbohydrate diet was consumed with exercise, the RQ changed from 0.85 to 0.90 before decreasing to 0.78, whereas, with a low-carbohydrate diet, the RQ increased from 0.79 to 0.82 before returning to 0.75. Their key conclusion was that the energy for muscular work was primarily derived from carbohydrates (144).

Intrinsic to metabolic transformation studies with exercise are calculations concerning mechanical efficiency. Using the recorded data and making various assumptions, Benedict and Cathcart estimated that the foot treadle experiments of Seguin and Lavoisier had a net mechanical efficiency of 7.7% (144). Hermann von Helmholtz (1821–1894) of Germany used the heat data from Edward Smith's walking studies and computed a gross efficiency value of 20.0%. In the first bicycle experiment involving Leo Zuntz in 1899, the net efficiency was 28.0%. Between 1900 and 1915, the most extensive and detailed studies concerning the mechanical efficiency of cycling, walking, and running in a variety of circumstances were conducted by Benedict with Carpenter or with Cathcart. They reported net efficiency values ranging from a low of 9.9% to a high of 25.2%, with most in the low 20s (144).

The Hematopoietic System

The concept that acute exercise would increase the number of erythrocytes and the concentration of hemoglobin began in 1894 with J. Mitchell in Philadelphia, when he observed higher red blood cell counts in subjects who ran before participating in a massage experiment (147). After the turn of the century, Zuntz and Schumberg made measurement of soldiers before and after 7-hour marches while covering 18 to 25 km and carrying packs of 22 to 31 kg. They found an average increase of 9% in the number of red blood cells (148). In 1904 at the University of Pennsylvania, Hawk had 22 subjects perform exercise experiments that included walking, sprinting, short-distance runs, long-distance runs, jumping, and bicycling. In all experiments, they found mean increases in erythrocytes that ranged from 10% to 23% (149). Eleven years later, Edward Schneider and Havens at Colorado College measured the influences of sprints, 2-mile runs, and a composite of running and sprints and found increases in red blood cell counts ranging from 3% to 23%, depending on the event (150). They also measured hemoglobin in their subjects and found increases ranging from 4% to 10%. Hawk explained the elevations as being the result of new corpuscles, release of corpuscles from storage sites, copious sweating, loss of fluids from the lungs, and movement of fluid into muscle (149). These investigators attributed the hemoconcentration effect of exercise to the passage of a protein-poor fluid from the vascular system into the interstitial space. Schneider and Havens studied the effect of 3 months of training for the 2-mile run by three members of the track team and reported two exhibited increases in erythrocyte numbers (5% and 18%) and hemoglobin concentration (4% and 9%) (150). Boothby and Berry had subjects exercise on a bicycle ergometer and found increases in red blood cells of 0% to 25% and 7% to 11% for hemoglobin. Rather than relate their results to work performed, they concluded that increases would result if sweating occurred because of the withdrawal of water from the cells (151).

In 1903, Christian Bohr (1855–1911) in Copenhagen demonstrated the S-shaped oxygen dissociation curve and a year later, Krogh showed that the curve was affected by the carbon dioxide content of the blood (152). In 1910, Joseph Barcroft in England found that the addition of acid to solutions of hemoglobin caused a shift in the curve similar to what was exhibited when carbon dioxide content was elevated (153). Two years later, Barcroft and associates used a 1910 equation determined by A. V. Hill to show that "severe" exercise (climbing 1000 feet in the mountains in 20 minutes) shifted the dissociation curve in the direction of greater acidity (to the right), whereas normal exercise (climbing 1000 feet in 45 minutes) had no noticeable effect on the curve (153). Although Barcroft showed in 1914 that temperature changes would also alter the curve in a manner found with increased levels of acidity (152), several decades would elapse before Barcroft and Rodolfo Margaria (1901–1983) would conduct the definitive studies associated with dynamic exercise. As to the effects of training on these measures, including blood volume, several decades would pass before they were effectively addressed.

Body Fluids and Temperature Regulatory Systems

Before 1919, no techniques were available to accurately measure plasma volume; intracellular, interstitial, and extracellular fluid volumes; or total body water—hence, changes in hemoconcentration, weight loss, sweat production, and urine formation were used to assess the effects of exercise. Not unexpectedly, weight loss was the method of choice. Perspiration was also assessed by the collection of sweat. Recall that in 1734, Bryan Robinson collected and weighed samples while his subjects continued to exercise (86). Sweat glands were first identified in 1664 by Steno, who reported that insensible perspiration and sweat "passed out" of them (154). By 1887, it was accepted that the evaporation of sweat would have a cooling effect on the body and serve an important role in thermal regulation (92), an idea advanced a century earlier by Lavoisier. The concept that

individuals exposed to exercise and heat should consume body fluids was advocated as early as 1866 for sportsmen by the trainer Archibald Maclaren (155), although the need to maintain fluid balance was promoted in 1912 by E. H. Hunt (156).

During the 1850s, it was considered prudent to exercise to the point when body temperature was increased, the skin was moist with sweat, and the cheeks were red, but not to the signs of fever. However, that perspective changed when the emphasis changed to learning of the effects with maximal exertion (94). In 1898, Pembrey and Nicol measured the surface temperatures from five different regions of the body while walking and found increases from 0.2° to 2.2°C. They recognized the unreliability of recordings of oral temperatures during dynamic exercise and recommended either securing rectal temperatures or urine temperatures after micturition. When rectal temperatures were measured during "heavy exercise," values ranging from 38.3° to 40°C (100° to 104°F) were found (157). Soon researchers in Europe and the United States were assessing body temperature changes (mostly rectal, but several insisted on oral) associated with marching soldiers, mountain climbers, cyclists, runners, skiers, and individuals performing various exercises. Because external environmental conditions will affect internal temperature measurements, efforts were made to study rectal temperature changes under standardized ambient conditions. At the turn of the century, Lagrange indicated that a rise in body temperature during exercise would increase the mechanical efficiency of muscle and recommended a "preliminary canter" for warming up (104). Investigations on the rectal temperature changes in 1904 Olympic marathon runners showed increases ranging from 1.15° to 1.9°C, with the highest value being 38°C (100.4°F) with a runner showing no distress (158). Benedict and Cathcart in 1913 (144) were among the first to carefully control conditions and to use a calorimeter to measure the heat produced with exercise. They demonstrated that "severe" exercise on a bicycle ergometer was associated with a rapid rise in body temperature (before peaking at 37.7°C and falling to a plateau of 37.4°C). They felt the rise in temperature during exercise was proportional to the intensity of the work performed and would be associated with an enhanced muscle blood flow (144).

The Renal System

Beginning in the Dark Ages, health status was assessed by examination of the urine for color, turbidity, sediments, smell, and taste (67). This practice persisted for centuries and partly explains why most of the early exercise literature on kidney function consists of uroscopy reports.

One of the first to analyze urine for functional insights was August Flint Jr. As mentioned previously, he collected urine from a pedestrian (Edward Weston) who was capable of walking 100 miles in less than 22 hours (100). Of interest was an increase in urinary water, nitrogenous products, sulfates, and phosphates, with no meaningful changes in chlorides. Because of the nature of the diet and types of fluids consumed, uncertainty existed on the importance of his findings. Eight years later in Germany, Justus von Leube (1803–1873) observed the presence of albumin in urine from soldiers after a strenuous march but felt it was a physiologic process (filtration through the pores of the glomerular membrane) (159). When the urinary results from a march of 100 km were analyzed, 40% of the soldiers had elevated protein levels. In fact, the urinary profile (protein, blood cells, and casts) was similar to that associated with a disease condition: acute parenchymatous nephritis. This resemblance gave rise to the concept that prolonged exercise was associated with "pathologic urine" (160). Urinalysis results were also used to assess the effects of the marathon on kidney function, and all of the Olympic runners tested exhibited evidence of albumin and most had casts, red blood cells, and acetone bodies. None had evidence of glucose being filtered (158). Not surprisingly, these results continued to fuel the controversy as to whether prolonged heavy exercise had a pathologic effect on the kidneys.

This concern was one factor that impelled the Athletic Committee at Harvard University to have Darling include kidney function in his assessment of the acute and chronic effects of competitive rowing. He found notable increases in urinary specific gravity, urea, albumin, and casts and concluded, "Finally, this investigation has demonstrated that the physiologic effects of training, on the heart and kidneys in particular, may approach unpleasantly near to pathologic conditions, and that there should be some competent supervision to insure that the safe limits, when those are determined, shall not be passed" (135, p. 233). Two years later (1901), he published a subsequent study on these same crew members in which he included minimal information on kidney changes (136). His summary stated, "It may be said that no ill effects, which can reasonably be attributed to training, were to be discovered nine months after stopping the training" (136, p. 559).

The Gastrointestinal System

Digestion was included in the Harvard crew study initiated by Darling. The concern was weak stomachs and the prostration caused by diarrhea. However, after repeated observations, he concluded that the issue was one of nutrition and eating habits rather than exertion (135). Other than infrequent episodes of indigestion after the cessation of training, there was no information or conclusion on this subject.

At the turn of the century, Walter Cannon (1871–1945) of Harvard University began his illustrious research career by studying the functioning of the gastrointestinal system. His interest in gastric hunger contractions motivated Anton J. Carlson (1875–1956) at the University of Chicago to study the effects of exercise on this phenomenon. In humans, he found little change when subjects were standing or walking, whereas running had an inhibitory effect (161). When he placed gastric fistulas in dogs and ran them on a treadmill at progressive speeds, the results were similar to what he had reported for humans.

The Endocrine System

At the time of the Byford manuscript, castration was known to affect the sexual characteristics and functions of males; Claude Barnard had shown that the liver released glucose into the blood as an "internal secretion"; and Thomas Addison of Guy's Hospital and Medical School in London had characterized a syndrome associated with the destruction of the adrenal cortex. Thus, any implication of an endocrine influence of exercise related to a vestige of the humoral doctrine of Hippocrates. Around the turn of the century, William Bayliss (1860–1924) and Ernst Starling (1866–1927) in London contributed to the birth of endocrinology when they reported that a chemical substance from intestinal tissue called secretin was responsible for stimulation of the secretion of fluids from the pancreatic gland (67).

Endocrinology evolved primarily because of animal experiments. In 1892, Jacobj of Germany demonstrated that the electrical stimulation of the splanchnic nerves supplying the adrenal glands released a substance that altered the amplitude of contractile tissue (162). Three years later, Oliver and Schafer discovered an adrenal extract that was similar to the one found after stimulating the splanchnic nerves (163). Cannon used this knowledge in planning his experiment with de la Paz and showed that the blood of cats excited by barking dogs contained epinephrine and increased concentrations of glucose (115). This information led to the splanchnic nerve experiment with Nice (164), demonstrating that stimulated fatigued tibialis anterior muscles increased their force production and contributed to the fight-or-flight concept associated with Cannon because he believed the increased epinephrine would enhance muscle power and blood flow in the process. When Cannon was conducting these experiments, others had shown with isolated preparations that epinephrine would increase heart rate, oxygen consumption, cardiac contractility, and coronary vasodilation; thus, it would appear during the recognition years that physiologists were advocating a key role for epinephrine in augmenting an exercise response. Surprisingly, that was not the case with Bainbridge. He considered the uncertainty and variability found with such measurements too great. In fact, he states, "It is very doubtful, therefore, whether the suprarenal glands, as regards the secretion of adrenalin, take any share in bringing about the circulatory and other changes occurring during exercise under ordinary conditions" (6, p. 132).

Because of the astute observations of Thomas Addison (1793–1860) in the middle of the nineteenth century, an association existed between the adrenal gland (cortex) and muscular weakness and fatigue. In fact, Charles Edouard Brown-Sequard (1817–1894) of London in 1856 proposed that the adrenal cortex detoxified the metabolites of muscular activity (165). However, almost 80 years would elapse before experimental exercise studies were undertaken with adrenalectomized animals and adrenal cortical extracts to investigate the basis of Addison's observations. In addition, it was well after the recognition years that exercise studies involving the pituitary, thyroid, and pancreatic glands were studied.

The Immune System

In ancient Rome, the term *immunity* described an exemption of service or duty to the state. When defined medically, it meant protection against infectious diseases. However, before it was defined, it was recognized and accepted that the first attack of a disease provided protection against a second incident. As the germ theory of disease was being accepted, immunology was born in the French laboratory of Louis Pasteur (1822–1895). In the 1880s, his acquired immunity results with chicken cholera and sheep anthrax were soon known by the scientific and medical community (166). Although the field was evolving, with discoveries related to the presence and actions of antigens and antibodies or the existence of cellular and autoimmunity, little interest or concern pertained to how exercise would alter immune responses. Of the attention given, most pertained to infections and the role of leukocytes in the process.

One of first studies on the effects of exercise on leukocytes (in 1835 physiology texts, they were known as white globules) was conducted by Zuntz and Schumburg in 1901 with soldiers (148). Their post-march results showed elevations in leukocyte counts, which were attributed to increases in neutrophils and lymphocytes. In the 1904 Hawk investigation on the effects of various athletic activities ($N = 13$) on blood constituents, leukocytes increased in all events by an average of 57% (149).

Compared to nonathletic subjects of that era, the athletes in the Hawk study had resting values (8,000 leukocytes per mL) that were noticeably higher (~11%). Schneider and Havens, in their study of track athletes, also found increases in leukocytes after running events that ranged from 3% to 23%. When they performed differential white cell counts, the polymorphonuclear cells increased by 9% to 45%, whereas the mononuclear cells exhibited decreases ranging from 14% to 55% (150). Collectively, these changes were attributed to the redistribution of cells and fluids with exercise and no attempt was made to relate them to the responses associated with infections. (However, some investigators who followed have made such an assertion.)

The interest in the relationship between physical fitness status and immunity against infectious diseases is, in part, related to a post–World War I observation by Professor Hans Zinsser in Boston, that athletic men serving in the American Overseas Expeditionary Force experienced a high incidence of influenza and death (presumably, higher than found with nonathletic soldiers) (167). Although this observation remained unresolved, modern insights on the relationship are presented in the chapter related to the immune system.

The Text of McKenzie

In 1910, while at the University of Pennsylvania as director of physical education, the renowned sculptor of sport, R. Tait McKenzie, MD, published the first of several editions of *Exercise in Education and Medicine* (168). The text was addressed to "students and practitioners of physical training; to teachers of the youth; to students of medicine and to its practitioners, with the purpose to give a comprehensive view of the space exercise should hold in a complete scheme of education and in the treatment of abnormal or diseased conditions" (168, p. 9). After defining exercise and sorting it into active and passive categories, McKenzie discussed exercises of effort, skill, and endurance while indicating that endurance exercises were associated with different types of fatigue. The emphasis on the physiology of exercise was predominately limited to changes associated with the muscular, respiratory, and cardiovascular systems, with minimal details on metabolic, hemopoietic, and excretory systems. Little, if any, of the information mentioned by Robinson, Seguin, and Lavoisier, Byford, Hartwell, Flint, or Kolb was included although the views mentioned by Lagrange were noted.

Summary of the Publications and Investigations of the Nineteenth and Early Twentieth Centuries

The Publications

When reflecting on the myriad publications associated with this time period, it is necessary to determine whether the authors are presenting their views or opinions of the times or the results of observations or experiments. Although the former provides insights on the era and the status of the knowledge base, only the latter can advance the scientific foundations of exercise physiology. Thus, the 1833 observations of Beaumont are important and markedly advanced our understanding of the role of the stomach in nonexercise and exercise conditions. Flint's textbook of physiology, which had several editions, was extremely valuable because (a) it provided "the state of the art" physiologic foundation for future physicians who might become faculty members in departments of physical education and (b) the text contained experimental results pertaining to exercise physiology that he and other investigators had collected. Kolb's 1893 text warrants mention because he presented extensive results that he had obtained on sportsmen, the majority of whom were rowers. His text covers matters of training, training effects, and training schedules and includes data on the amount of work being performed and the effects of fatigue and select responses from the respiratory and cardiovascular systems that raise minor questions as to their merit. His rectal temperature results of 40°C (104°F) may have impressed future Olympic officials that this value was an upper limit for future competitors. The publication of Byford views on the naming and importance of exercise physiology have historical significance but his physiologic concepts are more a reflection of views than results. One aspect of Hartwell's papers is they mention the important role of genetics in an exercise response.

The Establishment of Courses in Exercise Physiology

William Byford's article in 1855 introduced the term and the potential of exercise physiology but did nothing to stimulate physiology departments to consider, including exercise physiology within their academic offerings. As indicated by Roberta Park, after the Civil War, there was an intense interest by the American public in health and health education and an intent to include these topics with physical training, gymnastics, and sports within existing educational systems. Because physicians were responsible for the health of students and, in most institutions, the gymnasiums, they were available for instructional purposes. Subsequently, courses in exercise physiology were offered by several institutions with the one taught by George Wells Fitts, MD, in 1892 at The Lawrence Scientific School of Harvard University regarded as the model.

TEST YOURSELF

Provide a rationale for supporting a declaration that the discipline of exercise physiology emerged from the classrooms and laboratories of physical education departments rather than those of physiology departments.

The Experimental Investigations

It is acknowledged that these results did not occur in the manner they are being presented. The fact that the nervous system was involved with locomotion, heart rate, and respiratory responses was known from experimental results found by Nathan Zuntz, August Julius Geppert, and Jons Erik Johannson. However, it was the cardiorespiratory experiments of August Krogh and Johannes Lindhard in which their neural mechanism was associated with the "irradiation of impulses from the motor cortex" that led to the motor command activation concept that currently explains the role of the nervous system in the movement, respiratory, and circulatory responses.

The measurement of heart rate during exercise began with Galen, continued with Robinson, and effectively reported by Bowen in 1904 with cycling students. Blood pressure was first recorded in exercising horses by Etienne Marey before Leonard Hill, James McCurdy, and Wilbur Bowen reported their results with humans. Hill demonstrated the occurrence of postexercise hypotension while McCurdy reported the effects resistance exercise and, with Bowen, noted the effects of dynamic exercise on arterial pressures. Johannes Lindhard perfected a nitrous oxide rebreathing method to measure cardiac output during exercise and reported values of 28.6 L $\cdot$ min^{-1}. Although much debate on its validity has occurred since its use, Bengt Saltin makes the argument that research in the two decades has vindicated their methods and values. Lindhard also reported that stroke volume would be increased by exercise and training. Although measurements and discussions prevailed on the effects of exercise on the size of the heart, the methodology was lacking in precision to substantiate the results on the subject.

Edward Smith's efforts to use respiratory methods to demonstrate the harmful effects of treadmill exercises for prison inmates resulted in extensive data on work performed, respiratory frequency, and carbon dioxide expired volumes (as carbonic acid). A notable finding was that CO_2 production was linearly related to the intensity of exercise. From their experiments, Krogh and Lindhard postulated that the rapid response was related to the presence of hydrogen ions on the respiratory center. However, it was Marie Krogh who demonstrated that the diffusion of oxygen was increased by moderate to heavy exercise. After Antoine Lavoisier had demonstrated the measurement of oxygen intake during exercise, Francis Benedict conducted careful experiments in his Washington, DC, laboratory and showed that it was possible for an exercising human to record values over 3.0 L $\cdot$ min^{-1} with heavy exercise.

At the turn of the century, the histologic findings in dogs reported by B. Morpurgo demonstrated that chronic exercise would result in muscular hypertrophy because of an increase in sarcoplasm. Angelo Mosso developed an ergograph and quantified the fatigue process and indicated peripheral, as well as central fatigue, occurred with work. Theodore Hough's ergographic research with human muscles convinced him muscle soreness was associated with fatigue products and tissue damage. From the careful metabolic studies conducted by Francis Benedict and associates, the mechanical efficiency percentages of muscles performing work was generally in the low 20s.

During this time, different opinions prevailed between Justus Liebig (proteins), J. B. Auguste Chauveau (fats), and Nathan Zuntz (carbohydrates) on the substrates being utilized during exercise. Again, the investigations of Francis Benedict and Edward Cathcart demonstrated that carbohydrate transformations were the predominate energy source for an exercise response.

Studies by Nathan Zuntz, Edward Schneider, and P. B. Hawk demonstrated that acute and chronic exercise would increase the number of erythrocytes and hemoglobin concentrations but, because of the inability to accurately measure blood and plasma volumes, their findings have more historical than physiologic importance.

Perfection of surface and rectal thermometers made it possible for Pembrey and Nicol to record temperatures during moderate and heavy exercise. However, the increases did not exceed 38.4°C. With a laboratory capable of being a calorimeter, Benedict and Cathcart measured the heat produced, as well as the rectal temperature during "severe" exercise and reported a peak value of 37.7°C. When rectal temperatures were recorded on marathon runners at the 1904 Olympics, the highest temperature was 38.0°C.

Renal physiology was assessed by urinalysis results and the elevation in albumin began the concern, which continues to linger, that postexercise proteinuria has the remote potential to reflect kidney disorders. Walter Cannon's experiments demonstrated the adrenal extract that increased heart rate, oxygen consumption, glucose utilization, and retarded fatigue in animal experiments was epinephrine and likely would have the same effect in humans in fight-or-run situations. Experiments by Zuntz, Hawk, and Schneider demonstrated leukocytes would be elevated with acute exercise, but they had no insights on how these cells were to be associated with the immune system.

CHAPTER SUMMARY

With ancient humans, exercise was a way of life, a means of survival, and the mode of migration from the continent of Africa. With migration were the fears of the unknown, the ravages of disease, the search for supernatural protection and benevolence, the desire to be healthy, and the need to understand life and the structure and function of the human body. It is of interest that ancient inhabitants of the banks of the Indus and Yellow Rivers and the territory of ancient Greece had similar elements (but not identical) responsible for the formation of the human body, and that the transformations of the elements and their qualities were associated with humors which, when in equilibrium, were important for function and the acquisition of health with residents of India and, to a limited extent, ancient Greece. To the Chinese, these aspects were related to the proportions and balance between the yang and yin principles.

Susruta of India, a surgeon, prescribed moderate exercise as a means to achieve equilibrium among the humors which, in turn, would restore health and minimize the diseases associated with an imbalance. He also identified the effects of chronic exercise. Early in the dynasties, Chinese physicians and philosophers prescribed breathing exercises to help eliminate the "bad air" and, after the acceptance of the Yin-Yang doctrine, advocated exercises for its yang or health effect. Although sports and games were important for citizens of both India and China, there was no evidence of physiologic advice being provided to enhance performance. However, both cultures believed that excessive exercise was harmful and potentially lethal.

In the city-state of Sparta, exercise was intrinsic to its governance and included within the educational process because it enhanced the state's goal of becoming a warrior nation. The physiologic result was fitness for combat. For other regions of Greece, especially Athens, exercise (identified with gymnastics) was incorporated into the educational process for promoting a healthy body. In addition, moderate exercise was advocated by Greek physicians, notably Hippocrates, because physical activity could alter the equilibrium among humors and minimize or prevent the consequences of disease. One should not forget that the first detailed exercise prescription was written by Hippocrates for a patient with consumption.

Galen, who was 500 years after Hippocrates, championed his views concerning the benefits of exercise for health and its role in minimizing disease. Despite Hippocrates and Galen's disdain for trainers, after the fifth century BC, did provide physiologic concepts to enhance performance. However, there were few physicians or trainers who endorsed the concept of performing heavy exercise to achieve a trained state.

Physiology is an experimental science whose foundations are based on measurement and the same is true for exercise physiology. Thus, the physiologic effects of exercise from the time of Hippocrates to the seventeenth century were confined to observations and reports that were usually explained by health rather than by physiology. Although understandable, these observations pertained to the circulatory (pulse rates, pulse "force"), respiratory (breathing rates), muscular (mass, strength, endurance, tone), thermoregulatory (sweating, fever), and digestive systems (bowel movements, indigestion). The seventeenth century was identified as the demarcation point because during that time, measurements relevant to exercise physiology were made by Glisson, Borelli, Stensen, Santorio, Harvey, and Bernoulli.

Described as the Age of Enlightenment, the eighteenth century could be remembered as the era of Lavoisier, Floyer, Robinson, and Tissot. Lavoisier is recognized for providing the chemical foundation for respiration, metabolism, and body temperature while measuring oxygen consumption during exercise; Floyer for being the first to record the effects of exercise on heart rate; Robinson for his experiments and ideas pertaining to heart rate, muscle strength, blood flow, and temperature regulation; and Tissot because he provided a template for the exercise prescription.

The nineteenth century has been described as the beginning for both physiology and medicine. For exercise physiology, it generally occurred after formal instruction occurred in established educational institutions. Although its beginnings were not as auspicious or noteworthy as those of physiology or medicine, it was a start. The early decades of the twentieth century were identified as the recognition years, as a sufficient number of investigations in the United States and in Europe were concerned with the circulatory, respiratory, nervous, metabolic, muscular, and thermoregulatory systems to indicate that exercise physiology was being recognized as an emerging scientific discipline.

TEST YOURSELF

Provide a rationale for opposing a declaration that exercise physiology evolved and flourished because of its value in enhancing and improving performance.

A description of the study (in French and English) and a listing of the results can be found in Benedict and Cathcart (144, p. 6), Flint (100, p. 138), and with the original text (84). From his previous studies, including those on animals, Lavoisier knew that respirable air (he later named it *oxygine*) would enter the lung and leave it as chalky aeriform acids (carbon dioxide) in almost equal volumes. In addition, the respirable portion of the air had the property to combine with blood and to change its color to red. These studies led him to conclude that respiration was a slow combustion process between carbon and hydrogen that required oxygen and resulted in the formation of heat that dispersed throughout the body (he thought the combustion process occurred in the lungs). Therefore, to determine the effects on respiration of resting, food consumption, and exercise, he had the chemist Armand Seguin wear a copper mask to breath oxygen provided via a trough and to perform work using a foot treadle (nearby table). His wife, Marie-Anne Lavoisier (Fig. 1.12) served as a recorder, and a physician was present to assess the health status of Seguin (heart sounds and heart rate). The copper mask was held in place by wax or a cement-like substance.

The experiment had five phases. The first two were to measure resting oxygen consumption and carbon dioxide production in the fasting state at two external temperatures, about 26°C and 12°C. Then Seguin performed work with a foot treadle that lifted a 7.343 kg weight to a height of 613 pieds, or about 200 m in a 15-minute period. After he consumed a meal (believed to be his breakfast), resting measurements were repeated as was the work experiment. However, after the meal, Seguin lifted the same weight to an equivalent of 650 pieds, or about 211 m in the allotted time. Oxygen consumption was recorded in pounces

(1000 pounces = 19.8363 L) and expressed on an hourly basis. The results were as follows.

Condition	Cubic Pounces/hr	L/hr	L/min	Work Performed (kg/min)
Resting, 26°C, fasting	1210	24.002	0.400	
Resting, 12°C, fasting	1344	26.660	0.444	
Resting after food	1800–1900	37.689	0.628	
Work, fasting	3200	63.477	1.058	1469
Work after food	4600	91.428	1.524	1549

Ignoring the obvious problems in design and methodology (values are an approximation), Seguin and Lavoisier demonstrated for the first time in humans the transformations of energy with specific reference to the effects of external temperature, digestion, and exercise. By measuring oxygen consumption and having a physician record heart rates during the experiment (data not shown), they revealed an awareness of a relationship between the circulatory and metabolic systems well in advance of nineteenth-century investigators. To the exercise physiologist of today, oxygen consumption is the gold standard to assess and prescribe exercise; thus, we should not forget that it started with Lavoisier more than 200 years ago!

Seguin A, Lavoisier A. Premier Memoire sur la Respiration des Animaux. Mem Acad R Sci. 1789:566–584.

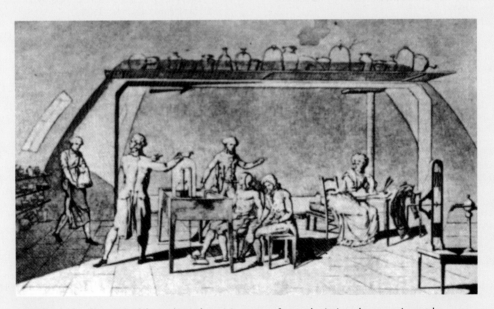

FIGURE 1.12 Sketch by Marie-Anne Lavoisier, one of two depicting the experiment by Lavoisier and Seguin. (From McKie D. *Antoine Lavoisier, Scientist, Economist, Social Reformer.* New York: Henry Schuman; 1952:353.)

REFERENCES

1. Sherrington C. *Man on His Nature*. New York: Macmillan; 1941:6–8.
2. Byford WH. On the physiology of exercise. *Am J Med Sci*. 1855;30:32–42.
3. Brock AJ. *Greek Medicine*. London: Dent & Sons; 1929.
4. Tipton CM. Historical perspective: the antiquity of exercise, exercise physiology and the exercise prescription for health. In: Simopoulos SP, ed. *Nutrition and Fitness: Cultural, Genetic, and Metabolic Aspects*. Basel: Karger; 2008:198–245.
5. Tipton CM. Contemporary exercise physiology: fifty years after the closure of the Harvard Fatigue Laboratory. *Exerc Sport Sci Rev*. 1998;26:315–339.
6. Bainbridge FA. *The Physiology of Muscular Exercise*. London: Longmans, Green; 1919.
7. Roy SB. *Mohenjardo*. New Delhi: Institute of Chronology; 1982.
8. Wilson HH. *Rig-Veda Samhita*. Vols. I-VII. New Delhi: Cosmos Publications; 1977.
9. Bahita SL. *A History of Medicine with Special Reference to the Orient*. New Delhi: Office of the Medical Council of India; 1977.
10. Kutambiah P. *Ancient Indian Medicine-Orient*. Madras: Longmans; 1962.
11. Ray P, Gupa H, Roy M. *Susruta Samhita*. New Delhi: Indian National Science Academy; 1980.
12. Bhishagratna KK. *The Sushruta Samhita*. Vol. II, 2nd ed. Varanasi, India: Chowkhamba Sankrist Series Office; 1963.
13. Tipton CM. Susruta of India: an unrecognized contributor to the history of exercise physiology. *J Appl Physiol*. 2008;104:1553–1557.
14. Bhishagratna KK. *The Sushruta Samhita*. Vol. I, 2nd ed. Varanasi, India: Chowkhamba Series Office; 1963.
15. Bhishagratna KK. *The Sushruta Samhita*. Vol. III, 2nd ed. Varanasi, India: Chowkhamba Series Office; 1963.
16. Raja V. Susruta of ancient India. *J Opthal*. 2003;51:2–7.
17. Das S. Susruta, the pioneer urologist of antiquity. *J Urol*. 2001;165:1405–1408.
18. Sharma RK, Dash VB. *Angivesa's Caraka Samhita*. Vol. I. Varanasi, India: Chowkhamba Series Office; 1977.
19. Sharma RK, Dash VB. *Angivesa's Caraka Samhita*. Vol. III. Varanasi, India: Chowkhamb Series Office; 1977.
20. Gordon BL. *Medicine throughout Antiquity*. Philadelphia: Davis; 1949.
21. Amoit JM. *Memoires concernant l' historie, les sciences, les arts, les moerus, les usages, des chinois par les missionnaires de Pekin*. Vol. IV Paris: Saint-de Beauvis vis-à-vis le College; 1779:1–519.
22. Veith I. *The Analysis of the Huang Ti Nei Chung SuWen* [The Yellow Emperor's Classic of Internal Medicine]. Berkeley: University of California Press; 2002.
23. Wong KC, Lien-Teh W. *History of Chinese Medicine*. 2nd ed. Shanghai: National Quarantine Service; 1936.
24. Harper DJ. *Early Chinese Medical Literature* (The Mawangdui Medical Manuscripts). London: Kegan Paul International; 1998.
25. Biers WR. *The Archaeology of Greece: An Introduction*. Ithaca: Cornell University Press; 1980.
26. Robinson RS. *Sources for the History of Greek Athletics*. Chicago: Ares Publishers; 1981.
27. Nicoll A. *Chapman's Homer: The Iliad*. Vol. I. New York: Bolingen Foundation Pantheon Books; 1956.
28. Mitchell H. *Sparta*. Westport, CT: Greenwood Press; 1985.
29. Wright FA. *Greek Athletics*. London: Cape; 1925.
30. Hooker JT. *Ancient Spartans*. London: Dent; 1980.
31. Barnes J. *The Presocratic Philosophers*. Vol. I. London: Routledge & Kegan; 1979.
32. Kirk GS, Raven JE, Schofield M. *The Presocratic Philosophers*. 2nd ed. Cambridge: Cambridge University Press; 1983.
33. Vogel CJ. *Pythagoras and the Pythagorean Society*. Assen: Royal Van Gorcum & Co; 1996.
34. Lambridis H. *Empedocles, A Philosophical Investigation*. Alabama: The University of Alabama Press; 1976.
35. Garrison FH. *An Introduction to the History of Medicine*. 2nd ed. Philadelphia: Saunders; 1917.
36. *Hippocrates*. Vol. I. Jones WH, trans-ed. Cambridge, MA: Harvard University Press; 1923.
37. Elliott JS. *Outlines of Greek and Roman Medicine*. Boston: Milford House; 1971.
38. Park R. *An Epitome on the History of Medicine*. Philadelphia: Davis; 1997.
39. Olivova V. *Sports and Games in the Ancient World*. London: Orbis Publishing Co; 1984.
40. Licht S. *Therapeutic Exercise*. New Haven: Elizabeth Licht Publisher; 1965.
41. Jowett B. *Book III: The Republic of Plato*. London: The Colonial Press; 1901.
42. Harris HA. *Greek Athletes and Athletics*. London: Hutchinson; 1964.
43. Miller SG. *Arete, Greek Sports from Ancient Sources*. Berkeley: University of California Press; 1991.
44. Woody T. Philostratus: concerning gymnastics. *Res Quart*. 1943;17:127–137.
45. Lund FB. *Hippocrates*. New York: Hoeber; 1936.
46. Haggard HW. *Mystery, Magic and Medicine, The Rise of Medicine from Superstition to Science*. Garden City, NY: Doubleday; 1933.
47. Rothschuh KE. *History of Physiology*. Huntington, NY: Krieger Publishing; 1973.
48. *Hippocrates*, Vol. IV. Jones WHS, trans-ed. Cambridge, MA: Harvard University Press; 1923.
49. *Hippocrates*, Vol. VI. Potter P, trans-ed. Cambridge, MA: Harvard University Press; 1988.
50. Levine EB. *Hippocrates*. New York: Twayne; 1971.
51. *Hippocrates*, Vol II. Jones WHS, trans-ed. Cambridge, MA: Harvard University Press; 1923.
52. Worthington ET. *Hippocratic Writings*. New York: Penquin Books; 1950.
53. Jowett B. *The Dialogues of Plato*. Vol. III, 3rd ed. London: Oxford University Press; 1931.
54. Edelstein L. *Ancient Medicine: Selected Papers of Ludwick Edelstein*. Baltimore: Johns Hopkins Press; 1967.
55. Longrigg, J. *Greek Medicine, A Source Book*. London: Duckworth & Co; 1998.
56. Scarborough J. *Roman Medicine*. Ithaca: Cornell University Press; 1969.
57. Webster G. *The Roman Imperial Army*. 3rd ed. Norman, OK: The University of Oklahoma Press; 1998.
58. Watson GR. *The Roman Soldier*. Bristol: Thames & Hudson; 1969.
59. Whipp BJ, Ward SA, Hassall MWC. Paleo-bioenergetics: the metabolic rate of marching Roman legionaries. *Br J Sports Med*. 1998;32:261–262.
60. Kohne E, Ewiglelben E, eds. *Gladiators and Caesars*. Berkeley: University of California Press; 2000.
61. Vegetius. *Epitome of Military Science*. Milner NP, trans-ed. Liverpool: Liverpool University Press; 1993.
62. Nutton V. *Ancient Medicine*. London: Routledge; 2004.
63. May MT. *Usefulness of the Parts of the Body: De Usu Partium*. Ithaca: Cornell University Press; 1958.
64. Berryman JW. Ancient and early influences. In: Tipton CM, ed. *Exercise Physiology: People and Ideas*. New York: Oxford University Press; 2003:1–38.
65. Green RM. *A Translation of Galen's Hygiene* (De sanitate tuenda). Springfield, MO: Charles C. Thomas; 1951.
66. Galen. *Selected Works*. Singer PN, trans-ed. New York: Oxford University Press; 1997.
67. Lyons AS, Petrucelli RJ. *Medicine: An Illustrated History*. New York: Harry Abrams; 1978.
68. Grunner OC. *A Treatise on the Canon of Medicine of Avicenna, Incorporating a Translation of the First Book*. New York: Augustus M. Kelley; 1970.
69. Krueger HC. *Avicenna's Poem on Medicine*. Springfield, MO: Charles C. Thomas; 1963.
70. Olser W. *The Evolution of Modern Medicine*. New York: Arno Press; 1922.
71. Mendez C. *Book of Bodily Exercise* (1553). Copyright Elizabeth Licht. Baltimore: Waverly Press; 1960.
72. Harvey W. *Exercitatio Anatomica De Motu Cordis et Sanguinis in Animalibus*. 3rd ed. Presented by Leake CD. Springfield, IL: Charles C. Thomas; 1941.
73. Lower R. A treatise on the heart on the movement and colour of the blood and on the passage of the chyle in the blood. London: Printed by John Redmayne for James Allestry at the sign of the Rose and Crown in the street commonly called Duck Lane; 1669. In: Gunther RT. *Early Science in Oxford*. Oxford: Printed for the Subscribers; 1932.
74. Frank RG Jr. *Harvey and the Oxford Physiologists*. Berkeley: University of California Press; 1980.

75. Boyle RA. Defense of the doctrine touching the spring and weight of the air. London: Printed by F.G. for Thomas Robinson Bookseller in Oxon; 1662.

76. Foster M. *Lectures on the History of Physiology During the Sixteenth, Seventeenth, and Eighteenth Centuries.* London: Dover Publications; 1970.

77. Mayow J. Medico-physical Works, Being a Translation of Tractatus Quinque Medico Physici; 1674. Edinburgh: Printed for James Thin, republished by the Alembic Club in London by Simpkin, Marshall, Hamilton, Kent; 1907.

78. Isler H. *Thomas Willis, 1621–1675, Doctor and Scientist.* New York: Hafner; 1968.

79. Bernoulli J. *Dissertations on the Mechanics of Effervescence and Fermentation and on the Mechanics of the Movement of the Muscles by Johann Bernoulli.* Philadelphia: American Philosophical Society; 1997.

80. Wilson LG. William Croone's theory of muscular contraction: notes and records. *Royal Society of London.* 1961;16:158–178.

81. Santorio S. *Medicina Statica, or, Rules of Health in Eight Sections of Aphorisms.* London: Printed for John Starkey; 1636.

82. Finney G. Fear of exercising the lungs related to iatro-mechanics 1675–1750. *Bull Hist Med.* 1971;45:341–366.

83. Berryman JW. Exercise and the medical tradition from Hippocrates through antebellum America: a review essay. In: Berryman JW, Park RJ, eds. *Sport and Exercise Sciences: Essays in the History of Sport Medicine.* Urbana: University of Illinois; 1992:1–57.

84. Seguin A, Lavoisier A. Premier Memoire sur las Respiration des Animaux. *Mem Acad R Sci.* 1789:566–584.

85. Floyer SJ. *The Physician's Pulse-Watch; or, An Essay to Explain the Old Art of Feeling the Pulse, and to Improve it by the Help of a Pulse Watch.* London: Printed for Sam Smith and Benj. Walford; 1707.

86. Robinson BA. *A Treatise of the Animal Oeconomy.* 2nd ed. Dublin: Printed by S. Powell for George Ewing and William Smith; 1734.

87. Hales S. *Statical Essays: Containing Haemastaticks.* New York: Hafner; 1964.

88. Keill J. *An Account of Animal Secretion, the Quantity of Blood in the Humane Body, and Muscular Motion.* London: Printed for George Strahan; 1708.

89. Hall AR. John Theophilus Desaguliers, 1663–1744. In: Gillispie CC, ed. *Dictionary of Scientific Biography.* Vol. V. New York: Charles Scribner & Sons; 1971:43–46.

90. Pearn J. Two early dynamometers: an historical account of the earliest measurements to study human muscular strength. *J Neurobiol Sci.* 1978;37:127–134.

91. Tissot J-C. *Gymnastique Médicinale et Chirurgicale.* Licht E, Licht S, trans-ed. New Haven: Elizabeth Licht; 1964.

92. Renbourn ET. The natural history of insensible perspiration: a forgotten doctrine of health and disease. *Med History.* 1960;4:135–152.

93. Sinclair J. *The Code of Health and Longevity; or, A Concise View of the Principles Calculated for the Preservation of Health and the Attainment of Long Life.* Edinburgh: Arch, Constable and Co; 1807.

94. Park RJ. Athletes and their training in Britain and America, 1800–1914. In: Berryman JW, Park RJ, eds. *Sport and Exercise Science.* Urbana: University of Illinois; 1992.

95. Beaumont W. Experiments and observations on the gastric juice and the physiology of digestion. In: Osler W, ed. *A Pioneer American Physiologist* (facsimile of the original edition of 1833 with a biographical essay). New York: Dover Publications; 1959.

96. Combe A. *The Principles of Physiology Applied to the Preservation of Health, and to the Improvement of Physical and Mental Education.* New York: Harpe; 1836.

97. Dunglison R. *On the Influence of Atmosphere and Locality; Change of Air and Climate; Seasons; Food; Clothing; Bathing; Exercise; Sleep; Corporeal and Intellectual Pursuits, etc. on Human Health; Constituting Elements of Hygiene.* Philadelphia: Carey, Lea & Blanchard; 1835.

98. Flint A. *A Textbook of Physiology.* 4th ed. New York: Appleton; 1896.

99. Flint A Jr. *On the Physiological Effects of Severe and Protracted Muscular Exercise: With Special Reference to Its Influence Upon the Excretion of Nitrogen.* New York: Appleton-Century-Crofts; 1871.

100. Flint A Jr. *On the Source of Muscular Power.* New York: Appleton; 1878.

101. Hartwell EM. On the physiology of exercise (part 1). *Boston Med Surg J.* 1887;116:297–302.

102. Hartwell EM. On the physiology of exercise (part 2). *Boston Med Surg J.* 1887;116:321–324.

103. Kolb G. *Physiology of Sport.* 2nd ed. London: Krohne & Sesemann; 1893.

104. Lagrange F. *Physiology of Bodily Exercise.* New York: Appleton; 1893.

105. Fitz GW. American physical education review, 1897;2:56. In: McArdle WA, Katch FI, Katch VL. *Exercise Physiology.* 5th ed. Philadelphia: Lippincott Williams & Wilkins; 2001.

106. McArdle WA, Katch FI, Katch VL. *Exercise Physiology.* 5th ed. Philadelphia: Lippincott Williams & Wilkins; 2001.

107. Park RJ. The rise and demise of Harvard's B.S. program in anatomy, physiology, and physical training: a case of conflicts of interest and scarce resources. *Res Quart Exerc Sport.* 1992;63:246–260.

108. Buskirk ER, Tipton CM. Exercise physiology. In: Massengale JD, Swanson RA, eds. *The History of Exercise and Sport Science.* Champaign, IL: Human Kinetics; 1997:367–438.

109. Geppert J, Zuntz N. Über die Regulation der Atmung. *Arch Ges Physiol.* 1888;42:189–244.

110. Johansson JE. Über die Einwirkung der Muskelthatigkeit auf die Athmung und die Herzthatigkeit. *Skan Arch Physiol.* 1893;5:20–66.

111. Krogh A, Lindhard J. The regulation of respiration and circulation during the initial stages of muscular work. *J Physiol (Lond).* 1904;31:112–133.

112. Herring HE. Über die Beziehung der extracardialen Herznerven zur Steigerung der Herzschlagzahl dei Muskelthatigkeit. *Pflugers Arch Ges Physiol.* 1895;40:429–492.

113. Bowen WP. Changes in heart-rate, blood pressure, and duration of systole resulting from bicycling. *Am J Physiol.* 1904;11:59–77.

114. Gasser HS, Meek WJ. A study of the mechanisms by which muscular exercise produces acceleration of the heart. *Am J Physiol.* 1914;34:48–71.

115. Cannon WB, de la Paz D. Emotional stimulation of adrenal secretion. *Am J Physiol.* 1911;28:64–70.

116. Park RJ. Physiologists, physicians, and physical educators: nineteenth century biology and exercise, hygienic and educative. *J Sport Hist.* 1987;14:28–60.

117. Mosso A. *Fatigue.* Drummond M, Drummond WB, trans-ed. London: George Allen & Unwin; New York: Putnam's Sons; 1915.

118. Waller A. The sense of effort: an objective study. *Brain.* 1891;14:179–249.

119. Hough T. Ergographic studies in muscular soreness. *Am J Physiol.* 1902;7:76–92.

120. Hough T. Ergographic studies in neuromuscular fatigue. *Am J Physiol.* 1901;5:240–265.

121. Ryffel JH. Experiment on lactic acid formation in man. *J Physiol (Lond).* 1910;39:xxix–xxxii.

122. Hill AV. The absolute mechanical efficiency of the contraction of an isolated muscle. *J Physiol (Lond).* 1913;46:435–469.

123. Morpurgo B. Über Activitats-Hypertrophie der wikurlichen Muskeln. *Virchows Arch.* 1897;150:522–544.

124. Hedvall B. Fatigue and training. *Skan Arch Physiol.* 1915;32:115.

125. Lowsley OS. The effects of various forms of exercise on systolic, diastolic and pulse pressures and pulse rate. *Am J Physiol.* 1911;27:446–466.

126. Hill L. Arterial pressure in man while sleeping, resting, working, bathing. *J Physiol (Lond).* 1898;22:xxvi–xxx.

127. McCurdy JH. The effect of maximum muscular effort on blood-pressure. *Am J Physiol.* 1901;5:95–103.

128. Hooker DR. The effect of exercise on venous blood pressure. *Am J Physiol.* 1911;28:235–247.

129. Rowell LB. The cardiovascular system. In: Tipton CM, ed. *Exercise Physiology: People and Ideas.* New York: Oxford University; 2003:98–137.

130. Zuntz N, Hagermann O. Untersuchungen über den Stoffwechsel des Pferdes bei Ruhe und Arbeit. *Landw Jb.* 1898;27(Erganz Bd 3):371–412.

131. Lindhard J. Über das Minutenvolumen des Herzens bei Ruhe und bei Muskelarbeit. *Pflugers Arch.* 1915;161:233–383.

132. Williamson CS. The effects of exercise on the normal and pathological heart: based on the study of one hundred cases. *Am J Med Sci.* 1915;149:492–503.

133. Chauveau A, Kaufman M. Expériences pour la détermination du coefficient de l'activité nutritive et respiratoirs des muscles en repos et en travail. *C R Acad Sci (Paris).* 1887;104:1126.

134. Krogh A. The supply of oxygen to the tissues and the regulation of the capillary circulation. *J Physiol (Lond).* 1919;52:457–474.

135. Darling E. The effects of training: a study of the Harvard University crew. *Boston Med Surg J.* 1899;141:229–233.

136. Darling E. The effects of training: second paper. *Boston Med Surg J.* 1901;144:550–559.

137. Chapman CB. Edward Smith (? 1818–1874) physiologist, human ecologist, reformer. *J Hist Med Allied Sci.* 1967;22:1–26.
138. Smith E. Inquiries into the quantity of air inspired throughout the day and night and under the influence of exercise, food, medicine, temperature. *Proc Royal Soc.* 1857;8:451–454.
139. Smith E. Experimental inquiries into the chemical and other phenomena of respiration, and their modifications by various physical agencies. *Phil Trans.* 1859;149:681–714.
140. Douglas CG, Haldane JS. The capacity of the air passages under varying physiological conditions. *J Physiol (Lond).* 1912;45:235–238.
141. Hough T. The influence of muscular activity upon the alveolar tensions of oxygen and carbon dioxide. *Am J Physiol.* 1912;30:18–36.
142. Douglas CG, Haldane JS. The regulation of breathing. *J Physiol (Lond).* 1908;38:420–440.
143. Krogh M. The diffusion of gases through the lungs of man. *J Physiol (Lond).* 1915;49:271–300.
144. Benedict FG, Cathcart EF. *Muscular Work.* Washington: Carnegie Institute of Washington; 1913.
145. Katzenstein G. Über die Einwirkung der Muskelthatigkeit auf den Stoffverbrauch des Menschen. *Pflugers Arch Ges Physiol.* 1891;49:330–404.
146. Chauveau A. Source et nature du potentiel directment utilisé dans le travail musculaire, d'après les échanges respiratoires, chez l'homme en état d'abstinence. *C R Acad Sci (Paris).* 1896;122:1163–1221.
147. Mitchell JK. The effect of massage on the number and hemoglobin value of red blood cells. *Am J Med Sci.* 1894;107:502–515.
148. Zuntz N, Schumberg W. *Studien zu einer Physiologie des Marsches.* Berlin: Hirschwald; 1901.
149. Hawk PB. On the morphological changes in the blood after muscular exercise. *Am J Physiol.* 1904;10:384–400.
150. Schneider EC, Havens LC. Changes in the blood after muscular activity and during training. *Am J Physiol.* 1915;36:239–259.
151. Boothby W, Berry FB. The effect of work on the percentage of haemoglobin and numbers of red corpuscles in the blood. *Am J Physiol.* 1915;37;378–382.
152. Krogh A. On the combination of hemoglobin with mixtures of oxygen and carbonic oxide. *Skand Arch Physiol.* 1910;23:217–223.
153. Barcroft J, Peters RA, Roberts FF, et al. The effect of exercise on the dissociation curve of blood. *J Physiol (Lond).* 1912;45:xiv.
154. Renbourn ET. The history of sweat and the sweat rash from the earliest times to the end of the 18th century. *J Hist Med Allied Sci.* 1959;14:202–227.
155. Maclaren A. *Training in Theory and Practice.* London: Macmillan; 1866.
156. Hunt EH. The regulation of body temperature in extremes of dry heat. *J Hygiene.* 1912;12:479–488.
157. Pembry MS, Nicol BA. Observations upon the deep and surface temperature of the human body. *J Physiol (Lond).* 1898;23:386–406.
158. Barauch JH. Physiological and pathological effects of severe exertion (the marathon race). *Am Phys Ed Rev.* 1912;16:1–11,144–150,200–205,262–268,325–334.
159. Von Leube W. Über die ausscheidung von eiweiss im harn ges gesunden Menschen. *Virchow Archiv Pathol Anat Physiol Klin Med.* 1878; 72:145–157.
160. Baldes, Heishelheim, Metzger. Untersuchungen über den einfluss grosser koperanstrengungen auf zirkulationapparat, nieren und nervensystem. *Muenchen Med Wschr.* 1906;53:1865–1866.
161. Carlson AJ. *The Control of Hunger in Health and Disease.* Chicago: University of Chicago; 1916.
162. Jacobj C. Beitrage zur physiologischen und pharmakologischen Kenntniss der Darmbewegungen mit besonder Beruksichtigung der Beziehung der Nebenniere zu denselben. *Arch Exp Pathol Pharmak.* 1892;29:71–211.
163. Oliver G, Schafer EA. The physiological effects of extracts of the suprarenal capsules. *J Physiol (Lond).* 1895;18:230–276.
164. Cannon WB, Nice LB. The effect of adrenal secretion on muscular fatigue. *Am J Physiol.* 1913;32:44–60.
165. Brown-Sequard CE. Recherches expérimentales sur la physiologie et la pathologie des capsules surrenals. *C R Acad Sci.* 1856;43:422–425.
166. Paul WE. *Fundamental Immunology.* 3rd ed. New York: Raven Press; 1993.
167. Jokl E. *Physiology of Exercise.* Springfield, IL: Charles C. Thomas; 1964.
168. McKinze RT. *Exercise in Education and Medicine.* Philadelphia: Saunders; 1910.

Exercise and Responses of Biologic Systems

CHAPTER 2

The Nervous System and Movement

V. Reggie Edgerton and Roland R. Roy

Abbreviations

5-HT	5-hydroxytryptamine	GTO	Golgi tendon organ
ATP	Adenosine triphosphate	LTD	Long-term depression
ATPase	Adenosine triphosphatase	LTP	Long-term potentiation
BDNF	Brain-derived neurotrophic factor	MLR	Mesencephalic locomotor region
CGRP	Calcitonin gene-related peptide	MVC	Maximum voluntary contraction
CNS	Central nervous system	NE	Norepinephrine
CPG	Central pattern generation	NGF	Nerve growth factor
EMG	Electromyography	PCSA	Physiologic cross-sectional area
fMRI	Functional magnetic resonance imaging	PET	Positron emission transmission

Introduction

The first portion of this chapter focuses on how the nervous system controls and generates movement, with an emphasis on posture and locomotion. In the second portion, neural adaptations to locomotion and other forms of exercise are discussed. Both of these topics are important in understanding the role that the nervous system has in modulating the response of the body to single and repetitive movements. Because this is the only chapter in this textbook focusing on the nervous system, most of the topics addressed are necessarily brief. Two strategies were used in selecting the topics to address. Some were selected because they seemed to be the most relevant from an exercise physiology perspective and these are discussed in some detail. Other topics were selected based on our perception of their particular interest and importance for further study. These topics are highlighted but not discussed in depth. Hopefully, these topics will stimulate individuals to examine them more thoroughly.

One could easily argue that the nervous system is more important than the muscular system from the standpoint of defining motor performance and understanding how the body generates, responds, and adapts to movement.

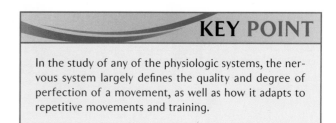

KEY POINT

In the study of any of the physiologic systems, the nervous system largely defines the quality and degree of perfection of a movement, as well as how it adapts to repetitive movements and training.

How is Movement Generated?

The maximum force generated by a single muscle fiber is proportional to the number of crossbridges that are arranged in parallel in one-half of a sarcomere and that are in the force-generating phase of crossbridge cycling at that instant. Essentially, the force generated by a muscle is directly related to the number of muscle fibers arranged in parallel that are activated by the nervous system. The maximum force potential of a muscle is determined by the maximum number of fibers in parallel that the nervous system can activate at the same time. Larger muscles usually have the potential to generate higher forces because they have more fibers in parallel. Of course, muscles also can increase their force potential when individual fibers become larger in cross-sectional area—that is, when the fibers hypertrophy. This increased force potential results from the larger fibers having more crossbridges in parallel that can be in a force-generating phase at any instant.

The Force-Generating Capability of a Muscle is a Function of its Physiologic Cross-Sectional Area

Factors other than the number and size of fibers affect the force potential of a muscle. For example, the angle of attachment of the fibers relative to the line of pull on the muscle tendon can have some impact on the force-generating capacity of the muscle. Muscle fibers can be arranged in series and these fibers also add to the mass and the displacement potential, but not the force-generating potential, of the muscle (Fig. 2.1). One can calculate the physiologic cross-sectional area (PCSA) of a muscle, which is directly

proportional to maximum force potential, using the following formula:

$$\text{PCSA} = \frac{\text{(muscle mass) (cosine of the angle of pinnation)}}{\text{(fiber length) (muscle density)}}$$

Thus, the mass of a muscle can contribute to its force and displacement and, therefore, velocity potential. In some muscles, most of the fibers are arranged *in parallel*, whereas in other muscles most fibers are arranged *in series*. Almost all muscles have fibers that are arranged in both manners. Thus, the relative force and displacement potential of a muscle of a given size is a function of the relative proportion of sarcomeres arranged *in parallel* or *in series*. Details of these structure–function relationships can be found elsewhere (1,2).

Relationship between PCSA and Size of Muscle Fibers

Theoretically, an increase in PCSA can be accomplished by adding sarcomeres *in parallel* within existing fibers (hypertrophy) or by adding new fibers *in parallel* (hyperplasia). The former case would be analogous to existing muscle

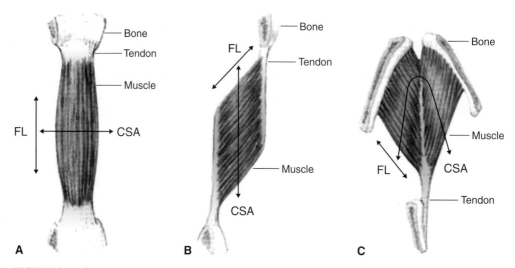

FIGURE 2.1 Examples of whole-muscle architecture demonstrating different muscle fiber arrangements. Average fiber length is shown by the line labeled *FL*. Average fiber cross-sectional area is shown by the line labeled *CSA*. Muscle contraction velocity is proportional to the length of the line *FL*, whereas contraction force is proportional to the length of line *CSA*. **A.** Longitudinal architecture designed to provide high contraction velocity. **B.** Pinnated architecture with fibers oriented at a fixed angle relative to the axis of force generation in order to provide high contractile force while conserving space. This muscle would generate more force and contract at a slower velocity than the muscle shown in **A**. **C.** Pinnated architecture with the fibers oriented at varying angles relative to the axis of force generation. This muscle would generate more force than the muscles in either **A** or **B**. On inspection, all three muscles would appear to be of similar size, but normalization of force or velocity to gross muscle size would be misleading. (Reprinted with permission from Lieber RL. Skeletal muscle adaptability. 1: Review of basic properties. *Dev Med Child Neurol.* 1986;28(3):390–397.)

fibers becoming larger in diameter or circumference. There are factors, however, other than PCSA—for example, the efficacy of each crossbridge in generating force and general changes in crossbridge dynamics that define the force output potential of a muscle.

Skeletal muscles in large animals, such as humans, have very complex designs. In most muscles, as noted previously, muscle fibers are not arranged strictly in either in a parallel or in a series fashion. The maximum force and displacement potential of a muscle, however, are rarely of real functional relevance. This is because almost all movements are generated by the nervous system recruiting a relatively small percentage of fibers in any given muscle.

KEY POINT

From a neural perspective, the force and displacement generated by a given muscle are functions of the number of fibers recruited within the muscle that are in series or in parallel, respectively, and the number of fibers recruited is a function of the number of motor units recruited for each of the motor pools involved in the movement.

How the Nervous System Decides How Many and Which Motor Units to Activate for Each Movement

Motor unit activation is determined "automatically" by the neural control mechanisms (discussed later). The force generated is modulated by recruiting muscle fibers in increments of motor units. A motor unit consists of an α-motoneuron and all the extrafusal muscle fibers that it innervates.

KEY POINT

The amount of force generated by a muscle at any particular instant is largely a function of (a) the number of motor units activated; (b) the frequency at which these motor units are activated; and (c) the total cross-sectional area of all of the muscle fibers controlled by those motor units.

Primarily, the number of muscle fibers in a given motor unit determines the total cross-sectional area of the motor unit. The size of the individual fibers also affects the total cross-sectional area, but this variable probably contributes <10% of the variance in the maximum force generated among motor units within a given motor pool (Fig. 2.2). When a regression line is plotted among fast and slow units, a smaller slope is seen among the slow units than among the fast units. This difference in the slopes is a reflection of the production of less force per cross-sectional area for slow than fast motor units.

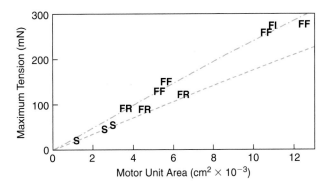

FIGURE 2.2   Relationship between the maximum tension and the total cross-sectional area of 11 glycogen-depleted motor units from the cat tibialis anterior identified as slow fatigue resistant (S), fast fatigue resistant (FR), fast fatigue intermediate (FI) and fast fatigable (FF). Regression lines represent the slow and the fast motor units. The correlations were 0.97 and 0.99 for the fast and slow motor units, respectively. (Modified from Bodine SC, Roy RR, Eldred E, et al. Maximal force as a function of anatomical features of motor units in the cat tibialis anterior. *J Neurophysiol.* 1987;57(6):1730–1745.)

Similarly, the phenotype of the muscle fibers of a given motor unit contributes to only a few percent of the range in forces generated among the motor units of a single muscle. All α-motoneurons that project to a given muscle collectively are called a *motor pool*. Each motor pool innervates different combinations of muscle fiber phenotypes, but each motor unit usually innervates only one fiber phenotype (Fig. 2.3). As noted previously, the wide difference in the force-generating capability of motor units is attributable largely to the difference in the number of fibers innervated by the motoneuron. Bodine-Fowler and associates (3) observed that, within a muscle, the cross-sectional area occupied by an individual motor unit—that is, the motor unit cross-sectional territory, in the predominantly fast tibialis anterior of the cat—was about 10% to 25% of the total muscle cross-section, with the slow motor units generally having the smallest territories (Fig. 2.4). Similar calculations for the homogeneously slow cat soleus muscle yielded motor unit territories that are somewhat larger, ranging between 40% to 75% of the muscle cross-section.

Motor unit types

The concept of muscle fiber phenotypes is widely recognized (see Chapters 4–8), but the concept of motor unit types is less recognized (Fig. 2.3). This is, in part, due to the absence of observations that specific molecular features of motoneuron types have been linked to specific molecular features of the muscle fibers of a motor unit (*i.e.*, the muscle unit). These phenotypic features of motor units depend largely on the properties of the muscle unit. There is, however, a long list of electrophysiologic and morphologic features that differentiate motoneuron types (Table 2.1).

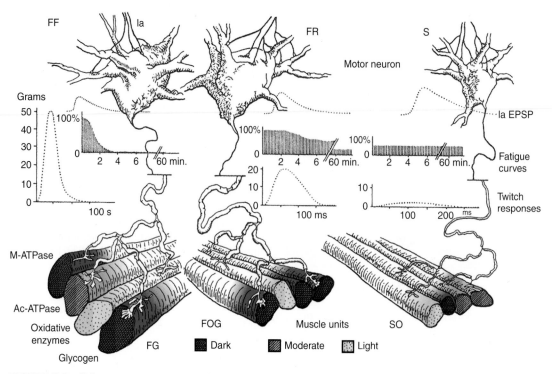

FIGURE 2.3 Schematic summarizing the most important features of the organization of the three major motor unit types identified in a typical predominantly fast mammalian muscle: FF, fast fatigable; FR, fast fatigue resistant; and S, slow fatigue resistant. The size of the motoneurons, axons, and muscle fibers are scaled appropriately for each motor unit type based on observations from a population of motoneurons. The density of Ia terminals and size of Ia excitatory postsynaptic potentials (EPSPs) are S > FR > FF, whereas the number of Ia terminals per motoneuron are approximately the same for each motor unit type. The shading of the muscle fibers denotes the relative staining intensity for each of the histochemical reactions identified in the fibers of the FF motor unit: M-ATPase, myofibrillar adenosine triphosphatase, alkaline preincubation; Ac-ATPase, myofibrillar ATPase, acid preincubation; oxidative, a representative marker of oxidative metabolic capacity; and glycolytic, a representative marker of glycolytic metabolic capacity. The M-ATPase staining is closely linked to the expression of specific myosin isoforms identified immunohistochemically. The fatigue resistance to repetitive stimulation and the isometric twitch contraction time are S > FR > FF. The neurons with the largest cell bodies also have the largest dendritic trees and axons. The largest axons have the fastest conduction velocities. The larger axons also branch intramuscularly more times and innervate more muscle fibers than the smaller axons. FG, fast glycolytic fiber; FOG, fast oxidative glycolytic fiber; SO, slow oxidative fiber. (Adapted with permission from Edington DW, Edgerton VR. *The Biology of Physical Activity.* Boston: Houghton Mifflin; 1976:53.)

Unlike the muscle unit phenotypes that can be classified based on specific profiles of protein isoforms, differences among motoneurons are largely linked to characteristics that fall on a continuous scale, such as soma size, number of dendrites, total surface area, input resistance, threshold for depolarization, and so forth.

Given the many features of motoneurons and the muscle fibers that they innervate, most motor units from a wide variety of animal species, including humans, fall within a general profile of one of three categories. These motor unit types have been identified according to their isometric contractile twitch speed and fatigability as fast fatigable, fast fatigue resistant, and slow fatigue resistant (4) (Fig. 2.3). A fourth category of motor units has been identified as fast intermediate but, in our view,

does not represent a qualitatively unique fast type (4). An alternative nomenclature combines a physiologic and a biochemical property of the muscle unit—that is, fast glycolytic, fast oxidative, glycolytic, and slow oxidative (5). A simpler and more commonly used nomenclature relative to muscle fiber properties has been based only on the basic myosin phenotype—slow (type I) or fast (type II)—there are several subtypes of the fast fibers (see Chapter 4).

Linked tightly to the force-generating properties of motor unit types are the speed-related properties. In fact, this is implied in the nomenclature noted previously. One of the explanations for these differences in velocities among different fiber phenotypes is the myosin isoform that is prominent among those muscle fibers innervated by

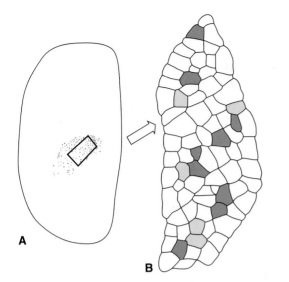

A

B

FIGURE 2.4   A. Distribution of depleted muscle fibers (*solid circles*) belonging to a single motor unit within a single muscle cross-section. The outlined region represents that area within the motor unit territory that was selected for analysis. **B.** Schematic representation of a single fascicle within the selected area of the motor unit. All fibers within the selected area were classified as being depleted or not depleted on the basis of periodic acid-Schiff staining, and slow or fast on the basis of myosin ATPase (alkaline preincubation) staining. Muscle fibers in the fascicle are identified as depleted motor unit fibers (*light blue*), slow, nondepleted fibers (*dark blue*), or fast, nondepleted fibers (*white*). (Modified from Bodine SC, Garfinkel A, Roy RR, et al. Spatial distribution of motor unit fibers in the cat soleus and tibialis anterior muscles: local interactions. *J Neurosci.* 1988;8(6):2142–2152.)

a given motoneuron (Fig. 2.3). It is also, however, apparent that there are other factors within muscle fibers that define their speed of shortening; for example, different combinations of myosin light chain, C-protein, and sarcoplasmic reticulum adenosine triphosphatase (ATPase) isoforms.

TEST YOURSELF

Is there a "master gene" that regulates the prominence of the different protein systems (excitation-contraction, relaxation, glycolytic pathways, oxidative phosphorylation, etc.) within and among muscle fiber phenotypes?

Motor unit types and recruitment

At this point, it should begin to be clear why the concept of motor unit types plays a central role in understanding how muscle force is modulated. Thus, an understanding of how different types of motor units are recruited in normal movements is key to understanding how movements are controlled and why there is a link between the intensity of an exercise and the duration that this intensity can be sustained. This comprehension is of fundamental importance when studying mechanisms related to exercise performance capacity and adaptability to a given type of exercise.

One of the most commonly used techniques to study how motor units are recruited is to identify the specific muscle fibers that have been depleted of glycogen following activation. An example of the range of staining levels for glycogen among fibers of a typical mixed, predominantly fast muscle (*i.e.,* the tibialis anterior of an adult cat) after repetitive stimulation of a single motor unit is shown in Fig. 2.5. Fibers belonging to the same motor unit can be depleted of glycogen (no staining) by isolating the motoneuron or its axon and then repeatedly electrically stimulating it. Note that there is a range of glycogen (staining) levels even among the muscle fibers that were not stimulated. In an animal with a diet containing sufficient carbohydrates, the lighter staining (for glycogen) fibers are typically slow, whereas the darker staining fibers are typically fast (*i.e.,* with the fast fatigue resistant muscle units having the highest levels of glycogen).

TABLE 2.1	Morphologic and Electrophysiologic Properties of Cat Motoneurons Innervating Different Motor Unit Types		
Motoneuron Property	**Slow**	**Fast Fatigue Resistant**	**Fast Fatigable**
Soma diameter (micrometers)	49	53	53
Total membrane area (micrometers)	249	323	369
Stem dendrite number	12.0	12.6	10.0
Input resistance (megaohms)	1.6–2.6	0.9–1.0	0.6
Rheobase (nanoamperes)	5.0	12.0	21.3
Threshold depolarization (millivolts)	14.4	18.5	20.1
After-hyperpolarization duration (milliseconds)	16.1	78.0	65.0
Minimum firing frequency (impulses/sec)*	10.0	1.4	22.0
Maximum firing frequency (impulses/sec)*	20	+++	70
Current/frequency slope (impulses/sec/nanoampere)	1.4	53.0	1.4
Late adaptation	+	369	+++
Membrane bistability	++	10	+

*Primary range of firing

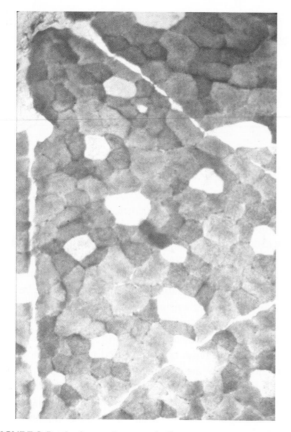

FIGURE 2.5 A photomicrograph illustrating the contrast between the staining intensity for the periodic acid-Schiff reaction (glycogen content) in depleted and surrounding nondepleted fibers of a motor unit in the cat tibialis anterior is shown. The motor unit fibers were depleted of glycogen by ventral root teasing of a single axon innervating the muscle and repetitive stimulation of the ventral root in an in situ preparation. Among the nondepleted fibers, the fast fibers typically stain darker than the slow fibers.

Note also that the wide range in fiber size among the glycogen-depleted fibers, all of which are innervated by the same motoneuron. This variation in fiber size reflects the facts that most fibers in the cat tibialis anterior taper to a smaller size over a substantial length of the fiber and that the size of a fiber within a motor unit differs no matter where, along its length, it is sectioned (6). Also, note that the glycogen-depleted fibers are spatially arranged within the cross-section of the muscle such that there are few adjacent depleted fibers. There seems to be some mechanism during development to prevent adjacent fibers from being innervated by the same motoneuron (7). The tissue section in Fig. 2.5 shows only a small proportion of the muscle fibers that were depleted and, thus, innervated by the same motoneuron. Fig. 2.4 shows the cross-section of a muscle along with the total region of the muscle cross-section that was occupied by a single motor unit (i.e., the motor unit territory). Although the physiologic significance of the spatial distribution of muscle fibers and the cross-sectional territory of a muscle unit are unknown, these probably reflect important features that the nervous system must take into account in the modulation of continuously changing forces during a movement.

Relationship between motor unit architecture and physiologic properties

There is some clear clinical relevance to the spatial distribution of muscle fibers of a single motor unit. For example, if one suspects damage to the peripheral nerves that occurs in some chronic overuse syndromes, the clinician may study the activation properties of single motor units using an indwelling recording electrode. In such a case, if the electrode is inserted into the middle of the region of this motor unit, the highest amplitude action potential will be recorded (highest density of fibers generating action potentials simultaneously). If the recording tip of the electrode is outside this region, an action potential is recorded, but its amplitude is smaller (lower density of activated fibers and a longer distance from the recording electrodes).

KEY POINT

All muscle fibers of the motor unit will generate an action potential at essentially the same time.

Summary

There will be a single action potential shape recorded by a single electrode for each activation signal generated by a given motoneuron. The importance of recording these action potentials that represent the electrical properties of a single motoneuron is that it provides one of the most readily available sites from which neurons from the nervous system can be observed in vivo.

Motor pools

As noted previously, all of the α–motoneurons that innervate fibers within the same muscle constitute a motor pool. A motor pool is usually distributed over several contiguous spinal cord segments. Within this cluster or pool, the size and type of α-motoneurons seem to be spatially distributed in a random fashion (8). For example, an α-motoneuron of a given type is as likely to occur in one region of the pool as another. A similar randomness of location within a motor pool seems to be true for the smaller γ-motoneurons that innervate the intrafusal muscle fibers of a primary sensory organ within the muscle (i.e., the muscle spindles [discussed later]).

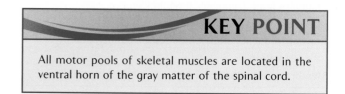

KEY POINT

All motor pools of skeletal muscles are located in the ventral horn of the gray matter of the spinal cord.

The axonal projections of these motoneurons exit the spinal cord as a ventral root. This ventral root contains thousands of axons from multiple motor pools. As these axonal projections from several spinal ventral roots extend peripherally, they merge to form a large peripheral nerves that project further peripherally and begin to subdivide into muscle nerves as they approach a given muscle. At the point that the single axon of each motoneuron reaches the muscle, the axon will divide into as many branches as necessary to innervate all of the muscle fibers of a given muscle unit. For example, if a motoneuron innervates 300 muscle fibers, it will have at least 300 branches. If it innervates only two muscle fibers, then the axon will branch only once (as occurs in some extraocular muscle units).

The nerve trunks formed by the merging of ventral roots also contain sensory axons that project from the periphery toward the spinal cord via dorsal roots. The peripheral nerves on the other hand are mixed in the sense that they have axons projecting action potentials both distally (peripherally) to the muscles (motor) and centrally (sensory) to the spinal cord.

The spinal cord can be readily divided into white and gray matter. The white matter contains few cell bodies and is composed primarily of ascending and descending axons. In general, the gray matter of the spinal cord contains cell bodies along with axons and dendrites. The neurons of the gray matter receive input from multiple sources, including the brain, higher segmental levels within the cord itself, and the sensory input from the periphery. An anatomical depiction of the complexity and the orientation of the axonal projections along a coronal slice within the spinal gray matter is shown in Fig. 2.6. In general, input from the brain and periphery will travel from the dorsal edge of the dorsal horn toward the ventral horn, eventually reaching a motoneuron within a given motor pool.

Size Principle of Recruitment within a Motor Pool

Among all of the attempts to understand how the nervous system controls movement, the efforts that resulted in the formulation of the size principle of motor unit recruitment have been the most significant. The motoneurons within a motor pool are generally distributed spatially within an elongated, core-shaped volume in a very predictable position within the gray matter of the ventral horn of the spinal cord. Although the motoneurons within this confined region are randomly distributed with respect to the type and size, there is an impressive consistency in the order of the sequence of activation of these motoneurons within each pool.

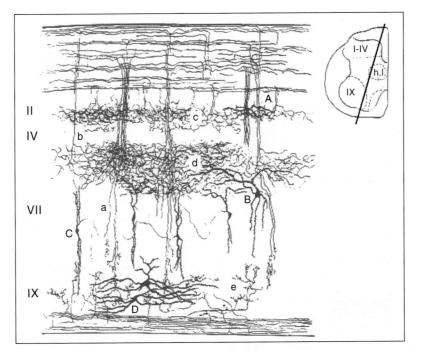

FIGURE 2.6 Coronal section of the spinal cord showing the complexity and the orientation of the axonal projections. Much of the supraspinal and peripheral input travels from the dorsum to activate interneurons and eventually the motoneurons located in the gray matter. (Modified from Scheibel M, Scheibel A. A structural analysis of spinal interneurons and Renshaw cells. In: Brazier MAB, ed. *UCLA Forum in Medical Science: The Interneuron*. Los Angeles: University of California Press; 1969:177.)

KEY POINT

The size principle states that, within a single motor pool, the motoneurons will be recruited in the order of ascending size, the smallest first and the largest last, regardless of the type of effort (9–11).

Defining the size of a motor unit

An obvious question is, which features of a motor unit best reflect its "size"? This has been the topic of numerous experiments and, although there is not complete agreement among scientists studying this issue, there is a consensus. The data presented in Table 2.1 show that the smallest motoneurons have the smallest soma membrane surface area, the fewest dendrites and branches, and innervate the fewest muscle fibers. The smallest motor units also generate the smallest amount of force because the number of muscle fibers determines, in large part, the amount of force generated by a given motor unit. The opposite is true for the largest motoneurons.

KEY POINT

Although a large number of parameters are highly correlated with motor unit recruitment order, the amount of force that a motor unit can generate is one of the most consistent to date (12) (see Fig. 2.3).

TEST YOURSELF

How does the size of the motoneuron determines order of recruitment?

KEY POINT

The most basic explanation for the size principle is that the net excitatory current needed to reach the activation threshold of a motoneuron is inversely related to the total surface area of the membrane of the motoneuron (13).

Summary

It seems that all sources of input to a given motor pool are more or less evenly distributed among the motoneurons; therefore, the smaller the motoneuron, the more likely that it will be excited when the motor pool is presented with a given level of depolarizing current from all of its synapses. The amount of input from a given source is generally evenly distributed among the motoneurons of a given motor pool. An analogy would be water spouts releasing water at the same rate placed over buckets differing in size—the smallest bucket would always be filled first (i.e., its threshold would be reached first).

Identifying motor units and their firing patterns using electromyography

The order of recruitment within a motor pool can be readily observed by recording the action potentials from muscles using electromyography (EMG). The firing patterns of single motor units can be recorded from electrodes placed on the skin overlying a specific muscle (surface EMG) or, more readily, from needle or fine wire electrodes placed in the muscle. Action potentials from single motor units can be discerned more easily when the active recording sites of the electrodes are very small and there is a small distance between electrodes. It is also easier to identify the action potentials from a single motor unit when small forces are produced—that is, when a small number of motor units are recruited (Fig. 2.7).

Action potentials belonging to the same motor unit can be identified by the similarity in their amplitude and shape. The uniqueness of the amplitude and shape for a given motor unit action potential is a function of the location of the active electrode recording site relative to the fibers within the motor unit. As the force exerted increases, motor units with larger action potentials (i.e., the larger motor units) will be recruited as dictated by the size principle. Generally, the larger motor units generate a higher amplitude action potential because the signal is derived from more muscle fibers than for the smaller motor units. Therefore, in general, under controlled isometric conditions, there is a direct relationship between the force and EMG amplitude during motor unit recruitment (Figs. 2.7 and 2.8). Often, the force threshold for derecruitment is lower than that for recruitment (Fig. 2.8). There is no clear explanation for this hysteresis effect, although it may be related to muscle fiber thixotropy or residual actomyosin bonds.

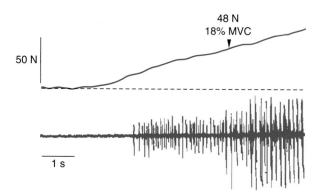

FIGURE 2.7   Recording of motor unit potentials in a human subject during a ramp force generated by the plantar flexors. Note that larger action potentials appear at selected levels of torque, representing the "force threshold" for that motor unit. Each action potential generated by a given motor unit will have a similar amplitude and shape. Only the amplitudes can be differentiated in this graph because of the slow time scale in plotting the graph. MVC, maximum voluntary contraction. (Unpublished observation, VR Edgerton.)

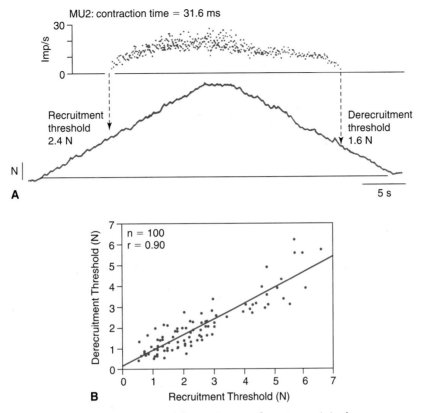

A.

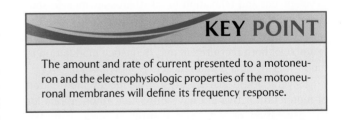

FIGURE 2.8   A. Recruitment and derecruitment of a motor unit in the extensor carpi radialis of human subjects during isometric imposed-ramp contraction and relaxation. Derecruitment threshold is lower than recruitment threshold. **B.** Relationship between recruitment and derecruitment thresholds for 20 extensor carpi radialis motor units. Note again that the derecruitment threshold is systematically lower than the recruitment threshold. (Modified from Romaiguère P, Vedel JP, Pagni S. Comparison of fluctuations of motor unit recruitment and de-recruitment thresholds in man. *Exp Brain Res.* 1993;95(3):517–522.)

Frequency modulation of motor units

In addition to the recruitment of more motor units, muscle force can be modulated by the frequency of activation of the motor units (Fig. 2.9). There have been a number of studies to determine the relative importance of these two mechanisms in modulating force, but there is no consensus on this issue. There seems to be a difference in their relative importance from muscle to muscle (14) and in the amount of force being exerted within a muscle. At the lower forces, recruitment seems to be more important, whereas, at the higher forces, frequency modulation may become most important. For example, if there are 100 motor units in a motor pool, motor unit 5 in the recruitment order would probably have its frequency modulated during a contraction force requiring only 10% of its maximum force potential. If the muscle force required was at 80% of maximum, however, unit 5 would have already been activated at its maximum frequency. Most of the frequency modulation is likely to occur among the motor units that have been most recently recruited or derecruited as the force is increasing or decreasing, respectively.

Another feature associated with frequency modulation is that motor units seem to have an initial (minimum) firing frequency of 5 to 10 Hz (*i.e.*, action potentials per second). The maximum frequencies vary among motor units, with the higher threshold units generating the higher frequencies within a burst of potentials, mostly in the range of 25 to 35 Hz. Single individual interspike intervals, however, typically can range from 5 to 100 ms.

> ### KEY POINT
>
> The amount and rate of current presented to a motoneuron and the electrophysiologic properties of the motoneuronal membranes will define its frequency response.

Once the current reaches a certain level, there will be no further frequency modulation of that unit. As more excitatory input is presented to the motor pool, however, additional motor units will be recruited. Fig. 2.10 shows the relationship between frequency of excitation and the

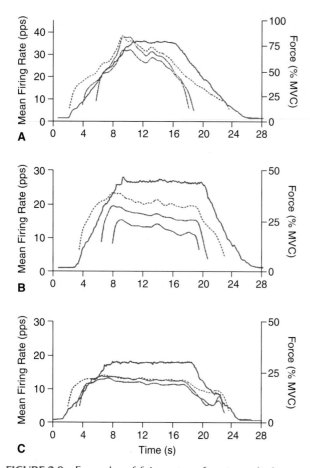

FIGURE 2.9   Examples of firing rates of motor units in tibialis anterior during isometric dorsiflexion of the ankle at (**A**) 80%, (**B**) 50%, and (**C**) 30% of maximum voluntary contraction (MVC). The force record (showing plateau) is the thick line. The other three lines in each of **A**, **B**, and **C** show mean firing rates of detected motor units. Note how firing rates decrease throughout the constant-force interval at all force levels. (Reprinted with permission from De Luca CJ, Foley PJ, Erim Z. Motor unit control properties in constant-force isometric contractions. *J Neurophysiol.* 1996;76(3):1503–1516.)

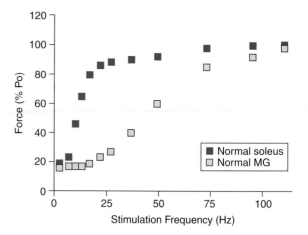

FIGURE 2.10   Relative force (% of maximum tetanic tension, Po)—frequency of stimulation relationships for a typical fast (medial gastrocnemius) and a typical slow (soleus) rat hind limb muscle are shown. Note that a higher frequency of stimulation is necessary to produce the same relative force in a fast vs. a slow muscle. The same relationship exists at the motor unit level. (Modified from Roy RR, Baldwin KM, Martin TP, et al. Biochemical and physiological changes in overloaded rat fast- and slow-twitch ankle exteriors. *J Appl Physiol.* 1985;59(2):639–646.)

is stimulated with a consistent frequency to serve as a control. When there is a prolonged interpulse interval in the middle of a train of impulses, the tension will drop significantly and continue at this lower level even though subsequent pulses are identical to those of the control condition. The significance of this observation is that this "catch" property provides a mechanism by which the nervous system can provide remarkably subtle changes in the excitation pattern to produce a significant modulation of force (16).

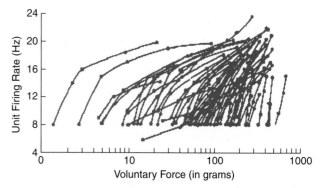

FIGURE 2.11   Firing frequencies of individual motor units in human extensor digitorum communis muscle. All units discharge in approximately the same frequency range, but for different ranges of voluntary force. Note that the frequency for the smaller, lower threshold motor units has peaked before many of the larger, high threshold motor units are recruited initially. (Modified from Stuart DG, Enoka RM. *Motoneurons, Motor Units, and the Size Principle.* New York: Churchill Livingstone; 1983:486.)

amount of force generated by a slow and a fast muscle. The curve for the fast muscle is shifted to the right compared to the slow muscle. This reflects the greater speed of force development and relaxation in fast than slow muscle and, therefore, the necessity for a higher frequency to reach the same relative force is greater in fast than slow muscle. An example of both recruitment and frequency modulation of motor units from a human muscle is shown in Fig. 2.11.

Several additional features of frequency modulation of motor unit activation have important implications for the generation of force and control of movement. For example, the "catch" principle that can be described as follows (15): the interval between two consecutive action potentials within a motor unit and the previous history of this interval duration within a given burst of action potentials can be critically important in defining the force generated by a motor unit. In Fig. 2.12 a motor unit

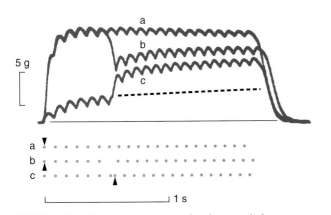

FIGURE 2.12 Tension responses of a slow medial gastrocnemius motor unit to three trains of 22 stimuli each, at a basic rate of 12.2 pps (interpulse interval, 82 ms). In each train, one or two stimulus intervals were altered. The tension traces are labeled (*a*, *b*, *c*), and the corresponding pulse sequences are similarly designated. The arrows at the first pulses in *a* and *b* indicate double stimulation with an interpulse interval of 10 ms. The arrow in *c* denotes a single pulse following the previous pulse with an interval shorter than that in the basic train but longer (about 26 ms) than the double stimuli in *a* and *b*. In trace *b*, note the drop in tension to a new level when one interval in the train was lengthened to about 117 ms. This sensitivity to single interspike intervals in the generation of force illustrates the criticalness in controlling single intervals in generating and maintaining a given force level. It demonstrates that a short interval at the beginning of a train of impulses can have a lasting effect during a train of impulses. This phenomenon is referred to as the "catch principle." (Modified from Burke RE, Rudomin P, Zajac FE 3rd. Catch property in single mammalian motor units. *Science.* 1970;168(927):122–124.)

Ballistic-type resistance training (involving maximal intentional rate of force development) markedly increases the incidence of "doublets" (*i.e.*, two successive action potentials with an unusually short interspike interval). Training with dynamic contractions results in more synchronous firing of motor units at the start of a brisk contraction (17). Although there are clear examples of short interpulse intervals occurring early in a burst, when the force ramp is very rapid, it remains unclear to what extent the nervous system can and does utilize this mechanism.

To understand how the central nervous system (CNS) modulates force, it is convenient to think of the relative and absolute forces generated by a motor pool relative to the percentage of the motoneurons activated within that motor pool. As discussed previously, motor units are generally assumed to be recruited according to the size principle. If all motor units were of the same size, then the relationship between the number of motor units recruited and the cumulative force from the active units would be linear. The forces generated during walking, or even running, are small relative to the maximum force that can be generated by a given motor pool. Although only ~20% of the

maximum force potential of the muscle may be required during running, more than 50% of the motor units in that motor pool are recruited (Fig. 2.13). There is also a high probability that the smaller motor units are in the slow type, the fast fatigue-resistant units are moderate in size, and the fast fatigable units are the largest units and recruited last (Fig. 2.3). This is not to mean, however, that this order and type relationship is rigid (see later). Although similar detail for human motor units is not available, there is indirect evidence that the same principles apply (18).

It is also useful to recognize that not all motor pools and muscles have the same proportion of motor unit types. There even is remarkable variability for any given muscle from individual to individual. Fig. 2.14 illustrates the range in tetanic forces, isometric twitch times, and fatigability among a population of motor units within the cat medial gastrocnemius motor pool.

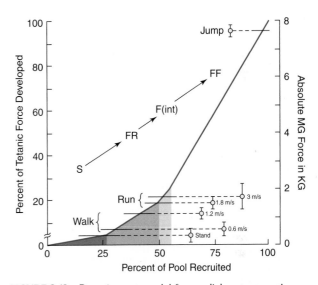

FIGURE 2.13 Recruitment model for medial gastrocnemius (MG) motor unit pool based on distributions of motor unit types and of maximum tetanic tension for individual motor units. The heavy solid curve indicates estimated percentage of maximum (fused tetanus) MG force (left ordinate) as a function of percentage MG pool recruited (abscissa) (see original reference for assumptions made). Intensity of shading beneath the curve denotes relative fatigue resistance of the motor unit groups in MG (*i.e.*, types S > FR > F(int) > FF). In generating the cumulative force for this graph, it is assumed that all motor units would be recruited in the order of increasing size. The labeled circles and brackets indicate mean ± SD MG forces during standing, locomotion at various speeds, and 120 cm jumps—all referred to right ordinate scaled in kilogram weight. It should be recognized that there is no clear line of demarcation of motor units of a certain size being of the same type. It is more accurate to view the graph as a progressively changing probability with the probability of the smaller motor units being slow and the largest motor units being fast fatigable units. FF, fast fatigable; FR, fast fatigue resistant; S, slow fatigue resistant. (Modified from Walmsley B, Hodgson JA, Burke RE. Forces produced by medial gastrocnemius and soleus muscles during locomotion in freely moving cats. *J Neurophysiol.* 1978;41(5):1203–216.)

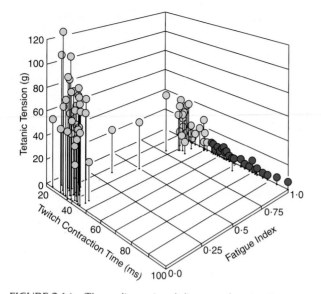

FIGURE 2.14   Three-dimensional diagram showing inter-relationships among four physiologic properties of 81 MG muscle units in a representative sample pooled from three different animals. *Light blue circles* denote units with "sag" in unfused tetani (type FF and FR); *dark blue circles*, those without "sag" (type S). Note that clustering of unit groups in different regions of the multidimensional space defined by the four parameters. (Modified from Burke RE, Levine DN, Tsairis P, et al. Physiological types and histochemical profiles in motor units of the cat gastrocnemius. *J Physiol (Lond)*. 1973;234(3):723–748.)

Changes in recruitment order

Even though the size principle seems to explain many features of motor unit recruitment, in some situations, other neural control factors are operating. It appears that in some physiologic states, the usual order of recruitment of motor units within a pool can be altered. For example, electrical stimulation of the skin over the index finger in humans can change the order of recruitment of motor units within the first dorsal interosseous muscle during isometric contractions (19). Changes in recruitment order have also been reported in very rapid contractions compared to very slowly increasing the force in an isometric contraction (20). A more significant change in recruitment order seems to occur when a muscle is activated in a rapid eccentric compared to a slow isometric contraction (21). It appears that in the eccentric mode, there is some selection of fast motor units in preference to the usually more excitable smaller slow motor units. Another apparent exception can be seen in a paw shake compared to locomotion in cats in the relative recruitment of the slow soleus and the fast medial gastrocnemius muscles (22). This, however, is a reversal of recruitment order of motoneurons across rather than within a motor pool.

There also is *some* evidence of an alternation (rotation) in motor unit recruitment in repetitive and prolonged movements (23). For example, Tamaki et al. (24) reported a rotation in the activation of the triceps surae muscles during low-level contractions, indicating that there were sudden

and frequent changes in the combinations of motor units and motor pools being recruited during these prolonged efforts. Perhaps, some level of rotation is inevitable given the inherent variability that occurs even in the most simple types of repetitive movements. This rotation of motor unit recruitment might play a role in lessening fatigue during prolonged contractions (25) (also see later).

There are some exceptions to the size principle that raise several important questions. In very rapid contractions, the order of the action potentials of a pair of motor units is probably trivial in terms of the functional consequences. There is always the question of how far apart the thresholds of the motor units (showing a change in recruitment order) are in excitability. If they have very similar thresholds, then they would readily rotate in order. Another fundamental issue relates to the definition of a motor pool.

> ### KEY POINT
>
> Many muscles are divided anatomically, and to some extent physiologically, into neuromuscular compartments (2,26).

For example, the cat lateral gastrocnemius muscle has four anatomically distinct compartments that can be independently recruited during locomotion as reflected by EMG recordings from each compartment (27). In humans, superficial and deep compartments in the tibialis anterior can be controlled somewhat independently—this is assumed to be reflected by the activation of different regions of the cerebral cortex when recruiting these two compartments (28). These anatomical and physiologic properties both neurally and muscularly suggest that there is likely to be some degree of flexibility in the order of recruitment within a single muscle.

Summary

Although there have been many disputes about the consistency of the size principle, it is our view that, with some exceptions, the order of recruitment is remarkably constant. In terms of a neural control strategy, this would seem to greatly simplify the control. It seems logical, given the predictability of the type and kind of work that the neuromotor system routinely performs, that a relatively fixed order can be a very significant advantage in survivability.

Limitations in the ability to maximally recruit all motor units within a motor pool

Can an individual recruit all motor units within a motor pool? Intuitively one may assume that the nervous system can routinely recruit even the highest threshold motor units within a motor pool. This, however, does not seem to always be the case (Fig. 2.15). For example, when five subjects were asked to generate a maximum voluntary elbow flexion on multiple occasions within a single day and over a period of 5 days, the maximum torque that could be generated was estimated to vary between 78% and 100%. This assessment was based on a technique called "twitch interpolation," whereby the muscle is electrically stimulated with a single maximum pulse during the maximum voluntary contraction (MVC). If the twitch adds force to the maximum voluntary effort, the contraction is interpreted as a submaximal effort. None of the subjects could produce a maximal effort on every occasion during a maximum voluntary effort. In fact, one subject could recruit all motor units on only one occasion of several attempts. Some studies use a short tetanus rather than a twitch and report that a twitch may not be enough to assure a maximum contraction. Other studies have reported near full voluntary activation if the subjects were allowed to become familiar with the testing maneuver, received visual feedback of the force record, and received enthusiastic verbal enouragement (29). As might be expected, when these types of visual, auditory, and motivational encouragement are provided and the best effort is reported in a series of maximum efforts, it will appear that "maximum" efforts are easier to generate (30–32). The relative ability to recruit all motor units within a motor pool does not also seem to be closely related to the level of training of the individual. Although some improvement can be observed with practice (32,33), there still remains a high incidence of some submaximal efforts when one is attempting to generate a maximum force.

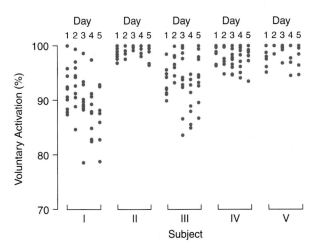

FIGURE 2.15 Ability to maximally activate elbow flexors during a maximum voluntary contraction (MVC) varies among trials on the same day among subjects. Five subjects were given 10 trials on each of five days. Voluntary activation was calculated as (1 − superimposed twitch in response to electrical stimulation during MVC/twitch at rest) × 100, a technique called twitch interpolation. (Modified from Allen GM, Gandevia SC, McKenzie DK. Reliability of measurements of muscle strength and voluntary activation using twitch interpolation. *Muscle Nerve.* 1995;18(6):593–600.)

Size Principle Across Motor Pools

There is some evidence for a size recruitment principle that operates across motor pools (34). For example, the recruitment order would be independent of the pools, but dependent on the size within the combined motor pools. This observation, however, still does not identify the neural mechanisms used to select different portions of multiple pools to be recruited for a given movement or task. A movement may require 10%, 50%, and 80% of the motor units recruited from three motor pools. The nervous system then may select 15%, 45%, and 80% of the motor units from these same motor pools to generate a slightly different movement.

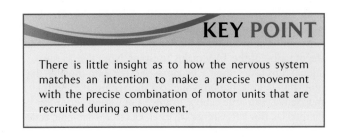

Relative levels of recruitment of motor unit types during routine movements

To identify the stimuli that may be responsible for inducing metabolic adaptations to exercise, it is important to understand some fundamental features of the strategy used by the CNS to execute movements varying in force, velocity, and duration. What neural control strategies allow an individual to run faster or run uphill, or to bicycle at a fast pedaling rate on the flat versus at a 5-degree incline?

Differential activation of extensors and flexors

During treadmill locomotion in intact quadrupeds (35), a hyperbolic relationship exists between the step cycle duration and the speed of locomotion (Fig. 2.16). Furthermore, as the speed of locomotion increases, the duration of the support phase of each step cycle decreases relatively more than the swing phase (36). These relationships also have been observed in low thoracic, chronically spinalized cats during assisted treadmill locomotion, and in the individual legs of decerebrate cats while walking on a split treadmill when each belt moves at a different speed (35,37).

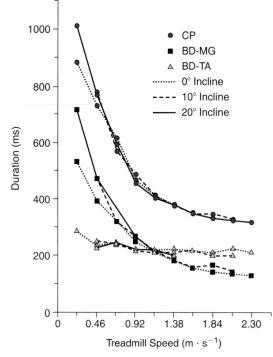

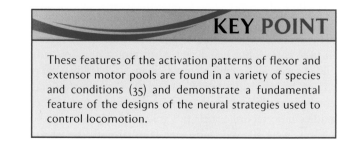

FIGURE 2.16 Cycle period (CP) and burst durations (BD) of an ankle extensor, the medial gastrocnemius (MG), and an ankle flexor, the tibialis anterior (TA), plotted against treadmill speed and incline for one cat. The duration of the MG is consistently about 200 ms shorter than the cycle period while the duration of the TA remains constant. Note that as the animal runs faster, the CP becomes shorter, with most of the reduction in cycle duration due to a shortening of extensor muscle BD with little change in the TA BD. (Modified from Pierotti DJ, Roy RR, Gregor RJ, et al. Electromyographic activity of cat hindlimb flexors and extensors during locomotion at varying speeds and inclines. *Brain Res.* 1989;481(1):57–66.)

In accordance with the assumption that the size principle is a predominant factor in determining the order of recruitment within a motor pool, the high threshold, fast-contracting fibers that can produce the highest tensions will be activated when the demands on the work rate are increased (Figs. 2.11 and 2.13). At higher speeds and/or inclines, the fast muscles can provide most of the additional power necessary to complete the work in the time available per step. Because of the greater rise of the animal's center of gravity, the extensor musculature must complete more work per step during the stance phase when the incline is increased. When speed is increased along with incline, more work (*i.e.*, more power) must be produced in shorter periods. EMG recordings indicate that the excitability of motor units of different types, sizes, and thresholds holds true, at least to some degree, across motor pools as it does within a motor pool (9). In contrast, changes in the duration of the swing phase of a step cycle are small and the inertial forces imposed on the leg are relatively constant over a range of speeds.

In adult cats, the horizontal distance that the hip travels during the support phase increases from about 16 to almost 30 cm over a range of speeds of locomotion from

0.1 to 0.9 m · s⁻¹ on the flat (37). It also has been reported, however, that the cat's joint angles at the hip, knee, and ankle remain relatively constant during a walk and a trot (38). These observations demonstrate that the strategy to control extensor muscles must differ from those of the flexor musculature, particularly during load-bearing locomotion. It remains unclear what features of which neural circuitry are responsible for the asymmetrical modulation of extensors and flexors as one runs faster.

KEY POINT

These features of the activation patterns of flexor and extensor motor pools are found in a variety of species and conditions (35) and demonstrate a fundamental feature of the designs of the neural strategies used to control locomotion.

A fundamental variable to control speed of locomotion at a given incline is the activation level of extensor motor pools. The levels of excitation of the extensor and flexor motor pools are important to consider with respect to the time and the distance the animal travels. These time-distance factors also have metabolic consequences. Hoyt and Taylor (39) demonstrated that the rate of energy consumption in horses at a gait increases linearly with stride frequency. Indeed, the integrated EMG per minute of the fast extensors increased linearly with speed. The additional effort required for locomotion at increased speeds and inclines seems to be supplied primarily by the fast extensor muscles. Although the mean EMG per minute of predominantly fast muscles increases with speed and incline, it actually decreases in the predominantly slower muscles. This results in a higher power output of type II fast muscles and a relative decrease in the power output of the type I slow muscles (40). Gregor and associates (41) reported a 20% decrease in the slow soleus and a 40% increase in the fast medial gastrocnemius in vivo tendon peak forces at comparable speeds and inclines. It appears that the soleus might be at a mechanical disadvantage in the latter stages of the stance phase, when the velocity of shortening required to produce force is very high. In addition, the soleus could become slightly unloaded due to a greater amount of force contributed by its fast major synergists during high velocity movements.

Type of contraction and energy cost

Whether a movement involves principally isometric, shortening, or lengthening, contractions has a significant effect on the fatigue properties and the neural control strategies. For example, the neural control strategies used by subjects differed significantly when they were asked to make repetitive maximum contractions at the knee in a concentric versus an eccentric mode (42). The level of activation progressively increased with repeated concentric contractions, whereas the activation level remained relatively constant

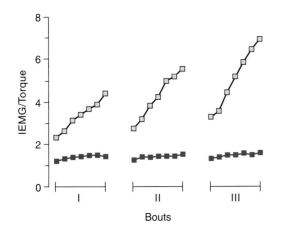

FIGURE 2.17 Integrated electromyography (IEMG)/torque ratio during concentric (CON) (□) and eccentric (ECC) (■) bouts of exercise. IEMG for the vastus lateralis and rectus femoris muscles were combined and averaged. Note the progressive increase in the ratio during CON but not ECC contractions from bouts I to III. There was a higher IEMG during the maximum CON than ECC contractions. (Modified from Tesch PA, Dudley GA, Duvoisin MR, et al. Force and EMG signal patterns during repeated bouts of concentric or eccentric muscle actions. *Acta Physiol Scand.* 1990;138(3):263–271.)

with repeated eccentric contractions (Fig. 2.17). This differential neural response is linked to the fact that energy expenditure is much lower during eccentric than concentric contractions (43). These features are likely related to the fundamentally different mechanical dynamics with respect to the metabolic cost per cross-bridge cycle and the duration of the force-generating stage of the cross-bridge interactions between these two contractile modes. Therefore, the nature of the movement will have a very predictable consequence with respect to fatigue, energy consumption, and even the type of substrates that are used in a given effort.

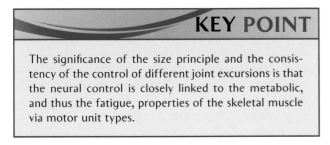

KEY POINT

The significance of the size principle and the consistency of the control of different joint excursions is that the neural control is closely linked to the metabolic, and thus the fatigue, properties of the skeletal muscle via motor unit types.

The Pattern of Glycogen Loss in Skeletal Muscle Fibers during Movement: Consistent with the Size Principle of Recruitment

As shown in Figure 2.5, the amount of glycogen in a skeletal muscle fiber can be semi quantitatively assessed using a dye that binds to glycogen—that is, the histochemical periodic acid-Schiff reaction. The amount of glycogen in a muscle fiber is determined by the rate of glycogen degradation (largely a function of the level of contractile activity

and the metabolic profile of the muscle fiber) and the rate of glycogen synthesis (44).

Taking these variables into account, one can gain considerable insight into the interactions among the metabolic properties of muscle fibers, muscle fiber phenotypes, and the recruitment strategies used by the nervous system. For example, in Fig. 2.18 the changes in the level of glycogen in four fiber phenotypes in response to different intensity levels of exercise performed over 60 to 80 minutes reflect a combination of metabolic and phenotypic properties, along with recruitment strategies. When subjects exercised at 43% of maximum oxygen uptake for 60 minutes there was a gradual loss of glycogen only in the type I fibers. At this low intensity of exercise, type II fibers were recruited minimally and, although they have a relatively low oxidative capacity, little glycogen loss was observed. When the subjects exercised at a slightly higher percentage (61%) of their maximum, some glycogen was lost from the type IIa fibers and, according to the size principle, these fibers would be expected to be recruited after the type 1 fibers. At the highest power output (91% of maximum), all fiber phenotypes were recruited to a significant degree. However, there still was slightly less glycogen loss in type II than type I fibers. Two points should be highlighted. First, these data are consistent with the orderly recruitment of motor units according to the size principle, even at very high power outputs. Second, although all fiber phenotypes lost glycogen at the highest power output, because of the glycogen sparing effect of the high-oxidative capacity of the type I fibers, one cannot conclude that type II fibers were recruited as often as type I fibers.

In a variation of this experiment, subjects worked intermittently to exhaustion at 75% of their maximum oxygen uptake (45). The level of glycogen depletion was consistent with the expected recruitment levels among fiber phenotypes—that is, the least depletion was observed in the fast type IIb (largest and least recruited) fibers and the most depletion in slow type I fibers. Although the subjects exercised to exhaustion, the type IIb and IIa fibers still had approximately half of their normal glycogen content. This indicates that considerable glycogen can remain in some muscle fibers even at exhaustion.

KEY POINT

It is extremely difficult to deplete all of the glycogen in all of the muscle fibers by exercising, and a significant level of glycogen depletion in most of the fibers only occurs when a sustained exercise is ~75% to 85% of maximum.

If the exercise intensity is greater, most fibers will not be depleted of glycogen unless the high intensity exercise is repeated a number of times. In other words, glycogen depletion as a factor in fatigue is likely to be important only in a limited number of exercise scenarios. In general, the

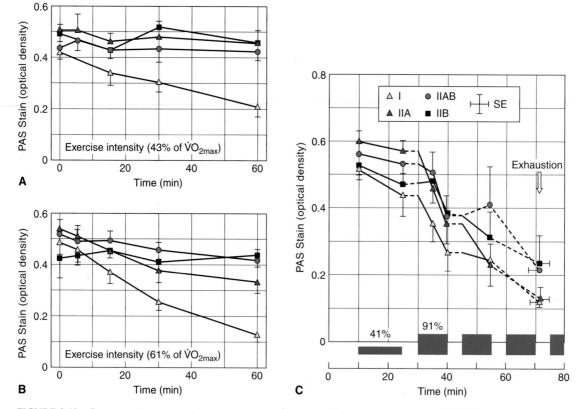

FIGURE 2.18 Decrease in average glycogen content (measured by periodic acid-Schiff [PAS] staining intensity) of individual fiber phenotypes in the vastus lateralis during bicycle ergometer exercise at several intensities: (a) 43%, (b) 61%, and (c) 91% of maximal oxygen consumption. The higher the rate of work, the higher the proportion of glycogen depletion in the larger motor units—that is, those motor units that require more excitatory input to reach their excitation threshold. (Modified from Vøllestad NK, Blom PC. Effect of varying exercise intensity on glycogen depletion in human muscle fibres. *Acta Physiol Scand.* 1985;125(3):395–405.)

results shown in Fig. 2.18 are consistent with a combination of two factors: (a) the relative probability of recruitment of a given muscle fiber phenotype; and (b) the relative differences in the oxidative capacity and glycogen sparing properties of the muscle fiber phenotypes.

Summary

Having addressed many of the details that define any given movement, all of these details and concepts can be reduced to two relatively simple variables. For any movement, the nervous system has to "decide" which motor pools and what proportion of these motor pools will be activated. How the nervous system makes this decision to recruit certain motor pools versus other motor pools and what portion of each motor pool to recruit remains a mystery. As described previously, the physiologic principle for defining the order of motor unit recruitment is largely explained by the "size principle." Briefly, this principle states that all of the motoneurons within a motor pool will be recruited in a relatively fixed order as determined by the size of the motor unit (i.e., the smaller motor unit is almost always recruited prior to the next larger motor unit).

Spinal Control of Posture and Locomotion

Historically, the level of control that the spinal cord can have in performing postural and locomotor tasks has been substantially underestimated. Some new insight is now being gained into the properties of the spinal cord that enable it to execute these tasks largely without supraspinal control. Some of the reflexes commonly used to test motor function will be examined, with a focus on the phenomenon of central pattern generation (CPG) within the spinal cord. Much of our understanding of how the spinal cord can control locomotion is based on studies of a wide range of vertebrates (35).

KEY POINT

Emphasis is on the concept of spinal automaticity—that is, the ability of the neural circuitry of the spinal cord to interpret complex sensory information and to make appropriate decisions to generate successful postural and locomotor tasks (46).

The mechanical and electrical events during locomotion are so closely linked that when the locomotion is being performed in a constant environment, the knowledge of the EMG activity of only one muscle provides extensive predictability of the activity patterns and the kinematic patterns of the limbs during locomotion. These observations suggest that individual muscles and joints are controlled by the nervous system not as individual components but as a highly interactive system with all of its components highly interdependent. The implications to locomotion are that the control system can essentially vary a single parameter to achieve locomotion over a range of speeds. This greatly simplifies the neural control by reducing the degrees of freedom that must be controlled to execute very complex but largely stereotypical movements, at least in a constant environment. It is this type of control that has led to the evolution of the concept of automaticity or the automatism of stepping.

KEY POINT

Although there is remarkable consistency in the overall activation patterns, an important point about the neural control mechanisms of locomotion is that the activity patterns of the muscles vary much more than the kinematics patterns. This means that the nervous system can generate multiple patterns of activity and still accomplish basically the same mechanical effects.

Central Pattern Generation

KEY POINT

CPG is a physiologic phenomenon in which an oscillatory motor output is generated in the absence of any oscillatory input (35). In mammalian systems, CPG represents an important component of the neural circuitry located in the lumbosacral spinal cord that generates and controls posture and locomotion.

There are other examples of CPGs in biologic systems (*e.g.*, those associated with breathing and chewing). Considerable progress has been made in understanding the circuitry that can generate CPGs by using more simple vertebrate systems such as the lamprey (47). This has been helpful to understanding neural control in humans because, in the evolution of the neural control of movement, the conservation of the circuitry and the neurotransmitters of the circuitry are remarkable. In this chapter, we focus on CPG in mammalian systems associated with locomotion.

A major challenge for biologists has been to identify the mechanisms for CPG. One general hypothesis is that the oscillatory output is generated by specific neurons that behave similarly to the pacemaker of the heart that generates the heartbeat. An alternative hypothesis is that the oscillatory behavior is a manifestation of the properties of a network of neurons (48). It seems reasonably clear that, even in invertebrate systems, multiple neurons are necessary to generate sustained oscillatory motor outputs.

Methods in studying central pattern generation

The importance of CPG can be illustrated under a range of experimental conditions. A method commonly used over the last 30 years has been to record from muscle nerves of a decerebrated (to avoid the effects of anesthesia) and completely spinalized (low thoracic, to avoid any supraspinal influences on the spinal circuitry) cat whose peripheral nerves have been severed and/or the muscles paralyzed (*e.g.*, with curare) to prevent any modulation from movement-related sensations. When this animal is given an appropriate pharmacologic stimulus, such as L-Dopa, combined with an inhibitor of dopamine reuptake (*e.g.*, monoamine oxidase), oscillatory efferent output can be sustained for hours (Fig. 2.19). The efferent output is highly coordinated and there is alternating ipsilateral as well as contralateral flexion and extension activity. Both motoneurons and interneurons are active throughout all layers of the gray matter of the spinal cord and over all of the lumbosacral segments in a step-like pattern (49).

KEY POINT

A highly significant point with respect to CPG is that a highly coordinated oscillatory pattern (resembling that observed during locomotion) can be generated by the circuitry within the spinal cord in the absence of input from the brain or the periphery.

Importance of sensory input to spinal neural circuits that can generate CPG

Without sensory input to provide cues associated with the environment, the functional significance of the CPG by itself is limited. If, on the other hand, the spinal cord has access to sensory information from peripheral receptors, then a wide range of useful and highly adaptable motor tasks can be performed without input from the brain (Fig. 2.20). For example, an adult cat completely spinalized (low thoracic level) can generate full weight-bearing stepping and readily adjusts the stepping pattern to the speed of a moving treadmill belt (50). It is

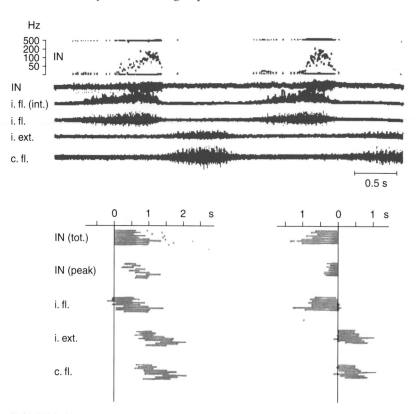

FIGURE 2.19   An example of the equivalent of two step cycles is illustrated at the top. These step cycles illustrate the phenomenon of fictive locomotion whereby oscillating efferent (motor) output from peripheral nerves leading to flexor and extensor muscles is generated by the spinal cord circuitry without any input from the brain (complete low thoracic spinal cord transection) or from the periphery (all muscle nerves are cut and the animal is paralyzed pharmacologically with curare). IN refers to the activity (frequency of action potentials) from a single interneuron in the lumbar spinal cord during the two cycles. Note the similarity in the timing and frequency modulation of the IN for both cycles. Also, note the similar timing relationship to the activity from an ipsilateral flexor (integrated and raw signal), ipsilateral extensor, and contralateral flexor muscle nerve. At the bottom, the relative timing of the IN and the muscles are shown for nine consecutive cycles, with the onset of the IN firing used as a common reference point for each cycle. The dot after each line illustrating IN activity marks the end of each cycle. Note the variation in the absolute times for the activities, but regardless of this variation in cycle duration the relationships between the on and off times are remarkably consistent. (Modified from Edgerton VR, Grillner S, Sjöström A, et al. Central generation of locomotion in vertebrates. In: Herman RM, Stein PSG, Stuart DG, eds. *Neural Control of Locomotion.* New York: Plenum; 1976:439–464.)

apparent that this stepping ability results from a combination of the processing of the sensory input and the CPG itself.

The spinal cord is smart

The circuitry responsible for CPG receives and interprets the sensory information in a highly dynamic way. That is, whether a group of muscles is excited or inhibited by a given afferent from a mechanoreceptor during locomotion often will depend on the stage of the step cycle. For example,

a stimulus applied to the dorsum of a cat's paw (as in a stumbling response) will excite the flexor muscles of the ipsilateral limb when applied during the swing phase, whereas the same stimulus will excite the extensor muscles when applied during the stance phase of the step cycle (51). This observation, and a series of other experiments demonstrating qualitatively similar capabilities of the spinal cord, has led to the concept that the spinal cord is "smart" (52,53). That is, the spinal cord receives sensory information and makes a decision as to what the appropriate response is at that time.

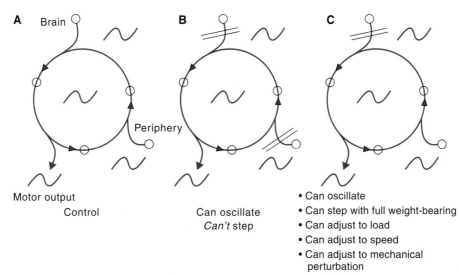

FIGURE 2.20 The motor output capabilities of the spinal cord are illustrated under three conditions. On the left, the control situation is shown whereby the spinal cord is able to receive normal input from the brain and the peripheral nerves transmitting proprioceptive input largely from mechanoreceptors. Movement capability in this case would be normal. The figure in the center represents the output potential when both brain and peripheral input are eliminated. As shown in Fig. 2.19, the spinal cord can generate oscillating efferent patterns that approximate those properties observed during actual locomotion. On the far right, the motor capacity of the spinal cord without input from the brain but with the peripheral input preserved has a greatly enhanced capability, including the ability to step over a range of speeds and loads and can even make adjustments when the legs are tripped. The spinal cord also can learn motor tasks as described in the text. (Unpublished observation, VR Edgerton and RR Roy.)

> ## KEY POINT
>
> In this context, it is logical to think of the spinal cord as interpreting the total ensemble of afferent information at any given time, as opposed to receiving input from each sensory receptor and responding to each receptor in a stereotypically reflex manner.

An analogy is the way we interpret a visual image. When we are observing an artistic painting, it is the total visual field of the painting that our brain interprets as opposed to processing each individual "pixel" of information independently and then deriving a final image. At any given instant in time, the spinal cord is receiving information from all receptors throughout the body and then "deciding" which neurons to excite.

> ## KEY POINT
>
> The "smart" and integrative features of CPGs provide a basis for the automaticity in the neural control of posture and locomotion.

For example, in the completely spinalized animal, the CPG neurons can predict the next "logical" sequence of neurons to activate based on the specific groups of neurons that were activated immediately prior to that point. The importance of CPG is not that it can continuously generate repetitive cycles, but that these networks can receive and interpret sensory input and then predict the next logical sequences of action.

> ## KEY POINT
>
> It is perhaps useful to think of the neurons that produce CPG as basically modulating the probability of a given set of neurons being active at any given time, whereas the peripheral sensory input modulates the probabilities of completing each component of a motor task successfully.

The degree of detail in motor output that can be generated by the spinal cord in combination with the information from the periphery can be appreciated by comparing the EMG and force signals from a battery of muscles from a cat before and after a complete spinal cord transection at a low thoracic level (Fig. 2.21). Although there are some differences in the EMG signals in chronically spinalized cats during bipedal stepping relative to that in intact controls, these are relatively minor and may be associated with only slight differences in the biomechanics of the hindquarters.

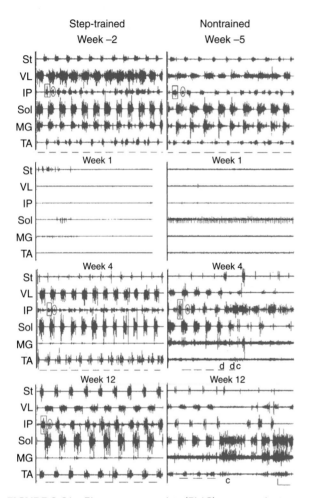

FIGURE 2.21 Electromyographic (EMG) activity during bipedal hind limb stepping in a step-trained and a nontrained cat before (–2 or –5 wk) and 1, 4, and 12 weeks after a complete low thoracic spinal cord transection. Raw EMG was recorded from selected hind limb muscles (St, semitendinosus; VL, vastus lateralis; IP, ilio-psoas; Sol, soleus; MG, medial gastrocnemius; TA, tibialis anterior) during stepping at a treadmill speed of 0.4 m · s⁻¹. Stance phase during full weight-bearing step cycles is indicated by the horizontal lines below the EMG records. c, a step failure (collapse); d, contact of dorsal surface of paw on treadmill belt (toes curled). □, IP bursts during swing (IP$_{sw}$); ○, stance (IP$_{st}$) in one step cycle. Horizontal calibration, 1 s, and vertical calibration, 1.0 mV for all muscles except for the Sol (2.0 mV). (Reprinted with permission from de Leon RD, Hodgson JA, Roy RR, et al. Locomotor capacity attributable to step training versus spontaneous recovery after spinalization in adult cats. *J Neurophysiol.* 1998;79(3):1329–1340.)

Sources of Peripheral Sensory Information

Overview

In this section we discuss mechanoreceptors that provide sensory information to the spinal cord about the physiologic and mechanical environment associated with the control of movement.

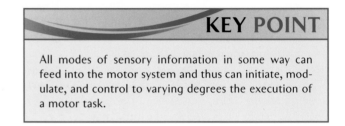

KEY POINT

All modes of sensory information in some way can feed into the motor system and thus can initiate, modulate, and control to varying degrees the execution of a motor task.

The following section addresses the sensory information associated with the mechanical (mechanoreceptors) and chemical (chemoreceptors) events associated with muscular activity. The different types of receptors probably provide ensembles or patterns of activity from specific receptors at specific locations and within a specific temporal characterization that have "meaning" to the spinal cord and the brain. With respect to proprioception, the mechanoreceptors, spindles, and Golgi tendon organs (GTOs) provide an abundance of sensory input for the spinal cord to integrate and interpret. An important component of the neural control of movement lies within the skeletal muscles, tendons, and joints where a wide range of mechanoreceptors provide the CNS with the kinematics and kinetic states of the movement.

The classic physiologist, Arthur Steinhaus, often stated that the muscles are the largest sensory organs in the human body. The brain and spinal cord constantly receive sensory input throughout one's life and it is readily apparent that the patterns and modes of input influence the immediate responses in the brain. It can be approximated that a single afferent from the hind limbs of a cat can generate action potentials at an average rate of 80/s and that there are ~10,000 large afferents in the hind limb musculature. Thus, during 1 second of locomotion, ~800,000 action potentials are conducted centrally. These action potentials diverge to conduct excitatory potentials to virtually all homonymous motoneurons and to many motoneurons innervating synergistic muscles. One could approximate that a conservative number of neurons receiving excitatory potentials would be ~10,000. Therefore, some 8 billion excitatory postsynaptic potentials could be generated per second from a single large afferent.

Not only are the brain and spinal cord receiving and integrating information continuously, they are receiving very complex patterns from sensory receptors (e.g., vision, audition, smell, taste, touch, and proprioception). Based on the number of sensory axons in peripheral nerves to all of the skeletal muscles and joints, more than one-half of the axons in the muscle nerves are sensory and most of the body mass is comprised of muscle. Thus, if one considers only the muscle nerves, one must expect that exercise and motor training can play a significant role in shaping how the CNS functions. Among these sensory axons are a number of types of mechanoreceptors that are capable of detecting changes in muscle length, force, and pressure. In addition, some nerve branches are essentially all or predominantly sensory and they project to tendons, joints, and skin. One of the most studied mechanoreceptors is the skeletal muscle spindle that provides proprioceptive information to the CNS (54). During exercise, the brain also receives input from axons that convey touch, sound, vision, smell, and taste and these sources of information influence the physiology of the CNS. There are many examples of ways these sensory systems affect our motor performance, reflecting the fact that each of these sensory modes has input to the motor system. A loud sound can increase voluntary strength. Cutaneous cues shape our reactions in maintaining posture and in the kinematics of locomotion. Vision is a major source of input for guiding virtually all movements. Sound can direct our posture and head position. Even olfactory input can initiate locomotor movements.

Muscle spindles

A muscle spindle consists of about four to six small muscle fibers surrounded by a collagenous sheath. The maximum diameter of the collagenous sheath usually approximates the size of the extrafusal muscle fibers. The muscle fibers within the capsule are striated, similar to the extrafusal muscle fibers—these are intrafusal muscle fibers. The ends of these intrafusal fibers commonly project beyond the clearly defined spindle capsule. The intrafusal fibers are innervated by γ-motoneurons and each intrafusal muscle fiber is surrounded by several sensory axons called primary and secondary spindle afferents (Fig. 2.22). These sensory axons generate action potentials when the length of the intrafusal fiber changes. Stretch of the intrafusal fibers can be caused by two events: (a) activation of the γ-motoneurons, which will cause shortening of the distal ends of the intrafusal fibers and, therefore, stretch the center where the annulospiral sensory nerve endings are; and (b) passively lengthening or shortening the intrafusal fibers because they lie parallel and are physically attached indirectly to the extrafusal muscle fibers. Very small changes in length can stimulate the primary (also referred to as Ia afferents) and secondary sensory fibers from the spindle. In general, the primary afferents from the muscles spindles demonstrate a more dynamic response, whereas the secondary fibers have a more static response to changes in length. The primary Ia fibers are the main afferents responding to a tendon tap and vibration (55).

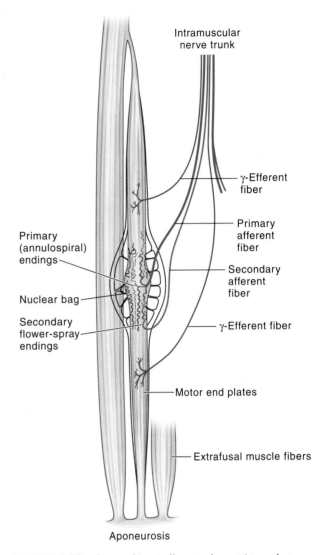

FIGURE 2.22 A muscle spindle attaches at its ends to connective tissues within a muscle. Sometimes two or even three spindles are interconnected in series. A connective tissue capsule surrounds three to eight intrafusal fibers located within each spindle. Motor end plates are located at the ends of each intrafusal fiber. These endplates represent the junction of the γ-motoneuron with the intrafusal muscle fiber and provide a mechanism for inducing the intrafusal fiber to shorten or place tension on the center of the muscle fiber. This increased tension triggers action potentials in the sensory endings—that is, annulospiral (primary) and flower spray (secondary) afferent fibers. These endings also can be activated by passively stretching the muscle and therefore the spindles. The afferent input projects to the spinal cord making synaptic contact on most motoneurons that project to that muscle. This input also projects to some motoneurons that innervate synergistic muscles, as well as to interneurons that inhibit motoneurons innervating antagonistic muscles. (Modified from Ross M, Romrell L, Kaye G. *Histology: A Text and Atlas.* 3rd ed. New York: Harper and Row; 1995:227.)

Afferents during locomotion

Some specific examples of how Ia fibers form muscle spindles in the ankle extensors (plantarflexors) of the cat function during locomotion are shown in Fig. 2.23. In Fig. 2.23A, the spindle was firing throughout the step cycle with the frequency being modestly higher during stance (*i.e.* E1 through E3). The E1 phase is the extension of the limb at the end of the swing phase prior to paw contact. The E2 phase begins at paw contact and extends to the end of the yield phase of stance. The E3 phase continues throughout the remainder of the stance phase. In Fig. 2.23B, again, the spindle Ia is activated throughout the step cycle but at a higher firing rate during E2 and E3. Also, the level of activation of the extensor muscle was higher in Fig. 2.23B than in Fig. 2.23A. In early E1 in Fig. 2.23B, a few pulses with a very short interpulse interval can be seen. Fig. 2.23C shows a similar pattern to that in Fig. 2.23A and B, but in the first step cycle shown the highest firing frequency occurred at mid E3, whereas in the next step, it occurred at mid E1. This emphasizes the variation in the details of the activation patterns of γ- and α-motoneurons, not only among different afferent fibers but even from step to step for the same afferent. This step-to-step variability is a steadfast feature of locomotor networks even under the most controlled conditions possible. All three of these examples illustrate the likelihood that the γ-motoneurons innervating the intrafusal muscle fibers were sufficiently active during all phases of the step cycle to sustain some sensitivity of the spindle to the intramuscular mechanical events (55).

One of the most common ways to demonstrate the responsiveness of muscle spindles to stretch is to tap the tendon to trigger a muscle contraction. Tapping the tendon induces a monosynaptic reflex by activating the spindle afferents that project to the dendrites of the motoneurons associated with the same muscle containing the spindle. Each spindle afferent sends axonal branches to nearly every motoneuron within that motor pool and to a significant proportion of the motoneurons that innervate synergistic muscles (56). In addition, the same Ia afferent from the spindle projects to interneurons that inhibit the motoneurons innervating antagonistic muscles (Fig. 2.24).

One can vibrate a muscle-tendon unit with a wide range of cycle frequencies such that the peak-to-peak change in length is <1 mm. This stretch will activate the Ia afferents that, in turn, will excite motoneurons innervating that muscle, and thus enhance its force generation even when the muscle is fatiguing during a MVC (Fig. 2.25).

The density of muscle spindles varies widely among muscles. Muscles or muscle regions having a high percentage of slow fibers usually have a relatively high incidence of spindles and thus are highly sensitive to length changes (57). The intrinsic muscles of the hip, for example, have a high spindle density, are extremely sensitive to length

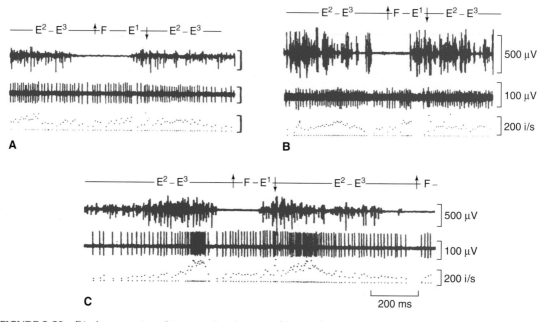

FIGURE 2.23 Discharge trains of intermediately active (**A** and **B**) and very active (**C**) ankle extensor spindle primary afferents during step cycles. *Upper traces:* lateral gastrocnemius electromyography (EMG); *lower traces:* afferent discharges and their instantaneous firing rate. All three afferents showed slightly different firing patterns, but each had a higher firing rate during stance. **C** represents the most extreme degree of presumed α-γ coactivation observed since the afferents were active during the phase of the cycle when the muscle was shortening. Note lack of correspondence between primary afferent firing rate and EMG amplitude. (Reprinted with permission from Prochazka A, Westerman RA, Ziccone SP. Discharges of single hindlimb afferents in the freely moving cat. *J Neurophysiol.* 1976;39:1090–1104.)

Supraspinal Input

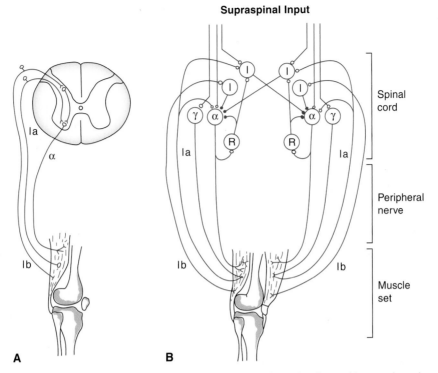

FIGURE 2.24 Spinal connections between sensory receptors located in muscle and α motoneurons. The Ia axon conveys afferent information from the muscle spindle to the CNS. The Ib axon represents a similar connection but from the tendon organ. **A.** Homonymous relationships: muscle spindles and tendon organs located in a muscle connect with the α motoneurons that activate the same muscle. Afferent and efferent axons that service muscles located on the right side of the body enter and exit the spinal cord on the right side, and vice versa. **B.** The same connections for an agonist–antagonist muscle set (*e.g.*, the hamstrings and quadriceps for the right leg) but this time emphasizing the complexity of the interneuronal connections. Also note the input from the brain to the same interneurons that receive peripheral afferent input from the muscles. *Open circles* represent excitatory connections; *filled circles* indicate inhibitory effects; α, alpha motoneuron; γ, gamma motoneurons; I, Ia inhibitory interneuron; Ia, muscle spindle afferent; Ib, tendon organ afferent; R, Renshaw cell. (Modified from Enoka R. *Neuromechanical Basis of Kinesiology.* Champaign, IL: Human Kinetics; 1988:139.)

changes and provide very important information for modulating the motor output during routine motor tasks such as stepping (58). These length sensors provide important cues as to when the stance and swing phases of a step should begin and terminate and when the body weight is being shifted from one leg to the other while standing.

Other mechanoreceptors

Another mechanoreceptor within the muscle tendon unit is the GTO. In spite of the name, most GTOs are within the muscle. They are able to detect small changes in force generated within the muscle. The high level of sensitivity to force of the GTOs contrasts with the traditional concept that they are activated only by high forces and that their function is to prevent tendon injury by inhibiting the muscle from generating excessive forces (54,59). The sensory information generated by GTOs will excite some muscles and inhibit others, with these effects being highly state-dependent. For example, the specific neurons that are excited or inhibited can change with the phase of a step cycle and probably other physiologic conditions. A third type of muscle mechanoreceptor is referred to as free nerve endings because there is no remarkable specialization at the ends of these axons. These free endings generate action potentials when excited by mechanical as well as biochemical or metabolic stimuli (metaboreceptors). Free nerve endings actually constitute most of the sensory endings from muscle. Their function is not well understood, although they are thought to be actively involved in muscle spasticity in individuals with a spinal cord injury.

From the perspective of the systems level, all of the muscle spindle afferents, GTOs, and free nerve endings serve as mechanoreceptors that provide important information associated with proprioception.

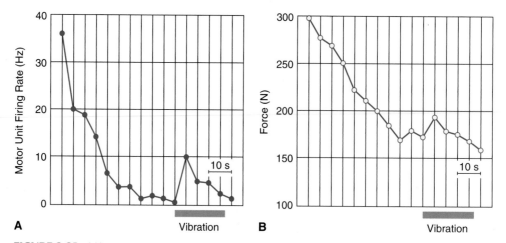

FIGURE 2.25 Vibration of the tibialis anterior temporarily counteracts (**A**) the decline in motor unit firing rates and (**B**) muscle force that occurs during a maximum voluntary contraction of foot dorsiflexors. (Modified from Bongiovanni LG, Hagbarth KE. Tonic vibration reflexes elicited during fatigue from maximal voluntary contractions in man. *J Physiol.* 1990;423:1–14.)

> ### KEY POINT
>
> Proprioception is a broad term often used to convey the idea that there are sensory receptors that provide precise information to the spinal cord and brain regarding the exact biomechanical state of the musculoskeletal system at any given time.

As noted previously, mechanoreceptors seem to have specialized in the periphery, which enables them to provide detailed information about the kinematics of a movement from a micro and macro perspective and also from a dynamic and static perspective.

> ### KEY POINT
>
> The combined effect of all of these mechanoreceptors projecting to the spinal circuits is to provide an ensemble of sensory information that provides the instructions needed for the spinal cord to control and modulate the kinematics of the movements in a very predictable way, thus minimizing the necessity for supraspinal (conscious) control of routine movements.

As noted previously, an important basic neurophysiologic concept with respect to proprioceptive input from the mechanoreceptors, as well as cutaneous receptors, is that their synaptic functional connectivity to the spinal circuitry is highly dynamic. The connectivity between these mechanoreceptors and specific interneuronal populations within the spinal cord vary according to the physiologic state. Even the efficacy of the monosynaptic input from muscle spindles to the motoneuron changes readily from one portion of the step cycle to another and according to whether a subject is running or walking (60,61).

Smart responses in the spinal cord of humans

Another excellent example of the ability of the spinal cord to receive complex proprioceptive input and to use this information in a functional way was shown by Harkema and associates (62) (Fig. 2.26). These authors demonstrated that the level of activation of an extensor muscle, the soleus, is modulated according to the amount of load that is placed on the lower limbs of a human subject. In the example on the left of Fig. 2.26, the increase in the level of activation, as illustrated by the EMG amplitude, is directly related to the load imposed on the limb. The results of a similar experiment on a subject who has a complete spinal cord injury (no voluntary control of any muscles below the lesion and no sensation from tissues below the lesion) are shown on the right of Fig. 2.26. The similarity of the relationship between the level of loading and the level of activation of the motor pool (EMG amplitude) in the uninjured and the complete spinal cord injured subjects demonstrates that the spinal cord circuitry is able to sense the level of load and activate the soleus and other motor pools accordingly. Two of several interpretations of how the spinal cord senses load "online" are (a) sensory receptors in the limbs (*e.g.*, soles of the feet, tendons, muscles, and joints) that specifically sense load; and (b) an ensemble of many types of sensory receptors at multiple locations within the limbs generate a highly recognizable "image" to inform the spinal circuitry of the biomechanical status of the weight bearing. The second interpretation is the one we favor. It is consistent with the concept that has been alluded to many times previously—that is, it is the ensemble of sensory input that

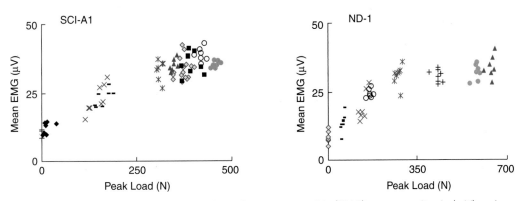

FIGURE 2.26 Relationships between soleus electromyographic (EMG) mean amplitude (mV) and limb peak load (N) for an ASIA A spinal cord injured (SCI-A1) and a nondisabled (ND-1) subject stepping on a treadmill with a harness suspended from overhead to provide a range of loading conditions. An ASIA A SCI subject is one commonly called complete—that is, there is no clinical evidence of any motor control below the lesion site or sensory information from below the lesion. Each data point represents one step and each symbol represents a series of consecutive steps at one level of body weight support. Note that as the subjects bear more body weight the EMG amplitude increases similarly in both the SCI and ND subjects. (Adapted with permission from Harkema SJ, Hurley SL, Patel UK, et al. Human lumbosacral spinal cord interprets loading during stepping. *J Neurophysiol.* 1997;77(2):797–811.)

has meaning and can be interpreted by the spinal cord circuitry so that an appropriate motor pattern can be generated (63,64). These data also demonstrate that the spinal cord can activate the motor pools in a precise and highly coordinated manner.

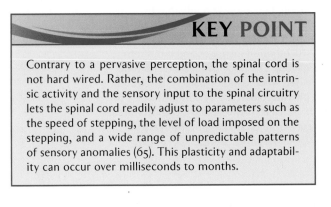

KEY POINT

Contrary to a pervasive perception, the spinal cord is not hard wired. Rather, the combination of the intrinsic activity and the sensory input to the spinal circuitry lets the spinal cord readily adjust to parameters such as the speed of stepping, the level of load imposed on the stepping, and a wide range of unpredictable patterns of sensory anomalies (65). This plasticity and adaptability can occur over milliseconds to months.

Some of the key points related to sensory processing by the spinal cord include:

1. Within the musculoskeletal and cutaneous tissues is an extensive network of mechanoreceptors and metaboreceptors that continuously update the spinal cord on the physiologic state of the peripheral tissues;
2. The mechanoreceptors provide highly integrated and perceptually meaningful information as well as an ensemble of this information to the spinal cord;
3. The spinal cord is smart enough to interpret and appropriately respond to the highly complex and meaningful sensory ensembles; and
4. The human spinal cord demonstrates this smartness and automaticity.

Supraspinal Control of Posture and Locomotion

Overview

In general, the functional organization of the neural control of locomotion in humans and quadrupeds is similar. Although the spinal cord has neuronal systems that alternate the activation patterns of the musculature to produce stance and swing phases during locomotion, the brain also has neuronal systems that can accomplish these tasks. These supraspinal neuronal networks are highly responsive to sensory information from the periphery. A hypothesis presented by Orlovsky, Deliagina, and Grillner (66) is that each limb is modulated by supraspinal input via groups of spinal neurons called "controllers." These controllers respond to a simple tonic drive from the brain by generating a relatively complex rhythmic pattern that activates the limb musculature in a coordinated pattern to generate locomotion. It is not clear what these controllers are anatomically, or how many there are, but one can imagine a number of such controllers that could interact in very predictable ways to control the individual joints in each limb. Shik and Orlovsky (36) proposed a two-level automatism control system for locomotion. One level provides nonspecific tonic input that determines the intensity of locomotion (speed and grade). The second level is responsible for making fine adjustments in the control of the limbs, including maintaining equilibrium. This level of the control system normally interacts with sources of sensory information, such as visual and proprioceptive inputs, to execute fine adjustments in the locomotor pattern (Fig. 2.27). Locomotion seems to be initiated by supraspinal centers that activate these limb controllers, with the reticulospinal neurons and the mesencephalic locomotor region (MLR) playing

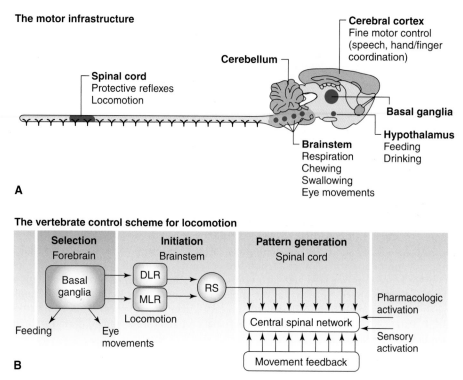

FIGURE 2.27 The motor infrastructure. **A.** Location of different networks (central pattern generators [CPGs]) that coordinate different motor patterns in vertebrates. These areas can coordinate the activation of different CPGs in a behaviorally relevant order. For instance, if the fluid intake area is activated, an animal will look for water, walk toward it, position itself, and start drinking. The cerebral cortex is important in particular for fine motor coordination involving hands and fingers and for speech. **B.** General control strategy for vertebrate locomotion. Locomotion is initiated by activity in reticulospinal neurons (RS) of the brainstem locomotor center, which produces the locomotor pattern in close interaction with sensory feedback. With increased activation of the locomotor center, the speed of locomotion increases and interlimb coordination can change (e.g., from a walk to a gallop). The basal ganglia exert a tonic inhibitory influence on motor centers that is released when a motor pattern is selected. Experimentally, locomotion can also be elicited pharmacologically by administration of excitatory amino-acid agonists and by sensory input. DLR, diencephalic locomotor area; MLR, mesopontine locomotor area. (Modified from Grillner S. The motor infrastructure: from ion channels to neuronal networks. *Nat Rev Neurosci.* 2003;4(7):573–586.)

important roles. There are differences in opinion regarding the relationship of the neural control of posture to that of locomotion. One hypothesis is that the control systems are rather distinct. An alternative hypothesis is that the neural programs for posture and locomotion are highly integrated and share extensively in the control of standing and stepping.

Descending pathways for controlling locomotion

The primary anatomical descending pathways for initiating locomotion are the corticospinal, reticulospinal, vestibulospinal, and rubrospinal tracts. The motor cortex gives rise to the corticospinal tract that decussates and influences the spinal circuitry associated primarily with the contralateral limbs. Some of these neurons have rhythmic firing patterns during locomotion. This rhythm seems to be generated by the spinal circuitry driven by CPG as well as by sensory feedback.

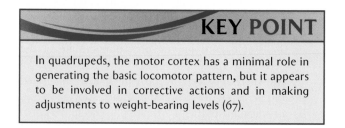

KEY POINT

In quadrupeds, the motor cortex has a minimal role in generating the basic locomotor pattern, but it appears to be involved in corrective actions and in making adjustments to weight-bearing levels (67).

The motor cortex, however, does play an important role in executing more skilled movements that are less repetitive and in adjusting the basic activation patterns during locomotion in a more variable environment. Although corticospinal neurons may provide instruction for refining or modifying locomotor movements, it is clear that the basic locomotor patterns can be relatively normal without corticospinal input (Fig. 2.28). In primates, including humans, lesions of the motor cortex or spinal cord may produce a greater disruption of the basic locomotor patterns than in lower mammalian species (68). Most of the dysfunction occurs in the distal musculature that controls the wrist, ankle, and digits.

The medial reticular formation of the pons and medulla gives rise to neurons that form the reticulospinal tract. These axons descend within the ventrolateral funiculi of the spinal cord and a single neuron can project to multiple levels of the spinal cord. The neurons that form the reticulospinal tract receive input from the brainstem including the MLR and from the cerebellum. The MLR, just rostral to the medial reticular formation (Fig. 2.29), provides input to the neurons that form the reticulospinal tract. Stimulation of the MLR (a 1-mm long strip of cells in the nucleus cuneiformis) can elicit locomotion. Stimulation of the MLR

region activates reticulospinal neurons that, in turn, can stimulate the spinal centers producing locomotion. Reticulospinal neurons become more active during locomotion than when the animal is at rest. The reticulospinal tract in cats is necessary to elicit locomotion when stimulating the MLR. Also, if the ventrolateral funiculi of the spinal cord are cut, a coordinated locomotor pattern cannot be initiated. A second area in the brainstem that can initiate locomotion and that also projects to reticulospinal neurons is the subthalamic locomotor region (66).

The exact manner in which these neurons induce locomotion is not known. Activity of neurons in the MLR, however, increases during locomotion. There is some evidence that the MLR region is controlled by inhibition and that the initiation of stepping may be induced by disinhibition (66). Neurons that form the reticulospinal, vestibulospinal, and rubrospinal tracts are rhythmically active during locomotion. Most of the vestibulospinal neurons are active at the beginning of stance. Most of the neurons forming the rubrospinal and reticulospinal tracts are maximally active during the swing phase of a step cycle.

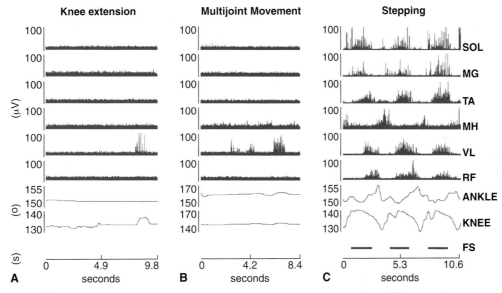

FIGURE 2.28 Single and multijoint movements and stepping from a clinically incomplete, but severely injured, subject with a spinal cord injury. When the subject is asked to extend the knee, little movement occurred (lower left of **A**) and EMG was recorded from one muscle. The subject was slightly more successful when instructed to move the limbs in a cycling motion. Electromyographic (EMG) activity (μV) from the soleus (SOL), medial gastrocnemius (MG), tibialis anterior (TA), medial hamstrings (MH), vastus lateralis (VL), and rectus femoris (RF); knee and ankle angles (°); and footswitches (black bars indicate stance phase) during an attempted single joint movement (**A**), multijoint movement (**B**), and during weight-bearing stepping at 0.28 m · s with 56% body weight support (BWS) (**C**). Minimal EMG was observed only in the VL during attempted knee extension (**A**), and only the MH became more active (although no clear EMG burst) during multi joint effort (**B**). Minimal movement of the knee or ankle occurred. This EMG pattern contrasts with the alternating bursts in each muscle during stepping (**C**). These results emphasize the fact that voluntary control from the brain is not essential for generating stepping. The TA was largely synchronized with the SOL and MG whereas the MH EMG was reciprocal to that in the VL and RF and with ankle muscles. (Modified from Maegele M, Muller S, Wernig A, et al. Recruitment of spinal motor pools during voluntary movements versus stepping after human spinal cord injury. *J Neurotrauma.* 2002;19:1217–1229.)

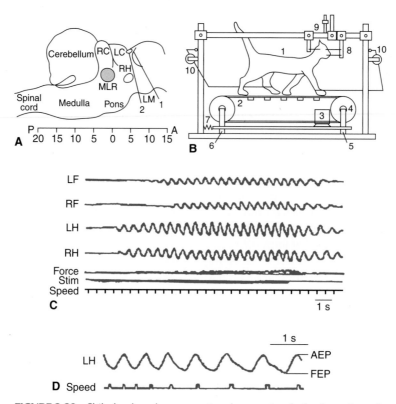

FIGURE 2.29   Shik developed a preparation that consisted of a decerebrated (**A**) animal placed in a frame over a treadmill belt. MLR, mesencephalic locomotor region; LM, corpus mammillare; LC, superior colliculus; RC, inferior colliculus; RH, red nucleus. (**B**). When the brainstem is sliced, so that the superior colliculus and the red nucleus lie just caudal to the slice, the animal can generate full weight-bearing stepping as shown in (**C**). Movements of the limbs are recorded by levers attached to the ankles as shown in (**C**). The timing of the brainstem stimulation is indicated by the thick horizontal line. Note that stepping begins several seconds after the stimulation is initiated and it continues for a number of seconds after the tonic stimulation is terminated. LF, left forelimb; RF, right forelimb; LH left hind limb; RH, right hind limb. An adjustment in stepping cycle rate accommodates the changing speed of the treadmill belt (**D**). AEP, anterior extreme position; FEP, posterior extreme position. (Modified from Orlovsky G, Deliagina T, Grillner S. *Neuronal Control of Locomotion: From Mollusc to Man.* Oxford University Press; 1999:166.)

KEY POINT

Thus, the vestibulospinal tract seems to facilitate extensor motoneurons, whereas the reticulospinal tract mainly facilitates flexor and inhibits extensor motoneurons. The rubrospinal and corticospinal tracts mainly facilitate flexor motoneurons (66).

Thus, these descending tracts seem to have a modulatory effect on the motoneurons during specific phases of the step cycle. It should be noted that the rhythm and firing of these descending tracts are due, in large part, to the influences from ascending input derived from the spinal cord circuitry. This phasic input (cyclic input associated with stepping) can occur independently of the afferent input from the periphery. For example, in paralyzed and decerebrated cats in which phasic afferent inflow from the periphery is precluded, phasic descending and ascending activity between the spinal cord and supraspinal centers is still present during spontaneous motor activity.

Summary

It seems that supraspinal centers such as the MLR can increase or decrease the force or velocity of contraction of a muscle by changing the level of excitatory and/or inhibitory input to the motoneuronal pools (35). If treadmill speed is kept constant, however, increased input to the midbrain in a decerebrate cat has no effect on the duration of the stance phase or step frequency (69). This suggests that the cycle duration is influenced by mechanical factors such as the position or the placement of the hind limb and, therefore, is mediated at least in part by proprioceptive signals.

Role of cerebellum in locomotion

The cerebellum also plays an important role in motor control. A major function of the cerebellum is to assist in the control of limb movements by modulating supraspinal motor centers. It mediates sensory feedback from the spinal cord and modifies the motor output accordingly. The cerebellum also receives information from CPGs of the limbs to modulate the motor output. In addition, the cerebellum compares different inputs and, based on these comparisons, provides a means of correcting intended movements (66).

Automaticity in Posture and Locomotion

This section addresses the relative importance of different supraspinal nuclei in initiating and controlling locomotion. It is apparent that these centers can control different muscle groups (*e.g.*, extensors vs. flexors). Each of these control centers has a strong gating function whereby its input is timed closely with the phase of the step cycle. Clearly, specific regions within the brainstem can initiate and control very complex motor behaviors, apparently with little or no necessity for "conscious" control, resulting in the generation of largely automatic responses.

It is often assumed that the initiation of a movement, even the more automatic ones such as stepping, is triggered by a conscious event in the motor cortex. Even a superficial examination of this assumption raises the question of what is consciousness. Actually, there seems to be a continuum of consciousness ranging from a totally simple reflex without any conscious awareness or capability of control to modulation of a task in which one is fully and continuously aware of every aspect of the movement. What is the level of consciousness when one begins to step compared to the level of automaticity during a simple monosynaptic reflex? Even the efficacy of a monosynaptic response can be modulated by conscious control by a rat, monkey, or human. A human with a low thoracic spinal cord injury and with no supraspinal control below the lesion can learn to stand and initiate steps using sensory information associated with unilaterally bearing weight and manipulating the hip position (70). This spinal stepping can be initiated consciously and voluntarily, although the subject initiates the process "reflexively." Thus, the subject manipulates the afferent inflow by controlling critical biomechanical as well as neurophysiologic signals by manipulating other parts of the body (71).

A variety of approaches have been used to identify how one initiates a movement. Functional MRI (fMRI) is being used to examine where within the CNS the decision is made to initiate a movement. A number of studies suggest that the "urge" to move precedes the actual initiation of movement by about 200 ms. Thus, there seems to be a readiness potential that precedes the subjective decisions. fMRI shows elevated blood flow in the dorsal prefrontal cortex, intraparietal sulcus, and supplementary motor area in preparation for a movement (72).

Automaticity Derived from the Brainstem to Control Locomotion

For example, once the decision to walk across a room is made, very little conscious effort is required to perform the details of that task. It seems that the CNS is designed so that much of the intricate decision making associated with posture and locomotion occurs automatically. Both supraspinal and spinal sources contribute to the pathways responsible for this automaticity. For example, a subthalamic cat, decerebrated just rostrally to the mammillary bodies, can walk in response to exteroceptive stimulation and can sometimes walk spontaneously. A cat decerebrated at the caudal border of the mammillary bodies cannot walk with or without exteroceptive stimulation. Therefore, the subthalamic locomotor region lies between these two transection levels. When the subthalamic locomotor region remains intact, the animal can walk by itself, go to a plate of food, and even kill and eat a mouse. Such a cat, however, cannot perform locomotion voluntarily.

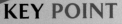

KEY POINT

There is a strong element of automaticity in the neural control of most movements, both from the brain and spinal cord (66,73).

Automaticity and Autonomic Function during Locomotion

Automaticity is also evident in the coordination of the neural control of locomotion with that of respiration and cardiovascular function. For example, not only does the stimulation of the MLR generate remarkably normal locomotion, it also leads to a modulation of cardiovascular and respiratory function that is appropriate for locomotion. When the MLR of a mesencephalic cat is stimulated and the limbs are stepping on a treadmill, a 20% to 35% higher arterial blood pressure, a 70% to 90% greater cardiac output, and an increase of 15% to 20% in heart rate relative to the resting conditions have been observed (74). In addition, pulmonary ventilation can increase threefold as a result of increased tidal volume and frequency of breathing. These observations demonstrate the highly integrated and automated nature of the neural system to control locomotion with some assurance that the cardiovascular and respiratory systems will be modulated accordingly. It would be interesting, however, to perform experiments whereby the MLR was stimulated in a paralyzed preparation to exclude the involvement of mechanisms directly linked to activation of the muscle tissue and the consequential metabolic impact of muscular contractions.

Levels of Automaticity

Clearly, there are a number of levels of automaticity (absence of conscious detailed control) of the neural control of posture and stepping. For example, decerebrated cats can run without hitting obstacles and jump over obstacles. When the MLR is stimulated, the decerebrated cat can generate locomotion and demonstrate awareness of spatial orientation. In animals that have a chronic lesion (several weeks) in the subthalamic locomotor region, locomotor behavior is nearly normal.

Spinal automaticity remains in the absence of supraspinal input, as occurs after a complete transection of the spinal cord. A large body of data demonstrates that the spinal cord is much more than a static conduit for communication between the brain and muscles. It was shown in the mid 1970s that kittens whose spinal cords were transected at a neonatal age can be trained to take steps on all four limbs (35,37). A significant level of automaticity was also evident when it was learned that stimulating the dorsum of the lumbosacral spinal cord in a tonic pattern generates stepping motions in paraplegic mammals (49,75) including humans (76). Also, rhythmic locomotor patterns can be induced by the spinal cord when selected regions of the brainstem are stimulated tonically even in the absence of sensory feedback from the spinal cord. The spinal cord can also generate patterns resembling locomotion in the absence of sensory feedback when the spinal cord is stimulated pharmacologically (*e.g.*, as with L-Dopa).

After a complete transection at a midthoracic level of the spinal cord, the automaticity generated from the lumbosacral spinal cord is attributable to two primary processes: (a) CPG (77); and (b) sensory input to the spinal cord from the periphery (63,78). When sensory input from cutaneous and proprioceptive sources is combined with CPG, the spinal circuitry is capable of executing a much wider range of complex motor tasks than when the output is generated by the spinal circuitry alone. How does the automaticity of posture and locomotion emerge from the interactions between the sensory inputs and the spinal circuits that generate CPG? For these two systems to work in synergy, each system must have intrinsic activation and inhibition patterns that are orderly, sequential, and coordinated. For example, the sequence of activation patterns associated with a step cycle can occur only with a critical level of synergy between the sources and modes of peripheral input and the cyclic events from CPG. The patterns of afferent information must interface with the CPG circuitry, as do two pieces of a jigsaw puzzle, at any given time "bin" (or segment of time) within a step cycle: (a) to inform the CPG of the current state of the step cycle; (b) to make the circuitry aware of which bin or bins preceded that instant; and (c) to predict which bin or bins should occur next. In this scenario, a bin consists of the afferent input and stage of activation-inhibition of the neurons that generate the CPG output at that instant. Again, the temporal patterns of ensembles of peripheral inputs must be matched at some critical level with that of the CPG for locomotion to continue effectively.

Automaticity and the Spinal Cord

In subjects with a complete spinal cord injury, the level of automaticity manifested is quite striking. From a systems standpoint, the specific combination of recruited motor pools and the net level of activation of this combination of motor pools at any given time within a step cycle must be highly precise if the subject is to step successfully. Equilibrium and balance must be sustained under highly dynamic conditions—that is, avoid falling when faced with a perturbation. Even when the precision of the activation patterns is not impressive at the individual motor pool level, the net effect—for example, successful stepping—can be remarkably consistent at the systems level.

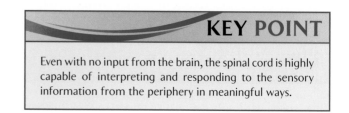

Spinal Learning

Although spinal cord plasticity can be modulated to alter its motor capacity after a complete spinal cord injury, one may argue that this behavior requires long periods of motor training and formation of new neuronal connections in the spinal cord. The state-dependent property of the spinal circuitry, which permits highly functional and integrated responses, however, can occur in acute, novel situations. For example, when an object is placed in front of a spinal cat stepping on a treadmill or during the swing phase of one hind limb, that limb will exhibit a greater degree of flexion during the following steps to avoid the perturbation (51). Hyperflexion induced by a stumbling stimulus during the swing phase of a step will persist for several steps even after the removal of the perturbation (53), suggesting that a learning and memory-type phenomenon may be taking place (Fig. 2.30). The persistent hyperreflexive action must be considered as more than a momentary adaptation because a memory trace is shown behaviorally in a number of these studies even after the perturbation requiring adaptation is removed.

More recent evidence of the "smartness" of the spinal cord was demonstrated when a robotic device was used to apply specific forces to rat hind limbs during certain phases of a step cycle. In one experiment, a downward force proportional to the velocity of stepping was applied unilaterally or bilaterally to the ankles of spinal rats. Step timing and kinematics were altered within a few minutes to allow locomotion to continue (79). In a separate but similar set of experiments, a robotically induced upward force proportional to the forward velocity of the swing (swing-phase force field) was exerted at the ankle of one limb during the swing phase, resulting in a visually obvious kinematics disturbance. After as few as 20 steps, the limb adjusted its output to become kinematically similar to that observed prior to the perturbation, although with different EMG patterns (80). Furthermore, with repetitive trials of ~20 steps followed by ~20 steps off of the swing-phase force field paradigm, the average swing duration

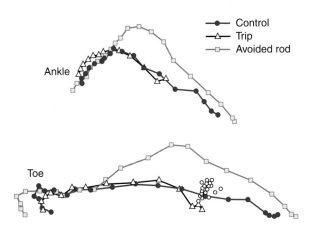

FIGURE 2.30 Swing trajectories of the foot (*lower traces*) and ankle (*upper traces*) of a spinal cat responding to the placement of a 1-cm diameter bar in the path of the foot during the swing phase of the step cycle. The control trace shows the trajectory before the placement of the bar. The trip trace shows the trajectory of the ankle and toe when the cat hit the bar. The remaining trace shows the trajectory when the foot completely cleared the bar. The bar position for each frame of the digitized video is shown by an *open circle*. Note the increased elevation of the foot well before it encountered the bar in the step and following the first step when the trip occurred. The rod was avoided in the first step after the tripping episode. (Adapted with permission from Hodgson JA, Roy RR, de Leon RB, et al. Can the mammalian lumbar spinal cord learn a motor task? *Med Sci Sports Exerc.* 1994;26:1491–7.)

during the force-field-on period decreased to force-field-off levels by the fourth bout (Fig. 2.31). The results of these studies show that, in essence, the spinal cord is solving problems in real time based on the continually changing state of incoming peripheral information to elicit a nearly constant behavior, even though the means to the endpoint differs.

The implication of these studies is that spinal learning takes place in a very short period, and a type of memory trace allows for quicker adaptation upon re-exposure to a given perturbation. Although the underlying cellular mechanisms are unknown, some of the molecules and processes involved in spinal learning are similar to those involved in hippocampal learning (81). Whether this phenomenon continues for longer periods (hours to days) is unknown. Indeed, the spinal cord can exhibit long-term potentiation (LTP) and long term depression (LTD) (synaptic changes that are recognized as vital in hippocampal learning) in dorsal horn neurons in the spinal cord in response to nociceptive stimuli (82). Whether spinal learning occurs via similar processes, the hippocampus remains to be determined.

From a teleologic perspective, one can question the concept of automaticity with respect to how useful these autonomic responses are. All sensory and motor systems, however, have evolved so that they can function within their known environments. Similar sensory and motor components among a wide range of animals with vastly different musculoskeletal structures have evolved in a manner that

enables many postural and locomotor tasks to occur quite automatically within Earth's gravitational fields (63). The automaticity aspect of these functions reflect the successful evolution that enables postural and locomotor responses to occur without relying on more complicated, and probably more unpredictable, delayed decision making by higher neural centers. A greater reliance on the brain would require additional time and would impose disadvantages in the execution of a variety of postural and locomotor tasks, particularly when the response time is critical for survival. In this sense, "evolutionary learning" has played a key role in the automaticity of neural control during the execution of motor tasks. This plasticity includes the ability to learn and forget motor tasks that are practiced (80,83–85).

KEY POINT

Thus, the nervous system, even without conscious control, not only demonstrates a sophisticated level of automaticity, but it is also smart and highly adaptable or plastic.

TEST YOURSELF

How similar are the mechanisms of spinal learning to those in the hippocampus?

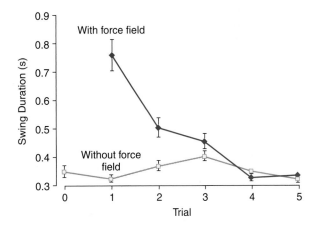

FIGURE 2.31 The changes in swing duration over five trials with and without an imposed perturbation (upward force field) for one representative rat. Note that the swing duration is elevated by more than twofold during the first perturbation and then quickly returns to levels observed without any perturbation. Swing durations were consistent across trials when the stepping was performed without any force field. Bars are SEM. (Modified from de Leon RD, Reinkensmeyer DJ, Timoszyk WK, et al. Use of robotics in assessing the adaptive capacity of the rat lumbar spinal cord. In: McKerracher L, Doucet G, Rossignol SE, eds. *Progress in Brain Research.* Amsterdam: Elsevier Science; 2002:141–149.)

Automaticity, Physiologic State, and Spinal Learning: Putting it All Together

In adult cats, a significant level of weight-bearing and coordinated bipedal stepping after the spinal cord is completely transected at a midthoracic level can recover with step training alone. In rats spinalized as adults, however, little weight-bearing stepping is recovered with step training alone. The recovery of full weight-bearing bipedal stepping is possible; however, if a combination of postinjury interventions having complementary effects are applied (86). These interventions capitalize on the automaticity of the spinal circuitry that can generate stepping and on the ability to acutely modulate the physiologic state of the spinal circuitry using (a) tonic epidural stimulation, (b) selected pharmacologic agonists (*e.g.*, serotonergic agonists

of 5-hydroxytryptamine $(5\text{-HT})_{1,2, \text{ and } 7}$ receptors), and/or (c) chronic modulation of the physiologic state of the spinal circuitry via step training for weeks. As noted previously, the automaticity of the locomotor circuitry, at least in complete spinal animals, can be attributed to its CPG potential to generate rhythmic and coordinated motor output and to the ability of the CPG circuitry to receive and interpret the ensemble of proprioceptive input derived from the load-bearing hind limbs. In fact, once the appropriate physiologic state of the circuitry is achieved with epidural stimulation and pharmacologic modulation, the sensory input from the hind limbs to the locomotor circuitry actually serves as the source of control of the stepping. This sensory control is illustrated in Figs. 2.32 and 2.33. No stepping is observed as long as the treadmill belt is stationary even in the presence of epidural stimulation and

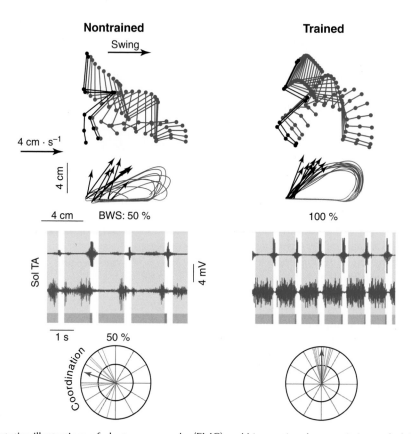

FIGURE 2.32 Representative illustrations of electromyography (EMG) and kinematics characteristics underlying bipedal hind limb locomotion recorded at 9 weeks postinjury for a nontrained spinal rat that did not receive pharmacologic or epidural stimulation interventions for the entire duration of the postinjury period until the day of testing and a spinal rat that was trained for 8 weeks with a combination of all interventions—that is, under the combination of quipazine *plus* 8-OHDPAT and epidural stimulation at spinal cord segment levels L2 *plus* S1. To illustrate hind limb movements during bipedal treadmill stepping at 4 cm · s⁻¹, a representative stick diagram decomposition of the hind limb movement during swing is shown for both rats together with successive (*n* = 10 steps) color-coded (stance, light blue; drag, black; swing, dark blue) trajectories of the limb endpoint. The nontrained and trained rats stepped with 50% and 100% body weight support (BWS), respectively. Vectors represent the direction and intensity of limb endpoint velocity at swing onset. A sequence of raw EMG activity from tibialis anterior (TA) and soleus (Sol) muscles is shown below the trajectory plots. In the middle graphs, the light and darker blue bars indicate the duration of stance and drag phases, respectively. Finally, a polar plot representation documents the coordination between the left and right hind limbs (thin dark line, single cycle; blue arrow, average of 10 cycles). A value of 50% (12 o'clock position) indicates that both limbs are moving perfectly out of phase, as occurs during well-balanced bipedal gait. (Adapted from Courtine G, Gerasimenko YP, van den Brand R, et al. Transformation of nonfunctional spinal circuits into functional and adaptive states after the loss of brain input. *Nature Neurosci.* 2009;12:1333–1342.)

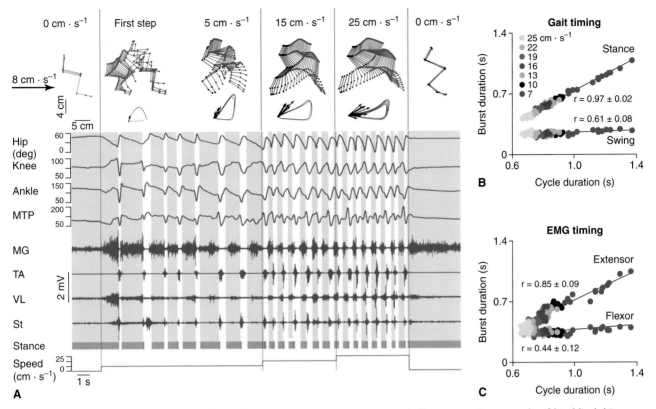

FIGURE 2.33 Effects of velocity-dependent afferent input on motor patterns. **A.** Representative example of hind limb kinematics and electromyography (EMG) activity recorded from a continuous sequence of steps during which the speed of the treadmill belt was changed gradually (0, 5, 15, 25, 0 cm · s⁻¹). Data are presented as in Fig. 2.32, except that changes in hind limb joint angles also are shown. Stick diagram decomposition of the first step is shown to demonstrate the smooth transition from standing to stepping. MG, medial gastrocnemius, TA, tibialis anterior, VL, vastus lateralis, St, semitendinosus. **B.** The durations of the swing and stance phases are plotted against the cycle duration. Color-coded labels indicate the measured treadmill belt speed during the performance of the represented gait cycles. **C.** The durations of flexor (TA) and extensor (MG) EMG bursts are plotted against the cycle duration. **B,C** are shown for a representative rat. Mean (± SEM) correlation values computed by averaging values obtained from linear regressions computed on each rat ($n = 6$) individually are reported in each plot. All rats were trained with a combination of the interventions for 3 weeks before the experimental testing. These data illustrate that the sensory input detects the speed of movement of the hind limbs and can essentially serve as a source of the neural control of stepping. (Adapted from Courtine G, Gerasimenko YP, van den Brand R, et al. Transformation of nonfunctional spinal circuits into functional and adaptive states after the loss of brain input. *Nature Neurosci.* 2009;12:1333–1342.)

serotonergic agonists. As soon as the treadmill belt starts to move backward, however, the animal begins to step forward with the rate of stepping depending on the speed of the treadmill belt. When the movement of the treadmill belt is stopped, the hind limbs stop stepping. By positioning the rat hind limbs so that they would have to step sideward or backward when the treadmill belt was moving, this concept of sensory control of stepping was tested further. Under these conditions, the kinematics of the hind limbs readily adapted to the direction of the treadmill belt.

is related to the level of automaticity that is built into the neuronal pathways that execute different types of movements. In general, there seems to be an underestimation of the importance of the level of automaticity within these neural circuits, with the automaticity triggered to a large extent by combinations of input from multiple sources of sensation. Furthermore, the details of these responses to specific combinations of sensory input are routinely modified based on our experiences.

Summary

It can be readily surmised from the previous discussion that our level of understanding of the basic principles of the control of posture and locomotion is rather limited. An important and evolving concept, however,

Central Nervous System and Fatigue

What is the nature of central fatigue? Fatigue is generally attributed to the muscle as discussed in detail in Chapter 6. Here, we consider fatigue in the performance of a motor task that is neurally based.

> ## KEY POINT
>
> Central fatigue can be considered as the failure to maintain the required or expected force or power output when these specific deficits cannot reasonably be explained by dysfunction within the muscle itself.

The site for this fatigue can be in the brain, spinal cord, or even at the neuromuscular junction. In some conditions, there can also undoubtedly be failing elements within the autonomic nervous system (see Chapter 7). Furthermore, the fatiguing components may lie within sensory pathways, at interneuronal synapses, or at the level of the motoneuron. CNS fatigue of sensorimotor function can be demonstrated during MVCs using the twitch or tetanic interpolation technique—that is, the force produced during a MVC can be enhanced by a single maximum stimulus or a brief train of electrical stimulation as described previously. Clearly, there is a state dependence of the excitability of neurons associated with motor control.

Motor Cortex and Motor Fatigue

Changes in neuronal excitability can occur in the human motor cortex in response to a fatiguing effort. The threshold for excitation and inhibition in the motor cortex declines after a few seconds of a maximal voluntary effort and recovers within 15 s even if the muscle is maintained in an ischemic state. A brief facilitation occurs immediately after fatiguing exercise but this is usually followed by a depression in the EMG responses to cortical stimulation lasting several minutes. Based on a number of studies of cortically evoked EMG during sustained contractions, synaptic failure may occur along the cortico motoneuronal pathway at any of several sites (87).

Evidence that the reduced excitability of the motor cortex to transcranial stimulation associated with fatigue that is physiologically relevant is indicated by the fact that cortical stimulation of a rested muscle does not generate a force that exceeds the normal MVC. After fatigue, however, cortical stimulation routinely generates a force that exceeds what can be produced voluntarily. In addition, after a fatiguing exercise, transcranial magnetic stimulation can activate only a portion of the spinal motoneurons suggesting a higher threshold for either the cortical neurons or the interneurons that project to a given motor pool (88). Most evidence suggests that fatiguing contractions do not change the threshold for excitation of corticospinal neurons. It is interesting to note that fatigue is more pronounced when the subjects are concentrating on their performance than when they are distracted or when performing with the eyes closed as opposed to open (89). Impaired motor performance is usually associated with increased perceived effort as well as the actual failure to produce the desired force. Each of these observations demonstrates that a significant element of neural fatigue can be at the conscious level. Clearly, our perception and cognition of performing a task under fatiguing conditions can affect the level to which we can activate a given motor pool (90).

Why might there be a reduction in corticospinal drive to the motoneurons as a result of performing a repetitive task? This may be due to a reduction in corticospinal impulses reaching the motoneurons and/or an inhibition of motoneuron excitability by neurally mediated afferent feedback from the muscles. The latter is referred to as the sensory feedback hypothesis (91). Specifically, this hypothesis states that feedback from mechanoreceptors inhibits motoneurons and reduces their firing rates. These mechanoreceptors (metaboreceptors) may be group III and IV free nerve endings, which are sensitive to muscle metabolites that accumulate during fatigue. Sedentary and dynamically exercised subjects performed fatiguing isometric plantarflexion contractions (30% MVC initially, and considered fatigued when there was a 30% decline in torque) (92). Surprisingly, at the end of the fatiguing task, the H-reflex amplitude had declined by 47% in the sedentary subjects and 67% in the trained subjects. Only a small change occurred in M-wave amplitude, indicating that the H-reflex decline was not due to neuromuscular propagation failure. The possible reasons for the different response were: (a) the trained subjects required less central drive to maintain the relatively simple task at 30% MVC, especially at the early time points; and/or (b) the trained subjects were able to relax more than the sedentary subjects when at rest. Thus, the endurance-trained subjects could maintain a submaximal contraction with a level of reflex inhibition that was greater than in sedentary subjects. It seems that this fatigue-related multifaceted reflex inhibition cannot be explained solely by small diameter afferents (groups III and IV) responding to the by-products of muscle contraction.

Motor Unit Rotation

In some way, the neural control system continuously adapts to changing physiologic conditions by alternating different combinations of motor units that are active. When subjects are asked to maintain a low constant plantarflexor load (10% MVC) for longer than 3 hours, surface EMG recordings show alternating periods of high and low activity in the three major plantarflexors (soleus and medial and lateral heads of the gastrocnemius) (24). These synergistic muscles rotate in a complementary manner to maintain a nearly constant torque. The number of alternating instances is more frequent as the duration of the effort increases—that is, when motor unit fatigue would be expected to be occurring. Similar alternating motor unit patterns during prolonged elbow flexion at 10% MVC have been observed (23).

Adaptation Strategies of the CNS during Fatigue

The adaptive strategy of the nervous system during repetitive, fatiguing contractions differs with the type of movement. For example, whereas repetitive maximum knee extensions in a concentric mode result in a significant loss of torque, repetitive eccentric contractions not only result in a significantly higher torque, but the maximum torques do not decline. The neural control differs for these conditions in that the vastus lateralis and rectus femoris activation levels are 25% to 40% higher during concentric than eccentric maximal efforts. Furthermore, the EMG levels relative to the amount of torque increases as fatigue progresses during concentric, but not eccentric, contractions (Fig. 2.17). These data show clear differences in the neural control properties of muscles depending on whether they are lengthening or shortening in a maximally activated state.

Role of Neurotransmitter Modulation in Fatigue

Underlying all of these physiologic changes are many biochemical changes that are tightly linked in ways that we understand very little at a systems level. Some examples of these changes readily demonstrate the complexity of the biochemical changes that modify motor performance during the onset of fatigue.

Most areas of the brain have elevated levels of norepinephrine (NE) and serotonin (5-HT) after training on a treadmill, and a single bout of exercise increases the release of NE (93,94). Elevated levels of 5-HT within the CNS are associated with fatigue. One mechanism to counter fatigue could be to decrease the release of 5-HT (93). For example, a reduction in the sensitivity to 5-HT after 6 weeks of treadmill training in rats has been observed, perhaps due to a reduction in $5\text{-}HT_{1a}$ receptors. Also, when 5-HT reuptake is inhibited pharmacologically, which increases the levels of 5-HT, there is increased fatigability and impaired cognition in humans. It is also interesting that when blood glucose levels in the brain are elevated, the levels of 5-HT decrease, most likely because of a decrease in its release. On the other hand, running increases the rate of synthesis of 5-HT in the brain that, in turn, could contribute to fatigability.

During locomotion, 5-HT is an important neurotransmitter in the spinal cord as it is in the brain. The cell bodies of these serotonergic spinal projections are, for the most part, in the brainstem. When rats were run on a treadmill for 60 minutes up a 5-degree slope, the peak levels of 5-HT in the ventral funiculus of the spinal cord increased about fourfold, whereas these levels slightly decreased in the ventral horn (gray matter) (95). There is also some evidence that training may decrease the sensitivity to 5-HT release by reducing the receptor density (96). Because 5-HT has been associated with fatigue, this reduced sensitivity to 5-HT may be a mechanism by which training could lead to greater resistance to fatigue (97). Clear evidence for a training-induced reduction in sensitivity to 5-HT in humans, however, has not been reported. The modulation of 5-HT receptors in response to exercise training also has been examined. Although 7 weeks of training on a treadmill had no effect on $5\text{-}HT_{1B}$ receptor mRNA in the striatum or hippocampus, the levels in the frontal cortex and cerebellum were reduced (98). It was observed that the sensitivity to $5\text{-}HT_{1B}$ receptors was reduced or eliminated in the hippocampus by the exercise training. Exercise training at a moderate intensity has been reported to increase the level of 5-HT transporters and the $5\text{-}HT_{2A}$ receptors in isolated platelet membranes. Platelet membranes were studied because they seem to serve as a convenient indicator of neuronal effects. Heavy exercise training, on the other hand, actually decreased the $5\text{-}HT_{2A}$ receptors in the platelet membranes (97).

Norepinephrine and Exercise

NE levels increase in whole brain in response to running and swimming. As expected, the increase in the brain is highly region specific. For example, 8 weeks of training results in a significant increase in NE and its metabolites in the pons, medulla, and spinal cord, but not in the frontal cortex and hippocampus of rats (94). More than half of the NE in the brain is in the pons and medulla. Several days of a running exercise increased tyrosine hydroxylase activity (a measurement of catecholamine activity) in the locus coeruleus and ventral tegmental area of the rat's brain (99).

It is speculated that the reduction in depression that have been reported in response to exercise training is related to the modulation in NE levels. Chronic exercise (wheel running) of rats also has been reported to prevent the depletion of NE that occurs when exposed to footshock. In addition, exercise reduced the latency before responding to a footshock, consistent with there being a NE-mediated modulation of the behavior (94). Changes in NE metabolism and function in response to training is also of interest because of its potential role in regulating cardiovascular function. Rats that are trained on a treadmill have a reduced affinity for and density of α_2-adrenergic receptor binding sites in the nucleus tractus solitarii. In addition, there is an increase in affinity of vasopressin receptors in the nucleus tractus solitarii. Both of these adaptations are important in the neural control of cardiovascular function (100).

Dynamic Exercise Training and the CNS

There is presently a surge in interest in the ways exercise affects the nervous system. As a result of this surging interest, a large number of papers report results that do not yet form a logical or consistent basis for formulating useful generalizations of their scientific or clinical significance. The results of many of these studies are interesting and intriguing and warrant continuing study. There is substantial evidence that the rate of axoplasmic transport in neurons is elevated in rats trained on a treadmill. The peak and average transport velocities, as well as the total amount of protein-bound radioactivity, for fast axonal transport in the sciatic nerve is higher in trained than untrained rats (101). The effects are most likely chronic adaptations in fast axonal transport because the measurements were made 21 to 22 days after the last exercise bout. The responses varied among different motor pools, with the increase apparently being related to the amount of overload imposed on the motor pool. In rats that were run on a treadmill with increasing intensity over 8 weeks (102) axonal transport of acetylcholinesterase was enhanced in the rat sciatic nerve. Swim training did not have this effect.

KEY POINT

Some of the reasons for this surge include the evidence accumulating that dynamic exercise can (a) enhance the recovery from traumatic neural injuries, (b) enhance learning, and (c) stimulate neurogenesis.

Each of these observations showing changes in neurotransmitters and their receptors with dynamic exercise and training demonstrate that the brain is adapting to different levels and kinds of activity in many complex ways. The studies to date have not led to any fundamentally new concepts regarding exercise or how the brain functions. They do show, as would be expected, that many if not most areas of the brain and spinal cord are very dynamically involved in most movements. How the changes noted previously relate to changes in functional capacity and in the perception of the quality of performance is a subject for further investigations as we learn more about how the CNS accommodates movement.

Summary

An important take-home message is that fatigue routinely occurs at varying sites and the consequences of this fatigue at each of these sites are unique. For example, one can experience fatigue by repeating the identical task many times and the manner in which these repeated movements are made will define the sites most susceptible to fatigue (e.g., neurotransmitter release, excitation-contraction coupling, adenosine triphosphate (ATP) levels in the muscle, etc.). Fatigue can also simply emerge as a result of a lack of adequate amounts and quality of sleep, although it is unknown why we even need to sleep to avoid this type of fatigue.

Muscle Atrophy and Movement Control

To execute fine motor control, the brain and spinal cord must generate a series of action potentials that will reach a very specific number and kind of motoneurons in a very specific sequence. In addition, the brain and spinal cord must "know" rather precisely the mechanical consequences of activation of a given set of motoneurons. Therefore, the brain and spinal cord assume the force- and speed-generating properties of the muscle fibers that are activated. Our understanding of how the adjustments or resynchronization of neural and muscular elements occurs, however, remains incomplete.

KEY POINT

During the performance of normal daily activities, there are continuous opportunities for the nervous and muscular systems to become familiarized with or update one another so that the nervous system can accurately predict the mechanical consequences of muscle hypertrophy or atrophy.

When the mechanical output is an error of consequence during the performance of a routine task, the nervous system assumed that a different mechanical output would have occurred. For example, if the nervous system is predicting a 10-G force from a motor unit but the muscle fibers have atrophied, the force and power will be less than expected. When this mismatching occurs, the nervous system is able to readily adjust by recruiting more motor units or by increasing the frequency of excitation of the active motor units. Because muscle atrophy often occurs gradually, as observed with aging and some neuromuscular diseases, these adjustments can be made more readily. There must be numerous neural and musculoskeletal mechanisms through which this compensation can occur.

Another indirect consequence of muscle atrophy on motor unit recruitment and movement performance is an increase in fatigability (Fig. 2.34). Often, it is assumed that increased fatigability of a muscle can be attributed to a decrease in the metabolic potential of individual muscle fibers. The loss of fatigue resistance attributable to these intrinsic properties of the muscle fibers, however, is often rather small, even after prolonged periods of decreased activity or inactivity (103).

The more dramatic effect of muscle atrophy on fatigability may be attributed to the fact that more motor units must be recruited and at a higher frequency of excitation for an atrophied muscle to perform a given motor task. The overall fatigability will be greater because the additional motor units recruited—those motor units having the higher threshold levels and lower fatigue resistance will be more fatigable.

> ## KEY POINT
>
> Consequently, muscle fiber atrophy imposes several critical adjustments in the totally integrated neural control of the motor system, that is, altered sensory feedback, additional recruitment of more motor units, and increased fatigability.

Long-Term Neuronal Influences on Motor Unit Properties and Fatigability

Multiple factors regulate fatigability. A fundamental, but partially unresolved, issue is what factors determine the fatigability of each motor unit. Fatigue resistance clearly is directly related to the mitochondrial content of the muscle unit (i.e., the fibers of the motor unit) (104). The mitochondrial content of a fiber is determined to a large extent by neural factors independent of activity. Mitochondrial content of any given motor unit, however, can be modulated upward with greater neuromuscular activity as occurs with prolonged, endurance type exercise. The levels of enzymes

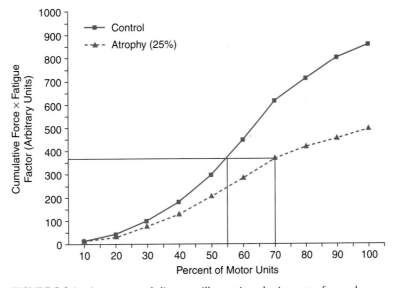

FIGURE 2.34   A conceptual diagram illustrating the impact of muscle atrophy without any further pathology on the functional output potential of that motor pool when performing a task lasting for several minutes. Two factors limit the performance in this case. There is the obvious deficit due to the 25% muscle loss and the proportional loss in force. Thus, to accomplish a given motor task, more motor units must be recruited. Recall that the higher in the recruitment order within a motor pool, the more fatigable the larger units will be. So the combined loss of force and the increased fatigability of the additional units that must be recruited to complete a task result in the individual fatiguing more rapidly even if there is no loss in the fatigability of the individual units. The plot demonstrates that with atrophy, 70% of the motor pool would have to be recruited to perform the same task as 55% of the motor pool in the absence of atrophy. (Unpublished figure, VR Edgerton and RR Roy.)

linked to oxidative phosphorylation are inversely related to the fatigability of the muscle, motor unit, or muscle fiber (105). Many other factors also affect the fatigability of a motor unit. For example, the rate at which ATP is utilized is hydrolyzed to adenosine diphosphate and P_i is determined, in part, by the myosin phenotype. For example, if a fiber has slow myosin, it will have a slow maximum rate of ATP hydrolysis and the fiber will be more resistant to fatigue. With respect to maintaining homeostasis, a general concept would be that the ratio of oxidative phosphorylation to ATP hydrolysis potential is directly related to the resistance to fatigue of a muscle, motor unit, or muscle fiber (also see Chapter 6).

The high fatigue resistance of the soleus muscle and its motor units is largely maintained after cross-reinnervation with a nerve that normally innervates a fatigable muscle (106), after spinal cord transection (107), after spinal cord isolation (108), and after chronic hind limb unloading (109). These results indicate that the fatigue properties of type I (slow) muscle fibers can be relatively independent on the amount of activation and loading and of phenotypic changes. After spinal cord injury in humans, the fatigue resistance of the soleus muscle is maintained for about 6 weeks but becomes more fatigable after about 1 year of complete paralysis (110).

Normal In Vivo Neuromuscular Activity Patterns

As alluded to several times earlier in this chapter, the nervous system not only controls the specific movements that occur but also it determines to a very large extent the properties of a muscle, such as size, speed, and fatigability. So, what is it about the activation patterns generated by the CNS that defines the muscle properties?

KEY POINT

There is an interactive effect between the daily activation and loading characteristics of a muscle in determining its mechanical and phenotypic properties.

The relationship between the total daily activity of a muscle and its mass, however, is highly nonlinear (Fig. 2.35). For example, the soleus muscle of a normal adult cat is active about 14% to 23% of the day during routine cage activity (111,112). When the muscle is made chronically inactive (<1% of normal activity) via spinal cord isolation, the mass is reduced to about one-third of normal (108). Therefore, one-third of the mass of

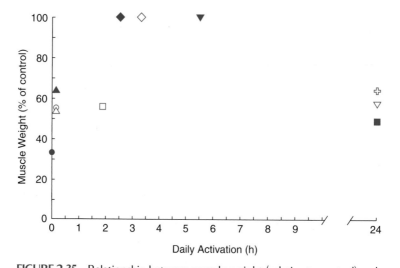

FIGURE 2.35 Relationship between muscle weight (relative to control) and the daily activation level of the muscle. Control soleus: cat (◇) and Rhesus monkey (▼). Four month spinal cord isolated (SI) cat soleus: SI only (●); SI plus shortening contractions (△); SI plus lengthening contractions (○); SI plus isometric contractions (▲). Six month spinal cord transected cat soleus: (□). Chronically electrically stimulated: rabbit tibialis anterior (TA) for 2 weeks at 10 Hz (⊕); rabbit TA for 6 weeks at 10 Hz (▽), and rabbit TA for 12 weeks at 10 Hz or rat TA for 8 weeks at 10 to 20 Hz (■). Note that as little as 9 min of contractions in the otherwise silent cat soleus muscle maintained a similar relative weight as continuous stimulation of the rabbit or rat TA for 2 to 12 weeks. These data suggest that there is an optimal amount of activation-load that will preserve the size of muscle fibers. (Modified from Roy RR, Zhong H, Hodgson JA, et al. Influence of electromechanical events in defining skeletal muscle properties. *Muscle Nerve.* 2002;26:238–251.)

this predominantly slow muscle is independent of its electrical activity and passive mechanical events. Only approximately 9 minutes of high-resistance isometric, shortening, or lengthening electrically evoked contractions per day (0.62% of the day) results in the maintenance of ~64%, 55%, and 55% of the mass of the otherwise inactive soleus muscle, respectively. In chronic complete low thoracic spinal cord transected cats, the soleus is active ~8% of the day (115 min per day) during routine cage activity and 56% of its mass is maintained (111). Note the similarity in the preservation of muscle mass in the spinal cord transected (~56%) and spinal cord isolated plus electromechanically stimulated (~55%–64%) cats despite daily activation durations of 115 (moderately low loading) compared to 9 (maximum loading) minutes. This comparison highlights the role of the loading dynamics in maintaining muscle mass. When electrically and mechanically "silenced" muscles are stimulated electrically with the same duration and pattern but under isometric, shortening or lengthening conditions, the relative preservation of the muscle mass is isometric > lengthening > shortening (113).

KEY POINT

These results demonstrate that the mechanical events, as well as the electrical events play a role in defining the mass of the muscle.

Daily EMG activity levels of selected hind limb muscles also have been assessed in Rhesus monkeys during normal cage activity (114). The soleus is a highly active muscle relative to the medial gastrocnemius, tibialis anterior, and vastus lateralis, regardless of how the activity is expressed or normalized (Fig. 2.36). However, as with the cat, one of the most active muscles—the soleus—is inactive for a large proportion of the day. Similar trends are observed when comparing the soleus and medial gastrocnemius activity in humans (115). When one looks at the details, however, there is not a close link between how active a muscle is and its predominant phenotype (116).

TEST YOURSELF

How are the mechanisms that control muscle fiber size related to the activity levels of the muscle fiber?

Plasticity of the Nervous System in Response to Activity: A Neural Darwinian Process

How does the nervous system continuously adapt to changing demands throughout life? Edelman (117) theorized that the brain is dynamically organized into cellular populations

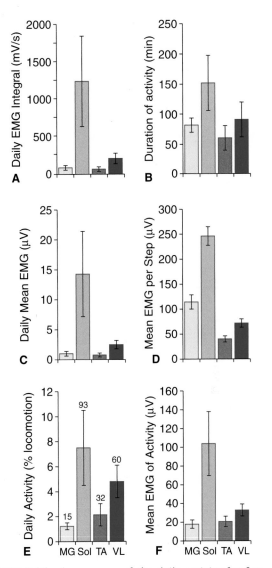

FIGURE 2.36 A summary of the daily activity for five monkeys housed in colony cages. **A.** The daily integral is the integral of electromyography (EMG) for the entire day. **B.** The duration of activity is the total time that EMG activity was detected in the muscle. **C.** The daily mean EMG is the daily integral divided by 24 hours (86,400 seconds). **D.** Mean EMG per step is the mean EMG amplitude calculated over the entire step. It was calculated from five steps of treadmill locomotion at 1.33 m · s^{-1}. **E.** Daily activity (% locomotion) is the percentage of the day that the Rhesus would have to spend walking at 1.33 m · s^{-1} to generate the daily EMG integral equivalent for each muscle, assuming that they participated in no other activity. The duration of the locomotion in minutes is shown above the bar for each muscle. **F.** The mean EMG of activity is the total daily activity divided by the duration of activity (*i.e.*, A/B). MG, medial gastrocnemius; Sol, soleus; TA, tibialis anterior; VL, vastus lateralis. Bars, SEM. (Modified from Hodgson JA, Wichayanuparp S, Recktenwalk MR, et al. Circadian force and EMG activity in hindlimb muscles of rhesus monkeys. *J Neurophysiol.* 2001;86:1430–1444.)

containing individually varied networks, the structure and function of which are selected by different means during development and behavior. The cellular populations are proposed to be collections of hundreds to thousands of strongly interconnected neurons acting as a functional unit.

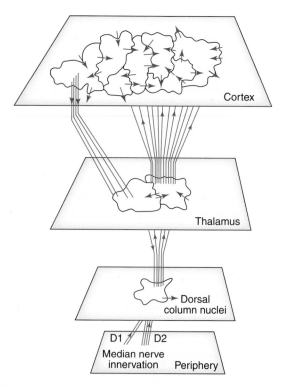

KEY POINT

The key functional elements of this concept of neuronal group selection are: (a) there is continuous spatial temporal representation of an object and a mechanism for continuous updating of the selection of neuronal groups that can generate a given motor synergy or pattern; and (b) these neuronal groups that generate a movement pattern can "degenerate" by selectively matching new sensory and motor processes.

This concept also assumes that different neuronal groups can accomplish the same function. From a neural Darwinian perspective, the adaptive nature of these functional units reflects neural projections that formed either during development (primary repertoire) or as a result of experience and via changing synaptic efficacy (secondary repertoire) (Fig. 2.37).

The concept of neuronal group selection, a key component of neural Darwinism, can play a dominating role in the execution of motor patterns controlled by the lumbosacral spinal cord. The neuronal group selection theory, although originally considered a supraspinal phenomenon, is as relevant to the circuitry within the spinal cord as it is to the brain. For example, the human spinal cord can generate motor synergies that can be categorized as being primary (formulated during development) and secondary (formulated from experience and learning) repertoires (Fig. 2.38). Experiments have demonstrated that the human lumbosacral spinal cord can match complex proprioceptive information with predictable motor repertoires such as stepping, standing, and limb flexion even after severe muscle atrophy and neural impairment. The execution of these motor tasks in subjects with a spinal cord injury with no supraspinal input demonstrate that dynamically organized cellular populations can generate synergies that are not confined to the brain. Furthermore, it appears that secondary repertoires can occur in the human spinal cord because the synaptic efficacy of the networks that generate stepping and standing can markedly improve with repetitive movements in which the sensory ensemble is appropriately matched (i.e., context dependent). In addition, these data are consistent with the neuronal group selection theory in that the motor tasks studied can be performed by functionally, but not morphologically, equivalent networks.

FIGURE 2.37 Schematic diagram of dynamic vertical and horizontal reentrant connectivity across a linked system of laminae and nuclei. Changes in any one level must result in readjustment of all "linked" levels. The concept is that different functional groups of neurons are forming throughout life and that this reorganization is activity-dependent. These functional groups form during development (primary) and in the adult (secondary). (Modified from Edelman GM. *Neural Darwinism: The Theory of Neuronal Group Selection.* New York: Basic Books; 1987:173.)

strong evidence that training of complete spinal humans on a treadmill belt using a weight-supporting device combined with overground training can increase the levels of motor pool activation, improve coordination of motor pool recruitment (Fig. 2.38), and reduce muscle atrophy (70). These improvements occur slowly, that is, after weeks or even months of training.

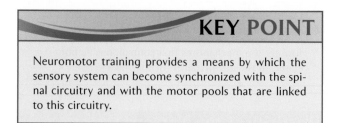

KEY POINT

Neuromotor training provides a means by which the sensory system can become synchronized with the spinal circuitry and with the motor pools that are linked to this circuitry.

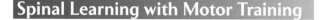
Spinal Learning with Motor Training

Neuromotor training has been a primary intervention that consistently improves the ability to step and stand even after the spinal cord is isolated from the brain (52,65). There is

A Simple Model of Spinal Learning: Flexor Withdrawal Response

Early evidence that spinal circuits respond to neuromotor training came from studies of simple hind limb motor reflexes in animals with a complete spinal cord transection.

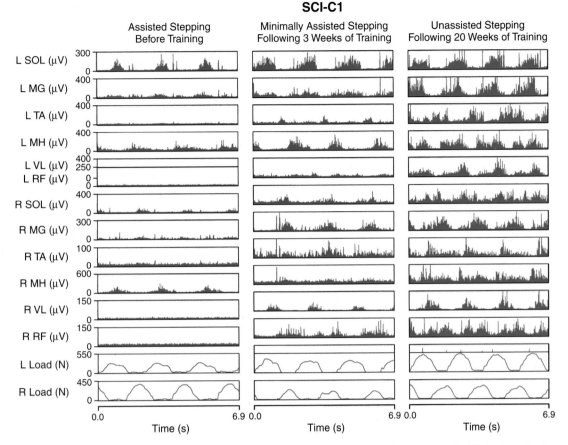

FIGURE 2.38 An example of the development of new functional neuronal groups, probably in the spinal cord, of a severely injured spinal cord subject. The fact that more motor pools can be activated with locomotor training, and the fact that shifts in the timing of the bursts can occur, illustrate the formation of secondary neuronal groups as illustrated in Fig. 2.35. L, left; R, right; SOL, soleus; MG, medial gastrocnemius; TA, tibialis anterior; MH, medial hamstrings; VL, vastus lateralis; RF, rectus femoris; μV, micro voltage. (Compliments of Susan Harkema, University of Louisville, Kentucky.)

Simple hind limb reflexes (*e.g.*, the hind limb withdrawal reflex) can be modulated via classical (118) or operant (119) conditioning techniques. An example of operant conditioning within the spinal cord is the prolonged dorsiflexion that occurs in a spinal rat after a series of electrical stimuli are presented to the paw. In this paradigm, when the paw drops below a threshold position, a stimulus is delivered to the leg. During 5 to 20 minutes a completely spinalized rat can be conditioned to avoid the stimuli by maintaining a more dorsiflexed position, even though there can be no conscious perception of the shock (115). In contrast, no conditioning occurs in yoked spinal rats that get shocked in a manner that is not associated with a specific foot position.

KEY POINT

All of these findings are consistent with the conclusion that spinal circuits can be trained to perform relatively simple hind limb motor tasks in the absence of any connection between the spinal cord and the brain.

Learning in the Spinal Cord of More Complex Motor Tasks

The works of Nesmeyanova (121) and Shurrager and Culler (122) were the first to suggest that complex postural and locomotor tasks can be improved after some training paradigm. It is now clear that hind limb stepping in spinal cats can be improved with daily practice of walking on a treadmill. Several laboratories (50,123,124) have demonstrated that adult spinal cats performed full weight-bearing hind limb stepping on a treadmill after as little as 2 to 3 weeks of locomotor training (Fig. 2.39). These data provided the most compelling behavioral evidence that the circuitry within the lumbosacral spinal cord that generates hind limb stepping can be modified by the sensorimotor experience. With training, there is a steady increase in the maximum treadmill speed achieved with full weight-bearing and in the number of plantar surface steps performed (84). In addition, locomotor training tended to normalize the characteristics of the locomotion based on similarities in EMG and kinematics patterns of trained spinal and intact cats. Normal flexor and extensor muscle activation relationships, EMG burst waveform shapes, and adjustments

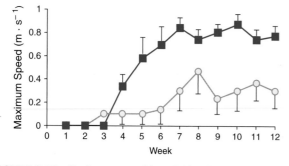

FIGURE 2.39 Performance of bipedal hind limb stepping on a treadmill after a complete transection of the spinal cord at a low thoracic level in step-trained and nontrained cats. Average maximum speeds for six step-trained (■) and six nontrained (○) cats are shown 1–12 weeks after spinal cord transection. The difference between the two lines represents the effects of training versus spontaneous recovery. Bars, SEM; *, significantly different from nontrained ($P < 0.05$). (Modified from de Leon RD, Hodgson JA, Roy RR, et al. Locomotor capacity attributable to step training versus spontaneous recovery after spinalization in adult cats. *J Neurophysiol.* 1998;79:1329–1340.)

in EMG burst durations across speeds of locomotion are preserved in trained spinal cats. With step training, the overall patterns of joint angle excursions during a step cycle, the sequence of flexion and extension movements in the hind limbs joints, and the force levels in the soleus muscle are similar, but not identical, during stepping in intact and spinal cats (Fig. 2.40).

That the activity in neural networks of the lumbar spinal cord is to a large extent determined by the pattern of activity in the hind limbs is further demonstrated by the effect of stand training in spinal cats. Spinal cats can be trained to perform full weight-bearing extension (maintaining posture) for long periods (83). Most stand-trained spinal cats, however, cannot generate even a few successful weight-supported steps. Thus, the spinal cord learns the specific motor task presented during the training sessions. Furthermore, when the step training is stopped for 12 weeks, the stepping ability is as poor as it was prior to any training—the spinal cord seems to forget the specific motor task if it is not practiced (Fig. 2.41). Although it is possible that these learned behaviors can occur only in the injured spinal cord, a more logical interpretation is that some aspects of these repetitive motor responses can be learned by neural networks in the spinal cord of uninjured individuals as well.

Supraspinally induced plasticity of the spinal monosynaptic reflex

Several studies showing an increase in both the firing threshold potential and the amplitude of the after-hyperpolarization potential of motoneurons after an H-reflex conditioning protocol provide evidence that the efficacy of the monosynaptic synapse can be modulated via some activity-dependent mechanisms. These studies show functional as well as

morphologic changes associated with the Ia fiber terminals on motoneurons as a result of supraspinal modulation of the excitability of these afferent synapses over weeks or even months. The changes in the monosynaptic efficacy in the spinal cord observed after several weeks persisted immediately after a complete midthoracic spinal cord transection (125). In addition, Beaumont and Gardiner (126) reported that slow type motoneurons of 12-week treadmill trained rats had greater after-hyperpolarizations than control rats.

> ## KEY POINT
>
> Thus, there are adaptations in the intrinsic properties of motoneurons as well as the synapses that modulate motoneuron excitability associated with motor learning and training.

Summary

Understanding the synaptic plasticity that underlies more complex motor tasks is a very difficult challenge. Our general interpretation of these findings is that the lumbar spinal circuitry can learn to step with exposure to repetitive step training. In the absence of any training, the patterns of motor output are generated in response to the stimuli associated with the movement of the treadmill. The probability that the correct patterns (*i.e.,* synchronization of ipsilateral and contralateral events) will be generated in nontrained animals over a series of consecutive step cycles is low.

> ## KEY POINT
>
> The effect of training, therefore, is to repetitively activate the appropriate extensor and flexor networks in a specific temporal and spatial pattern so that the probability of generating successful responses will be improved.

A Continuously Adapting Synaptic Milieu for Motor Control

Even when one is completely rested and when there is little or no likelihood of fatigue, there will be variation in the motor task from one effort to the next. After years of practicing to make a free throw in basketball, one is rarely successful 95% of the time. In fact, the percentage is about 75% even for professional athletes. In addition to this baseline level of variability under the most optimal and constant conditions, further variations are imposed by continuously changing physiologic states. The term *physiologic states,*

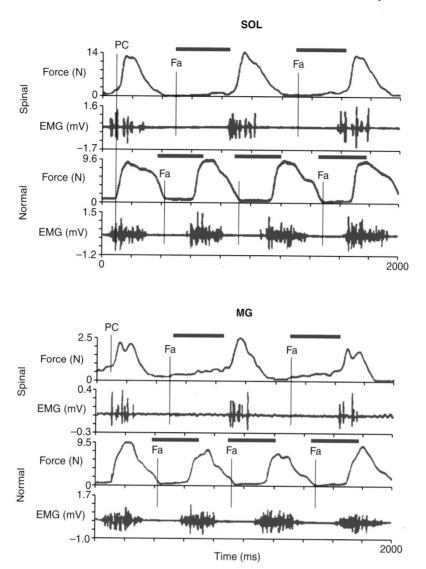

FIGURE 2.40   Force and electromyography (EMG) records from the soleus (SOL) and medial gastrocnemius (MG) muscles of a spinal (complete transection at T12) and a control cat stepping on a treadmill belt moving at a moderate speed. The force was recorded using implanted strain gauges on the tendons of the muscles. Note that the timing of the EMG and force patterns are similar for the spinal and control cats. However, there are some obvious differences as well. For example, the force pattern in the soleus is shorter in the spinal cat. Also note that although the peak force levels are similar in the soleus, the peak force in the MG of the spinal cat is much less than in the control. This reflects a limitation in the level of recruitment of the motor pools consisting of the larger, less excitable motor units. This is also indicated in the intensity of the EMG signals of the MG of the spinal versus control cat. PC, time of paw contact; Fa, point of ankle flexion. The *thick horizontal line* indicates time for stance in the contralateral limb. (Modified from Lovely RG, Gregor RJ, Roy RR, et al. Weight-bearing hindlimb stepping in treadmill-exercise adult spinal cats. *Brain Res.* 1990;514:206–218.)

as used here, encompasses a time scale ranging from milliseconds to years. In this sense, the nervous system is changing constantly, at least physiologically, and some features change more rapidly than others. These continuously fluctuating properties reflect changing probabilities of excitation and inhibition of neuronal synapses between multiple supraspinal centers and the neuromuscular junctions. Given

that millions of synaptic events shape every instant of a motor task, some variations in the pattern of activation of the net ensemble of motoneurons activated from effort to effort might be expected. Although some of the changes in the efficacy of excitation of some synapses might be viewed from a perspective of fatigue, this seems unlikely unless one's definition of fatigue includes any activity or

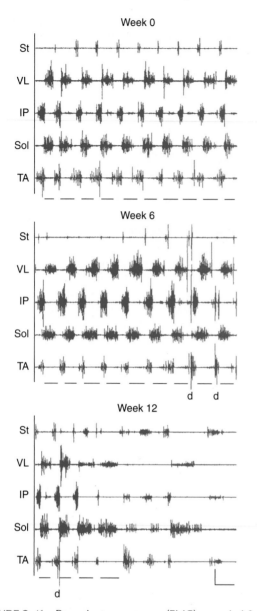

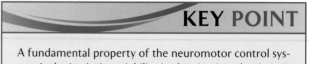

state-dependent phenomenon. The key point is that the history of the synaptic effects plays a role in defining the probabilities of excitation at some point thereafter.

KEY POINT

A fundamental property of the neuromotor control system is the intrinsic variability in the circuitry that is activated during a motor task (127) (also see Fig. 2.23).

Examples are used to illustrate these general concepts. These examples represent synaptic plasticity ranging from the cerebral cortex to the neuromuscular junction. Two of the most studied synapses in mammalian physiology have been the neuromuscular junction and the monosynaptic stretch reflex. The reason for focusing on these synapses is their accessibility for experimentation. Implications of changing synaptic efficacy of other synapses; however, often can be implied by indirect methods and with clever experimental designs. In most cases, it is difficult to ascertain which synapses are responsible for the experimental observations, particularly for in vivo models. Although there may be a scientific urge to pinpoint the synapse to which a change in performance in vivo can be attributed, it is likely that the changes reflect highly interactive dynamics involving synaptic efficacy at multiple levels (128).

Effects of Mental Practice and Cross Education on Motor Performance

One can mentally rehearse a motor task so that maximum strength and motor skill will improve (129). Although synaptic efficacy at supraspinal sites may be important to these changes in performance, some effects may be at the spinal cord level. For example, there is an elevated level of excitation of the relevant motor pools to the extent that both motor units and mechanoreceptors are activated in muscles during mental practice. Even when there is no apparent activation of motor units during mental practice; however, there tends to be an elevated level of excitability of the motor pools associated with the mentally practiced motor task. But, even in the case where there is some activity in a muscle during mental practice, the synaptic events needed to excite a large number or even all of the motor units within a pool do not occur.

FIGURE 2.41   Raw electromyogram (EMG) recorded from selected hind limb muscles of one spinal cat during tests of stepping at a treadmill speed of 0.4 m · s⁻¹ after step training (week 0) and after the cessation of step training (weeks 6 and 12). St, semitendinosus; VL, vastus lateralis; IP, ilio-psoas; Sol, soleus; TA, tibialis anterior. Lines drawn under the EMG records indicate the stance phases in which full weight-bearing occurred on the plantar surface of the paw. Horizontal calibration, 1 s; vertical calibration 1 mV for all muscles except for the Sol, 2 mV. Note that only after a 12-week absence of motor training was there a significant degradation in the coordination of the lower limb motor pools. (Modified from de Leon RD, Hodgson JA, Roy RR, et al. Retention of hindlimb stepping ability in adult spinal cats after the cessation of step training. *J Neurophysiol.* 1999;81:85–94.)

KEY POINT

It seems that with mental practice there is a sufficient level of net excitatory input to a population of motoneurons and interneurons, although at a subliminal or subthreshold level, such that a lingering memory trace can be formed (129).

Cross Education Training

Another example of training-induced synaptic adaptations is improvement in strength in an untrained limb when the contralateral limb is trained. Although some of this cross-education effect may occur at a supraspinal level, the improvement in strength in both limbs by voluntarily activating the muscles of only one limb also may be due to changes in the spinal cord. The presence of this cross-education effect has been demonstrated in a variety of muscles and in response to isometric, concentric, and eccentric training (130–132). The primary contralateral muscles that are affected are the homologous muscles. The magnitude of the effect has varied considerably among the many experiments studying this phenomenon. These cross-education effects seem to be highly specific for the mode of training and testing. In response to training by voluntary isometric or concentric contractions, the gains in strength in the contralateral limb vary from about 5% to 25% (132). Training eccentrically results in greater contralateral effects, with the gains being as high as 75% of the ipsilateral effect (130). Electrical stimulation has an even greater contralateral effect when tested in the same mode as used during the training (131).

In most of the studies of contralateral training effects, it seems reasonably clear that the activity level in the untrained muscles during training is relatively low and usually no muscle hypertrophy is observed. It also seems that both supraspinal and spinal circuits contribute to these cross-education effects (133). Obviously not all of the motoneurons of the motor pools that actually execute a movement need be activated to improve the performance of that movement.

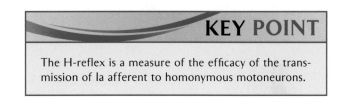

KEY POINT

Perhaps it is only necessary to activate neural circuits that set up the execution of a movement and the activation of these planning circuits can improve the performance of an intended task.

Summary

It is becoming more generally recognized that the learning of a motor skill occurs at multiple sites throughout the nervous system. The concept that motor learning is restricted to the cerebellum is no longer viable. Learning-related phenomena seem to occur within and among neural networks throughout the nervous system, including the spinal cord. It also seems likely that the mechanisms underlying these learning phenomena are similar within and among these different networks.

Adaptations of Muscle Afferents

Short- and Long-Term Changes in the H-reflex

Many of the properties of the sensory input from the neuromuscular system are activity dependent. The excitability of the monosynaptic stretch reflex or its electrical analog, the H-reflex, can change from millisecond to millisecond and it can adapt over weeks or months by either increasing or decreasing its sensitivity to stretch. Testing monosynaptic efficacy by electrically stimulating the peripheral nerve enables one to control the excitatory signals (the number of sensory axons excited) more accurately than by actually controlling it mechanically (i.e., using a muscle-tendon tap).

KEY POINT

The H-reflex is a measure of the efficacy of the transmission of Ia afferent to homonymous motoneurons.

Modulation of the H-reflex within a Step Cycle

The clearest example of the acute plasticity of the monosynaptic reflex is its modulation during a single step. For example, during walking, the H-reflex rises during the stance phase, falls during the onset of the swing phase, and then gradually rises during the latter portion of the swing phase of each step. During running, the H-reflex falls during the stance phase at the interval between the end of stance and beginning of the swing phase. The H-reflex increases to its highest level at the end of the swing and the beginning of stance (Fig. 2.42) (61). In these experiments, using the H-reflex as an indicator of the excitability of monosynaptic reflexes under different conditions or at different times, it is essential that the same number of sensory axons be stimulated for the conditions being compared. Given this assumption, how many motoneurons reach the threshold for excitation for a given number of sensory axons stimulated? Because the number of motoneurons activated differs over the course of a step cycle, the synaptic efficacy of the sensory projections is also changing. This is due to the modulation of other synaptic inputs directly onto the Ia terminals. These synaptic inputs can increase or decrease the efficacy of the monosynaptic reflex and this input can come from supraspinal or spinal neurons. Because the H-reflex is modulated during stepping in humans with a complete spinal cord injury, it is apparent that the spinal circuits can mediate the H-reflex in the absence of supraspinal input. This does not mean, however, that there is no supraspinal modulation as the work of Wolpaw and colleagues (125) shows.

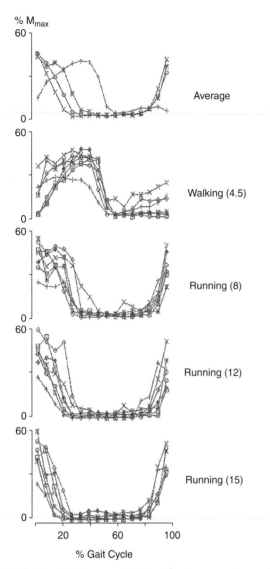

% M_{max}

Average

Walking (4.5)

Running (8)

Running (12)

Running (15)

% Gait Cycle

FIGURE 2.42 H-reflex modulations. In the top tracings, the modulation of the soleus H-reflex is shown as the average from seven subjects during walking at 4–5 km · h^{-1} (+), running at 8 km · h^{-1} (*), running at 12 km · h^{-1} (−) and running at 15 km · h^{-1} (x). Each tracing shows data for each subject and for each velocity investigated. Each of the seven subjects is represented by a specific symbol. All data are expressed as a percentage of M_{max}. The gait cycle was divided into 16 time slices and normalized with heel strike at 0% and 100%. Each cycle starts at foot contact. Note that in all cases, the H-reflex amplitude rises rapidly just prior to foot contact and is suppressed during the swing phase. Walking differs from running in that the facilitation state persists for almost half of the cycle duration compared to a shorter duration of facilitation at the fastest running speeds (see average plots). Also note that during walking there tends to be less facilitation prior to foot contact compared to running. These data are consistent with the view that the stretch reflex contributes significantly to the dynamics of stepping, perhaps by taking advantage of the considerable amount of elastic energy that can be stored in muscle-tendon units. (Modified from Simonsen EB, Dyhre-Poulsen P. Amplitude of the human soleus H reflex during walking and running. *J Physiol.* 1999;515:929–939.)

Changes in the H-reflex due to Repetition and Training

The stretch reflex gain (greater response per stimulus input) has been reported to be elevated (134) or depressed (135,136) during and after submaximal fatiguing contractions. These apparent contradictory results could be due to the muscle studied, the manner in which the reflex was quantified, and other factors. In response to resistance training and an increase in strength, the H-reflex excitability is elevated during MVC (137). The H-reflex also is elevated in humans following jump, resistance, or endurance training (137). This elevated H-reflex could be due to greater presynaptic excitatory drive from higher centers to the monosynaptic synapses—although, smaller H-reflexes have been reported in athletes trained for explosive power, such as volleyball players, sprinters, and ballet dancers (138). These results should be viewed cautiously because the H-reflex amplitudes are a function of the percentage of the motor unit types. Because athletes tend to migrate to events that take advantage of their predominance of fiber phenotypes, this also may be accompanied by basic differences in the H-reflex. For example, is it the training or the selection of certain phenotypes that explains a given athlete's physiologic properties?

Interestingly, chronic exposure to microgravity reduces the threshold for excitation of the monosynaptic reflex and raises the gain of this reflex. Observations to date leave it unclear what the mechanisms following different activity paradigms may be. Also, the eventual functional significance of these modulations in controlling a motor task remains unclear.

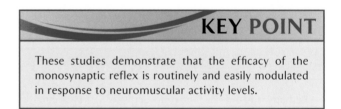

KEY POINT

These studies demonstrate that the efficacy of the monosynaptic reflex is routinely and easily modulated in response to neuromuscular activity levels.

Modulation of Other Spinal Reflexes

Other spinal reflexes also can be modulated by input that changes the excitability of a synaptic circuit. Extremely acute changes in smaller muscle afferents (groups III and IV) occur with the onset of fatigue. Group III and IV afferents fire at higher rates during fatiguing contractions and modulation of these afferents may contribute to changes in blood pressure and heart rate. For example, when the ulnar nerve of human subjects is stimulated to generate isometric forces, blood pressure rises and is directly and closely linked to a decrease in isometric force. The sensitivity of the muscle afferents to the force generating status is further illustrated when the hand is elevated. Under these conditions, the muscle force declines more and the blood pressure increases proportionally more than with the hand not elevated. An important point here is the highly integrative nature of the muscle afferents: not only do they sense changing kinematics and kinetics, they also induce a correspondingly appropriate compensatory action in the cardiovascular system (139).

Firing Patterns of Afferents during Locomotion

Recordings from spindle primary afferents (group Ia fibers) during locomotion demonstrate a range of firing behaviors. These afferents are large and have a low threshold for activation when the axons are electrically stimulated. Examples of these are shown in Fig. 2.23.

The slightly smaller group Ib fibers have their receptors (GTOs) toward the end of the muscle fascicles and near aponeuroses and tendons. These mechanoreceptors are activated during low force contractions as well as at high forces, similar to the group Ia fibers. It is a common misconception that the group Ib fibers associated with the GTOs are very insensitive to modest forces and that their function is to detect very high forces and, in response, provide a strong inhibition of the motoneurons to that muscle to prevent excessive forces. It appears that the GTOs represent another mechanoreceptor that provides unique input to the spinal cord and brain about the routine modulation of forces in the musculotendinous structures (57).

The even smaller group III and IV afferent fibers also seem to provide important information about the environment of the muscle. It is well known that these small afferents mediate reflexes from the muscle that can modulate heart rate, blood pressure, myocardial contractility, and ventilation. For example, when muscles in an anesthetized animal are stimulated via the ventral root, arterial pressure, heart rate, and ventilation will increase. This response, however, is eliminated if the dorsal roots, which carry the sensory information from the muscle to the spinal cord and brain, are cut (140). Subsequent experiments have demonstrated that the large afferents (i.e., group I and II afferents) play little or no role in these cardiovascular and ventilatory responses and that the reflex component can be attributed largely to the group III and IV afferents (141). Furthermore, it appears that the group III and IV afferents differ in their sensitivity to mechanical perturbations. Most group III fibers (almost 80% in the cat) respond vigorously within a second after a contraction of the triceps surae muscle complex, whereas about 40% of the group IV fibers respond to a similar stimulus. Perhaps more importantly is that almost all of the group III fibers slowed or terminated their response as the tension declined, but the response tended to increase in group IV fibers as the contraction continued. Also group IV afferent excitation is not closely linked to the oscillations in force generation after the first few contractions of a longer series of contractions.

These observations led to the hypothesis that group III and particularly, group IV afferents were sensors of the metabolic status of the muscle (i.e., metaboreceptors). Muscle ischemia alone resulted in an increase in afferent activity in almost 50% of the group IV compared to about 10% of the group III fibers (142). It appears that infusion of lactic or arachidonic acid (without an adjustment in pH) will increase excitation of group III and IV afferents (143).

Input to the spinal cord from group III and IV afferents also seems to have an influence on the fatigue response and H-reflexes during submaximal contractions. For example, metabolic/chemical changes in fatigued muscles can activate group III and IV afferents that, in turn, can increase presynaptic inhibition and reduce afferent feedback to the active motor pools, resulting in a decrease in the H-reflex (135,136). In addition, input to the spinal cord by small diameter afferents can depress the excitability of motoneurons that innervate elbow extensors, whereas there is an increase in the excitability of motoneurons innervating elbow flexors (144). Furthermore, these effects are longer under ischemic conditions—that is, when the input from the fatigue sensitive afferents was prolonged. Some failure of voluntary activation of a muscle associated with fatigue also can be associated with supraspinal mechanisms and group III and IV afferents may have a role as they may act to limit circuits that generate cortical output (145). In effect, small diameter afferents can have a differential effect on specific muscle groups during fatiguing contractions through presynaptic inhibition or inhibition of cortical output.

In effect, muscles are exquisite sensors of mechanical and chemical events. There are thousands of mechanoreceptors and metaboreceptors in each muscle. About half of most peripheral nerves are sensory and half motor. Furthermore, combinations of sensors can provide precise information about the levels and locations of forces and displacements.

> ## KEY POINT
>
> Many of these mechanoreceptors and metaboreceptors combined, both within and among muscles, provide extensive detail about the functional state of the whole body.

Regions of the Brain Activated during Dynamic Exercise

Because the motor system receives input from so many sensory sources, one would expect that most of the areas of the brain become activated during exercise. This seems to be the case but, to date, a consistent pattern of activation relative to resting conditions has not emerged. Vissing et al. (146) reported 40% increases in the total radiolabeled glucose uptake in the rat brain during running (85% of max VO_2, 28 m · min^{-1}). The greatest increase was observed in the cerebellum (110%), whereas the motor cortex (39%), basal ganglia (30%), and substantia nigra (37%) also had significant increases. All of these areas of the brain are linked to the coordination of motor functions. The auditory and visual cortex had increases of 32% and 42%, respectively, suggesting enhanced neuronal activity associated with the sound of the treadmill and the constant visual input associated with running on a treadmill belt in a relatively confined cubicle. Other areas of the brain, including those associated with autonomic function—subthalamic nuclei (47%), posterior hypothalamic nuclei (74%), and hippocampus (29%)—had substantial increases in glucose uptake.

> ## KEY POINT
>
> The major point is that significant increases in the metabolic properties occur in many areas of the brain during most motor tasks—in this case, locomotion.

Despite the limitations in techniques to gain insight into how the CNS controls motor function, it is apparent that most of the brain participates in these fundamental tasks. A major advantage of the glucose uptake approach is that in vivo experiments can be performed. But information about the changes in glucose uptake only gives clues to which areas of the brain are involved. It provides no insight to how the physiologic properties of these areas are changing. Advances in molecular biology have led to a number of techniques that permit one to ask, What are the cellular events that underlie changes in behavior? Using new in vivo imaging technologies, it is now possible to repetitively monitor specific mRNA expressions in vivo over weeks using the microPET (positron emission transmission). In this technology the energy emitted from radioligands can be detected and localized. These radioligands are designed to have short half-lives and are relatively expensive to generate. Future studies are likely to provide extremely valuable information on how the CNS functions as a totally integrated system during exercise.

Because most of the known cell-to-cell interactions in the brain and spinal cord in the form of action potentials are generated by neurons, most of the emphasis in trying to understand neural function during exercise has focused on these cells. Another population of cells in the CNS, however, plays important supportive roles that largely remain unclear. These cells are called glia, meaning glue. They have been described as cells that provide the medium within which the neurons rest. Most of the cells in the brain are glial cells, not neurons. These glial cells probably play a major role in defining the patterns of glucose uptake and the general physiologic state of its surrounding neurons. It is generally assumed (without good evidence to support it) that changes in the glucose uptake of the glia will occur primarily in the areas where the neurons are electrically active. Glia also may play an important role in the modulation of neurotrophic factors during exercise.

Changes in Neural Control Properties after Dynamic and Resistive Training

Changes in Cortical Function with Training

> ## KEY POINT
>
> Neural adaptations can contribute to strength increments and efficiency of motion simply by improving muscular coordination.

Resistance training of the fingers increases muscular strength and the stability of sensorimotor coordination during a difficult motor task—that is, the muscles are recruited in a more consistent manner (the variation in the timing, amplitude, and duration of muscle activity being lower) after than before training (147). It is not clear at all, however, where the neural adaptations occur. Synaptic effectiveness of neural connections between areas within the primary cortex can be modified through physical activity (148). It also appears that motor learning may be associated with physiologic adaptations in the primary cortex, contributing to more efficient execution of the learned movements. Use-dependent changes occur in the movement representations in the primary motor cortex of squirrel monkeys (149). Also, there are changes in the activity levels in secondary motor areas when a motor task involving sequential movements is learned (150). Dettmers and associates (151) reported that neural activity increases in the primary motor cortex and caudal supplementary motor area as greater levels of isometric force are produced.

> ## KEY POINT
>
> Training for a specific motor task also may improve performance in related tasks (positive transfer) by reducing the extent of cortical activation and, thus, the activation of the neural elements that may interfere with or are not necessary for the optimal execution of the movement.

When resistance training produces muscle hypertrophy, fewer motor units are needed to generate a given level of torque. This could reduce the level of activation of the motor areas and improve performance. A reduction in activity at several supraspinal sites (e.g., dorsal premotor area, parietal cortex, and lateral cerebellum) may occur with the acquisition of a motor skill (152).

Resistance training can induce relatively long-lasting changes in the functional properties of the corticospinal pathway in humans. The magnitude of the compound EMG, commonly called motor evoked potentials (MEP), in response to transcranial magnetic stimulation (TMS) is smaller after resistance training. The magnitude of muscular responses to TMS reflects the level of transsynaptic excitation of the corticospinal cells. The peak MEP also occurs at a lower percentage of MVC after resistance training, suggesting that the level of contraction at which the entire population of motor units receiving the transcranial volley was recruited is lower after training.

Changes in the Areas of Activation in the Brain with Resistance Training

It has been demonstrated that, as a subject changes the level of force exerted, unique regions of the brain are activated (153). There is growing interest in the possibilities of associating the performance of specific motor tasks with activation of specific regions of the brain and spinal cord. fMRI studies have shown that the area of the primary cortex activated during a specific sequence of finger movements increases after 3 weeks of daily practice (154) and the size of the hand area in the motor cortex increases after 2 hours of piano practice for 5 days (155). Elite racquet players show heightened excitability of the cortical projection to the hand (156). Patten and Kamen (157) used a dorsiflexion force-modulation training regimen (a motor leaning paradigm) to improve force accuracy and surprisingly found an increase in maximum voluntary force in young individuals. The increase in strength is related to a lower force threshold for motor unit recruitment and higher motor unit discharge rates, indicative of adaptations at the spinal segmental level (increased excitability of the agonist motoneuron pools) and, thus, a more complete recruitment of available motor units (158). These results also are consistent with observations that the volume of muscle activated can increase within 2 weeks of resistance training (159). We now know that motoneuron excitability can increase in a range of muscles, including the extensor digitorum brevis, soleus, brachioradialis, and hypothenar, after weeks or months of strength training (160).

The greater excitability of motoneurons after training theoretically should result in higher levels of motor pool activation as reflected in the whole muscle EMG signal. The activation levels of motor pools as measured using integrated EMG increases after strength training, involving weight lifting, isometric contractions, isokinetic eccentric contractions, and explosive jumping. Therefore, with strength training subjects can more fully activate their prime movers during MVCs. Reflex potentiation has been observed to increase after strength training and also to be enhanced in weight lifters (161) and elite sprinters (162). All of these results are consistent with significant adaptations in the sensorimotor pathways resulting from training, activity, and learning.

Changes in Motor Unit Synchronization with Training

Motor unit synchronization increases during the performance of attention-demanding tasks (163). The amount of synchronization of low threshold motor units varies with the type of contraction. Semmler and colleagues (164) demonstrated a striking difference between the level of synchronization of motor units in the first dorsal interosseous during shortening and lengthening contractions. They observed a 50% higher level of synchronization in eccentric than concentric contractions and, thus, considerably more common input on the motoneurons during eccentric than concentric contractions. Synchronization of motor units is more evident in the hand muscles of weightlifters (165), increases with strength training (161), but is less in some musicians (165).

> ## KEY POINT
>
> Motor unit synchronization, a measure of the correlation between the discharge times of action potentials by two or more motor units, is another sign of neural adaptation with training.

Training the dorsiflexors with rapid dynamic contractions at 30% to 40% maximum for 12 weeks also increases the force of motor units in the tibialis anterior distributed across the entire pool (based on spike-triggered averaging), without a change in recruitment order (17). Training also increased the average instantaneous discharge rate from 69 to 90 Hz and there was an increase in the number of doublets. Thus, the increase in strength (MVC) and speed could be linked to an increased motor unit initial discharge rate. Synchronization may increase the rate of force development, but does not necessarily influence the maximum force capability (166). This increase in synchronization may result from (a) an increase in the number or strength of common presynaptic inputs onto populations of motoneurons; and/or (b) descending corticospinal tract neurons with branched-stem axons (167). In summary, typical interpulse intervals of motor units can change with training. Recall that changing a single interpulse interval can significantly improve the force generated by a motor unit (i.e., the catch property). In addition, there is evidence that the interaction of motor units can become more synchronized with training and that this level of synchronization is a function of the type of muscular effort.

Training of a motor task results in a more efficient recruitment of neurons in the spinal circuitry to perform that motor task. One manifestation of the greater efficiency is that there are neurons activated in a defined period of stepping, based on the activity marker gene expression of c-fos. The location and number of active (c-fos

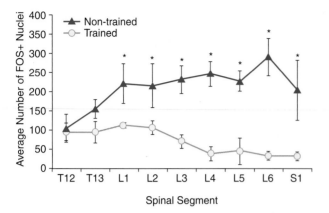

FIGURE 2.43 Spinal rats were run on a treadmill for one hour, returned to their cages for one hour and then intracardially perfused with % paraformaldehyde. Activated neurons were identified using c-fos immunohistochemistry. The average number of FOS+ nuclei per spinal segment was greater in nontrained than trained rats in spinal segments L₁ to S₁. Values are means ± SEM. S, significantly higher in nontrained versus trained at $P < 0.05$. (Adapted from Ichiyama RM, Courtine G, Gerasimenko YP, et al. Step training reinforces specific spinal locomotor circuitry in adult spinal rats. *J Neurosci.* 2008;28:7370–7375.)

positive) spinal neurons was determined in untrained and step-trained spinal rats after a 1-hour bout of bipedal stepping that was facilitated by epidural stimulation (168). The number of active neurons was lower in the step-trained than untrained spinal rats in almost every spinal segment studied (Fig. 2.43). These results provide further evidence that the spinal cord learns with step training by reinforcing the efficacy of selected sensorimotor pathways that control locomotion. In other words, it seems that there are fewer and more select pathways activated after step training.

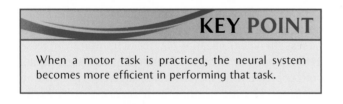

KEY POINT

When a motor task is practiced, the neural system becomes more efficient in performing that task.

Exercise, Nerve Growth Factors, and Learning

Activity Levels, Brain-Derived Neurotrophic Factor Expression, and Learning

There is substantial evidence that dynamic exercise can facilitate learning a spatial task in rats. Similar evidence has been reported in comparisons of the ability to learn and recall in humans who are physically active versus those that are inactive. Some understanding of the possible mechanisms of the exercise-induced facilitation of learning

is emerging. Rats that are allowed to run at will in a wheel connected to their cage have significantly elevated brain-derived neurotrophic factor (BDNF) protein levels in the hippocampus and spinal cord within 3 days than those of rats that are housed in a standard cage without access to running wheels (169,170). BDNF mRNA also is elevated in the hippocampus and spinal cord in these voluntarily exercised rats.

BDNF plays a critical role in the cascade of biochemical reactions thought to be important for LTP. LTP and LTD are thought to be important in many forms of learning, although there is some evidence that they are not essential. BDNF also is associated with many of the cellular events associated with synaptic plasticity in general. For example, synapsin 1, a member of a family of nerve terminal-specific phosphoproteins that are associated with synaptic vesicle turnover, and growth associated protein, which is related with synaptic reorganization, are linked to BDNF and both are upregulated in the hippocampus and spinal cord in response to exercise (Fig. 2.44).

Exercise, BDNF Expression, and Neurogenesis

Several genes linked to BDNF are upregulated in animals that have access to a running wheel compared with those that do not. Animals that are exercised in a running wheel or housed in an enriched environment can learn a water maze task more quickly than animals housed in a standard sedentary cage. The number of new neurons (i.e., those labeled with bromodeoxyuridine) in the dentate gyrus can double in response to wheel running exercise compared with those of mice that swim for the same period. An increase in the number of surviving bromodeoxyuridine neurons also was observed in mice that trained in a Morris water maze four times per day for 4 days compared with rats that did not train (171). There is some evidence that the exercise-induced neurogenesis and improved learning depend on the N-methyl-D-aspartate receptors (172). Also consistent with these observations is that BDNF and its TrkB receptor are reduced in the hippocampus when rats are deprived of habitual running.

There is also evidence that 12 weeks of dynamic exercise (forced running) may reduce neural damage after an injury (reduce the size of a neural infarct) via a neurotrophic mechanism (173). Dynamic exercise training also increases the nerve growth factor (NGF) receptor. It is known that the septo-hippocampal axis is activated with exercise (174) and that wheel running in rodents evokes hippocampal theta activity (activation of medial septum GABAergic afferents during running could contribute to BDNF gene upregulation). NE and 5-HT levels also may play an important role in the exercise-induced modulation of BDNF in the hippocampus (175). Thus, it appears that an enriched environment that includes exercise increases hippocampal BDNF

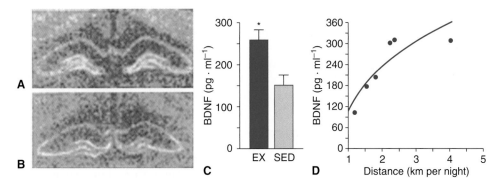

FIGURE 2.44   Effects of exercise on hippocampal brain-derived neurotrophic factor (BDNF) mRNA and protein levels. **A.** In situ hybridization shows that the expression of BDNF mRNA in the rat dentate gyrus (DG), hilus, CA1–CA3 regions, and cortex is greater following exercise (7 days of voluntary wheel-running) than in sedentary animals (**B**). **C.** ELISA quantification of BDNF protein levels in the hippocampus in sedentary (SED) and exercising (EX) animals, after five days of wheel-running (*$P < 0.05$). **D.** Rats and mice acclimate rapidly to the running wheel and progressively increase their extent of daily running. BDNF protein levels correlate with running distance (average over 14 days running; $R^2 = 0.771$). (Reprinted with permission from Cotman CW, Berchtold NC. Exercise: a behavioral intervention to enhance brain health and plasticity. *Trends Neurosci.* 2002;25:295–301.)

mRNA and protein that is regulated by neuronal activity and neurotransmitter input that converge on BDNF-expressing neurons.

Experiments also have been designed to determine whether there is a more specific interaction between neuronal circuits that are involved in performing more precise motor skills and the ability to perform the skill itself. Rats that live in an enriched environment as opposed to a standard cage environment develop more astrocytes, but no neurons or oligodendrocytes in the cerebral cortex. New neurons, however, were formed in the hippocampus. There is some evidence that insulin-like growth factor-1 plays a role in mediating this neurogenesis. Rats trained for a specific motor skill for a month have more synapses per Purkinje cell from both parallel fibers and climbing fibers in the cerebellum than rats that have been exercised in a wheel or sedentary rats (176). More mitochondria were observed in Purkinje cells following motor skill training. Rats that lived in a cage with a running wheel for a month had more capillary growth in the motor areas of the cerebral cortex than sedentary rats and they had a higher blood flow rate in the same area when they exercised. Other experiments have attempted to differentiate the neural adaptations associated with exercise in general from those associated with actually learning a specific motor task. For example, rats that learned a task showed greater synaptogenesis than rats that were more active but did not learn the task (177).

Pharmacologic treatments were used to remove either serotonergic or noradrenergic input and then the rats were allowed to run in voluntary cages for 7 days (100). Systemic deletion of the NE system eliminated the exercise increase in BDNF mRNA in all hippocampal subfields except one and in the dentate gyrus, whereas

a 5-HT lesion did not alter the BDNF mRNA response to dynamic exercise.

Dynamic Exercise-Induced Changes in Growth Factors in the Spinal Cord

Numerous studies have demonstrated a direct link between the modulation of NGFs and exercise. Some of these NGFs appear to be synthesized within muscles and/or the CNS.

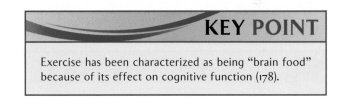

KEY POINT

Exercise has been characterized as being "brain food" because of its effect on cognitive function (178).

Treadmill exercise can improve cognitive function in normal and injured rats and this improved function is modulated, at least in part, by NGFs in the hippocampus (179). Endurance training also has been linked with elevated plasma levels of BDNF (180). There is growing evidence that one or more neurotrophic factors play an important role in mediating improved function after a wide range of neurologic disorders. Improved cognitive performance has been observed in rats after a traumatic brain injury and this effect can be mediated by BDNF (181). There is substantial evidence that physical exercise helps to ameliorate depression (182). BDNF also seems to play a role in the recovery of skilled motor tasks in response to a neural injury (183).

BDNF levels also are increased in the spinal cord as well when rats or mice are allowed to run voluntarily in a wheel.

In a number of examples, the BDNF and neurotrophin-3 (NT-3) differ in their response to exercise. For example, after running in a wheel for 7 days, the NT-3 levels in the hippocampus are reduced. NT-3 levels in the spinal cord, cerebellum, and hippocampus are less responsive to exercise than is BDNF (169).

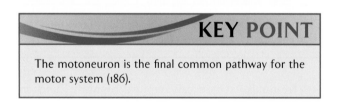

TEST YOURSELF

How dependent are the modulatory controls of neural plasticity mediated by NGFs dependent on neuromuscular activity?

Fibroblast Growth Factor and Dynamic Exercise

Fibroblast growth factor-2 mRNA and protein (immuno) levels also increase in the hippocampus (but not the striatum or the cerebral cortex) after 4 nights of running and then return to control levels after 7 nights of running (184). The time course suggests that exercise could be beneficial at the early stages of a training program. The point is that the hippocampus is important for cognitive function (trophic factor involvement in cognition). Fibroblast growth factor (a known angiogenic factor) also may be involved with the angiogenesis in the brain associated with exercise (185). In many cases growth factors are likely to be mediators for the positive effects of exercise on the brain.

Plasticity of Motoneurons to Varying Levels of Neuromuscular Activity

KEY POINT

The motoneuron is the final common pathway for the motor system (186).

Exercise involves a substantial increase in the number of action potentials generated by at least some of the motoneurons innervating the musculature and with resistance training the target size of individual motoneurons increases (i.e., muscle fiber hypertrophy ensues). Thus, it may be expected that motoneurons adapt their size and/or metabolic properties to reflect the increase in the volume and/or oxidative capacity of their target cells and the increase in their activation levels. Some motoneuron properties, however, are generally resistant to chronic adaptations in neuromuscular activity levels; for example, motoneuron size and metabolic properties have been reported to be generally unaffected

in response to hind limb unloading, spaceflight, spinal cord transection, spinal cord isolation, nerve block via tetrodotoxin administration, functional overload, and muscle nerve stimulation (187–189). After endurance training, small adaptations have been observed in mitochondrial enzyme activities in motor pools that are innervating muscles composed primarily of fibers of the slow phenotype (190). In other studies, there were no or only small changes in oxidative phosphorylation enzyme activity and soma size of motoneurons of slow and fast motor pools in response to endurance training or functional overload (191–193).

More substantial changes seem to occur in the physiologic properties of motoneurons in response to changes in neuromuscular activity levels. In rats that were allowed to run spontaneously for 12 weeks in wheels, the mean resting membrane potential became more hyperpolarized, the spike trigger voltage decreased, and the mean amplitude of the afterhyperpolarization increased in slow but not fast motoneurons (126). Munson and associates (194) also have reported that motoneurons innervating the medial gastrocnemius are more excitable (lower rheobase) and have a higher input resistance (smaller) and a longer duration of afterhyperpolarization after 6 months of chronic electrical stimulation—reflecting that the motoneurons acquired electrophysiologic characteristics that are more typical of slow motoneurons.

Chronic spinal cord injury in cats, which reduces the activity levels of soleus motoneurons by 75% (111), results in a shortening of the afterhyperpolarization and an elevation of rheobase, consistent with the motoneurons changing toward a fast type (107). Also, some muscle fibers in the cat soleus change to a fast phenotype after a complete spinal cord transection (195). In contrast, shifts toward slower electrophysiologic properties in sciatic nerve (196) and triceps surae (197) motoneurons (e.g., decrease of rheobase and increased in input resistance) have been reported after a complete spinal cord transection or spinal cord isolation (198) in adult rats. In both of these rat models, there is an increase in the proportion of fibers having a fast phenotype in several of the muscles innervated by these motoneurons (198). Therefore, it seems that some activity-linked mechanisms may induce some slow motor units to become faster in their physiologic and biochemical properties in cats, but the motoneurons do not appear to follow this pattern in rats. It seems likely that some of the phenotype-related changes might be modulated by neurotrophic factors. For example, calcitonin gene-related peptide (CGRP) (199) and BDNF (169) levels increase in response to exercise in a running wheel. Also, chronic infusion of BDNF into the gastrocnemius in the rat decreases motoneuronal rheobase after 5 days (200), suggesting that trophic substances from the active muscles can influence the motoneuron properties.

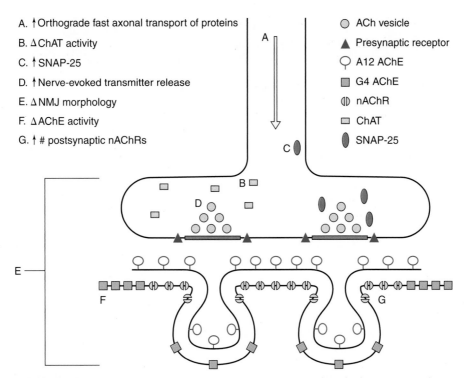

A. ↑ Orthograde fast axonal transport of proteins

B. Δ ChAT activity

C. ↑ SNAP-25

D. ↑ Nerve-evoked transmitter release

E. Δ NMJ morphology

F. Δ AChE activity

G. ↑ # postsynaptic nAChRs

○ ACh vesicle

▲ Presynaptic receptor

♀ A12 AChE

■ G4 AChE

◖◗ nAChR

□ ChAT

◖ SNAP-25

FIGURE 2.45 A summary of endurance exercise training-induced adaptations at the mammalian neuromuscular junction (NMJ). Each letter in the schematic of the NMJ (*A–G*) corresponds to an adaptation, which is described in the upper left-hand corner of the figure. The symbols located to the upper right of the schematic represent the various proteins and components found at the NMJ. (Modified from Gardiner P. *Neuromuscular Aspects of Physical Activity*. Champaign, IL: Human Kinetics; 2001:132.)

Adaptation of the Neuromuscular Junction to Changing Levels of Dynamic and Resistive Exercise

The neuromuscular junction for many years has served as a useful model for understanding use-dependent synaptic function and adaptability (Fig. 2.45). Although it is generally recognized that there is a significant margin for the amount of neurotransmitter that can be released from the neuromuscular junction, it seems that repetitive activation can induce significant changes in function and morphology. Resistance training (*i.e.*, climbing up a grid with attached weights for 7 weeks) produced a number of adaptations in the neuromuscular junctions in the soleus muscle (201). For example, endplate perimeter length and area increase and the membrane area containing the acetylcholine receptors within the endplate region is enlarged, even when there is no change in the muscle fiber size or phenotype. Dynamic exercise training of an endurance nature also increases neurotransmitter release at the neuromuscular junction (202–204). Crocket and associates (205) found that moderate endurance exercise increased the acetylcholinesterase-positive staining area at the endplates of the white vastus muscle in rats. Also, the muscles of endurance-trained rats have larger and more complicated neuromuscular

junctions (*i.e.*, more nerve terminal sprouts and growth configurations) than controls (183,206,207). Voluntary wheel running markedly upregulates total acetylcholinesterase mRNA and protein at the neuromuscular junction of the rat extensor digitorum longus, with a lesser increase in the soleus (208). After spinal cord transection or spinal cord isolation, there is a disassembly of a subset of neuromuscular synapses in flexor but not extensor muscles below the level of the lesion (209). Motorized cycling exercise diminished their incidence, suggesting an activity-dependent effect.

A single bout (30 minutes) of running downhill can result in an increase in the numbers of CGRP-positive motoneurons of selected motor pools such as the triceps surae (210). Other motor pools including the anterior crural, however, did not change with the same exercise paradigm. It is not clear how the duration, intensity, and kind of neuromuscular activity relate to the induction of a CGRP response in motoneurons. The function of CGRP in the motor system appears to include establishing and maintaining the neuromuscular junction and is present when there is axonal sprouting (211). These data are consistent with the sprouting at the motor terminals in the soleus muscle after a single 9-hour bout of voluntary wheel running in mice (212). The reverse may not be true—that is, that CGRP is always a positive indicator of axonal sprouting.

It was clear when these three classic articles were published that there was an important link between the specific motor pool and the type of muscle that it normally innervated. It was also known that there were slow and fast muscles in all mammals and probably all animals. Earlier, Wuerker and Henneman (213) suggested that muscle fibers were homogeneous within a motor unit and alluded to the findings of Buller and associates (193,194) showing a neural effect on muscle properties. These researchers transected the nerves to the slow soleus muscle and the fast flexor digitorum longus muscle and then crossed the nerves so that they would reinnervate the opposite muscle. About 1 to 6 months after cross-reinnervation, they examined whether there was any evidence of plasticity in the spinal cord.

Some of the personal details of the situation surrounding this initial experiment, which is a classic one of its own, are interesting, to say the least. Based on my (VRE) personal conversations with Buller, the story goes like this. Sir John Eccles, who was at the Australian National University in Canberra at that time, was one of the most famous physiologists in the world. He received the Nobel Prize in physiology several years later (1963) for his work on the electrophysiology of spinal neurons. Buller, who had just completed his PhD in England and was considered to be among the most outstanding young physiologists in England was given the opportunity to study with Eccles. So he boarded a freighter heading for Australia. After about a 2-week journey, Eccles met him and took him directly to the laboratory where the first cross-reinnervation experiments were being performed.

Part of the irony is that the experiments were done to examine the plasticity of the synapses of the spinal cord, not the muscle. The original intent was to determine whether the afferent projections to a given motor pool would realign as a result of the nerves innervating a foreign muscle. The way that Buller describes that first night goes like this. The cat had been prepared for the experiment and electrodes had been placed on the muscle nerves. When the normally slow soleus muscle was stimulated, it visibly had a fast twitch. (A standard procedure in studying motoneurons is to stimulate the peripheral nerve to record the antidromic spikes and, thus, identify which muscle the motoneurons innervated.) Eccles immediately became excited by this observation. The reader should realize that one can readily see the difference in the twitch properties of a predominantly slow versus a predominantly fast muscle in a cat and, certainly, Eccles had plenty of experience. At this point in the experiment, Eccles elected to take a quick nap before proceeding with the experiments. This was commonly done when performing very long experimental procedures. Before he began his nap, however, he instructed the young Buller to find a force transducer and record the muscle properties. But Buller did not know what a force transducer looked like. He began going through the lab drawers to find one, but eventually swallowed his pride and awakened Eccles to ask what a force transducer looked like.

As history has shown, in effect, these observations of the muscle properties after cross-reinnervation defined, at least to a very large extent, that the motoneurons in some way controlled the gene expression of thousands of myonuclei within each muscle unit. Although it remains today somewhat unclear how this neural dominance on muscle gene expression is accomplished, it is clear that this modulation or control is mediated by both activity-dependent and activity-independent factors. At this time, slow and fast myosins had been isolated and a direct relationship between myosin ATPase and muscle speed was often assumed.

With respect to the size principle, these researchers' observation provided the backdrop for the idea that the specific motoneuron–muscle fiber linkage was very important in ways other than being a way to activate the muscle. The articles by Henneman and coworkers concluded that slow motor units tended to be small (generating low force) and fast units tended to generate the highest forces. This range in forces among motor units within a motor pool was linked to the size of the axons as measured by conduction velocity as well as by the input resistance to current. Finally, the crucial observation was that the order in which these motor units became excited when stimulating via afferent inputs was constant and was directly related to the size of the unit. They also demonstrated in this series of papers that the size was a determining factor regardless of the source of the excitation (using excitatory reflexes). These studies also showed a constant relationship between size and the level of inhibitory input: the larger the unit, the more susceptible it was to inhibition.

Thousands of articles have challenged this principle. Although some exceptions have been noted over many years, these many challenges have contributed to its robustness, importance, and significance rather than the reverse. For a number of years, our laboratory performed experiments designed to determine whether in some types of efforts the order of recruitment of motor units within a motor pool could be altered. But in the end, Henneman and coworkers were much more right than wrong. In essence, a neural control system that would have to select which and how many motor units to activate for every movement would be enormously large and complex. As it turns out, having many degrees of freedom in choosing which motor units are activated is neither feasible nor necessary.

Subsequent to the initial papers on the size principle a number of other papers further clarified many details of the motoneuron–muscle fiber relationship, most of which demonstrate the centrality of the size principle. The concept of the size principle set the plate for a series of observations. The Henneman papers make this motoneuron–fiber phenotype linkage obvious. Histochemical, biochemical, and physiologic analyses of slow and fast muscles; the size principle; and cross-reinnervation experiments made it clear that the muscle fiber biochemical and physiologic properties were determined in large part by the motoneuron. It also became clear that the fast muscles could be divided into a fatigable and a nonfatigable population and that the observed electrophysiologic properties of motoneurons were consistent with this subdivision. But still there was no direct link of a muscle fiber phenotype to a specific motoneuron type until the technique of glycogen depletion came on the scene. At almost the same time, Kugelberg and Edstrom (216) and our laboratory (217) reported that glycogen depletion (or phosphorylase depletion) could be observed in individual muscle fibers following repetitive stimulation. Kugelberg and Edstrom electrically stimulated muscle nerves in situ and found that the larger, fast, and low oxidative fibers were preferentially depleted of glycogen. This work showed the feasibility of using glycogen depletion to identify muscle fibers that had been active. Given the ease with which the large low oxidative fibers were depleted of glycogen and phosphorylase with stimulation, they suggested that these fibers must be used sparingly over short periods and, thus, would be innervated by motoneurons with very high thresholds. Thus, these motor units would be recruited only during strong, quick contractions and innervated by phasically discharging motoneurons. In fact, when we exercised rodents on a treadmill the slow, high oxidative fibers were selectively depleted as might be expected according to the size principle.

These two results are actually what we would expect in that electrical stimulation of a muscle nerve will selectively activate the larger, faster axons. But, more important, when the stimulus is maximal (activates all axons) the large, low oxidative fibers are more susceptible to glycogen depletion and, therefore, will be depleted more quickly than the high oxidative fibers (as long as blood flow is adequate). The crucial experiment that confirmed a close relationship among the size of a motor unit, the physiologic properties of the muscle, and the biochemical properties of the muscle fibers was performed by Burke and colleagues (218) when they linked the motoneuron properties and the muscle unit properties of the same motoneurons using glycogen depletion techniques. In this case, they depleted the muscle fibers by individual motoneurons and definitively linked the electrophysiology of motoneurons with the physiology and biochemistry of the muscle unit.

Henneman E, Somjenn G, Carpenter DO. Functional significance of cell size in spinal neurons. J Neurophysiol. 1965;28:560–580.

Henneman E, Olson CB. Relations between structure and function in the design of skeletal muscles. J Neurophysiol. 1965;28:581–598.

Henneman E, Somjen G, Carpenter DO. Excitability and irritability of motor neurons of different sizes. J Neurophysiol. 1965;28:599–620.

CHAPTER SUMMARY

Movements are produced by modulating the activation of specific combinations of motor pools and by controlling the level of activation within each of these motor pools. The "final common pathway" is the motor unit: a motoneuron and all of the muscle fibers that it innervates. The order of recruitment of motor units within each motor pool is defined largely by the size principle—that is, the recruitment order within and, to some degree, across synergistic motor pools is normally from the smallest to the largest units. The size of a motor unit is directly related to the size of the motoneuron, dendritic tree, axons, the number of muscle fibers innervated by the motoneuron, and the force generated by the motor unit. Modulation of the forces derived from a motor pool are determined by the number of motor units that are recruited and the frequency of excitation of those motor units, with the frequency modulation being sensitive to a single interspike interval (catch property).

The motor units that are the most excitable are likely to be slow fatigue resistant, those that are moderately excitable are likely to be fast fatigue resistant, and those that are the least excitable are likely to be predominantly fast fatigable motor units. Therefore, to a major degree, the size principle defines the metabolic and physiologic responses to an exercise of a given duration and intensity. For example,

according to the size principle the patterns of glycogen depletion during an exercise will reflect the recruitment of motor units.

The three primary components of the nervous system that regulate posture and locomotion can be conveniently categorized into those neuronal systems: (a) within the brain, (b) within the spinal cord that are associated with CPG, and (c) involved with providing sensory input to the nervous system. The primary descending systems from the brain that control posture and locomotion are the reticulospinal, rubrospinal, vestibulospinal, and corticospinal tracts. There are several areas in the brainstem that receive information associated with locomotion and posture that can generate stepping and standing when stimulated tonically. One of the primary areas that can generate these motor tasks is referred to as the MLR.

There is an extensive level of automaticity in generating posture and locomotion. CPG of locomotion refers to the generation of alternating patterns of flexion and extension that mimic those patterns that occur during locomotion, but without any alternating or rhythmic input from either the brain or the periphery. This alternating output from CPG is referred to as fictive locomotion.

In preparations that eliminate supraspinal input, the spinal cord can interpret sensory information derived from the limbs as an ensemble that provides a precise "picture" of the position of the limbs at any given time during posture or locomotion. Therefore, the spinal cord can respond to these ensembles of input without assistance from the brain, and generate effective weight-bearing locomotion and standing posture. In addition, the spinal neural networks that generate standing and locomotion can learn to produce these tasks more effectively when they are trained to perform that specific task. The sensory information provided to the spinal cord is derived in large part from a variety of mechanoreceptors located in muscles, tendons, ligaments, and skin.

Fatigue while performing a motor task can have a central as well as muscular origin. Central fatigue refers to the failure to maintain the required or expected force or power output when these deficits cannot be explained by a muscle dysfunction. The site for this fatigue can be in the brain, spinal cord, or neuromuscular junction. Exercise training can induce adaptations at any of these sites to enhance performance.

The neuromotor system is in a constant state of adaptation, similar to what is conceptually described as neural Darwinism. There is extensive modulation of synaptic efficacy throughout the nervous system as a result of varying levels of physical activity and there seems to be a "specificity" of the exercise effect. Neurotrophic growth factors most likely play a major role in the adaptive process of the nervous system to exercise.

REFERENCES

1. Lieber RL. *Skeletal Muscle Structure and Function*. Baltimore: Williams & Wilkins; 1992:303.
2. Roy RR, Edgerton VR. Skeletal muscle architecture and performance. In: Komi PV, ed. *Strength and Power in Sport: Encyclopedia of Sports Medicine*. Oxford: Blackwell Scientific Publications; 1992:115–129.
3. Bodine-Fowler S, Garfinkel A, Roy RR, et al. Spatial distribution of muscle fibers within the territory of a motor unit. *Muscle Nerve*. 1990;13:1133–1145.
4. Burke RE, Levine DN, Tsairis P, et al. Physiological types and histochemical profiles in motor units of the cat gastrocnemius. *J Physiol*. 1973;234:723–748.
5. Peter JB, Barnard RJ, Edgerton VR, et al. Metabolic profiles of three fiber types of skeletal muscle in guinea pigs and rabbits. *Biochemistry*. 1972;11:2627–2633.
6. Ounjian M, Roy RR, Eldred E, et al. Physiological and developmental implications of motor unit anatomy. *J Neurobiol*. 1991;22:547–559.
7. Bodine SC, Garfinkel A, Roy RR, et al. Spatial distribution of motor unit fibers in the cat soleus and tibialis anterior muscles: local interactions. *J Neurosci*. 1988;8:2142–2152.
8. Ishihara A, Roy RR, Edgerton VR. Succinate dehydrogenase activity and soma size of motoneurons innervating different portions of the rat tibialis anterior. *Neuroscience*. 1995;68:813–822.
9. Henneman E, Mendell LM. Functional organization of motoneuron pool and its input. In: Mountcastle JM, Brooks VB, eds. *Handbook of Physiology, Section 1, Vol. II, The Nervous System, Motor Control, Part 1*. Bethesda, MD: American Physiological Society; 1981:423–507.
10. Henneman E, Olson CB. Relations between structure and function in the design of skeletal muscles. *J Neurophysiol*. 1965;28:581–598.
11. Henneman E, Somjen G, Carpenter DO. Functional significance of cell size in spinal motoneurons. *J Neurophysiol*. 1965;28:560–580.
12. Cope TC, Clark BD. Motor-unit recruitment in the decerebrate cat: several unit properties are equally good predictors of order. *J Neurophysiol*. 1991;66:1127–1138.
13. Pinter MJ, Curtis RL, Hosko MJ. Voltage threshold and excitability among variously sized cat hindlimb motoneurons. *J Neurophysiol*. 1983;50:644–657.
14. Kukulka CG, Clamann HP. Comparison of the recruitment and discharge properties of motor units in human brachial biceps and adductor pollicis during isometric contractions. *Brain Res*. 1981;219:45–55.
15. Burke RE, Rudomin R, Zajac FE III. Catch property in single mammalian motor units. *Science*. 1970;168:122–124.
16. Burke RE, Rudomin P, Zajac FE III. The effect of activation history on tension production by individual muscle units. *Brain Res*. 1976;109:515–529.
17. Van Cutsem M, Duchateau J, Hainaut K. Changes in single motor unit behaviour contribute to the increase in contraction speed after dynamic training in humans. *J Physiol*. 1998;513 (pt 1):295–305.
18. Enoka RM, Fuglevand AJ. Motor unit physiology: some unresolved issues. *Muscle Nerve*. 2001;24:4–17.
19. Stephens JA, Garnett R, Buller NP. Reversal of recruitment order of single motor units produced by cutaneous stimulation during voluntary muscle contraction in man. *Nature*. 1978;272:362–364.
20. Desmedt JE, Godaux E. Fast motor units are not preferentially activated in rapid voluntary contractions in man. *Nature*. 1977;267:717–719.
21. Nardone A, Romano C, Schieppati M. Selective recruitment of high-threshold human motor units during voluntary isotonic lengthening of active muscles. *J Physiol*. 1989;409:451–471.
22. Smith JL, Betts B, Edgerton VR, et al. Rapid ankle extension during paw shakes: selective recruitment of fast ankle extensors. *J Neurophysiol*. 1980;43:612–620.
23. Fallentin N, Jorgensen K, Simonsen EB. Motor unit recruitment during prolonged isometric contractions. *Eur J Appl Physiol Occup Physiol*. 1993;67:335–341.
24. Tamaki H, Kitada K, Akamine T, et al. Alternate activity in the synergistic muscles during prolonged low-level contractions. *J Appl Physiol*. 1998;84:1943–1951.
25. Bawa P, Pang MY, Olesen KA, et al. Rotation of motoneurons during prolonged isometric contractions in humans. *J Neurophysiol*. 2006;96:1135–1140.
26. Bodine SC, Roy RR, Meadows DA, et al. Architectural, histochemical, and contractile characteristics of a unique biarticular muscle: the cat semitendinosus. *J Neurophysiol*. 1982;48:192–201.
27. English AW. An electromyographic analysis of compartments in cat lateral gastrocnemius muscle during unrestrained locomotion. *J Neurophysiol*. 1984;52:114–125.
28. Akima H, Ito M, Yoshikawa H, et al. Recruitment plasticity of neuromuscular compartments in exercised tibialis anterior using echo-planar magnetic resonance imaging in humans. *Neurosci Lett*. 2000;296:133–136.
29. Garfinkel S, Cafarelli E. Relative changes in maximal force, EMG, and muscle cross-sectional area after isometric training. *Med Sci Sports Exerc*. 1992;24(11):1220–1227.
30. Herbert RD, Dean D, Gandevia SC. Effects of real and imagined training on voluntary muscle activation during maximal isometric contractions. *Acta Physiol Scand*. 1998;163:361–368.
31. Huber A, Suter E, Herzog W. Inhibition of the quadriceps muscles in elite male volleyball players. *J Sports Sci*. 1998;16:281–289.
32. Knight CA, Kamen G. Adaptations in muscular activation of the knee extensor muscles with strength training in young and older adults. *J Electromyogr Kinesiol*. 2001;11(6):405–412.
33. Pensini M, Martin A, Maffiulette NA. Central versus peripheral adaptations following eccentric resistance training. *Int J Sports Med*. 2002;23(8):567–574.
34. Cope TC, Sokoloff AJ. Orderly recruitment among motoneurons supplying different muscles. *J Physiol Paris*. 1999;93:81–85.
35. Grillner S. Control of locomotion in bipeds, tetrapods, and fish. In: Brookhart JM, Mountcastle JM, eds. *Handbook of Physiology, Section 1, Vol. II, The Nervous System, Motor Control, Part 1*. Bethesda, MD: American Physiological Society; 1981:1179–1236.
36. Shik ML, Orlovsky GN. Neurophysiology of locomotor automatism. *Physiol Rev*. 1976;56:465–501.
37. Halbertsma JM. The stride cycle of the cat: the modelling of locomotion by computerized analysis of automatic recordings. *Acta Physiol Scand Suppl*. 1983;521:1–75.
38. Goslow GE Jr, Reinking RM, Stuart DG. The cat step cycle: hind limb joint angles and muscle lengths during unrestrained locomotion. *J Morphol*. 1973;141:1–41.
39. Hoyt D, Taylor R. Gait and the energetics of locomotion in horses. *Nature*. 1981;292:239–240.

40. Whiting WC, Gregor RJ, Roy RR, et al. A technique for estimating mechanical work of individual muscles in the cat during treadmill locomotion. *J Biomech.* 1984;17:685–694.

41. Gregor RJ, Roy RR, Whiting WC, et al. Mechanical output of the cat soleus during treadmill locomotion: in vivo vs in situ characteristics. *J Biomech.* 1988;21:721–732.

42. Tesch PA, Dudley GA, Duvoisin MR, et al. Force and EMG signal patterns during repeated bouts of concentric or eccentric muscle actions. *Acta Physiol Scand.* 1990;138:263–271.

43. Ryschon TW, Fowler MD, Wysong RE, et al. Efficiency of human skeletal muscle in vivo: comparison of isometric, concentric, and eccentric muscle action. *J Appl Physiol.* 1997;83:867–874.

44. Vollestad NK, Vaage O, Hermansen L. Muscle glycogen depletion patterns in type I and subgroups of type II fibres during prolonged severe exercise in man. *Acta Physiol Scand.* 1984;122:433–441.

45. Vollestad NK, Blom PC. Effect of varying exercise intensity on glycogen depletion in human muscle fibres. *Acta Physiol Scand.* 1985;125:395–405.

46. Edgerton VR, Tillakaratne N, Bigbee A, et al. Plasticity of spinal circuitry after injury. *Ann Rev Neurosci.* 2004;27:145–167.

47. Parker D, Grillner S. Neuronal mechanisms of synaptic and network plasticity in the lamprey spinal cord. *Prog Brain Res.* 2000;125:381–398.

48. Feldman JL, Mitchell GS, Nattie EE. Breathing: rhythmicity, plasticity, chemosensitivity. *Annu Rev Neurosci.* 2003;26:239–266.

49. Edgerton VR, Grillner S, Sjostrom A, et al. Central generation of locomotion in vertebrates. In: Herman RM, Grillner S, Stein PSG, Stuart DG, eds. *Neural Control of Locomotion.* New York: Plenum Publishing Corporation; 1976:439–464.

50. Lovely RG, Gregor RJ, Roy RR, et al. Effects of training on the recovery of full-weight-bearing stepping in the adult spinal cat. *Exp Neurol.* 1986;92:421–435.

51. Forssberg H. Stumbling corrective reaction: a phase-dependent compensatory reaction during locomotion. *J Neurophysiol.* 1979;42:936–953.

52. Edgerton VR, Leon RD, Harkema SJ, et al. Retraining the injured spinal cord. *J Physiol.* 2001;533:15–22.

53. Hodgson JA, Roy RR, de Leon R, et al. Can the mammalian lumbar spinal cord learn a motor task? *Med Sci Sports Exerc.* 1994;6:1491–1497.

54. Hutton RS, Atwater SW. Acute and chronic adaptations of muscle proprioceptors in response to increased use. *Sports Med.* 1992;14:406–421.

55. Prochazka A. *Proprioceptive Feedback and Movement Regulation.* New York: Oxford University Press; 1996:89–127.

56. Nelson SG, Mendell LM. Projection of single knee flexor Ia fibers to homonymous and heteronymous motoneurons. *J Neurophysiol.* 1978;41:778–787.

57. Botterman B, Binder M, Stuart D. Functional anatomy of the association between motor units and muscle receptors. *Am Zool.* 1978;18:135–152.

58. Andersson O, Forssberg H, Grillner S, et al. Phasic gain control of the transmission in cutaneous reflex pathways to motoneurones during 'fictive' locomotion. *Brain Res.* 1978;149:503–507.

59. Nichols TR. Receptor mechanisms underlying heterogenic reflexes among the triceps surae muscles of the cat. *J Neurophysiol.* 1999;81:467–478.

60. Capaday C. The special nature of human walking and its neural control. *Trends Neurosci.* 2002;25:370–376.

61. Simonsen EB, Dyhre-Poulsen P. Amplitude of the human soleus H reflex during walking and running. *J Physiol.* 1999;515 (pt 3):929–939.

62. Harkema SJ, Hurley SL, Patel UK, et al. Human lumbosacral spinal cord interprets loading during stepping. *J Neurophysiol.* 1997;77:797–811.

63. Edgerton VR, Roy RR, de Leon RD. Neural darwinism in the mammalian spinal cord. In: Grau JW, Patterson MM, eds. *Spinal Cord Plasticity: Alterations in Reflex Function.* Boston: Kluwer Academic Publishers; 2001:185–206.

64. Prochazka A, Gorassini M. Ensemble firing of muscle afferents recorded during normal locomotion in cats. *J Physiol.* 1998;507 (pt 1):293–304.

65. Edgerton VR, de Guzman CP, Gregor RJ, et al. Trainability of the spinal cord to generate hindlimb stepping patterns in adult spinalized cats. In: Shimamura M, Grillner S, Edgerton VR, eds. *Neurobiological Basis of Human Locomotion.* Tokyo: Japan Scientific Societies Press; 1991:411–423.

66. Orlovsky G, Deliagina T, Grillner S. *Neuronal Control of Locomotion: From Mollusc to Man.* Oxford: Oxford University Press; 1999.

67. Grillner S. The motor infrastructure: from ion channels to neuronal networks. *Nat Rev Neurosci.* 2003;4:573–586.

68. Vilensky JA, Moore AM, Eidelberg E, et al. Recovery of locomotion in monkeys with spinal cord lesions. *J Mot Behav.* 1992;24:288–296.

69. Shik ML, Orlovskii GN, Severin FV. Organization of locomotor synergism. *Biofizika.* 1996;11:879–886.

70. Harkema SJ. Neural plasticity after human spinal cord injury: application of locomotor training to the rehabilitation of walking. *Neuroscientist.* 2001;7:455–468.

71. Wernig A, Muller S. Laufband locomotion with body weight support improved walking in persons with severe spinal cord injuries. *Paraplegia.* 1992;30:229–238.

72. Eagleman DM. Neuroscience. The where and when of intention. *Science.* 2004;303:1144–1146.

73. Baev K. *Biological Neural Networks: The Hierarchical Concept of Brain Function.* Boston: Birkhauser; 1998.

74. Sirota MG, Shik ML. The cat locomotion elicited through the electrode implanted in the mid-brain. *Sechenov Physiological Journal of the USSR.* 1973;59:1314–1321.

75. Gerasimenko YP, Avelev VD, Nikitin OA, et al. Initiation of locomotor activity in spinal cats by epidural stimulation of the spinal cord. *Neurosci Behav Physiol.* 2003;33:247–254.

76. Dimitrijevic MR, Gerasimenko Y, Pinter MM. Evidence for a spinal central pattern generator in humans. *Ann N Y Acad Sci.* 1998;860:360–376.

77. Grillner S, Ekeberg A, El Manira A, et al. Intrinsic function of a neuronal network—a vertebrate central pattern generator. *Brain Res Brain Res Rev.* 1998;26:184–197.

78. Prochazka A, Gritsenko V, Yakovenko S. Sensory control of locomotion: reflexes versus higher-level control. *Adv Exp Med Biol.* 2002;508:357–367.

79. Timoszyk WK, De Leon RD, London N, et al. The rat lumbosacral spinal cord adapts to robotic loading applied during stance. *J Neurophysiol.* 2002;88:3108–3117.

80. de Leon RD, Reinkensmeyer DJ, Timoszyk WK, et al. Use of robotics in assessing the adaptive capacity of the rat lumbar spinal cord. In: McKerracher L, Doucet G, Rossignol S, eds. *Progress in Brain Research.* Netherlands: Elsevier Science B.V.; 2002:141–149.

81. Jindrich DL, Joseph MS, Otoshi CK, et al. Spinal learning in the adult mouse using the Horridge paradigm. *J Neurosci Meth.* 2009;182:250–254.

82. Garraway SM, Hochman S. Serotonin increases the incidence of primary afferent-evoked long-term depression in rat deep dorsal horn neurons. *J Neurophysiol.* 2001;85:1864–1872.

83. de Leon RD, Hodgson JA, Roy RR, et al. Full weight-bearing hindlimb standing following stand training in the adult spinal cat. *J Neurophysiol.* 1998;80:83–91.

84. de Leon RD, Hodgson JA, Roy RR, et al. Locomotor capacity attributable to step training versus spontaneous recovery after spinalization in adult cats. *J Neurophysiol.* 1998;79:1329–40.

85. de Leon RD, Hodgson JA, Roy RR, et al. Retention of hindlimb stepping ability in adult spinal cats after the cessation of step training. *J Neurophysiol.* 1999;81:85–94.

86. Courtine G, Gerasimenk YP, van den Brand R, et al. Transformation of nonfunctional spinal circuits into functional and adaptive states after the loss of brain input. *Nature Neurosci.* 2009;12:1333–1342.

87. Gandevia SC, Petersen N, Butler JE, et al. Impaired response of human motoneurones to corticospinal stimulation after voluntary exercise. *J Physiol.* 1999;521 (pt 3):749–759.

88. Andersen B, Westlund B, Krarup C. Failure of activation of spinal motoneurones after muscle fatigue in healthy subjects studied by transcranial magnetic stimulation. *J Physiol.* 2003;551:345–356.

89. Asmussen E, Mazin B. Recuperation after muscular fatigue by "diverting activities." *Eur J Appl Physiol Occup Physiol.* 1978;38:1–7.

90. Todd G, Taylor JL, Gandevia SC. Measurement of voluntary activation of fresh and fatigued human muscles using transcranial magnetic stimulation. *J Physiol.* 2003;551:661–671.

91. Enoka RM, Stuart DG. Neurobiology of muscle fatigue. *J Appl Physiol.* 1992;72:1631–1648.

92. Garland SJ. Role of small diameter afferents in reflex inhibition during human muscle fatigue. *J Physiol.* 1991;435:547–558.

93. Davis JM, Bailey SP. Possible mechanisms of central nervous system fatigue during exercise. *Med Sci Sports Exerc.* 1997;29:45–57.

94. Dishman RK. Brain monoamines, exercise, and behavioral stress: animal models. *Med Sci Sports Exerc.* 1997;29:63–74.

95. Gerin C, Becquet D, Privat A. Direct evidence for the link between monoaminergic descending pathways and motor activity, I: a study with microdialysis probes implanted in the ventral funiculus of the spinal cord. *Brain Res.* 1995;704:191–201.

96. Dwyer D, Browning J. Endurance training in Wistar rats decreases receptor sensitivity to a serotonin agonist. *Acta Physiol Scand.* 2000;170:211–216.

97. Weicker H, Struder HK. Influence of exercise on serotonergic neuromodulation in the brain. *Amino Acids.* 2001;20:35–47.

98. Chennaoui M, Drogou C, Gomez-Merino D, et al. Endurance training effects on 5-HT(1B) receptors mRNA expression in cerebellum, striatum, frontal cortex and hippocampus of rats. *Neurosci Lett.* 2001;307:33–36.

99. Tumer N, Demirel HA, Serova L, et al. Gene expression of catecholamine biosynthetic enzymes following exercise: modulation by age. *Neuroscience.* 2001;103:703–711.

100. De Souza CG, Michelini LC, Fior-Chadi DR. Receptor changes in the nucleus tractus solitarii of the rat after exercise training. *Med Sci Sports Exerc.* 2001;33:1471–1476.

101. Jasmin BJ, Lavoie PA, Gardiner PF. Fast axonal transport of labeled proteins in motoneurons of exercise-trained rats. *Am J Physiol.* 1988;255:C731–C736.

102. Jasmin BJ, Lavoie PA, Gardiner PF. Fast axonal transport of acetylcholinesterase in rat sciatic motoneurons is enhanced following prolonged daily running, but not following swimming. *Neurosci Lett.* 1987;78:156–160.

103. Roy RR, Baldwin KM, Edgerton VR. The plasticity of skeletal muscle: effects of neuromuscular activity. In: Holloszy J, ed. *Exercise and Sports Sciences Reviews.* Baltimore: Williams and Wilkins; 1991:269–312.

104. Martin TP, Bodine-Fowler S, Roy RR, et al. Metabolic and fiber size properties of cat tibialis anterior motor units. *Am J Physiol.* 1988;255:C43–C50.

105. Burke RE, Edgerton VR. Motor unit properties and selective involvement in movement. *Exerc Sport Sci Rev.* 1975;3:31–81.

106. Edgerton VR, Goslow GE Jr., Rasmussen SA, et al. Is resistance of a muscle to fatigue controlled by its motoneurones? *Nature.* 1980;285:589–590.

107. Cope TC, Bodine SC, Fournier M, et al. Soleus motor units in chronic spinal transected cats: physiological and morphological alterations. *J Neurophysiol.* 1986;55:1202–1220.

108. Roy RR, Zhong H, Hodgson JA, et al. Influences of electromechanical events in defining skeletal muscle properties. *Muscle Nerve.* 2002;26:238–251.

109. Winiarski AM, Roy RR, Alford EK, et al. Mechanical properties of rat skeletal muscle after hind limb suspension. *Exp Neurol.* 1987;96:650–660.

110. Shields RK. Fatigability, relaxation properties, and electromyographic responses of the human paralyzed soleus muscle. *J Neurophysiol.* 1995;73:2195–2206.

111. Alaimo MA, Smith JL, Roy RR, et al. EMG activity of slow and fast ankle extensors following spinal cord transection. *J Appl Physiol.* 184;56:1608–1613.

112. Hensbergen E, Kernell D. Daily durations of spontaneous activity in cat's ankle muscles. *Exp Brain Res.* 1997;115:325–332.

113. Roy RR, Zhong H, Monti RJ, et al. Mechanical properties of the electrically silent adult rat soleus muscle. *Muscle Nerve.* 2002;26:404–412.

114. Hodgson JA, Wichayanuparp S, Recktenwald MR, et al. Circadian force and EMG activity in hindlimb muscles of rhesus monkeys. *J Neurophysiol.* 2001;86:1430–1444.

115. Edgerton VR, McCall GE, Hodgson JA, et al. Sensorimotor adaptations to microgravity in humans. *J Exp Biol.* 2001;204:3217–3224.

116. Hodgson JA, Roy RR, Higuchi N, et al. Does daily activity level determine muscle phenotype? *J Exp Biol.* 2005;208:3761–3770.

117. Edelman GM. *Neural Darwinism: The Theory of Neuronal Group Selection.* New York: Basic Books Inc.; 1987.

118. Durkovic RG, Damianopoulos EN. Forward and backward classical conditioning of the flexion reflex in the spinal cat. *J Neurosci.* 1986;6:2921–2925.

119. Buerger AA, Fennessy A. Learning of leg position in chronic spinal rats. *Nature.* 1970;225:751–752.

120. Grau JW, Joynes RL. Pavlovian and instrumental conditioning within the spinal cord: methodological issues. In: Patterson JWE, ed. *Spinal Cord Plasticity: Alterations in Reflex Function.* Boston, MA: Kluwer Academic Publishers; 2001:13–54.

121. Nesmeyanova T. *Experimental Studies in Regeneration of Spinal Neurons.* New York: John Wiley & Sons; 1977.

122. Shurrager P, Culler E. Conditioning in the spinal dog. *J Exp Psychol.* 1940;26:133–159.

123. Barbeau H, Rossignol S. Recovery of locomotion after chronic spinalization in the adult cat. *Brain Res.* 1987;412:84–95.

124. Lovely RG, Gregor RJ, Roy RR, et al. Weight-bearing hindlimb stepping in treadmill-exercised adult spinal cats. *Brain Res.* 1990;514:206–218.

125. Wolpaw JR, Tennissen AM. Activity-dependent spinal cord plasticity in health and disease. *Annu Rev Neurosci.* 2001;24:807–843.

126. Beaumont E, Gardiner P. Effects of daily spontaneous running on the electrophysiological properties of hindlimb motoneurones in rats. *J Physiol.* 2002;540:129–138.

127. Kording KP, Wolpert DM. Bayesian integration in sensorimotor learning. *Nature.* 2004;427:244–247.

128. Scheidt RA, Dingwell JB, Mussa-Ivaldi FA. Learning to move amid uncertainty. *J Neurophysiol.* 2001;86:971–985.

129. Yue G, Cole KJ. Strength increases from the motor program: comparison of training with maximal voluntary and imagined muscle contractions. *J Neurophysiol.* 1992;67:1114–1123.

130. Hortobagyi T, Lambert NJ, Hill JP. Greater cross education following training with muscle lengthening than shortening. *Med Sci Sports Exerc.* 1997;29:107–112.

131. Hortobagyi T, Scott K, Lambert J, et al. Cross-education of muscle strength is greater with stimulated than voluntary contractions. *Motor Control.* 1999;3:205–219.

132. Zhou S. Chronic neural adaptations to unilateral exercise: mechanisms of cross education. *Exerc Sport Sci Rev.* 2000;28:177–184.

133. Lee M, Gandevia SC, Carroll TJ. Unilateral strength training increases voluntary activation of the opposite untrained limb. *Clin Neurophysiol.* 2009;120:802–808.

134. Leonard CT, Kane J, Perdaems J, et al. Neural modulation of muscle contractile properties during fatigue: afferent feedback dependence. *Electroencephalogr Clin Neurophysiol.* 1994;93(3):209–217.

135. Duchateau J, Hainaut K. Behaviour of short and long latency reflexes in fatigued human muscles. *J Physiol.* 1993;471:787–799.

136. Duchateau J, Balestra C, Carpentier A, et al. Reflex regulation during sustained and intermittent submaximal contractions in humans. *J Physiol.* 2002;541(3):959–967.

137. Aagaard P. Training-induced changes in neural function. *Exerc Sport Sci Rev.* 2003;31:61–67.

138. Casabona A, Polizzi MC, Perciavalle V. Differences in H-reflex between athletes trained for explosive contractions and non-trained subjects. *Eur J Appl Physiol Occup Physiol.* 1990;61:26–32.

139. Gandevia SC. Mind, muscles and motoneurones. *J Sci Med Sport.* 1999;2:167–180.

140. Coote JH, Hilton SM, Perez-Gonzalez JF. The reflex nature of the pressor response to muscular exercise. *J Physiol.* 1971;215:789–804.

141. McCloskey DI, Mitchell JH. Reflex cardiovascular and respiratory responses originating in exercising muscle. *J Physiol.* 1972;224:173–186.

142. Kaufman MP, Rybicki KJ. Discharge properties of group III and IV muscle afferents: their responses to mechanical and metabolic stimuli. *Circ Res.* 1987;61:I60–165.

143. Rotto DM, Kaufman MP. Effect of metabolic products of muscular contraction on discharge of group III and IV afferents. *J Appl Physiol.* 1988;64:2306–2313.

144. Martin PG, Smith JL, Butler JE, et al. Fatigue-sensitive afferents inhibit extensor but not flexor motorneurons in humans. *J Neurosci.* 2006;26(18):4796–4802.

145. Taylor JL, Gandevia SC. A comparison of central aspects of fatigue in submaximal and maximal voluntary contractions. *J Appl Physiol.* 2008;104:542–550.

146. Vissing J, Andersen M, Diemer NH. Exercise-induced changes in local cerebral glucose utilization in the rat. *J Cereb Blood Flow Metab.* 1996;16:729–736.

147. Carroll TJ, Barry B, Riek S, et al. Resistance training enhances the stability of sensorimotor coordination. *Proc R Soc Lond B Biol Sci.* 2001;268:221–227.

148. Cohen LG, Ziemann U, Chen R, et al. Studies of neuroplasticity with transcranial magnetic stimulation. *J Clin Neurophysiol.* 1998;15:305–324.

149. Nudo RJ, Milliken GW, Jenkins WM, et al. Use-dependent alterations of movement representations in primary motor cortex of adult squirrel monkeys. *J Neurosci.* 1996;16:785–807.

150. Jenkins IH, Brooks DJ, Nixon PD, et al. Motor sequence learning: a study with positron emission tomography. *J Neurosci*. 1994;14:3775–3790.

151. Dettmers C, Ridding MC, Stephan KM, et al. Comparison of regional cerebral blood flow with transcranial magnetic stimulation at different forces. *J Appl Physiol*. 1996;81:596–603.

152. van Mier H, Tempel LW, Perlmutter JS, et al. Changes in brain activity during motor learning measured with PET: effects of hand of performance and practice. *J Neurophysiol*. 1998;80:2177–2199.

153. Cramer SC, Weisskoff RM, Schaechter JD, et al. Motor cortex activation is related to force of squeezing. *Hum Brain Mapp*. 2002;16:197–205.

154. Karni A, Meyer G, Jezzard P, et al. Functional MRI evidence for adult motor cortex plasticity during motor skill learning. *Nature*. 1995;377:155–158.

155. Pascual-Leone A, Nguyet D, Cohen LG, et al. Modulation of muscle responses evoked by transcranial magnetic stimulation during the acquisition of new fine motor skills. *J Neurophysiol*. 1995;74:1037–1045.

156. Pearce AJ, Thickbroom GW, Byrnes ML, et al. Functional reorganisation of the corticomotor projection to the hand in skilled racquet players. *Exp Brain Res*. 2000;130:238–243.

157. Patten C, Kamen G. Adaptations in motor unit discharge activity with force control training in young and older human adults. *Eur J Appl Physiol*. 2000;83:128–143.

158. Suzuki S, Hayami A, Suzuki M, et al. Reductions in recruitment force thresholds in human single motor units by successive voluntary contractions. *Exp Brain Res*. 1990;82:227–230.

159. Akima H, Takahashi H, Kuno SY, et al. Early phase adaptations of muscle use and strength to isokinetic training. *Med Sci Sports Exerc*. 1999;31:588–594.

160. Sale DG. Neural adaptation to resistance training. *Med Sci Sports Exerc*. 1988;20:S135–S145.

161. Milner-Brown HS, Stein RB, Lee RG. Synchronization of human motor units: possible roles of exercise and supraspinal reflexes. *Electroencephalogr Clin Neurophysiol*. 1975;38:245–254.

162. Upton A, Radford P. Motoneuron excitability in elite sprinters. In: Komi PV, ed. *Biomechanics V-A*. Baltimore: University Park Press; 1975:82–87.

163. Schmied A, Pagni S, Sturm H, et al. Selective enhancement of motoneurone short-term synchrony during an attention-demanding task. *Exp Brain Res*. 2000;133:377–390.

164. Semmler JG, Kornatz KW, Dinenno DV, et al. Motor unit synchronisation is enhanced during slow lengthening contractions of a hand muscle. *J Physiol*. 2002;545:681–695.

165. Semmler JG, Nordstrom MA. Motor unit discharge and force tremor in skill- and strength-trained individuals. *Exp Brain Res*. 1998;119:27–38.

166. Taylor AM, Steege JW, Enoka RM. Motor-unit synchronization alters spike-triggered average force in simulated contractions. *J Neurophysiol*. 2002;88:265–276.

167. Farmer SF, Bremner FD, Halliday DM, et al. The frequency content of common synaptic inputs to motoneurones studied during voluntary isometric contraction in man. *J Physiol*. 1993;470:127–155.

168. Ichiyama RM, Courtine G, Gerasimenko YP, et al. Step training reinforces specific spinal locomotor circuitry in adult spinal rats. *J Neurosci*. 2008;28:7370–7375.

169. Gomez-Pinilla F, Ying Z, Opazo P, et al. Differential regulation by exercise of BDNF and NT-3 in rat spinal cord and skeletal muscle. *Eur J Neurosci*. 2001;13:1078–1084.

170. Neeper SA, Gomez-Pinilla F, Choi J, et al. Exercise and brain neurotrophins. *Nature*. 1995;373:109.

171. van Praag H, Kempermann G, Gage FH. Running increases cell proliferation and neurogenesis in the adult mouse dentate gyrus. *Nat Neurosci*. 1999;2:266–270.

172. Kitamura T, Mishina M, Sugiyama H. Enhancement of neurogenesis by running wheel exercises is suppressed in mice lacking NMDA receptor epsilon 1 subunit. *Neurosci Res*. 2003;47:55–63.

173. Cotman CW, Berchtold NC. Exercise: a behavioral intervention to enhance brain health and plasticity. *Trends Neurosci*. 2002;25:295–301.

174. Lee TH, Jang MH, Shin MC, et al. Dependence of rat hippocampal c-Fos expression on intensity and duration of exercise. *Life Sci*. 2003;72:1421–1436.

175. Ivy AS, Rodriguez FG, Garcia C, et al. Noradrenergic and serotonergic blockade inhibits BDNF mRNA activation following exercise and antidepressant. *Pharmacol Biochem Behav*. 2003;75:81–88.

176. Anderson BJ, Alcantara AA, Greenough WT. Motor-skill learning: changes in synaptic organization of the rat cerebellar cortex. *Neurobiol Learn Mem*. 1996;66:221–229.

177. Swain RA, Harris AB, Wiener EC, et al. Prolonged exercise induces angiogenesis and increases cerebral blood volume in primary motor cortex of the rat. *Neuroscience*. 2003;117:1037–1046.

178. Ploughman M. Exercise is brain food: the effects of physical activity on cognitive function. *Dev Neurorehabil*. 2008;11:236–240.

179. Gomez-Pinilla F, Vaynman S, Ying Z. Brain-derived neurotrophic factor functions as a metabotrophin to mediate the effects of exercise on cognition. *Eur J Neurosci*. 2008;28:2278–2287.

180. Zoladz JA, Pilc A, Majerczak J, et al. Endurance training increases plasma brain-derived neurotrophic factor concentration in young healthy men. *J Physiol Pharmacol*. 2008;59 (suppl 7):119–132.

181. Griesbach GS, Hovda DA, Gomez-Pinilla F. Exercise-induced improvement in cognitive performance after traumatic brain injury in rats is dependent on BDNF activation. *Brain Res*. 2009;1288:105–115.

182. aan het Rot M, Collins KA, Fitterling HL. Physical exercise and depression. *Mt Sinai J Med*. 2009;76:204–214.

183. Ying Z, Roy RR, Zhong H, et al. BDNF-exercise interactions in the recovery of symmetrical stepping after a cervical hemisection in rats. *Neuroscience*. 2008;155:1070–1078.

184. Gomez-Pinilla F, Dao L, So V. Physical exercise induces FGF-2 and its mRNA in the hippocampus. *Brain Res*. 1997;764:1–8.

185. Black JE, Isaacs KR, Anderson BJ, et al. Learning causes synaptogenesis, whereas motor activity causes angiogenesis, in cerebellar cortex of adult rats. *Proc Natl Acad Sci U S A*. 1990;87:5568–5572.

186. Sherrington C. *The Integrative Action of the Nervous System*. New Haven: Yale University Press; 1906.

187. Edgerton VR, Bodine-Fowler S, Roy RR, et al. Neuromuscular adaptation. In: Shepherd JT, Rowell LB, eds. *Handbook of Physiology. Section 12. Exercise: Regulation and Integration of Multiple Systems*. New York: Oxford University Press; 1996:54–88.

188. Roy R, Edgerton VR, Ishihara A. Influence of endurance training and detraining on motoneurone and sensory neurone morphology and metabolism. In: Astrand RJS, editor. *Endurance in Sport, Encyclopaedia of Sports Medicine*. Oxford: Blackwell Scientific Publishers; 2000:136–157.

189. Roy RR, Matsumoto A, Zhong H, et al. Rat α- and γ-motoneuron soma size and succinate dehydrogenase activity are independent of neuromuscular activity level. *Muscle Nerve*. 2007;36:234–241.

190. Nakano H, Masuda K, Sasaki S, et al. Oxidative enzyme activity and soma size in motoneurons innervating the rat slow-twitch and fast-twitch muscles after chronic activity. *Brain Res Bull*. 1997;43:149–154.

191. Chalmers GR, Roy RR, Edgerton VR. Motoneuron and muscle fiber succinate dehydrogenase activity in control and overloaded plantaris. *J Appl Physiol*. 1991;71:1589–1592.

192. Gerchman LB, Edgerton VR, Carrow RE. Effects of physical training on the histochemistry and morphology of ventral motor neurons. *Exp Neurol*. 1975;49:790–801.

193. Seburn K, Coicou C, Gardiner P. Effects of altered muscle activation on oxidative enzyme activity in rat alpha-motoneurons. *J Appl Physiol*. 1994;77:2269–2274.

194. Munson JB, Foehring RC, Mendell LM, et al. Fast-to-slow conversion following chronic low-frequency activation of medial gastrocnemius muscle in cats. II. Motoneuron properties. *J Neurophysiol*. 1997;77:2605–2615.

195. Roy RR, Talmadge RJ, Hodgson JA, et al. Training effects on soleus of cats spinal cord transected (T12–T13) as adults. *Muscle Nerve*. 1998;21:63–71.

196. Petruska JC, Ichiyama RM, Jindrich DL, et al. Changes in motoneuron properties and synaptic inputs related to step training after spinal cord transection in rats. *J Neurosci*. 2007;27:4460–4471.

197. Button DC, Kalmar JM, Gardiner K, et al. Does elimination of afferent input modify the changes in rat motoneurone properties that occur following chronic spinal cord transection? *J Physiol*. 2008;586:529–544.

198. Roy RR, Zhong H, Siengthai B, et al. Activity-dependent influences are greater for fibers in rat medial gastrocnemius than tibialis anterior muscle. *Muscle Nerv*. 2005;32:473–482.

199. Gharakhanlou R, Chadan S, Gardiner P. Increased activity in the form of endurance training increases calcitonin gene-related peptide content in lumbar motoneuron cell bodies and in sciatic nerve in the rat. *Neuroscience*. 1999;89:1229–1239.

200. Gonzalez M, Collins WF 3rd. Modulation of motoneuron excitability by brain-derived neurotrophic factor. *J Neurophysiol*. 1997;77:502–506.

201. Deschenes MR, Judelson DA, Kraemer WJ, et al. Effects of resistance training on neuromuscular junction morphology. *Muscle Nerve*. 2000;23:1576–1581.

202. Andonian MH, Fahim MA. Endurance exercise alters the morphology of fast- and slow-twitch rat neuromuscular junctions. *Int J Sports Med*. 1988;9:218–223.

203. Deschenes MR, Maresh CM, Crivello JF, et al. The effects of exercise training of different intensities on neuromuscular junction morphology. *J Neurocytol*. 1993;22:603–615.

204. Waerhaug O, Dahl HA, Kardel K. Different effects of physical training on the morphology of motor nerve terminals in the rat extensor digitorum longus and soleus muscles. *Anat Embryol (Berl)*. 1992;186:125–128.

205. Crockett JL, Edgerton VR, Max SR, et al. The neuromuscular junction in response to endurance training. *Exp Neurol*. 1976;51:207–215.

206. Rosenheimer JL. Effects of chronic stress and exercise on age-related changes in end-plate architecture. *J Neurophysiol*. 1985;53:1582–1589.

207. Stebbins CL, Schultz E, Smith RT, et al. Effects of chronic exercise during aging on muscle and end-plate morphology in rats. *J Appl Physiol*. 1985;58:45–51.

208. Sveistrup H, Chan RY, Jasmin BJ. Chronic enhancement of neuromuscular activity increases acetylcholinesterase gene expression in skeletal muscle. *Am J Physiol*. 1995;269:C856–C862.

209. Burns AS, Jawaid S, Zhong H, et al. Paralysis elicited by spinal cord injury evokes selective disassembly of neuromuscular synapses with and without terminal sprouting in ankle flexors of the adult rat. *J Comp Neurol*. 2007;500:116–133.

210. Homonko DA, Theriault E. Calcitonin gene-related peptide is increased in hindlimb motoneurons after exercise. *Int J Sports Med*. 1997;18:503–509.

211. Sala C, Andreose JS, Fumagalli G, et al. Calcitonin gene-related peptide: possible role in formation and maintenance of neuromuscular junctions. *J Neurosci*. 1995;15:520–528.

212. Wernig A, Salvini TF, Irintchev A. Axonal sprouting and changes in fibre types after running-induced muscle damage. *J Neurocytol*. 1991;20:903–913.

213. Wuerker RB, Henneman E. Reflex regulation of primary (annulospiral) stretch receptors via gamma motoneurons in the cat. *J Neurophysiol*. 1963;26:539–550.

214. Buller AJ, Eccles JC, Eccles RM. Differentiation of fast and slow muscles in the cat hind limb. *J Physiol*. 1960;150:399–416.

215. Buller AJ, Eccles JC, Eccles RM. Interactions between motoneurones and muscles in respect of the characteristic speeds of their responses. *J Physiol*. 1960;150:417–439.

216. Kugelberg E, Edstrom L. Differential histochemical effects of muscle contractions on phosphorylase and glycogen in various types of fibres: relation to fatigue. *J Neurol Neurosurg Psychiatry*. 1968;31:415–423.

217. Edgerton VR, Simpson D, Barnard RJ, et al. Phosphorylase activity in acutely exercised muscle. *Nature*. 1970;225:866–867.

218. Burke RE, Levine DN, Zajac FE III. Mammalian motor units: physiological-histochemical correlation in three types in cat gastrocnemius. *Science*. 1971;174:709–712.

CHAPTER 3

The Skeletal-Articular System

Ronald F. Zernicke, Gregory R. Wohl,
and Jeremy M. LaMothe

Abbreviations

BMC	Bone mineral content		y	Perpendicular distance from the wall
BMD	Bone mineral density		$(du/dy)_w$	Velocity gradient of blood flow at the wall
DXA	Dual energy x-ray absorptiometry			
ER-α	Estrogen receptor alpha		V_{SGP}	Streaming potential
HRT	Hormone replacement therapy		ζ	Zeta potential
QCT	Quantitative computed tomography		ϵ	Dielectric permittivity of the bulk fluid
τ_w	Fluid-imposed wall shear stress		σ	Conductivity of the bulk fluid
μ	Blood viscosity coefficient		η	Viscosity of the bulk fluid
u	Velocity component of the fluid flow parallel to the longitudinal direction of the wall		P_{eff}	Effective driving pressure due to mechanical deformation

Introduction

The skeletal-articular system comprises connective tissues that serve primarily mechanical roles in locomotion and in protection of vital organs. Bones provide support for movement as levers and pivots for muscle-driven motion and ligaments, tendons, and menisci at the joints blend muscular forces into controlled skeletal motions. Normally, these musculoskeletal tissues function at loads well below their mechanical limits, while possessing safety factors seven- to 10-fold greater than normal physiologic use to minimize the likelihood of failure and sustain normal function. Although generally perceived as inert tissues, skeletal-articular tissues are patently dynamic and adapt to changes in their physiologic environment such as exercise.

The turnover (replacement of old tissue with new tissue) of musculoskeletal tissues can be influenced by dynamic and resistance exercises. In particular, exercise can substantially influence bone morphology. Although

the precise nature of the exercise stimuli that orchestrates adaptive responses remains elusive, it is generally accepted that tissue strain (change in dimension of a loaded tissue normalized to the original dimension of the tissue) influences tissue adaptation. Specifically, strain magnitude, frequency, rate, and gradients all influence adaptive responses. Potentially, cells in skeletal-articular connective tissues sense stimuli arising from exercise via cell deformations, or indirectly via exercise-induced interstitial fluid flow, and orchestrate adaptive responses. Of the skeletal-articular tissues, bone is by far the most studied. Bone loss (*e.g.*, osteoporosis) in aging individuals has significant implications for quality of life and mobility in individuals and for cost of health care to society. A substantial amount of skeletal-articular research focuses on the effects of exercise on bone adaptation. Physical activity can dramatically enhance bone mass. Consequently, the effects of exercise on bone mass have significant clinical implications, and understanding the precise nature of the stimuli influencing bone may allow identification of exercise regimens that more effectively counter age-related bone loss.

In this chapter, we describe the basic structure and biochemistry of bone, ligament, tendon, and meniscus, and the response of these connective tissues to exercise stimuli. To examine the effects of exercise on the skeletal-articular tissues, we present the effects of mechanical stimuli on connective tissue adaptation and mechanisms by which connective tissues adapt to their mechanical environment. Included in the exposition are explanations of how components of loading (*e.g.*, strain magnitude, rate, frequency, and gradient) influence skeletal-articular tissue adaptation and, further, how the cells interpret their mechanical milieu through different means of mechanical transduction. Understanding how physical forces interact with skeletal-articular tissues may lead to a clearer view of how skeletal-articular structure and function can be optimized for normal function and for prevention of tissue damage and may help to develop effective nonpharmacologic treatments to combat skeletal-articular pathologies characterized by low bone mass.

Skeletal-Articular Physiology

The biochemical composition of the skeletal-articular tissues complements their mechanical roles in the body.

Ligaments and tendons are collagenous bands central to guiding and producing controlled movements, respectively. Ligaments tether bones across a joint (Fig. 3.1) and—in tandem with articular geometry—control the relative motion of the joint. Tendons connect muscles to bones and transmit muscular forces to the bones. Menisci are fibrocartilage structures that help maintain joint components in appropriate position, reduce joint stress by bearing load, and enhance rotation in synovial joints. In the knee, for example, menisci are avascular crescent- and triangular-shaped structures firmly attached to the tibia with ligaments (Fig. 3.2).

Compared to other organ systems, skeletal-articular tissues have low cellularity, and extracellular matrix constitutes the majority of tissue volume. The extracellular matrix of the soft connective tissues is 70% to 75% water, and collagen comprises 60% to 70% of the dry mass. In ligaments and tendons, the quintessential collagen molecule is tropocollagen. Five parallel tropocollagen molecules tightly stagger together to form microfibrils (Fig. 3.3). Sequentially, microfibrils, collate to form subfibrils, which aggregate to form fibrils and, finally, fibers; fibers aggregate to form fiber bundles (1). Fiber bundles are collated into fascicles. A tendon (ligament) is a collection of fascicles grouped by a sheath termed the paratenon (or epiligament). Water plays a significant role in the mechanical behavior of ligaments and ten-

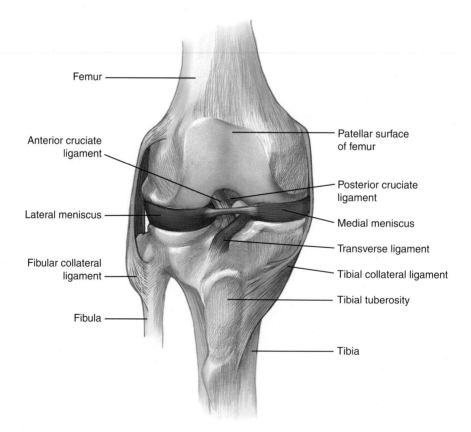

FIGURE 3.1   Frontal section of the knee including ligaments, bones, and menisci. (Asset provided by Anatomical Chart Co.)

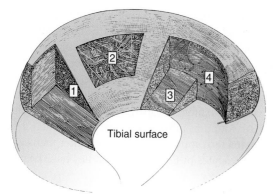

FIGURE 3.2 Reconstruction of the fiber pattern of the meniscus. At the tibial surface (*1*), collagen fibers are predominantly in the radial direction. Tangential to the femoral meniscal surface, fibers are predominantly woven together (*2*). Fibers are prominently organized circumferentially through the center of the meniscus (*3*). Through the thickness of the meniscus, parallel to its edge, fibers are predominantly radial (*4*). Collagen bundles from the radial fibers curl up into the body of the meniscus. (Adapted from Bullough PG, Munuera L, Murphy J, et al. The strength of the menisci of the knee as it relates to their fine structure. *J Bone Joint Surg Br.* 1970;52:564–567.)

dons. Noncollagenous proteins called proteoglycans bind the water in the matrix, creating a gel-like matrix about the tightly packed collagen fibers. The proteoglycans and collagenous network resist fluid flow during loading, contributing to the viscoelastic mechanical behavior of the tissues.

Similar to ligaments and tendons, the meniscal extracellular matrix is 70% to 75% water. In menisci, there are two distinct zones, the outer, superficial layer, and the deep, inner zone (2). Type I collagen predominates in menisci. In the deep zone, collagen fibers are aligned circumferentially to resist stresses engendered during compressive loading in the knee, whereas the collagen fibers in the superficial layer are more randomly organized (Fig. 3.2). Proteoglycans also bind water in the meniscus, but the avascular inner two-thirds produce more proteoglycans than the vascularized outer third.

In addition to mechanical support, bones are center for hematopoiesis and are the body's largest calcium reservoir, which can be mobilized via bone resorption when serum calcium drops. Bone has unique tissue properties that are dependent on the interactions among an organic

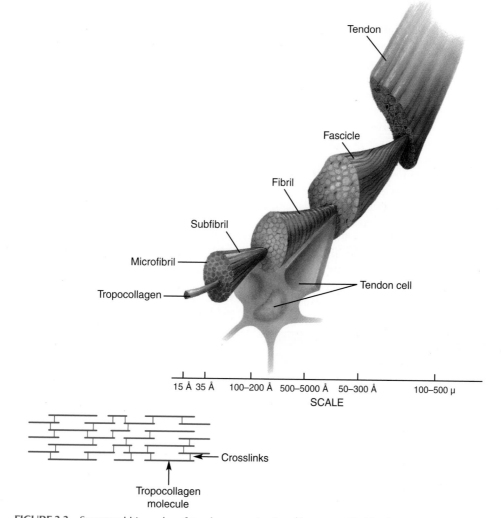

FIGURE 3.3 Structural hierarchy of tendon organization. (Asset provided by Anatomical Chart Co.)

phase (~25% by mass), inorganic phase (~70%), and water (~5%). As with ligaments and tendons, the organic phase comprises mostly type I collagen (the mechanical function of which is to resist tensile forces) and numerous noncollagenous proteins (*e.g.*, glycosaminoglycans) (3). Also, like the other connective tissues, bone cells constitute a minor portion of the organic component. Bone is unique in that the compressive forces are principally supported by the inorganic mineral component of bone. Plate-like calcium hydroxyapatite crystals, $Ca_{10}(PO_4)_6OH_2$, precipitate in the unmineralized organic matrix (osteoid) within and between the collagen fibrils. Collagen fibril organization and size, as well as the presence of some noncollagenous proteins, can regulate the size and timing of crystal growth. Water is present in spaces between hydroxyapatite crystals.

TEST YOURSELF

What effect would an abnormally low amount of collagen have on bone mechanical properties?

There are many levels of bone porosity. On a gross structural level, bone can be highly porous with large pores between bone fragments (called trabeculae) visible to the naked eye or relatively compact with small pores not visible to the naked eye. Highly porous bone is called trabecular (or cancellous) bone and exists in flat bones (*e.g.*, skull), in cuboidal bones (*e.g.*, vertebrae), occasionally under ligament insertions, and at the end of long bones (Fig. 3.1). Bone marrow pervades the spaces between trabeculae, and trabecular bone is sheathed by a layer of more compact bone. The more compact bone is called cortical (or compact) bone. Cortical bone has small pores associated with vascular structures and nerves (*e.g.*, Haversian canals; ~40 μm radius), osteocyte lacunae (~10 μm radius), and canaliculi (~200 nm radius), housing the osteocytes and their processes, respectively, and pores associated with gaps in the mineral structure (~10 nm radius). As with the soft connective tissues, on a gross structural level, bone fluid saturates all levels of porosity, which adds to bone's viscoelastic behavior and likely is important in adaptation to exercise.

TEST YOURSELF

What is the significance of tubular, hollow long bones when a solid bone would have a greater mechanical strength?

Skeletal-Articular Tissue Turnover

Cell populations in connective tissues maintain a fine balance of extracellular matrix components, turning over damaged matrix, and repairing or building new matrix in response to injuries or mechanical stimuli. In ligaments and tendons, *fibroblasts* are the primary cell population, aligned in a columnar arrangement along the long axis of the tissue. In menisci, there are morphologically two distinct cell populations. Cells in the superficial layer are ovoid- or fusiform-shaped, whereas cells in the deeper zones are round or polygonal. Regardless of their morphologic characterization, it is unclear whether meniscal cells are chondrocytes or fibroblasts, and they have been called *fibrochondrocytes*.

The soft, fibrous connective tissues are relatively avascular. Ligament and tendon vascular elements are limited mainly to the outer surface. Similarly, vascularity in mature menisci is limited to the outer third of the crescent. The low cellularity and vascularity have mechanical and biologic implications. Biologically, a low vascularity restricts the metabolic capacity of the fibroblasts and fibrochondrocytes during matrix turnover, and the adaptive response of these soft connective tissues to stimuli is less vigorous than in bone. Furthermore, ligaments, tendons, and menisci respond poorly to injury—the repaired tissue rarely achieves normal structure or function and commonly degenerates. Mechanically, cells and blood vessels constitute holes that weaken the tissue structure. Minimizing these "structural defects" improves mechanical efficiency for tissue size. Thus, fibrous connective tissues are optimized for mechanical function, and tissue turnover during normal activity is generally sufficient to maintain healthy tissues over a lifetime.

In contrast to the fibrous soft tissues, bone is the most dynamic of the skeletal-articular tissues and can completely turnover in as little as 3 years, depending on location in the body. Bone is formed and maintained by cells of two different origins (3). *Osteoblasts*, mononuclear cells of stromal origin, secrete unmineralized matrix as the first phase of bone formation. Occasionally, osteoblasts become quiescent on the bone surface after matrix secretion and are called *bone lining cells*, or they become encased in matrix and differentiate into *osteocytes*. Osteocytes maintain connections with adjacent osteocytes throughout the bone matrix, as well as bone lining cells, via cellular processes in the interconnecting canaliculi. Giant multinuclear cells of hematogenic origin, called *osteoclasts*, degrade and remove bone by first adhering to a bone surface. To dissolve the inorganic and organic components of bone, mineral, protons and proteolytic enzymes are secreted across the osteoclast cell membrane adjacent to sites of adhesion to the bone matrix.

Turnover of the bone tissue occurs through two main processes—*modeling* and *remodeling* (Fig. 3.4). In the process of modeling, osteoblasts and osteoclasts can work independently of each other on both the periosteal surface (*i.e.*, outer surface of bone, apposed

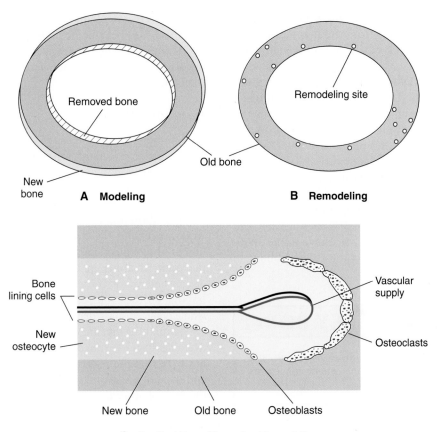

A Modeling

Removed bone

New bone

Old bone

B Remodeling

Remodeling site

Bone lining cells

New osteocyte

Vascular supply

Osteoclasts

New bone

Old bone

Osteoblasts

C Cortical Bone Haversian Remodeling

FIGURE 3.4 Diagrammatic representation of modeling and remodeling in a bone diaphyseal cross-section (original bone shown as dark blue). **A.** During modeling, bone is removed from one surface (*e.g.*, the endosteum—*hatch mark*) and, by a separately regulated process, formed on another surface (*e.g.*, the periosteum—*light blue*). Modeling can change the size or shape of the bone. **B.** During remodeling, osteoclasts remove existing bone (*white circles* within cortex) and the resorption is normally coupled immediately with subsequent bone formation. **C.** In cortical bone remodeling, the osteoclasts tunnel through the cortex forming Haversian canals. A vascular supply is closely associated with the remodeling as the process requires a significant amount of energy, nutrients, and waste removal. The osteoblasts follow, creating and depositing new osteoid matrix, and many of the osteoblasts become embedded in the matrix as osteocytes, or remain on the surface as bone lining cells. In the remodeling of trabecular bone, osteoclasts create pits (Howships lacunae) on the surface of the trabeculae. As with cortical remodeling, that is typically coupled with subsequent bone formation.

to the periosteum) and the endocortical surface (*i.e.*, inner surface of bone, bordering the marrow cavity). Modeling can occur on trabecular surfaces as well. This process involves cellular activation and bone formation and/or resorption, is more common during growth, and changes the size and shape of bones. Remodeling is a more locally coupled process of activation-resorption formation in which osteoclasts are activated and resorb bone in focal regions (~200 μm in diameter), followed immediately by the activation of osteoblasts to fill in the cavity with newly synthesized organic matrix that later mineralizes.

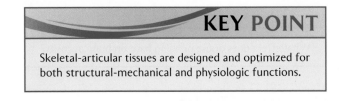

KEY POINT

Skeletal-articular tissues are designed and optimized for both structural-mechanical and physiologic functions.

Factors in Tissue Adaptation

The structure of musculoskeletal tissues is determined by an intricate blend of genetic constraints and epigenetic conditions. Genetics can influence up to 80% of peak bone mineral density (BMD) and the remaining influences are a summation of environmental conditions. In humans, bone strength is typically approximated using bone mass, density, size, and geometry. Dual energy x-ray absorptiometry (DXA) and quantitative computed tomography (QCT) are used to measure bone mineral content (BMC), apparent areal (DXA) and volumetric (QCT) bone density, as well as cross-sectional area of bone (QCT). DXA or QCT (indirect measures), however, do not give the full picture of the quality and quantity of bone, as the microarchitecture of cancellous and cortical bone also influences bone strength. DXA is further limited in that bone cross-sectional area and shape influence bone strength. Systemic factors, such as diet and hormones, can interact with local factors (*e.g.*, mechanical loading) and collectively affect the ability of bone to adapt to exercise.

> ### KEY POINT
>
> Epigenetic factors (*e.g.*, exercise, disuse, nutrition, and hormones) are superimposed on the genetic constraints influencing skeletal-articular tissues.

Tissue Response to Mechanical Stimuli

Genetics play a significant role in the shape and size of the musculoskeletal tissues, but the structure of connective tissues is also determined, in part, by the mechanical environment. Chronic exercise can lead to bone hypertrophy. Conversely, chronic immobilization may lead to bone atrophy, which can manifest as shape alterations (such as a loss of long bone curvature) and decreased density. The sensitivity of the skeleton to these mechanical stimuli is a function of particular characteristics of the mechanical stimuli itself and can also be influenced by a host of variables including genetic, dietary, hormonal, and ontogenetically related considerations.

> ### TEST YOURSELF
>
> What effect does disuse or aging have on bone porosity?

Ligament and Tendon

Although studies describing the mechanical and biochemical properties of ligaments and tendons are extensive, there are a paucity of details on how these collagenous structures respond to exercise and immobilization. These deficiencies can partly be explained by reports—as recent as a few decades ago—suggesting that ligaments and tendons were essentially inert and unresponsive to exercise (4). It has become obvious, however, that ligaments and tendons can be responsive to exercise, although the majority of adaptation data pertain to ligament, rather than tendon.

Catabolic stimuli

Joint immobilization can cause significant changes in ligament, which can lead to substantial decrements in ligament stiffness and strength (5,6). Histologically and biochemically, immobilization can induce notable changes (7–10). Immobilization decreases the number of small diameter collagen fibrils and the mean collagen fibril density, meanwhile increasing the number of large diameter collagen fibrils. Immobilization disrupts the parallel orientation of the collagen fibrils in ligament, decreases glycosaminoglycan and water content, and increases collagen cross-linking. Furthermore, collagen turnover increases and the whole collagen mass decreases.

Similar to ligament, immobilization increases the overall collagen turnover in tendon (11). Reports indicate, however, that the relative quantity of tendon components and overall tendon mass do not change (11–13). Despite the lack of substantial biochemical change, immobilization can significantly decrease tendon stiffness, failure load, and ultimate strength (12,13). The loss of tendon and bone mechanical integrity during immobilization demonstrates the dramatic interplay between the tissues in response to altered loading. After 4 weeks of immobilization, Achilles tendon failure typically occurs at the point of insertion into bone, whereas at 8 weeks, failure typically occurs by means of calcaneal fracture (13). If the Achilles tendon is severed (simulated injury), the glycosaminoglycan content, fibroblast number, and number of small collagen fibers increase, but these changes are minimal if the tendon is sutured (14). Thus, tensile load appears to be necessary to maintain tendon biochemical and biomechanical properties.

Anabolic stimuli

Normal daily activity (without training) is sufficient to maintain 80% to 90% of a ligament's mechanical potential and, thus, exercise or training can enhance the mechanical potential by 10% to 20% (5). Following chronic exercise, significant increases occurred in the strength and stiffness of the anterior cruciate ligament in exercised rats; those increases were greater when endurance exercises were conducted more frequently and for a shorter duration (15). Biochemically, exercise can increase collagen concentration, glycosaminoglycan content, collagen turnover, and collagen nonreducible cross-links (16). Furthermore, ligaments in exercised rats have more small diameter collagen fibers than in rats that have not been exercised (17). Together, these biochemical alterations may account for the observed increase in stiffness and load-bearing capabilities of exercised ligaments. Although the effects of training on ligaments can be moderate, injured ligaments that have been exercised consistently have improved biochemical and mechanical properties relative to injured, unexercised ligaments.

TEST YOURSELF

Does every ligament have the capacity for repair?

Similar to ligament, tendon can exhibit adaptive responses to exercise. Exercise can increase the number of active fibroblasts (18) and collagen synthesis in growing tendon (19). Mice exercised on a treadmill for 1 week showed increases in the number and size of the collagen fibrils as well as the total cross-sectional area of the digital flexor tendons (20). Following 7 weeks of exercise training, the average collagen fibril diameter was smaller than sedentary controls, and that reduction appeared to be caused by a splitting of the collagen fibrils. By 10 weeks of training, the flexor tendons' cross-sectional areas were similar to control values. In another long-term exercise experiment, immature swine were exercised at a moderate level for 1 year, after which there were no significant differences in tendon biomechanical properties or cross-sectional areas between exercisers and controls (21). Other models reported enhanced biomechanical properties following chronic exercise training. A long-term exercise regimen resulted in increased tendon stiffness in guinea fowl (22). Chronic exposure to repetitive loading can produce tendon hypertrophy. Runners who trained ≥ 80 km $\cdot$ wk^{-1} had significantly larger Achilles tendon cross-sectional area relative to age-matched nonrunners (23). Conversely, in a randomized control trial, an exercise intervention ($\sim$9 months of running) did not alter the mechanical properties of the triceps-surae aponeurosis complex or the cross-sectional area of the Achilles tendon (24). Thus, although some reports suggest that exercise does not influence tendon geometrical or mechanical properties, other reports indicate that tendon, like other musculoskeletal tissues, adapts its geometrical or mechanical properties to physical stimuli.

Meniscus

Meniscal adaptation to exercise is poorly understood. Until the 1970s, menisci were thought to have no functional role in the knee, and meniscectomy was advocated for meniscal injury. Damage or removal of the menisci can lead to joint degradation. Partial meniscectomy is the gold standard treatment for meniscal bucket-handle tears, but can lead to articular cartilage degradation and subsequent osteoarthritis (25). Despite the importance of menisci in proper joint function, there is a relative paucity of data regarding their adaptive responses to disuse and training. An interest in tissue engineering for surgical replacement of damaged menisci has spurred increased research in the mechanotransductive mechanisms of meniscal fibrochondrocytes.

Catabolic stimuli

As with ligament and tendon, immobilization can be a catabolic stimulus for the meniscus. In comparison to periarticular bone, which experienced significant atrophy after 8 weeks of immobilization, menisci in the canine hind limb showed no outward sign of atrophy (26). Biochemically, however, significant changes were reported. Aggrecan is one of the major proteoglycans of the meniscus and is largely responsible for its viscoelastic compressive properties. Aggrecan gene expression decreased and water content increased when beagles were immobilized for 4 weeks (27,28). Data suggest that the amount of nutrient delivery to the tissue is strongly related to the degree of tissue surface exposed to synovial fluid (29), and cyclic loading during exercise may improve nutrient delivery to the tissue. Thus, immobilization may impair cell function via starvation. Ochi and colleagues (30) examined the penetration of a tracer with immobilization and remobilization. Horseradish peroxidase was injected into the knee joints of rabbits, and legs were immobilized with a cast. In nonimmobilized knee joints, the tracer pervaded the entire meniscus. After 8 weeks of immobilization, however, the tracer was restricted to the superficial layer, and degenerative changes were seen in the deep layer of the meniscus as early as 6 weeks. Meniscal permeability was recovered with remobilization, but the degenerative changes remained, even after 4 weeks of remobilization. Mechanical stimulus is also essential during developmental stages for normal meniscal formation; in absence of mechanical loading by skeletal muscle, menisci formed in the early embryonic stages do not mature and degrade in later embryonic stages (28,31). Immobilization can also impair the normal healing process. With meniscal injury, blood flow to the meniscus significantly increases, and immobilization during recovery prevents blood flow enhancement (32). Static loading is also catabolic to the meniscus. Although exogenous growth factors induce proteoglycan and protein synthesis, the addition of static compressive loading on meniscal explants inhibits the anabolic effects (33), and can reduce expression of matrix molecules decorin, and type I and II collagen while increasing expression of matrix metalloproteinase-1 (collagenase) (34).

Anabolic stimuli

The effects of exercise on meniscal biomechanics and biochemistry are not as well documented as the effects of exercise on other skeletal articular tissues. Anabolic and catabolic changes have been reported for exercise, with the nature of the change likely related to exercise intensity. Strenuous exercise can delay the formation of collagen pyridinoline cross-links in menisci in skeletally immature chickens and cause premature decrements in dermatan sulphate proteoglycans (35). In one of the more prominent studies detailing the adaptive response of menisci to exercise (36), rats were trained to run on a motor-driven treadmill 5 days a week for 12 weeks. The potential for the exercise to elicit an adaptive response was apparent as there was a 65% increase in gastrocnemius succinate dehydrogenase.

In response, the posterior lateral horn of the meniscus, which likely received principally compressive stress during locomotion, had significantly greater concentrations of collagen, proteoglycans, and calcium. Increases in collagen and proteoglycan would augment the meniscus' ability to bear mechanical loading (37). Although collagen fiber orientation was not measured, it is also likely relevant to a meniscus' capacity for load-bearing. Longitudinal collagen fibers ensure tension resistance in the meniscus while transverse fiber bundles unite the longitudinal fibers and thus retain the shape of the meniscus (38).

Mechanical loading of meniscal explants and cultured fibrochondrocytes has shed some light on the cellular signals triggered by mechanical loading. Dynamic compression of porcine meniscal explants induced increases in protein and proteoglycan synthesis, as well as nitric oxide (NO), a cytokine involved in matrix metabolism and inflammation in intraarticular tissues (28). Similarly, dynamic cyclic compression of cultured human meniscal fibrochondrocytes induces an increase in the expression of type I collagen and tissue inhibitors of matrix metalloproteinases (1 and 2) (39). Similar to bone, mechanotransductive signalling in meniscal cells is associated with fluid flow-induced shear stresses. Oscillatory fluid flow caused an increase in intracellular calcium levels and induced increases in sulphated glycosaminoglycan production in cultured rabbit meniscal cells (40). Mechanical loading with exercise causes a redistribution of fluid in the tissue (41,42). The location of the fibrochondrocyte within the meniscus likely affects its response to mechanical loading (43). Cells from the inner meniscus exhibit a more chondrocytic phenotype (increased expression of type II collagen and aggrecan and less type I collagen) than those from the outer meniscus.

TEST YOURSELF

Why do meniscal fibrochondrocytes have a differential response to static versus dynamic loading?

Bone

The salutary effects of exercise on bone are well known, but more dramatic examples of bone mechanosensitivity are exemplified when mechanical stimuli are removed. The Space Studies Board of the American National Research Council has stated that, along with radiation exposure, the most significant obstacle to prolonged space missions remains the osteopenia associated with microgravity (44). In space flight, bone loss has been reported to approach 1.6% per month in regions such as spine and femoral neck and long bone metaphyses (45). The implications of significant increases in fracture risk during long missions in space are apparent, especially upon reexposure to Earth's gravitational field. As with microgravity, prolonged bed rest or immobilization can dramatically impair bone formation rates and increase resorption with a net loss in BMD. A more extensive account of the potent effects of microgravity is provided by Schneider and Convertino (Chapter 26).

Positive effects of exercise

Bone formation in response to dynamic and resistance exercises can lead to an increase in bone cross-sectional area. Thus, the forces generated from exercises will be applied over a greater area of bone, and that will lead to a reduction in bone mechanical stresses (stress is force per unit area). "Wolff's law" ostensibly describes the ability of bone to alter its morphology in accordance with the prevailing mechanical milieu. The originator of that concept, however, was von Roux, and it is simpler and more appropriate to refer to the "functional adaptation" of bone. Long-term, chronic exercise can augment BMD and increase bone strength. Larger, stronger bones can decrease bone stresses generated during normal physiologic activities. Thus, exercise-induced adaptations may enhance the safety factor of bone (ratio of ultimate load at which the bone fractures to typical peak load).

Bone formed in response to exercise can be adaptive at two different levels—structural and material. Structurally, bone accretion through modeling will alter geometry. If exogenous loads differ in direction from the loads normally applied to the bone, the cross-sectional shape of the bone may be altered to optimize the mechanical properties of the bone in response to this new loading regime. Cross-sectional geometry can be altered by a modeling phenomenon termed a *modeling drift*. By adding bone to the periosteal surface, farther from the cross-sectional neutral axis or centroid, the bone will become more resistant, respectively, to bending or torsion. Cross-sectional moment of inertia numerically represents the distribution of material about the neutral axis of bending and how this structure resists bending. Polar moment of inertia numerically represents the distribution of material about the centroid axis and how the structure resists torsion. Such a functional adaptation appears to occur during aging, even in the absence of specified exercise regimes. Although BMD and mineral content decrease with age, the cross-sectional moments of inertia in long bones increase by endocortical resorption and periosteal apposition which partially preserves bone strength. These geometrical changes can be influenced by exercise. Vainionpää et al. (46) conducted a prospective randomized trial on 120 women, 35 to 40 years old. Women were randomized to a high-impact exercise group three times per week or control group and were followed for 12 months. Women in the exercise group had a significant gain in midfemur circumference as detected by spiral quantitative computed tomographic imaging, and gains were positively correlated with number of impacts and the impact intensity (46).

At the material level, newly accreted bone may have different properties than older, existing bone. Initially, there is a lag (~1–2 weeks) from when the osteoid is first laid down to about 65% of its complete mineralization. Recently formed bone is less mineralized than older bone. Over the next few months, the bone tissue, normally, will become completely mineralized. Following complete mineralization, evidence suggests that the material properties of newer bone do not differ from preexisting bone (47). Nevertheless, the degree of active remodeling can affect the amount of bone incompletely mineralized at any given time and, hence, the net BMC.

TEST YOURSELF

Is it always advantageous to have a greater mineralized bone?

Numerous studies report the relations between exercise and bone mass (Fig. 3.5). Cross-sectional studies and longitudinal studies, generally, show that exercise significantly increases BMD. Cross-sectional studies, however, can be riddled with confounding variables. On average, cross-sectional studies contain younger and more male subjects than longitudinal studies. Furthermore, it remains unclear how much genetics play a role in the differences between exercise and sedentary population groups; subjects in cross-sectional studies may be self-selected for sports and vigorous physical activity. While genetics may be responsible for up to 70% to 80% of an individual's bone mass, mechanical loads associated with exercise and physical activity are key to a healthy skeleton. Unilateral loading studies (*e.g.*, of athletes in racquet sports) are useful

in that by using the lesser active appendage as an internal control, genetic and lifestyle effects are eliminated. Many studies have shown that racquet sports significantly augment bone growth in the playing limb when compared to the contralateral limb (48).

Longitudinal studies are particularly germane in assessing if exercise-induced gains are maintained. Gunter et al. (49) conducted a longitudinal study where prepubertal children were randomized to a jumping exercise regimen or a stretching regimen for 7 months. Children in the jumping group had 3.6% more BMC than the children in the stretching group. More than 8 years after the initial exercise regimen, children in the jumping group had 1.4% more BMC than those in the stretching group, which suggested that exercise-induced gains can be maintained long after cessation of exercise. Although children have a greater osteogenic potential than adults and the elderly, exercise-induced gains are possible in all age groups. Women between 65 to 70 years of age who exercised three times per week for 48 weeks had significantly greater BMD of the femoral neck and trochanter and significantly improved body sway compared to the control group who did not exercise (50).

In human studies, bone gains, in response to exercise, are commonly assessed DXA. DXA uses the principle of x-ray beams being differently attenuated by tissues of varying densities. Based on the differential attenuations, tissues can be separated into bone versus soft tissue. DXA is fast, relatively precise, and only exposes patients to low radiation doses (51). Bone strength is determined by the bone material characteristics and geometry, but DXA is unable to quantify the latter. DXA is two-dimensional and cannot resolve three-dimensional bone geometry. Furthermore, DXA may not be able to resolve small amounts of bone accretion in response to exercise. Small quantities of new bone, if placed correctly, can dramatically increase biomechanical properties. DXA-measured BMD increase of 5.4% corresponded to a 64% increase in ultimate force and a 94% increase in the energy to failure of the rat ulna (52).

Small amounts of new bone can significantly increase resistance to bending because stress in a loaded beam is inversely proportional to the cross-sectional moment of inertia. The cross-sectional moment of inertia is proportional to the radius of the section to the fourth power. Thus, small increments of bone accreted on the outer (periosteal) surface can translate into large increases in mechanical properties. QCT has the benefit of being able to discern alterations in bone geometry due to bone accretion in addition to changes in BMD.

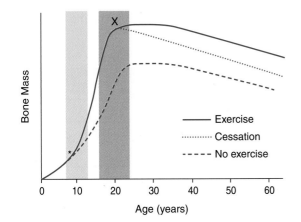

FIGURE 3.5 Theoretical relation between exercise and bone mass. The velocity of bone mass accrual increases during peripuberty (*light gray rectangle*) and decreases when peak bone mass is achieved (*dark gray rectangle*). Commencement of exercise (*) is associated with an enhanced peak bone mass. Cessation of exercise (*X*) is associated with a more rapid loss of bone with aging. (Adapted from Modlesky CM, Lewis RD. Does exercise during growth have a long-term effect on bone health? *Exerc Sport Sci Rev.* 2002;30:171–176.)

TEST YOURSELF

Are there any disadvantages to using QCT to quantify bone?

The relation is complex between chronic exercise and bone adaptation. In designing an exercise regimen for increasing bone mass, five training principles are classically considered (53): (a) *specificity*, (b) *overload*, (c) *reversibility*, (d) *initial values*, and (e) *diminishing returns*. Bone adaptation is a site-specific phenomenon and, therefore, exercise regimens should *specifically* target the bone of interest. Jumping exercises will stimulate gains in hip but not wrist BMD. In contrast to cardiovascular and muscular systems, bone has a "lazy zone" of imposed loading (via exercise) within which bone mass is maintained but no osteogenic activity is stimulated (54). Loading stimuli arising from exercise modes, such as cycling, may lie within this range, whereas, stimuli from impact loading can *overload* (exceed) the upper threshold of this range and stimulate osteogenic adaptation. Accordingly, adaptive osteogenesis varies with exercise mode. Generally, weightlifters have greater bone strength relative to marathon runners although confounding factors, such as diet, may also play a role in the relatively poor bone mass of runners. As Borelli noted in the late seventeenth century, muscle insertions often lie close to the center of joint rotation, and thus muscles work at an incredible mechanical disadvantage. Because of that disadvantage, large local forces are transmitted to bones. Joint reaction forces during postural maintenance as well as during physical activity routinely exceed several multiples of body weight. Thus, excluding trauma, forces due to muscles are among the largest forces that weight-bearing bones experience. Bone can adapt in response to such forces.

Adaptive gains in bone mass from exercise may be *reversible*; cessation of exercise can be coupled with an attenuation of exercise-induced gains in bone mass (53). That further supports the need for exercise to *maintain* bone mass—particularly in aging populations. The osteogenic potential of an exercise regime also depends on the *initial* bone mass; there is an inverse relation between initial bone mass and the osteogenic potential of a specific exercise regime. Thus, those with low bone mass have the most to gain through exercise. Osteogenesis in response to elevated mechanical loading is greater in the initial stages relative to latter stages. That is the phenomenon of *diminishing returns*. Adaptation in immature rat tibiae in response to jumping was seen after five jumps per day and did not substantially increase when rats jumped up to 40 times per day (55). Similar to exercise effects on muscles, a few brief bouts of exercise over a given duration can be more osteogenic than one long exercise bout. If the daily duration of physical activity is to be decreased, the duration of each exercise bout should be shortened, but eliminating exercise bouts diminishes the osteogenic potential of the exercise (56).

Systemic effects arising from exercise can modify exercise-induced changes in bone structure. Although the data regarding bone blood flow in response to exercise are sparse, acute exercise can increase bone blood flow. Vascular flow in lower appendages has been inversely correlated with the rate of bone loss at the hip and calcaneus in older women—which may be linked to reduced physical activity level and osteoporosis (57).

Acute dynamic exercise alters intestinal and renal calcium absorption and secretion (see Chapters 12 and 22). Additional calcium is absorbed through the small intestine in response to exercise, and that calcium is required for new bone growth and replenishes the ions excreted in sweat.

An increase in bone mass in response to exercise may underpin the development of nonpharmacologic treatments for osteoporosis. Osteoporosis adversely affects quality of life and burdens the health care system. In 2005 in the United States alone, there was estimated to be more than 2 million osteoporotic fractures, which cost approximately $17 billion (58). Of osteoporotic fractures, 90% of hip fractures and 50% of spine fractures resulted from unexpected falls (54). With an increase in global life expectancy, osteoporosis-related fractures have the potential to become a significantly greater problem. Exercise-induced bone formation may mitigate significant morbidity and mortality related to osteoporosis by four different mechanisms: (a) exercise in growing individuals could increase peak bone mass attained and optimize bone structure—younger bones have a greater adaptive response to exercise; (b) exercise in adulthood may slow age-associated bone loss; (c) exercise-induced bone accrual throughout adulthood and old age may counterbalance age-associated bone loss and result in net bone gains; and (d) exercise can significantly improve musculoskeletal coordination thereby reducing the risk of unexpected falls.

TEST YOURSELF

What is an example of improved musculoskeletal coordination and how could that influence the probability of a fall?

Negative effects of exercise

Traumatic injury aside, exercise is not always beneficial for bone. Extremely intense exercise can adversely affect the skeletal system. Prolonged bouts of extremely intense exercise can produce microdamage (i.e., microscopic cracks within bone matrix). Each load cycle by itself may be too small to cause microdamage, but the cumulative effect of some thousands of load cycles can lead to microdamage accumulation within bone in what is termed a *stress reaction* or *stress fracture*. A stress reaction is a site of increased cellular activity, whereas a stress fracture is a crack that

TEST YOURSELF

How do you determine the optimal exercise protocol for a specific bone?

propagates in bone. Stress fractures are painful, may or may not be evident in radiographs, and are of significant medical concern. Up to 73% of U.S. Marine recruits experience stress fractures (59). Risk factors for stress fractures include low bone density, inadequate muscle function, overtraining, inadequate equipment, female gender, and amenorrhea (60).

TEST YOURSELF

How would inadequate muscle function or muscle fatigue have a negative effect on bone?

Females involved in extremely intense exercise can develop the *female athlete triad*: eating disorder(s), amenorrhea, and osteoporosis (see also Milestone of Discovery). When energy availability (total energy intake minus total energy expenditure) falls below 20 to 30 kCal $\cdot$ kg^{-1} lean body mass/day reproductive dysfunction (amenorrhea) can result (61). Prolonged hormonal disruptions can lead to reduction in BMD, termed *osteopenia*, which in turn elevates the risk of developing osteoporosis years later (62). Weakened bones are especially dangerous for competitive athletes, as active competition elevates the risk of fracture above that in sedentary women.

Up to 26% of total adult skeletal calcium is accumulated through 2 years of peak skeletal growth during adolescence (63). Peak skeletal growth precedes peak height growth velocity and occurs earlier for girls (12.5 years) than boys (14 years) (64). Mineral accrual can be substantially altered with exercise during growth. Reportedly, there is a 9% and 17% increase in total body BMC for active boys and girls, respectively, relative to nonactive children (65). However, extremely strenuous exercise during periods of rapid adolescent growth could interrupt normal growth and, as a result, body stature may be stunted.

Interactions with Exercise

The potential for exercise to increase bone mass is related to more than the nature of the mechanical stimuli. The requisite genetic, dietary, hormonal, and developmental conditions must be satisfied for exercise to mount a positive adaptive response. In some cases, if these conditions are unsatisfied, exercise that would normally exert positive effects can have negligible or negative effects.

Genetics

Heritability is deemed the most important determinant of BMD, as up to 80% of peak bone mass is typically attributed to genetics. Some of the genes controlling peak BMD have been revealed. Osteocalcin (most abundant noncollagenous protein in bone) and vitamin D receptor gene polymorphisms have been linked to BMD differences among individuals (66,67). Evidence suggests that genes controlling BMD may interact with exercise to augment or attenuate exercise effects on bone adaptation. It has recently been shown that vitamin D receptor and interleukin-6 gene polymorphisms affect skeletal adaptation to exercise (68,69).

Diet

Some of the key dietary factors in bone health include minerals (most notably calcium), vitamin D, protein, and fat. Although diet and exercise can influence bone independently, a poor diet reduces the available nutritional building blocks and can diminish positive exercise-related effects on bone. The data about the relation between calcium intake and exercise, however, are equivocal and poorly understood. Analysis of exercise intervention trials that included information on dietary calcium intake reveal that exercise produces increases in BMD only when calcium intake exceeds 1000 mg $\cdot$ d^{-1}, with this effect more pronounced in the lumbar spine, rather than the radius (70). It is generally accepted that chronic exercise and dietary calcium can improve bone mass to a greater extent than calcium intake alone. The body uses calcium in numerous biologic processes and functions, and it is imperative to maintain appropriate serum calcium balance. Bone's dual mechanical-biologic roles can sometimes be in opposition, particularly if dietary calcium is low; bone will be resorbed to elevate serum calcium levels, thereby decreasing mechanical integrity.

Vitamin D increases intestinal absorption of calcium, and thus diets rich in vitamin D may augment bone formation in response to exercise. Protein is also important as a tissue building block, and diets high in protein have enhanced the osteogenic effect of strenuous exercise in young growing rats (71). Dietary fatty acids can influence bone at both local and systemic levels. Saturated fatty acid triglycerides form soaps with calcium in the intestine and can reduce intestinal absorption of dietary calcium (72). Corwin and colleagues (73) reported a negative association between saturated fat intake and femoral neck BMD in men and women using National Health and Nutrition Examination Survey III (1988–1994) data ($n = 14,850$). After adjusting for age, sex, weight, height, race, total energy and calcium intake, smoking, and weight-bearing exercise, the greatest effects were seen in men under the age of 50 in the femoral neck—those with the highest intake of saturated fat had lower femoral neck BMD. At the bone tissue level, prostaglandins involved in bone remodeling processes are formed from n-6 fatty acid precursors in the cells. Diets high in saturated fatty acids alter the fatty acid profile of cells in the bone and may alter the bone's ability to respond to mechanical stimuli.

Monosaccharide glucose and disaccharide sucrose are simple carbohydrates that can have influences on bone (74). With substantial ingestion of glucose, for example, calcium excretion although the urine is increased (75). Lemann and colleagues (1970) showed that glucose consumption affected urinary calcium excretion, either through increased glomerular filtration rate or reduced net renal tubular reabsorption in the kidney (76). When a large amount of simple carbohydrates in the diet are coupled with saturated fats, bone mechanics and mineralization can be negatively influenced (71,77,78). In particular, cortical bones that had been exposed to a high fat and simple carbohydrate diet had significantly lower maximal strength and failure properties. Likely because of its greater bone turnover and higher metabolic rate, cancellous bone (*e.g.*, vertebrae) was more adversely affected than cortical bone.

Dietary choices favoring items high in quality protein of animal or plant origin, polyunsaturated fatty acids, fruits and vegetables high in potassium and fiber, and dairy products or other beverages fortified with calcium and vitamin D are essential to ensure adequate vitamin and mineral availability to the skeleton (74). Primary sources of calcium in the diet are cheese, milk, yogurt, kale and turnip greens, broccoli, tofu, and calcium-fortified foods such as orange juice (79). Appropriate nutrition, in sufficient amount and substance, is vital for skeletal health.

Hormones

Studies of male and female osteoporoses consistently show a close relation between hormones (*e.g.*, growth hormone and estrogen) and BMD (Chapter 19). However, the interaction between hormones and exercise and their effects on BMD remain largely equivocal. The loss of sex steroids in men and women with old age is coupled with substantial bone losses. Recently, it was shown that osteoblasts require estrogen receptor alpha (ER-α) to mount effectively an osteogenic response to mechanical loading (80). ER-α expression is positively correlated with serum estrogen concentration and, therefore, age-related decrements in sex steroid concentrations could decrease the expression of ER-α and, hence, mechanical sensitivity. Hormone replacement therapy (HRT) can increase BMD following menopause, but has been linked with a number of comorbidities such as heart disease, breast cancer, and stroke. Exercise has been suggested to be a nonpharmacologic method to augment BMD in postmenopausal women. However, there is not widespread agreement that absolute gains in BMD can be achieved by exercise alone in estrogen-deficient women. Some studies report that exercise and HRT can interact to bring about a synergistic increase in BMD, and it has been suggested that the synergistic increases in BMD in response to HRT and exercise is due to a decreased bone turnover (81).

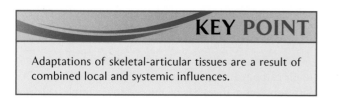

KEY POINT

Adaptations of skeletal-articular tissues are a result of combined local and systemic influences.

TEST YOURSELF

Genetics, mechanical loading, diet, and hormones: what is the relative capacity of each for determining bone structure and mechanical properties?

Development and aging

Skeletons of all ages are sensitive to exercise, but responsiveness to exercise changes with age. Throughout growth (adolescence, in particular), it is generally accepted that the adaptability of the skeleton is much greater than after maturity. In female squash players, significant differences in BMD between the playing and nonplaying arm were greater if training was started before menarche (48). Emerging data (82–87) suggest that the "critical period" for exercise to be most efficacious during growth is just before puberty—but that remains a wide range within the context of growth. The data suggest a significant posttraining advantage for premenarcheal (all maturity groups within premenarche pooled), but not postmenarcheal girls (88), and for early pubertal, but not prepubertal girls (89). Complementing those findings, McKay and coworkers have reported their comprehensive longitudinal studies examining how exercise interventions in schools can be effective for enhancing bone development (*e.g.*, Macdonald et al. [87]). A 16-month randomized controlled trial, using a school-based daily jumping program, in addition to 15 minutes of daily classroom physical activity, increased the bone strength index, assessed with peripheral QCT at the distal tibia in prepubertal boys. This jumping intervention took less than 3 minutes of classroom time and used various jumping styles (*e.g.*, countermovement jumps and side-to-side jumps) to generate unique strain environments (87,90). More extensive exercise programs have also proven effective (84–86). A 12-minute program, 3 days per week, of diverse weight-bearing activities that were blended into physical education classes produced up to 5% greater increase in lumbar spine and femoral neck BMC in pre- and early pubertal girls compared with controls after 2 years (84). Similarly, prepubertal boys had 4% greater gain in their femoral neck BMC (86).

In the aggregate, those studies suggest that exercise is most effective in stimulating bone growth if initiated some time before or during early puberty, rather than after puberty (90); this timing presents as a "window of opportunity" as noted by MacKelvie and colleagues (84). Heaney (91) reiterated that adolescence is a critical time for bone development, as boys and girls gain approximately 40% of their peak bone mass between the ages of 12 and 16, and 35% of total BMC is laid down in the 2 years around peak height velocity (63).

Differences in skeletal adaptability with age likely stem from the differing bone cell activities with age. During skeletal growth, osteoblasts covering the periosteal surface act to expand bone size (considered periosteal expansion), whereas osteoclasts cover and act primarily at the endocortical surface, resorbing bone and enlarging the marrow cavity (considered endocortical expansion). Changes in bone shape that arise from osteoblasts and osteoclasts acting independent of each other are termed *modeling*. During puberty, both of these surfaces may be undergoing bone apposition. After peak BMD is reached at skeletal maturity (20–30 years of age), skeletal maintenance is dominated by *remodeling*, which typically does not alter skeletal shape. Presumably, it is easier to stimulate existing modeling bone cells to alter bone shape than recruit a new population of bone cells, as would have to be done in mature bones. During growth, humoral factors necessary for proper skeletal development (*e.g.*, insulin-like growth-factor 1) are abundant. With age, physiologically active concentrations of growth factors decline, potentially blunting exercise-induced osteogenesis.

TEST YOURSELF

Assuming bone mass is conserved, what happens to the bending stiffness of a long bone that experiences simultaneous endocortical and periosteal expansion?

Aging beyond skeletal maturity is associated with a loss of BMD. Cortical bone thinning is caused by an imbalance between endocortical expansion and periosteal apposition, where expansion is favored. Cortical thinning is less apparent in males than females because the difference between periosteal apposition and endocortical expansion rates are less in males. Cortical bone becomes heavily remodeled, trabeculae become less numerous, and trabeculae thin with age. The increased fracture risk due to compromised bone structure is compounded by diminished muscular coordination that can lead to an increased risk of falling; hence, age is associated with a dramatic increase in risk of fracture. In terms of recommended "best exercises" for helping to maintain BMD and effective neuromotor coordination in postmenopause women, aerobic, weightbearing, and resistive exercises have all been shown to have positive effects on BMD (*e.g.*, lumbar spine) (92,93).

TEST YOURSELF

What happens to the buckling strength of trabeculae as connectivity is decreased?

Mechanisms of Bone Adaptation

Exercise, as well as many other factors, can modulate bone adaptation. The mechanisms regulating adaptation, however, remain elusive. Bone cells may respond directly to mechanical deformation or indirectly to other stimuli generated by mechanical load or exercise (*e.g.*, pressure-driven fluid flow; see *Mechanical Transduction*), but either way, strain magnitude, frequency, rate, and gradient can all influence bone adaptation.

Proposed Strain Components

In vivo, there is considerable interaction among strain (change in length/original length) components, and the probability of synergistic effects modulating adaptation is high. For clarity, however, the following discussion assumes all other parameters are held constant with the parameter of interest varied.

Magnitude

Bone adaptation is roughly proportional to the magnitude of strain induced during loading. This suggests that bone adaptation is linearly related to strain magnitude. This is true, however, only after a threshold strain is surpassed. Accordingly, exercises with large ground reaction forces (*e.g.*, gymnastics) have greater potentials for osteogenic adaptation (82). Newly formed bone can be positioned effectively to minimize large strain magnitudes (*i.e.*, periosteal surfaces). It has been proposed that strain magnitudes must be within a specified range to maintain healthy bone tissue. If strain magnitudes decline below that range, disuse adaptation ensues (bone loss/osteopenia). If strain magnitudes rise above that range, adaptation to increased loading ensues (bone gain).

For a given strain magnitude to stimulate bone growth, a threshold number of daily load cycles must be reached (Fig. 3.6).

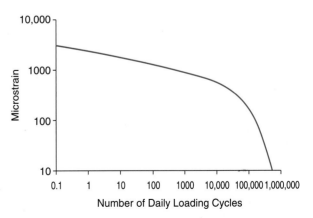

FIGURE 3.6 Strain threshold required for osteogenesis as a function of the number of daily loading cycles. Stimuli above the line are osteogenic. (Adapted from Qin YX, Rubin CT, McLeod KJ. Nonlinear dependence of loading intensity and cycle number in the maintenance of bone mass and morphology. *J Orthop Res.* 1998;16:482–489.)

Frequency

Generally, bone adaptation is also proportional to frequency of loading stimulation. Daily, bones experience thousands of small strains (<10 $\mu\epsilon$) and only a few larger strains (>1000 $\mu\epsilon$ [94]). Sustained muscular contractions, such as those during postural regulation, subject bone to high-frequency (e.g., 30 Hz), low-magnitude vibrations. As the frequency of stimulation increases, the daily number of loading cycles also increases and, thus, high-frequency stimuli require only low-magnitude strains to surpass the threshold for osteogenesis (Fig. 3.6). Recently, it was shown in animal models that brief exposure (<1 hr) to high-frequency vibrations ($\sim$30 Hz) produced an osteogenic response (95,96). The therapeutic potential in preventing bone loss has been demonstrated in human studies with high-frequency (30 Hz) vibration stimuli for short durations (<10 min) (97–100). Two treatments per day resulted in reduced bone loss in the lumbar spine and femoral neck of postmenopausal women, compared to a placebo group (98,100). Treatments (<10 min $\cdot$ d^{-1}) have also been shown to be effective at increasing bone mass in the femur (cortical) and lumbar spine (cancellous) in young women (15–20 years) with low bone mass (97,100); and in the proximal tibia of adolescent children with musculoskeletal disorders (e.g., cerebral palsy and muscular dystrophy) (99,100).

TEST YOURSELF

Are strain magnitude and frequency mutually exclusive mechanisms driving bone adaptation?

Rate

Static stimuli (strains held at a constant level; strain rate = 0) are not osteogenic and may induce catabolic effects. To be osteogenic, dynamic stimuli are needed for osteogenesis—strains must change with respect to time (strain rate > 0). Impact exercises are more osteogenic than nonimpact exercises. In addition to the larger magnitude strains present with impact, impact exercises are also characterized by higher strain rates. Larger strain rates cause intracortical bone fluid to flow with greater velocity. Fluid velocity could positively correlate with the adaptive potential of transduction mechanisms, including fluid shear stresses and streaming potentials (see *Transduction Mechanisms*).

Gradient

With exercise, bone is primarily deformed by a combination of axial loading and bending. As a result, strains differ spatially throughout bone. Strain gradient refers to the change in strain magnitude, as a function of position on the bone. In the absence of large intramedullary pressures, intracortical strain gradients are proportional to pressure gradients (101). Intracortical fluid flow would be greatest where the strain gradient is greatest. Current hypotheses suggest that fluid flow within bone mediates bone adaptation (see *Transduction Mechanisms*). In avian models, strain gradients were correlated with sites of exercise-induced bone formation, supporting the view that fluid flow could mediate bone adaptation (101,102). Furthermore, strain gradients produce electrokinetic potentials across the bone, which could also influence bone adaptation (103).

Mechanical Transduction

For exercise to stimulate bone adaptation, four steps must be completed in what is referred to as *mechanotransduction* (104): (a) *Mechanocoupling*, in which biophysical forces are converted into cellular vernacular. Once mechanical signals are comprehensible to cells, biologic responses (e.g., release of autocrine and paracrine mediators) emanate in (b) *biochemical coupling*. Because bone cells do not exist in isolation (c) *cell-to-cell signalling* is a prerequisite for coordinated function. Lastly, individual cell biologic responses are orchestrated into a (d) *effector response*, which results in bone homeostasis (i.e., bone formation and/or bone resorption).

Cell populations (signal pathways)

For mechanotransduction to occur, physical stimuli must be perceived by biologic entities. In the case of bone, four groups of cells exist that conceivably could be linked by mechanocoupling—osteoclasts, osteoblasts, bone lining cells, and osteocytes. Osteoblasts and osteoclasts are transient, as they, respectively, are present when actively forming or resorbing bone. It is unlikely that transient cell populations transduce the continual forces bones are exposed to into effector responses. Osteoclasts eventually undergo apoptosis. Unlike osteoclasts, the fate of an osteoblast is tripartite. Osteoblasts can undergo apoptosis, become entombed in bone matrix (osteocytes), or lie quiescently on the bone surface as bone lining cells. Osteocytes and bone lining cells make up 95% of all bone cells. In addition to their abundance and long-lived existence, osteocytes and bone lining cells are ideally situated to perceive mechanical stimuli. Both bone lining cells and osteocytes subsist throughout the entire cortex. When osteoblasts terminally differentiate into osteocytes, long slender processes appear and extend through microscopic channels (canaliculi) in the bone matrix. Processes from osteocytes and bone lining cells maintain connection with one another via gap junctions, and attachments to the communal pericellular matrix. Hence, cellular connections are maintained throughout the entire bone cortex. Two extensive communication systems exist between cells (105), namely, *intercellular communication* via gap junctions and cytoskeletal connections that create a syncytium of mechanosensory cells, and *extracellular communications* that are mediated by fluid filing the spaces between osteocytes, their processes, and the adjacent bone matrix. Thus, osteocytes are ideally situated to perceive exercise-induced physical phenomena. Furthermore, because osteocytes maintain connections

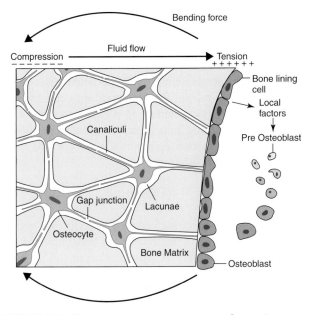

FIGURE 3.7   Diagrammatic representation of a section of bone in bending. Bone fluid in regions of compressive stress develops high hydrostatic pressures and bone fluid in regions of tensile stress develops low hydrostatic pressures. To equalize this pressure differential, bone fluid flows from regions of high to low pressure. Fluid can flow through the lacunocanalicular system and aid in nutrient transport and waste removal. Furthermore, fluid flow can exert shear stresses and streaming potentials on osteocytic membranes, potentially causing the cells to initiate an adaptive response. Mechanotransductive signals are transmitted throughout the network of osteocytes via cell processes connected by gap junctions. Those connections terminate on bone lining cells. Bone lining cells can subsequently release local factors (*e.g.*, IGF-1) that stimulate the differentiation of preosteoblasts into osteoblasts, which can form new bone matrix.

with the marrow and periosteal surface, augmented osteoblast recruitment is easily envisaged (Fig. 3.7). This is critical because osteogenic adaptation is marked by an increase in osteoblastic activity or osteoblast differentiation. Because osteocytes neither secrete bone matrix nor differentiate into osteoblasts, they must signal effector cells such as osteoblasts and preosteoblasts.

The role of osteocytes in adaptation is evident when their function or viability is compromised. Reilly et al. (106) demonstrated that destruction of the pericellular matrix of an osteocyte was associated with a decreased release of prostaglandins in response to mechanical loading. If osteocytes are killed, bone quality is attenuated. Tatsumi et al. (107) developed a transgenic mouse model with inducible ablation of osteocytes using targeted expression of diphtheria toxin receptors. After a single exposure to diphtheria toxin, 80% of osteocytes were killed, and the bones of these mice were fragile with striking features of the aging skeleton (107). Mice lacking osteocytes were resistant to unloading-induced bone loss. Together, these results support the proposed role of osteocytes in sensation of mechanical stimuli and coordination of skeletal turnover.

TEST YOURSELF

Do osteocytes communicate with osteoclasts?

Transduction mechanisms

Osteocytes may perceive and transduce biophysical stimuli via a number of different mechanisms, none of which are mutually exclusive.

BONE CELL STRAIN/STRETCH RECEPTORS, CYTOSKELETON Perturbations in cell shape may regulate cellular processes including growth, differentiation, and mechanotransduction. Regulation of these processes is mediated through the cytoskeleton in which an interconnected network of microfilaments (tensile bearing), microtubules (compressive bearing), and intermediate filaments can link cell surface proteins to the nucleus (108). Cell surface proteins mediating mechanotransduction could include integrins, mechanosensitive ion channels, or humoral receptors. Signals from stimulation of these proteins could be transferred to the nucleus to influence cellular processes.

In vivo, deformations of bone during maximal exercise rarely exceed 3000 $\mu\epsilon$ (0.3% strain). However, in vitro studies typically demonstrate that bone cells, as do many other cell types (109), require strains considerably larger than 0.3% to elicit an adaptive response. Thus, it is questionable if in vivo strains and deformations of bone cells caused by exercise are large enough to mediate bone cell mechanotransduction. Most in vitro studies have ignored the anatomical connections osteocytes have with their pericellular matrix. In a theoretical model, Wang et al. (110) calculated that these $\alpha_v\beta_3$ integrin connections between osteocytes and their lacunar and canalicular walls amplify the signal osteocytes receive to within the range shown to open stretch-activated cation channels. Hence, measured bone surface strains may not reflect the strain magnitudes experienced by bone cells.

PIEZOELECTRICITY Piezoelectricity, a direct result of matrix deformation, refers to the ability of a range of materials to convert mechanical deformations into electric fields. Fukada and Yasuda (111) discovered that bone is piezoelectric and concluded bone piezoelectricity was due to collagen, as they observed similar piezoelectric effects in tendon. Bone collagen molecules consist of three interwoven tropocollagen polypeptide chains. Polypeptide chains aggregate into microfibrils, which then aggregate into fibrils with a diameter of 0.2 μm and a length of several micrometers. During fibril formation, bone mineral is incorporated in fibril structure, and most of the bone mineral resides there. That arrangement yields an asymmetric positive and negative charge, with the arrangement producing a net dipole moment aligned parallel to bone's long axis (111). As the deformation of a piezoelectric material increases, so does the asymmetric charge arrangement. Thus, net dipoles are exacerbated in a linear fashion with deformation magnitude. Because electromagnetic fields can affect bone cell dynamics and fracture healing, alterations in the mechanical milieu of bone cells via piezoelectric fields may induce adaptive responses. Although piezoelectric effects in isolation have not recently been considered major factors in tissue adaptation, piezoelectricity may indirectly influence bone cell activities by regulating bone microstiffness, streaming potentials, or sensitivity to mechanical loading (112).

FLUID FLOW   Pressure-driven fluid flow, an indirect stimulus resulting from bone matrix deformation, is increasingly recognized as a critical stimulant affecting bone adaptation. As bones are deformed, hydrostatic and dynamic pressure gradients develop. Bone fluid flows from regions of high hydrostatic pressure (compression) to regions of low hydrostatic pressure (tension; Fig. 3.7). Fluid flow generates three distinct signals, all of which may be perceived by bone cells: shear flow, ion flow, and nutrient flow. Osteocytes may orient themselves in accordance with these mechanical stimuli (113) and respond differently to different fluid flow profiles (114).

Shear flow   As fluid flows through bone pores, fluid shear stresses are imposed on both the matrix wall and cell membranes. With canaliculi of 6 to 7 nm in diameter, wall shear stresses have a magnitude of 0.8 to 3.0 Pa (115); shear stresses are tangential forces generated by velocity gradients (or shear rate) in fluid flow. Equations describing hemodynamic wall shear stresses in blood vessels are extendable to the flow of extracellular fluid within bone:

$$\tau_w = \mu \cdot (du/dy)_w \qquad [1]$$

where τ_w is the fluid-imposed wall shear stress, μ is the blood viscosity coefficient, u is the velocity component of the fluid flow parallel to the longitudinal direction of the wall, y is the perpendicular distance from the wall, and $(du/dy)_w$ represents the velocity gradient of blood flow at the wall. The nanogeometry of bone matrix may also influence osteocyte fluid shear stresses (116). Fluid shear stresses stimulate an adaptive response in endothelial cells (117,118). Vascular endothelial cells release vasoactive substances in response to hemodynamic forces. Shear stresses as small as 0.2 to 0.5 Pa can initiate endothelial cell responses that control local blood pressure. Sensor cells in the endothelium produce paracrine signalling factors in response to changes in wall shear stresses. Signalling factors travel to the effector cell (vascular smooth muscle cell) and result in vasodilation or vasoconstriction (104). Cerebral pressure is regulated in that manner. As arterial pressure builds, shear stresses increase and vessels are stimulated to vasoconstrict. That helps maintain constant cerebral blood flow over a wide range of arterial pressures (117). Given the variety of cells that are able to sense shear stresses, it is not surprising bone cells are sensitive to fluid shear stresses. Both osteoblasts and osteocytes produce signaling factors such as nitric oxide, prostaglandin E_2 (PGE$_2$),

and adenosine triphosphate in response to 1 Pa fluid shear stress, and upregulate gap junction formation (119–121).

Ion flow   When ionic solutions flow across charged surfaces, electric potentials emanate. These potentials are governed by the Helmholtz-Smoluchowski equation, which describes the electric potential in a capillary tube filled with an ion-containing fluid. From that relation, a generalized equation for streaming potentials in bone has been derived (equation 2) (122):

$$V_{SGP} = \{\zeta\epsilon/(4\pi\sigma\eta)\}P_{eff} \qquad [2]$$

where V_{SGP} is the streaming potential, ζ is the zeta potential, ϵ is the dielectric permittivity of the bulk fluid, η is the viscosity of the bulk fluid, σ is the conductivity of the bulk fluid, and P_{eff} is the effective driving pressure due to mechanical deformation. The zeta potential may be influenced by matrix piezoelectricity (112). Fixed negative charges in bone matrix electrostatically attract bone extracellular fluid cations toward the solid/fluid interface. With an effective driving pressure parallel to the pore longitudinal axis, fluid flows parallel with the driving pressure (122). That produces a "streaming current" that develops a nonzero potential between the two ends of the bone pore. In response to this nonzero potential, an electrical field originates in 180-degree opposition to the streaming current. Due to the electrical field, ions flow opposite to the direction of the pressure-driven streaming current. Thus, the streaming current ion movement is countered, and a steady state is achieved. In that steady state, the potential difference between the two ends of the pore is referred to as the "streaming potential." Streaming potentials can alter a bone cell's electrical environment. The electrical milieu of a bone cell may influence its cellular activities, thereby regulating adaptive response.

TEST YOURSELF

What interplay exists between bone piezoelectric effect and streaming potentials?

Nutrient flow   Convective mixing of the media surrounding bone cells (bone extracellular fluid) displaces essential nutrients and wastes. Presumably, altering metabolite concentrations will affect cell activities and thereby provide a mechanism by which local adaptation can be coordinated. Experimentally, Knothe Tate and colleagues demonstrated that diffusive transport is sufficient to transport small molecules (MW 300–400 Da), such as amino acids, to osteocytes in the mid cortex within minutes. Diffusion alone, however, may not be sufficient to transport larger molecules (MW 1800 Da) evenly throughout the cortex. Convective transport mediated by pressure-driven fluid flow may by necessary to supply osteocytes with proteins to prevent osteocyte starvation and regulate adaptive processes (123).

Convective transport increases with higher loading magnitude and decreases with higher loading frequency. Transport is also a function of bone microarchitecture. Goulet and colleagues (124) developed a complex model based on a human tibia to illustrate how mechanical loading and bone microarchitecture influenced fluid flow. After 10 loading cycles, there was a ninefold increase in fluid flow in the compressive region, relative to diffusion alone, and fluid exchange was greatest at the junction between the vascular pores and the lacunocanicular porosity (124).

KEY POINT

Cells in skeletal-articular tissues "sense" and respond to their biophysical, biochemical, and bioelectrical environments.

CHAPTER SUMMARY

Skeletal articular tissues allow our body to produce movements. Ligaments tether bones together, tendons transmit muscular forces to bones, menisci guide joints in their proper orientation and attenuate joint stresses, and bones actuate motion by acting as a system of rigid pivots and levers. The complex tissue properties of skeletal articular tissues emerge from an intricate interaction of water, organic, and mineral (bone) phases. These properties, in conjunction with the organization of these tissues into functional units, enable them to serve unique biologic, physical, and anthropologic roles. Biologically, bone is a center for hematopoiesis and serves as the largest calcium reservoir in the body—a reservoir that is sensitively adjusted to metabolic demands. Physically, skeletal tissues coordinate motion and bones also provide protection for vital organs. The biologic and physical roles of bone

A MILESTONE OF DISCOVERY

Low estrogen levels, as found with postmenopause and amenorrhea, are linked to low bone mineral density (BMD). Physical activity can inhibit or potentially reverse bone loss in postmenopausal women, but as late as 1984, the interrelation between exercise and amenorrhea remained clouded. Amenorrhea (low estrogen level and an abnormally low number of menstrual cycles) has a greater prevalence in athletes—particularly at the elite level—than in the general population. The training regimens for endurance amenorrheic athletes far exceed the intensity of those effective for an osteogenic response in postmenopausal women. Prior to this pioneering study by Drinkwater and her colleagues, it was generally accepted that the intense physical activity of endurance amenorrheic athletes would exert a protective effect against bone loss. Their findings dismissed that prevailing view.

In their study, amenorrhea was defined as having had no more than one menstrual flow in the past 12 months. Fourteen amenorrheic athletes enrolled in the study and, from a large cohort, 14 matched eumenorrheic (normal menstrual cycle) athletes were selected. In order of priority, matches were based on sport, age, weight, height, and the frequency and duration of daily exercise. Women with a history of eating disorders were eliminated from the study. The experimental design maximized the potential for amenorrhea to be secondary to the athlete's physical exercise (athletic amenorrhea). Venous blood samples were assayed for estradiol, progesterone, testosterone, and prolactin. Distal radius and lumbar spine BMD was determined by photon absorptiometry. Dietary journals and questionnaires chronicled dietary information, menstrual history, and athletic activities.

The physical characteristics, training regimens, and diets were not significantly different between amenorrheic and eumenorrheic women—with one exception: amenorrheic women ran significantly greater distances than eumenorrheic women (see the table to the right). Of greatest importance,

however, was that the average BMD in the lumbar vertebrae of amenorrheic athletes was nearly 14% lower than that of matched eumenorrheic athletes (see the table) and was equivalent to that of women 51.2 years of age. Because BMD is related to bone strength, decrements in bone density and mass may have substantial implications for fracture risk, especially in elite athletes. Furthermore, the bone losses in amenorrheic athletes might not be fully recoverable even upon resumption of normal menses.

This significant study revealed the first quantitative link between "athletic amenorrhea" and low bone density. That linkage was central to characterizing the *female athlete triad*, which comprises disordered eating behavior, amenorrhea, and low bone density. With the discovery of those three interrelated factors, scientists, physicians, coaches, and athletes began to realize the very significant clinical and performance consequences of the female athlete triad.

Characteristics of Amenorrheic and Eumenorrheic Athletes

	Amenorrheic	Eumenorrheic	P
Age (yr)	24.9 ± 1.3	25.5 ± 1.5	NS
Length of participation in sport (yr)	7.0 ± 1.6	6.6 ± 1.1	NS
Miles run per week	41.8 ± 5.2	24.9 ± 3.0	<0.01
Vertebral bone mineral density (g · cm^{-2})	1.12 ± 0.04	1.30 ± 0.03	<0.01
Mean estradiol (pg · mL^{-1})	38.58 ± 7.03	106.99 ± 9.80	<0.01
Peak estradiol (pg · mL^{-1})	67.75 ± 13.77	205.39 ± 20.6	<0.01

Drinkwater BL, Nilson K, Chesnut CH, et al. Bone mineral content of amenorrheic and eumenorrheic athletes. N Engl J Med. 1984;311:277–281.

can be at odds, but bone's role in calcium metabolism will supersede its mechanical role. The mineral content of bone that contributes substantially to its physical role also heightens the preservation of bone in the fossil record, thus providing anthropologists insight into processes of evolution.

Although skeletal articular tissues can appear as static tissues on gross morphologic scales, they are highly dynamic and adapt their metabolism in response to the prevailing mechanical environment. Bone is, by far, the most dynamic and most studied of the skeletal articular tissues. Bone is consistently maintained by a highly dynamic group of cells. Osteoclasts degrade and osteoblasts deposit bone matrix. Occasionally osteoblasts become buried in their matrix where they survive as osteocytes, which are key links in the mechanosensory chain. Bone cell activities can be modulated by exercise. Mechanical loading through dynamic, resistance exercise can significantly influence bone morphology. Chronic exercise, generally, will lead to bone accretion. Disuse or lack of mechanical loading has a profound and negative effect on bone morphology, leading to decrements in bone density, alterations in bone shape, and reduced mechanical integrity. Different exercise modalities can influence bone differently—the net result of the exercise stimulus is a complex blend of cellular and systemic interactions with local mechanical loading. Although the effects of physical activity on ligament, tendon, and meniscus are not as well documented as the effects on bone, the general principle that physical activity and exercise have potent effects on the skeletal system is supported in all skeletal articular tissues.

The precise nature of the stimuli underlying adaptation to exercise remains elusive, but experimental data reveal that strain magnitude, frequency, rate, and gradients can all influence bone adaptation. Osteocytes likely perceive these stimuli via direct and indirect stimuli, with the prime candidates for mechanotransduction being bone fluid flow and shear stress effects on cytoskeletal conformation, piezoelectric fields, and streaming potentials. Understanding how skeletal tissues perceive and respond to physical stimuli may lead to the development of optimal physical loading or exercise regimes that are effective alternatives to pharmacologic therapies to combat low bone mass.

ACKNOWLEDGMENTS

The development of this chapter has been supported, in part, by the Canadian Institutes for Health Research, the Natural Sciences and Engineering Research Council of Canada, the Alberta Heritage Foundation for Medical Research, Alberta Provincial CIHR Training Program in Bone and Joint Health, the Wood Professorship in Joint Injury Research, and the University of Michigan.

REFERENCES

1. Kastelic J, Galeski A, Baer E. The multicomposite structure of tendon. *Connect Tissue Res.* 1978;6:11–23.

2. Sweigart MA, Athanasiou KA. Toward tissue engineering of the knee meniscus. *Tissue Eng.* 2001;7:111–129.

3. Jee WSS. Integrated bone tissue physiology: anatomy and physiology. In: Cowin SC, editor. *Bone Mechanics Handbook.* Boca Raton: CRC Press; 2001. p. 1–53.

4. Butler DL, Grood ES, Noyes FR, et al. Biomechanics of ligaments and tendons. *Exerc Sport Sci Rev.* 1978;6:125–181.

5. Frank CB. Ligament injuries. In: Zachazewski JE, Magee DJ, Quillen WS, editors. *Athletic Injuries and Rehabilitation.* Philadelphia: Saunders; 1996. p. 9–26.

6. Tipton CM, Matthes RD, Sandage DS. In situ measurement of junction strength and ligament elongation in rats. *J Appl Physiol.* 1974;37:758–761.

7. Akeson WH. An experimental study of joint stiffness. *Am J Orthop.* 1961;43-A:1022–1034.

8. Akeson WH, Amiel D, LaViolette D. The connective-tissue response to immobility: a study of the chondroitin-4 and 6-sulfate and dermatan sulfate changes in periarticular connective tissue of control and immobilized knees of dogs. *Clin Orthop.* 1967;51:183–197.

9. Woo SL, Matthews JV, Akeson WH, et al. Connective tissue response to immobility. Correlative study of biomechanical and biochemical measurements of normal and immobilized rabbit knees. *Arthritis Rheum.* 1975;18:257–264.

10. Amiel D, Woo SL, Harwood FL, et al. The effect of immobilization on collagen turnover in connective tissue: a biochemical-biomechanical correlation. *Acta Orthop Scand.* 1982;53:325–332.

11. Klein L, Dawson MH, Heiple KG. Turnover of collagen in the adult rat after denervation. *J Bone Joint Surg Am.* 1977;59:1065–1067.

12. Loitz BJ, Zernicke RF, Vailas AC, et al. Effects of short-term immobilization versus continuous passive motion on the biomechanical and biochemical properties of the rabbit tendon. *Clin Orthop.* 1989;265–271.

13. Matsumoto F, Trudel G, Uhthoff HK, et al. Mechanical effects of immobilization on the Achilles' tendon. *Arch Phys Med Rehabil.* 2003;84:662–667.

14. Flint M. Interrelationships of mucopolysaccharides and collagen in connective tissue remodelling. *J Embryol Exp Morph.* 1982;27:481–495.

15. Cabaud HE, Chatty A, Gildengorin V, et al. Exercise effects on the strength of the rat anterior cruciate ligament. *Am J Sports Med.* 1980;8:79–86.

16. Tipton CM, James SL, Mergner W, et al. Influence of exercise on strength of medial collateral knee ligaments of dogs. *Am J Physiol.* 1970;218:894–902.

17. Binkley JM, Peat M. The effects of immobilization on the ultrastructure and mechanical properties of the medial collateral ligament of rats. *Clin Orthop.* 1986:301–308.

18. Zamora AJ, Marini JF. Tendon and myo-tendinous junction in an overloaded skeletal muscle of the rat. *Anat Embryol (Berl).* 1988;179:89–96.

19. Curwin SL, Vailas AC, Wood J. Immature tendon adaptation to strenuous exercise. *J Appl Physiol.* 1988;65:2297–2301.

20. Michna H. Morphometric analysis of loading-induced changes in collagen-fibril populations in young tendons. *Cell Tissue Res.* 1984;236:465–470.

21. Woo SL, Ritter MA, Amiel D, et al. The biomechanical and biochemical properties of swine tendons—long term effects of exercise on the digital extensors. *Connect Tissue Res.* 1980;7:177–83.

22. Buchanan CI, Marsh RL. Effects of long-term exercise on the biomechanical properties of the Achilles tendon of guinea fowl. *J Appl Physiol.* 2001;90:164–171.

23. Rosager S, Aagaard P, Dyhre-Poulsen P, et al. Load-displacement properties of the human triceps surae aponeurosis and tendon in runners and non-runners. *Scand J Med Sci Sports.* 2002;12:90–98.

24. Hansen P, Aagaard P, Kjaer M, et al. The effect of habitual running on human Achilles tendon load-deformation properties and cross-sectional area. *J Appl Physiol.* 2003;95:2375–2380.

25. Cox JS, Nye CE, Schaefer WW, et al. The degenerative effects of partial and total resection of the medial meniscus in dogs' knees. *Clin Orthop.* 1975:178–183.

26. Klein L, Heiple KG, Torzilli PA, et al. Prevention of ligament and meniscus atrophy by active joint motion in a non-weight-bearing model. *J Orthop Res.* 1989;7:80–85.

27. Djurasovic M, Aldridge JW, Grumbles R, et al. Knee joint immobilization decreases aggrecan gene expression in the meniscus. *Am J Sports Med.* 1998;26:460–466.

28. Weinberg JB, Fermor B, Guilak F. Nitric oxide synthase and cyclooxygenase interactions in cartilage and meniscus: relationships to joint physiology, arthritis, and tissue repair. *Subcell Biochem.* 2007;42:31–62.

29. Amiel D, Abel MF, Kleiner JB, et al. Synovial fluid nutrient delivery in the diathrial joint: an analysis of rabbit knee ligaments. *J Orthop Res.* 1986;4:90–95.

30. Ochi M, Kanda T, Sumen Y, et al. Changes in the permeability and histologic findings of rabbit menisci after immobilization. *Clin Orthop.* 1997:305–315.

31. Mikic B, Johnson TL, Chhabra AB, et al. Differential effects of embryonic immobilization on the development of fibrocartilaginous skeletal elements. *J Rehabil Res Dev.* 2000;37:127–133.

32. Bray RC, Smith JA, Eng MK, et al. Vascular response of the meniscus to injury: effects of immobilization. *J Orthop Res.* 2001;19:384–390.

33. Imler SM, Doshi AN, Levenston ME. Combined effects of growth factors and static mechanical compression on meniscus explant biosynthesis. *Osteoarthritis Cartilage.* 2004;12:736–744.

34. Upton ML, Chen J, Guilak F, et al. Differential effects of static and dynamic compression on meniscal cell gene expression. *J Orthop Res.* 2003;21:963–969.

35. Pedrini-Mille A, Pedrini VA, Maynard JA, et al. Response of immature chicken meniscus to strenuous exercise: biochemical studies of proteoglycan and collagen. *J Orthop Res.* 1988;6:196–204.

36. Vailas AC, Zernicke RF, Matsuda J, et al. Adaptation of rat knee meniscus to prolonged exercise. *J Appl Physiol.* 1986;60:1031–1034.

37. Mow VC, Holmes MH, Lai WM. Fluid transport and mechanical properties of articular cartilage: a review. *J Biomech.* 1984;17:377–394.

38. Egner E. Knee joint meniscal degeneration as it relates to tissue fiber structure and mechanical resistance. *Pathol Res Pract.* 1982;173:310–324.

39. Suzuki T, Toyoda T, Suzuki H, et al. Hydrostatic pressure modulates mRNA expressions for matrix proteins in human meniscal cells. *Biorheology.* 2006;43:611–622.

40. Eifler RL, Blough ER, Dehlin JM, et al. Oscillatory fluid flow regulates glycosaminoglycan production via an intracellular calcium pathway in meniscal cells. *J Orthop Res.* 2006;24:375–384.

41. Kessler MA, Glaser C, Tittel S, et al. Recovery of the menisci and articular cartilage of runners after cessation of exercise: additional aspects of in vivo investigation based on 3-dimensional magnetic resonance imaging. *Am J Sports Med.* 2008;36:966–970.

42. Kessler MA, Glaser C, Tittel S, et al. Volume changes in the menisci and articular cartilage of runners: an in vivo investigation based on 3-D magnetic resonance imaging. *Am J Sports Med.* 2006;34:832–836.

43. Gupta T, Haut Donahue TL. Role of cell location and morphology in the mechanical environment around meniscal cells. *Acta Biomater.* 2006;2:483–492.

44. Osborn M. *A Strategy for Reserach in Space Biology and Medicine in the New Century.* Washington DC: National Academy Press; 1998.

45. Vico L, Collet P, Guignandon A, et al. Effects of long-term microgravity exposure on cancellous and cortical weight-bearing bones of cosmonauts. *Lancet.* 2000;355:1607–1611.

46. Vainionpaa A, Korpelainen R, Sievanen H, et al. Effect of impact exercise and its intensity on bone geometry at weight-bearing tibia and femur. *Bone.* 2007;40:604–611.

47. Woo SL, Kuei SC, Amiel D, et al. The effect of prolonged physical training on the properties of long bone: a study of Wolff's Law. *J Bone Joint Surg Am.* 1981;63:780–787.

48. Haapasalo H, Kannus P, Sievanen H, et al. Long-term unilateral loading and bone mineral density and content in female squash players. *Calcif Tissue Int.* 1994;54:249–255.

49. Gunter K, Baxter-Jones AD, Mirwald RL, et al. Impact exercise increases BMC during growth: an 8-year longitudinal study. *J Bone Miner Res.* 2008;23:986–993.

50. Park H, Kim KJ, Komatsu T, et al. Effect of combined exercise training on bone, body balance, and gait ability: a randomized controlled study in community-dwelling elderly women. *J Bone Miner Metab.* 2008;26:254–259.

51. Genant HK. Current state of bone densitometry for osteoporosis. *Radiographics.* 1998;18:913–918.

52. Robling AG, Hinant FM, Burr DB, et al. Improved bone structure and strength after long-term mechanical loading is greatest if loading is separated into short bouts. *J Bone Miner Res.* 2002;17:1545–1554.

53. Drinkwater BL. C. H. McCloy Research lecture: does physical activity play a role in preventing osteoporosis? *Res Q Exerc Sport.* 1994;65:197–206.

54. Beck BR, Snow CM. Bone health across the lifespan—exercising our options. *Exerc Sport Sci Rev.* 2003;31:117–122.

55. Umemura Y, Ishiko T, Yamauchi T, et al. Five jumps per day increase bone mass and breaking force in rats. *J Bone Miner Res.* 1997;12:1480–1485.

56. Turner CH, Robling AG. Designing exercise regimens to increase bone strength. *Exerc Sport Sci Rev.* 2003;31:45–50.

57. Vogt MT, Cauley JA, Kuller LH, et al. Bone mineral density and blood flow to the lower extremities: the study of osteoporotic fractures. *J Bone Miner Res.* 1997;12:283–289.

58. Burge R, Dawson-Hughes B, Solomon DH, et al. Incidence and economic burden of osteoporosis-related fractures in the United States, 2005–2025. *J Bone Miner Res.* 2007;22:465–475.

59. Greaney RB, Gerber FH, Laughlin RL, et al. Distribution and natural history of stress fractures in U.S. Marine recruits. *Radiology.* 1983;146:339–346.

60. Bennell KL, Brukner PD. Epidemiology and site specificity of stress fractures. *Clin Sports Med.* 1997;16:179–196.

61. Loucks AB. Energy availability, not body fatness, regulates reproductive function in women. *Exerc Sport Sci Rev.* 2003;31:144–148.

62. Khan KM, Liu-Ambrose T, Sran MM, et al. New criteria for female athlete triad syndrome? As osteoporosis is rare, should osteopenia be among the criteria for defining the female athlete triad syndrome? *Br J Sports Med.* 2002;36:10–13.

63. Bailey DA, Martin AD, McKay HA, et al. Calcium accretion in girls and boys during puberty: a longitudinal analysis. *J Bone Miner Res.* 2000;15:2245–2250.

64. Martin AD, Bailey DA, McKay HA, et al. Bone mineral and calcium accretion during puberty. *Am J Clin Nutr.* 1997;66:611–615.

65. Bailey DA, McKay HA, Mirwald RL, et al. A six-year longitudinal study of the relationship of physical activity to bone mineral accrual in growing children: the university of Saskatchewan bone mineral accrual study. *J Bone Miner Res.* 1999;14:1672–1679.

66. Gustavsson A, Nordstrom P, Lorentzon R, et al. Osteocalcin gene polymorphism is related to bone density in healthy adolescent females. *Osteoporos Int.* 2000;11:847–851.

67. Morrison NA, Qi JC, Tokita A, et al. Prediction of bone density from vitamin D receptor alleles. *Nature.* 1994;367:284–287.

68. Nakamura O, Ishii T, Ando Y, et al. Potential role of vitamin D receptor gene polymorphism in determining bone phenotype in young male athletes. *J Appl Physiol.* 2002;93:1973–1979.

69. Dhamrait SS, James L, Brull DJ, et al. Cortical bone resorption during exercise is interleukin-6 genotype-dependent. *Eur J Appl Physiol.* 2003;89:21–25.

70. Specker BL. Evidence for an interaction between calcium intake and physical activity on changes in bone mineral density. *J Bone Miner Res.* 1996;11:1539–1544.

71. Zernicke RF, Salem GJ, Barnard RJ, et al. Adaptations of immature trabecular bone to exercise and augmented dietary protein. *Med Sci Sports Exerc.* 1995;27:1486–1493.

72. Atteh JO, Leeson S. Effects of dietary saturated or unsaturated fatty acids and calcium levels on performance and mineral metabolism of broiler chicks. *Poult Sci.* 1984;63:2252–2260.

73. Corwin RL, Hartman TJ, Maczuga SA, et al. Dietary saturated fat intake is inversely associated with bone density in humans: analysis of NHANES III. *J Nutr.* 2006;136:159–165.

74. Lorincz CR, Manske SL, Zernicke RF. Bone health, Part 1: nutrition. *Sports Health: A Multidisciplinary Approach.* 2009;1:253–260.

75. DeFronzo RA, Cooke CR, Andres R, et al. The effect of insulin on renal handling of sodium, potassium, calcium, and phosphate in man. *J Clin Invest.* 1975;55:845–855.

76. Lemann J Jr, Lennon EJ, Piering WR, et al. Evidence that glucose ingestion inhibits net renal tubular reabsorption of calcium and magnesium in man. *J Lab Clin Med.* 1970;75:578–585.

77. Li KC, Zernicke RF, Barnard RJ, et al. Effects of a high fat-sucrose diet on cortical bone morphology and biomechanics. *Calcif Tissue Int.* 1990;47:308–313.

78. Salem GJ, Zernicke RF, Barnard RJ. Diet-related changes in mechanical properties of rat vertebrae. *Am J Physiol.* 1998;262:R318–R321.

79. Kunstel K. Calcium requirements for the athlete. *Curr Sports Med Rep.* 2005;4:203–206.

80. Lee K, Jessop H, Suswillo R, et al. Endocrinology: bone adaptation requires oestrogen receptor-alpha. *Nature.* 2003;424:389.

81. Kohrt WM, Snead DB, Slatopolsky E, et al. Additive effects of weight-bearing exercise and estrogen on bone mineral density in older women. *J Bone Miner Res.* 1995;10:1303–1311.

82. Khan K, McKay HA, Haapasalo H, et al. Does childhood and adolescence provide a unique opportunity for exercise to strengthen the skeleton? *J Sci Med Sport.* 2000;3:150–164.

83. Petit MA, McKay HA, MacKelvie KJ, et al. A randomized school-based jumping intervention confers site and maturity-specific benefits on bone structural properties in girls: a hip structural analysis study. *J Bone Miner Res.* 2002;17:363–372.

84. MacKelvie KJ, Khan KM, McKay HA. Is there a critical period for bone response to weight-bearing exercise in children and adolescents? A systematic review. *Br J Sports Med.* 2002;36:250–257; discussion 257.

85. MacKelvie KJ, Khan KM, Petit MA, et al. A school-based exercise intervention elicits substantial bone health benefits: a 2-year randomized controlled trial in girls. *Pediatrics.* 2003;112:e447.

86. MacKelvie KJ, Petit MA, Khan KM, et al. Bone mass and structure are enhanced following a 2-year randomized controlled trial of exercise in prepubertal boys. *Bone.* 2004;34:755–764.

87. Macdonald HM, Kontulainen SA, Khan KM, et al. Is a school-based physical activity intervention effective for increasing tibial bone strength in boys and girls? *J Bone Miner Res.* 2007;22:434–446.

88. Heinonen A, Sievanen H, Kannus P, et al. High-impact exercise and bones of growing girls: a 9-month controlled trial. *Osteoporos Int.* 2000;11:1010–1017.

89. Mackelvie KJ, McKay HA, Khan KM, et al. A school-based exercise intervention augments bone mineral accrual in early pubertal girls. *J Pediatr.* 2001;139:501–508.

90. Manske SL, Lorincz CR, Zernicke RF. Bone health, Part 2: physical activity. *Sports Health: A Multidisciplinary Approach.* 2009;1:341–346.

91. Heaney RP. Calcium, dairy products and osteoporosis. *J Am Coll Nutr.* 2000;19:83S–99S.

92. Bonaiuti D, Shea B, Iovine R, et al. Exercise for preventing and treating osteoporosis in postmenopausal women. *Cochrane database of systematic reviews.* 2002;2002:CD000333.

93. Martyn-St James M, Carroll S. High-intensity resistance training and postmenopausal bone loss: a meta-analysis. *Osteoporos Int.* 2006;17:1225–1240.

94. Fritton SP, McLeod KJ, Rubin CT. Quantifying the strain history of bone: spatial uniformity and self-similarity of low-magnitude strains. *J Biomech.* 2000;33:317–325.

95. Rubin C, Turner AS, Mallinckrodt C, et al. Mechanical strain, induced noninvasively in the high-frequency domain, is anabolic to cancellous bone, but not cortical bone. *Bone.* 2002;30:445–452.

96. Xie L, Rubin C, Judex S. Enhancement of the adolescent murine musculoskeletal system using low-level mechanical vibrations. *J Appl Physiol.* 2008;104:1056–1062.

97. Gilsanz V, Wren TA, Sanchez M, et al. Low-level, high-frequency mechanical signals enhance musculoskeletal development of young women with low BMD. *J Bone Miner Res.* 2006;21:1464–1474.

98. Rubin C, Recker R, Cullen D, et al. Prevention of postmenopausal bone loss by a low-magnitude, high-frequency mechanical stimuli: a clinical trial assessing compliance, efficacy, and safety. *J Bone Miner Res.* 2004;19:343–351.

99. Ward K, Alsop C, Caulton J, et al. Low magnitude mechanical loading is osteogenic in children with disabling conditions. *J Bone Miner Res.* 2004;19:360–369.

100. Judex S, Gupta S, Rubin C. Regulation of mechanical signals in bone. *Orthod Craniofac Res.* 2009;12:94–104.

101. Gross TS, Edwards JL, McLeod KJ, et al. Strain gradients correlate with sites of periosteal bone formation. *J Bone Miner Res.* 1997;12:982–988.

102. Judex S, Gross TS, Zernicke RF. Strain gradients correlate with sites of exercise-induced bone-forming surfaces in the adult skeleton. *J Bone Miner Res.* 1997;12:1737–1745.

103. Otter MW, Palmieri VR, Wu DD, et al. A comparative analysis of streaming potentials in vivo and in vitro. *J Orthop Res.* 1992;10:710–719.

104. Duncan RL, Turner CH. Mechanotransduction and the functional response of bone to mechanical strain. *Calcif Tissue Int.* 1995;57:344–358.

105. Burger EH, Klein-Nulend J, van der Plas A, et al. Function of osteocytes in bone—their role in mechanotransduction. *J Nutr.* 1995;125:2020S–2023S.

106. Reilly GC, Haut TR, Yellowley CE, et al. Fluid flow induced PGE2 release by bone cells is reduced by glycocalyx degradation whereas calcium signals are not. *Biorheology.* 2003;40:591–603.

107. Tatsumi S, Ishii K, Amizuka N, et al. Targeted ablation of osteocytes induces osteoporosis with defective mechanotransduction. *Cell Metab.* 2007;5:464–475.

108. Wang N, Naruse K, Stamenovic D, et al. Mechanical behavior in living cells consistent with the tensegrity model. *Proc Natl Acad Sci U S A.* 2001;98:7765–7770.

109. Smalt R, Mitchell FT, Howard RL, et al. Mechanotransduction in bone cells: induction of nitric oxide and prostaglandin synthesis by fluid shear stress, but not by mechanical strain. *Adv Exp Med Biol.* 1997;433:311–314.

110. Wang Y, McNamara LM, Schaffler MB, et al. A model for the role of integrins in flow induced mechanotransduction in osteocytes. *Proc Natl Acad Sci U S A.* 2007;104:15941–15946.

111. Fukada E, Yasuda I. On the piezoelectric effect of bone. *Journal of the Physical Society of Japan.* 1957;12:1158–1162.

112. Ahn AC, Grodzinsky AJ. Relevance of collagen piezoelectricity to "Wolff's Law": a critical review. *Med Eng Phys.* 2009.

113. Vatsa A, Breuls RG, Semeins CM, et al. Osteocyte morphology in fibula and calvaria—is there a role for mechanosensing? *Bone.* 2008;43:452–458.

114. Ponik SM, Triplett JW, Pavalko FM. Osteoblasts and osteocytes respond differently to oscillatory and unidirectional fluid flow profiles. *J Cell Biochem.* 2007;100:794–807.

115. Weinbaum S, Cowin SC, Zeng Y. A model for the excitation of osteocytes by mechanical loading-induced bone fluid shear stresses. *J Biomech.* 1994;27:339–360.

116. Anderson EJ, Knothe Tate ML. Idealization of pericellular fluid space geometry and dimension results in a profound underprediction of nano-microscale stresses imparted by fluid drag on osteocytes. *J Biomech.* 2008;41:1736–1746.

117. Lansman JB. Endothelial mechanosensors. Going with the flow. *Nature.* 1988;331:481–482.

118. Barakat AI, Davies PF. Mechanisms of shear stress transmission and transduction in endothelial cells. *Chest.* 1998;114:5S–563S.

119. McAllister TN, Du T, Frangos JA. Fluid shear stress stimulates prostaglandin and nitric oxide release in bone marrow-derived preosteoclast-like cells. *Biochem Biophys Res Commun.* 2000;270:643–648.

120. Genetos DC, Kephart CJ, Zhang Y, et al. Oscillating fluid flow activation of gap junction hemichannels induces ATP release from MLO-Y4 osteocytes. *J Cell Physiol.* 2007;212:207–214.

121. Cherian PP, Siller-Jackson AJ, Gu S, et al. Mechanical strain opens connexin 43 hemichannels in osteocytes: a novel mechanism for the release of prostaglandin. *Mol Biol Cell.* 2005;16:3100–3106.

122. Kowalchuk RM, Pollack SR. Stress-generated potentials in bone: effects of bone fluid composition and kinetics. *J Orthop Res.* 1993;11:874–883.

123. Knothe Tate ML, Niederer P, Knothe U. In vivo tracer transport through the lacunocanalicular system of rat bone in an environment devoid of mechanical loading. *Bone.* 1998;22:107–117.

124. Goulet GC, Hamilton N, Cooper D, et al. Influence of vascular porosity on fluid flow and nutrient transport in loaded cortical bone. *J Biomech.* 2008;41:2169–2175.

125. Bullough PG, Munuera L, Murphy J, et al. The strength of the menisci of the knee as it relates to their fine structure. *J Bone Joint Surg Br.* 1970;52:564–567.

126. Modlesky CM, Lewis RD. Does exercise during growth have a long-term effect on bone health? *Exerc Sport Sci Rev.* 2002;30:171–176.

127. Qin YX, Rubin CT, McLeod KJ. Nonlinear dependence of loading intensity and cycle number in the maintenance of bone mass and morphology. *J Orthop Res.* 1998;16:482–489.

CHAPTER 4

The Muscular System: Structural and Functional Plasticity

Vincent J. Caiozzo

Abbreviations

a	Constant used in the Hill equation, having units of force	$ML \cdot s^{-1}$	Muscle lengths per second
ADP	Adenosine diphosphate	mRNA	Messenger RNA
ATP	Adenosine triphosphate	O_2	Molecular oxygen
ATPase	Adenosine triphosphatase	P	Tension
b	Constant used in the Hill equation, having units of velocity	P_0	Maximal isometric tension
		P_t	Twitch tension
cTnC	Cardiac isoform of troponin-C	pCa^{++}	Concentration of Ca^{++} using an inverse log scale
DHPR	Dihydropyridine receptor		
dP/dt	Change in tension as a function of time	pCa^{++}_{50}	Concentration of Ca^{++} that produces 50% of P_0
ε	Strain		
E	Elastic modulus	PEVK	Region of titin molecule believed to act as a molecular spring
EO	Extraocular MHC isoform		
F_0	Subunit of the mitochondrial proton pump that acts as proton channel	P_i	Inorganic phosphate
		PLB	Phospholamban
F_1	Subunit of the mitochondrial proton pump	½ RT	One-half relaxation time
F-actin	Filamentous actin	ROS	Reactive oxygen species
FDL	Flexor digitorum longus	RyR	Ryanodine receptor
FFA	Free fatty acids	S1 fragment	Subfragment-1 the globular head of the MHC
FG	Fast glycolytic fiber type		
FOG	Fast oxidative glycolytic fiber type	S2 fragment	Subfragment-2
fTnC	Fast isoform of troponin-C	SERCA	Ca^{++}-ATPase pump of the sarcoplasmic reticulum of which there are two isoforms known as SERCA1 and SERCA2a
G-actin	Globular actin		
Hz	Hertz; cycles per second		
k	Stiffness	SO	Slow oxidative fiber type
L_0	Optimal muscle length at which P_0 occurs	SR	Sarcoplasmic reticulum
		SRS	Short range stiffness
mDa	Megadaltons	σ	Stress
MHC	Myosin heavy chain	TPT	Time-to-peak tension
MLC	Myosin light chain	V	Velocity
MLC_1	Essential light chain of which there is both a slow ($sMLC_1$) and fast ($fMLC_1$) isoform	V_{muscle}	Shortening velocity of whole muscle
		V_0	Maximal unloaded shortening velocity as determined by the slack test
MLC_2	Regulatory light chain of which there is both a slow ($sMLC_2$) and fast ($fMLC_2$) isoform		
		V_{max}	Maximal shortening velocity as determined by extrapolation of the force–velocity relationship
MLC_3	Fast essential light chain that is also referred to as $fMLC_3$		

Introduction

Within the field of physiology, there are a number of fundamental principles. Some of these key principles are (a) homeostasis, (b) the linkage between gene expression and physiology, and (c) structure–function relationships. It is this latter principle that forms the foundation of the current chapter. The concept of structure–function relationships extends across the organism-to-molecule spectrum. At the organism level, one can think about a number of examples. For instance, the structural relationship between the glenoid fossa and the head of the humerus gives the shoulder six degrees of motion—a motion that is uncommon among other joints. At the molecular level, one can think about the structure of myosin heavy chains (MHCs) and how this translates into certain functional properties like the force–velocity relationship.

The discipline of exercise physiology really represents a subdiscipline or an extension of the field of physiology; and, as such, the fundamental principles are essentially the same except that they are examined typically under conditions where physical activity has been altered. In this context, a great deal of interest has been given to understanding the effects of both activity and inactivity on the structural and functional properties of skeletal muscle during the past 30 to 35 years.

Of any cell/tissue type, skeletal muscle certainly exhibits some of the clearest structure–function relationships. Given this perspective, one of the key objectives of this chapter is to provide a backdrop for some of the more detailed discussions that follow in successive chapters. The current chapter is organized into three distinct sections. The first section provides an overview of some of the key structural properties of skeletal muscle (macroscopic to molecular anatomy). The second part of the chapter addresses the linkage between structure and function and the topic of skeletal muscle plasticity as influenced by altered physical activity. The final section of this chapter examines issues of muscle plasticity from a comparative perspective and introduces the concept of symmorphosis, a concept related to the optimality of design.

The Macroscopic and Molecular Anatomy of Skeletal Muscle

Overview

This section provides a brief overview of some of the key anatomical and structural features of skeletal muscle (Figs. 4.1 to 4.3). For the purposes of this chapter, however, the main story is illustrated in Figure 4.2. There are three fundamental processes that ultimately determine the amount of work and power that can be produced across a broad spectrum of activities. The three fundamental processes are (a) Ca^{++} cycling, (b) crossbridge cycling, and (c) cellular respiration. From a temporal perspective, it is only the first of these two

processes that is important during activities that are relatively short in duration. However, as the duration of physical activity begins to extend beyond several minutes, cellular respiration becomes progressively more important in meeting the energetic demands of both crossbridge cycling and Ca^{++} cycling. Therefore, extensive structural information about each of these three processes is included in Figure 4.2.

The Macroscopic Anatomy of Skeletal Muscle

As with most tissues, the structural anatomy of skeletal muscle is quite complex; however, the degree of structural organization in skeletal muscle is unsurpassed by any other tissue. This complexity is illustrated in both Figs. 4.1 and 4.2, which provide a macroscopic to microscopic perspective. Skeletal muscles are composed of individual cells also known as muscle fibers. The numbers and sizes of these fibers can differ significantly from one muscle to another. Skeletal muscles that are typically responsible for generating large forces contain thousands of individual muscle fibers, whereas those muscles that are involved in fine motor control typically have far fewer fibers. Muscle fibers are packaged into small bundles of fibers (~10–40 fibers per bundle) that are known as fascicles, and these fascicles are encased in a connective tissue sheath known as the endomysium.

From an architectural perspective, muscles are often classified on the basis of the orientations of the muscle fibers' longitudinal axes relative to that of the entire muscle. For instance, longitudinal muscles are composed of muscle fibers whose longitudinal axis runs parallel to that of the whole muscle. Good examples of this type of architecture are the rectus abdominis and the sartorius muscles. In fusiform muscles, the fibers run parallel to the longitudinal axis throughout most of the muscle, but taper at the ends of the muscle. The soleus and brachioradialis muscles are typical of this architecture. Muscles can also exhibit a so-called pennate (unipennate, bipennate) architecture whereby the longitudinal axis of the individual muscle fibers runs diagonal to that of the whole muscle. A good example of a bipennate muscle is the gastrocnemius muscle. The muscle fibers of angular or fan-shaped muscles radiate from a narrow attachment at one end and fan out, resulting in a broad attachment at the other end as is seen in muscles like the pectoralis major.

As noted previously, the primary theme of this chapter is related to structure–function relationships, and, in this context, muscle architecture can be an important determinant of muscle function. For instance, muscles that have a fusiform architecture will have muscle fibers that are typically longer than those found in bipennate muscles. The functional consequence of such an architectural design is that the fusiform muscle will be able to shorten and lengthen to a greater degree than the bipennate muscle and, assuming similar crossbridge cycling rates, will be able to generate much higher shortening velocities. Conversely, the structural advantage of the bipennate design is that it optimizes the physiologic cross-sectional area of

Key Features

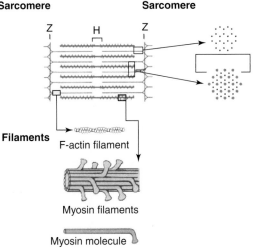

Muscle

Epimysium   Fascicle   Muscle   Tendon

Muscles are really a tissue, composed of many different cell types. Some of these include muscle fibers (cells), vascular cells, fibroblasts, and satellite cells.

Fascicle

Part of a fascicle

Muscle fiber (cell)

Perimysium

Skeletal muscle fibers (cells) are organized into bundles known as fascicles. Each bundle contains tens of fibers.

Muscle fiber (cell)

Nucleus

Myofibril

Part of a muscle fiber   Striations

Each skeletal muscle fiber is an individual cell, and they are primarily composed of a large number of cylinders known as myofibrils. Human muscle fibers have cross-sectional areas that range from ~3000–6000 mm^2. The majority of the cell volume is occupied by myofibrils, with the SR and mitochondrial volumes accounting for ~10% of the cell volume.

Myofibril

Sarcomere

Z   Z

Myofibril

H zone   A band   I band

Each myofibril runs the entire length of the fiber, and they are made up of repeating contractile units known as sarcomeres that are in series with one another. Each myofibril has a cross-sectional area of ~1–2 μm^2. Therefore, there are ~5000 myofibrils in a muscle with a cross-sectional area of 5000 μm^2. Myofibrils make-up ~85%–90% of the total cell volume.

Sarcomere   **Sarcomere**

Z   H   Z

Sarcomeres are building blocks used to assemble myofibrils. Sarcomeres are sometimes referred to as contractile units of skeletal muscle. Number of sarcomeres in parallel determines the maximal force, whereas the number in series determines length excursion and shortening velocity. Typical sarcomere is 2.5 mm long, and there are ~40,000 in series in a muscle fiber 100 mm in length.

Filaments

F-actin filament

Myosin filaments

Myosin molecule

The major filaments associated with the sarcomere are the thick and thin filaments. Each thin filament is composed of an actin filament and its associated regulatory contractile proteins (Tm, TnT, TnI, and TnC). Each thick filament is primarily composed of ~300 native myosin molecules.

FIGURE 4.1   Illustration of macroscopic to microscopic anatomy of skeletal muscle.

the muscle, meaning that there are a greater number of muscle fibers and sarcomeres in parallel. Therefore, the bipennate design is better optimized for the production of force rather than high shortening velocities.

Molecular Anatomy of the Myofibril

Looking at Figs. 4.1 and 4.2, it is clear that the structure of skeletal muscle at the molecular level is quite complex. Each muscle fiber is made up of thousands of myofibrils that are

arranged in parallel to one another. Each myofibril has a cross-sectional area of approximately 1 to 2 μm^2 and, therefore, a muscle fiber with a cross-sectional area of ~1000 μm^2 would contain about ~1000 myofibrils (for simplicity, the relative volumes of the sarcoplasmic reticulum [SR] and mitochondria are not included in this estimate). Typically, the cross-sectional area of a muscle fiber can range from ~1000 to 7000 μm^2. Each myofibril runs the entire length of a muscle fiber and consists of a repeating series of striations that are due to the arrangement of so-called sarcomeres in series.

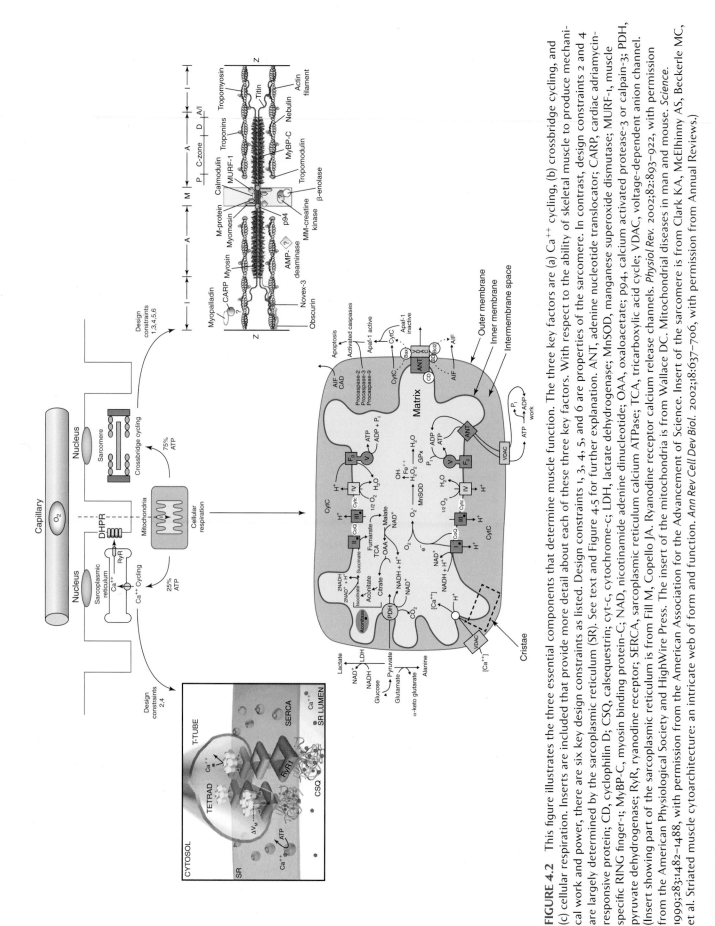

FIGURE 4.2   This figure illustrates the three essential components that determine muscle function. The three key factors are (a) Ca^{++} cycling, (b) crossbridge cycling, and (c) cellular respiration. Inserts are included that provide more detail about each of these three key factors. With respect to the ability of skeletal muscle to produce mechanical work and power, there are six key design constraints as listed. Design constraints 1, 3, 4, 5, and 6 are properties of the sarcomere. In contrast, design constraints 2 and 4 are largely determined by the sarcoplasmic reticulum (SR). See text and Figure 4-5 for further explanation. ANT, adenine nucleotide translocator; CARP, cardiac adriamycin-responsive protein; CD, cyclophilin D; CSQ, calsequestrin; cyt-c, cytochrome-c; LDH, lactate dehydrogenase; MnSOD, manganese superoxide dismutase; MURF-1, muscle specific RING finger-1; MyBP-C, myosin binding protein-C; NAD, nicotinamide adenine dinucleotide; OAA, oxaloacetate; p94, calcium activated protease-3 or calpain-3; PDH, pyruvate dehydrogenase; RyR, ryanodine receptor; SERCA, sarcoplasmic reticulum calcium ATPase; TCA, tricarboxylic acid cycle; VDAC, voltage-dependent anion channel. (Insert showing part of the sarcoplasmic reticulum is from Fill M, Copello JA. Ryanodine receptor calcium release channels. *Physiol Rev.* 2002;82:893–922, with permission from the American Physiological Society and HighWire Press. The insert of the mitochondria is from Wallace DC. Mitochondrial diseases in man and mouse. *Science.* 1999;283:1482–1488, with permission from the American Association for the Advancement of Science. Insert of the sarcomere is from Clark KA, McElhinny AS, Beckerle MC, et al. Striated muscle cytoarchitecture: an intricate web of form and function. *Ann Rev Cell Dev Biol.* 2002;18:637–706, with permission from Annual Reviews.)

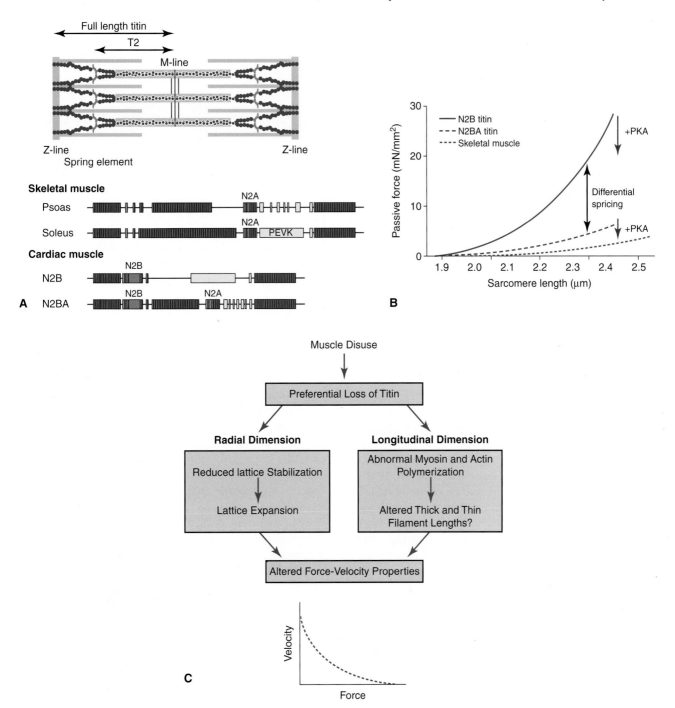

FIGURE 4.3   A. Key features of titin and its association with the thick and thin filament. As noted in the text, titin can be thought to represent a third filament, complementing the function of the thick and thin filaments. Note that the spring elements of titin are located in the I-band. The various domains are also shown in (**A**) and note the key differences between slow (soleus), fast (psoas), and cardiac isoforms. (*Dark blue*, Ig domain; *light blue*, PEVC domain; blue represents unique sequences.) **B.** Relationship between passive force and sarcomere length. Note the importance of the different isoforms and how this influences the passive mechanical properties of a sarcomere. **C.** Effects of muscle disuse on titin and how this has the potential to influence both the radial and longitudinal structure of a sarcomere. By reducing the stabilization of the lattice, losses in titin will presumably result in greater distances between thick and thin filaments with the potential to influence both force production and maximal shortening velocity.

Sarcomeres are often referred to as the contractile units of skeletal muscle and each sarcomere is approximately 2.5 μm in length. In a muscle fiber that is 100 mm in length (as in the human brachioradialis muscle), each myofibril would consist of ~40,000 sarcomeres in-series. If it is assumed that each myofibril has a cross-sectional area of 1 μm^2 and that the muscle fiber has a cross-sectional area of 5000 μm^2, then the muscle fiber contains ~200,000,000 sarcomeres!

TEST YOURSELF

Think about a muscle fiber with more than 200,000,000 sarcomeres and describe the underlying mechanisms that are responsible for synchronizing their actions with one another. What would happen if all sarcomeres were not activated simultaneously? Although the on/off status of sarcomeres might be synchronized, describe the behavior of sarcomeres under different types of conditions (e.g., hoping). Also, describe some cutting-edge approaches for studying sarcomere dynamics in vivo.

From a very basic perspective, sarcomeres consist of Z-lines, thin filaments, and thick filaments. The interdigitation of thick and thin filaments along with the presence of Z-lines is responsible for the striation pattern of skeletal muscle. As shown in Figure 4.1, the Z-lines are dense thin structures that are found in the middle of the I-band. In reality, each Z-line represents an anchor point to which thin filaments are attached. The I-band represents a region where there is no overlap of the thin filaments (by thick filaments), yielding a relatively light band. The A-band is composed of the thick filament and is strongly birefringent, producing a dark band on microscopic inspection. The length of the A-band is equivalent to the length of the thick filament. Normally, there is a partial overlap between the thick and thin filaments and, as a result, there is a lighter region in the middle of the A-band known as the H-zone.

Changes in sarcomere length and, as a result, muscle fiber length are due to the sliding of the thick and thin filaments relative to one another. In its most simplistic sense, this model states that contraction takes place not because of changes in the individual lengths of thick and thin filaments, but rather by the sliding of thin filaments past thick filaments. This model of contraction is known as the sliding-filament hypothesis (1).

Molecular Anatomy of the Sarcomere

The ultrastructure of the sarcomere is quite complex (see Figs. 4.1 and 4.2), and the numbers of thick and thin filaments found within a given sarcomere basically illustrates this point. Each Z-line has a cross-sectional area of ~1 to 2 μm^2, and attached to each Z-line are ~3000 to 6000 individual thin filaments (thin filament density of ~3000/μm^2).

In turn, there are approximately ~1000 to 2000 thick filaments (thick filament density of ~1000/μm^2) associated with the larger number of thin filaments. This yields a thin-to-thick filament ratio of 3:1.

KEY POINT

When one begins to consider the factors that are responsible for keeping sarcomeres in register, maintaining the organization of the sarcomere during force production and load bearing, and regulating the necessary pool of proteins, it is clear that the sarcomere is incredibly complex.

For many years, the numbers of proteins thought to be associated with the sarcomere were relatively few. However, over the course of the past 10 years, the list of proteins associated with the sarcomere has grown significantly (see Fig. 4.2 and Table 4.1). For a better appreciation of this, the reader is referred to the excellent article by Clark et al. (2). From a fundamental perspective, the proteins associated with the sarcomere can be categorized into three groups: (a) contractile proteins, (b) regulatory contractile proteins, and (c) structural and costameric proteins.

Actin and myosin are often referred to as contractile proteins, given their central role in the contractile process. Individual monomers of actin (globular form of actin; G-actin) bind to one another to form so-called actin filaments (F-actin). The thick filament is composed primarily of MHC molecules packed in an anti-parallel arrangement. A more detailed description of myosin is provided later in the section *Anatomy of the Molecular Motor*.

Regulatory contractile proteins are defined as those that turn on/off the contractile apparatus and those that can modulate the activity of the MHC. In skeletal muscle, the regulatory contractile proteins involved in turning on/off the contractile apparatus are associated exclusively with the actin filament and these proteins include tropomyosin, troponin-T, troponin-I, and troponin-C. Collectively, the thin filament is composed of the actin filament and these (i.e., tropomyosin, troponin-T, troponin-I, and troponin-C) regulatory contractile proteins. The myosin light chains (MLCs) are also classified as regulatory contractile proteins and they are associated with the lever arm of the MHC (see *Anatomy of the Molecular Motor*). Although there is some debate over the precise role of MLCs in skeletal muscle, several studies have shown that they can modulate the kinetics of crossbridge cycling (3,4).

Structural and costameric proteins play several essential roles. Electron micrographs demonstrate that sarcomeres are organized in a very orderly fashion such that the Z-lines of adjoining sarcomeres seem to be in register with one another. Intermediate filaments like desmin and vimentin are believed to play key roles in aligning the Z-line of adjacent sarcomeres. Other proteins like synemin are also

TABLE 4.1   Overview of Key Proteins Involved With the Sarcomere and Cytoskeletal–Extracellular Matrix Interactions in Skeletal Muscle

Classes and Types of Sarcomeric Proteins	Molecular Wt (kDa)	Isoforms	Location	Function
Contractile Proteins				
Myosin heavy chain	~200	~9	Thick filament	Molecular motor; binds to actin; generates force and length change
Embryonic				
Neonatal				
Slow type Iβ cardiac				
Slow type Iα cardiac				
Fast type IIA				
Fast type IIX				
Fast type IIB				
Extraocular/type IIL				
Superfast type IIM				
Actin	~42		Thin filament	Binds myosin and translates force and/or length changes
Regulatory contractile proteins				
Tropomyosin	~37	>3	Thin filament	Regulates interaction between actin and myosin; stabilizes thin filament
Troponin-T	~30	>6	Thin filament	Couples troponin complex to actin?
Troponin-I	~22	2	Thin filament	Influences position of tropomyosin
Troponin-C	~18	2	Thin filament	Binds Ca^{++}; influences position of tropomyosin
Cardiac/slow TnC				
Fast TnC				
Myosin light chain-1	~22	2	Thick filament	Influences V_{max}
Slow MLC1				
Fast MLC1				
Myosin light chain-2	~20	2	Thick filament	Influences tension–pCa^{++} relationship
Slow MLC2				
Fast MLC2				
Myosin light chain-3	~18	1	Thick filament	Influences V_{max}
Fast MLC3				
Structural proteins associated with thin filament				
CapZ-α, CapZ-β	~36, ~32	2	Z-line	Caps free end of actin, regulates actin filament length; binds to α-actinin
Tropomodulin	~40	2	Thin filament	Caps pointed end of actin filament
Nebulin	~600–900	+2	I-band	Anchors actin to Z-line; molecular ruler of actin filament length?
Associated with thick filament				
Myosin binding protein-C	~140	2	Thick filament	Binds to lever arm and rod region; titin binding site
Myomesin	~185	2	M-line	Binds to myosin and titin; may play a role in linking myosin and titin
MurF-1	~40		M-line	May play key role in degradation
Calpain-3; p94		2	M-line	Binds to titin
Titin	~3000–4000	+2	Spans A-I bands	Molecular spring? Sarcomere template?

(continued)

TABLE 4.1	Overview of Key Proteins Involved With the Sarcomere and Cytoskeletal–Extracellular Matrix Interactions in Skeletal Muscle *(continued)*			
Classes and Types of Sarcomeric Proteins	Molecular Wt (kDa)	Isoforms	Location	Function
Associated with Z-line				
α-Actinin	~97	2	Z-line	Major protein of Z-line
LIM	~23	+2	Z-line	Binds α-actinin, zyxin, β-spectrin
FATZ	~32		Z-line	Binds calcineurin to Z-line
Intermediate filaments				
Desmin	~53		Z-line	Longitudinal and lateral alignment of sarcomeres
Skelemin	~200		M-band	M-line integrity
Vimentin	~53		Z-line	Periodicity of Z-lines
Costameric proteins				
Ankyrin	17–440	Many	Costamere	Localization
α-Dystrobrevin	~87	2	Costamere	Membrane stabilization; transmembrane signaling involved with NOS
α/β-Dystroglycan	~156, 43	2	Costamere	Prevents injury to sarcolemma
Dystrophin	427		Costamere	Stabilizes cytoskeleton and sarcolemma
α-Fodrin	85		Costamere	Attachment of cytoskeleton to ECM; signaling
Integrins	~90 and 150	Many	Costamere	Stabilization of cytoskeleton
α-Sarcoglycan	~240		Costamere	Binds dystrophin and α-dystrobrevin; associated with NOS
α/β-Spectrin	~250	+2	Costamere	Stabilization of sarcomere
Syntrophins	~57–60	3	Costamere	NOS?
Talin	~235		Costamere-MTJ	Role in stabilizing link between muscle fiber and tendon fibrils?
Vinculin	116	3	Costamere, MTJ	Role in stabilizing link between muscle fiber and tendon fibrils?

ECM, extracellular matrix; FATZ, γ-filamin-, α-actinin-, and telethonin-binding protein of the Z-disc; MLC, myosin light chain; MTJ, myotendinous junction; NOS, nitric oxide synthase.

thought to be involved in the alignment of sarcomeres. Structural proteins also play a key role in developing a mechanical linkage between sarcomeres and the extracellular matrix. These sites of connectivity between the sarcomere–cell membrane–extracellular matrix have been referred to as costameres, and there is a growing list of proteins associated with these complexes (see Table 4.1). Some of these proteins include dystrophin and the integrins.

Titin as a third filament

The existence of both the thin and thick filaments has been known for ~50 years. During the past 15 to 20 years, however, it has been clear that there is a third filamentous structure composed of titin, which is the third most common sarcomeric protein. Although myosin and actin account for the main contractile features of skeletal muscle, it is titin that seems to play a key role in dictating the passive elastic properties of skeletal muscle. In this context, slow muscles appear to have longer Ig and PEVK regions (the so-called spring regions of titin that are located in the I-band; see Fig. 4.3A and B) and this is thought to result in lower passive force in the slower muscle fibers. Just as intriguing is the role that titin plays in defining the overall lattice structure of the sarcomere and how titin may be a major target of muscle disuse. Figure 4.3C illustrates a scheme developed by Fukuda et al. (5), which highlights the central role that titin may play in modulating the loss of function that occurs with muscle disuse. Specifically, titin has the potential to influence both the radial dimensions of the lattice and the length of thick and thin filaments.

Anatomy of the Molecular Motor

The term *myosin molecule* is used commonly in conjunction with descriptions of the molecular motor. As has been documented in a number of publications (6–8), the myosin molecule is really in reference to the so-called native molecule, which is a hexameric complex that is composed of six proteins. The primary nomenclature used to describe each of these six proteins is based on their molecular weights. Two of the six proteins that make up the native myosin molecule are known as MHCs because they have the heaviest molecular weights (~200 kDa) of any of the proteins making up the native myosin molecule. Each MHC is associated with one essential MLC (MLC_1 or MLC_3) and one regulatory MLC (MLC_2). Each MHC is made up of (a) a long rod region; (b) subfragment-2 (S2); and (c) a globular head (also known as subfragment-1; S1). The rod region of the MHC is important from a structural perspective because it determines the packing of MHCs within the thick filament, with each thick filament composed of ~300 individual MHCs. In contrast, the globular head is directly involved in binding to actin and generating force and/or length steps. The globular head consists of three domains known as (a) the catalytic domain, (b) the converter domain, and (c) the lever arm. The catalytic domain contains sites involved with binding actin, binding adenosine triphosphate (ATP), and hydrolyzing ATP. The converter region is currently thought to be involved with the transduction of energy, whereas the lever arm transports the load. Mutations within the globular head are believed to play a key role in serious cardiomyopathies such as familial hypertrophic cardiomyopathy. Each MHC has one essential and one regulatory light chain bound to the S1 fragment. Finally, consider that within a single fiber from a human brachioradialis muscle, there are ~200,000,000 sarcomeres; that each sarcomere consists of ~1000 thick filaments; and that each thick filament consists of ~300 individual MHCs. The dimensions of the system reflect its complexity: ~10^{13} to 10^{14} individual MHC molecules per single fiber.

The diversity of the native myosin molecule is further complicated by the presence of isoforms for both the MHCs and MLCs. From a mechanical perspective, it has been known for quite some time that muscles could be categorized as slow and fast. During the course of the past 20 years, it has been shown (at various levels) that the speed related properties of skeletal muscle are due primarily to the existence of different MHC isoforms and that the kinetics of crossbridge cycling can be secondarily modulated by MLC isoforms (3,4). The various MHC isoforms that have been identified to date are shown in Table 4.1. As shown in this table, the main nomenclature used to classify fiber types is linked to the MHC isoform composition of that fiber. This seems quite appropriate given that the ultimate design constraint of the skeletal muscle is the force–velocity relationship and that the shape of this relationship is really dependent on the kinetics of crossbridge cycling. In small adult mammals, the primary MHC isoforms found throughout most of the body are known as the slow type I, fast type IIA, fast type IIX, and fast type IIB MHC isoforms (in order of their ATPase activity). In humans, it is

currently thought that only the first three MHC isoforms are expressed. The absence of the fastest MHC isoform (type IIB) in adult human skeletal muscle seems to be consistent with some allometric (scaling) considerations that might govern the speed of limb movement. Other adult MHC isoforms have been found in muscles associated with the larynx (EO/type IIL), mastication (superfast type IIM), and movement of the eyes (EO). Two developmental MHC isoforms have been found in mammalian skeletal muscle and these are referred to as the embryonic (E) and neonatal (NEO) MHC isoforms. Finally, the hearts of both small mammals and humans are known to express two cardiac MHC isoforms: the β- and α-cardiac MHC isoforms. The β-cardiac MHC isoform is also known as the slow type I MHC isoform. Collectively, a total of eight to nine different MHC isoforms have been reported in skeletal muscle.

Several nomenclatures have been developed for describing the various MLCs. The most prevalent terminology is based simply on electrophoretic migration of the MLCs, giving rise to the terms MLC_1, MLC_2, and MLC_3. Both MLC_1 and MLC_3 can also be categorized as so-called essential light chains, implying that their presence is "essential" for myosin ATPase activity. In reality, the term *essential light chain* is a misnomer in skeletal muscle because the absence of these MLCs does not inhibit the ability to hydrolyze ATP. From a historical perspective, MLC_2 was initially classified as a regulatory light chain, meaning that its phosphorylation influenced or regulated crossbridge cycling. Clearly, in smooth muscle, the phosphorylation of MLC_2 is critical; however, in skeletal muscle, it appears to be relatively unimportant. As with the MHCs, there are also MLC isoforms. There are both slow and fast isoforms of MLC_1 ($sMLC_1$; $fMLC_1$) and MLC_2 ($sMLC_2$, $fMLC_2$), whereas only one type (a fast isoform) of MLC_3 ($fMLC_3$) isoform has been identified.

In thinking about the various types of MHC and MLC isoforms and how they might be arranged within a native myosin molecule, it becomes obvious that there are many possible combinations, as was discussed in some detail by Pette and Staron (7). It should also be noted that there are fast and slow isoforms of other sarcomeric proteins such as tropomyosin, troponin-T, troponin-I, and troponin-C (see Table 4.1). (For further development of this idea, see later section *Muscle Fiber Types and Polymorphism*.)

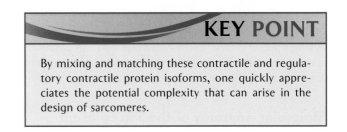

KEY POINT

By mixing and matching these contractile and regulatory contractile protein isoforms, one quickly appreciates the potential complexity that can arise in the design of sarcomeres.

The sequence of a crossbridge cycle is shown in Figure 4.4. In the first frame, myosin is detached from actin. Subsequently, the head of the MHC is attached to actin and releases inorganic phosphate (P_i), leading to the power stroke (change

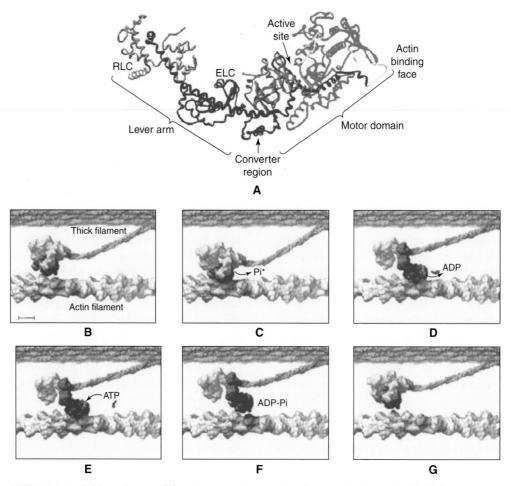

FIGURE 4.4   Ribbon diagram (**A**) and stop-motion movie of a crossbridge cycle (**B–G**). Note in Figure 4.3A that the globular head of the myocin heavy chain (MHC) consists of three key regions known as the motor domain, converter region, and lever arm. The motor domain has also been referred to as the catalytic domain, given that it is involved in the hydrolysis of adenosine triphosphate (ATP). RLC, regulatory light chain; ELC, essential light chain; ADP, adenosine diphosphate; P_i, inorganic phosphate. (Figure is from Vale RD, Milligan RA. The way things move: looking under the hood of molecular motor proteins. *Science.* 2000;288:88–95, with permission from the American Association for the Advancement of Science.)

in position of head between Fig. 4.4C and D). Following completion of the power stroke, adenosine diphosphate (ADP) is released, and subsequently ATP binds to the nucleotide-binding site (Fig. 4.4E). The hydrolysis of ATP ultimately leads to the globular head of the MHC returning to its original position. The magnitude of crossbridge cycling that occurs during a single contraction is enormous, and can approach rates equivalent to 10^{17} to 10^{18} crossbridge cycles per gram of muscle per second, quite an astonishing number!

Molecular Anatomy of the Sarcoplasmic Reticulum

The ability of skeletal muscle to perform repetitive shortening–lengthening contractions involves four fundamental processes: (a) excitation, (b) coupling, (c) contraction, and (d) relaxation. Of these four processes, the second and fourth are governed by the structure-function properties of the SR that are involved in Ca^{++} cycling.

As illustrated in Figure 4.2, the calcium release channels of the SR are in proximity to the t-tubule and this region of the SR is often referred to as the terminal cisternae. Collectively, one t-tubule and the terminal cisternae on both sides of the t-tubule are referred to as a triad. The calcium release channels of the SR are also known as ryanodine receptors (RyRs) because they selectively bind the plant alkaloid, ryanodine.

The conformational state of the RyR in skeletal muscle is regulated by the voltage-gated Ca^{++} channels found in the membrane of the t-tubule. These voltage-gated Ca^{++} channels are also known as dihydropyridine receptors (DHPRs) because they selectively bind a class of drugs with this name. The exact mechanism by which the DHPRs regulate the conformational state of the RyRs is unknown, but it is thought that there is some type of physical contact between the two proteins. As illustrated in Figure 4.2, the physical arrangement between the DHPRs and RyRs appears to be quite complex. Note that the DHPRs are arranged in so-called tetrads within the membrane of the t-tubule and that every other RyR is associated with a tetrad in fast skeletal muscle. Depolarization of the t-tubule membrane is thought to produce a conformational change in the DHPR, which then acts via direct physical contact on the RyR. The connection between the DHPR and RyR may be mediated by a cytoplasmic loop of the DHPR. One of the important features of this form of communication between the tetrad and RyR is speed, allowing Ca^{++} to be released almost immediately following depolarization.

After repolarization of the sarcolemma, the calcium-release channels (RyRs) of the SR close and Ca^{++} is sequestered via calcium ATPase pumps in the SR, otherwise known as SERCAs. The SR Ca^{++} ATPase pumps are located primarily along the longitudinal region of the SR. As with many proteins associated with the sarcomere, there are isoforms of the SERCAs, with SERCA2a found in slow skeletal muscle and SERCA1 found in fast skeletal muscle (see section entitled *Muscle Fiber Types* for the discussion of functional differences).

Molecular Anatomy of the Mitochondria

From a hierarchical perspective that simply revolves around the mechanical activity of skeletal muscle, one might think of the mitochondria as a slave to the energetic needs of the contractile apparatus and the SR. In reality, the mitochondria are involved in many other processes, some of which include the production of reactive oxygen species (ROS) and the initiation of apoptosis (programmed cell death). Both of these processes may be important in mediating muscle fiber size. Figure 4.2 illustrates some of the key features involved in these three processes (ATP production, production of ROS, and initiation of apoptosis).

The main morphologic features of the mitochondria are the (a) outer membrane; (b) the inner membrane; (c) the intermembrane space, which is located between the outer and inner membranes; (d) the cristae, which are the folds of the inner membrane that help to maximize inner membrane surface area; and (d) the matrix.

As the length of physical activity increases beyond a few seconds in duration, so does the demand on the mitochondria to provide ATP to the contractile apparatus and the SR. The production of ATP by the mitochondria involves an extensive set of biochemical and biophysical events that ultimately involves the transfer of energy from electrons to ATP. From a biochemical perspective, the Krebs cycle enzyme system (matrix) plays a key role in providing electrons that are in a high-energy state to the electron transport chain (located within the inner membrane). The electron transport chain consists of four complexes (see Fig. 4.2) that are known simply as complexes I through IV, and these participate in a set of biophysical events: (a) that move electrons from one metal ion to another; and (b) result in a drop in the energy levels of electrons, transferring (remember the first law of thermodynamics) that energy into a proton gradient across the inner membrane. The large electrochemical H^+ gradient then causes H^+ to move from the intermembrane space into the matrix via ATP synthase. The ATP synthase is composed of two major subunits known as F_0 and F_1. The F_0 subunit functions as a proton channel (see Fig. 4.2), allowing H^+ to move along their electrochemical gradient and back into the matrix. The energy stored in the proton gradient is then used to drive the synthesis of ATP via the F_1/V_1 subunit of the ATP synthase (see Fig. 4.2). The newly synthesized ATP is then exported (in exchange for ADP and inorganic phosphate) out of the mitochondria and into the sarcoplasm via the adenine nucleotide transporter (see Fig. 4.2). Ultimately, this process is dependent on the presence of O_2 given that it plays the central role in maintaining electron transport via the oxidation of cytochrome-a_3.

Collectively, the steps described here are referred to as oxidative phosphorylation, and the two major sources of fuel involved in providing electrons to the electron transport chain are pyruvate (derived from carbohydrate breakdown) and free fatty acids (FFAs). Both pyruvate and FFAs are derived from exogenous and endogenous sources. With respect to pyruvate, the major exogenous sources of carbohydrates are the circulating levels of glucose in the blood and the glycogen stored in the liver. Glycogen is also stored in muscle fibers themselves, representing a large endogenous source of carbohydrates. With respect to FFAs, the majority is found in the adipose fat stores of the body (i.e., there is a large exogenous source of FFAs). However, evidence is accumulating that an important source of FFA is derived from triglyceride stores maintained within the muscle fibers themselves.

The mitochondria in skeletal muscle are primarily located between myofibrils, and these mitochondria are typically referred to as interfibrillar or core mitochondria. These mitochondria appear to be strategically located such that there is virtually no diffusional limitation regarding the supply of ATP to the contractile apparatus. Other mitochondria are also located just below the sarcolemma and these are typically referred to as subsarcolemmal mitochondria. Currently, the functional significance of their location is unknown.

Because the mitochondria are one of the more plastic organelle systems in skeletal muscle fibers, there has been a great deal of interest in identifying a single index that can be used as a measure of cellular respiration. Some have used various biochemical markers such as succinate dehydrogenase or citrate synthase activity. Others have quantified key electron transport proteins such as cytochrome-c. Finally, some have applied morphometric measurements of mitochondrial volume density, an expression of mitochondrial volume per unit of cell volume.

TEST YOURSELF

Calculate the mass, number of moles, and number of molecules of ATP that are hydrolyzed per minute under resting conditions (assume oxygen consumption rate of 0.3 L · min⁻¹). Perform similar calculations for an individual working at a metabolic rate equivalent to an oxygen consumption rate of 3.5 L · min⁻¹. The number of ATP molecules hydrolyzed per minute should be a pretty impressive number!

Muscle Fiber Types and Polymorphism

Historical Perspective on Muscle Fiber Type Nomenclature

Many of the classic articles on muscle fiber types were written in the late 1960s and early 1970s. Some of the most highly cited of these articles were those by Brooke and Kaiser (9) and Barnard et al. (10). Brooke and Kaiser (9) employed histochemical techniques that differentiated muscle fibers on the basis of the pH lability of the myofibrillar ATPase activity of myosin. Using this approach, these investigators identified fibers as slow type I, fast type IIA, and fast type IIB. Subsequently, this nomenclature was applied to the classification of MHC isoforms and it is the dominant nomenclature currently used. This seems reasonable given that (a) the force–velocity relationship defines the maximum boundary of all forms of physical activity; and (b) the shape of the force–velocity relationship is determined primarily by the MHC isoform composition. During the early 1990s, the nomenclature developed by Brooke and Kaiser (9) was expanded to include the presence of fast type IIX fibers, which evolved from the discovery of the fast type IIX MHC isoform (8,11). The approach employed by Barnard et al. (10) attempted to develop acronyms that were more descriptive, incorporating information about both the mechanical and biochemical properties of the muscle fiber. This approach gave rise to the terms slow oxidative (SO), fast oxidative glycolytic (FOG), and fast glycolytic (FG).

Fiber Type Differences

Some of the key differences between fiber types can be found in a classic publication by Saltin and Gollnick (12), and these are summarized in Table 4.2. The brief discussion that follows below addresses these differences with respect to (a) contractile proteins, (b) Ca⁺⁺ cycling and the SR, and (c) the mitochondria.

Myosin is the molecular motor of skeletal muscle and, as such, the two main functions of myosin are to generate force and/or length changes. The forces and the rate of length change (i.e., velocity) are determined by the manner

in which sarcomeres are arranged (i.e., numbers in parallel and in series) and the type of myosin. The numbers of sarcomeres in parallel determines (to a large extent) the maximal force that a muscle fiber can generate, whereas the numbers of sarcomeres in series is a key factor that determines both excursion and the maximal shortening velocity of a muscle fiber. A broad survey of human skeletal muscles suggests that fast and slow muscle fibers do not differ markedly from one another with respect to cross-sectional area (an indirect measure of the number of sarcomeres in parallel [12]). In contrast, fast muscle fibers, in rodents, are usually much larger than slow fibers (the soleus muscle seems to be an exception to this rule). Importantly, the myofibrillar volume density seems to be very similar in both slow and fast human skeletal muscle. This basically means that slow and fast skeletal muscle fibers have the same number of sarcomeres per unit of cross-sectional area and, as a consequence, should be capable of producing the same amount of force when normalized to cross-sectional area (i.e., specific tension). Stated simply, the intrinsic ability to generate force should not be strongly dependent on fiber type. Interestingly, some single fiber studies have reported fiber type differences regarding specific tension; however, no attempt has been made to correlate such findings with whole muscle mechanics. In contrast to specific tension, the shortening velocity of skeletal muscle is highly dependent on fiber type due to the presence of slow and fast MHC isoforms, and the existence of these isoforms is responsible for approximately a threefold to fivefold difference in maximal shortening velocity.

KEY POINT

Myosin is the molecular motor of skeletal muscle and, as such, the two main functions of myosin are to generate force and/or length changes.

The ability to rapidly release and sequester Ca⁺⁺ is primarily dependent on the properties of the SR. Therefore, the SR plays a central role in determining the rates of activation, relaxation, and, as a result, the maximal frequency of oscillatory work that can be achieved. In human skeletal muscle, the SR accounts for ~2% to 6% of the cell volume, and the volume is the greatest in the fast type II fibers (~5%–6% cell volume). This finding is consistent with the more rapid relaxation rates found in fast fibers.

The release of Ca⁺⁺ from the SR is determined by the properties and types of RyRs. A number of RyRs have been identified and classified as RyR1, RyR2, and RyR3. The dominant form found in both slow and fast skeletal muscle is RyR1. RyR2 plays the central role in cardiac muscle and RyR3 appears to be ubiquitously distributed in a number of tissues/cell types. Unlike the other two isoforms, RyR1 plays a fundamental role in excitation–contraction coupling in the absence of extracellular Ca⁺⁺, and this has been referred to as

TABLE 4.2	Key Properties of Fiber Types With Emphasis on Human Skeletal Muscle		
Structural or Functional Property	Slow Type I	Fast Type IIA	Fast Type IIX
Speed-related contractile properties			
TPT	Slow	Fast	Fastest
½ RT	Slow	Fast	Fastest
K_{TR}	Slow	Fast	Fastest
V_{max}	Slow	Fast	Fastest
V_o	Slow	Fast	Fastest
Force-related contractile properties			
P_o	Same?	Same?	Same?
E	?	?	?
Tension-pCa^{++} relationship	Left	Right	Right
Pca^{++}_{SO}	High	Low	Low
Fatigue-related contractile properties	Fatigue resistant	Moderately fatigable	Highly fatigable
Contractile-related proteins			
MHC isoform	Slow type I	Fast Type IIA	Fast Type IIX
Essential MLC isoform	sMLC₁	fMLC₁	fMLC₃
Regulatory MLC isoform	sMLC₂	fMLC₂	fMLC₂
Myosin ATPase activity	Lowest	Intermediate	Highest
TnC isoform	cTnC	fTnC	fTnC
TnT isoform	sTnT	fTnT	fTnT
TnI isoform	sTnI	fTnI	fTnI
Tropomyosin	β-TM	α-TM	α-TM
SR-related proteins			
Ca^{++} release channel isoform (RyR)	RyR₁	RyR₁	RyR₁
Ca^{++} release channel number	Lowest	High	High
SERCA isoform	SERCA2a	SERCA1	SERCA1
SERCA number	Lowest	High	High
Phospholamban	Present	Absent	Absent
Parvalbumin	Low	High	High
Mitochondrial-related systems			
Respiratory capacity			
Per-unit muscle mass	Highest	Intermediate	Lowest
Per-unit mitochondrial mass	Same?	Same?	Same?
Proton conductance			
Per-unit mitochondrial mass	Same	Same	Same
Per-unit of surface area	Low	High	High
Capacity to handle reactive oxygen species			
MnSOD activity	Highest	Intermediate	Lowest
GPx activity	Highest	Intermediate	Lowest
Apoptosis	Unknown	Unknown	Unknown
Morphometric-related properties			
Cross-sectional area	Same	Same	Same
Myofibrillar volume density	Same	Same	Same
SR volume density	Lowest	Intermediate	Largest
Mitochondrial volume density	Largest	Intermediate	Smallest

(continued)

TABLE 4.2   Key Properties of Fiber Types With Emphasis on Human Skeletal Muscle (continued)

Structural or Functional Property	Slow Type I	Fast Type IIA	Fast Type IIX
Substrate-related properties			
Triglyceride	Highest	Intermediate	Lowest
Glycogen	Lowest	Intermediate	Highest
ATP	Same	Same	Same
CP	Lowest	Higher	Higher
Enzymatic activity properties			
Phosphorylase	Lowest	Intermediate	Highest
PFK	Lowest	Intermediate	Highest
LDH	Lowest	Intermediate	Highest
Triosephosphate dehydrogenase	Lowest	Intermediate	Highest
SDH	Highest	Intermediate	Lowest
CS	Highest	Intermediate	Lowest
Blood flow-related properties			
Capillary density	Highest	Intermediate	Lowest
Capillary length density per cell volume	Highest	Intermediate	Lowest
Krogh cylinder volume	Smallest	Intermediate	Highest
Mitochondrial volume: capillary volume	Same?	Same?	Same?
Myoglobin	Highest	Intermediate	Lowest

In some instances animal data have been included, since it is difficult to perform some of these analyses on human skeletal muscle. ½ RT, one-half relaxation time; ATP, adenosine triphosphate; CP, creatine phosphate; CS, citrate synthase; E, elastic modulus; K_{TR}, time constant for the redevelopment of tension; LDH, lactate dehydrogenase; MHC, myosin heavy chain; MLC, myosin light chain; P_o, maximal isometric tension; P_t, twitch tension; PFK, phosphofructokinase; RyR, ryanodine receptor; SDH, succinate dehydrogenase; SERCA, sarcoplasmic reticulum Ca^{++} ATPase pump; TnC, troponin-C; TnI, troponin-I; TnT, troponin-T; TPT, time peak tension; V_{max}, maximal shortening velocity; V_o, maximal unloaded shortening velocity.

skeletal-type excitation–contraction coupling. The greater release rate found in fast skeletal muscle (as compared to slow) is primarily due to differences in the numbers of RyR1 receptors, with fast skeletal muscle having up to a 10-fold difference. This results from (a) a twofold to threefold difference in SR volume density; and (b) a twofold to threefold difference in the numbers of RyR1 per unit of SR.

As mentioned previously, both fast (SERCA1) and slow (SERCA2a) SERCA isoforms are found in skeletal muscle. Given this observation, the question arises whether the rapid relaxation rates found in fast skeletal muscles are simply due to a greater SR volume density and/or the presence of a faster Ca^{++}–ATPase pump (i.e., SERCA). Current data suggests that both SERCA1 and SERCA2a have similar enzymatic properties, and this has given rise to the concept that the relaxation rate of skeletal muscle is highly correlated with SR volume density. It should be noted, however, that the activity of SERCA2a can be modified by the presence of phospholamban (PLB). In a dephosphorylated state, PLB acts to inhibit the Ca^{++}–ATPase activity of SERCA2a, whereas dephosphorylation of PLB causes it to dissociate from SERCA2a, allowing the Ca^{++}–ATPase activity of SERCA2a to increase.

The mitochondrial volume density, in humans, is about twofold to threefold different between slow type I and fast type II fibers. Mitochondrial volume density in human slow type I fibers is typically ~6%, whereas it only is ~2% to 3% in fast type II fibers. There are also corresponding differences in key enzymes. For instance, succinate dehydrogenase activity (the only membrane bound enzyme of the Krebs cycle) is ~1.5- and threefold higher in slow type I fibers as compared to fast type IIA and fast type IIX fibers, respectively. Citrate synthase activity also follows a similar pattern. Interestingly, in rodent skeletal muscle, fast type IIA fibers (or FOG) have a higher oxidative capacity than slow type I (or SO) fibers.

Polymorphism

For many years, it was believed that muscle fibers expressed only one type of MHC isoform. This helped to keep the concept of a "muscle fiber type" simple. One of the most significant concepts to evolve during the past 10 to 15 years has been the recognition that there can be an extensive proportion of so-called hybrid or polymorphic fibers in both human and nonhuman species. Pette and Staron (11) were at the forefront of this issue, and it is now known that muscle fibers can express anywhere from 1 to 4 adult MHC isoforms in smaller mammals and 1 to 3 in larger mammals such as humans (11,13,14). If muscle fibers are classified strictly on the basis of the MHC isoforms expressed in a given fiber, then there are 15 different possible combinations in the muscle fibers of small mammals (where four adult isoforms are expressed) and seven combinations in human (where three adult isoforms can be found). If one considers muscles such as the posterior cricoarytenoid muscle of the larynx that also expresses the EO/type IIL MHC isoform, then the number of potential combinations of MHC isoforms increases to 31. The theoretical number of molecular motors is quite impressive when the possible combinations of MHC isoform are coupled with that for MLC proteins. If all of the individual components involved with Ca^{++} cycling, crossbridge cycling, and cellular respiration are considered, it is surprising that nature has been kind enough to allow us to think that there are discrete fiber types.

Muscle Fiber Type Plasticity and the I ↔ IIA ↔ IIX ↔ IIB Transition Model

Each muscle appears to have its own unique pattern of muscle fibers that can vary by (a) type, (b) region, and (c) degree of polymorphism. Studies during the past 20 years have shown that the adaptation of muscle fiber composition to altered physiologic states is muscle dependent. For instance, some muscles like the plantar flexors of the ankle seem to be more inclined to undergo atrophy and MHC isoform transitions as compared to the dorsiflexors of the ankle. Additionally, this concept has been refined further to indicate that adaptation is fiber type specific. As with most generalizations, however, such rules do not always apply and it should be noted that the same fiber types within a given muscle can respond differently to the same stimulus. As an example, it appears that there are different populations of the slow type I fibers in the rat soleus muscle that differ in their sensitivity to mechanical unloading and thyroid state (10).

One area of muscle plasticity that needs further attention is related to the fiber type dependence of plasticity. In rats, the plasticity of MHC isoform expression is much greater in the slow type I fibers than in fast type II fibers. For instance, it has been shown that the majority of slow type I fibers in the soleus muscle can be converted into fast muscle fibers, whereas it is very difficult to perturb the majority of fast fibers in rat muscles to become heavily biased in the slow direction.

As mentioned previously, Pette and Staron (11) performed a series of studies examining transitions in single fiber MHC isoform expression via electrophoretic techniques. As a result of these studies, this group of investigators proposed that muscle fibers were obligated to follow a transition scheme that can be described as follows: I ↔ IIA ↔ IIX ↔ IIB. According to this scheme, a muscle fiber undergoing a transition from a slow type I to fast type IIX phenotype would be obligated to first express the fast type IIA MHC isoform. More recently, however, other studies (13–15) found various combinations of MHC isoforms that

are not consistent with this obligatory transition scheme. For instance, Caiozzo et al. (15) found pools of I/IIB and I/IIX/IIB fibers in muscles that were manipulated via mechanical unloading and hyperthyroidism. Additionally, it has recently been reported that muscles like the diaphragm can contain pools of I/IIX fibers (13). These types of observations are further supported by those of Talmadge and colleagues (14,16) who observed significant pools of I/IIX fibers following hind limb suspension or spinal cord transection. Thus, skeletal muscle fibers clearly have the ability to undergo MHC isoform transitions that do not adhere to the obligatory scheme. The question is whether such asynchronous transitions are an exception to the rule. This obviously requires much more investigation, especially at the myonuclear level (see the following section for further comment).

> ### KEY POINT
>
> Thus, skeletal muscle fibers clearly have the ability to undergo MHC isoform transitions that do not adhere to the obligatory scheme.

Myonuclear Plasticity

One of the remarkable features of skeletal muscle is the extensive multinucleation that is present in each muscle fiber. A typical skeletal muscle fiber has from 100 to 200 myonuclei per mm of length. Therefore, in small mammals like rats, there are ~3000 to 6000 nuclei per fiber in a muscle like the soleus. This is quite a remarkable number of nuclei. Imagine how many myonuclei there are in a skeletal muscle fiber of the human brachioradialis muscle, where the fibers have lengths >100 mm (10,000–20,000 myonuclei). One of the great challenges ahead is to understand the degree of coordination between individual myonuclei. Do all myonuclei have exactly the same gene expression program, or are there slight to large variations from one myonucleus to another? Does polymorphism arise because all myonuclei coexpress exactly the same set of sarcomeric protein isoforms, or is it possible that polymorphism exists because one myonucleus may express a set of sarcomeric protein isoforms that differs from its neighboring myonucleus? Several observations suggest that the gene expression programs of myonuclei can vary along the length of the fiber. For instance, it is known that the myonuclei associated with the neuromuscular junction express genes responsible for the localization of acetylcholine receptors (17). Additionally, Peuker and Pette (18) reported the existence of segmental variations in the MHC mRNA isoform expression and, consistent with this observation, Edman et al. (19) found segmental differences in ATPase activity. If segmental variation does occur along the length of muscle fibers, then this finding will surely excite and confuse us further regarding our concept of a fiber type. Ultimately, however, it will allow us to definitively determine if there truly is an I $\leftrightarrow$ IIA $\leftrightarrow$ IIX $\leftrightarrow$ IIB transition scheme.

The observation that skeletal muscle fibers are capable of exhibiting a wide repertoire of MHC polymorphism gives rise to some interesting functional issues and these are addressed in the section titled *The Force–Velocity Relationship in the Shortening Domain.*

Linking Structure to Function

Overview

When skeletal muscles are excited, they convert chemical energy into mechanical energy. The forces and/or length changes a muscle produces are determined by a number of key factors and, from a conceptual perspective, investigators like Rome and Linstedt (20) and Josephson (21) referred to these various factors as "design constraints" or "primary/secondary determinants." There are four primary design constraints that determine the performance of skeletal muscle fibers under isometric and shortening conditions (see Fig. 4.5). These four factors are (1) the length–tension relationship, (2) the degree and rate of activation, (3) the force–velocity relationship in the shortening domain, and (4) the degree and rate of relaxation. During lengthening contractions, the mechanical properties of skeletal muscle are not only determined by the extent of activation but also the (5) force–velocity relationship in the lengthening domain and (6) the passive stiffness (k) of skeletal muscle (see Fig. 4.5).

As noted throughout much of this section, many of the processes associated with factors 1 through 4 are highly malleable. With respect to this point, Booth and Baldwin (22) published an extensive review examining the effects of altered contractile activity on the mRNA levels of various contractile and metabolic genes (see Table 24.4 from their publication [22]).

This section of the chapter is organized into three distinct sections. The first will introduce the reader to "muscle mechanics 101" and will focus on mechanical measurements that illustrate the importance of (a) the degree of activation, (b) sarcomere length, and (c) the loading conditions imposed on the muscle. The second section addresses the plasticity of the force–velocity relationship both in the shortening and lengthening domains. The underlying basis for the emphasis on the force–velocity relationship is that it reflects the intrinsic properties of the molecular motor and, as such, sets the theoretical limits for muscle performance under all conditions. The third section introduces the work loop concept. Work loops offer an interesting perspective because the performance of skeletal muscle during a work loop (oscillatory length change) is dependent on the integration of all six design criteria noted previously. In this last section on work loops, special attention will be given to the importance of activation, relaxation, and passive k.

When thinking about mechanical models of contracting muscles, it is common to think about three components (see Fig. 4.6): (a) the contractile element (CE), (b) the series elastic element (SEC), and (c) the so-called parallel elastic element (PEC). The CE accounts for both the length–tension and force–velocity relationships of muscle. The SEC represents all of the elastic elements in series with the CC, and this takes into consideration the elasticity of the contractile apparatus itself, tendon fibrils, and tendons themselves. The PEC consists of elastic elements (*e.g.*, extracellular matrix, sarcolemma), which are in parallel to the CE. In large part, this approach evolved from Hill's classic 1938 article (23) and has come to be popularly known as the Hill model. Although very useful for thinking about muscle mechanics, it should be noted that the Hill model has some key shortcomings. As just one example, it does not properly model the behavior of skeletal muscle during lengthening contractions, failing to properly predict phenomenon such as (a) short-range stiffness (SRS) , (b) yield, and (c) postyield forces.

Muscle Mechanics 101

The relationship between activation, stimulation frequency, and force production

The term *activation* is typically used to describe the degree to which the contractile apparatus has been activated or turned on. In reality, the degree of activation reflects the number of attached crossbridges and, in turn, this is dependent primarily on the binding of Ca^{++} to TnC.

When a single muscle fiber is stimulated using a single brief stimulus, the muscle fiber will produce a mechanical event known as a "twitch." A twitch will generate a relatively small amount of force (typically 15%–25% of P_0) due to a complex interplay between Ca^{++} cycling, force production, and stretching of the series elastic component. In addition, because a twitch results from a single stimulus, its duration is brief and, in this context, the duration of a twitch sets the theoretical limits regarding the oscillatory frequencies at which a muscle can operate (see section titled *The Concept of Work Loops*). Usually, twitch measurements are made under conditions where muscle length is held constant (*i.e.*, isometric conditions) and this simplifies the potential complexity of making such measurements, especially since measures of twitch tension and relaxation are dependent on muscle length and shortening velocity.

Typically, three measurements are made from an isometric twitch (see Table 4.3), and these include measures of (a) twitch tension (P_t); (b) time-to-peak tension (TPT); and (c) one-half relaxation time (½ RT). Measures of P_t provide insight regarding the force that a muscle/muscle fiber can produce; however, P_t is a submaximal measure. With respect to Figure 4.5, a key determinant of P_t is the number of sarcomeres in parallel (factor 3). In contrast to P_t, both TPT and ½ RT are often referred to as speed-related properties. TPT reflects processes involved with

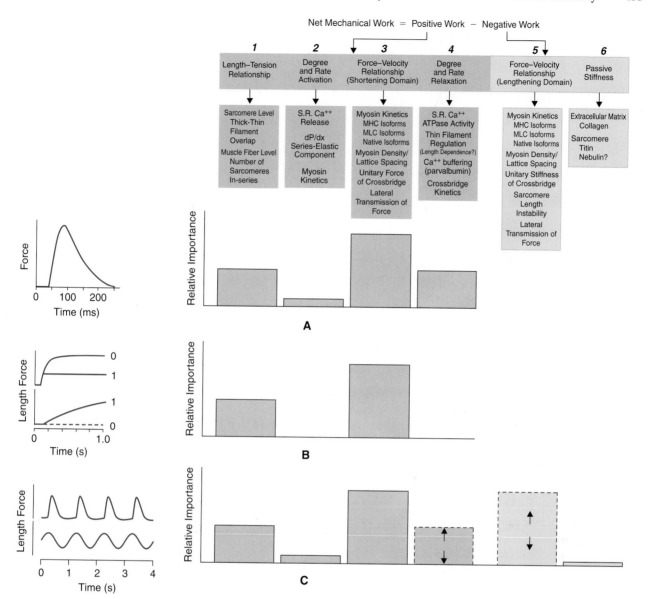

FIGURE 4.5   This figure illustrates the six key design constraints that determine the amount of force, work, and power that can be produced under any contractile condition. These six factors include (*1*) the length–tension relationship; (*2*) the rate and extent of activation; (*3*) the force–velocity relationship in the shortening domain; (*4*) the rate of relaxation; (*5*) the force–velocity relationship in the lengthening domain; and (*6*) the passive stiffness of skeletal muscle. Note that there are a series of three bar graphs aligned below these six factors, and the purpose of these bar graphs is to illustrate the importance of each of these factors under different contractile conditions. An isometric twitch is shown in **A**. The four factors that determine the kinetics of the twitch are factors 1 to 4, with factor 3 being the dominant factor. **B**. Two examples of isotonic contractions that are used to determine the force–velocity relationship. Typically, the muscle is fully activated when these types of measurements are made, and relaxation kinetics are irrelevant to such measures. Hence, factors 1 and 3 are the critical factors that determine the shape of the force–velocity relationship. **C**. Length and force records during a work loop experiment. The advantage of the work loop is that it provides a more realistic measure of work and power that a muscle can produce as compared to similar measures made from force–velocity curves (also see Table 4.3). Note that each design criteria plays a role during work loops. As mentioned in the text, the force–velocity relationship sets the theoretical limits of muscle performance under all conditions and, as such, it always has the greatest relative importance. The *arrows* shown in the bars for factors 4 and 5 are meant to indicate that the importance of these two factors can vary significantly depending on the length (which influences relaxation kinetics in slow skeletal muscle) and activation pattern (which might affect the amount of negative work required to relengthen the muscle).

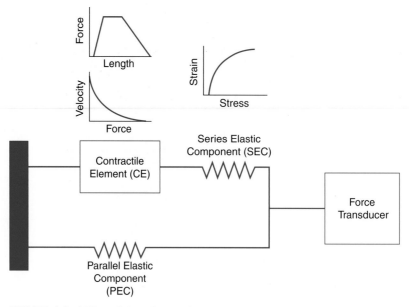

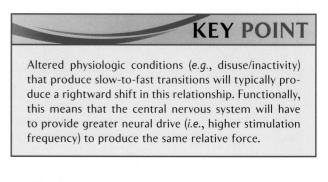

FIGURE 4.6   Hill model used to explain mechanical properties of skeletal muscle. The mechanical properties accounted for by the CE include the length–tension and force–velocity relationships. The SEC component accounts for the stress-strain characteristics of activated muscle.

activation (factor 2) and the rate of crossbridge cycling (factor 3). TPT will be very short in muscles and muscle fibers where Ca^{++} is rapidly released from the SR and crossbridge cycling is fast. One-half relaxation time is dependent primarily on the kinetics of the sarcoplasmic reticulum Ca^{++} ATPase pumps and their numbers (factor 4).

Mechanical unloading of slow skeletal muscle produces a slow → fast transition that influences the numbers RyRs, myosin isoform composition, and SERCA isoform composition. As a consequence, this causes significant reductions in both TPT and ½ RT.

The response of skeletal muscle to repetitive stimuli is much more complex than that described for a twitch and depends on the stimulation frequency. If the frequency is such that the muscle or muscle fiber completely relaxes between individual stimuli, then the muscle or muscle fiber will generate a series of individual twitches and peak tension will be approximately equal to P_t. If the frequency of stimulation is increased so that relaxation is not complete prior to the onset of the succeeding stimulus, then the force generated during the second stimulus will add onto the residual force from the preceding contraction, leading to a summation in force. This type of response is referred to as an unfused tetanus (*i.e.*, partial relaxation between individual stimuli). If stimulation frequency is increased further such that there is no relaxation between individual stimuli, then this will result in fused tetanus (*i.e.*, no relaxation between individual stimuli). It is under these conditions that the muscle generates maximal isometric tension (P_0). The relationship between stimulation frequency and force reflects a complex set of events that involves the release of Ca^{++} from the SR, the binding of Ca^{++} to TnC, crossbridge

cycling, and stretch of the series elastic component. As shown in Table 4.3, the force–frequency relationship has a sigmoidal shape, and fast muscles and muscle fibers have force–frequency relationships that are shifted to the right of those for slow muscles and muscle fibers.

The force–frequency relationship represents a complex interplay between the Ca^{++} bound to TnC and the series elastic component. The binding of Ca^{++} to TnC is determined by a complex set of events involved with Ca^{++} cycling (*i.e.*, Ca^{++} release and Ca^{++} sequestration) and the binding of Ca^{++} to TnC. The Ca^{++} binding properties of TnC are often described by plotting the relationship between tension and $[Ca^{++}]$, and the $[Ca^{++}]$ is described using an inverse log plot analogous to that used to describe pH. A pCa^{++} of 7.0 is equivalent to a 0.0000001 M concentration of Ca^{++}. Troponin-C has both high and low affinity binding sites for Ca^{++}, and the numbers of these are dependent on the isoform of TnC. The slow/cardiac isoform of TnC (cTnC) has one high and one low affinity binding site for Ca^{++}. In contrast, the fast isoform of TnC (fTnC) has two high and two low affinity Ca^{++} binding

TABLE 4.3   Muscle Mechanics

Name of Mechanical Measurement	Mechanical Measurements	Functional Significance	Key Structures	Malleability
Isometric twitch		TPT is often used as an index of the speed characteristics of a muscle. Reflects activation of contractile apparatus as well as cross-bridge kinetics. ½ RT is used as an index of relaxation. Reflects sequestration of Ca^{++} by SR	Whole muscle Ca^{++} release by SR MHC isoforms Ca^{++} uptake by SR (SERCA isoforms) Single fiber Same as for whole muscle.	Both TPT and ½ RT can be significantly altered, and this is true especially for slow muscles undergoing slow-to-fast transition. ½ RT is probably more sensitive to altered physiologic conditions than is TPT. Additionally, ½ RT is sensitive to muscle/fiber length, while TPT is relatively insensitive.
Force–frequency relationship		This represents the relationship between stimulation frequency and force production. Stimulation frequency controls pCa^{++} and modulates force via the tension–pCa^{++} relationship.	Whole muscle SR Ca^{++} release SR Ca^{++} uptake TnC isoform Skinned single fiber TnC isoform	Whole muscle Shape of force–frequency relationship in slow skeletal muscle can be manipulated by producing a slow-to-fast transition via mechanical unloading or altered thyroid state. This results in a curve shifted to the right and reflects an increase in the kinetics of the SERCA. As noted in numerous places throughout the text, it is difficult to produce a fast-to-slow transition that results in a significant shift in the force–frequency relationship.
Tension–pCa^{++} relationship				Skinned single fiber The tension–pCa^{++} curve primarily reflects the binding of Ca^{++} to troponin-C. The cardiac or slow form of TnC (cTnC) has two binding sites for Ca^{++}. One of these is a high affinity site for Ca^{++} and always has Ca^{++} bound to it. The second site has a low affinity for Ca^{++}, and it is this site that regulates the actions of TnC. Muscles that undergo a cTnC → fTnC transition will exhibit a right shift in the tension–pCa^{++} relationship, because the fast form of TnC has two high- and two low-affinity binding sites.

(continued)

TABLE 4.3   Muscle Mechanics (continued)

Name of Mechanical Measurement	Mechanical Measurements	Functional Significance	Key Structures	Malleability
Afterload technique for determination of force–velocity relationship		Force–velocity relationship describes the force that a muscle can generate at any given shortening velocity. The top panel illustrates various afterloads, while the middle panel shows the corresponding length–time records. A given velocity is simply the slope of a given length–time record. The resultant force–velocity relationship is shown in the bottom panel. The force–velocity relationship sets the theoretical boundary for muscle performance. Muscles can work on or below this relationship, but they cannot operate above it.	Whole muscle Muscle architecture MHC isoforms MLC isoforms Lattice spacing Single fiber Same except for architecture	The force–velocity relationship is quite malleable. A decrease in physical activity will result in a loss of sarcomeres in parallel (atrophy). This will lead to a loss of force production. Typically, a slow-to-fast MHC isoform transition occurs concomitantly with muscle atrophy. The net result is an increase in V_{max}. The increase in V_{max} partially offsets the reduction in force production such that loss in maximal power is partially attenuated. Resistance training produces an increase in the number of sarcomeres in parallel, and as a consequence the muscle will be able to produce more force. It has been shown in both rodents and humans that resistance training also produces a faster-to-fast transition (e.g., IIX → IIA). Such shifts, however, do not result in large changes in V_{max}.

(continued)

TABLE 4.3	Muscle Mechanics (continued)			
Name of Mechanical Measurement	**Mechanical Measurements**	**Functional Significance**	**Key Structures**	**Malleability**
Slack test	(Force vs Time plot; Length vs Time plot with L1, T1; Length vs Time plot with $\Delta L/\Delta t = V0$)	Provides measure of maximal unloaded shortening velocity (V_o). Ratio of $V_o:V_{max}$ in whole muscle may reflect heterogeneity of MHC isoform composition among individual fibers. In muscles where most fibers are slow (*e.g.*, soleus muscle), the $V_o:V_{max}$ will be high. In fast muscles, the $V_o:V_{max}$ ratio will be lower.	Whole muscle MHC isoforms MLC isoforms Lattice structure Muscle architecture Single fiber MHC isoforms MLC isoforms Lattice structure	The V_o of fibers undergoing slow-to-fast transition will exhibit large increases in V_o. The V_o of fast fibers is difficult to alter given an apparent inability to make significant fast-to-slow transitions in MHC isoform composition.
Ramp stretch or isovelocity lengthening contraction	(Force vs Stress plot, $SRS = \Delta P/\Delta L$ or $E = \sigma/\varepsilon$; Length vs Strain plot; Force vs Stress plot with Strain axis)	The mechanical properties during lengthening contractions have not been extensively studied, especially under altered physiologic conditions. Stiffness of skeletal muscle may play an important role in joint stability. Modulus represents the slope of the relationship between stress and strain. Hence, it is normalized to the dimensions of the muscle. Yield strain may be an important parameter with respect to protection of joints and joint ligaments to injury.	Whole muscle Muscle architecture Number of functional crossbridges Unitary stiffness of individual crossbridges Single fiber Dimensions of fiber Number of functional crossbridges Unitary stiffness of individual crossbridges	Stiffness: Stiffness is simply the slope of the relationship between force and length. Hence, it is dependent on cross-sectional area and muscle length. Disuse of skeletal muscle typically produces a loss of sarcomeres in parallel and as a consequence, cross-sectional area. This results in a decrease in isometric tension and a loss of stiffness. Resistance training, in contrast, increases the number of sarcomeres in parallel and the isometric tension of a muscle or muscle fiber. As a result, the muscle is stiffer when activated and lengthened. Additionally, atrophy seems to produce alterations in the lattice structure that appear to reduce the unitary stiffness of individual crossbridges. This reflects a so-called material property known as elastic modulus, which attempts to normalize stiffness to the geometric properties of a muscle.

(continued)

TABLE 4.3   Muscle Mechanics (continued)

Name of Mechanical Measurement	Mechanical Measurements	Functional Significance	Key Structures	Malleability
Work loop	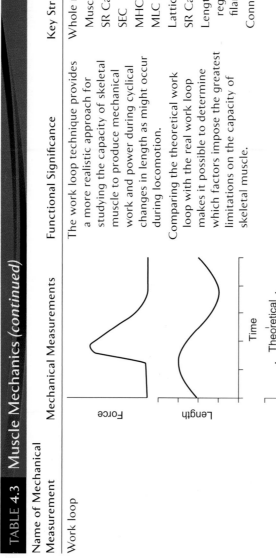	The work loop technique provides a more realistic approach for studying the capacity of skeletal muscle to produce mechanical work and power during cyclical changes in length as might occur during locomotion. Comparing the theoretical work loop with the real work loop makes it possible to determine which factors impose the greatest limitations on the capacity of skeletal muscle.	Whole muscle Muscle architecture SR Ca++ release SEC MHC isoforms MLC isoforms Lattice spacing SR Ca++ uptake Length-dependent regulation of thin filament Connective tissue Single fiber Same except for connective tissue	Virtually every one of the key structures is malleable. This is true especially for factors controlling the shape of the force–velocity relationship and relaxation kinetics. Key structural features that determine the shape of the force–velocity relationship include architectural features such as the number of sarcomeres in parallel. The types of MHC and MLC isoforms are also critical in determining the shape of the force–velocity relationship. Relaxation kinetics are also very important in determining the amount of mechanical work that can be realized. Hence, the SR is a key structural feature.

sites. Under resting conditions, the high affinity sites are saturated with Ca^{++}, whereas Mg^{++} is bound to the low affinity sites. Immediately following excitation, Ca^{++} is quickly released from the SR, causing the concentration of free Ca^{++} to rapidly rise. The Ca^{++} then displaces Mg^{++} from the low affinity sites and causes tropomyosin to undergo a conformational change such that the myosin binding sites on actin become exposed, allowing myosin to bind and generate force. Because the cardiac isoform of TnC has only one low affinity binding site for Ca^{++}, the tension–pCa^{++} relationship of slow type I fibers is shifted to the left of that for fast type II fibers. The pCa^{++}_{50} is defined as the Ca^{++} required to produce 50% of P_0 and it reflects the binding properties of TnC. Hence, the pCa^{++}_{50} of slow type I fibers is greater than that of fast type II fibers because less Ca^{++} is required to saturate the low affinity sites of the cTnC isoform. Given this perspective, altered physiologic conditions that produce transitions in TnC isoforms will produce corresponding shifts in the tension–pCa^{++} relationship and pCa^{++}_{50}.

The length–tension relationship (factor 1)

It has been known for more than 100 years that the force a muscle or muscle fiber can generate is dependent on its length. The length–tension relationship is shown in Figure 4.7. Ultrastructural studies of mammalian skeletal muscle have shown that each thin filament is ~1 μm in length, whereas each thick filament has a length of ~1.6 to 1.7 μm. According to the sliding filament hypothesis, the force that a sarcomere can produce is dependent on the overlap between thick and thin filaments. For instance, at a sarcomere length of ~3.6 μm, there is no overlap between the thick and thin filaments and, as a consequence, there is an inability to produce force. At a sarcomere length of 2.2 μm, in contrast, the overlap between the thick and thin filaments is optimal and force production is maximized.

Typically, three regions of the length–tension relationship are described. The ascending limb extends from a sarcomere length of approximately 1.3 to 2.0 μm. In this region, the amount of isometric tension increases in direct proportion to the increase in sarcomere length. The plateau region extends from ~2.0 to 2.5 μm in mammalian fibers and, in this range, there is an optimal overlap between the thick and thin filaments. Beyond a sarcomere length of 2.5 μm, the isometric force that can be produced decreases as a linear function of sarcomere length, reflecting a progressive decrease in overlap between the thick and thin filaments. The changes in striation patterns during shortening contractions played a central role in developing the sliding filament hypothesis. Table 4.4 summarizes the changes in the striation pattern that occur during isometric shortening and lengthening contractions.

The length–tension relationship of the sarcomere is thought to represent a static design criteria (20), implying that it does not change with various types of

interventions such as mechanical unloading. It should be noted, however, that spastic conditions might alter some aspects of the length–tension relationship. In contrast to the length–tension relationship of a sarcomere, that of individual muscle fiber is quite malleable. For instance, it is well known that muscles that are immobilized in a lengthened position will increase the number of sarcomeres in-series, leading to the longitudinal growth of the fiber. Conversely, immobilization in a shortened position will reduce the number of sarcomeres in series and will result in a shorter muscle fiber. As a consequence, such manipulations have the potential for influencing the overall length–tension relationships of muscle fibers and whole muscles. Normal types of physical activity/inactivity probably have little impact on the length–tension relationships of sarcomeres, muscle fibers, or whole muscles. In some abnormal states like those seen with contractures, however, there may be significant alterations in the length–tension relationship at all three levels (i.e., sarcomere, muscle fiber, muscle [24,25]).

> ## TEST YOURSELF
>
> Explain the central role of the length–tension relationship in developing the sliding filament hypothesis as developed by Huxley. Provide a contemporary explanation for all sarcomeres having a similar blueprint with respect to their dimensions. What are some of the key proteins thought to be involved in this process?

The force–velocity relationship (factors 3 and 5)

A fully activated muscle will shorten at a slow velocity when it contracts against a heavy load (see Table 4.3). In contrast, the shortening velocity will be much greater when this same muscle contracts against a light load. This inverse relationship between force and shortening velocity is simply known as the force–velocity relationship, and, under conditions where the muscle shortens during the contraction, this relationship is hyperbolic in nature (see Fig. 4.8).

Fully activated muscles can also be forcibly lengthened by imposing a force on the muscle that exceeds P_0. These types of contractions are often referred to as eccentric contractions; however, for the purposes of this chapter, they will be referred to as lengthening contractions. The shape of the force–velocity relationship in the lengthening domain is often represented as shown in Figure 4.8. However, as noted later, the mechanics in the lengthening domain are determined by three variables (force, velocity, and time) and, as such, the shape of the force–velocity relationship in the lengthening domain is three-dimensional.

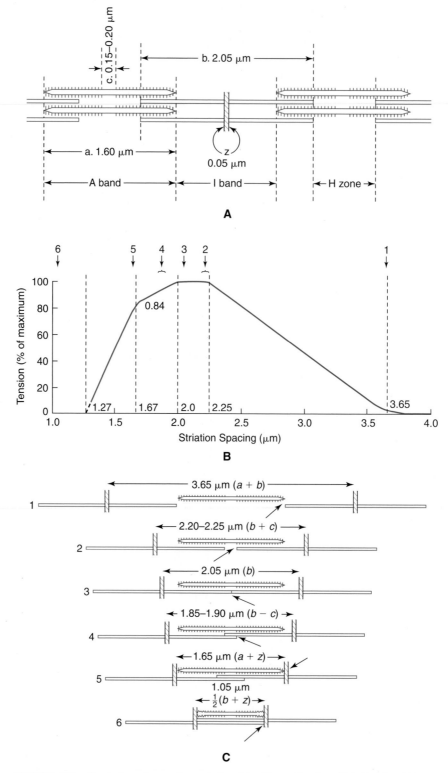

FIGURE 4.7   Classic length–tension relationship. (From Gordon AM, Huxley AF, Julian FJ. The variation in isometric tension with sarcomere length in vertebrate muscle fibres. *J Physiol.* 1966;184:170–92, with permission of The Physiological Society and Blackwell Publishing Co.)

TABLE 4.4	Effects of Types of Contractions on the Lengths of Various Bands, Zones, and Lines					
Type of Contraction	Z-line	I-band	A-band	H-zone	M-line	Sarcomere Length
Isometric	↔	↔	↔	↔	↔	↔
Shortening (isotonic)	↔	↓	↔	↓	↔	↓
Lengthening (eccentric)	↔	↑	↔	↑	↔	↑

↔, no change in length; ↓ decrease in length; ↑ increase in length.

The force–velocity relationship accounts for two of the six design constraints noted previously and, of any of these six, the force–velocity relationship sets the theoretical limit of muscle performance. Muscles can either operate on or below the force–velocity relationship, but they cannot operate above it. Hence, the other design constraints are really modulators of muscle performance. The force–velocity relationship is not important just because it describes the relationship between force and velocity. Rather, this relationship is also important

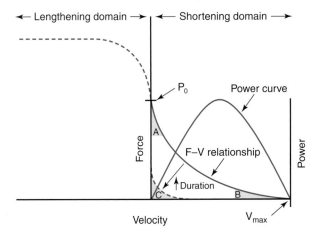

FIGURE 4.8 Illustration of the shortening and lengthening domains of the force–velocity (F–V) relationship. Three areas of activity have been identified in the shortening domain. Activities performed in region *A* require the muscle to produce contractions that generate high forces and slow velocities of shortening. Contractions in region *B* produce high shortening velocities and low forces. From a temporal perspective, muscle activity in either region can only be supported for short periods of time. Hence, when the duration of activity increases, the forces and velocities that a muscle generates will move onto submaximal F–V curves as shown in region *C*. The F–V relationship in the lengthening domain is typically represented as shown in this figure. However, as noted in the text, the F–V relationship in the lengthening domain is much more complicated and is three-dimension in nature, having axes of force, velocity, and time. Although muscle fiber type plays an important role in determining the shape of the F–V relationship in the shortening domain, it is unclear how important muscle fiber type is in determining the shape of this relationship in the lengthening domain. P_0, maximal isometric tension; V_{max}, maximal shortening velocity as determined by extrapolation of the force–velocity relationship.

because it (a) reflects the complexity of crossbridge cycling, (b) determines the work and power that can be produced under any contractile condition, and (c) determines the metabolic cost and mechanical efficiency of contractile activity.

One important feature of the force–velocity relationship that cannot be overemphasized is that it is a functional measurement that reflects important structural information. For instance, in the high force region of the force–velocity relationship (region *A* in Fig. 4.8), the maximal isometric force (P_0) that a muscle can produce is (a) dependent on the number of sarcomeres that are in parallel with one another and (b) independent of myosin isoform composition. At the other end of the force–velocity spectrum (region *B* in Fig. 4.8), maximal shortening velocity (V_{max}) is determined by the myosin isoform composition and not the number of sarcomeres in parallel. Figure 4.9A illustrates the importance of MHC isoform composition on the shape of the force–velocity relationship. The fast muscle (in this case a rat plantaris muscle) has a V_{max} that is considerably greater than that of the slow muscle (a rat soleus muscle). It should be emphasized that the impact of MHC isoform composition is not restricted solely to V_{max} itself, but instead impacts the entire spectrum of the force–velocity relationship, with the exception of P_0. Interestingly, however, the beneficial effect of the faster MHC isoform profile becomes progressively smaller as the loading condition approaches P_0.

The Force–Velocity Relationship Determines the Maximal Power that a Muscle Can Produce under Any Loading Condition

Mechanical power is determined by the force and velocity of a given contraction. Mechanical power is zero at either end of the force–velocity relationship where shortening velocity or force are zero. Maximal power typically occurs around 0.25 to 0.3 P_0. As noted previously, the MHC isoform composition of a muscle can have a big impact on the force that can be produced at any given shortening velocity. It follows then that the MHC isoform composition of a muscle also influences the shape of the power curve (see Fig. 4.9A). It should be noted that the data shown in Figure 4.9A contrasts the differences between fast and slow muscles while performing single maximal contractions. However, in many instances, muscles are required to undergo cyclic deformations in

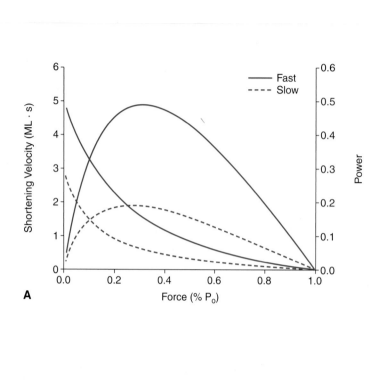

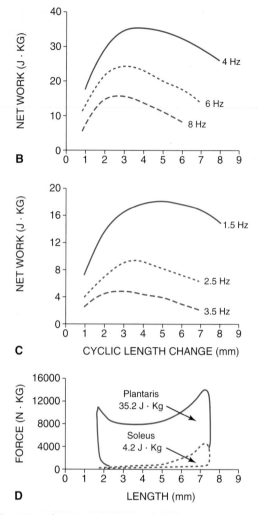

FIGURE 4.9   Force–velocity and work loop data for slow (rat soleus muscle) and fast (rat plantaris muscle). The force–velocity data illustrate the impact of myosin heavy chain (MHC) isoform composition on the shapes of force–velocity relationships. Importantly, it should be noted that the impact extends throughout the entire force–velocity relationship, with the exception of P_o. Because mechanical power is the mathematical product of force multiplied by velocity, mechanical power must also be dependent on MHC isoform composition. As noted in the text, however, the differences in mechanical work and power are much larger between slow and fast muscles when they are required to perform oscillatory work. The larger than expected difference is due to differences in relaxation kinetics, which can be substantial. This is illustrated by the data shown in **B–D.**

length (oscillatory work), and under such circumstances, the ability to produce mechanical work is not only dependent on the shape of the force–velocity relationship but also the relaxation kinetics of the muscle. These considerations are addressed in the section *The Concept of Work Loops.*

Plasticity of the Force–Velocity Relationship in the Shortening Domain (Factor 3)

The shape of the force–velocity relationship of *single fibers* is really dependent on a complex distribution of crossbridges, whereby a crossbridge can act as either a positive or negative force generator. Huxley (1) developed a model describing this complexity in 1957. This model proposes that, at slow velocities, crossbridges attach and act as positive force generators, detaching before they are swept into the region where they act as negative force generators. At

higher shortening velocities, however, a greater proportion of the crossbridges that initially attach and generate a positive force will be swept into the negative force generating region before they can detach, causing a reduction in net force production by the muscle fiber. Shifts in isoforms induced by altered neural, mechanical, or hormonal conditions can alter the MHC isoform composition of a muscle fiber and, by doing so, influence the proportion of crossbridges acting as positive or negative force generators at any given velocity of contraction. This, in turn, alters the shape of the force–velocity relationship of the *single fiber.*

At the *whole muscle level,* the shape of the force–velocity relationship is really a composite of the force–velocity relationships of each individual muscle fiber. Hill (26) developed a statistical model that provided a mathematical approach for understanding the complexity of the force–velocity relationship. In his model, Hill utilized 82 fibers that were distributed in a manner consistent with a probability curve, yielding 10 different pools of fibers. The Hill equation of the force–velocity relationship states:

$$(P + a)\,(V + b) = b\,(P_0 + a) \qquad [1]$$

In this common form of the Hill equation, P_0 is maximal isometric tension, P is isotonic tension, V is shortening velocity, and a and b are constants with dimensions of force and velocity, respectively. The curvature of the force–velocity relationship is represented by a/P_0. Equation 1 can be normalized to P_0 and V_{max} as follows (27):

$$(P/P_0 + a/P_0)\,(V/V_{max} + b/V_{max})$$
$$= b/V_{max}\,(1 + a/P_0) \qquad [2]$$

Equation 2 can be rewritten using the substitutions of $P/P_0 = P'$, $V/V_{max} = V'$, and $a/P_0 = b/V_{max} = 1/G$ such that:

$$P' = (1 - V')/(1 + VG) \qquad [3]$$

This equation can then be used as shown in Table 4.5 to determine the force–velocity of any individual pool of fibers by (a) determining the relative shortening velocity for that pool of fibers and using this to solve Equation 3 and (b) determining the relative overall force and adjusting for the proportion of fibers in that pool. The V' for any pool of fibers (V'_{fiber}) is determined by dividing the maximal shortening velocity of that group of fibers ($V_{0, fiber}$) by the shortening velocity of the whole muscle (V_{muscle}). Note that in the example given in Table 4.5A, the whole muscle shortening velocity is equivalent to 0.05 fiber lengths $\cdot$ s^{-1} (FL $\cdot$ s^{-1}).

TABLE 4.5 Application of Hill's 82-Fiber Model

n	p_{fiber}	$V_{0,fiber}$	V_{muscle}	V_{fiber}	P'_{fiber}
1	0.012	2.4	0.05	0.0208	0.0110
3	0.037	2.2	0.05	0.0227	0.0328
7	0.085	2.0	0.05	0.0250	0.0757
13	0.159	1.8	0.05	0.0278	0.1387
17	0.207	1.6	0.05	0.0313	0.1785
17	0.207	1.4	0.05	0.0357	0.1749
13	0.159	1.2	0.05	0.0417	0.1302
7	0.085	1.0	0.05	0.0500	0.0676
3	0.037	0.8	0.05	0.0625	0.0274
1	0.012	0.6	0.05	0.0833	0.0084
					$\Sigma = 0.8453$

Panel A

n	p_{fiber}	$V_{0,fiber}$	V_{muscle}	V'_{fiber}	P'_{fiber}
1	0.012	2.4	1.10	0.4583	0.0023
3	0.037	2.2	1.10	0.5000	0.0061
7	0.085	2.0	1.10	0.5500	0.012
13	0.159	1.8	1.10	0.6111	0.0179
17	0.207	1.6	1.10	0.6875	0.0173
17	0.207	1.4	1.10	0.7857	0.0107
13	0.159	1.2	1.10	0.9167	0.0028
7	0.085	1.0	1.10	>1	0.000
3	0.037	0.8	1.10	>1	0.000
1	0.012	0.6	1.10	>1	0.000
					$\Sigma = 0.0692$

Panel B

Calculations are shown for whole muscle shortening velocities (V_{muscle}) of 0.05 (panel A) and 1.10 (panel B) FL $\cdot$ s^{-1}.

n, number of fibers in a given pool; p_{fiber}, number in the pool divided by the number of fibers ($n = 82$); $V_{0,fiber}$, maximal unloaded shortening velocity of fibers; V_{muscle}, shortening velocity of muscle; V'_{fiber}, relative shortening velocity for a given pool of fibers, defined as $V_{0,fiber}$ divided by V_{muscle}; P'_{fiber}, relative amount of force produced by a given pool of fibers, expressed as P divided by P_0. The amount of force produced by the whole muscle is the sum of the individual values for P'_{fiber}.

Example calculation for the fastest pool of fibers, given $p_{fiber} = 0.012$; $V_{0,fiber} = 2.4$ FL $\cdot$ s^{-1}; $V_{muscle} = 0.05$ FL $\cdot$ s^{-1}; $a/P_0 = 0.25$; $G = 4$.

$$P'_{fiber} = [(1 - V'_{fiber})/(1 + V'_{fiber} \times G)] \times p_{fiber}$$
$$P'_{fiber} = [(1 - 0.0208)/(1 + 0.0208 \times 4)] \times 0.012 = 0.0110$$

In this example, all of the fibers have a $V_{0,fiber}$ that exceeds this shortening velocity, and hence each fiber can contribute to overall force production. In contrast, when the muscle is shortening at a velocity equivalent to 1.10 FL $\cdot$ s^{-1} (see Table 4.5B), the three slowest pools of fibers are unable to contribute to overall force production.

One of the utilities of Hill's 82-fiber statistical model is that it can be used to predict alterations in the force–velocity relationship of whole muscle based on changes in (a) cross-sectional area as is associated with hypertrophy and atrophy and (b) myosin isoform composition. A slow-to-fast myosin isoform transition can be modeled, for instance, by altering the distribution of the 82 fibers such that they are distributed in the four slowest pools of fibers. The predicted effect is quite evident—that is, a reduction in the V_{max} of the muscle. The effects of hypertrophy/atrophy can be described by multiplying P'_{fiber} by a constant. For example, if a muscle atrophied by 50%, then each P'_{fiber} value would be reduced by this proportion.

The application of Hill's approach has been extended to (a) model differences in the force–velocity relationships of hind limb muscles in the rat (13) and (b) explain the effects of myosin isoform transitions (28). The requirements for modeling the whole muscle force–velocity relationship in this fashion are dependent on (a) a statistical model, (b) knowledge about the distribution of myosin isoforms at the single fiber level, and (c) some assumptions regarding the maximal shortening velocity of slow type I, fast type IIA, fast type IIX, and fast type IIB fibers. The first requirement (a statistical model) involves the application of a model like that of Hill's or that described by Josephson and Edman (29). The second requirement (i.e., knowledge about single fiber myosin isoform composition) entails a large amount of electrophoretic single fiber analyses. This can be performed at the native, MHC, and/or MLC levels. The third requirement (i.e., regarding V_{max}) can be met by actually making such measurements or by using published data (as was done in Caiozzo et al. [13]). It should be stated that the publications of Reiser et al. (30), Bottinelli et al. (3,31), Larsson and Moss (32), and Edman et al. (33) have been pivotal in establishing the relationships between MCH and MLC isoforms and maximal shortening velocity as defined by V_{max} or V_0.

With respect to modeling, the force–velocity relationships of different muscles in the rat, it should be stressed that there are few true slow muscles like the soleus. Rather, most muscles are composed of various pools of mono- and polymorphic fast fibers. This is even true for so-called red regions of muscles like the medial gastrocnemius. The modeling of force–velocity relationships of rodent's hind limb muscle suggests that there is a high degree of convergence, meaning that the differences in force–velocity relationships are subtle and not dramatic (13).

The application of Hill's model has also been used to examine transitions in MHC isoform composition. Mechanical overload (e.g., compensatory overload; resistance training) has been shown to produce a fast → slow

transition in myosin isoform phenotype in both human and nonhuman species. Compensatory overload of the rat plantaris muscle typically produces a large increase in the percentage of fibers expressing the slow type I MHC isoform. On this basis, one might predict that V_{max} would be reduced in accordance with the increased percentage of fibers expressing the slow type I MHC isoform. Single fiber electrophoretic analyses reveal, however, that there is not a large increase in fibers that exclusively express the slow type I MHC isoform. Rather, the upregulation of the slow type I MHC isoform results in polymorphic fibers that are typically dominated by a large proportion of fast MHC isoforms. In one study (28), the modeling of the force–velocity relationship using Hill's approach suggested that V_{max} of the whole muscle should be decreased mildly (~10% to 15%) by compensatory overload, and this was close to the actual 14% decrease that was observed. Whether by design or coincidence, MHC isoform shifts that produce polymorphism (rather than monomorphic changes) seem to minimize the functional consequences of MHC isoform transitions (28).

Factors such as mechanical unloading (e.g., as accompanies cast immobilization) and altered thyroid hormone status will produce shifts in the contractile and regulatory contractile protein isoform profiles such that muscles/muscle fibers will become faster. For instance, cast immobilization may lead to a transition from the slow type I to the fast type IIX MHC isoform. From a functional perspective, this will lead to an increase in V_{max}.

KEY POINT

Although it is commonly thought that strength training is an effective tool for increasing sprint speed, it should be noted that this seems to produce fast-to-slow transitions in MHC isoform expression.

TEST YOURSELF

Using the explanation in text and the data shown in Table 4.5, determine the force–velocity relationship of the fibers having a $V_{0,fiber}$ of 2.4. Perform a similar analysis for the fibers having a $V_{0,fiber}$ of 0.6. For each group of fibers, determine their V_{max}. Using the given $V_{0,fiber}$, determine the V_0/V_{max} ratio. What does this indicate with respect to the utility of V_{max}?

V_0: A Measure of Maximal Unloaded Shortening Velocity

The maximal shortening velocity of a skeletal muscle/muscle fiber can be measured using several different approaches. One method involves extrapolation of the force–velocity relationship to where it intersects the y-axis (see example in Table 4.3 and Fig. 4.8). This predicted that maximal shortening velocity is typically referred to as V_{max}. Often, however, V_{max} does not provide an accurate estimate of a muscle's true maximal shortening velocity. There are several reasons for this. First, the force–velocity relationship is a composite that reflects the individual force–velocity relationships of all of the fibers. Hence, the shape of a muscle's force–velocity relationship can be biased by the slowest fibers such that V_{max} underestimates the true maximal shortening velocity (28). Additionally, the force–velocity relationship is typically modeled as though it perfectly fits a rectangular hyperbola, which it does not. Indeed, Hill noted that the force–velocity relationship deviated from a rectangular hyperbola in the low force region (13). The degree to which V_{max} underestimates the true maximal shortening velocity is dependent on the muscle fiber composition of a muscle, and in muscle where there is a large proportion of slow fibers and a small pool of fast fibers, the underestimation will be the greatest.

Another approach that is commonly used to measure maximal shortening velocity is the slack test (see Table 4.3). Using this approach, the muscle is fully activated and allowed to rise onto its isometric plateau. A rapid decrease in muscle length is then imposed on the muscle such that the velocity of the length step greatly exceeds the maximal shortening velocity of the muscle. This maneuver imposes a slack in the muscle and allows the muscle to contract against zero external load until the slack is taken up. The time required to take up the slack is defined as the interval between the onset of the length step and the reappearance of force. By performing a series of quick releases that vary in the length steps, a plot can be made that describes the relationship between length step amplitude versus the time required to take up slack (see Table 4.3). The slope of this relationship then defines maximal unloaded shortening velocity (V_0).

Changes in Maximal Shortening Velocity without Concomitant Changes in MHC Isoform Expression

Key studies (3,4,30) have clearly established a relationship between MHC isoform expression and maximal shortening velocity. However, it should be noted that McDonald et al. (34) have consistently observed that mechanical unloading of slow type I fibers produces an increase in maximal shortening velocity (as defined by either V_{max} or V_0) without a concomitant slow-to-fast transition in MHC isoform expression. There are several possible explanations for these findings. First, unloading may produce an isoform transition that cannot be identified by current methods. Second, mechanical unloading of skeletal muscle produces significant alterations in the ultrastructure of skeletal muscle. For instance, it appears as though mechanical unloading may selectively reduce the density of thin filaments. The altered lattice structure that accompanies mechanical unloading

may affect the interaction between actin and myosin such that it influences crossbridge cycling and increases maximal shortening velocity.

The Plasticity of the Force–Velocity Relationship in the Lengthening Domain (Factor 5)

Although a great deal of attention has been given to the mechanical properties of skeletal muscle under isometric and shortening conditions, much less has been directed toward understanding the mechanical properties of skeletal muscles while actively lengthened. This is especially true with respect to conditions where the physiologic conditions have been altered (e.g., altered loading state).

The force–velocity relationship in the lengthening domain is often represented as shown in Figure 4.8. However, the response of activated skeletal muscle to a lengthening contraction is much more complex than that shown in this figure, as is evident in Table 4.3. In the example of a ramp stretch shown in Table 4.3, the muscle is fully activated and allowed to rise onto its isometric plateau. Note that when a ramp stretch equivalent to a strain rate of ~0.6 ML · s^{-1} is imposed on the muscle, there is a very rapid rise in force above the isometric baseline. After a strain of approximately 1% to 2%, there is a dramatic yield in the force record such that force continues to rise, but at a slower rate. This single example illustrates several key points. First, during the initial phase of stretch, tension rises even though the lengthening velocity is constant. This response is quite different than that seen under shortening conditions and it indicates that, in the lengthening domain, the force–velocity relationship cannot simply be described by a planar curve as it is in the shortening domain. Rather, in the lengthening domain, the force–velocity relationship is three-dimensional with axes of lengthening velocity, force, and time. Second, a further complication in understanding the force–velocity relationship in the lengthening domain is the yield that occurs after a strain of approximately 1% to 2%. This yield might occur because (a) there is a rapid detachment of crossbridges, and/or (b) so-called weaker sarcomeres "pop." Currently, it is not clear which potential mechanism accounts for this yield.

In performing ramp stretches like those shown in Table 4.3, a number of mechanical measurements can be made. Some of these include stiffness (k) and elastic modulus (E). k is simply the slope of the relationship between force and length ($\Delta P/\Delta L$), and the initial slope of this relationship during a ramp stretch has been defined as short-range stiffness (SRS). Because the force a muscle fiber can generate is dependent on the number of sarcomeres in parallel, k is a function of structural properties like cross-sectional area. Therefore, a muscle with a physiologic cross-sectional area twice that of another muscle will have a SRS that is also twice as great. In contrast to k, E is an expression of k that is normalized relative to the architecture/geometry of the muscle. In other words, E is the slope of stress (force/cross-sectional area; σ) versus strain (relative change in length; $\Delta L/L_o$; ϵ) relationship, and E is thought to represent a so-called material property—meaning that it represents an intrinsic property of the material. Given the example, the muscle with twice the physiologic cross-sectional area will have an E that is the same as the smaller muscle.

To date, few studies have attempted to examine the importance of muscle fiber type on the shape of the force–velocity relationship in the lengthening domain. As noted, such studies are complicated given that this relationship in the lengthening domain is three-dimensional in nature and there appears to be a yield in the force record after a strain of ~1% to 2%. In focusing on the preyield force record (for simplicity), it is not clear whether there should be a dependence on fiber type. It could be argued that the slower crossbridge cycling rate found in slow type I fibers will cause these slower crossbridges to be strained to a greater extent (at any given velocity) prior to detachment and that this will result in a more rapid rise in force during the initial phase of stretch (i.e., the preyield phase). Alternatively, although faster crossbridges may detach at a faster rate, they will also reattach at a faster rate, thereby offsetting or minimizing any potential influence of fiber type dependence. Obviously, more studies are needed to clarify whether the lengthening domain of the force–velocity relationship is dependent on fiber type.

TEST YOURSELF

When a muscle is fully activated and undergoes a ramp stretch, there is an initial phase where force/tension rises very rapidly and then a sudden yield occurs. The subsequent phase has a much slower slope. What events at the sarcomere level might account for the sudden yield? Provide some possible explanations that account for the differences in these two slopes.

Muscles constantly undergo cyclic activity where they are loaded during the lengthening phase. In some instances, activation during the lengthening phase is necessary for motor control, and, in others, the forcible lengthening of skeletal muscle may play an important role in protecting joints from ligamentous injury. Ligaments are often referred to as "static" joint stabilizers, whereas muscles are thought to function as "dynamic" joint stabilizers. Hypothetically, muscles that undergo atrophy and, as a consequence, have a reduction in k presumably will act as poorer joint stabilizers and place the involved joint at greater risk for injury. Alternatively, muscles that hypertrophy in response to resistance training will have a greater k and provide the involved joint with greater protection. It has been postulated that the higher incidence of knee ligament injuries in

women may be due to weaker quadriceps that, in turn, act as poorer joint stabilizers (35).

To date, few studies have examined the effects of mechanical unloading (as might result from cast immobilization) on SRS, E, and the force–velocity relationship in the lengthening domain. k is thought to be a structural property, as noted, but in reality, it is not only dependent on the physiologic cross-sectional area but also the E. It might be presumed that mechanical unloading simply affects k by reducing the number of sarcomeres in parallel. This, however, is not the case as E also appears to be influenced by such perturbed physiologic conditions. The effects of mechanical unloading on E can be quite substantial, reducing E by 50% or more. The possible mechanisms responsible for such a large loss in E might include (a) a decrease in unitary crossbridge k, and/or (b) a reduction in the density of attached crossbridges. With respect to this second mechanism, there are a number of alterations that might be responsible for the loss in E. First, there might be a number of dysfunctional myofibrils undergoing degeneration/disarray due to protein degradation. Second, thin filaments may have been altered such that their lengths are short or they are not attached to the Z-line. Third, there may be selective thin filament loss as reported by Riley et al. (36).

The Concept of Work Loops

The mechanical measurements described thus far result from experimental conditions where the muscle produces single submaximal (twitch, force-frequency, tension-pCa^{++}) or maximal contractions (force–velocity relationship). The ability of skeletal muscle to produce mechanical work and power can be calculated from the force–velocity relationship, but these are measures of so-called instantaneous mechanical work and power (see Figs. 4.8 and 4.9A). Typically, force–velocity and power curves are derived from conditions where the contractile apparatus is fully activated. Hence, such measures of instantaneous mechanical work and power do not take into account issues related to activation and relaxation that must occur during cyclic activity. In this framework, the work loop technique popularized by Josephson (21) represents an approach for studying the mechanical properties of skeletal muscle during cyclic shortening–lengthening contractions.

An example of a work loop is shown in Table 4.3, and, in this example, the muscle undergoes a series of cyclic changes in length. The net mechanical work produced during a work loop can be calculated as:

$$\begin{array}{ccc} \text{Net Mechanical} & = & \text{Positive Mechanical} & - & \text{Negative Mechanical} \\ \text{Work} & & \text{Work} & & \text{Work} \\ & & \text{(Shortening domain)} & & \text{(Lengthening domain)} \end{array} \quad [4]$$

Although this formula is very basic, the factors that dictate the amount of positive and negative mechanical work produced during single or repetitive contractions are numerous and quite complex in nature. This complexity is illustrated in Figure 4.5 and involves the integration of all six design criteria noted previously. If activation and relaxation were instantaneous events, then the mechanical work and power a muscle could produce under any work loop condition would simply be defined by the so-called theoretical work loop. A theoretical work loop can be developed by first determining the force–velocity relationship and then using this data to predict the force developed at any given velocity throughout the shortening phase of the work loop. Because neither activation nor relaxation are instantaneous events, however, the amount of mechanical work and power that can be realized will always be less than that predicted from the theoretical work loop. This point is nicely illustrated in Figure 4.9B–D. For instance, the force–velocity data shown in Figure 4.9A would suggest that the difference in maximal power is approximately 2.5-fold. However, under work loop conditions, the difference in mechanical work (and, as a consequence, power) is much more substantial. For instance, the soleus muscle oscillating at 3.5 Hz is capable of producing about 4 J · kg^{-1}. This is in contrast to the fast plantaris muscle that is capable of producing almost nine times more work under very similar conditions. This difference is not only due to the differences in the force–velocity relationship, but also due to differences between the relaxation kinetics of the two muscles.

KEY POINT

A basic question remains as to how important rates of activation and relaxation are limiting the production of mechanical work and power during cyclic activity?

TEST YOURSELF

Determine the amount of mechanical work that a muscle should be able to theoretically produce while performing sinusoidal work given the following information:

$$P_0 = 2.0 \text{ N}$$

$$V_{max} = 100 \text{ mm} \cdot \text{s}^{-1}$$

$$a/P_0 = 0.25$$

$$\text{Frequency} = 4 \text{ Hz}$$

$$\text{Amplitude of shortening} = 4 \text{ mm}$$

Contrast this with a muscle that has a V_{max} of 200 mm · s^{-1}. Will the amount of work performed by the faster muscle simply be twice as much?

The Rate of Activation (Factor 2)

Activation is a term that is applied to turning on the contractile apparatus, and the speed with which it occurs can be defined by measures such as dP/dt. As indicated in Figure 4.2, this involves a complex set of events that primarily includes the release of Ca^{++} from the SR and the binding of Ca^{++} to TnC and the rate of crossbridge cycling. From a temporal perspective, the release of Ca^{++} from the SR occurs quite rapidly such that the rise in tension substantially lags behind the rise in Ca^{++}.

The potential limitations that activation and relaxation can impose on the production of mechanical work and power during cyclic activity are really dependent on the frequency of length change. At a low frequency of 0.5 Hz, for example, the shortening phase (1000 ms in duration) is sufficiently long that neither the rate of activation nor relaxation imposes significant limitations. However, at a higher frequency of 4 Hz, the shortening phase becomes temporally compressed (125 ms in this example) such that processes involved in turning the contractile apparatus on (activation) and off (relaxation) may impose significant limitations.

In looking at the time course of a twitch in skeletal muscle fibers (especially slow type I fibers), TPT is often much shorter than that for complete relaxation. Such observations suggest that the rate of relaxation may impose a greater limitation on the production of mechanical work as compared to the rate of activation. Consistent with this perspective, it appears as though factors controlling the rate of activation account for a relatively small amount of unrealized work (i.e., ~5%–10%) in slow muscles like the soleus. Hence, even in slow skeletal muscles, the rate of activation does not impose a large limitation in producing mechanical work.

The Rate of Relaxation (Factor 4)

The rate of relaxation can be studied from a variety of different perspectives. For instance, the rate of relaxation can be described using measurements like ½ RT. Alternatively, the rate of relaxation has also been studied using measures of −dP/dt. The main factors responsible for controlling the rate of relaxation are shown in Figure 4.5, and it is known that most (if not all of these) can be influenced by changes in neural, mechanical, and hormonal status.

Typically, the rate of relaxation is measured under isometric conditions; and, as a consequence, it is not clear what the true physiologic relevance of such measurements might be. As noted previously, we have used the work loop approach to provide an alternative perspective regarding the importance of relaxation kinetics, and our findings suggest that under some conditions the rate of relaxation may limit the production of mechanical work and power by ~50%. It has also been shown that this modulatory influence of relaxation kinetics can be dramatically altered by interventions such as mechanical unloading and hyperthyroidism. Each of these interventions significantly increases the rate of relaxation such that a muscle can produce much more work under certain work loop conditions (6).

It should be emphasized that the rate of relaxation also seems to be length dependent in slow muscles/muscle fibers (but not fast fibers) such that at lengths beyond L_0 ½ RT increases substantially. This length dependence of relaxation may be due to the presence of the cTnC isoform.

Physiologic perturbations such as mechanical unloading are known to increase the rate of relaxation in slow skeletal muscles and muscle fibers. For instance, Schulte et al. (37) observed that 28 days of hind limb unloading produced a large increase in the fast SERCA isoform at both the protein and mRNA levels, and this led to a 170% increase in Ca^{++} ATPase activity.

Conditions such as immobilization and mechanical unloading produce significant amounts of atrophy and, as a consequence, markedly reduce the ability of skeletal muscle to produce mechanical work and power. However, it is important to stress that the mechanical unloading of slow skeletal muscle fibers produces compensatory effects that are manifested in a slow → fast MHC isoform transition and an increased rate of Ca^{++} sequestration. The first effect via its influence on the force–velocity relationship partially minimizes the loss of peak power predicted to occur from a reduction in the ability to produce force. The second effect (i.e., increased rate of Ca^{++} sequestration) means that the muscle can effectively operate and produce mechanical work at higher than normal cycling frequencies.

The Passive Stiffness of Skeletal Muscle (Factor 6)

During cyclic locomotor activity, the work required to lengthen a muscle is dependent on (a) the degree of activation, (b) the force–velocity relationship in the lengthening domain, and (c) the passive k of the muscle. If the muscle is completely relaxed, then the first two factors can be ignored and the work required to lengthen the muscle is simply dependent on the passive k of the muscle. The passive k of skeletal muscle can be measured by several different means. One of these involves performing cyclic sinusoidal length changes with the muscle or muscle fiber in a passive state. This type of approach provides a more realistic and instantaneous measure of passive k as compared to other techniques like the stretch–release technique, whereby measurements of passive k are made under static conditions. The stretch–release approach involves small stepwise increments/decrements in stretch, and typically a step change in length is held for several minutes to allow for stress relaxation. The slope of the force deformation curve represents k, and, if normalized to cross-sectional area and length, then E under passive conditions can be determined.

Currently, the passive k and E of skeletal muscle are thought to be due to the connective tissue content of skeletal muscle and the presence of sarcomeric proteins like titin. Titin is sometimes referred to as a molecular spring, and it is a giant molecule (27,000 amino acids) with a molecular weight of ~3 mDa. Titin extends from the Z-line into the M-line, and it is the I-band segment of titin that is thought to possess the properties of a molecular spring. In this region, there are three key segments that have been identified as the (a) PEVK region, (b) the immunoglobulin (Ig) segments that flank the PEVK region, and (c) N2A segments. A number of different titin isoforms have been identified, and these are believed to be partially responsible for differences in the passive properties of various types of muscles (slow, fast, cardiac).

Few studies, to date, have examined the effects of altered mechanical loading on the passive properties and titin content of single fibers. In one of the few studies in this area, Toursel et al. (38) reported that mechanical unloading of the soleus muscle actually produced a decrease in E under passive conditions. With respect to titin, this might occur as a result of transitions in titin isoforms or a reduction in the amount of titin per unit volume. Toursel et al. (38) observed that the reduction in E occurred in the absence of titin isoform transitions. Interestingly, there was a reduction in the titin:MHC ratio, and this finding is consistent with the hypothesis that the reduction in the passive E may have been partially/completely due to a selective loss of titin per unit volume.

Structure–Function Relationships: Lessons Learned from Comparative Physiology

The field of comparative physiology, given its interest in organismal function, shares many common interests with that of exercise physiology and provides a potentially beneficial perspective for thinking about structure–function relationships and their plasticity. In this section, design constraints are considered further, but from a comparative approach. When combined with the previous sections, this provides an important backdrop for discussing symmorphosis and the concept of optimality.

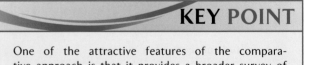

KEY POINT

One of the attractive features of the comparative approach is that it provides a broader survey of structure–function relationships and, as such, may provide better insight into the actual rules of muscle plasticity.

As stated previously, the briefest mechanical event that a muscle can produce is an isometric twitch and this is simply the response to a single stimulus. The amplitude and time course of a twitch are defined by factors 1 to 4 shown in Figure 4.5. The duration of a twitch can be quite short in some vertebrates, whereas in others it can be much longer. For instance, in sonic muscles of some fish (used for mating), the total twitch duration is very short ($\sim$10–20 ms) and the muscles can operate at frequencies of 100 to 200 Hz. Similarly, the shaker muscles of rattlesnakes also have short twitch durations and can operate at frequencies of $\sim$90 Hz. Human skeletal muscle fibers, in contrast, have isometric twitch durations that are much longer (*e.g.*, $\sim$250 ms), and as a consequence are confined to operate at low frequencies (*e.g.*, $\sim$2–5 Hz).

As eloquently addressed by Rome and Linstedt (39), the simple contrast between sonic and shaker muscles brings forth some important design considerations that can be summarized as follows: Ultimately, the performance of a muscle is largely dependent on the distribution of SR, myofibrillar, and mitochondrial volumes. These general design considerations can be illustrated using the following examples. Muscles that operate at high frequencies are obligated to have fast Ca^{++} cycling kinetics and, as a result, a relatively large proportion of cell volume must be dedicated to the SR (in some instances >25% of the cell volume). If such muscles are active for long periods of time, then a significant amount of the cell volume must also be dedicated to the mitochondria. In such muscles, the myofibrillar volume will be relatively small and the muscles will be incapable of generating large forces when normalized to cross-sectional area. Alternatively, if the muscles are active for only short durations, then a much greater proportion of the cell volume can be occupied by myofibrils, allowing the muscle to generate moderate to large forces. The myofibrillar volume density will be greatest in muscles optimized to produce force but, in these muscles, the tradeoff is that they will not be able to operate at high oscillatory frequencies or support high levels of metabolic activity. Finally, muscles that are required to support high metabolic levels for prolonged periods of time (like flight muscles) must have large mitochondrial volumes (*e.g.*, 35% of the total cell volume), and this will correspondingly impose limitations on the SR and myofibrillar volumes and the functions they support.

KEY POINT

Most human skeletal muscles appear to be optimized for myofibrillar volume, suggesting that the generation of force may have been a prime factor in the evolution of human muscles.

Herein lies one of the unique aspects of contractile protein isoforms given the three-compartment model (*i.e.*, SR, myofibril, mitochondria). The presence of contractile protein isoforms confirms a level of functional plasticity that can occur in the absence of changes in compartment volumes.

Symmorphosis and the Concept of Optimality

Collectively, the tradeoffs for space were referred to by Rome and Linstedt (39) as the "zero sum game." Some might extend this concept to basically state that muscles and muscle fibers are perfectly adapted to the physiologic tasks that they perform. In this context, Weibel, Taylor, and Hoppeler (40) proposed the concept of "optimality" of design in physiologic structures—the concept of symmorphosis. This was defined as the perfect matching of structure to functional need, such that no excess capacity was maintained. In terms of energetic efficiency, the metabolic cost of building and maintaining structures superfluous to maximal performance should be prohibitive. Given the perspective described relative to the three-compartment model, the concept of symmorphosis would postulate, for instance, that mitochondrial volume density is perfectly matched to the energetic requirements of the SR and myofibrils. Certainly, the adjustment of muscle structure to higher functional demands (*i.e.*, training), and the reverse when training ceases, suggests a cost-to-benefit relationship may help shape "optimization" of muscle.

The notion of economical design in animals is not a recent one, but the formulation of symmorphosis has been a stimulus to much interesting research. It is an appealing and seemingly intuitive concept of design and the discussion of the applicability of economy of structural costs to the evolution of organisms is a very fruitful area of investigation. However, as Diamond and Hammond (41) remarked, "The concept is worth posing not because we believe it to be literally true, but because only by posing [it]. . . can one hope to detect where it breaks down, and to identify the interesting reason for its breakdown."

TEST YOURSELF

From a comparative perspective, describe how gait frequency, fiber type, and sarcoplasmic reticulum scale with body mass within mammals. Relate your findings to so-called work loops and the ability to realize mechanical work and power.

ACKNOWLEDGMENTS

The authors would like to acknowledge the insight and comments of Dr. Kenneth M. Baldwin. This work was supported in part by National Institutes of Health grants AR 46856 (VJC) and NIH F32 AR47749 (BCR).

It is widely recognized that the structural and functional properties of skeletal muscles are under the influence of neural, mechanical, and hormonal factors. Although the specific rules of muscle plasticity remain to be completely elucidated, there have been significant strides made on a number of fronts. Much of what has evolved emanated from landmark studies like that of Buller, Eccles, and Eccles. In this classic study, these investigators utilized a "cross-innervation" or "cross-union" paradigm whereby the slow soleus muscle of cat was reinnervated with the motor nerve innervating the fast flexor digitorum longus (FDL) muscle, and the FDL was reinnervated with the motor nerve from the soleus muscle. On the contralateral side, the motor nerves innervating a given muscle were simply cut and the ends were resutured together. By contrasting the cross-innervated group with the reinnervated group, Buller, Eccles, and Eccles were able to account for changes induced by cross-innervation (Fig. 4.10).

Remarkably, these investigators observed that the cross-innervated slow soleus muscle adopted the functional properties of a fast muscle while the cross-innervated fast FDL developed slower contractile properties. This occurred without any corresponding changes in the properties of the motor neurons. On the surface, these findings appear to agree with the "frequency" hypothesis, which simply states that the low firing frequency of motor neurons innervating the soleus muscle would cause the FDL to transition to a slower muscle, and the converse would be true of the high firing frequency of the motor neurons innervating the FDL. Interestingly, Buller, Eccles, and Eccles did not interpret these findings to support the frequency hypothesis. Rather, they reasoned that if the frequency hypothesis were correct, then the complete cessation of stimulation should produce an even slower phenotype, which it did not. Their reasoning was apparently based on directional changes in firing frequency (*i.e.*, progressively lower firing frequencies produce progressively slower phenotypes and vice versa).

Buller, Eccles, and Eccles also tested the "aggregate" hypothesis, which stipulated that the slow tonic firing pattern of the soleus motor nerve would result in a greater aggregate of impulses and, as a result, a slower phenotype, whereas the phasic firing pattern of the a fast motor nerve would produce a smaller aggregate and thereby faster contractile properties. The cross-innervation findings were certainly consistent with this hypothesis. However, Buller, Eccles, and Eccles observed that a complete lack of activation (as studied by spinal isolation) actually caused a fast muscle to become slower and not faster as predicted by the aggregate hypothesis. Having rejected both the frequency and aggregate hypotheses, these investigators proposed the "chemical" hypothesis, which stated that motor neurons control the contractile properties of skeletal muscle by releasing a "chemical" (latter referred to as trophic) substance that traverses the neuromuscular junction and then spreads along the length of the muscle fiber. Some 45 years later, it is still unclear whether a trophic substance is produced by motor neurons; however, it is clear that this landmark study shaped several generations of scientific investigation and provided critical evidence to demonstrate that skeletal muscle possessed a plasticity that was previously unrecognized.

Buller AJ, Eccles JC, Eccles RM. Interaction between motoneurones and muscles in respect of the characteristic speeds of their responses. J Physiol. 1960;150:417–39.

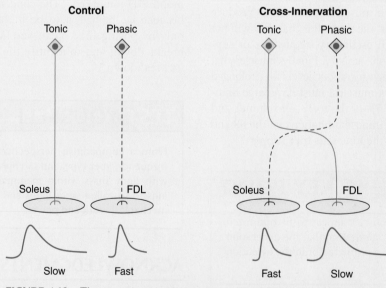

Control

Tonic   Phasic

Soleus   FDL

Slow   Fast

Cross-Innervation

Tonic   Phasic

Soleus   FDL

Fast   Slow

FIGURE 4.10   The cross-innervation experiment of Buller, Eccles, and Eccles in which the motor nerve to the flexor digitorum longus muscle (FDL) was changed to innervate the soleus muscle, whereas the motor nerve to the soleus muscle was altered so it would innervate the FDL muscle.

REFERENCES

1. Huxley AF. Muscle structure and theories of contraction. *Prog Biophys Biophys Chem*. 1957;7:255–318.
2. Clark KA, McElhinny AS, Beckerle MC, et al. Striated muscle cytoarchitecture: an intricate web of form and function. *Ann Rev Cell Dev Biol*. 2002;18:637–706.
3. Bottinelli R. Functional heterogeneity of mammalian single muscle fibres: do myosin isoforms tell the whole story? *Pflugers Arch*. 2001;443:6–17.
4. Bottinelli R, Betto R, Schiaffino S, et al. Unloaded shortening velocity and myosin heavy chain and alkali light chain isoform composition in rat skeletal muscle fibres. *J Physiol Lond*. 1994;478:341–349.
5. Fukuda N, Granzier HL, Ishiwata S, et al. Physiological functions of the giant elastic protein titin in mammalian striated muscle. *J Physiol Sci*. 2005;58:151–159.
6. Caiozzo VJ. Plasticity of skeletal muscle phenotype: mechanical consequences. *Muscle Nerve*. 2002;26:740–768.
7. Pette D, Staron RS. Cellular and molecular diversities of mammalian skeletal muscle fibers. *Rev Physiol Biochem Pharmacol*. 1990;116:1–76.
8. Schiaffino S, Reggiani C. Myosin isoforms in mammalian skeletal muscle. *J Appl Physiol*. 1994;77:493–501.
9. Brooke MH, Kaiser KK. Muscle fiber types: how many and what kind? *Arch Neurol*. 1970;23:369–379.
10. Barnard RJ, Edgerton VR, Furukawa T, et al. Histochemical, biochemical, and contractile properties of red, white, and intermediate fibers. *Am J Physiol*. 1971;220:410–414.
11. Pette D, Staron RS. Transitions of muscle fiber phenotypic profiles. *Histochem Cell Biol*. 2001;115:359–372.
12. Saltin B, Gollnick PD. Skeletal muscle adaptability: significance for metabolism and performance. In: Peachey L, ed. *Handbook of Physiology*. American Physiological Society; 1983:555–631.
13. Caiozzo VJ, Baker MJ, Huang K, et al. Single-fiber myosin heavy chain polymorphism: how many patterns and what proportions? *Am J Physiol Regul Integr Comp Physiol*. 2003;285:R570–R580.
14. Talmadge RJ, Roy RR, Edgerton VR. Persistence of hybrid fibers in rat soleus after spinal cord transection. *Anat Rec*. 1999;255:188–201.
15. Caiozzo VJ, Haddad F, Baker M, et al. MHC polymorphism in rodent plantaris muscle: effects of mechanical overload and hypothyroidism. *Am J Cell Physiol*. 2000;278:C709–C717.
16. Talmadge RJ, Roy RR, Edgerton VR. Distribution of myosin heavy chain isoforms in non-weight-bearing rat soleus muscle fibers. *J Appl Physiol*. 1996;81:2540–2546.
17. Hall ZW, Ralson E. Nuclear domains in muscle cells. *Cell*. 1989;l59:771–772.
18. Peuker H, Pette D. Quantitative analyses of myosin heavy-chain mRNA and protein isoforms in single fibers reveal a pronounced fiber heterogeneity in normal rabbit muscles. *Eur J Biochem*. 1997;247:30–36.
19. Edman KAP, Reggiani C, Schiaffino S, et al. Maximum velocity of shortening related to myosin isoform composition in frog skeletal muscle fibres. *J Physiol Lond*. 1988;395:679–694.
20. Rome LC, Linstedt SL. Mechanical and metabolic design of the muscular system in vertebrates. In: Dantzler WH, ed.

21. Josephson RK. Dissecting muscle power output. *J Exp Biol*. 1999;202 Pt 23:3369–75.
22. Booth FW, Baldwin KM. *Muscle Plasticity: Energy Demand and Supply Processes*. New York: Oxford University Press; 1996.
23. Hill AV. The heat of shortening and the dynamic constants of muscle. *Proc R Soc London Ser B*. 1938;126:136–95.
24. Friden J, Lieber RL. Spastic muscle cells are shorter and stiffer than normal cells. *Muscle Nerve*. 2003;27:157–64.
25. Lieber RL, Friden J. Spasticity causes a fundamental rearrangement of muscle-joint interaction. *Muscle Nerve*. 2002;25:265–70.
26. Hill AV. *First and Last Experiments in Muscle Mechanics*. New York (NY): Cambridge University Press; 1970.
27. Woledge RC, Curtin NA, Homsher E. *Energetic Aspects of Muscle Contraction*. New York: Academic Press; 1985.
28. Caiozzo VJ, Baker MJ, Baldwin KM. Novel transitions in myosin isoforms: separate and combined effects of thyroid hormone and mechanical unloading. *J Appl Physiol*. 1998;85:2237–48.
29. Josephson RK, Edman KAP. The consequences of fibre heterogeneity on the force-velocity relation of skeletal muscle. *Acta Physiol Scand*. 1988;132:341–52.
30. Reiser PJ, Kasper CE, Moss RL. Myosin subunits and contractile properties of single fibers from hypokinetic rat muscles. *J Appl Physiol*. 1987;63:2293–3300.
31. Bottinelli R, Schiaffino S, Reggiani C. Force-velocity relations and myosin heavy chain isoform compositions of skinned fibres from rat skeletal muscle. *J Physiol*. 1991;437:655–672.
32. Larsson L, Moss RL. Maximum velocity of shortening in relation to myosin isoform composition in single fibres from human skeletal muscles. *J Physiol*. 1993;472:595–614.
33. Edman KA, Reggiani C, Schiaffino S, et al. Maximum velocity of shortening related to myosin isoform composition in frog skeletal muscle fibres. *J Physiol*. 1988;395:679–694.
34. McDonald KS, Blaser CA, Fitts RH. Force-velocity and power characteristics of rat soleus muscle fibers after hindlimb suspension. *J Appl Physiol*. 1994;77:1609–1616.
35. Wojtys EM, Huston LJ, Schock HJ, et al. Gender differences in muscular protection of the knee in torsion in size-matched athletes. *J Bone Joint Surg Am*. 2003;85-A:782–789.
36. Riley DA, Bain JL, Thompson JL, et al. Decreased thin filament density and length in human atrophic soleus muscle fibers after spaceflight. *J Appl Physiol*. 2000;88:567–572.
37. Schulte LM, Navarro J, Kandarian SC. Regulation of sarcoplasmic reticulum calcium pump gene expression by hindlimb unweighting. *Am J Physiol*. 1993;264:C1308–C1315.
38. Toursel T, Stevens L, Granzier H, et al. Passive tension of rat skeletal soleus muscle fibers: effects of unloading conditions. *J Appl Physiol*. 2002;92:1465–1472.
39. Rome LC, Lindstedt SL. The quest for speed: muscles built for high-frequency contractions. *News Physiol Sci*. 1998;13:261–268.
40. Weibel ER, Taylor CR, Hoppeler H. The concept of symmorphosis: a testable hypothesis of structure-function relationship. *Proc Natl Acad Sci U S A*. 1991;88:10357–10361.
41. Diamond J, Hammond K. The matches, achieved by natural selection, between biological capacities and their natural loads. *Experientia*. 1992;48:551–557.

Comparative Physiology. New York (NY): Oxford University Press; 1997:1587–1651.

CHAPTER 5

The Muscular System: The Control of Muscle Mass

Richard Tsika

Abbreviations

Akt	Cytosolic protein kinase recruited to the membrane when PI(3)K is activated (also known as PKB)	MuRF1	Muscle ring finger 1
		MuRF3	Muscle ring finger 3
		MyHC	Myosin heavy chain
ATPase	Adenosine triphosphatase	NFAT	Nuclear factor of activated T-cell
Atrogin-1	E3 ubiquitin ligase also called muscle atrophy F-box (Atrogin-1)	nNOS	Neuronal nitric oxide synthase
		$p70^{S6K}$	Kinase that phosphorylates the S6 subunit of ribosomes
bp	Base pair		
CaMK	Calcium-calmodulin protein kinase	PHAS-1	Phosphorylated heat- and acid-stable protein-1; also known as 4E-BP1
CaN	Calcineurin		
Cb1-b	Casitas b-lineage lymphoma-b; an E3 ubiquitin ligase	PI(3)K	Phosphatidylinositol-3-OH kinase
		Purα/Purβ	Purine-rich; α and β isoforms, single-stranded DNA and RNA binding proteins
CsA	Cyclosporin A		
FoxO	Forkhead box O; a transcription factor	PKD1	Polycystic kidney disease 1; cytosolic protein kinase involved in calcium regulation of cell signaling
GDF-8	Growth differentiation factor-8; also termed myostatin		
		Ras	Monomeric GTP-binding protein
GSK-3β	Glycogen synthase kinase-3β	Sm	Slow myosin
HDAC	Histone deacetylase	Sp1	Specific protein 1
HS	Hind limb suspension	Sp3	Specific protein 3
IGF-1	Insulin-like growth factor-1	TEAD-1	Transcriptional enhancer factor-1
MAPK	Mitogen-activated protein kinase	V_{max}	Maximum unloaded shortening velocity
MCK	Muscle creatine kinase	Work	Force × distance
MEF2	Myocyte enhancer factor-2	YB-1	Y-box binding protein; single-stranded DNA and RNA binding protein
MOV	Mechanical overload		
mTOR	Mammalian target of rapamycin		

Introduction

An extraordinary characteristic of adult skeletal muscle is its intrinsic ability to adapt to a broad range of physiologic stimuli, such as those produced by various exercise paradigms. For example, increased skeletal muscle workload (force × distance) as imposed by various weight training regimens has a profound effect on both mass (hypertrophy) and strength (force production) (1,2). This type of adaptation in response to weight training is so well known it is legendary. Milo of Crotona, a sixth century BC Greek athlete, reportedly acquired the strength to carry a bull around a stadium by lifting the bull daily from the time it was a newborn calf, thereby gradually accommodating to the increased load as the calf increased in weight (3). Conversely, decreased muscle loading associated with inactivity resulting from normal aging processes, immobilization due to injury, various systemic diseases, and the less frequently encountered exposure to zero gravity (space travel) leads to the undesirable decline in muscle mass (atrophy) and function (1,4). Because of obvious ethical considerations, rigorous biochemical and molecular studies concerning altered muscle-loading conditions have used animal models as opposed to human subjects. Nevertheless, the relentless advancements made in biotechnology over the past decade, including the powerful genetic methodology of transgenesis, allowed scientists to unravel complex molecular mechanisms underlying the biochemical and physiologic adaptations that occur in muscle following alterations in load-bearing activity. This chapter focuses on some of the most recent and remarkable discoveries that form just the beginning of our insight into the control of muscle mass.

Hypertrophy

Hypertrophy of adult skeletal muscle is a complex biologic response wherein the cross-sectional area of each fiber in a given muscle increases (Fig. 5.1A–D). This enlargement in adult rodent (rat and mouse) muscle size does not involve an increase in muscle fiber (individual cell) number, a process referred to as hyperplasia. Because adult skeletal muscle fibers are terminally differentiated, they have lost the ability to proliferate and, thus, any increase in size due to increased workload must occur without increased numbers of cells.

General Physiologic and Biochemical Properties of Skeletal Muscle

The differentiation and maturation of skeletal muscle fibers into distinct phenotypes involve transcriptional activation of

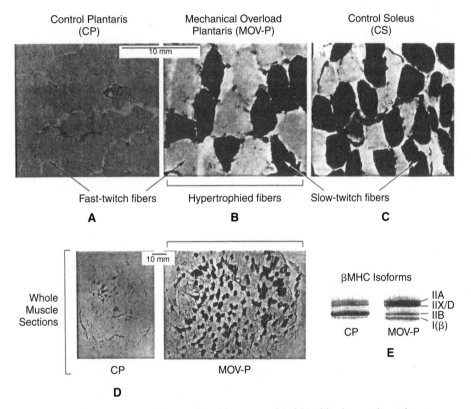

FIGURE 5.1   Cross-section of control and hypertrophied hind limb muscle with corresponding isomyosin profile. **A–C.** Muscle sections subjected to acid-stable myosin ATPase histochemistry, which results in the dark staining of only slow-twitch fibers. A 10-mm bar shows the approximate magnification for all three panels. **A.** Control plantaris. **B.** Hypertrophied plantaris that resulted from mechanical overload (MOV). **C.** Control soleus. (Reprinted with permission, Wiedenman JL, Tsika GL, Gao L, et al. Muscle specific and inducible expression of 293-base pair beta-myosin heavy chain (βMyHC) promoter in transgenic mice. *Am L Physiol.* 1996;271:R688–R695.) **D.** Cross-sections of both control and hypertrophied whole plantaris muscle. **A–D.** Approximate doubling of fiber size in the hypertrophied plantaris when compared to control sections. In addition to increased fiber size, the MOV-induced hypertrophied sections show that some fibers undergo a fast-to-slow phenotypic transition. **E.** Further evidence of this fiber-type switch: induction of the βMyHC (type I isoprotein), an increase in type IIa and IIx/d isoproteins, and a decrease in the fast type IIb isoprotein in the MOV-P muscle extract.

numerous unlinked muscle-specific genes encoding cytoskeletal, calcium-handling, metabolic, and contractile proteins that when assembled create an elaborate machine capable of accommodating a large array of functional demands (1,5). A distinguishing feature of skeletal muscle is its intricate organization of contractile proteins into striated myofibrils composed of repeating units called sarcomeres, the smallest force-producing unit of a myofibril. Although each sarcomere displays the same precise structural organization, the amount and type of contractile protein comprising a given sarcomere can differ based on the differential use of fiber type–specific contractile protein isoforms. The functional implications of the differential use of contractile protein isoforms are exemplified by the sarcomeric myosin heavy chain (MyHC) gene family (5–7). For example, in the adult rat and mouse, four MyHC isoforms (fast type IIb, IIx/d, IIa, and slow type I [also referred to as βMyHC]) are differentially expressed, and this expression pattern has been shown to contribute to the histochemical (myofibrillar adenosine triphosphatase [ATPase]) and immunohistochemical (anti-MyHC) classification of four primary fiber types, termed IIb, IIx/d, IIa, and slow type I.* In addition, hybrid fibers that coexpress multiple MyHC isoforms have been identified and the relative population of these fibers increases in response to perturbations, such as increased and decreased muscle loading states (1,4). Each muscle fiber type displays unique functional properties with respect to size, metabolism, fatigability, and intrinsic properties. The notion that each MyHC serves a physiologic role is underscored by the classic finding that actin-activated myosin ATPase and maximum unloaded shortening velocity (V_{max}) are highly correlated to the amount and type of native isomyosin or MyHC comprising a given muscle or muscle fiber (8). Consistent with the latter concept, a functional analysis of skeletal muscle obtained from mice with either MyHC IIa or MyHC IIx/d gene inactivation (gene targeting) revealed altered contractile properties that were unique to each MyHC null mutation (7).

Summary

Evidence gathered from other studies on both animal and in vitro models have provided ample evidence that the amount and type of MyHC in a muscle's contractile apparatus has functional significance, as well as producing the physiologic consequences of alterations in MyHC composition, whether induced by physiologic stimuli, disease, or mutation (natural or by gene targeting) (1,5–8).

KEY POINT

The amount and type of contractile protein comprising a given sarcomere can differ based on the differential use of fiber type–specific contractile protein isoforms.

---

*The MyHC IIb gene is present in the human genome, but it is not clear if this MyHC protein is expressed at detectable levels.

Experimental Models

Over the years several animal models have been developed for the purpose of elucidating the cellular, biochemical, and molecular mechanisms involved in skeletal muscle remodeling in response to increase muscle loading. These models include stretch, resistance exercise, and compensatory overload (2). Evidence gathered from these studies has revealed that although the contractile activity and magnitude of work overload imposed differs between these diverse models, all skeletal muscles adapt with varying degrees of hypertrophic growth, increased strength, and a fast-to-slow phenotype transition (2). The compensatory overload model produces the most profound changes in skeletal muscle hypertrophy and phenotype and, because of this feature, this model has been frequently used to characterize physiologic and biochemical adaptations to increase muscle loading (Fig. 5.2). More recently, this model has been combined with transgenesis to elucidate in vivo complex integrated biologic responses such as cell signaling and transcriptional regulation (9,10). Thus, compensatory overload is the focus of this section, where sustained adaptations induced by chronic workload is concerned. In some cases, acute adaptations will be discussed. For a detailed description of the stretch or resistance exercise models of muscle hypertrophy and the adaptations associated with each of these models, consult the outstanding reviews of Booth and Baldwin (1), Timson (2), and Baldwin and Haddad (4).

The compensatory overload model and skeletal muscle adaptations

In the rodent (mouse, rat) model of compensatory overload, a chronic increase in muscle loading is induced by the

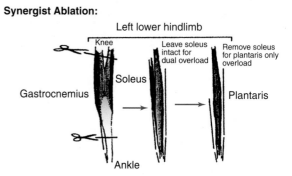

Synergist Ablation:

Removes 85%: Gastrocnemius (mixed), Soleus (type I)
Retains 15%: Plantaris (type II)

Imposes:
Chronic weight-bearing activity

Induces:
Hypertrophy of all muscle fibers
Fiber type transitions:

Fast-glycolytic   Slow-oxidative

Type IIB ⟶ IIX/D ⟶ IIA ⟶ Type I

FIGURE 5.2 Mechanical overload (MOV) model. Significant features of MOV used to induce both skeletal muscle hypertrophy and fiber phenotype fast-to-slow changes.

surgical removal of a given muscle's synergists (Fig. 5.2). For example, compensatory overload of the rodent fast-twitch plantaris muscle involves the surgical removal of its synergists, the soleus and gastrocnemius (2). In this case, the imposition of chronic loading demands that the remaining fast-twitch plantaris muscle (used in high-force locomotor activity) takes over the functional duties normally performed by the slow-twitch soleus (used for chronic postural maintenance) and mixed-fiber typed gastrocnemius (locomotor movements) muscles. Because this model requires the plantaris muscle to perform the duties of the soleus and gastrocnemius muscles and to develop a sustained increase in force, it has also been referred to as functional overload or mechanical overload (MOV). In this chapter, this model is called MOV. The MOV model can be used to induce hypertrophy and fiber phenotype switches in both slow-twitch muscle (*e.g.*, soleus) and fast-twitch muscle (*e.g.*, plantaris). Even though the soleus muscle is already primarily comprised of type I fibers (85% type I in rats; 50%–70% type I in mice), the direction of the fiber type shift remains fast-to-slow twitch. However, because the adult rodent fast-twitch plantaris muscle is comprised primarily of fast type II fibers (95%), it is the preferred muscle with which to study load-induced enlargement and fast-to-slow phenotype switches.

MOV is a physiologic stimulus associated with a rapid increase in muscle mass. Notably, the rapid enlargement that occurs within the first week after MOV is accompanied by inflammatory edema and, therefore, assessments of true muscle hypertrophy (protein accretion) during this early time should be viewed with caution (2). Nevertheless, a steady-state hypertrophy of the adult MOV plantaris muscle appears to occur between 6 and 9 weeks after overload (1,11). This enlargement is achieved by an increase in the rate of protein synthesis, primarily resulting in an increase in the cross-sectional area (sarcomeres in parallel) of all existing fibers, whereas models of stretch hypertrophy largely result in increased muscle length (primarily sarcomeres in series) (2). The MOV-induced protein accretion is coincident with increases in essential contractile proteins that, when assembled into sarcomeres (smallest force-generating units of striated muscle), enhance the force-generating capacity of the hypertrophied plantaris muscle. The adaptation in contractile properties within the MOV plantaris muscle includes increases in absolute peak tension and maximal tetanic isometric force, while the unloaded shortening velocity (V_{max}) is decreased (8). Consistent with a decrease in V_0, the actin-activated myosin ATPase activity is also decreased (1,2). The latter adaptations are consistent with a fast-to-slow fiber type transition, which has been confirmed by histochemical staining for myofibrillar ATPase, MyHC immunohistochemistry, and electrophoretic separation of native myosin and MyHC isoforms (Fig. 5.1) (1,4). Concurrent with a fast-to-slow phenotype remodeling, a change in innervation pattern or total electrical activity of the MOV muscle has been observed (12).

KEY POINT

The MOV model can be used to induce hypertrophy and fiber phenotype switches in both slow-twitch muscle (*e.g.*, soleus) and fast-twitch muscle (*e.g.*, plantaris).

TEST YOURSELF

You have developed a transgenic mouse that expresses a transgene encoding the βMyHC only in fast-twitch muscles such as the plantaris. You have confirmed that the βMyHC protein is expressed and incorporated within the sarcomeres of the plantaris muscle. (a) Would this affect the contractile properties of the plantaris muscle? (b) If so, what contractile properties would be affected? (c) As opposed to making transgenic mice, is there an animal model that would increase βMyHC expression in the plantaris?

MOV as a complex externally imposed stimulus which activates numerous signals

Because MOV is a complex external stimulus associated with the activation of numerous signals, it is not possible to accurately replicate all its effects using cell culture systems. This is illustrated by the fact that adult-stage muscle phenotypes, fiber type transitions, and equivalent loading conditions cannot be duplicated with myogenic cells in culture. Further limitations are that many control mechanisms associated with hormonal (endocrine), circulatory, neural input, and important communication between different cell types are not represented in permanent cell lines or primary cells in culture. Thus, the elucidation of the regulatory mechanisms that control skeletal muscle adaptations in response to MOV requires the use of rat or mouse models. Also, with intact animals, any adaptation that occurs in response to MOV is the result of an integrated physiologic response that includes input (independent and convergent signals) from but not limited to:

1. Increased levels of load bearing
2. Increased electrical activation (as measured by electromyography [EMG] signal)
3. Autocrine (*e.g.*, insulin-like growth factor-1 [IGF-1], prostaglandins) signals
4. An acute immune response associated with cytokine secretion (interleukin-6, leukemia inhibitory factor)
5. Growth factors
6. Rapid and transient induction (1–48 hours) of EMG thought to be involved in the growth response
7. Decreased expression (within first 2 days) of enzymes representative of a glycolytic profile (α-glycerophosphate dehydrogenase, Glyceraldehyde-3-phosphate dehydrogenase, and muscle creatine kinase) that may represent a metabolic signal for a switch to a more oxidative (slow) phenotype

8. Activation of integrin signaling cascades within the first week
9. Regulation of myostatin
10. Activation of satellite cells and putative endogenous muscle stem cells (2,9,12–14)
11. Transduction of extracellular signals that activate intracellular signaling pathways and nuclear transcription
12. Likely other as yet unidentified stimuli (Fig. 5.3).

It is clear from this list that the identification of precise regulatory mechanisms controlling load-induced skeletal muscle remodeling (hypertrophy and phenotype) will be a challenging task because this process involves the differential expression of hundreds of genes representing numerous subcellular systems. Regardless of inherent complications with intact animal model usage, the importance of these models lies in the fact that they are not discrete and, thus, are relatively likely to mimic human activity that requires sustained increases in force development (load). Despite difficulties, significant advances have been made in defining cell signaling pathways activated by MOV (see *Intracellular Signal Transduction Pathways*) and the involvement of satellite cells in the development of skeletal muscle hypertrophy.

Satellite cells are mitotically quiescent, mononucleated cells that reside between the surrounding basal lamina and the sarcolemma of differentiated muscle fibers (14). These quiescent cells have been shown to be responsible for the majority of postnatal skeletal muscle growth, repair, and regeneration following injury or damage. When satellite cells are activated due to injury or exercise they proliferate extensively, undergo self-renewal, and differentiate into new muscle fibers by fusing to themselves or into the existing muscle fibers. Because satellite cells display lineage-specific differentiation (muscle cell) and self-renewal, two characteristics of stem cells, they can be considered adult skeletal muscle stem cells. The capability of self-renewal is an important property of satellite cells as it assures that the resident satellite cell pool of a myofiber is restored after activation and is available for subsequent cycles of damage-induced degradation and regeneration of skeletal muscle.

When activated in response to MOV, these cells proliferate and eventually their progeny fuse to existing muscle fibers and provide additional nuclei that are necessary to maintain the ratio of nuclei to cytoplasmic volume. Because adult skeletal muscle cells cannot divide, they require the activation and incorporation of satellite cells to undergo hypertrophic growth in response to increased load-bearing stimuli such as MOV (14). Experiments have shown that irradiation of

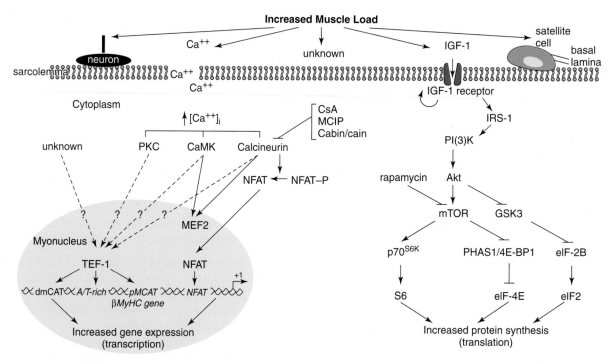

FIGURE 5.3 IGF-1/PI(3)K/Akt/mTOR and the Ca^{++}-dependent signaling pathways calcineurin (CaN) and calcium-calmodulin protein kinase (CaMK). These signaling pathways may be involved in growth (IGF-1/PI(3)K/Akt/mTOR), phenotype changes (CaN and CaMK), or possibly both. Intracellular signaling pathways recently shown to be associated with load-induced hypertrophic growth and fiber type transitions are shown (muscle remodeling). Akt, cytosolic protein kinase recruited to the membrane when PI(3)K is activated; CsA, cyclosporin A; eIF-2B, eukaryotic translation initiation factor 2B; eIF-4E, eukaryotic translation initiation factor 4E; GSK-3, glycogen-synthase kinase-3; IGF-1, insulin-like growth factor-1; IRS-1, insulin receptor substrate 1; MCIP-1, modulatory calcineurin-interacting protein; MEF2, myocyte enhancer factor-2; mTOR, mammalian target of rapamycin; βMyHC, beta-myocin heavy chain; NFAT, nuclear factor of activated T-cell; PHAS-1, phosphorylated heat- and acid-stable protein-1(also known as 4E-BP1); PI(3)K, phosphatidylinositol-3-OH kinase; p70 S6K, kinase that phosphorylates the S6 subunit of ribosomes; TEF-1, transcriptional enhancer factor-1.

skeletal muscle to destroy the satellite cell population elimi-nates MOV-induced hypertrophy and increased numbers of myonuclei (15). On the other hand, although irradiation blocked MOV-induced skeletal muscle hypertrophy, it did not alter the fast-to-slow transition in MyHC gene expres-sion. This raises the question to what extent satellite cells participate in the MOV-induced, fast-to-slow phenotype transition. Although numerous signals have been implicated in satellite cell activation, those directly involved in the MOV response are not well defined. Some evidence supports a role for IGF-1 and a macrophage response involving secretion of cytokines (14). Additional work will be required to precisely delineate MOV-induced signals involved in satellite cell acti-vation and to resolve issues regarding cross talk between signaling pathways involved in hypertrophic growth versus phenotype transitions.

TEST YOURSELF

What ability has the adult skeletal muscle lost by being terminally differentiated? How does it make up for this loss? Explain your answer in detail.

Why are satellite cells considered adult stem cells? What is the location of satellite cells and what signals activate them?

Molecular Pathways for Skeletal Muscle Hypertrophy

All eukaryotic cells have the innate ability to respond to a broad range of extracellular stimuli ultimately resulting in a suitable physiologic response. This action occurs via the integration of multiple intracellular signaling pathways and gene networks to modulate the activity of transcription factors and cellular proteins involved in protein synthesis and degradation (Fig. 5.3).

Intracellular signal transduction pathways

A well-known response to external signals is the activation of intracellular protein kinases and phosphatases, which modu-late the phosphorylation status of a multitude of intracellular and nuclear molecules. Ultimately, these modifications alter the function of the target protein. For example, phosphoryla-tion or dephosphorylation can alter the DNA-binding activity of a transcription factor, its subcellular location, its stability, or whether it forms dimers. In addition to phosphorylation and dephosphorylation, other posttranslational modifications such as ubiquitination, glycosylation, lipidation, acetylation, or sumoylation have been shown to alter a given protein's activity. This section addresses some of the most intensely studied intracellular signaling pathways thought to control skeletal muscle hypertrophy and phenotype.

CALCINEURIN (CAN): A CA^{++}-DEPENDENT SIGNALING PATHWAY CaN is a cytoplasmically located calcium- and calmodulin-dependent serine-threonine protein phosphatase.

The functional role of CaN was first delineated in T-cells, where increased levels of intracellular calcium were found to mediate the interaction between calmodulin and CaN, leading to CaN activation. Mechanistically, cytoplasmic nuclear factor of acti-vated T-cell (NFAT) proteins are dephosphorylated by activated CaN, allowing their translocation into the nucleus, where they act combinatorial with other transcription factors to activate target gene transcription (16,17). Since calcium is known to regulate many cellular processes in striated muscle, the ques-tion arose whether the CaN signaling pathway also functioned in striated muscle. The work of Molkentin and colleagues (18) provided the first evidence that CaN was involved in the devel-opment of cardiac hypertrophy. This was followed by the obser-vation of Chin and associates (19), whose work implicated a role for this enzyme in determining skeletal muscle fiber type. The latter conclusion was based on the finding that treatment of rats with cyclosporin A (CsA), an inhibitor of CaN activity, led to a decrease in the proportion of slow fibers populating the soleus muscle while the proportion of fast fibers increased. Addition-ally, cell culture experiments implicated the CaN-NFAT path-way in modulating both skeletal muscle phenotype and the development of IGF-1-induced hypertrophy (16,17).

Since these initial observations, numerous research teams have investigated the role of CaN in determining skeletal muscle fiber type gene expression and the induc-tion of hypertrophy. This work has led to a proposed model postulating that calcium-mobilizing signals evoked by stimuli—such as chronic low-frequency motor nerve stimulation, MOV, or voluntary wheel running—induce a sustained low-amplitude elevation in intracellular calcium levels and this, in turn, stimulates both the CaN and cal-cium-calmodulin protein kinase (CaMK) signaling path-ways. Activation of these two signaling pathways leads to induction of hypertrophic growth and the transcriptional activation of slow fiber genes mediated by downstream modulators comprising various members of the NFAT and myocyte enhancer factor-2 (MEF2) transcription fac-tor families (16,17). The transcriptional activity of nuclear MEF2 is enhanced by CaN in two ways: (a) by its dephos-phorylation and (b) by direct interaction with nuclear DNA-bound NFAT. CaMK and polycystic kidney disease 1 (PKD1) are also thought to activate the transcriptional activity of DNA-bound MEF2 by disrupting MEF2's asso-ciation with class II histone deacetylases (HDACs), which act to suppress the transcriptional activation function of MEF2. Disruption of the class II HDAC-MEF2 interaction results in the ubiquitination and proteasomal degradation of class II HDACs (20,21). However, this overall model is not without controversy.

Although an initial series of studies provided evidence implicating a primary role for CaN in mediating skeletal mus-cle hypertrophy and phenotype, a number of recent studies have shown that although this pathway may play a central role in the development of many forms of cardiac hyper-trophy, it is not necessarily required for the development of skeletal muscle hypertrophy or fiber-type shifts (17). To more clearly resolve whether CaN plays a role in skeletal muscle hypertrophy and/or phenotypic transitions, gene targeting mice that lack greater than 80% of their total skeletal muscle CaN were generated (22). These mice were found to display a dramatic impairment in the fast-to-slow fiber type transition in response to MOV; however, hypertrophic growth was not altered indicating that CaN is not required for MOV-induced skeletal muscle hypertrophy (22).

KEY POINT

All muscle skeletal muscle cells can mount a suitable physiologic response to chronic use. This action occurs via the integration of multiple intracellular signaling pathways and gene networks to modulate the activity of transcription factors and cellular proteins involved in protein synthesis and degradation.

Summary

Because NFAT and MEF2 have been implicated in the activation of slow muscle gene expression, a more complete knowledge of their downstream gene targets will be necessary for understanding their role in modulating fast and slow phenotype switches in response to various physiologic perturbations. Likewise, continued investigations will also be required to fully elucidate additional downstream effectors (transcription factors) of CaN signaling and for a more complete picture of how CaN signaling integrates with other signaling pathways involved in both hypertrophic growth and phenotype transitions.

CALCIUM-CALMODULIN PROTEIN KINASE (CaMK): A Ca^{++}-DEPENDENT SIGNALING PATHWAY The activity of CaMK, like CaN, is regulated by intracellular calcium although the amount and type of calcium signal differs. Whereas CaN is activated by sustained low-amplitude calcium signals, CaMK is presumably activated by short-duration, high-amplitude calcium signals (16,17). As previously described, CaMK is thought to enhance MEF2 transcriptional activity by disrupting its interaction with HDACs which function as transcriptional repressors. In addition, new evidence has revealed that PKD1 also functions in this capacity (20). The activation of MEF2 has been tied to skeletal muscle fiber–type gene expression based on a number of observations:

1. MOV, chronic low-frequency nerve stimulation, voluntary wheel running, and overexpression of an activated CaN protein resulted in decreased nuclear MEF2 phosphorylation (16,17) (supports role for CaN)
2. Electrophoretic mobility shift assays, which are designed to examine DNA–protein interaction, have shown that the degree of MEF2 protein binding at MEF2 elements does not change in response to these perturbations (16) (indicates a release of HDAC transcriptional repression supporting a role for CaMK)

3. Increased nuclear degradation of HDACs (21) (a collaborative role for PKD1 with CaMK and CaN)
4. These same perturbations activated a MEF2-dependent reporter transgene in transgenic mice (termed MEF2-sensor mice [16]) and this effect was blocked by treatment with CsA and by transgenic expression of modulatory calcineurin-interacting protein-1 (a peptide inhibitor of CaN now termed RCAN1) (16) (supports a role for CaN and CaMK)

However, conclusions concerning MEF2 involvement in regulating slow fiber gene expression based on the results obtained with the MEF2-sensor transgenic mice must be viewed with caution because it was recently shown that all four TEAD-1 (also referred to as transcriptional enhancer factor-1 [TEF-1]) family members avidly bind the desmin MEF2 element used in the MEF2 sensor transgene (see *Transcriptional Regulation of the βMyHC Gene in Response to MOV* [23]). Here again, more work needs to be done to sort out roles for this pathway in the transduction of exercise-induced signals into growth or phenotypic transitions.

TEST YOURSELF

You have isolated a new gene that is expressed only in skeletal muscle. Stimulation of intracellular signaling pathway X has been shown to activate a downstream mediator (transcription factor) that confers muscle-specific expression to other muscle genes.

Should you assume that the same signaling pathway and transcription factor confers muscle-specific expression to your gene?

How might stimulation of a given signaling pathway alter the activity of a DNA-bound transcription factor?

RAS-MITOGEN-ACTIVATED PROTEIN KINASE (MAPK) PATHWAY The important influence of neural input on modulating muscle phenotype has been recognized since the early studies of Buller and associates (24), which demonstrated that fast muscles take on slow-twitch contractile properties following cross-innervation with a slow motor neuron and vice versa. To determine the signaling pathways involved in this process, Murgia and colleagues (25) investigated the role of the monomeric GTP-binding protein (Ras)-MAPK pathway, previously shown to be activated by electrostimulation of muscle. Use of several Ras mutants allowed these researchers to show that the Ras-MAPK pathway mimics the effects of slow nerve innervation, thereby implicating its role in regulating nerve-dependent slow muscle gene expression (25). A constitutively activated Ras mutant was found to activate the ERK pathway (a MAPK pathway), which reproduced the effect of slow motor nerve input by activating slow myosin (Sm) expression and decreasing fast myosin expression in denervated regeneration muscle. In contrast, Sm expression was blocked in innervated muscle that overexpressed a dominant negative mutant of Ras (interferes with Ras signaling). This observation is relevant to many exercise models and specifically to the overload model because MOV is associated with an increase in motor nerve activity (as measured by EMG signal) and increased Sm expression. It is interesting that several recent investigations have shown that NFAT transcription factors differentially translocate to the nucleus depending on the electrical stimulation patterns used, and that NFATc1, in particular, seems to act as a repressor of fast muscle gene expression in slow muscle (26,27). Additional research will be required to determine if the increased motor nerve activity associated with MOV differentially modulates the NFAT transcription factors to facilitate a fast-to-slow fiber type transition.

INSULIN-LIKE GROWTH FACTOR-1 (IGF-1)/PHOSPHATIDYLINOSITOL-3-OH KINASE (PI(3)K)/AKT (PROTEIN KINASE B)/ MTOR (MAMMALIAN TARGET OF RAPAMYCIN) PATHWAY (IGF-1/PI(3)K/AKT/MTOR) IGF-1 has been shown to serve important functional roles during myogenesis and, in adult muscle, respond to muscle injury and growth-inducing stimuli such as MOV. In particular, one isoform of IGF-1 is upregulated in skeletal muscle only in response to mechanical stimuli and, thus, has been termed *mechano growth factor* (28). Studies on transgenic mice have shown that IGF-1 overexpression results in skeletal muscle hypertrophy, and IGF-1 has also been shown to stimulate satellite cell proliferation which may contribute to its hypertrophic effect on muscle (Fig. 5.3).

Observations that IGF-1 has the potential to improve skeletal muscle regenerative capacity in injured, diseased (*mdx* [muscular dystrophy]), and aged mice have prompted considerable interest in deciphering the downstream signaling pathway or pathways activated by IGF-1 leading to skeletal muscle hypertrophy. Briefly, the signaling pathway downstream from IGF-1 binding to its membrane receptor (a receptor tyrosine kinase) involves the serial activation of several downstream kinases (PI[3]K, Akt [cytosolic protein kinase recruited to the membrane when PI{3}K is activated; also known as PKB], mTOR, and p70^{S6K}) leading to increased protein synthesis, a necessary step in the development of skeletal muscle hypertrophy (Fig. 5.3). Studies utilizing myogenic cells in culture have reported that IGF-1 signaling involves the calcium-activated CaN pathway (29); however, the findings of others dispute this observation by showing that treatment of cells with CsA did not block IGF-1-mediated hypertrophy of myotubes (29). Instead, the latter studies provided strong evidence for a PI(3)K-Akt-mTOR pathway by showing increased phosphorylation of these downstream IGF-1 effectors following treatment of cells with IGF-1 and by demonstrating that CsA treatment did not block this response nor could a calcium ionophore induce this response (29). The involvement of this pathway in inducing skeletal muscle hypertrophy was further supported by animal studies wherein the levels of Akt phosphorylation were found to be increased in response to MOV, and treatment with the mTOR inhibitor rapamycin nearly eliminated hypertrophy of the MOV-plantaris muscle (29). The overexpression of a constitutively active form of Akt in adult

mouse skeletal muscle was also found to induce hypertrophy and to prevent atrophy (29). In addition, constitutively active PI(3)K, the upstream activator of Akt, was also shown to prevent muscle atrophy (29). Further support for the involvement of the Akt pathway in muscle growth comes from transgenic gain of function experiments wherein skeletal muscle restricted overexpression of constitutively active Akt1 resulted in enhanced growth of adult skeletal muscle (29). Conversely, in loss of function studies, mice carrying the targeted deletion of Akt1$^{-/-}$ (or Akt1$^{-/-}$ × Akt2$^{-/-}$) showed growth retardation and a striking amount of muscle atrophy (30). In summary, activation of the Akt pathway led to activation of mTOR, which in turn activates its targets, p70^{S6K}, and inhibits PHAS-1/4E-BP1 (phosphorylated heat- and acid-stable protein-1; also known as 4E-BP1), which are necessary steps for increased protein synthesis and, thus, skeletal muscle hypertrophy.

> ## KEY POINT
>
> IGF-1 has been shown to serve important functional roles during myogenesis and, in adult muscle, respond to MOV.

MYOSTATIN Myostatin, or growth differentiation factor-8 (GDF-8), is a member of the transforming growth factor-β family, and like other members of this family, it is also secreted. The expression of myostatin is primarily restricted to muscle from early embryonic development to adult life. The targeted deletion of myostatin resulted in a highly muscled mouse phenotype that resembled a phenotype observed in two breeds of cattle (Belgian Blue and Piedmontese) as early as 1807 (31). This naturally occurring phenotype in cattle was described as an inheritable condition of hyperplasia (increase in cell number) as opposed to hypertrophy (increase in cell size as seen with MOV) in 1982 and hence termed *doubling muscling*. A loss of function mutation in the human myostatin gene has also been shown to enhanced muscle growth. The finding that the absence of biologically active myostatin, whether due to a natural gene mutation (frameshift mutation due to 11-nucleotide deletion in cattle) or via gene targeting, led to increased muscle mass indicated that myostatin is a negative regulator of muscle growth.

Because of myostatin's obvious potential therapeutic value as a countermeasure of muscle-wasting diseases, studies have been undertaken to determine whether the absence of biologically active myostatin would be effective in maintaining muscle mass in several mouse models of muscular dystrophy, and whether the postnatal absence of biologically active myostatin would induce skeletal muscle hypertrophy. Indeed, the inhibition of myostatin activity was found to have a favorable effect on maintaining muscle mass in dystrophic mice, and to induce a moderate level of skeletal muscle hypertrophic growth in postnatal skeletal muscle (32–36). As satellite cells are thought to be the primary cellular source of postnatal muscle growth, the hypertrophic growth resulting from the postnatal absence of myostatin has been attributed to satellite cell proliferation and incorporation into existing fibers. However, new evidence suggests that postnatal skeletal muscle hypertrophy of wild type and dystrophic mouse muscle due to myostatin deficiency can occur without the involvement of satellite cells (36). This finding is important because it indicates that the absence of postnatal myostatin may be an effective countermeasure against disease-induced muscle wasting without depleting the satellite cell pool due to repetitive cycles of damage-induced degradation and regeneration. However, additional work will be required to confirm this intriguing observation and to elucidate signaling components of the myostatin pathway to be used as targets to block myostatin's negative influence on muscle growth.

TEST YOURSELF

Do the same signaling pathways regulate hypertrophic growth and phenotype shifts? Do you think there is cross talk between intracellular pathways so that hypertrophic growth and phenotype shifts occur concurrently? How does hypertrophic growth that is induced by MOV differ from that induced by a decrease in active myostatin in postnatal skeletal muscle?

Transcriptional control of skeletal muscle hypertrophy

An important aspect of understanding how skeletal muscle hypertrophy and phenotype are controlled undoubtedly involves the transcriptional regulation of muscle genes representing contractile proteins that constitute, in part, the protein accretion necessary for enlargement and for increased force development. Although the protein products of these muscle genes must be assembled in precise stoichiometric amounts to produce sarcomeres, a common genetic regulatory program for controlling muscle gene transcription has not been identified. An explanation may be derived from the following observations: (a) Most muscle genes are in different parts of the genome which may not be transcriptionally activated by the same signals; (b) although some promoter and enhancer regions of muscle genes share conserved DNA-regulatory elements (sites of protein binding, also called cis-acting element), not all muscle genes contain these regulatory elements within their control regions; (c) the existence of a conserved element within a gene's control region does not necessarily imply a functional role for this element under all physiologic conditions (Fig. 5.4).

GENERAL SKELETAL MUSCLE TRANSCRIPTIONAL REGULATION
Although no genetic regulatory program comprised of a common set of cis-acting elements and trans-acting factors that regulates all muscle genes has been elucidated, recent

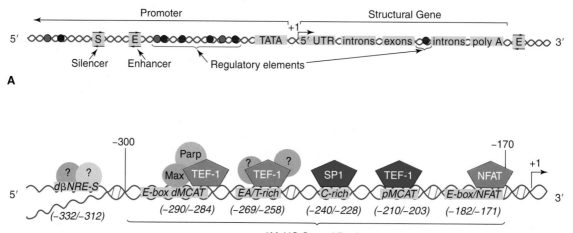

FIGURE 5.4 The modular nature of gene control regions is depicted. **A.** The general structure of a gene and the hypothetical location of regulatory regions that can influence its expression in a manner specific to tissue, developmental stage, and perturbation. The modular arrangement of regulatory regions and elements allows for the integration of combinatorial signals in a gene-specific manner. **B.** A minimal human beta-myocin heavy chain (βMyHC) promoter previously shown to direct the expression of a reporter gene in a pattern that mimics the expression pattern of the endogenous βMyHC promoter throughout development and in response to mechanical overload. Numerous studies on the βMyHC promoter have identified the presence of a strong positive muscle-specific control region (−300/−170) that is highly conserved in sequence and location across species. The regulatory elements comprising this control region and their cognate binding factors are shown. This region contains highly conserved distal muscle-CAT (dMCAT; −290/−284), A/T-rich (βA/T-rich −269/−258; also called GATA), C-rich (−248/−225, not shown: −160/−140, −61/−41), proximal MCAT (pMCAT; −210/−203), and E-box/NFAT elements (−182/−171). In addition, a negative element resides immediately upstream from the dMCAT element and is termed negative regulatory element-sense strand (dβNRE-S) (−332/−312). NFAT, nuclear factor of activated T-cell; SP1, specific protein1; TEF-1, transcriptional enhancer factor-1.

efforts have revealed some common aspects of transcriptional control that seem to be shared by all muscle genes. It is now clear that the initiation and maintenance of skeletal muscle cell differentiation, growth, and adult specification (fiber type) involves the activation of subsets of genes by the combinatorial action of sequence-specific DNA-binding transcription factors and chromatin remodeling enzymes. The DNA sequences that regulate gene expression are generally located 5′ to its start site of transcription (also termed *CAP site,* +1) and are composed of a mosaic pattern of regulatory elements that can be distributed distally or appear clustered in the proximal promoter. However, these regulatory modules can also be located 3′ to the structural gene or within introns (Fig. 5.4A).

Ample evidence supports the notion that the modular arrangement of clustered or discrete *cis*-acting elements provide an elegant mechanism by which the location, time, and magnitude of gene expression can be precisely regulated during development and in response to various physiologic and pathophysiologic stimuli (37). For example, activation of tissue-specific gene transcription involves the assembly of unique combinations of transcription factors at distinct sets of cis-acting DNA elements within promoter and enhancer regions. These DNA–protein interactions become a dynamic foundation for transcription. *Cis*-acting elements within these regulatory regions appear to be arranged such that either independent and/or simultaneous signals can be accommodated through the recruitment of transcriptional cofactors. Such an arrangement of elements also facilitates protein–protein interactions between bound factors. The multiprotein complexes that assemble at these various regulatory modules involve the collaborative interaction of transcription factors that are expressed ubiquitously (*e.g.,* specific protein 1 (Sp1), MEF2, NFAT, serum response factor), in a tissue specific-manner (*e.g.,* MyoD, GATA4), or activated by intrinsic or extrinsic signals. Other features that add specificity to complex gene regulation:

1. The existence of overlapping *cis*-acting elements (composite elements)
2. The relatedness in nucleotide composition between various *cis*-acting DNA-regulatory elements
3. *Cis*-element sequence similarity does not always predict which transcription factor will bind
4. Sequences flanking a regulatory element can have profound effects on transcription factor binding
5. The possible combinatorial interactions which can occur between different classes of transcription factors
6. The involvement of coactivator and corepressor protein factors that can function via protein–protein interactions to bring about altered transcriptional specificity and efficiency
7. The posttranslation modifications of transcription factors, coactivators, and corepressors, which may include, but not be limited to, phosphorylation, glycosylation, lipidation, ubiquitination, SUMOylation, acetylation, methylation, and ribosylation.

As can be seen in (Fig. 5.4B), all of the aforementioned regulatory features exist in the 5′-flanking region of the βMyHC gene. In addition, the βMyHC is a quintessential marker of the slow muscle phenotype and is very responsive to load; thus, it represents an excellent model gene system to illustrate transcriptional regulation in response to MOV.

KEY POINT

The modular arrangement of clustered or discrete *cis*-acting elements provides an elegant mechanism by which the location, timing and magnitude of gene expression can be precisely regulated in response to various physiologic such as muscle overload.

TRANSCRIPTIONAL REGULATION OF THE βMYHC GENE IN RESPONSE TO MOV One of the most physiologically significant changes that occurs in the rodent MOV plantaris muscle is a striking induction of βMyHC expression, a MyHC that is virtually nonexistent in this muscle. This adaptation has been documented by measured increases in endogenous βMyHC mRNA, protein, and βMyHC transgene expression (1,4,38,39). A transgenic analysis of both the mouse and human βMyHC promoters has delineated a minimal 293-base pair (bp) human βMyHC promoter that mimicked the expression pattern of the endogenous βMyHC gene during early development (fetal heart and hind limb), in adult type I fibers, and in response to MOV (38,39). Transgenic mutagenesis studies revealed that the dMCAT and NFAT elements were not required for MOV responsiveness or basal slow fiber expression; however, the βA/T-rich element was found to be required for constitutive (basal) slow muscle expression and possibly, MOV responsiveness of the minimal 293-bp βMyHC transgene (23,40,41). Analysis of protein–DNA interaction studies using EMSAs provided support for the notion that the βA/T-rich element contributes to MOV induction as enriched binding of two distinct nuclear proteins was detected only when using MOV-plantaris (MOV-P) nuclear extract (41). Because the nucleotide sequence of the βA/T-rich element comprises a composite GATA/MEF2-like element, it was expected that this element would bind members of either the GATA or MEF2 transcription factor families; however, binding of these transcription factors was not detected in an EMSA analysis when using control or MOV nuclear extracts (41). In a subsequent study, TEAD-1 was identified as the cognate βA/T-rich binding factor by using the βA/T-rich element as bait in a yeast-1-hybrid screen of a MOV-plantaris cDNA library (23). The determination of TEAD-1 as the enrich βA/T-rich binding factor was completely unexpected as TEAD-1 was previously thought to bind only MCAT elements. Nevertheless, the functional significance of TEAD-1 binding to the βA/T-rich element was demonstrated in transient expression assays wherein overexpression of each of the four TEAD-1 family members was shown to trans-activate βMyHC reporter genes and TEAD-1 dependent heterologous promoters in cultures of myogenic cells (21).

In addition to the βA/T-rich element, the TEAD-1 proteins were shown to bind a broad subset of A/T-rich and MEF2 sites as well as the pal-Mt in the control region of other genes representative of the slow phenotype. Several of these regulatory elements displayed enriched TEAD-1 binding in EMSAs only when using MOV-plantaris nuclear extract. Of particular interest was the finding that the desmin pal-Mt element, which overlaps the desmin MEF2 element used to construct the MEF2-sensor transgene, bound TEAD-1 protein as opposed to MEF2 when using a variety of muscle nuclear extracts including MOV-plantaris (23). Importantly, upregulation of the desmin MEF2-dependent transgene (MEF2-sensor mice) has been used in numerous studies as a marker of enhanced MEF2 transcriptional activation (recall that MEF2 is a downstream target of the CaN/CaMK/PKD1 pathways) in response to several exercise paradigms, including electrical stimulation, voluntary wheel running, and MOV (16,17). It is intriguing to imagine that in adult skeletal muscle MEF2 and TEAD proteins may compete for MEF2 site occupancy, depending of the activity state of a given skeletal muscle. For example, MOV may induce TEAD protein binding at the desmin MEF2-Mt element, whereas voluntary wheel running or motor nerve pacing may induce MEF2 activity.

To extend the previously described findings, an analysis of striated muscle restricted TEAD-1 overexpression in transgenic mice was undertaken to determine whether TEAD-1 functions as a modulator of slow gene expression (42). TEAD-1 overexpression was shown to induce a transition toward a slow skeletal muscle contractile protein phenotype (MyHC, troponin complex, and sarcoplasmic reticulum), slower shortening velocity (V_{max}), and longer contraction and relaxation times in the adult fast-twitch extensor digitalis longus muscle (42). An unexpected, but intriguing finding in this study was that a sustained increase in nuclear TEAD-1 leads to the activation of glycogen synthase kinase-3α/β (GSK-3α/β) resulting in a decrease in nuclear NFATc1 and NFATc3 indicating that the transition toward a slower contractile protein phenotype was accomplished in a seemingly NFAT-independent manner (42).

Summary

These findings indicate that TEAD-1 can induce a transition toward a slower contractile phenotype independent of activation of the calcium-regulated pathways (CaMK, CaN, and PKD1), conceivably via direct TEAD-1 element binding and combinatorial interactions with adjacently bound transcriptional regulators and coactivators (42). Clearly, additional work will be required to clarify whether TEAD or MEF2 proteins occupy these MEF2 binding sites in fast versus slow skeletal muscle and under various conditions of muscle activity. In any event, the specific binding of TEAD-1 to a variety of MEF2, A/T-rich, and MCAT elements under control and MOV conditions (23), its involvement in altering

the activity of key cellular signaling proteins (GSK-3-α/β), and to induce a slower contractile protein phenotype strongly suggests that TEAD proteins may serve a broader than previously thought role in striated and smooth muscle gene regulation under basal and hypertrophic conditions.

TEST YOURSELF

While performing transient expression assays in cultured myogenic cells, you find that the expression of a muscle-specific reporter gene initially increases, then decreases as you increase that amount of transcription factor X. (a) What could account for this effect?

Cis-acting regulatory element Z has been shown to confer muscle-specific expression to other muscle genes and is bound by transcription factor Z'. (b) Although this regulatory element is present in the control region of a gene you have recently isolated, should you assume that it confers muscle-specific expression to your gene and that transcription factor Z' binds to your element? (c) Do you think that a given transcription factor is activated by the same signal transduction pathways in response to all perturbations that alter hypertrophic growth and phenotype transitions?

Atrophy

Atrophy is defined as the decrease in the cross-sectional area of muscle fibers without the loss of number of muscle fibers (Fig. 5.5).

Experimental Models

The response of adult skeletal muscle to non–weight-bearing (NWB) activity has been extensively studied using several models that include ground-based hind limb suspension (HS), limb immobilization with muscle in a shortened position, bed rest, spinal cord isolation or transection, and space flight. Several excellent reviews provide a more comprehensive description of the experimental models used to impose muscle disuse and the physiologic consequences of muscle inactivity (1,4,43). This section will provide current information on the mechanistic basis underlying muscle atrophy and phenotype switches in response to NWB activity induced by HS.

The non–weight-bearing model and skeletal muscle adaptations

Although both fast- and slow-twitch muscle fibers are sensitive to NWB activity, muscles (soleus) or muscle regions composed predominantly of slow-twitch type I fibers, which function primarily during postural and low-intensity locomotor activity, have been shown to be more susceptible. In general, this is evidenced by a rapid loss in muscle mass

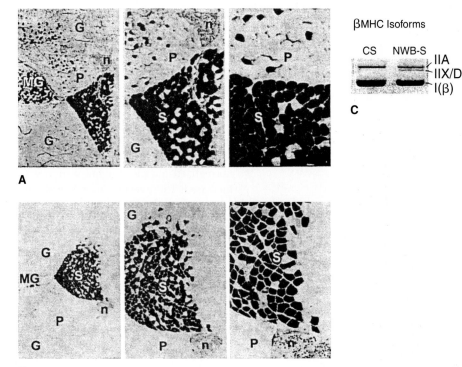

βMHC Isoforms

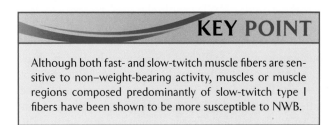

FIGURE 5.5   Cross-section of control and non–weight-bearing (NWB) hind limb muscle with corresponding isomyosin profile. *Right to left.* Sections at increasing magnification of hind limb skeletal muscles subjected to acid-stable ATPase histochemistry. **A.** Control muscles include the gastrocnemius (G), the medial portion of the gastrocnemius (MG), plantaris (P), and soleus (S). The major nerve that runs parallel and directly adjacent to the bone is labeled *n*. **B.** The same skeletal muscles, G, MG, P, and S, subjected to 2 weeks of hind limb suspension (HS)-induced NWB. Fiber size has been significantly reduced in the NWB muscles when compared to control tissues and some fibers have undergone a slow-to-fast fiber type transition distinguished by a decrease in the number of dark stained fibers. **C.** A reduced amount of βMyHC (type I fibers) and type IIa isoproteins and an induction of the type IIx/d isoprotein in the NWB-S muscle, which is consistent with slow-to-fast fiber type transition.

(cross-sectional area), a decrease in bone density, and an altered protein phenotype that correlates with a slow-to-fast change in proteins representing various subcellular systems, such as sarcomeres, glycolytic and oxidative enzymes, sarcoplasmic reticulum, and T-tubules. This shift toward a fast-twitch phenotype is characterized in part by an increase in maximum unloaded shortening velocity (V_0), faster contraction and relaxation times, and a greater susceptibility to fatigue (1,4). Furthermore, recent quantitative EMG measurements provided evidence that the total amount and pattern of electrical activity is significantly decreased in the NWB rat soleus and plantaris muscles throughout the period of hind limb unweighting (44). Thus, it is not surprising that chronically innervated postural muscles such as the soleus are most susceptible to the effects of NWB activity (Fig. 5.6).

Prevention of skeletal muscle atrophy: countermeasures

Over the last decade, in an attempt to identify and test potential countermeasures for NWB atrophy and phenotype changes, numerous studies have shown the direct relationship between various types and combinations of postural loading to the preservation of muscle mass. The underlying common result in all of these studies is that successful countermeasures contain some form of mechanical loading, such as surgically induced MOV, intermittent weight-bearing activity, centrifugation to reload muscles, or some combination of either hind limb unweighting with MOV or administration of anabolic adjuvants.

> **KEY POINT**
>
> Although both fast- and slow-twitch muscle fibers are sensitive to non–weight-bearing activity, muscles or muscle regions composed predominantly of slow-twitch type I fibers have been shown to be more susceptible to NWB.

SIMULTANEOUS IMPOSITION OF OVERLOAD AND NON–WEIGHT-BEARING   In this countermeasure model, the rat fast-twitch plantaris muscle was mechanically overloaded and simultaneously subjected to HS so that for 6 weeks the animals were never allowed to bear weight. Whereas MOV alone results in plantaris hypertrophy of

Hindlimb suspension:

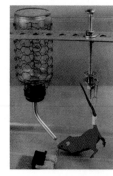

Imposes:
Chronic non–weight-bearing activity

Induces:
Atrophy of all hindlimb muscles (predominantly type I)

Fiber type transitions:

Slow oxidative	Fast glycolytic

Type I ⟶ Type IIA ⟶ IIX/D ⟶ IIB

FIGURE 5.6 Significant features of the non–weight-bearing (NWB) hind limb suspension (HS) model used to induce both skeletal muscle atrophy and fiber phenotype slow-to-fast changes. The HS model is a noninvasive model that induces near maximum NWB changes in muscle mass and phenotype within 2 weeks in either rats or mice. If it is done correctly, the animal has ability to feed and drink ad libitum and can rotate 360 degrees. Here this is accomplished with a simple sewing bobbin and a paper clip attached to a bolt and a series of locking nuts (46). Because the tail is an important component of thermoregulation, as much as possible it should remain exposed. Here athletic tape applied over thick soft cotton gauze that does not exceed an inch in width placed at the base of the tail. Not shown: with mice, four suspension stations easily fit into a double-sized breeding cage, which allow mice to socialize without climbing, so their hind limbs do not bear weight. Animals' hind limbs suspended in this manner remain healthy and active throughout the experimental period.

80% to 100% and NWB alone results in an approximate 20% atrophy, the combined models resulted in a modest 18% increase in normalized plantaris weight. In addition, native Sm content (5%), which is normally completely repressed under NWB conditions, was restored to levels that were slightly above those observed for controls (45). In a similar study, only 2 weeks of the simultaneous imposition of MOV and HS counter the loss in absolute and normalized mouse soleus weight but did not prevent decreased βMyHC transgene expression (4). The latter finding emphasizes that the hypertrophic stimulus of MOV was not an efficient countermeasure against the NWB-induced phenotype switch, a switch that assuredly contributes to the NWB soleus muscle's diminished functional capacity. Furthermore, these results suggest that there is a mechanistic divergence in the control of gene transcription leading to phenotypic transitions versus hypertrophic growth.

SEQUENTIAL OVERLOAD, NON–WEIGHT-BEARING When two diverse models of muscle usage (MOV for 12 weeks immediately followed by 7 weeks of NWB) were combined sequentially, a significant increase (27%) in normalized rat plantaris weight and a slight increase in Sm content were observed, indicating that the effects of loading could not be completely regressed by NWB (11).

By linking two diverse models of muscle usage (MOV induced by synergist ablation and NWB induced by HS) either simultaneously or sequentially, both Sm content and normalized muscle weights were not only preserved but increased. These results are presumably due to two factors: (a) The imposition of a chronic stretch induced a mechanical load imposed by the antagonistic muscles (tibialis anterior). Support for this notion comes from the observation of a 29% decrease in the weight of the tibialis anterior muscle (muscles in shortened position show accelerated degradation). (b) Although these rats (MOV plus NWB) were not allowed to bear weight, these animals continued to use their hind limbs in kicking movements during which their hind limbs were fully extended. This type of activity may have contributed to the low-level chronic mechanical stress, thereby preserving muscle mass and Sm content. Other paradigms involving intermittent periods of mechanical loading such as artificially induced gravity by centrifugation, intermittent periods of ground support (four times/day for 10 min for 7 days) and treadmill running have resulted in partial attenuation of soleus muscle atrophy.

ANABOLIC STEROIDS OR GROWTH HORMONE AND NON–WEIGHT-BEARING Combining anabolic steroids, a well-known adjuvant used to induce muscle growth, with NWB revealed that anabolic steroids enhanced both body and plantaris muscle weights in both control and HS rats (47). Further increases were observed when anabolic steroid administration was combined with the simultaneous perturbation of MOV and NWB induced by HS (48). In contrast, results using the soleus revealed that anabolic steroid treatment in combination with HS provided no apparent influence on muscle weight, or protein accumulation, nor did they appear to preferentially affect the percentages of myosin isoform content (47,48). Studies using intermittent loading (ladder climbing resistance exercise) have shown that the independent effects of either intermittent resistance exercise or growth hormone provided at best minimal countermeasure effects for sparing muscle mass. However, the combination of these two perturbations appeared to have strong interactive effects in preserving muscle mass and protein content (4).

In the absence of muscle loading, growth hormone treatment alone did not prevent soleus muscle atrophy during a 4-day space flight. Furthermore, it was shown that transgenic mice harboring a transgene that specifically targeted IGF-1 overexpression to skeletal muscle had normal body weights, whereas skeletal myofibers were hypertrophied (15%–20%). Interestingly, when these same transgenic mice were subjected to 14 days of HS, targeted overexpression of IGF-1 to skeletal muscle was not sufficient to attenuate NWB-induced muscle atrophy (4). Importantly, these studies illustrate that a hypertrophic stimulus may not necessarily serve as an efficient countermeasure against NWB atrophy.

Summary

By reviewing the literature, it becomes clear that considerable effort has been spent trying to identify suitable countermeasures to prevent or attenuate muscle atrophy as a result of NWB activity. Although mechanical load appears to be important for maintaining muscle mass, the use of countermeasures employing muscle loading to prevent muscle atrophy may not always be possible or, in the case of astronauts, may be too time consuming. Nevertheless, the continued quest to find a countermeasure coupled with the advancements in biotechnology has led to some progress in deciphering the mechanistic basis (signaling molecules and transcription factors) underlying muscle atrophy, thereby identifying potential protein targets for pharmacologic intervention.

TEST YOURSELF

In tests of various countermeasures thus far, what component has been found to be important for maintaining muscle mass? What might be some practical issues that need to be considered when designing effective countermeasures to prevent skeletal muscle atrophy?

Molecular Pathways for Skeletal Muscle Atrophy

It is well known that various forms of muscle inactivity or disuse, as experienced with disease, injury, aging, space travel, and sedentary lifestyle, results in the loss of both muscle mass and functional capacity. This entails a dramatic molecular remodeling, regardless of how muscle disuse commenced. The combination of mechanisms required to precisely orchestrate increased synthesis of newly required proteins, decreased synthesis of proteins no longer needed, and upregulation of degradation pathways requires the integrated input from numerous signaling pathways that ultimately influence transcriptional regulation.

KEY POINT

In response to HS several important mechanisms select for decreased protein translation, increased protein degradation, and thus skeletal muscle atrophy.

Intracellular signal transduction

The obvious value of elucidating the mechanistic basis controlling the amount and type of protein regulated in response to stimuli that result in skeletal muscle atrophy and changes in phenotype has focused the attention of many researchers on a variety of signaling pathways. As a result, a plethora of data has emerged (1,4) and accumulated research generally supports the notion that although the rate of protein synthesis is decreased in response to disuse, it appears that the majority of the observed loss in skeletal muscle mass is the result of increased protein degradation (1).

EVIDENCE FOR AKT SIGNALING IN DECREASED PROTEIN SYNTHESIS (AKT/MTOR/P70^{S6K} PATHWAY) AND INCREASED PROTEIN DEGRADATION: AKT/FOXO   Because the Akt signaling pathway and its downstream targets, GSK-3β and mTOR, as well as the mTOR effectors p70^{S6K} and PHAS-1/4E-BP1, were found to be instrumental in regulating muscle hypertrophy via increased protein synthesis, this signaling pathway represented a logical place to begin investigation into the mechanistic basis underlying decreased skeletal muscle mass following inactivity (Fig. 5.3). In support of this notion, HS was found to reduce total Akt protein, as well as phospho-Akt and phospho-p70^{S6K} protein levels in the rat gastrocnemius muscle while the levels of eIF4E-bound PHAS-1/4E-BP1 were increased, a scenario favoring decreased protein synthesis (29). Importantly, these modifications in response to HS were reverted in the gastrocnemius muscles of rats recovering from HS. On the other hand, activation of Akt signaling by transgenic overexpression of IGF-1 has been shown to block skeletal muscle atrophy in a variety of model systems, and to repress the expression of two muscle-specific E3 ubiquitin ligases termed *muscle ring finger 1 (MuRF1)* and *atrogin-1* (mechanism discussed later). In further support for the involvement of Akt in regulating skeletal muscle atrophy is the finding that constitutively active Akt blocked denervation-induced skeletal muscle atrophy. Activated Akt has been shown to phosphorylate the forkhead box O (FoxO) transcription factors inducing their export from the nucleus thereby interfering with the transcriptional regulation of the two skeletal muscle-specific ubiquitin E3 ligases, MuRF1 and atrogin-1. Conversely, reduced Akt activity as a result of atrophy inducing stimuli such as HS is associated with increased nuclear FoxO1 and transcriptional induction of MuRF1 and atrogin-1. Thus, it is not surprising that transgenic overexpression of FoxO1-induced MuRF1 and atrogin-1 gene expression that presumably lead to skeletal muscle atrophy, whereas the knockdown of FoxO1 by siRNA blocked the upregulation of these E3 ligases and the associated atrophy (33,34). In addition to Akt, recent evidence has shown that during HS, FoxO transcription factors can be regulated by neuronal nitric oxide synthase (nNOS). In response to HS, nNOS was shown to dislocate from the sarcolemma to the cytoplasm, where it generates

NO resulting in the regulation of the FoxO transcription factors and ultimately, the upregulation of MuRF1 and atrogin-1 leading to increased protein degradation by the ubiquitin-proteosome system and skeletal muscle atrophy (49). The nNOS null mice displayed a reduced level of skeletal muscle atrophy in response to HS. Collectively, these data reveal an important mechanism associated with HS that selects for decreased protein translation, increased protein degradation, and, thus, skeletal muscle atrophy.

EVIDENCE FOR INCREASED PROTEIN DEGRADATION: UBIQUITIN–PROTEOSOME PATHWAY Although there are several degradation pathways (lysosomal, cytosolic calcium dependent) operating in skeletal muscle, the ATP-dependent ubiquitin–proteasome pathway is thought to be the primary degradation pathway used in response to NWB induced by HS (Fig. 5.7).

Ubiquitin is a small protein that is recognized by the proteosome when it is bound in a multi-ubiquitin complex with the protein selected for degradation. The proteosome is a large structure comprised of 19S ubiquitin recognition subunits and a 20S core protein degradation subunit, which degrades targeted substrates into smaller peptides (29,50). Ubiquitination and subsequent degradation of substrates are both ATP-dependent processes. The exact mechanism that activates the ATP-dependent ubiquitin–proteasome pathway in NWB muscle has not been delineated; however, numerous studies have shown that various catabolic stimuli (sepsis, cancer, dexamethasone) are associated with increased levels of proteins in this pathway and upregulation of ubiquitin mRNA and E3 ubiquitin-protein ligases. Available evidence supports the notion that increases in mRNAs encoding pathway components in response to catabolic-inducing signals is regulated at the level of gene transcription. For example, glucocorticoid treatment of cultured L6 rat myotubes has been shown

to transcriptionally induce the UbC gene, which encodes ubiquitin C. Expression of the UbC gene was shown to involve activation of the MAP kinase-signaling pathway and enriched binding of the ubiquitously expressed SP1 transcription factor at several Sp1 elements (Fig. 5.8) (50). Whether or not the MAP kinase/Sp1 pathway is activated in NWB muscle remains to be determined.

Recent research has led to the identification of the distinct ubiquitin proteins ligases termed MuRF1 and atrogin-1/MAFbx. Both are E3 ligases; however, MuRF1 has been shown to act as a monomeric E3 ligase, whereas atrogin-1/MAFbx contains an F-box and is a component of an SCF type E3 ligase complex. Interestingly, their expression is restricted to striated muscle and is rapidly upregulated in response to several models of inactivity, including HS (27). In a test of the function of atrogin-1, its overexpression in cultures of differentiated myogenic cells resulted in smaller myotubes. A further test of the role of these two ubiquitin ligases in vivo was undertaken by generating genetically altered mice that carried null mutations of these gene loci. Mice carrying null mutations of either MuRF1 or atrogin-1 were found to partially prevent losses in muscle mass (36%–56%, respectively) in response to muscle inactivity (29). In addition to MuRF1 and atrogin-1, the E3 ubiquitin ligase Casitas b-lineage lymphoma-b (Cbl-b) is induced in unloaded skeletal muscle. Cbl-b was shown to mediate ubiquitination of the IGF-1 signaling intermediate insulin receptor substrate 1 targeting it for proteosomal degradation, thereby, impairing IGF-1 signaling, which lead to FoxO3-induced atrogin-1 gene expression and ultimately, skeletal muscle atrophy (51). As expected, Cbl-b deficient mice did not display a significant degree of unloading induced skeletal muscle atrophy in response to HS. In addition to the involvement of E3 ligases during HS, recent work has shown that mice deficient in MuRF1 and muscle ring finger 3 (MuRF3) develop skeletal muscle pathology

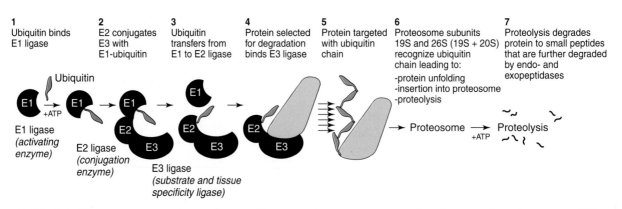

FIGURE 5.7 Ubiquitin–proteosome mechanism. Ubiquitination–proteasome-mediated protein degradation is an ATP-dependent, highly selective process with multiple component. Ubiquitin acts as a target signal for the proteosome when it is in a polyubiquitin chain bound to the protein selected for degradation. Three types of ubiquitin ligases are involved: (a) E1 ligase is the activating ligase that binds ubiquitin; (b) E2 ligase is a conjugating enzyme that combines the E2/E3 ligase complex to the E1-ubiquitin complex; and (c) The E3 tissue and substrate specific ligase. Proteosome subunits 19S recognize polyubiquitin chains and initiate a process of protein unfolding, insertion into the core (20S) proteosome, and proteolysis. This results in degradation of targeted protein into small peptides. Peptides undergo further degradation via endopeptidases and exopeptidases.

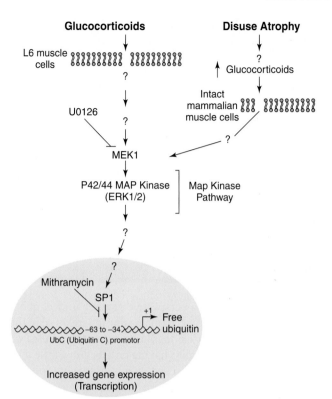

FIGURE 5.8 Mitogen-activated protein (MAP) kinase/specific protein 1 (SP1) pathway regulation of ubiquitin C (UbC) showing components shown to be involved in the production of increased levels of free ubiquitin. In response to treatment of glucocorticoids using L6 cells in culture, U0126 was shown to block MEK1 activation of extracellular signal-regulated kinase 1 (ERK1), which indicates that members of the MAP kinase signaling pathway are involved in glucocorticoid stimulated regulation of ubiquitin. Mithramycin was shown to block SP1 binding to the UbC promoter region (−63 to −34), showing specificity of SP1 involvement in upregulating ubiquitin gene transcription. Although these experiments have only been done in cell culture to date, it is possible that this pathway is activated in intact mammalian muscle to produce the increased levels of ubiquitin necessary for greater protein degradation requirements leading to reduced muscle mass.

characterized by subsarcolemma accumulation of MyHC (βMyHC and fast type IIa MyHC) indicating a role for MuRF1 and MuRF3 in the maintenance of basal contractile protein turnover (52). In line with this observation, MuRF1 was shown to specifically be involved in thick filament (MyHC, MyLC1 and MyLC2, myosin binding protein-C), but not thin filament, protein degradation (53).

Summary

In vivo functional studies have provided evidence that the ubiquitin ligases, MuRF1, MuRF3, atrogin-1, and Cbl-b play a significant role in targeting protein substrates for degradation via the ATP-dependent ubiquitin–proteosome pathway during skeletal muscle atrophy and in the maintenance of basal contractile protein turnover.

TEST YOURSELF

What are some of the common causes of skeletal muscle atrophy? Degradation of skeletal muscle occurs primarily via what pathway? What is the function of an E3 ligase? Does degradation of skeletal muscle occur only under conditions that involve changes in growth and phenotype? There are changes in gene transcription that occur in response to atrophic stimuli, does this involve proteins involved in degradation?

Transcriptional control of skeletal muscle atrophy

It is clear that the regulation of protein synthesis and degradation are key processes controlling muscle growth, hypertrophy, and atrophy. Transcriptional regulation was initially thought to play only a minor role, if any, in the remodeling of NWB skeletal muscle. However, recent evidence suggests that transcription is an important control point at which myofibrillar protein phenotype transitions are regulated, along with the expression of various components of the ubiquitin–proteosome pathway. This section discusses transcriptional regulation of the βMyHC gene because this gene has been the most extensively studied under NWB conditions.

TRANSCRIPTIONAL REGULATION OF THE βMYHC GENE NWB imposed by HS is associated with a striking shift in MyHC isoform expression that favors an increased proportion of fast MyHC and a decrease in slow type I MyHC (βMyHC) (1,4,46,54). The decrease in βMyHC expression observed in the NWB rodent soleus muscle has been measured at the protein and mRNA levels, suggesting that transcription, in part, serves a regulatory role in modulating βMyHC expression. This notion was first confirmed in vivo when the analysis of transgenic mice harboring two different transgenes comprised of either 5600 or 600 bp of βMyHC promoter region demonstrated a significant decrease in expression following 14 days of HS (46). Since that initial observation, other reports using direct DNA injection into NWB rat soleus muscle have shown decreased expression of βMyHC reporter genes (4), and increased expression of proteins representative of the fast phenotype (MyHC IIb, PGAM-M). Additional transgenic and DNA–protein interaction studies showed that although the 600 bp of βMyHC promoter region was sufficient to direct decreased βMyHC transgene transcription in response to NWB, mutation of three highly conserved cis-acting elements (dMCAT, C-rich, and pMCAT [also termed βe3]; Fig. 5.4B) within the βMyHC control region did not interfere with this process (46). A further search for the cis-element or elements responsible for NWB decreased expression led to the identification of a negative element that displayed binding only on the sense strand and was thus termed: distal beta negative regulatory element sense strand (dβNRE-S, −332 to −311) (Fig. 5.4B) (54). In DNA–protein interaction studies, this element demonstrated highly enriched binding of two distinct nuclear proteins only when NWB-soleus nuclear extract was used. Further, these two proteins were found to be antigenically distinct from cellular nucleic acid-binding protein and YB-1, two single-stranded DNA-binding proteins previously shown to bind this element when using heart nuclear extract. Further work identified these two single-stranded binding proteins as Purα and Purβ (purine-rich; α and β isoforms) and demonstrated that they negatively regulate βMyHC gene expression in transient expression assays (55). Subsequent transgenic analysis revealed that additional regulatory element or elements located downstream from the dβNRE-S element were also involved in NWB-induced decreased βMyHC transgene expression (Fig. 5.4B). Three closely spaced consensus GC-rich Sp-protein binding elements were identified under NWB conditions and shown to bind the negative acting transcription factor Sp3, which was also shown to physically interact with Purα and Purβ to negatively regulate βMyHC gene expression (55,56). It was also revealed that although the pMCAT element appeared to play an important role in regulating decreased expression of rat βMyHC reporter genes, it was not involved in NWB-induced human βMyHC transgene expression (57).

KEY POINT

Recent evidence suggests that transcription is an important control point at which myofibrillar protein phenotype transitions are regulated, along with the expression of various components of the ubiquitin–proteosome pathway during periods of disuse.

Summary

Several important insights into the mechanisms controlling βMyHC transcription in response to NWB activity become apparent:

1. Decreased expression of the βMyHC gene involves transcriptional regulation
2. βMyHC DNA-regulatory elements responsive to NWB were distinct and segregated from those identified to be MOV responsiveness showing that the molecular mechanisms controlling gene expression during atrophy versus hypertrophy are different
3. The presence of a regulatory element does not necessarily infer a function for all genes, or for the same gene in different species.

Unfortunately, only a paucity of transcriptional regulation data is available regarding muscle atrophy; however, recently several laboratories—sparked by the discovery of the muscle ligases MuRF1, atrogin-1, and Cbl-b—have begun to investigate this important topic. A great deal of effort will need to be devoted to identifying transcriptional control mechanisms involved during the regulation of atrophy in response to various modes of muscle inactivity.

TEST YOURSELF

What happens to satellite cells during skeletal muscle atrophy? Considering the function of satellite cells, are they necessary for a fiber-type shift? Are the signaling pathways, DNA-regulatory elements, and transcription factors involved in skeletal muscle hypertrophy also involved in atrophy?

Drawing on your knowledge of previous sections within this chapter, how would the posttranslational modification of transcription factor alter their function? Can adult skeletal muscle undergo hypertrophic growth without the involvement of satellite cells?

CHAPTER SUMMARY

This chapter provides a perspective of current ideas about cellular and molecular mechanisms that are involved in the control of skeletal muscle mass and phenotype. Research in this area is in its infancy, having only begun a little over a decade ago. Nevertheless, several important concepts can be gleaned from this research:

1. No single signaling pathway, transcription factor, or DNA regulatory element (a silver bullet) will universally account for the unique adaptations that occur in both muscle size and phenotype in response to altered states of muscle loading.
2. It is inappropriate to declare that the molecular responses to one perturbation are universal for all exercise modes or species.
3. Because hundreds of proteins and genes are involved in the physiologic adaptations occurring during exercise, it is difficult to precisely assign any single mechanism exclusively to growth or phenotype changes.
4. Although it is clear that skeletal muscle hypertrophy and atrophy involve signaling pathways that coordinately regulate protein synthesis and degradation, transcriptional regulation also plays an important role in the regulation of muscle mass.
5. Despite the massive effort expended, controversy still exists over the precise role that the calcium-dependent CaMK and calcineurin pathways play in the control of skeletal muscle phenotype and mass.
6. The modular arrangement of DNA-regulatory elements (promoter or enhancer/silencer regions) optimizes combinatorial interactions between DNA-bound transcription factors and allows responsiveness to independent or multiple stimuli (single and converging signaling pathways) in the control of skeletal muscle gene transcription.
7. Posttranscriptional modification of proteins plays a vital role in regulating cellular signaling, gene transcription, protein degradation, and synthesis.
8. Exercise adaptations involve one or more complex mechanisms (see discussion on MEF2 sensor mice) and, thus, conclusions need to remain conservative.

A MILESTONE OF DISCOVERY

Although in 1961 regeneration of skeletal muscle following injury was recognized, the mechanistic basis underlying this process remained largely unknown. The first mechanistic insight into skeletal muscle regeneration came from Alexander Mauro's electron microscopy studies of frog muscle, which discovered a new muscle cell type primarily comprised of a nucleus (with little cytoplasmic volume) external to the mature skeletal muscle fiber. This cell would have appeared to be a peripheral nucleus in the muscle fiber if it were not for its position between the skeletal muscle fiber plasma membrane and the basal lamina; this unique location likely underlies the name *satellite cells* given by Mauro. Although experimental evidence concerning the function of satellite cells was completely absent at this time, Mauro advanced several insightful hypotheses concerning their role during skeletal muscle regeneration. To fully appreciate the accuracy of his insight, the following excerpts are provided:

". . . more in keeping with conventional notions of cytology, is that the satellite cells are remnants from the embryonic development of the multinucleate muscle cell which results from the process of fusion of individual myoblasts. Thus the satellite cells are merely dormant myoblast that failed to fuse with other myoblasts and are ready to recapitulate the embryonic development of skeletal muscle fiber when the main multinucleate cell is damaged" (p. 493).

". . . satellite cells are "wandering" cells that have penetrated the basement membrane and are lying underneath it ready to be mobilized into activity under the proper conditions" (p. 494).

". . . cardiac muscle has not revealed . . . satellite cells. It is exciting to speculate whether the apparent inability of cardiac muscle cells to regenerate is related to the absence of satellite cells" (p. 494).

We now know that satellite cells first appear at about day 17 during mouse embryonic development and reside between the basal lamina and the mature muscle fiber as an inactive myoblast. When satellite cells are activated, they (a) recapitulate the developmental program that resembles a program initiated in muscle progenitor cells during myogenesis; and (b) proliferate and replenish the satellite cell pool, fuse to generate myotubes that mature into myofibers, and migrate to sites of muscle damage, where they fuse and participate in the regenerative process.

As yet, a cardiac cell equivalent to the skeletal muscle satellite cell has not been identified and damaged heart muscle is, for the most part, incapable of undergoing an extensive regenerative process (58). Mauro's discovery of satellite cells has stimulated decades of research. This research has directly extended our fundamental knowledge of the role satellite cells play in the repair of mature skeletal muscle and their involvement in adult muscle hypertrophy. Because of their unique features, these cells have been used in transplantation studies with the goal to repair damaged cardiac muscle or to ameliorate skeletal muscle disease states such as muscular dystrophy. Furthermore, this research has led to the exciting identification of putative stem cells in several adult tissues, including skeletal muscle, and in some cases these stem cells have been postulated to find their way to areas of damaged muscle via the circulation. Collectively, this ongoing work holds tremendous promise for future remedies expected to rectify an assortment of debilitating myopathies.

Mauro A. Satellite cell of skeletal muscle fibers. J Biophys Biochem Cytol. 1961;9:493–495.

The future challenge for researchers will be to extend existing correlative observations into causative mechanisms that control skeletal muscle mass and phenotype. As future work emerges, these delineations will undoubtedly become less tangled and more comprehensive, an understanding worth obtaining because our collective health is at stake.

ACKNOWLEDGMENTS

The author's laboratory is supported by the University of Missouri-Columbia and by the National Institutes of Health for investigating molecular mechanisms involved in skeletal muscle hypertrophy (R01-AR41464-017) and atrophy (R01-AR45217-010). The author would like to apologize to many colleagues whose work has not been referenced due to space limitations.

REFERENCES

1. Booth FW, Baldwin KM. Exercise: regulation and integration of multiple systems. In: Rowell LB, Shepherd JT, eds. *Muscle Plasticity: Energy Demand and Supply Processes. Handbook of Physiology.* New York: Oxford University; 1996:1075–1123.
2. Timson BF. Evaluation of animal models for the study of exercise-induced muscle enlargement. *J Appl Physiol.* 1990;69:1935–1945.
3. Crowther NB. Weightlifting in antiquity: achievement and training. In: McAuslen I, Walcot P, eds. *Greece and Rome,* vol. XXIV. Oxford, UK: Oxford University; 1977:111–120.
4. Baldwin KM, Haddad F. Plasticity in skeletal, cardiac, and smooth muscle. Invited review: effects of different activity and inactivity paradigms on myosin heavy chain gene expression in striated muscle. *J Appl Physiol.* 2001;90:345–357.
5. Schiaffino S, Reggiani C. Molecular diversity of myofibrillar proteins: gene regulation and functional significance. *Physiol Rev.* 1996;76:371–432.
6. Weiss A, Leinwand LA. The mammalian myosin heavy chain gene family. *Annu Rev Cell Dev Biol.* 1996;12:417–439.
7. Sartorius CA, Lu BD, Acakpo-Satchivi L, et al. Myosin heavy chains IIa and IId are functionally distinct in the mouse. *J Cell Biol.* 1998;141:943–953.

8. Barany M. ATPase activity of myosin correlated with speed of muscle shortening. *J Gen Physiol.* 1967;5:197–218.

9. Tsika GL, Wiedenman JL, Gao L, et al. Induction of β-MHC transgene in overloaded skeletal muscle is not eliminated by mutation of conserved elements. *Am J Physiol Cell Physiol.* 1996;271:C690–C699.

10. Tsika RW, Hauschka SD, Gao L. M-creatine kinase gene expression in mechanically overloaded skeletal muscle of transgenic mice. *Am J Physiol.* 1995;269:C665–C674.

11. Tsika RW, Herrick RE, Baldwin KM. Time course adaptation in rat skeletal muscle isomyosins during compensatory growth and regression. *J Appl Physiol.* 1987;63:2111–2121.

12. Gardiner PF, Michel RN, Browman F, et al. Increased EMG of rat plantaris during locomotion following surgical removal of its synergists. *Brain Res.* 1986;380:114–121.

13. Carson JA, Wei L. Invited review: integrin signaling's potential for mediating gene expression in hypertrophying skeletal muscle. *J Appl Physiol.* 2000;88:337–343.

14. Hawke TJ, Garry DJ. Invited review: Myogenic satellite cells: physiology to molecular biology. *J Appl Physiol.* 2001;91:534–551.

15. Adams GR, Caiozzo VJ, Haddad F, et al. Cellular and molecular responses to increased skeletal muscle loading after irradiation. *Am J Physiol.* 2002;283:C1182–C1195.

16. Crabtree GR, Olson EN. Review: NFAT signaling: choreographing the social lives of cells. *Cell.* 2002;109:S67–S79.

17. Olson EN, Williams RS. Calcineurin signaling and muscle remodeling. *Cell.* 2000;101:689–692.

18. Molkentin JD, Lu JR, Antos CL, et al. A calcineurin-dependent transcriptional pathway for cardiac hypertrophy. *Cell.* 1998;93:215–228.

19. Chin ER, Olson EN, Richardson JA, et al. A calcineurin-dependent transcriptional pathway controls skeletal muscle fiber type. *Genes Dev.* 1998;12:2499–2509.

20. Kim M-S, Fielitz J, McAnally J, et al. Protein kinase D1 stimulates MEF2 activity in skeletal muscle and enhances performance. *Mol Cell Biol.* 2008;28:3600–3609.

21. Potthoff MJ, Wu H, Arnold M, et al. Histone deacetylase degradation and MEF2 activation promote the formation of slow-twitch myofibers. *J Clin Invest.* 2007;117:2459–2467.

22. Parsons S, Millay D, Wilkins B, et al. Genetic loss of calcineurin blocks mechanical overload-induced skeletal muscle fiber type switching but not hypertrophy. *J Biol Chem.* 2004;279:26192–26200.

23. Karasseva NG, Tsika G, Ji J, et al. Transcription enhancer factor 1 binds multiple muscle MEF2 and A/T-rich elements during fast-to-slow skeletal muscle fiber type transitions. *Molec Cell Biol.* 2003;23:5143–5164.

24. Buller AJ, Eccles JC, Eccles RM. Interactions between motoneurones and muscles in respect of the characteristic speeds of their responses. *J Physiol.* 1960;150:417–439.

25. Murgia MA, Serrano AL, Calabria E, et al. Ras is involved in nerve-activity-dependent regulation of muscle genes. *Nature Cell Biol.* 2000;2:142–147.

26. Rana ZA, Gundersen K, Buonanno A, Activity-dependent repression of muscle genes by NFAT. *Proc Natl Acad Sci U S A.* 2008;105:5921–5926.

27. Calabria E, Ciciliot S, Moretti I, et al., NFAT isoforms control activity-dependent muscle fiber type specification. *Cell Biol.* 2009;106:13335–13340.

28. Goldspink G. Gene expression in muscle in response to exercise. *J Muscle Res Cell Motil.* 2003;24:121–126.

29. Glass DJ. Review: molecular mechanisms modulating muscle mass. *Trends in Molec Med.* 2003;9:344–350.

30. Peng XD, Xu PZ, Chen ML, et al. Dwarfism, impaired skin development, skeletal muscle atrophy, delayed bone development, and impeded adipogenesis in mice lacking Akt1 and Akt2. *Genes Devel.* 2003;17:1352–1365.

31. McPherron AC, Lawler AM, Lee SJ. Regulation of skeletal muscle mass in mice by a new TGF-β superfamily member. *Nature.* 1997;387:83–90.

32. Wagner K, McPherro A, et al. Loss of myostatin attenuates severity of muscular dystrophy in *mdx* mice. *Ann Neurol.* 2002;52:832–836.

33. Kamei Y, Miura S, Suzuki M, et al., Skeletal muscle FOXO1 (FKHR) transgenic mice have less skeletal muscle mass, down-regulated type I (slow twitch/red muscle) fiber genes, and impaired glycemic control. *J Biol Chem.* 2004;279:41114–41123.

34. Sandri M, Sandri C, Gilbert A, et al., Foxo transcription factors induce the atrophy-related ubiquitin ligase atrogin-1 and cause skeletal muscle atrophy. *Cell.* 2004;117:399–412.

35. Bogdanovich S, Krag TO, Barton ER, et al. Functional improvement of dystrophic muscle by myostatin blockade. *Nature.* 2002;420:418–421.

36. Amthor H, Otto A, Vulin A, et al. Muscle hypertrophy driven by myostatin blockade does not require stem/precursor-cell activity. *Proc Natl Acad Sci USA.* 2009;106:7479–7484.

37. Firulli AB, Olson EN. Modular regulation of muscle gene transcription: a mechanism for muscle cell diversity. *Trends in Genet.* 1997;13:364–369.

38. Tsika GL, Wiedenman JL, Gao L, et al. Induction of β-MHC transgene in overloaded skeletal muscle is not eliminated by mutation of conserved elements. *Am J Physiol Cell Physiol.* 1996;271:C690–C699.

39. Wiedenman JL, Tiska GL, Gao L, et al. Muscle specific and inducible expression of 293-base pair beta-myosin heavy chain promoter in transgenic mice. *Am J Physiol.* 1996;271:R688–R695.

40. Vyas DR, McCarthy JJ, Tsika GL, et al. Multiprotein complex formation at the β myosin heavy chain distal muscle CAT element correlates with slow muscle expression but not mechanical overload responsiveness. *J Biol Chem.* 2001;276:1173–1184.

41. Vyas DR, McCarthy JJ, Tsika RW. Nuclear protein binding at the β-myosin heavy chain A/T-rich element is enriched following increased skeletal muscle activity. *J Biol Chem.* 1999;274:30832–30842.

42. Tsika R, Schramm C, Simmer G, et al. Overexpression of TEAD-1 in transgenic mouse striated muscles produces a slower skeletal muscle contractile phenotype. *J Biol Chem.* 2008;283:36154–36167.

43. Morey-Holton ER, Globus RK. Invited review: Hindlimb unloading rodent model: technical aspects. *J Appl Physiol.* 2002;92:1367–1377.

44. Riley DA, Slocum GR, Bain JLW, et al. Rat hindlimb unloading: soleus histochemistry, ultrastructure, and electromyography. *J Appl Physiol.* 1990;69:58–66.

45. Tsika R, Herrick RE, Baldwin KM. Interaction of compensatory overload and hindlimb suspension on myosin isoform expression. *J Appl Physiol.* 1987;62:2180–2186.

46. McCarthy JJ, Fox AM, Tsika GL, et al. βMyHC transgene expression in suspended and mechanically overloaded/suspended soleus muscle of transgenic mice. *Am J Physiol Reg Integ Comp Physiol.* 1997;41:R1552–R1561.

47. Tsika RW, Herrick RE, Baldwin KM. Effect of anabolic steroids on skeletal muscle mass during hindlimb suspension. *J Appl Physiol.* 1987;63:2122–2127.

48. Tsika RW, Herrick RE, Baldwin KM. Effect of anabolic steroids on overloaded and overloaded suspended skeletal muscle. *J Appl Physiol.* 1987;63:2128–2133.

49. Suzuki N, Motohashi N, Uezumi A, et al. NO production results in suspension-induced muscle atrophy through dislocation of neuronal NOS. *J Clin Invest.* 2007;117:2468–2476.

50. Price SR. Increased transcription of ubiquitin-proteasome system components: molecular responses associated with muscle atrophy. *Int J Biochem Cell Biol.* 2003;35:617–628.

51. Nakao R, Hirasaka K, Goto J, et al. Ubiquitin ligase Cbl-b is a negative regulator for insulin-like growth factor 1 signaling during muscle atrophy caused by unloading. *Mol Cell Biol.* 2009;29:4798–4811.

52. Fielitz J, Kim MS, Shelton JM, et al. Myosin accumulation and striated muscle myopathy result from the loss of muscle RING finger 1 and 3. *J Clin Invest.* 2007;117:2486–2495.

53. Cohen S, Brault JJ, Gygi SP, et al. During muscle atrophy, thick, but not thin, filament components are degraded by MuRF1-dependent ubiquitylation. *J Cell Biol.* 2009;185:1083–1095.

54. McCarthy JJ, Vyas DR, Tsika GL, et al. Segregated regulatory elements direct β-myosin heavy chain expression in response to altered muscle activity. *J Biol Chem.* 1999;274:1427–1429.

55. Ji J, Tsika GL, Rindt H, et al. Purα and Purβ collaborate with Sp3 to negatively regulate β-myosin heavy chain gene expression during skeletal muscle inactivity. *Mol Cell Biol.* 2007;27:1531–1543.

56. Tsika G, Ji J, & Tsika R. Sp3 proteins negatively regulate β myosin heavy chain gene expression during skeletal muscle inactivity. *Mol Cell Biol.* 2004;24:10777–10791.

57. Tsika RW, McCarthy J, Karasseva N, et al. Divergence in species and regulatory role of β-myosin heavy chain proximal promoter muscle-CAT elements. *Am J Cell Physiol.* 2002;283:C1761–C1775.

58. Bergmann O, Bhardwaj RD, Bernard S, et al. Evidence for cardiac renewal in humans. *Science.* 2009;324:98–102.

CHAPTER 6

The Muscular System: Fatigue Processes

Robert H. Fitts

Abbreviations

ADP	Adenosine diphosphate	mV	Millivolts
AM	Actomyosin	MVC	Maximal voluntary contraction
AP	Action potential	N-M	Neural-muscular
ATP	Adenosine triphosphate	PC	Phosphocreatine
a/P_o	Describes the degree of curvature of the Hill force–velocity curve, where a is a force constant	pCa	Negative log of the calcium concentration
Ca^{2+}_i	Intracellular calcium transient	PDE4D3	Phosphodiesterase 4D3
CaM	Calmodulin	pH	Negative log of the hydrogen ion concentration
CaMKII	Ca^{2+}-dependent kinase, calmodulin kinase II	P_i	Inorganic phosphate
$CK^{-/-}$	Creatine kinase deficient	PKA	Protein kinase A; cAMP-dependent protein kinase
CNS	Central nervous system	P_o	Peak isometric tetanic tension
DHPR	L-type voltage-gated Ca^{2+} channel or 1,4-dihydropyridine receptor	PP1	Protein phosphatase 1
$+dP/dt$	Peak rate of tension development	RLC	Regulatory light chain of myosin
$-dP/dt$	Peak rate of tension decline	ROS	Reactive oxygen species
E-C	Excitation-contraction	RyR1	Type 1 ryanodine-sensitive Ca^{2+} release channel of the SR
FFA	Free fatty acids	SR	Sarcoplasmic reticulum
H_2O_2	Hydrogen peroxide	T-SR	Junction of the T-tubular membrane with the sarcoplasmic reticulum
Hz	Stimulation frequency per second		
$[K^+]_e$	Extracellular potassium	V_m	Membrane potential
$[K^+]_i$	Intracellular potassium	V_{max}	Maximal velocity of muscle or fiber shortening determined by the Hill plot
k_{tr}	Rate constant of tension redevelopment following a rapid release and reextension of a muscle fiber	V_o	Maximal velocity of muscle or fiber shortening determined by the slack test
LFF	Low-frequency fatigue	ΔC	Concentration gradient across the SR

Introduction

In 1983, Edwards (1) defined muscle fatigue as the inability to maintain the required power output, and thus the degree of fatigue is dependent on the extent of decline in both force and velocity. The 1990, a National Heart, Lung, and Blood Institute workshop on respiratory muscle (2) defined fatigue as "a condition in which there is a loss in the capacity for developing force and/or velocity of a muscle, resulting from muscle activity under load which is reversible by rest." The last phrase distinguishes fatigue from muscle weakness or damage where the capacity for rested muscle to generate force is impaired. This definition implies that fatigue can exist before performance declines

171

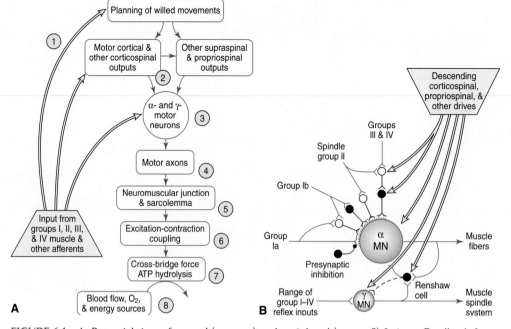

FIGURE 6.1   A. Potential sites of central (nos. 1–4) and peripheral (nos. 5–8) fatigue. Feedback from skeletal muscle (no. 1) is shown acting at three levels in the central nervous system. **B.** Summary of inputs to α- and γ-motor neurons for an agonist muscle. Cells with solid circles are inhibitory. Presynaptic inhibition is shown acting selectively on the afferent paths to motoneurons. (Figure modified from Gandevia SC. Spinal and supraspinal factors in human muscle fatigue. *Physiol Rev.* 2001;81(4):1725–1789, with permission of the author and copyright permission of The American Physiological Society.)

or task failure occurs (3). In this chapter, fatigue is defined as described by Edwards (1) with the clarifier that the process is reversible. Clearly, the etiology of muscle fatigue is an important question because the decline in force, velocity, and power that define fatigue often lead to serious limitations in muscle and whole body performance (4–6). Despite the obvious importance of this field and considerable research, the cellular causes of muscle fatigue remain controversial. The etiology of muscle fatigue is dependent on the individual's age, state of fitness, the fiber type composition of the involved muscles, dietary status, and the intensity, duration, and characteristics of the exercise (3–5). For example, the factors causing fatigue during prolonged exercise differ from those precipitating fatigue in high intensity contractile activity, and fatigue occurs earlier in a position versus a force maintenance task (3,5). The problem is complex because muscle fatigue might result from deleterious alterations in the muscle itself (peripheral fatigue) and/or from changes in the nervous system (central fatigue). In addition, because fatigue often results from the effects of multiple factors acting at various sites, and in some cases interacting synergistically, it has been difficult to unequivocally identify the causative factors (4,5,7). In 1984, Bigland-Ritchie (8) identified the major potential sites of fatigue as:

1. Excitatory input to higher motor centers
2. Excitatory drive to lower motor neurons
3. Motor neuron excitability
4. Neuromuscular transmission
5. Sarcolemma excitability
6. Excitation-contraction (E-C) coupling
7. Contractile mechanisms
8. Metabolic energy supply and metabolite accumulation

As shown in Figure 6.1A these sites represent all of the steps involved in voluntary force production. Although data exist to support a role for each of these sites in the fatigue process, in highly motivated athletes, sites 5 to 8 seem to be most important (5,9,10). Although the cellular etiologies of fatigue with high intensity compared to prolonged exercise are clearly different, both result in losses in force, velocity, and power. In this chapter, the functional changes that characterize fatigue are described, and this is followed by a consideration of the cellular mechanisms thought to be responsible for fatigue. Some examples of how fatigue is altered by programs of exercise training are discussed.

The Effect of Fatigue on Muscle Mechanics

Animal and human studies have shown that force, velocity, and power decline with fatigue, with the degree of change dependent on the fiber composition of the muscle.

The studies on muscle fatigue in animals have used isolated single fibers (both living and skinned fiber preparations), whole muscles in vitro, and anesthetized in situ preparations (5,7,11–13). Human studies on the other hand have for the most part been performed using in vivo exercise paradigms and muscle tests, and/or organelle isolated from muscle biopsies (3,5,10,14–17). Two general types of contraction (isometric and isotonic) have been evaluated and, for the most part, the alterations in contractile function with fatigue have been observed to be similar regardless of the species studied (5). When both peak force and velocity were compared, it has been generally observed that force declined sooner and to a greater extent than velocity (18). Because peak power is dependent on both, it was compromised to a greater extent than either force or velocity. When different muscles are compared, slow oxidative muscles like the soleus are more resistant to fatigue than fast muscles such as the tibialis anterior. Consistent with this, slow motor units, containing oxidative type I fibers, are more resistant to fatigue than motor units composed of fast type II fibers. Within fast motor units, the type IIx units showed resistance to fatigue that was intermediate between the highly fatigable type IIb and the relatively fatigue-resistant type IIa motor units (5).

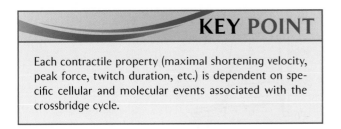

> ## KEY POINT
>
> Each contractile property (maximal shortening velocity, peak force, twitch duration, etc.) is dependent on specific cellular and molecular events associated with the crossbridge cycle.

Although the molecular details of the crossbridge cycle are not yet fully understood, a kinetic model of actin and myosin interaction in skeletal muscle has been developed (Fig. 6.2) (19,20). When myosin initially binds to actin, the actomyosin ($AM \cdot ADP \cdot P_i$) is in a weakly bound, low-force state and with the subsequent release of inorganic phosphate (P_i) (step 5; Fig. 6.2) the crossbridge transforms into a strongly bound, high-force state ($AM' \cdot ADP$). The latter is thought to be the dominant form during a maximal isometric contraction. The rate of transition (difference between the forward and backward rate constants of step 5; Fig. 6.2) is thought to limit the peak rate of force development ($+dP/dt$). In contrast, the maximal unloaded shortening velocity (V_0) is highly correlated with and likely limited by the actomyosin adenosine triphosphate (ATP) hydrolysis rate which, in turn, appears limited by the adenosine diphosphate (ADP) dissociation step (Fig. 6.2, step 7). This kinetic scheme has proven useful in assessing the cellular mechanisms of muscle fatigue for those factors acting at the crossbridge (5).

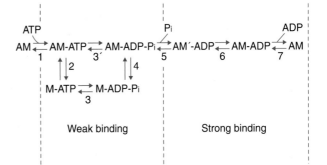

FIGURE 6.2   Schematic model of actomyosin adenosine triphosphate (ATP) hydrolysis reaction during contraction in skeletal muscle, where A is actin and M is the myosin head (myosin S1). Scheme is adapted from current models of ATP hydrolysis. ADP, adenosine diphosphate; P_i, inorganic phosphate. (Figure reprinted from Metzger JM, Moss RL. pH modulation of the kinetics of a Ca2(+)-sensitive cross-bridge state transition in mammalian single skeletal muscle fibres. *J Physiol.* 1990;428:751–764, with copyright permission of The Physiological Society.)

Summary

The etiology of muscle fatigue is complex as it results from multiple factors acting at various sites within the muscle (peripheral fatigue) and/or the central nervous system (CNS; central fatigue). The extent and time course of muscle fatigue is influenced by the individual's age, state of fitness, and the type of exercise performed.

Isometric Twitch and Tetanic Contractile Properties

During exercise, limb skeletal muscles go through a shortening and lengthening cycle and for a portion of the cycle may contract isometrically. The alpha motor neuron activation frequency varies from 10 to 50 Hz for slow and from 30 to >100 Hz for fast motor units—with force output dependent on the activation frequency as well as the number of recruited units. It is clear that muscles are never activated with single action potential (AP) or twitch contractions. However, the evaluation of isometric twitch properties before and after fatigue has proven useful in identifying the cellular sites of fatigue. Figure 6.3A shows representative isometric twitches recorded before and immediately following fatigue produced by in situ stimulation (2,100 ms fused contractions per second for 5 minute) of rat slow-twitch soleus muscles. As shown, twitch tension is generally depressed following fatiguing contractile activity. However, because twitch tension is influenced by muscle temperature (which increases during contractile activity), dP/dt, and the duration of the intracellular Ca^{2+} transient Ca^{2+}_i, it does not always reflect the degree of fatigue-induced decline in either the number of crossbridges that can be activated or the force per bridge. Other features of a postfatigued twitch

SOLEUS

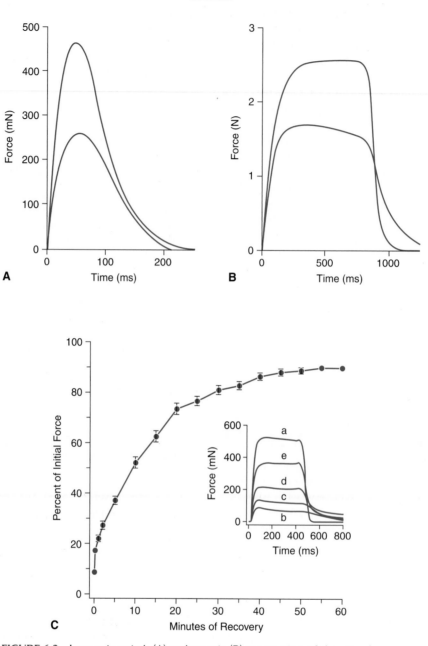

FIGURE 6.3   Isometric twitch (**A**) and tetanic (**B**) contraction of the rat soleus before and immediately following 5 min of in situ stimulation (2/s, 100 ms trains at 150 Hz for 5 min). Control and fatigued values were, respectively: Twitch tension (P_t) 462 and 260 mN; contraction time (CT) 43 and 54 ms; one-half relaxation time ($\frac{1}{2}$ RT) 60 and 74 ms; tetanic tension (P_o) 2.57 and 1.71 N; peak rate of tetanic tension development (+dP/dt) 25.0 and 22.1 N/s; peak rate of tetanic tension decline (−dP/dt) 27.5 and 7.6 N/s. (**C**) Recovery of force production of frog semitendinosus (percent of initial force) after stimulation. Values are means ± SE. Inset represents tetanus records at (a) prefatigued and at (b) 10 s, (c) 60 s, (d) 5 min, and (e) 20 min of recovery. Peak tetanic tension returned to prefatigued value by 45 min.
(**C** reprinted from Thompson LV, Balog EM, Riley DA, et al. Muscle fatigue in frog semitendinosus: alterations in contractile function. *Am J Physiol.* 1992;262(6 pt 1):C1500–C1506, with copyright permission of The American Physiological Society.)

are prolonged contraction and one-half relaxation times, and reductions in the (+dP/dt) and peak rate of tension decline (−dP/dt). In addition, when fatigue is produced in vitro, one generally observes a prolonged twitch duration (total time for contraction and relaxation). With in situ stimulation, the prolonged contraction and one-half relaxation times are usually prolonged, but the total twitch duration may remain unaltered (Fig. 6.3A). Relaxation appears to slow in direct proportion to the degree of fatigue and is exacerbated in conditions where intracellular acidosis develops (pH <6.9). The changes in the twitch with fatigue are a reflection of the Ca^{2+}_i, which has a reduced amplitude, a slower onset and rate of decline, and a prolonged duration in fatigued muscle fibers (11). The reduced P_t is a direct result of the decline in the amplitude of the Ca^{2+}_i. The amount of Ca^{2+} released in response to a single stimulus (twitch response) or even low frequency activation (10–20 Hz) places the muscle fiber on the steep region of the negative log of the calcium concentration (pCa–force relationship (Fig. 6.4), such that a small decline in the amplitude of the Ca^{2+}_i elicits a large drop in force.

Peak isometric tetanic tension (P_0) before and immediately following fatigue for the slow type I soleus muscle is shown in Figure 6.3B. The decline in P_0 (34% in this example) is a universal observation for all fatigued muscles and muscle fibers—by definition, a fatigued muscle

must have a reduced P_0. The decline in P_0 with fatigue can only be explained by a decline in the force per crossbridge and/or to the number of crossbridges in the high-force states (AM′·ADP, AM-ADP, and AM states shown in Fig. 6.2). Figure 6.4 summarizes the mechanisms involved in the reduction of isometric force with fatigue. The initial decline in force (mechanism 1, Fig. 6.4) occurs as a result of a reduction in maximal isometric force (inhibition of step 5, Fig. 6.2). Simultaneously, there is a right shift of the Ca^{2+}–force relationship (mechanism 2, Fig. 6.4), but this has no immediate consequence because the amplitude of the Ca^{2+}_i is still high. However, late in fatigue, the amplitude of the Ca^{2+}_i declines (mechanism 3, Fig. 6.4) and force is depressed by the combined effect of mechanisms 2 and 3. A combination of mechanisms 1 to 3 causes peak tension to decline along the dotted line shown in Figure 6.4.

In nonfatigued muscles, +dP/dt is limited by the rate of crossbridge transition from the low- to the high-force state, which depends on the difference between the forward and reverse rate constants of step 5, Figure 6.2. With contraction, the forward rate constant is accelerated by both cytoplasmic Ca^{2+} and the number of strongly bound crossbridges, both of which decrease with fatigue. In high intensity exercise, the decline in +dP/dt with fatigue could also be mediated by an increase in H^+ and P_i. The observation that +dP/dt divided by P_0 ([+dP/dt]/P_0) was not altered by fatigue suggests that the reduced +dP/dt resulted primarily from the decline in P_0 which in turn was caused by the fatigue-induced reduction in the number of strongly bound, high-force crossbridges. Of course the latter is dependent on the concentration of cytoplasmic Ca^{2+}, negative log of the hydrogen ion concentration (pH), and P_i (see *Crossbridge Mechanism of Fatigue*). In contrast, −dP/dt declines considerably more than force and, in the example shown in Figure 6.3B, the values were 28% and 66% of prefatigued for −dP/dt and P_0, respectively. The depression in −dP/dt with fatigue is even greater in fast muscles. This suggests a slower dissociation of actin from myosin in fatigued muscle cells, which could reflect a direct effect on the crossbridge detachment rate and/or a reduced rate of Ca^{2+} reuptake by the sarcoplasmic reticulum (SR) pumps. The rate of Ca^{2+} dissociation from troponin is thought to be too fast to be rate limiting (7). Relaxation from a tetanus generally occurs in three phases where force initially shows no change following the final AP (phase 1), then exhibits a slow, linear drop (phase 2), and finally a rapid exponential decline (phase 3). With fatigue each of these phases is slowed and the distinction between them is less clear (7). During phase 2 the sarcomere length remains constant and the force decline is thought to reflect the rate of crossbridge detachment. The time course of the decline in force is delayed compared to the predicted force, which is determined from the known relationship between the intracellular Ca^{2+} content and force in the steady state (pCa–force relationship).

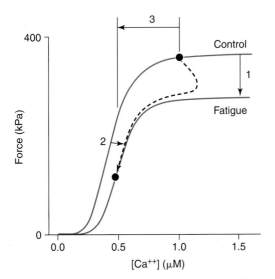

FIGURE 6.4   A plot of tetanic force versus intracellular calcium ($[Ca^{2+}]_i$) summarizing the mechanisms involved in the reduction of isometric force in fatigue: (1) reduced maximal force; (2) reduced myofibrillar Ca^{2+} sensitivity; and (3) reduced tetanic $[Ca^{2+}]_i$. The normal pattern during fatigue is schematically illustrated by the dashed line. The arrow shows the direction of time. (Figure reprinted from Allen DG, Lannergren J, Westerblad H. Muscle cell function during prolonged activity: cellular mechanisms of fatigue. *Exp Physiol.* 1995;80(4):497–527, with permission of The Physiological Society.)

KEY POINT

It has been hypothesized that the delay between the predicted force and measured force reflects the crossbridge detachment time. The observation that this delay increases in fatigued muscle fibers suggests that the slowed relaxation is caused in part by a reduced crossbridge dissociation rate (7).

Summary

The isometric twitch is a reflection of the Ca^{2+}_i which has reduced amplitude, a slower onset and rate of decline, and a prolonged duration in fatigued muscle fibers. The decline in P_0 with fatigue results from fewer high force crossbridges and/or less force per crossbridge, and to a right shift in the Ca^{2+}–force relationship which manifests late in fatigue as the amplitude of the Ca^{2+}_i declines. The slowed rate of relaxation ($-dP/dt$) with fatigue appears at least in part caused by a reduced rate of crossbridge detachment.

Force–Velocity and Force–Power Relationship

Since the work of A. V. Hill (21), it has been known that the force–velocity relationship is hyperbolic with the maximal velocity of shortening (V_{max}) obtained at zero load. The curvature of the relationship is described by the a/P_0 ratio, where a is a force constant of the Hill equation, and a higher ratio reflects less curvature (21). Fast-twitch muscles are characterized by a high V_{max} and a/P_0 ratio where the former is limited by the myofibrillar ATPase activity. Hence, V_{max} reflects the crossbridge cycle speed, which is considerably higher in fast-twitch compared to slow-twitch muscle. Figures 6.5A and B shows representative force-velocity curves for the rat slow-twitch soleus and fast-twitch plantaris. To compare the two muscles, V_{max} is expressed in muscle lengths (ML) per second. In this example, the fast plantaris showed a twofold higher V_{max} than the soleus. V_{max} is known to underestimate the true V_0 obtained by the slack test method where slow type I fibers have been shown to be approximately two- and threefold slower than the fast type IIa and IIx fiber types, respectively (22–24).

With the development of muscle fatigue, force usually declines sooner and to a greater extent than shortening velocity (18,24). In the example shown, the soleus P_0 fell by 34% (Fig. 6.3B) compared to an 8% drop in V_{max} (Fig. 6.5A). Although force always declines first, the reduction in V_{max} may ultimately drop by an amount equal to that observed for force (7). However, muscles contracting in vivo never experience zero loads, thus it is important to assess whether or not the curvature as reflected by the

a/P_0 ratio changes with fatigue. In fast muscles, the a/P_0 ratio is three- to fourfold higher compared to slow muscle (compare solid lines Figs. 6.5A and B, where the ratio was 0.129 and 0.521 for the soleus and plantaris, respectively). Consequently, individuals with a high percentage of fast-twitch fibers can generate higher velocity and power at a given relative load than those with predominantly slow-twitch fibers. There is little data assessing the affect of fatigue on the a/P_0 ratio. Because the extremes of the force–velocity relationship (V_{max} and P_0) in response to a given contractile paradigm are more resistant to change in slow compared to fast muscles, one might expect a similar difference in the stability of the a/P_0 ratio. For leg muscles of the rat, this appears to be the case, in the data shown in Figure 6.5—the a/P_0 ratio was relatively unaltered by fatigue in the soleus (0.129 vs. 0.117), but declined to 0.147 in the plantaris. The susceptibility to a fatigue-induced decline in the a/P_0 ratio is not entirely explained by fiber type. Jones et al. (24) observed a 50% depression in this ratio with fatigue in the human adductor pollicis, a muscle with 80% slow fibers (25). However, the contractile properties of the adductor pollicis resemble the mixed quadriceps (~50% type I muscle), and are considerably different from the slow soleus.

KEY POINT

These data suggest that with fatigue, relatively fast contracting muscles lose their ability to maintain relatively high velocities at moderate loads. The importance of this is that peak power is obtained at moderate loads and velocities (generally between 25% and 40% of V_{max} and P_0).

To prevent muscle fatigue and a deterioration of performance one must maintain peak power. Although peak power can be determined from the force–velocity relationship, few studies have actually assessed peak power or its change with fatigue. In human muscle, peak power varies with fiber type with a ratio of 10:5:1 for the type IIx, IIa, and I fibers, respectively. Recovery from fatigue generally shows a fast (complete in <2 min) and a slow component (1–2 hours) with the former particularly apparent in fast muscles (Fig. 6.3C). Due to the rapid recovery phase, it is difficult to acquire postfatigue power curves. Nonetheless, it can be accomplished and representative data are shown in Figs. 6.5C and D for the soleus and plantaris muscles, respectively. With fatigue, the reduced peak power results from a decline in both the tension and velocity where the latter is particularly important in fast muscles due to the decline in the a/P_0 ratio (24). As fatigue develops, peak power declines and is obtained at progressively lower shortening velocities making only slower movements effective.

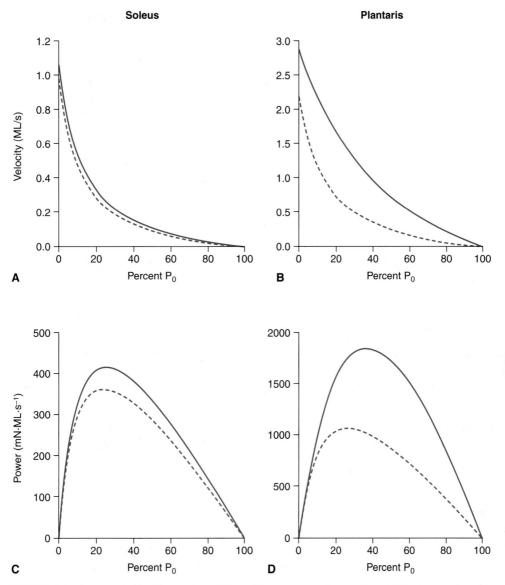

FIGURE 6.5   Force–velocity (traces **A** and **B**) and force–power (traces **C** and **D**) relationships for rat soleus (**A** and **C**) and plantaris (**B** and **D**) muscles before (——) and immediately following fatigue (-----) produced by in situ stimulation (2/s, 100 ms trains at 150 Hz [soleus] or 200 Hz [plantaris] for 5 min). Control and fatigued values were, respectively: soleus (**A**) maximal shortening velocity (V_{max}) 1.06 and 0.98 muscle lengths per second (ML · s^{-1}); a/P_o 0.129 and 0.117; plantaris (**B**) V_{max} 2.91 and 2.22 ML · s^{-1}; a/P_o 0.521 and 0.147; soleus (**C**) peak power 415 and 361 mN · ML · s^{-1}; and plantaris (**D**) peak power 1848 and 1072 mN · ML · s^{-1}.

Summary

Muscle fatigue is greater in fast compared to slow muscles with force declining earlier and to a greater extent than velocity. The force loss results from fewer high force crossbridges, a right shift in the Ca21–force relationship, and to a reduction in the amplitude of Ca21 transient. Power is compromised to a greater extent than either force or velocity, and in muscles with moderate to fast velocities is further reduced by a fatigue-induced decline in the a/P_o ratio.

TEST YOURSELF

What factors affect the extent and time course of fatigue and what alterations in mechanical properties are responsible for the fatigue-induced decline in peak power in slow and fast fibers?

Central Fatigue

Since the early part of the twentieth century, it has been recognized that changes in the afferent input to the central nervous system (CNS) or events within the CNS itself can contribute to fatigue. This component of fatigue has been referred to as "central fatigue." The relative importance of central versus peripheral fatigue is still unsettled and clearly depends on the work situation (competitive sport vs. every day activities) and the motivation of the individual. Most agree that central fatigue likely plays a minor role in limiting the performance of the highly trained athlete, but is likely more important in repetitive tasks performed in the work place (3,5,9,10). Merton (26) and others (10) used electrical stimulation of motor nerves to demonstrate that voluntary activation could maximally activate a muscle and that central fatigue did not exist during a maximal voluntary contraction (MVC).

KEY POINT

The cellular sites responsible for central fatigue have not been elucidated, but could involve alterations in:
1. Afferent inputs from group I, II, III, and IV muscle afferents
2. Supraspinal centers particularly regions of the cortex involved in planning of willed movements
3. Motor cortical and other corticospinal outputs
4. Other supraspinal and propriospinal outputs
5. α- and γ-motor neurons or their axons (Fig. 6.1A)

The latter conclusion was based on the observation that a twitch produced by nerve stimulation during an MVC did not elicit additional force (twitch interpolation technique), even when significant peripheral fatigue had developed. Since the initial studies of Merton (26), the resolution of the recording systems has improved and the twitch interpolation technique has been applied to numerous muscles. It is now generally accepted that the extent to which voluntary activation can produce peak force varies between muscles and the type of contraction (3,10). For example, it has been demonstrated that it is more difficult to elicit maximal force by voluntary activation in the ankle plantar flexors than the ankle dorsiflexors. With improved recording techniques, twitch interpolation has established the occurrence of central fatigue in several muscle groups including elbow flexors, ankle plantar and dorsiflexors, and quadriceps muscles (10). In addition, it occurs to a greater extent in repetitive isometric and shortening contractions compared to sustained contractions (3).

The identification of specific sites involved in central fatigue is problematic as it is difficult to separate factors mediated by changes in afferent inputs from suprasegmental alterations. The problem is exacerbated by the fact that the intrinsic properties of α-motoneurons can contribute to motor output. Figure 6.1B shows a summary of inputs to the α- and γ-motoneurons and demonstrates the complexity of the circuits affecting α-motoneuron excitability. It is well established that during a sustained maximal

voluntary effort the firing rate of α-motoneuron declines. This response was termed "muscular wisdom" as it was thought not to cause but rather protect against fatigue by matching the motor nerve firing rate to the slowed force transient of the fatiguing muscle. Bigland-Ritchie et al. (27) hypothesized that the reduced firing rate resulted from an increased activation of group III and IV muscle afferents that were activated by metabolic factors, such as, an increase in extracellular K^+. This hypothesis was supported by their observation that the firing rate did not recover during 3 min of rest while muscle blood flow was occluded, but did upon resumption of blood flow.

Proponents of a significant role for central fatigue suggest that the decline in α-motoneuron firing rate is excessive and results in reduced force caused by either too low a firing rate and/or a reduction in the number of active motor neurons (10). The supporting evidence is that a significant twitch interpolation can be observed and that motor cortical stimulus can increase the force output of the fatigued muscle. It seems likely (although not proven) that there is a net decline in α-motoneuron facilitation due to the combined effects of reduced Ia (muscle spindle) afferent input and increased activation of group III and IV muscle afferents activating inhibitory interneurons (Fig. 6.1B). In addition, with a maintained excitatory activation of an α-motoneuron, firing rate decreases due to altered ionic currents (increased K^+ and decreased Na^+) that are intrinsic properties of the motor neuron. Collectively, these changes would reduce the likelihood of an MVC producing optimal activation of the α-motor neuron pool. The observation that an extrinsic motor cortical stimulus can increase the force output of a muscle suggests that pathways proximal to the corticospinal outputs (Fig. 6.1A) contribute to central fatigue.

Summary

Given the current state of knowledge, it is not possible to determine the relative importance of central fatigue in limiting human performance. The increase in force in response to peripheral motor nerve or CNS motor cortical paths suggests at most a 10% contribution to the fatigue-induced decline in force. However, in certain repetitive contractile activities, such as might be experienced in the workplace, the contribution of central fatigue could be as high as 25% (3).

KEY POINT

Research is needed to establish that the observed changes in CNS function are causative and not simply correlative with fatigue, and identify the exact cellular sites involved in central fatigue.

Substrates and Fatigue with High Intensity Exercise

Fatigue caused by peripheral cellular events may have a site of origin at the crossbridge, E-C processes, and/or cell metabolic pathways. With high-intensity exercise, the muscle high-energy phosphates, ATP, and phosphocreatine (PC) decrease, whereas P_i, ADP, lactate, and the H^+ ion all increase as fatigue develops. All of these changes have been suggested as possible fatigue-inducing factors (4,5,7).

To avoid fatigue, adequate tissue ATP levels must be maintained, as this substrate supplies the immediate source of energy for force generation by the myosin cross-bridges. ATP is also needed in the functioning of the sodium-potassium pump (Fig. 6.6, no. 5), which is essential in the maintenance of a normal sarcolemma and T-tubular AP. Additionally, ATP binds to a cytoplasmic regulatory site on the SR Ca^{2+} release channel and is a substrate of the SR ATPase and thus is required in the process of Ca^{2+} release and reuptake by the SR (Fig. 6.6, nos. 4 and 6). A disturbance in any of these processes could lead to muscle fatigue (5).

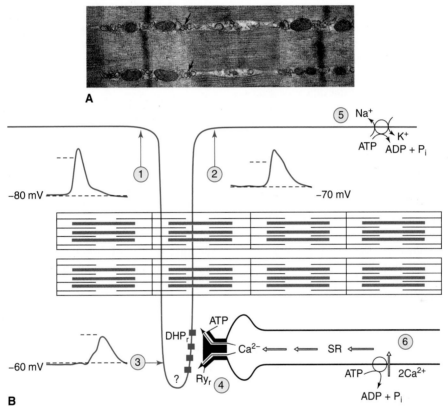

FIGURE 6.6   A. Electron micrograph (EM) showing a myofilament from a rat flexor digitorum brevis muscle fiber. The arrows show the position of the triads (T-tubule plus the sarcoplasmic reticulum terminal cisternae) at the A-I junctions providing two triad junctions for each sarcomere. **B.** A schematic representation of E-C coupling showing a representative sarcolemma action potential (AP) at rest (no. 1) and following fatigue (no. 2) with resting potentials of −80 and −70 mV, and AP amplitudes of 84 and 73 mV, respectively. It is unknown how fatigue affects the AP in the depths of the T-tubule. The displayed AP record (no. 3) showing a resting potential of −60 mV and AP amplitude of 58 mV (*i.e.,* spike potential reaching −2 mV) represents hypothesized rather than real values for a T-tubular AP. The SR Ca^{2+} release channel (ryanodine receptor) is shown as no. 4, whereas nos. 5 and 6 represent the sarcolemma Na^+-K^+ pump and the SR ATPase pump, respectively. The question mark (?) indicates that the composition of the extracellular fluid in the depths of the T-tubule in a fatigued muscle is currently unknown. The dotted line to the left of each AP represents the zero overshoot potentials. (The figure is a modification of that originally published in Fitts RH. Chapter 26, Cellular, molecular, and metabolic basis of muscle fatigue. In: Rowell LB, Shepherd JT, eds. *Handbook of Physiology, Section 12, Exercise: Regulation and Integration of Multiple Systems.* New York: Oxford University Press; 1995:1151–1183, while the AP records are data acquired in a study by Metzger JM, Fitts RH. Fatigue from high- and low-frequency muscle stimulation: role of sarcolemma action potentials. *Exp Neurol.* 1986;93(2):320–333. The EM in part A was provided by DA Riley.)

It is well established that whole cell ATP content declines during intense contractile activity and that in fast fibers it can drop from ~6 to 1.2 mM (5,28). However, even the latter would be more than 50-fold higher than that required for full crossbridge activation, and sufficient for normal Na^+-K^+ pump, SR pump, and Ca^{2+} release channel function. Consequently, for low ATP to be a factor in fatigue its distribution would have to show considerable compartmentalization where the ATP content around ion pumps and SR Ca^{2+} channels was below the cell average. As will be discussed in the section on E-C coupling, there is some evidence that compartmentalization of ATP does exist and that low ATP may inhibit SR Ca^{2+} release (29). Nonetheless, a cause and effect relationship between low cell ATP and muscle fatigue has not been demonstrated. In fact, the classic experiments of Karlsson and Saltin (17) illustrate the absence of a correlation between changes in ATP and performance. In this research, the needle biopsy technique was used to evaluate substrate changes after exercise to exhaustion at three different exercise intensities. After 2 min of exercise, ATP and PC were depleted to the same extent at all loads; however, fatigue occurred only with the highest workload. These results are equivocal since the biopsy was acquired some seconds after exercise ceased and the sample represented an average tissue ATP that might not reflect the concentration existing at the crossbridges, sarcolemma, or the SR. However, in vitro studies, in which the muscles were quick frozen while contracting, also failed to show a correlation between ATP and force (5).

Although PC is known to decline with heavy exercise, the time course of decline differs from that observed for tension, making a casual relationship unlikely (5). PC facilitates the movement of high-energy phosphates from the mitochondria to the sites of utilization, a process called the PC-ATP shuttle. A critically low PC level may disrupt this shuttle system and slow the rate of ADP rephosphorylation to ATP. This could lead to a critically low ATP at various subcellular sites. The interpretation of whole muscle determinations of ATP and PC are further complicated as compartmentalization may exist between as well as within fibers. Consequently, a high mean value postfatigue may not be representative of the most fatigued cells. Although low ATP may inhibit ion pumps and SR Ca^{2+} release, it seems unlikely that ATP content surrounding the crossbridges would be low enough to directly inhibit force production (28,29). The prevailing evidence suggests that fatigue produced by other factors reduces the ATP utilization rate before ATP becomes limiting at the crossbridge (5).

The role of an increased ADP in the development of muscle fatigue is not well understood. In resting muscle, the majority of the ADP is bound to F-actin and the activity of the creatine kinase reaction (ADP + PC ↔ ATP + creatine) maintains free ADP <10 µM (29). With intense exercise, the depletion of PC and the increase in creatine shifts the equilibrium of the creatine kinase reaction to higher ADP. The ADP increase would activate the myokinase reaction (2 ADP ↔ ATP + AMP) limiting the ADP increase to ~200 µM. However, it has been calculated that with PC depletion and the

relatively low activity of myokinase, ADP could rise from about 10 µM to 2 to 3 mM during heavy contractile activity (30). Although high ADP has been shown to increase force and depress velocity (7), the primary effect of mM ADP may be on the SR pump (see *SR ATPase Pump*).

Intense stimulation of skeletal muscle activates glycolysis producing a high rate of lactic acid production. The acid immediately dissociates into lactate and free H^+ and cell pH declines from 7.0 to values as low as 6.2 (5). In the early part of the twentieth century, lactic acid was linked to fatigue, and following the work of A. V. Hill in the late 1920s the lactic acid theory of muscle fatigue was highly popular. It is now generally thought that the component of fatigue correlated with lactate results from the effects of an increased free H^+ (low pH) rather than lactate or the undissociated lactic acid.

The H^+ ion could elicit fatigue by inhibiting:

1. Crossbridges
2. Ca^{2+} binding to troponin
3. Na^+-K^+ pumps
4. SR pumps
5. Glycolysis

Numbers 1 and 2 will be considered in the section *Crossbridge Mechanism of Fatigue*, and 3 and 4 in the section *Excitation-Contraction Coupling*. Regarding the possibility of number 5, two observations support the hypothesis that an elevated H^+ ion concentration inhibits glycolysis. First, lactate formation during muscle stimulation stopped when the intracellular pH dropped to 6.3 (28). Secondly, during a 60-second measurement period, Hermansen and Osnes (16) found no change in the pH of the most acidic homogenates of fatigued muscle, whereas the pH values of the homogenates from resting muscle showed a marked fall due to significant glycolysis. However, the observations that the changes in ATP were not correlated with either work capacity or force during recovery argues against an important role for H^+ inhibition of glycolysis in the fatigue process. If the inhibition of glycolysis was causative in fatigue, the decline in tissue ATP would likely reach limiting levels. Consequently, a significant correlation between force and ATP would exist during the development and recovery from fatigue.

TEST YOURSELF

With intense exercise what changes would you expect to see in muscle ATP, ADP, PC, and creatine? What metabolic reactions are critical to the observed changes?

Excitation-Contraction Coupling

The major components of a muscle cell involved in E-C coupling include the neural-muscular (N-M) junction, the surface membrane, the transverse (T)-tubules, and the SR membranes including the Ca^{2+} release channels (ryanodine

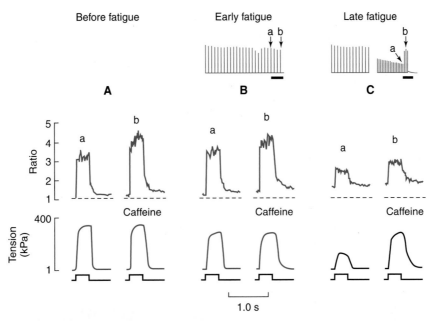

FIGURE 6.7   Application of 10 mM caffeine in control (**A**) and during two successive fatigue runs (**B** and **C**). Bars below tension records in top panels indicate caffeine exposure during fatiguing stimulation; caffeine was applied after 22 fatiguing tetani (**B**) and when tetanic tension was depressed to 0.36 P_o by 187 tetani (**C**). Fluorescence ratio and tension records from tetani elicited (a) before application of caffeine and (b) in presence of caffeine are shown in middle and bottom panels. Dashed lines represent resting ratio in control prefatigued fiber; stimulation periods are displayed below tension records. Note that tetanic ratio increase induced by caffeine in late fatigue was accompanied by a substantially enhanced tension production, whereas tension was not markedly affected by increased ratios in the other two states. (Figure reprinted from Westerblad H, Allen DG. Changes of myoplasmic calcium concentration during fatigue in single mouse muscle fibers. *J Gen Physiol.* 1991;98(3):615–635, with copyright permission of The Rockefeller University Press.)

receptor) and the Ca^{2+} pump proteins. Except for the N-M junction all have been suggested to play a role in muscle fatigue—particularly fatigue induced by high intensity contractile activity. Although the amount of transmitter released from the motor nerve endings may decline with high frequencies of activation, transmission block at the N-M junction has not been observed (5,26). The primary observations supporting a role for E-C coupling failure in muscle fatigue are: (a) the drop in force with electrical stimulation in single fibers is associated with a decline in the amplitude of the Ca^{2+} transient; and (b) direct release of Ca^{2+} from the SR by caffeine increases intracellular Ca^{2+} and to a large extent reverses the decline in force (Fig. 6.7).

Sarcolemma and T-tubular Membrane Action Potential

In nonfatigued muscle, the surface (sarcolemma) membrane AP propagates down into the T-tubules where the depolarization triggers a voltage-driven conformational change in an intramembranous T-tubular protein, the L-type voltage-gated Ca^{2+} channel, or 1,4- dihydropyridine receptor (DHPR). This T-tubular charge movement in turn triggers Ca^{2+} release from

adjacent type 1 ryanodine-sensitive Ca^{2+} release channel of the SR (RyR1) producing a uniform activation of the entire fiber (4,5). With heavy exercise, it is well documented that the resting potential of skeletal muscle fibers depolarizes by 10 to 20 millivolts (mV), and that the AP amplitude and duration are depressed and prolonged. A schematic representation of this change is shown in Figure 6.6 where points 1 and 2 show pre- and postfatigue APs, respectively. In this example, fatigue has resulted in a 10-mV depolarization of the resting membrane potential V_m and the amplitude of the AP has been reduced from 84 to 73 mV. It has been suggested, but not proven, that these changes in the sarcolemma and T-tubular V_m and APs induce fatigue by either preventing propagation of the AP into the depths of the fiber or inhibiting the T-tubular charge sensor which in turn reduces SR Ca^{2+} release (Fig. 6.6, no. 4). The problem is likely to be exacerbated in centrally located myofibrils (5). This hypothesis, termed the membrane mechanism of muscle fatigue (31), would allow contractions at reduced rates and forces while preventing catastrophic changes in cellular homeostasis that might lead to cell damage. The primary support for this theory comes from the observations that high frequency stimulation can (a) produce a spatial gradient of Ca^{2+} with higher concentrations near the fiber surface, and

(b) induce central core wavy myofibrils due to activation of peripheral but not centrally located fibrils (5,7). The extent of wavy myofibril formation has been shown to increase in parallel with the development of muscle fatigue, and be prevented by direct release of Ca^{2+} from the SR by caffeine.

The fatigued-induced depolarization of the sarcolemma and T-tubule resting V_m is caused by the combined effect of an increase in extracellular potassium $[K^+]_e$ and decrease in intracellular potassium $[K^+]_i$. With intense contractile activity, $[K^+]_e$ can increase from a few mM to 10 or more mM—a value that would be expected to dramatically reduce peak force (32). The loss of intracellular K^+ with contractile activity is considerably greater than can be attributed to the K^+ efflux during the APs, which suggests that an increased K^+ conductance contributes to the buildup in extracellular K^+ and thus V_m depolarization as fatigue develops. The extent of V_m depolarization with fatigue is less than what would be predicted from the observed change in $[K^+]_e$ and $[K^+]_i$ (32). This suggests that changes in the conductance and/or distribution of other ions, for example, Cl^- as well as activation of the Na^+-K^+ pump may prevent excessive depolarization of fatigued fibers. Nonetheless, the fatigue-induced depolarization contributes to the reduced AP amplitude and conduction velocity by decreasing the Na^+ conductance. It is clear from these data that despite activation by elevated intracellular Na^+ and catecholamine stimulation, the sarcolemma and T-tubular Na^+-K^+ pumps (Fig. 6.6, no. 5) fail to keep pace with the K^+ efflux and Na^+ influx during high-frequency activation (32,33). The insufficient pump activity is not due to a decline in pump density but rather to inactivation that might result from a reduced ATP/ADP + P_i ratio, an elevated H^+ in the intracellular fluid surrounding the membrane pumps and/or to reactive oxygen species (ROS) oxidation of the pump protein (32). Support for the latter comes from the observation that the intravenous infusion of the antioxidant N-acetylcysteine reduced the inactivation of the Na^+-K^+ pump and prolonged the time to fatigue in adult males exercising at 92% of their peak oxygen consumption (34). Pump inactivation might be exacerbated in the depths of the fiber where the T-tubular Na^+-K^+ pump density is low and diffusion limitation likely increases $[K^+]_e$. The extent of V_m depolarization and decline in the AP amplitude in the depths of the T-tubules has not been established, but it is plausible the V_m would be more depolarized and the AP amplitude less compared to the sarcolemma (Fig. 6.6, no. 3). As depicted by the question mark in Figure 6.6, the ionic conditions in the T-tubular lumen following intense contractile activity are unknown. It is particularly important to know what happens to lumen K^+ and Ca^{2+}. If either lumen K^+ or Ca^{2+} build up, the AP propagation could be blocked from reaching the depths of the fiber (5). Additionally, depolarization to values more positive than −60 mV would cause inactivation of the DHPR (6).

Intense exercise is known to reduce intracellular pH from 7.0 to values as low as 6.2 (5). Although large drops in intracellular pH (to values <6.7) are causative in fatigue (see *Crossbridge Mechanism of Fatigue*), moderate declines between 7.0 and 6.8 may protect against fatigue by reducing Cl^- conductance (32). The resulting decline in Cl^- influx with fiber activation allows for a greater Na^+-dependent AP amplitude, more SR Ca^{2+} release, and higher force (32).

Nielsen et al. (35) demonstrated that heavy one-legged exercise-training for 7 weeks reduced the rate of $[K^+]_e$ increase in the trained compared to the control leg. These authors also found an increased Na^+-K^+ ATPase pump protein, and hypothesized that the slower increase in $[K^+]_e$ in the trained leg was caused by a greater reuptake of K^+ due to a higher activity of the muscle Na^+-K^+ ATPase pumps. Consistent with the membrane mechanism of muscle fatigue, the trained leg showed a 28% longer time to fatigue during an incremental exercise test, and at the point of fatigue the $[K^+]_e$ levels were similar in the two legs.

TEST YOURSELF

With intense contractile activity, what causes the observed depolarization of the V_m and reduced AP amplitude, and what is the evidence that these changes contribute to fatigue?

The T-tubular Charge Sensor

The T-tubular DHPR (charge sensor) is stabilized by the negative resting potential and mM extracellular Ca^{2+} found in nonfatigued fibers, and inactivated by depolarization or zero extracellular Ca^{2+} (5). Currently, it is unknown how T-tubular lumen Ca^{2+} changes with fatigue. An increase in intracellular Ca^{2+} would be expected to activate the T-tubular Ca^{2+}-ATPase pump and increase lumen Ca^{2+}. However, T-tubular Ca^{2+} channels are opened by the AP depolarization and the electrochemical gradient favors Ca^{2+} influx. Small increases in T-tubular Ca^{2+} (~5 mM) would shift the activation potential ~15 mV more positive and help prevent depolarization-induced inactivation by stabilizing the charge sensor. The former would not contribute to fatigue as threshold would still be reached by −20 mV and even the most fatigued muscle fibers show AP spikes near zero. Fatigued fibers do exhibit a positive shift in the activation threshold (36), which supports the hypothesis that extracellular Ca^{2+} increased. The available evidence suggests that the T-tubular charge sensor is robust and unlikely to be inactivated even in highly fatigued muscle fibers. A significant decline in the amplitude of the Ca^{2+}_i was observed in the absence of any change in T-tubular charge movement (37). The result did not rule out a partial inactivation of the charge sensor by cell depolarization in fatigued cells as charge movement and Ca^{2+} release were measured at a −80 mV holding potential. The result does indicate that problems in SR Ca^{2+} release persisted in the fatigued cells with a normal T-tubular charge.

The SR Ca²⁺ Release Channel

During the past quarter century, considerable progress has been made in understanding the molecular mechanism by which T-tubular charge induces SR Ca^{2+} release. The important proteins at the T-tubular membrane with the sarcoplasmic reticulum T-SR junction have been identified, and it is now clear that the DHPR (T-tubular charge sensor) lies directly opposite and interacts with the RyR1 (29) (Fig. 6.6, no. 4). The exact mechanism of transduction across the T-SR junction and the stoichiometric relationship between DHPR and the RyR1 in mammalian muscle has not been established. In the toadfish swimbladder, the ratio is 1:2 indicating that only one-half of the Ca^{2+} release channels are regulated by the T-tubular charge sensor (5). The mechanism of regulation of the channels not facing DHPR is unknown. Unlike frog muscle, it appears that these channels are not activated by Ca^{2+} released from the neighboring voltage-regulated SR channels—a process termed *Ca²⁺-induced Ca²⁺ release*—but rather may depend on allosteric interaction between neighboring RyR1 (38).

A consistent observation is that the amplitude of the Ca^{2+} transient decreases as fatigue develops. Although the problem may be caused, in part, by a blockage of the T-tubular AP or reduced T-tubular charge movement, considerable support exists for the hypothesis that the primary problem involves a direct inhibition of Ca^{2+} release from the SR Ca^{2+} release channel (RyR1). The intracellular Ca^{2+} content depends on the relative activity of Ca^{2+} release from the SR, and Ca^{2+} removal processes. The latter consists of the activity of the SR Ca^{2+} pump and Ca^{2+}-binding proteins, particularly parvalbumin in fast muscles. Calcium release (or flux) from the SR is dependent on channel permeability and the concentration gradient between SR lumen and intracellular fluid (ΔC). The permeability is regulated by interplay between opening of the SR calcium release channels and channel inactivation.

A fatigue-induced decline in the amplitude of the Ca^{2+} transient could be caused by a reduction in ΔC or by factors that decrease channel activation (either directly or by inhibiting T-tubular charge) or increase channel inactivation. In addition, considering that force is related to intracellular Ca^{2+}, which in turn is dependent on the Ca^{2+} release, and removal fluxes, any influences that decrease removal of Ca^{2+} will tend to prolong the Ca^{2+} transient and slow relaxation.

Concentration gradient across the SR

The ΔC depends on the SR Ca^{2+} content—a reduction in SR Ca^{2+} decreases ΔC and thus release. Eberstein and Sandow (39) showed in the early 1960s that fatigue did not completely deplete the SR of Ca^{2+} as caffeine, a compound that acts directly on the SR to induce Ca^{2+} release, reversed the tension loss in fatigued fibers. Later this was directly confirmed by the simultaneous measurement of force and intracellular Ca^{2+} following caffeine administration to a single fiber (Fig. 6.7C). The reduction of SR Ca^{2+} during continuous contractile activity is likely due in part to an increased binding of Ca^{2+} to the intracellular Ca^{2+}-binding proteins parvalbumin (fast fibers only) and the SR pump. Consequently, during activation free Ca^{2+} would be removed more slowly. Additionally, the SR Ca^{2+} pump rate may be slowed in fatigued muscle fibers, further reducing SR Ca^{2+} stores, and decreasing ΔC and Ca^{2+} release. These mechanisms would increase the resting intracellular Ca^{2+} (5,11). The net effect is that Ca^{2+} would be displaced from the release pool (SR store) to the removal pool where it is unavailable for release. These events would explain the observed prolongation in the Ca^{2+} transient (11,40), twitch duration (5,7), and the relaxation time following a tetanic contraction in fatigued muscle (Fig. 6.3).

Besides the redistribution on Ca^{2+} from the SR to intracellular buffers, evidence suggests that the gradient or ΔC for SR Ca^{2+} can be further reduced during heavy exercise by P_i precipitation of SR Ca^{2+} (13,29,41). It is well documented that intense contractile activity leads to increases in intracellular P_i that can approach 30 mM (4,5,30). The hypothesis is that P_i enters the SR and, at concentrations above 6 mM, begins to form an insoluble precipitate of calcium phosphate (CaP_i). This reduces the amount of releasable Ca^{2+} (lowers ΔC) and depresses the amplitude of the Ca^{2+} transient, which contributes to the development of muscle fatigue. More recently, this result was extended to the mechanically peeled fiber where elevated cytosolic P_i was shown to reduce the AP mediated force response, which is indicative of a depressed SR Ca^{2+} release (42). Figure 6.8 provides a concise summary of the role of P_i in reducing SR Ca^{2+} release. The traces shown in Fig 6.8A were taken from the experiment of Fryer et al. (41) and demonstrate the depressive effect of 50 mM P_i exposure on a subsequent caffeine contracture. Figure 6.8B presents a schematic representation of how P_i reduced the releasable pool of SR Ca^{2+} by lowering free Ca^{2+} as well as the fraction bound to calsequestrin (see Figure 6.8 legend). According to Duke and Steele (43) the Ca-P_i precipitation may be reduced and less likely to contribute to fatigue in PC depleted cells. Their data suggest that the dominant influence of P_i in PC depleted cells is the activation of SR Ca^{2+} efflux via pump reversal. This P_i-induced pump reversal required high ADP, which only occurred in PC depleted cells. Rather than inhibiting Ca^{2+} release, this effect would contribute to the progressive increase in resting Ca^{2+} and prolongation of muscle relaxation observed during the development of fatigue.

> ## KEY POINT
>
> The relative importance of these competing mechanisms to the development of muscle fatigue will depend on the degree of increase in P_i and ADP, as well as the extent of PC depletion.

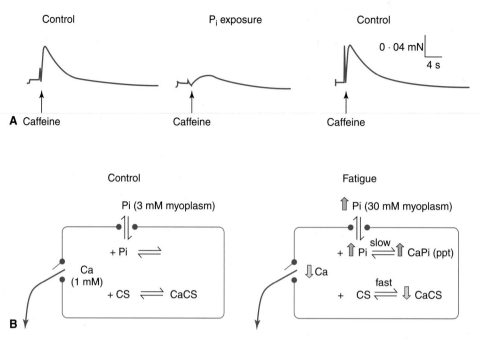

FIGURE 6.8   A. Force records from skinned fibers with intact SR. Caffeine was used to release SR Ca²⁺ producing the contractures shown; thus, the size of the contracture is an indication of the Ca²⁺ available for release in the SR. In the middle record, the muscle was exposed to 50 mM P_i for 20 s, the P_i was then washed off and caffeine applied. **B.** Schematic diagram of Ca²⁺ and P_i movements across the SR membrane and binding sites within the SR. Under control conditions $[P_i]_{myo} = [P_i]_{SR} = 3$ mM and $[Ca^{2+}]_{SR} = 1$ mM. Thus, $[Ca^{2+}]_{SR} \times [P_i]_{SR} = 3$ mM² and because this is below the solubility product of CaP_i (which is 6 mM²) none of this product is present. Ca²⁺ in the SR, however, binds rapidly and reversibly to calsequestrin (CS) so that there is a large pool of CaCS which buffers $[Ca^{2+}]_{SR}$. When the SR Ca²⁺ release channel opens, a large flux of Ca²⁺ into the myoplasm occurs because $[Ca^{2+}]_{SR}$ is high and is maintained high by the buffering of CaCS. In fatigue $[P_i]_{myo}$ is 30 mM and P_i enters the SR via anion channels. Once $[P_i]_{SR}$ exceeds 6 mM, the product of $[Ca^{2+}]_{SR} \times [P_i]_{SR}$ exceeds the solubility product of CaP_i and precipitation of CaP_i starts to occur slowly in the SR. As a consequence $[Ca^{2+}]_{SR}$ and CaCS fall and when the SR Ca²⁺ release channels are open the flux is smaller both because $[Ca^{2+}]_{SR}$ is lower and the buffering of $[Ca^{2+}]_{SR}$ by CaCS is reduced. Dissociation of CaP_i is assumed to be too slow to contribute to Ca²⁺ release. Heavy arrows indicate changes of key concentrations during fatigue. (Figure and figure legend were originally published by Allen DG, Westerblad H. Role of phosphate and calcium stores in muscle fatigue. *J Physiol.* 2001;536(pt 3):657–665, and are reprinted here with copyright permission of The Physiological Society. The data in **A** was adapted from Fryer MW, Owen VJ, Lamb GD, et al. Effects of creatine phosphate and P(i) on Ca²⁺ movements and tension development in rat skinned skeletal muscle fibres. *J Physiol.* 1995;482(pt 1):123–140.)

There is evidence that fibers can sustain some decline in ΔC without a change in Ca²⁺ release. Posterino and Lamb (44) observed a constant contractile force in skinned rat extensor digitorum longus fibers in response to AP activation where SR Ca²⁺ load was varied between 1 and 4 mM. A possible explanation is the observation of Royer et al. (45) that the evacuability of the SR increased as the SR Ca²⁺ load decreased due both to an increased SR permeability (P) and reduced buffer power (B) of the luminal Ca²⁺ buffering protein calsequestrin. With intense contractile activity, SR Ca²⁺ release decreases, however, an increased P/B ratio helps reduce the decline in Ca²⁺ release that is attributable to the reduced ΔC.

Inhibition of SR Ca²⁺ channel opening by ions and substrates

The observation that fatigued muscles exposed to caffeine (Fig. 6.7) show recovery of Ca²⁺ release and force demonstrates that SR Ca²⁺ stores were not depleted and that a reduced ΔC cannot totally explain the inhibition of SR Ca²⁺ release. Studies utilizing SR vesicles and isolated SR calcium release channels have demonstrated channel activity to be modulated by intracellular ions and substrates to include glycogen, ATP, Mg²⁺, H⁺, and Ca²⁺. A reduced pH has been shown to inhibit channel open probability with near zero activation at pH 6.2. However, when intact fibers were made acidotic the amplitude of the Ca^{2+}_i was increased, and low pH had no effect on SR Ca^{2+} release in skinned fibers. These data suggest that the low pH is unlikely to affect the SR Ca^{2+} release channel or the amplitude of the Ca^{2+}_i during in vivo contractile activity. Currently, the hypothesis with the most experimental support is that the SR Ca^{2+} release channel is inhibited during fatigue by the combined effect of an increased Mg^{2+} and a reduced ATP (7,11,29). The most convincing evidence comes from skinned muscle fiber studies where potential fatigue factors can be individual or collectively altered. Using this technique, Blazev and Lamb (46) observed that a decline in cell ATP to 0.5 mM had no effect, but when combined with an increased Mg^{2+} (3 mM) significant inhibition of Ca^{2+} release was observed. Because much of the intracellular Mg^{2+} is bound to ATP, the drop in cell ATP with intense exercise is mirrored by an increase in free Mg^{2+}. Allen et al. (7) used changes in Mg^{2+} to model cell ATP in single mouse fibers and found a linear relationship between the fall in ATP and the amplitude of the Ca^{2+}_i. A decline in the amplitude of the Ca^{2+}_i could be caused by a reduced SR Ca^{2+} release flux and/or to an increase in the intracellular Ca^{2+} buffer capacity. However, the latter seems unlikely in that intracellular acidosis and the reduction in strongly bound crossbridges associated with heavy activity would both reduce Ca^{2+} buffering by reducing Ca^{2+} affinity for troponin C (7). With the exception of conditions that elicit low-frequency fatigue (LFF), activity-induced depression in SR Ca^{2+} release recovers rapidly by a process that can be blocked by metabolic inhibitors, observations consistent with the low ATP, high Mg^{2+} hypothesis. Because even in the most fatigued cells ATP content remained above 1.2 mM, the hypothesis requires that ATP be compartmentalized with lower levels surrounding the SR release channels. The data of Han et al. (47) provide support for this hypothesis. They demonstrated that skeletal muscle triads contain a compartmentalized glycolytic reaction sequence, and that the ATP formed in the triadic gap appears restricted and unavailable for reactions elsewhere in the cell. The likelihood of compartmentalization would increase in fatigue PC content and the effectiveness of the PC-shuttle declined.

Studies employing creatine kinase deficient ($CK^{-/-}$) mice have provided evidence that the fatigue-induced decline in SR Ca^{2+} release can be explained by the combined effect of Ca-P_i precipitation within the SR and low ATP, high Mg^{2+} inhibition of the SR release channel (11,29). This conclusion is based on the observation that $CK^{-/-}$, but not control mice, showed a rapid decline in Ca^{2+}_i and force in response to heavy contractile activity, whereas with less intense stimulation the $CK^{-/-}$ mice were less fatigable than control mice. The $Ca^{-/-}$ mice would be unable to buffer the decline in ATP, thus, increasing the direct inhibition of low ATP on the SR release channel. However, intracellular P_i would remain low preventing the Ca-P_i-mediated reduction in SR Ca^{2+} release.

With intense stimulation, fibers show a rapid decline in SR Ca^{2+} release and in the fraction of Ca^{2+} that can be directly released by caffeine or other drugs. However, in glycogen depleted fibers the Ca^{2+}_i falls rapidly but the SR Ca^{2+} store is not depleted. Furthermore, recovery of both peak force and Ca^{2+}_i is slowed in fibers bathed in glucose free solutions (48). The reduced Ca^{2+} release in the low glycogen fibers was observed in the presence of high ATP. These observations suggest that cell glycogen or some intermediate of glycogen metabolism is required for optimal regulation of the SR Ca^{2+} release channel. Glycogen is known to be associated with the T-SR junctional complex and some critical level may be necessary for the maintenance of the structural integrity of the complex.

It is not known whether or not the inhibition of SR Ca^{2+} release with fatigue can be delayed or reduced by programs of exercise training. However, based on the known metabolic adaptations, exercise training should prove beneficial. The exercise training–induced increase in muscle mitochondria would allow a given tissue respiratory rate to be established with less of a rise in cell ADP, P_i, and Mg^{2+}, while maintaining a higher ATP (49). With heavy exercise, this should reduce the likelihood of a Ca-P_i mediated reduction in SR Ca^{2+} release or a direct inhibition of release by the combined affects of high Mg^{2+} and low ATP.

KEY POINT

During prolonged exercise, any mechanisms inhibiting SR Ca^{2+} release that is coupled to glycogen depletion would be delayed by endurance exercise training due to the slower rate of muscle glycogen depletion in the muscle of the trained individual (14,49).

TEST YOURSELF

Intense contractile activity has consistently been shown to reduce SR Ca^{2+} release. By what mechanisms could an increase in fiber Pi and free Mg^{2+} cause the reduced release?

SR ATPase pump

Fatigue is known to be associated with a prolonged relaxation time due to a reduced rate of SR Ca^{2+} reuptake. With heavy exercise, the inhibited SR pump function has been linked to the combined affects of the increase in H^+, P_i, and ADP. Low pH is known to inhibit the SR ATPase and Ca^{2+} pump rate with the latter declining by twofold between pH 7.1 and 6.6 and by additional twofold between 6.6 and 6.1 (7). Further support for a role for low pH in prolonging muscle relaxation time comes from the observation that iodoacetic acid-poisoned muscles underwent a 50% fall in tension with stimulation, but no change in pH or relaxation time (5). However, clearly other factors are involved as myophosphorylase-deficient subjects showed a slowed relaxation with no change in pH.

High P_i appears to inhibit the SR pump and increase Ca^{2+} leak through the SR Ca^{2+} release channel to the intracellular fluid. The latter is thought to be responsible for the increase and slowing in Ca^{2+}_i observed early in fatigue in control (Fig. 6.7B), but not $CK^{-/-}$ muscle fibers (11). In a series of papers, Macdonald and Stephenson (30,50,51) showed 1 mM ADP to reduce the amplitude and prolong the duration of AP elicited twitches in rat fast EDL fibers, and inhibit the SR Ca^{2+} pump rate and accelerate the pump leak rate in slow and fast fibers. High ADP apparently increased the Ca^{2+}-Ca^{2+} exchange function of the SR which moved Ca^{2+} from the SR lumen (high concentration) to the myoplasm (low concentration). This Ca^{2+} movement was not caused by a reversal of the SR pump as ATP was not synthesized, but by pump slippage allowing Ca^{2+} leak into the cytosol. The reduced SR pump rate could be, in part, due to the reduced free energy of ATP hydrolysis as the ATP/ADP + P_i ratio declines with fatigue (5).

In summary, alterations in E-C coupling from changes in the surface membrane and T-tubular AP to inhibition of SR Ca^{2+} release and reuptake have been shown to contribute to fatigue during intense contractile activity. The activity-induced increase in $[K^+]_e$ and intracellular sodium and decreased $[K^+]_i$ depolarize the V_m, reduce Na^+ conductance and the AP amplitude, and lead to a depressed SR Ca^{2+} release. Ion stimulation of the Na^+-K^+ pump is limited by other factors such as ROS oxidation of the pump and a reduced free energy of ATP hydrolysis. Finally, the decline in SR Ca^{2+} release is exacerbated by high P_i-induced precipitation of SR Ca^{2+}, Mg^{2+} inhibition of the RyR1 channel, and an increases SR pump leak attributed to high ADP.

TEST YOURSELF

What factors are responsible for triggering SR Ca^{2+} release in skeletal muscle, and why is release reduced in fatigued fibers?

Low-Frequency Fatigue

After certain contractile paradigms (elicited both in vivo in humans and in vitro in animals), muscle force required several hours to days to recover and the delayed recovery was especially apparent at low activation frequencies (52,53). The etiology of this condition, termed *low-frequency fatigue* (LFF), is still not understood. Because the amplitude of the Ca^{2+} transient is depressed and recovery slow, the mechanism is thought to involve a structural alteration of either the SR Ca^{2+} release channel and/or associated proteins (52,53). This structural change reduces the amplitude of the Ca^{2+} transient for all stimulation frequencies, but due to the shape of the pCa–force relationship a major depression of force is only observed at low frequencies. Bruton et al. (52) reviewed the literature in this field and concluded that short-term increases

in intracellular Ca^{2+} in the vicinity of the triads might initiate low-frequency fatigue (LFF). The primary evidence for this was the observation that mM Ca^{2+} abolished E-C coupling in isolated peeled single fibers, while caffeine contractures were maintained. Although the mechanism likely requires an elevated intracellular Ca^{2+}, the exact process involved is unclear. The most likely candidates are Ca^{2+} mediated events involving calmodulin (CaM), calcium-activated proteases, or ROS (52).

A logical site for LFF induction is the RyR1 the Ca^{2+} channel of the SR and the largest known channel with a molecular weight in excess of 2,000 kDa (54). The RyR1 is part of a multiprotein complex that includes accessory proteins involved in phosphorylation/dephosphorylation of the channel (cAMP-dependent protein kinase A [PKA], Ca^{2+} calmodulin dependent protein kinase [CaMKII], phosphodiesterase 4D3 [PDE4D3], and protein phosphatase 1 [PP1]), the Ca^{2+} binding proteins CaM and S100A1 involved in modulation of Ca^{2+} activation of the channel, and FK 506-binding protein FKBP12 thought to stabilize the channel and coordinate opening (Fig. 6.9). The channel also interacts with the SR membrane proteins junctin and triadin which, in turn, bind to the SR luminal Ca^{2+} binding proteins calsequestrin and histone-rich calcium binding protein (HRC).

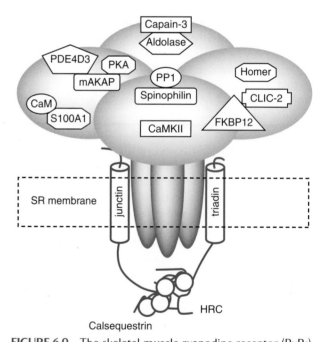

FIGURE 6.9 The skeletal muscle ryanodine receptor (RyR1) and associated proteins. Each of the four RyR1 monomers binds one of each of the accessory proteins except for calsequestrin and histidine-rich calcium binding protein (HRC). For clarity, only one of each of the proteins is shown. CaM, calmodulin; CaMKII, Ca^{2+}/calmodulin-dependent protein kinase; PKA, protein kinase A; PDE4D3, phosphodiesterase 4D3; FKBP12, FK506-binding protein 12 kDa; PP1, protein phosphatase 1; mAKAP, cAMP kinase anchoring protein; SR, sarcoplasmic reticulum; CLIC-2, chloride intracellular channel. (Figure reprinted from Balog EM. Excitation-contraction coupling and minor triadic proteins in low-frequency fatigue. *Exerc Sport Sci Rev.* 2010;38(3):135–142.)

It is well established that CaM plays a dual role in the regulation of the SR Ca^{2+} release channel (52). CaM binding activates or inhibits channel opening at low and high cytoplasmic Ca^{2+}, respectively. In a nonfatigued fiber, this process likely contributes to the cyclic activation and inactivation of the release channel. There is no evidence linking Ca^{2+}-CaM to an altered RyR1 function during LFF (52). However, the possibility exists that elevated cytoplasmic Ca^{2+} associated with fatigue leads to an altered CaM binding, such that the channel is harder to activate. An increased cytoplasmic Ca^{2+} might lead to a prolonged elevation in CaMKII and to an excess phosphorylation of the DHPR and/or the RyR1 (29). Prolonged β-adrenergic activity with exercise may also lead to an increased PKA activity and hyperphosphorylation of the RyR1. In addition, inhibition of PP1 and/or PDE4D3 could also lead to excess phosphorylation. Excess phosphorylation of the RyR1 might directly reduce RyR1 open probability or mediate the dissociation of the channel stabilizing protein FK 506-binding protein (29).

In addition to accessory proteins that bind directly to the RyR1and regulate Ca^{2+} release, alteration in the triadic proteins junctophilin-1 and -2, JEP-45, and Mg-29 could mediate LFF (54). These proteins are thought to play a role in maintaining the structural arrangement and link between the DHPR and the RyR1, and disruption of one or more of these proteins could reduce functional coupling and, thus, the amount of Ca^{2+} released for a given T-tubular charge movement. To date, there is no direct evidence for the involvement of these proteins in LFF. However, the loss of junctophilin-1 and junctophilin-2 has been observed to reduce force following eccentric contractions, and muscles from Mg-29 knockout animals and LFF muscles show similar force–frequency relationships (54).

Reactive Oxygen Species

ROS such as hydrogen peroxide (H_2O_2) and superoxide anion are produced during oxidative metabolism and their rate of production increases with the work intensity in skeletal muscle. For decades scientists have hypothesized that ROS play a role in LFF as well as more rapidly reversible muscle fatigue by oxidation of critical cell proteins such as the Na^+-K^+ pump, myofilaments, DHPR, and RyR1 (29,32). Presumably, the speed of recovery and/whether or not LFF results both depend on the site and/or extent of oxidation. The primary support for ROS induced fatigue is the observation that the antioxidant *N*-acetylcysteine reduces protein oxidation and delays the onset of fatigue (32,55). Studies in the mid-1990s suggested that ROS inhibited SR Ca^{2+} release in skinned fibers thus contributing to fatigue (52). One mechanism might be ROS oxidation of a critical RyR1 cysteine residue. However, Andrade et al. (56) found that brief exposures to H_2O_2 had no effect on the amplitude of the Ca^{2+} transient, but significantly increased force. This response was biphasic as longer exposures to H_2O_2 caused a small increase in myoplasmic Ca^{2+} with large declines in force. The latter effect was completely reversible by the reductant dithiothreitol (DTT). The authors concluded that the main effect of ROS was to alter the myofibrillar Ca^{2+} sensitivity, and that the effect on SR Ca^{2+} release was minor. This hypothesis gained support from the work of Moopanar and Allen (57) who, using an in vitro mouse model, found ROS to reduce myofibrillar Ca^{2+}-sensitivity. It seems likely that ROS alter multiple proteins and that the primary site(s) of action may be qualitatively and quantitatively different in fatigued induced in vivo compared to in vitro.

KEY POINT

Currently, there is insufficient data to categorically identify specific sites or mechanisms by which ROS induce fatigue.

Summary

LFF is characterized by a reduced SR Ca^{2+} release that appears to result from a structural alteration in the RyR1. The structural alteration in the RyR1 may result from a excess activation of CaMKII and/or PKA or inhibition of PP1 and/or PDE4D3 causing hyperphosphorylation of the RyR1. Alternatively, LFF may be mediated by Ca^{2+} activated protease and/or ROS alteration of critical proteins such as the DHPR, RyR1, triadic proteins, and the SR pump.

TEST YOURSELF

What is the evidence that LFF results from a reduced SR Ca^{2+} release, and why with that etiology is force only reduced at low frequency of activation?

Crossbridge Mechanism of Fatigue

Muscle contraction involves the hydrolysis of ATP to produce energy for crossbridge cycling with a resulting increase in ADP, P_i, and H^+. All three increase in proportion to the intensity of the work performed and due to the creatine kinase reaction show an inverse relation to PC. The initial decline in force with intense stimulation of individual muscle fibers (Fig. 6.7B) occurs with no change in the amplitude of the Ca^{2+}_i and is thought to be mediated by the combined effects of an increase in P_i and H^+ (7). Both ions have been shown to directly reduce the peak force of single skinned fibers (58) (Fig. 6.10) presumably by either inhibiting or reversing the crossbridge transition from the low- to the high-force state (Fig. 6.2, step 5) and/or reducing the force per crossbridge (59). There is no conclusive evidence as to which mechanism is most

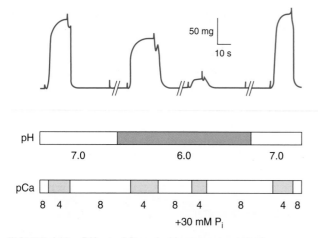

FIGURE 6.10   Effect of P_i and pH on maximal Ca^{2+}-activated force, pCa 4.0, of skinned muscle fiber. The recording shows the typical effects of pH 6.0 alone and pH 6.0 in combination with 30 mM P_i on maximal force of a fast-twitch skeletal muscle fiber. Calibration bars show 50 mg and 10 s, and spikes on record are solution exchange artifacts. For concision, record shown is not continuous but has been truncated at interrupted lines. (Figure reprinted from Nosek TM, Fender KY, Godt RE. It is diprotonated inorganic phosphate that depresses force in skinned skeletal muscle fibers. *Science.* 1987;236(4798):191–193, with copyright permission of AAAS.)

important, and it may differ between ions and muscle temperature. Due to the observation that isolated single fibers are not stable at temperatures much above 20°C, the majority of single fiber studies have been performed at 15°C. At that temperature, a drop in fiber pH has been shown to reduce the force per crossbridge in both fast- and slow-twitch fibers, while the number of strong (high force) crossbridges was reduced only in fast fibers (19). Metzger and Moss (19) observed that for the fast fiber type, the rate constant of tension redevelopment (k_{tr}) following a rapid slack and reextension of fiber length was depressed at pH 6.2 compared to 7.0 at suboptimal (pCa >5.0), but not maximal levels of Ca^{2+} activation. From this, they concluded that protons have a direct depressant effect on the forward rate constant for the transition between the weak and strong binding states of the crossbridge (Fig. 6.2, step 5). In contrast, P_i is thought to reduce P_0 and increase k_{tr} by accelerating the reversal of step 5 (Fig. 6.2). In addition to reducing the number of strong binding (high force) crossbridges, P_i may also reduce the force per bridge (5,59).

An increased H^+ not only depresses force, but also inhibits the myofibrillar ATPase activity, which contributes to the fatigue-induced drop in V_0. Thus, H^+ affects at least two steps in the crossbridge cycle (Fig. 6.2, steps 5 and 7), whereas an increase in P_i depresses force (step 5) but has no effect on V_0 (step 7). As can be seen in Figure 6.10, the effects of H^+ and P_i on fiber force are additive with considerably greater depression in force observed with both ions than with either one alone (58).

The fatigue-induced decline in peak power (Fig. 6.5) can at least, in part, be attributed to the direct effects of H^+ and P_i on crossbridge kinetics (Fig. 6.2, steps 5 and 7) and the resulting depression of force and velocity (59). It is also possible that the reduced a/P_0 ratio sometimes observed in fatigued muscle (Fig. 6.5B) and a contributing factor in reduced power is caused by the increase in H^+ and/or P_i. However in fast skeletal muscle, it is not due to H^+ alone as the a/P_0 ratio of single fast type II fibers studied at pH 6.2 and 30°C was unaltered compared to control conditions (23).

In addition to a direct effect on peak force, both H^+ and P_i shift the pCa–force relationship to the right such that higher free Ca^{2+} is required to reach a given tension. For low pH, this effect is mediated, in part, by competitive inhibition of Ca^{2+} binding to troponin-C. The observation that high Ca^{2+} (pCa 4.5) cannot eliminate the effect and that rigor tension is reduced by 33% at pH 6.2 compared to 7.0, suggests that factors in addition to competitive inhibition of Ca^{2+} binding to troponin-C are involved. The decline in the number of high force crossbridges (caused by both H^+ and P_i) reduces the thick filament mediated cooperativity between regulatory thin filament sites and this is thought to directly contribute to the right shift in the pCa–force relationship. This effect is shown as point 2 in Figure 6.4. Because the amplitude of the Ca^{2+}_i transient is known to decline with fatigue (point 3, Figs. 6.4 and 6.7), the right shift in the pCa–force relationship exacerbates the fatigue-inducing effects of H^+ and P_i. Recently, Debold et al. (60) found that the P_i-induced right shift in the pCa–force relationship was twofold greater at high (30°C) compared to low (15°C) temperature with the effect qualitatively similar in fast and slow fibers. Thus, at cytosolic Ca^{2+} concentrations known to exist in fatigued fibers, these results demonstrate that the force depressing effects of high P_i (and although not yet determined likely low pH) are greater as temperature increases. In additional, at less than maximal Ca^{2+} concentrations, the pH and P_i-induced right shift in the pCa–force relationship would also contribute to the decline in k_{tr} (and presumably +dP/dt) as the forward rate constant of step 5 (Fig. 6.2) would be slowed by the reduction in the number of strong binding, high-force crossbridges (19). In the fast fiber types, a drop in cell pH could also directly depress k_{tr} by inhibiting the forward rate constant of step 5 (Fig. 6.2).

In contrast, a rise in ADP would increase force by reducing the rate of step 7 (Fig. 6.2), thus increasing the number of crossbridges in the high force states (AM'·ADP and AM·ADP). Because step 7 is thought to be rate limiting to the overall crossbridge cycle speed, an increase in ADP contributes to the decline in fiber V_0.

In recent years, the importance of low pH in the etiology of muscle fatigue has been questioned (48,61). The challenge to the hypothesis that low pH contributes to fatigue has come from the observations that the inhibitory effects of low pH on P_0 and V_0 are reduced as the temperature increases from 10° to 30°C. However, these studies have not considered the effects of low pH on peak power or the combined effects of a reduced Ca^{2+} release, low pH and an elevated P_i. Knuth et al. (23) demonstrated that low pH significantly reduced the peak power of slow and fast fibers at both 15°C and 30°C. Importantly, Karatzaferi et al. (62) recently showed that low pH (6.2) combined with high P_i (30 mM) significantly inhibited fast fiber power measured at 30°C by 55%. Surprisingly, at high but not low temperature peak power was further depressed to 70% inhibition relative to control fibers by phosphorylation of the regulatory myosin light chain (RLC). Because RLC phosphorylation of fast fibers normally occurs with contraction, one can conclude that low pH coupled with high P_i contributes significantly to the fatigue-induced loss of peak power in fast type II fibers.

Regarding programs of regular exercise training, there is no evidence on whether or not exercise training causes any direct effects on the interaction between putative fatigue factors and either steps of the crossbridge cycle or the pCa–force relationship. However, endurance exercise training is known to increase mitochondrial content in all fiber types (see Chapter 18) and, consequently during exercise, trained individuals show less of an increase in muscle ADP, adenosine monophosphate, and P_i and a reduced glycolysis (49). The latter would also reduce the increase in cell lactate and H^+ at the same absolute or even relative workload. One would also expect to see higher cell ATP and less of an increase in Mg^{2+}. All of these changes would reduce muscle fatigue by limiting the known deleterious effects of low ATP and high Mg^{2+}, H^+, P_i, and ADP.

Summary

During intense exercise, the drop in fiber pH and rise in P_i would combine to depress force, velocity, and peak power. Although the depressive effects of both low pH and high P_i on force at saturating Ca^{2+} (pCa <5) are less at high compared to low temperature, the right shift in the pCa–force relationship (Fig. 6.4, pt. 2) caused by these ions is greater as temperature increases. Thus, force in fatigued fibers experiencing suboptimal Ca^{2+} would be more affected by low pH and high P_i as temperature increased. Importantly, the decline in peak power caused by the combined effects of low pH and high P_i are significant at known in vivo muscle temperatures, and in fast fibers are exacerbated by the greater change in these ions and phosphorylation of the myosin RLC.

TEST YOURSELF

High P_i can induce fatigue at multiple sites. What are these sites and how are they altered by muscle temperature?

Prolonged Exercise and Fatigue

Despite more than a century of research, the etiology of fatigue with prolonged endurance exercise is not fully understood. Hypoglycemia and/or high core temperature can limit endurance exercise, but with adequate carbohydrate and water intake during exercise fatigue from these factors can generally be prevented (14). At submaximal workloads the inability to continue exercise is frequently correlated with and perhaps, caused by muscle glycogen depletion. With exercise intensities below 50% or above 90% of one's maximal oxygen consumption, ample muscle glycogen remains at exhaustion (14). In addition to glycogen depletion, SR function has frequently been found to be compromised following prolonged exercise.

Glycogen Depletion

Since the development of the needle biopsy technique, multiple studies have found a correlation between muscle glycogen depletion, and fatigue with endurance exercise. Despite this a cause-and-effect relationship has not been demonstrated. However, the observation that regular exercise training reduces the rate of glycogen utilization, delays glycogen depletion, and increases exercise time to exhaustion supports the hypothesis that muscle glycogen depletion is an important factor in fatigue. Although muscle glycogen is an important fuel source, it is not clear why cell metabolism could not proceed with free fatty acids (FFA; blood and cellular) and blood glucose as substrates for energy. Carbohydrate feedings throughout exercise prevents hypoglycemia and delays fatigue by 30 to 60 minute, but does not alter the rate of muscle glycogen depletion or prevent fatigue (14). During prolonged exercise, after the first two hours, the primary carbohydrate fuel source switches from muscle glycogen to blood glucose. With blood glucose as the primary carbohydrate fuel source, Coyle (14) found that even trained cyclists could not maintain exercise intensities above 74% of maximal O_2 consumption. This suggests that the metabolism of bloodborne substrates (both glucose and FFA) is simply too slow to maintain heavy exercise intensities. An increased reliance on fat oxidation would further reduce an individual's work capacity as less ATP is generated per liter of oxygen consumed.

It seems unlikely that glycogen depletion is the sole cause of fatigue with prolonged exercise, but rather that it triggers additional events leading to fatigue. One hypothesis is that a certain level of muscle glycogen metabolism is required to maintain Krebs cycle intermediates at a level adequate for the optimal production of nicotinamide adenine dinucleotide and electron transport rate. Consistent with this is the observation that the concentration of Krebs cycle intermediates declined with prolonged exercise (63). Besides reducing carbon chain precursors for the production of Krebs cycle intermediates, glycogen depletion has been shown to be associated with an increased production of branch chain amino acids (BCAA) from Krebs cycle intermediates (64). The increase in BCAA aminotransferase reactions induced by glycogen depletion would contribute to the reduction in Krebs cycle intermediates.

With prolonged exercise and the resulting glycogen depletion, there is an increased reliance on FFA metabolism. Maintenance of high oxidation rates may be limited by the muscle cell's ability to translocate FFA into the mitochondria. The enzyme catalyzing this step, carnitine acyltransferase I (CAT I), is thought to be limiting for FFA oxidation (see Chapter 15). In the latter stages of endurance exercise, this step may be unable to keep up with the increased demand for fat oxidation. Support for this possibility comes from the observation that carnitine administration delayed fatigue in the isolated soleus muscle (65).

KEY POINT

It is well documented that regular exercise training delays fatigue during endurance exercise, and that the rate of muscle and liver glycogen depletion with exercise is slowed due to reduced carbohydrate and increased fat metabolism in trained individuals (49). It is generally thought that this glycogen sparing effect is important in delaying muscle fatigue, but as discussed here the exact mechanism(s) linking glycogen depletion with the inability to continue exercise has not been established.

SR Function

Of all the intracellular organelles, the SR seems particularly vulnerable to deleterious changes with prolonged exercise. Except for conditions that elicit LFF, there is little or no information on whether prolonged exercise inhibits SR Ca^{2+} release. In contrast, there is considerable data (in animals and humans) showing a reduced SR pump function. SR vesicles isolated from muscles fatigued by prolonged exercise show a reduced Ca^{2+} uptake rate, which is generally but not always related to reduced SR ATPase activity (5,15,66). A reduced SR Ca^{2+} uptake with no change in ATPase activity suggests either an uncoupling of the transport or a leaky vesicle whereby Ca^{2+} fluxes back into the intracellular fluid. This plus the observation of a reduced SR yield (67) suggests that the SR may be structurally damaged perhaps by the activation of proteases. The disruption in SR function appears more related to the degree of activity and not necessarily glycogen depletion. In rats swum to exhaustion, glycogen depletion was observed in muscles representative of all fiber types, but SR Ca^{2+} uptake was depressed in vesicles isolated from the slow type I soleus and fast type IIa deep region of the vastus lateralis, but not the fast type IIb/IIx superficial region of the vastus lateralis (67). Presumably the latter muscle was recruited less during the endurance swim. It is still possible that glycogen somehow stabilizes the SR membranes and that following glycogen depletion other factors lead to its disruption.

Other Factors

Glycogen depletion and a compromised SR function may not be exclusive factors mediating fatigue during prolonged exercise. A controversial area is whether or not prolonged exercise leads to mitochondrial swelling and a reduced oxidative capacity. There is structural and functional data to support and refute this hypothesis (5). Studies on skinned fibers isolated from human muscle following exhaustive bicycle exercise showed an increased respiration in the absence of ADP, but no change in maximal ADP-stimulated respiration (68). This observation suggests that fatigue-induced changes in mitochondria are unlikely to limit ATP production or performance.

The myofibrils seem relatively resistant to fatigue induced by prolonged exercise (5,67). Myofibrils isolated from fast and slow muscles of rats swum to exhaustion showed no change is ATPase activity, and despite a 26% drop in peak force, the maximal shortening velocity of the soleus was unaltered (67). However, force and power loss resulting from eccentrically induced muscle fiber damage can be easily mistaken for fatigue. The former can occur during either high intensity or endurance exercise and does involve disruption of myofibrils (5). From a performance standpoint, it's irrelevant whether the loss of power was caused by fiber damage or fatigue, except that the former requires a considerably longer recovery period (days as opposed to hours).

CHAPTER SUMMARY

The mechanisms of muscle fatigue are complex and dependent on the type of exercise (high-intensity versus endurance; repetitive versus sustained), one's age, state of fitness, and the fiber type composition of the muscle studied. As shown in Figure 6.1, it is clear that fatigue is not caused by a single entity, but rather from various factors acting at multiple sites of both central and peripheral origin. This chapter reviewed both central and peripheral factors, and provided evidence that, in well-motivated athletes, peripheral events within the muscle are most important in eliciting fatigue. However, with repetitive activities such as those experienced in industrial work place settings, central fatigue may contribute up to 25% of the total fatigue.

In short-duration, heavy-contractile activity, fatigue is, in part, mediated by the combined effects of an elevated H^+, P_i, and ADP acting at the crossbridge to reduce force, velocity, and power. The decline in power is exaggerated in fast fibers due to larger reductions in fiber pH and increases in P_i as well as the phosphorylation of the myosin RLC. Late in fatigue, the process is dominated by a precipitous fall in SR Ca^{2+} release which, when combined with the right shift in the pCa-force relation, causes a large drop in force. The inhibition of SR Ca^{2+} release is caused, in part, by activity-induced increase in $[K^+]_e$ and intracellular sodium and decreased $[K^+]_i$ that depolarize the V_m and reduce Na^+ conductance and the AP amplitude. Modest declines in fiber pH (i.e., between 7.0 to 6.8) seem to protect against this mechanism of fatigue by decreasing Cl^- influx, thus, limiting the decline in AP amplitude. Ion stimulation of the Na^+-K^+ pump is limited by other factors such as ROS oxidation of the pump and a reduced free energy of ATP hydrolysis. Finally, the decline in SR Ca^{2+} release is exacerbated by high P_i-induced precipitation of SR Ca^{2+}, Mg^{2+} inhibition of the RyR1 channel, and an increases SR pump leak attributed to high ADP.

A reduced SR Ca^{2+} release is also of prime importance in the etiology of LFF, a special condition in which force is reduced in response to low but not high activation frequencies. The etiology of LFF is unknown but may be caused by Ca^{2+} activated proteases and/or ROS-mediated modifications of critical proteins such as the DHPR, RyR1, triadic proteins, SR pump, and myofibrils.

Fatigue from prolonged exercise is highly correlated with and likely at least in part caused by muscle glycogen depletion. With reduced glycogen, muscles depend more on blood borne substrates (glucose and FFA) and this necessitates a reduced work rate. Carbohydrate supplementation can delay but not prevent fatigue, and, thus, other factors must contribute to fatigue. It may be that glycogen depletion limits the production of Krebs cycle intermediates, which leads to a reduced nicotinamide adenine dinucleotide production and electron transport rate. Prolonged exercise may disrupt organelles with the SR appearing particularly susceptible, as depression in both SR ATPase activity and Ca^{2+} uptake are known to occur. It will be important to understand the nature of the decline in SR Ca^{2+} release with heavy exercise and LFF, and the relationship of muscle glycogen depletion to the onset of other important factors (such as an altered SR pump function) in mediating fatigue during prolonged exercise.

KEY POINT

Programs of regular exercise training are known to delay the onset and reduce the extent of fatigue that occurs with both short duration heavy and moderate intensity prolonged exercise. However, additional research is needed to determine whether or not exercise training can reduce either the fatigue-inducing effects of H^+ and P_i at the crossbridge or the factors involved in the inhibition of SR function.

A MILESTONE OF DISCOVERY

For more than 100 years, muscle fatigue had been characterized by a loss of peak force and a prolonged relaxation transient, and for the first 70 years of the twentieth century, the leading hypothesis was that fatigue resulting from high-intensity contractile activity was caused by lactic acid. The first indication that calcium (Ca^{2+}) release from the sarcoplasmic reticulum (SR) and the resulting intracellular Ca^{2+} calcium transient (Ca^{2+}_i) might be involved in the fatigue process came in 1963. At that time, Eberstein and Sandow (39) observed that caffeine, a compound stimulating direct release of Ca^{2+} from the SR, could reverse the tension loss of fatigued fibers. This result, along with the observation of Lüettgau and colleagues (36) that fatigued fibers exposed to high K^+ responded with high force contractures, demonstrated that muscle fatigue was not caused by depletion of releasable Ca^{2+} from the SR. Two years prior to the milestone work of Westerblad and Allen (40), Allen et al. (12) dissected single fibers from Xenopus lumbrical muscles, and microinjected the fibers with the photoprotein aequorin to measure the myoplasmic free calcium concentration (Ca^{2+}_i) in rested and fatigued cells. The important observations were that the characteristic reduction in force and slowing of relaxation in the fatigued fibers was associated with a decline in the amplitude and a slowing of the rate of decline in the aequorin light signal. This was the first indication that fatigue may be mediated by a decline in SR Ca^{2+} release. About the same time, Lännergren and Westerblad (69) developed the single fiber technique in mammals utilizing a mouse foot muscle. They observed that fatigue occurred in 3 phases: an early 10% drop in tension (phase 1), a plateau period (phase 2), and finally a rapid decline in force (phase 3). Westerblad and Allen (40) studied the same preparation to test the hypotheses that phase 1 was independent of SR Ca^{2+} release, whereas phase 3 was a direct result of a decline in the amplitude of the Ca^{2+}_i. They were the first to utilize the fluorescent indicator Fura-2 to measure the amplitude of the Ca^{2+}_i. Figure 6.7 demonstrates the important results that were: (a) early fatigue occurred while the amplitude of the Ca^{2+}_i increased (Fig. 6.7B); and (b) the precipitous drop in tension late in fatigue was caused by a reduced Ca^{2+}_i (Fig. 6.7C). This point was proven by the application of caffeine, which increased the amplitude of the Ca^{2+}_i and restored force (Fig. 6.7C). Another important finding was that the sensitivity of the myofilaments to Ca^{2+} was reduced such that in fatigued fibers less force was obtained at a given Ca^{2+} concentration. This group and others have since shown that the early fatigue is associated with increases in H^+, P_i, and ADP acting directly on the crossbridge (Fig. 6.2). Perhaps, the most important consequence of this work was that it focused the attention of this field on the role of E-C coupling (and, in particular, SR Ca^{2+} release) in mediating fatigue. Subsequent studies have looked for the factor(s) inhibiting SR Ca^{2+} release and an extensive list has been studied (low ATP, high Mg^{2+}, ROS). A disappointment is that to date no factor has been unequivocally linked to the inhibition of the SR Ca^{2+} release.

Westerblad H, Allen DG. Changes of myoplasmic calcium concentration during fatigue in single mouse muscle fibers. J Gen Physiol. 1991;98:615–635.

ACKNOWLEDGMENTS

The author expresses his appreciation to Janell Roma-towski, who helped in the preparation of the figures, and to his former graduate students who participated in the laboratory's muscle fatigue research. The author's research has been sponsored by NASA and NIH.

REFERENCES

1. Edwards RH. Biochemical basis of fatigue in exercise performance: catastrophe theory of muscular fatigue. In: Knuttgen HG, ed. *Biochemistry of Exercise*. Champaign, IL: Human Kinetics; 1983:3–28.
2. National Heart, Lung and Blood Institute Workshop summary. Respiratory muscle fatigue. Report of the Respiratory Muscle Fatigue Workshop Group. *Am Rev Respir Dis.* 1990;142(2):474–480.
3. Enoka RM, Duchateau J. Muscle fatigue: what, why and how it influences muscle function. *J Physiol.* 2008;586(1):11–23.
4. Allen DG, Lamb GD, Westerblad H. Skeletal muscle fatigue: cellular mechanisms. *Physiol Rev.* 2008;88(1):287–332.
5. Fitts RH. Cellular mechanisms of muscle fatigue. *Physiol Rev.* 1994;74(1):49–94.
6. Fitts RH, Balog EM. Effect of intracellular and extracellular ion changes on E-C coupling and skeletal muscle fatigue. *Acta Physiol Scand.* 1996;156(3):169–181.
7. Allen DG, Lannergren J, Westerblad H. Muscle cell function during prolonged activity: cellular mechanisms of fatigue. *Exp Physiol.* 1995;80(4):497–527.
8. Bigland-Ritchie B. Muscle fatigue and the influence of changing neural drive. *Clin Chest Med.* 1984;5(1):21–34.
9. Enoka RM, Stuart DG. Neurobiology of muscle fatigue. *J Appl Physiol.* 1992;72(5):1631–1648.
10. Gandevia SC. Spinal and supraspinal factors in human muscle fatigue. *Physiol Rev.* 2001;81(4):1725–1789.
11. Allen DG, Kabbara AA, Westerblad H. Muscle fatigue: the role of intracellular calcium stores. *Can J Appl Physiol.* 2002;27(1):83–96.
12. Allen DG, Lee JA, Westerblad H. Intracellular calcium and tension during fatigue in isolated single muscle fibres from Xenopus laevis. *J Physiol.* 1989;415:433–458.
13. Allen DG, Westerblad H. Role of phosphate and calcium stores in muscle fatigue. *J Physiol.* 2001;536(pt 3):657–665.
14. Coyle EF. Carbohydrate metabolism and fatigue. In: Atlan G, Beliveau L, Bouissou P, eds. *Muscle Fatigue: Biochemical and Physiological Aspects*. Paris: Masson; 1991:153–164.
15. Gollnick PD, Korge P, Karpakka J, et al. Elongation of skeletal muscle relaxation during exercise is linked to reduced calcium uptake by the sarcoplasmic reticulum in man. *Acta Physiol Scand.* 1991;142(1):135–136.
16. Hermansen L, Osnes JB. Blood and muscle pH after maximal exercise in man. *J Appl Physiol.* 1972;32(3):304–308.
17. Karlsson J, Saltin B. Lactate, ATP, and CP in working muscles during exhaustive exercise in man. *J Appl Physiol.* 1970;29(5):596–602.
18. Edman KA, Mattiazzi AR. Effects of fatigue and altered pH on isometric force and velocity of shortening at zero load in frog muscle fibres. *J Muscle Res Cell Motil.* 1981;2(3):321–334.
19. Metzger JM, Moss RL. pH modulation of the kinetics of a Ca2(+)-sensitive cross-bridge state transition in mammalian single skeletal muscle fibres. *J Physiol.* 1990;428:751–764.
20. Geeves MA, Fedorov R, Manstein DJ. Molecular mechanism of actomyosin-based motility. *Cell Mol Life Sci.* 2005;62(13):1462–1477.
21. Hill AV. The heat of shortening and the dynamic constants of muscle. *Proceedings of the Royal Society of London Series B—Biological Sciences.* 1938;126(843):136–195.
22. Nyitrai M, Rossi R, Adamek N, et al. What limits the velocity of fast-skeletal muscle contraction in mammals? *J Mol Biol.* 2006;355(3):432–442.
23. Knuth ST, Dave H, Peters JR, et al. Low cell pH depresses peak power in rat skeletal muscle fibres at both 30 degrees C and 15 degrees C: implications for muscle fatigue. *J Physiol.* 2006;575(pt 3):887–899.
24. Jones DA, de Ruiter CJ, de Haan A. Change in contractile properties of human muscle in relationship to the loss of power and slowing of relaxation seen with fatigue. *J Physiol.* 2006;576(pt 3):913–922.
25. Round JM, Jones DA, Chapman SJ, et al. The anatomy and fibre type composition of the human adductor pollicis in relation to its contractile properties. *J Neurol Sci.* 1984;66(2–3):263–272.
26. Merton PA. Voluntary strength and fatigue. *J Physiol.* 1954;123(3):553–564.
27. Bigland-Ritchie BR, Dawson NJ, Johansson RS, et al. Reflex origin for the slowing of motoneurone firing rates in fatigue of human voluntary contractions. *J Physiol.* 1986;379:451–459.
28. Fitts RH. Mechanisms of muscular fatigue. In: Poortmans JR, ed. *Principles of Exercise Biochemistry*. Basel, Karger: Medicine Sport Science; 2004:279–300.
29. Allen DG, Lamb GD, Westerblad H. Impaired calcium release during fatigue. *J Appl Physiol.* 2008;104(1):296–305.
30. Macdonald WA, Stephenson DG. Effect of ADP on slow-twitch muscle fibres of the rat: implications for muscle fatigue. *J Physiol.* 2006;573(pt 1):187–198.
31. Lindinger MI, Sjogaard G. Potassium regulation during exercise and recovery. *Sports Med.* 1991;11(6):382–401.
32. McKenna MJ, Bangsbo J, Renaud JM. Muscle K+, Na+, and Cl disturbances and Na+-K+ pump inactivation: implications for fatigue. *J Appl Physiol.* 2008;104(1):288–295.
33. de Paoli FV, Overgaard K, Pedersen TH, et al. Additive protective effects of the addition of lactic acid and adrenaline on excitability and force in isolated rat skeletal muscle depressed by elevated extracellular K+. *J Physiol.* 2007;581(pt 2):829–839.
34. McKenna MJ, Medved I, Goodman CA, et al. N-acetylcysteine attenuates the decline in muscle Na+,K+-pump activity and delays fatigue during prolonged exercise in humans. *J Physiol.* 2006;576(pt 1):279–288.
35. Nielsen JJ, Mohr M, Klarskov C, et al. Effects of high-intensity intermittent training on potassium kinetics and performance in human skeletal muscle. *J Physiol.* 2004;554(pt 3):857–870.
36. Grabowski W, Lobsiger EA, Luttgau HC. The effect of repetitive stimulation at low frequencies upon the electrical and mechanical activity of single muscle fibres. *Pflugers Arch.* 1972;334(3):222–239.
37. Gyorke S. Effects of repeated tetanic stimulation on excitation-contraction coupling in cut muscle fibres of the frog. *J Physiol.* 1993;464:699–710.
38. Ríos E, Zhou J. Control of dual isoforms of Ca2 release channels in muscle. *Biol Res.* 2004;37(4):583–591.
39. Eberstein A, Sandow A. Fatigue mechanisms in muscle fibers. In: Gutmann E, Hnik P, eds. *The Effect of Use and Disuse on Neuromuscular Function*. Prague, Czech: Academic Science; 1963:515–526.
40. Westerblad H, Allen DG. Changes of myoplasmic calcium concentration during fatigue in single mouse muscle fibers. *J Gen Physiol.* 1991;98(3):615–635.
41. Fryer MW, Owen VJ, Lamb GD, et al. Effects of creatine phosphate and P(i) on Ca2+ movements and tension development in rat skinned skeletal muscle fibres. *J Physiol.* 1995;482(pt 1):123–140.
42. Dutka TL, Cole L, Lamb GD. Calcium phosphate precipitation in the sarcoplasmic reticulum reduces action potential-mediated Ca2+ release in mammalian skeletal muscle. *Am J Physiol Cell Physiol.* 2005;289(6):C1502–C1512.
43. Duke AM, Steele DS. Interdependent effects of inorganic phosphate and creatine phosphate on sarcoplasmic reticulum Ca2+ regulation in mechanically skinned rat skeletal muscle. *J Physiol.* 2001;531(pt 3):729–742.
44. Posterino GS, Lamb GD, Stephenson DG. Twitch and tetanic force responses and longitudinal propagation of action potentials in skinned skeletal muscle fibres of the rat. *J Physiol.* 2000;527 (pt 1):131–137.
45. Royer L, Pouvreau S, Rios E. Evolution and modulation of intracellular calcium release during long-lasting, depleting depolarization in mouse muscle. *J Physiol.* 2008;586(pt 19):4609–4629.
46. Blazev R, Lamb GD. Low [ATP] and elevated [Mg2+] reduce depolarization-induced Ca2+ release in rat skinned skeletal muscle fibres. *J Physiol.* 1999;520(pt 1):203–215.
47. Han JW, Thieleczek R, Varsanyi M, et al. Compartmentalized ATP synthesis in skeletal muscle triads. *Biochemistry.* 1992;31(2):377–384.

48. Westerblad H, Allen DG, Bruton JD, et al. Mechanisms underlying the reduction of isometric force in skeletal muscle fatigue. *Acta Physiol Scand.* 1998;162(3):253–260.

49. Holloszy JO, Coyle EF. Adaptations of skeletal muscle to endurance exercise and their metabolic consequences. *J Appl Physiol.* 1984;56(4):831–883.

50. Macdonald WA, Stephenson DG. Effects of ADP on sarcoplasmic reticulum function in mechanically skinned skeletal muscle fibres of the rat. *J Physiol.* 2001;532(pt 2):499–508.

51. Macdonald WA, Stephenson DG. Effects of ADP on action potential-induced force responses in mechanically skinned rat fast-twitch fibres. *J Physiol.* 2004;559(2):433–447.

52. Bruton JD, Lannergren J, Westerblad H. Mechanisms underlying the slow recovery of force after fatigue: importance of intracellular calcium. *Acta Physiol Scand.* 1998;162(3):285–293.

53. Westerblad H, Bruton JD, Allen DG, et al. Functional significance of Ca2+ in long-lasting fatigue of skeletal muscle. *Eur J Appl Physiol.* 2000;83(2–3):166–174.

54. Balog EM. Excitation-contraction coupling and minor triadic proteins in low-frequency fatigue. *Exerc Sport Sci Rev.* 2010;38(3):135–142.

55. Ferreira LF, Reid MB. Muscle-derived ROS and thiol regulation in muscle fatigue. *J Appl Physiol.* 2008;104(3):853–860.

56. Andrade FH, Reid MB, Allen DG, et al. Effect of hydrogen peroxide and dithiothreitol on contractile function of single skeletal muscle fibres from the mouse. *J Physiol.* 1998;509(pt 2):565–575.

57. Moopanar TR, Allen DG. Reactive oxygen species reduce myofibrillar Ca2+ sensitivity in fatiguing mouse skeletal muscle at 37 degrees C. *J Physiol.* 2005;564(pt 1):189–199.

58. Nosek TM, Fender KY, Godt RE. It is diprotonated inorganic phosphate that depresses force in skinned skeletal muscle fibers. *Science.* 1987;236(4798):191–193.

59. Fitts RH. The cross-bridge cycle and skeletal muscle fatigue. *J Appl Physiol.* 2008;104(2):551–558.

60. Debold EP, Romatowski J, Fitts RH. The depressive effect of Pi on the force-pCa relationship in skinned single muscle fibers is temperature dependent. *Am J Physiol Cell Physiol.* 2006;290(4):C1041–C1050.

61. Cairns SP. Lactic acid and exercise performance: culprit or friend? *Sports Med.* 2006;36(4):279–291.

62. Karatzaferi C, Franks-Skiba K, Cooke R. Inhibition of shortening velocity of skinned skeletal muscle fibers in conditions that mimic fatigue. *Am J Physiol Regul Integr Comp Physiol.* 2008;294(3):R955.

63. Sahlin K, Katz A, Broberg S. Tricarboxylic acid cycle intermediates in human muscle during prolonged exercise. *Am J Physiol.* 1990;259(5 pt 1):C834–C841.

64. Wagenmakers AJ, Beckers EJ, Brouns F, et al. Carbohydrate supplementation, glycogen depletion, and amino acid metabolism during exercise. *Am J Physiol.* 1991;260(6 pt 1):E883–E890.

65. Brass EP, Scarrow AM, Ruff LJ, et al. Carnitine delays rat skeletal muscle fatigue in vitro. *J Appl Physiol.* 1993;75(4):1595–1600.

66. Tupling R, Green H, Grant S, et al. Postcontractile force depression in humans is associated with an impairment in SR Ca(2+) pump function. *Am J Physiol Regul Integr Comp Physiol.* 2000;278(1):R87–R94.

67. Fitts RH, Courtright JB, Kim DH, et al. Muscle fatigue with prolonged exercise: contractile and biochemical alterations. *Am J Physiol.* 1982;242(1):C65–C73.

68. Tonkonogi M, Harris B, Sahlin K. Mitochondrial oxidative function in human saponin-skinned muscle fibres: effects of prolonged exercise. *J Physiol.* 1998;510(pt 1):279–286.

69. Lannergren J, Westerblad H. Force decline due to fatigue and intracellular acidification in isolated fibres from mouse skeletal muscle. *J Physiol.* 1991;434:307–322.

70. Thompson LV, Balog EM, Riley DA, et al. Muscle fatigue in frog semitendinosus: alterations in contractile function. *Am J Physiol.* 1992;262(6 pt 1):C1500–C1506.

71. Metzger JM, Fitts RH. Fatigue from high- and low-frequency muscle stimulation: role of sarcolemma action potentials. *Exp Neurol.* 1986;93(2):320–333.

The Autonomic Nervous System

Douglas R. Seals

Abbreviations

ANS	Autonomic nervous system	NPY	Neuropeptide Y
CNS	Central nervous system	PE	Plasma epinephrine
EMG	electromyographic	PNE	Plasma norepinephrine
GABA	Gamma-amino butyric acid	R-R interval	Period between successive R waves of the electrocardiogram, period between heart beats, inverse of HR
HRV	Heart rate variability		
MSNA	Muscle sympathetic nerve activity		
NE	norepinephrine	SNS	Sympathetic nervous system

Introduction

The primary goal of this chapter is to describe the changes in autonomic nervous system (ANS) activity that produce the physiologic adjustments necessary to maintain homeostasis in response to conventional forms of acute large-muscle dynamic exercise and the peripheral and central nervous system (CNS) mechanisms that mediate those changes in ANS activity. A secondary aim is to describe the influence of chronically performed exercise on the changes in ANS activity evoked during acute submaximal exercise and the CNS mechanisms involved. The possible effects of habitual exercise on ANS activity and ANS-mediated physiologic function under resting conditions also will be considered. To achieve these objectives, the chapter is divided into four sections:

- A description of the methods needed to understand the data on exercise and the ANS
- A discussion of the ANS adjustments to acute exercise
- A discussion of the ANS adaptations to chronic exercise
- An overall summary

Through its efferent parasympathetic and sympathetic nervous system (SNS) arms, the ANS is an important tool that the CNS uses to maintain organismic homeostasis at rest and during challenges imposed by acute changes in physiologic state, such as physical exercise. This homeostatic regulatory control is achieved primarily through cardiovascular, metabolic, and thermoregulatory adjustments produced by specific changes in the activity of the vagus nerves to the heart and the sympathetic nerves to the heart, other internal organs, and arterial blood vessels. The physiologic effects of the ANS depend on both (a) the change in the activities of the autonomic nerves and their release of neurotransmitters and (b) the responsiveness of the peripheral tissues to these neurochemical stimuli (1). The importance of the ANS in mediating the physiologic adjustments to exercise has been established by experiments in which the ANS has been eliminated by pharmacologic blockade of peripheral adrenergic receptors or by surgical ablation of ANS structures (2–4).

Cardiovascular Effects

The influence of the ANS on cardiovascular and thermoregulatory control during exercise is reviewed in detail elsewhere (1,5,6). Decreases in cardiac vagal nerve activity to the sinoatrial node and ventricular muscle of the heart during exercise reduce the tonic suppressive influence of the vagus nerve on heart rate and ventricular contractility, respectively. Complementary activation of sympathetic nerves to these cardiac tissues, along with SNS stimulation of epinephrine release from the adrenal medulla, further increases heart rate and ventricular contractility during exercise, primarily via stimulation of the β-adrenergic receptor signaling pathway (there is a modest α-adrenergic contribution to left ventricular contractility). Together, these changes in ANS activity serve to increase heart rate, left ventricular stroke volume, and cardiac output. The latter, in turn, plays a critical role in supporting systemic arterial blood pressure (and therefore vital organ perfusion); augmenting blood flow to the heart, respiratory muscles, and active locomotor muscles to help meet their increased metabolic (oxygen and energy substrate) demands; and increasing blood flow to the cutaneous circulation for heat dissipation. Activation of sympathetic nerves to arterial resistance vessels (arterioles) in response to exercise produces region-specific vasoconstriction via stimulation of α-adrenergic receptor signaling, thus mediating the redistribution of the increased cardiac output away from tissues in which metabolic rate is not elevated (*e.g.*, gut, liver, kidneys) while contributing to the augmentation of active muscle blood flow. This vasoconstriction also serves to maintain both cardiac output (by supporting, along with the active muscle pump, cardiac filling pressure) and systemic vascular resistance (conductance), thus supporting systemic arterial perfusion pressure in the face of marked vasodilation in active muscle.

Metabolic Effects

As reviewed in detail previously (1,5,7), activation of the sympathoadrenal system has physiologically significant effects on metabolism during exercise. These effects are mediated both by the direct influences of SNS activity and circulating epinephrine on target tissues in the periphery and by the indirect effects of the SNS (*e.g.*, inhibition of insulin release, stimulation of glucagon release) on those tissues. The influence of the sympathoadrenal system on metabolism during exercise includes the following:

- Stimulation of β-adrenergic–mediated lipolysis in adipose tissue with a consequent increase in circulating free fatty acid concentrations
- Stimulation of hepatic glycogenolysis via activation of glycogen phosphorylase and hepatic gluconeogenesis via activation of phosphoenolpyruvate carboxykinase (in combination with glucagon release from the pancreas)
- Modulation of substrate metabolism in active skeletal muscle (β-adrenergic–stimulated glucose uptake and utilization and glycogenolysis; fat and protein utilization) and, as a consequence, lactate release from muscle
- Potential role for α-adrenergic modulation of lipolysis and hepatic gluconeogenesis

Maximal Aerobic Capacity and Exercise Performance

The importance of the ANS in determining maximal aerobic exercise capacity and the ability to perform

submaximal exercise has been studied in both experimental animals and human subjects. Surgical ablation of ANS structures and pharmacologic blockade of autonomic receptors have been used to study these issues in human subjects (discussed later) and/or experimental animals. The key findings on this topic have been reviewed in detail previously by Tipton (8). In dogs, surgical disruption of the cardiac vagus nerve and sympathetic nerves are associated with reductions in work performance (8). Similarly, Robinson (9) reported in 1953 that pharmacologic blockade of the effects of the cardiac vagus nerve reduces maximal oxygen consumption (by about 10% on average) and exercise performance in humans, although a subsequent systematic investigation reported no effects of this procedure on oxygen consumption or exercise work time (10). Pharmacologic blockade of the sympathetic β-adrenergic system in untrained young adults causes marked reductions in heart rate, but only ~5% to 15% reductions in maximal oxygen consumption as a result of compensatory adjustments in other mechanisms (2,11). Submaximal and maximal dynamic exercise performance appear to be reduced by 10% to 50% during β-adrenergic receptor blockade (8). In endurance exercise–trained runners, the reductions in maximal oxygen consumption during exercise with β-adrenergic receptor blockade are greater than those observed in untrained subjects under the same conditions (12). These impaired exercise responses upon removal of the sympathetic β-adrenergic system are associated with reductions in cardiac output and leg blood flow, although metabolic changes resulting in enhanced muscle fatigue also may be involved (8). Thus, a substantial body of experimental evidence supports a critical role for the sympathetic β-adrenergic system and, to a lesser extent, the cardiac vagus nerve in determining maximal aerobic capacity and the ability to perform both submaximal and maximal dynamic exercise.

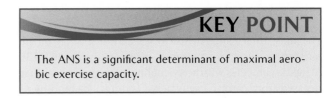

KEY POINT

The ANS is a significant determinant of maximal aerobic exercise capacity.

Exercise Training

These collective ANS adjustments to acute physical activity can be modified after a period of regular performance of exercise. Such adaptations are most clearly expressed during performance of the same absolute submaximal workload of large-muscle dynamic exercise after aerobic endurance training. Tonic (resting) ANS activity and/or the physiologic response to a given level of ANS activity during exercise also may be influenced by habitually performed exercise.

Summary

The ANS plays an essential role in producing physiologic adjustments to acute exercise that serve to maintain homeostasis while allowing optimal performance of submaximal and maximal physical activity. Habitual exercise results in changes in ANS activity during performance of standardized submaximal exercise and at rest that contribute to the physiologic adaptations to exercise training.

TEST YOURSELF

Which of the physiologic functions that are influenced by the ANS are related to your personal research interests? Will you need to consider these effects in your study?

Measurement of Autonomic Nervous System Activity

To properly interpret the experimental evidence upon which our understanding of ANS physiology during exercise is based, we begin with a brief discussion of the methods for assessing ANS activity, particularly in human subjects. These measurements of cardiac vagal and SNS–adrenal medullary activity have been performed during both actual exercise and simulated exercise (*e.g.*, electrical stimulation of motor areas in the brain, peripheral muscle contraction, and intent to perform exercise during muscle paralysis).

Assessment of Cardiac Vagal Activity

Cardiac vagus nerve (vagal) influences on the heart at rest and during exercise have been studied using two main experimental approaches.

Muscarinic receptor antagonists

The most direct approach involves administration of the muscarinic receptor antagonist atropine sulfate (4,9,13). Atropine competes with acetylcholine, the neurotransmitter released from cardiac vagus nerve endings, for binding to postjunctional muscarinic receptors in the heart, including the sinoatrial node and ventricular muscle. When atropine is administered prior to the beginning of exercise, baseline heart rate is increased as a result of removal of the tonic suppressive effect imposed by the cardiac vagus nerve. Any direct or indirect (*e.g.*, heart rate–related) anti-inotropic (*i.e.*, reduced forcefulness of contraction) effect of vagal activity on the left ventricle also is removed, but this is difficult to demonstrate under normal (intact) in vivo conditions, likely because the consequent reduced filling period (due to the increase in heart rate) decreases preload (*i.e.*, decreased Frank Starling effect) and negates any augmentation of

intrinsic contractility. The increase in baseline heart rate with administration of atropine therefore represents the tonic influence of the cardiac vagus nerve on cardiac chronotropic (frequency of contraction related) function. Thus, any increases in heart rate observed during subsequent exercise can be reasonably interpreted as being mediated by nonvagal ANS (*i.e.*, sympathoadrenal system) mechanisms. A less commonly used variation of this approach involves giving atropine during, rather than before, exercise (14,15). Under these conditions, the increase in heart rate upon acute administration of atropine would be interpreted as reflecting the influence of the cardiac vagus at that specific intensity and/or duration of exercise. The strength of this overall experimental approach involving the use of atropine is the ability to directly block the actions of the vagus nerve in mediating cardiac function, especially the control of heart rate. Limitations include:

- The side effects of atropine, which particularly in humans, necessitate doses that produce incomplete blockade of muscarinic receptors.
- Changes in baseline heart rate produced by administration of atropine that can make the interpretation of heart rate responses to exercise more difficult.
- The risks to human subjects of inducing cardiac events as a result of the changes in sympathovagal balance, especially in patients with existing disease or other high-risk groups (*e.g.*, elderly subjects).
- Potential problems with interpretation of results based on the fact that at low doses atropine possesses "vagomimetic" properties, whereas at higher doses its actions are "vagolytic."

Heart rate variability

A second approach for assessing the influence of the cardiac vagus nerve on the modulation of heart rate is to measure heart rate variability (HRV)—that is, the beat-to-beat variation in the length of cardiac cycles (14,16,17). This can be done using either time (usually expressed as the absolute length and standard deviation of the R-R intervals) or frequency (power spectral analysis of R-R interval frequency content) domain analyses. In general, the interpretation is that the greater the HRV, the greater the modulatory influence of the cardiac vagus nerve on heart rate. Greater HRV would be reflected either by an increased standard deviation of R-R intervals or an increased power at the respiratory frequency (high-frequency power of the R-R intervals, 0.15–0.50 Hz). The primary advantage of the HRV approach is its noninvasive nature, making it attractive to use in high-risk subject groups and/or under laboratory conditions in which the clinical support required to safely oversee the administration of cardiovascular drugs such as atropine is not available. The primary disadvantage of these measures is their indirect nature; that is, that nonvagal influences could affect the values obtained, especially during exercise with its concomitant changes in hemodynamic function and breathing, both of which can affect HRV (18). Measurement errors, superimposed motion, interpretation of heart rate compared with R-R interval–based expressions of the data, physiologic artifacts, and the dependence of some methods on steady-state exercise conditions (*i.e.*, questionable use during transitions and/or high heart rates) represent additional limitations of using HRV approach during exercise.

Assessment of Sympathoadrenal Activity

Initially, indirect approaches based on changes in cardiovascular function from resting conditions in response to exercise were used to estimate the activation of the sympathoadrenal during exercise. These included increases in heart rate, arterial blood pressure, and regional vascular resistance (inactive limbs and internal organs). Although the latter continues to be a useful marker of exercise-evoked increases in SNS vasoconstrictor activity to resistance vessels, a general limitation of all such methods is the fact that these and other cardiovascular functions are or can be, under certain conditions, influenced by mechanisms independent of the SNS.

Plasma norepinephrine concentrations

With the development of sensitive radioenzymatic assays in the 1970s and later high-performance liquid chromatography it became possible to estimate SNS activation during exercise from measurements of plasma norepinephrine (PNE) concentrations (1,5). Norepinephrine is the primary neurotransmitter released from postganglionic SNS neurons in response to sympathetic nerve discharge. Thus, increases in PNE from baseline resting conditions have been used to assess the activation of the SNS in response to various types, intensities, and durations of acute exercise (1,5). In general, this approach appears to yield accurate estimates of SNS activity, particularly during moderate to maximal intensities of large-muscle dynamic exercise that produce marked increases in PNE. However, PNE is the product of a complex process that involves norepinephrine (NE) release from postganglionic sympathetic nerve terminals in response to sympathetic nerve discharge (including prejunctional modulation of that release), NE uptake back into those nerve terminals (80%–90% of total release), extraneuronal metabolism of NE, diffusion of the remaining NE into the plasma compartment, and clearance of NE from the systemic circulation (19,20). As such, inaccuracies can occur in comparisons of individuals or groups that differ in any step in this process. Moreover, about 50% of the PNE obtained from antecubital vein blood samples (the most common sampling site) is derived from the NE released by the sympathetic nerves in the arm and, therefore, may not accurately reflect average systemic (whole body) SNS activity (19). Nevertheless, most of the available experimental data providing insight into the activation of the SNS during exercise is based on PNE.

Plasma norepinephrine spillover

A more accurate method of assessing SNS activity using circulating concentrations of NE involves determination of rates of NE spillover (appearance) into the plasma compartment (19,20). These values are obtained from measurements of arterial and venous PNE, extraction of NE by the tissues (using tritiated NE), and plasma flow and they are independent of any effects on NE clearance. NE spillover can be determined from measurements obtained from the systemic circulation (*i.e.*, whole body or total NE spillover) or from specific regional circulations (heart, kidneys, liver, gut, limbs). The limitations of this approach include the following:

- Invasiveness of the blood sampling required, typically requiring both arterial and venous catheters (although blood from arterialized hand veins also has been used); moreover, for regional NE spillover measurements, the venous catheter must be in a vein draining the organ or tissue of interest
- Costs of tritiated NE
- Need to measure regional or systemic plasma flow

In some regional circulations, simple arteriovenous differences in PNE have been used to estimate SNS activity (19,20); however, such measures do not take into account the influence of NE uptake into tissues, which could theoretically confound the results obtained. In experimental animals, regional SNS activity also has been assessed with measurements of NE turnover using isotope labeling and extraction and analysis of specific tissues or organs (21).

Neuropeptide Y

Neuropeptide Y (NPY) is a cotransmitter stored in sympathetic nerve endings that is released only during high frequencies of sympathetic nerve discharge. It has a much longer half-life and is believed to produce stronger and more sustained vasoconstriction than NE (22). Thus, increases in plasma concentrations and/or spillover of NPY would be interpreted as reflecting high levels of SNS activation during exercise (23,24).

Neural recording of sympathetic nervous system activity

The only direct method of assessing peripheral SNS activity during exercise is through recordings of the discharge rates of postganglionic sympathetic nerves. In humans, the technique of positioning the tip of a microelectrode in a peripheral nerve has been used to record SNS activity to skeletal muscle arterioles or the skin in primarily inactive limbs during exercise (25), whereas recordings of SNS activity have been obtained from internal organs in experimental animals. The key advantage of this overall approach is that it yields direct intraneural recordings of actual SNS activity rather than estimating SNS activity from neurochemical plasma markers or cardiovascular functions that are influenced by SNS activity. These recordings of peripheral SNS activity are believed to reflect SNS outflow from the CNS. Disadvantages of human subject microneurography include the following:

- Inability to assess SNS activity to internal organs
- Difficulty in maintaining neural recordings, even from inactive limbs, during conventional forms of

large-muscle dynamic exercise because of excessive body movement, which tends to dislodge the electrode from its recording site

- Expense associated with the hardware and software necessary for data acquisition and analysis
- Substantial investigator training, experience, and skill required to obtain interpretable recordings on a consistent basis
- Invasiveness of the procedure, which causes temporary local side effects in a small percentage of subjects

Whole nerve recordings of SNS activity from internal organs in experimental animals require highly invasive surgery to isolate and position the recording electrode on the internal organ nerve in question, postsurgical care and recovery of the animal, and considerable investment in equipment and investigator skill.

Low-frequency power of heart rate variability

Measurements of the low-frequency power of HRV also have been used to assess cardiac sympathetic modulation of heart rate (as well as overall cardiac SNS tone) (20). However, although noninvasive and convenient, there is considerable controversy as to the validity of these measurements as reflecting cardiac sympathetic modulation of heart rate (20). As such, the use of low-frequency power of HRV for this purpose has not received widespread support from informed investigators in the field.

Plasma concentrations and secretion of epinephrine

Release of epinephrine from the adrenal medulla has most commonly been assessed by measurement of plasma epinephrine (PE) concentrations via radioenzymatic assay or high-performance liquid chromatography (19,26). The strength of this approach is that PE accurately reflects the circulating concentrations of this hormone available to bind to β-adrenergic receptors in the systemic circulation both under resting baseline conditions and during exercise. Thus, if the circulating concentrations of epinephrine are most important for providing insight into the research question being addressed, measurement of PE is appropriate. However, the same limitation associated with interpretation of PNE applies to these measurements. That is, PE reflects the balance between the respective rates at which epinephrine is released from the adrenal medulla and the clearance of epinephrine from the plasma compartment (19,26). Therefore, accurate determinations of actual epinephrine release from the adrenal medulla during exercise cannot be made from PE. This is the case particularly when individuals or groups in a study sample differ in PE clearance. Rather, precise assessment of epinephrine secretion from the adrenal medulla at rest and during exercise requires measurement of total PE kinetics using tritiated epinephrine (26).

Adrenergic receptor antagonists

As is the case with the use of atropine to block cardiac vagal influences, various drugs can be used to block the peripheral effects of sympathoadrenal system activation during exercise, most commonly β- and α-adrenergic receptor antagonists (*e.g.*, propranolol, phentolamine) (8,20). As with atropine, these drugs can be administered either before (most common) or during exercise to assess the involvement of the sympathoadrenal system in mediating the physiologic responses observed. That is, any differences in the cardiovascular or other physiologic adjustments to exercise in the presence compared with the absence of these receptor antagonist agents are interpreted as indicating the specific contribution of the sympathoadrenal stimulus (neuronally released NE, circulating NE and epinephrine) and peripheral adrenergic (β- and/or α-adrenergic receptor) signaling pathway in question. Again, the ability to block sympathoadrenal system activation of specific peripheral adrenergic signaling pathways is the primary advantage of this approach. The primary disadvantages include the following:

- Changes in baseline cardiovascular function produced by administration of these cardiac and/or vasoactive agents, which can make interpretation of resting-to-exercise changes in cardiovascular function challenging
- Side effects of the drugs
- Acute circulatory risks of these agents
- Clinical support requirements for administering the drugs to human subjects

Assessment of Overall Autonomic Nervous System Effects: Surgical Ablation of Parasympathetic (Vagal) and Sympathetic Nervous System Structures

This experimental approach has been reviewed previously by Tipton (8). A classic approach to determining the importance of specific anatomical structures, including the ANS, in producing specific physiologic functions involves surgical ablation (lesioning) of those structures. Using this approach, the physiologic adjustments to exercise are established in the intact (control) state and after removal of ANS structures of interest. Any difference in a physiologic response in the presence compared with the absence of the structure in question is interpreted as evidence that the structure is required for the normal expression of the response during exercise. The strength of this approach is the ability to remove the effect of a specific structure and directly determine the effect of its absence on a particular physiologic response to exercise. Two obvious limitations of this model are the facts that it only can be used in experimental animals (although naturally occurring human genetic- and disease-based research models of ANS lesions exist) and the inability to study the same animal under control (intact) and experimental (lesioned) conditions in a balanced order. Another limitation is the possibility that other structures compensate for the absence of the ablated structure (redundancy of control). In this scenario, the physiologic response to exercise in the experimental (ablation) condition is normal, and the conclusion might be made that the structure in question is not normally involved in the neural regulation of the response. However, the structure may indeed normally be involved in the control of the exercise response, but this contribution cannot be shown because of redundant control mechanisms. Therefore, the appropriate interpretation for this type of outcome of an experiment using this approach is that the structure in question "is not necessary" to produce the response during exercise—that is, that the response does not depend on that structure. In other words, if the response is abolished after elimination of the structure, the interpretation of the experiment is definitive. If the response remains intact in the absence of the structure, the interpretation is not definitive. This same limitation also applies to the use of adrenergic receptor antagonists described earlier.

Transgenic Animals

Finally, use of transgenic animals represents a relatively new experimental approach to altering elements of the ANS, such as adrenergic receptors (27), that play a role in physiologic function (see Chapter 27). ANS structures and/or elements of their signaling pathways can be eliminated (knock-out models) or, alternatively, overexpressed. In these models, genetically modified animals are compared with intact control (wild type) animals. Any differences in the responses to exercise would be attributed to the absence or overexpression of the ANS structure or pathway in question. The strength of such approaches is the ability to directionally modify a specific ANS influence. The primary limitation is the possibility that other systems may adapt to help compensate for the genetic modification, thus altering their normal contributions to physiologic control and masking the usual effect of the genetically altered influence.

Summary

A number of models, techniques, and measurements have been used to assess ANS changes with acute and chronic exercise.

KEY POINT

Understanding the strengths and weaknesses of these experimental approaches is critical for proper interpretation of the research literature in this area.

TEST YOURSELF

Which, if any, of these techniques are available and/or could be used at your institution to address research issues of interest?

ANS Changes during Acute Dynamic Exercise

Conventional Vagal Modulation of Heart Rate Exercise Using a Large Muscle

At the onset of dynamic exercise cardiac vagal modulation of heart rate is reduced, presumably reflecting a decrease in efferent cardiac vagus nerve activity. This concept is consistent with at least two lines of experimental evidence:

1. Cardiac vagal–related expressions of HRV decrease from rest with the initiation of exercise (14,17,28) (Fig. 7.1).
2. Administration of atropine prior to exercise eliminates the abrupt increase in heart rate observed with the initiation of exercise (4,29) (Fig. 7.2).

Together, this evidence indicates that reduced cardiac vagal modulation of heart rate (reduced efferent cardiac vagus nerve activity) is the key mechanism involved in mediating the tachycardia associated with the onset of exercise.

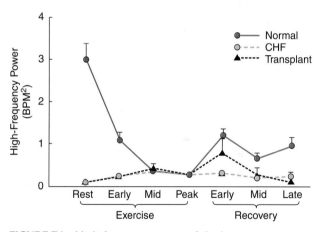

FIGURE 7.1   High-frequency power of the heart rate variability in groups of normal adult humans and patients with congestive heart failure (*left*) or heart transplantation (*right*) at rest prior to continuous incremental exercise; during the second to third minutes of the initial and lightest intensity of continuous incremental leg cycling exercise (early); during a workload about halfway from the lightest to the peak workload (mid); during the peak workload attained; and during early (minutes 1–2), middle (minutes 4–5), and late (minutes 8–9) postexercise recovery. Note in particular (a) the marked reduction in high-frequency power from rest to the initial few minutes of light exercise, reflecting a striking reduction in cardiac vagal modulation of heart rate evoked by the initiation of exercise, and (b) the further stepwise reductions in cardiac vagal modulation of heart rate with increasing exercise intensity and duration in the normal subjects. The patients lacked significant cardiac vagal modulation of heart rate at rest, during exercise, and during postexercise recovery. BPM, beats per minute; CHF, congestive heart failure. (Modified with permission from Arai Y, Saul JP, Albrecht P, et al. Modulation of cardiac autonomic activity during and immediately after exercise. *Am J Physiol.* 1989;256:H135.)

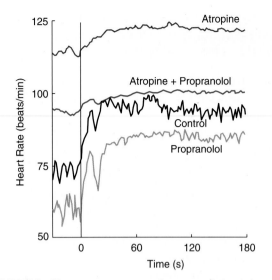

FIGURE 7.2 Heart rate responses from rest (left of the 0 time point) during the initial 3 minutes of light dynamic leg-cycling exercise (50 W) in healthy young men under control (no drug) conditions and after pretreatment with atropine alone (removes cardiac vagal influence), propranolol alone (removes β-adrenergic receptor signaling pathway), or combined atropine and propranolol. Blockade of the vagal influence with atropine caused a marked increase in heart rate at rest but significantly blunted the normal increase in heart rate at the onset of exercise, suggesting that vagal withdrawal mediates the tachycardia normally observed with the initiation of exercise. In contrast, propranolol lowered resting heart rate but did not influence the heart rate response to exercise, suggesting that increases in cardiac sympathetic nerve activity and β-adrenergic receptor signaling do not contribute to the tachycardia produced upon initiation of exercise. (Modified from Fagraeus L, Linnarsson D. Autonomic origin of heart rate fluctuations at the onset of muscular exercise. *J Appl Physiol.* 1976;40:680.)

Exercise intensity

Increasing exercise intensity is associated with a progressive, even exponential reduction in cardiac vagal modulation of heart rate, presumably reflecting a progressive reduction in cardiac vagal nerve activity. The experimental evidence supporting this conclusion includes the following:

1. Progressively greater reductions in cardiac vagal–related expressions of HRV increase with increasing intensities of exercise (14,28,30) (Figs. 7.1 and 7.3).
2. When compared with normal intact (control) conditions, after pretreatment with atropine, the increase in heart rate from rest in response to incremental exercise is either abolished or reduced during mild to moderate intensity workloads, but is progressively less affected with further increases in workload to maximum (4,9,29) (Figs. 7.4 and 7.5).

Reductions in cardiac vagal–related expressions of HRV from baseline (resting) levels have been observed experimentally at exercise intensities as low as about 20% of maximal

oxygen consumption (4,14,28). It is likely, however, that reductions in cardiac vagal modulation of heart rate occur at any exercise intensity that evokes an increase in heart rate above resting levels. Much of the reduction in cardiac vagal modulation of heart rate from resting levels appears to occur by intensities of exercise associated with increases in heart rate up to about 100 beats per minute (4,22,28). However, based on the following facts, it appears that at least some cardiac vagal modulation of heart rate is retained even during heavy submaximal intensities of dynamic exercise:

- Heart rate increases significantly during strenuous exercise after administration of atropine (9,14,15)
- Significant HRV remains during higher intensity exercise in dogs (14) (Fig. 7.3)

As emphasized by O'Leary and colleagues (15), the retention of at least some cardiac vagal modulation of heart rate during heavy submaximal exercise may be advantageous in that it would provide the ability to evoke a rapid arterial baroreflex–mediated increase in heart rate and cardiac output in the case of hypotension (the arterial baroreflex requires cardiac vagal withdrawal to produce rapid tachycardia). At maximal exercise intensities in humans there is no obvious remaining cardiac vagal modulation of heart rate based on these observations:

- Atropine administration has no effect on maximal heart rate (9) (Fig. 7.5).

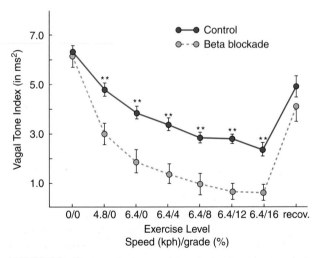

FIGURE 7.3 Changes in the vagal tone index based on analysis of heart rate variability from rest during incremental treadmill running in healthy mongrel dogs under control conditions and after pretreatment with propranolol, a nonspecific β-adrenergic receptor antagonist. Note, in particular, in the normal (control) condition (a) that progressive reduction in cardiac vagal tone index from rest during exercise of increasing intensity, suggesting an important role for cardiac vagal withdrawal in mediating the progressive tachycardia observed with increasing exercise intensity; and (b) that significant vagal tone remains during heavy submaximal exercise. (Modified from Billman GE, Dujardin JP. Dynamic changes in cardiac vagal tone as measured by time-series analysis. *Am J Physiol.* 1990;258:H898.)

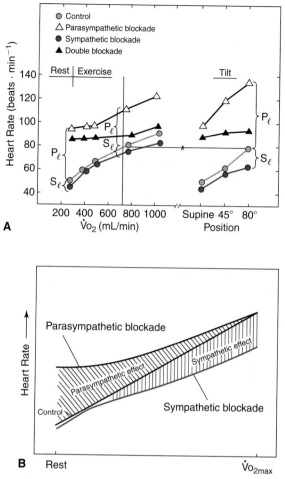

A

- Relatively little HRV exists during peak cycling exercise in healthy humans (28) (Fig. 7.1).

Prolonged submaximal exercise

There is little or no direct information on cardiac vagal modulation of heart rate during prolonged (>30 min) dynamic exercise performed at a fixed submaximal intensity. Based on the facts that (a) some reserve for cardiac vagal modulation of heart rate remains up to heavy submaximal intensities of exercise (9,14,15) and (b) heart rate continues to rise above early steady-state levels during prolonged submaximal exercise (6), one might reasonably predict that at least part of this progressive tachycardia with sustained exercise is mediated by further reductions in cardiac vagal modulation of heart rate. Recent observations showing progressively greater reductions in HRV during prolonged fixed intensity of submaximal running exercise in dogs support this postulate (31) (Fig. 7.6).

TEST YOURSELF

What changes in cardiac vagal modulation of heart rate are likely to occur during the types of exercise that you or someone you know typically perform?

B

FIGURE 7.4 A. Heart rate during dynamic leg-cycling exercise of increasing intensity in primarily healthy young men under control (no drug) conditions and after pretreatment with atropine alone (parasympathetic blockade—removes cardiac vagal influence), propranolol alone (sympathetic blockade—removes β-adrenergic receptor signaling pathway), or combined atropine and propranolol (double blockade) (*left side, top*). Blockade of the vagal influence with atropine caused a marked increase in heart rate at rest but significantly blunted the normal increase in heart rate with increasing exercise intensities, suggesting that vagal withdrawal mediates the tachycardia normally observed with light to moderate intensity exercise. In contrast, propranolol lowered resting heart rate slightly, did not influence the heart rate response to mild to moderate submaximal exercise (suggesting that increases in cardiac sympathetic nerve activity and/or circulating epinephrine and β-adrenergic receptor signaling do not contribute to the tachycardia occurring at these exercise intensities), but reduced heart rate at heavier submaximal exercise intensities, suggesting an important role for this mechanism in mediating the tachycardia under these conditions. **B.** The relative influences of cardiac vagal withdrawal (parasympathetic effect) and sympathetic β-adrenergic stimulation (sympathetic effect) in mediating the increases in heart rate observed during exercise of increasing intensity. (Modified with permission from Robinson BF, Epstein SE, Beiser GD, et al. Control of heart rate by the autonomic nervous system. Studies in man on the interrelation between baroreceptor mechanisms and exercise. *Circ Res.* 1966;19:400–411.)

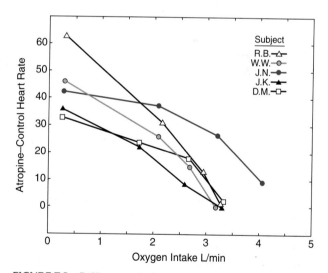

FIGURE 7.5 Differences in heart rate during treadmill running in five healthy men during cardiac vagal blockade (pretreatment with atropine) compared with control (intact cardiac vagal tone). Note (a) the differences in heart rate between vagal blockade and control become less with increasing exercise intensities, demonstrating progressive cardiac vagal withdrawal; and (b) in four of the five men, there was no observable vagal influence remaining at maximal exercise (*far right data points on individual lines*). (Modified from Robinson S, Pearcy M, Brueckman F, et al. Effects of atropine on heart rate and oxygen intake in working man. *J Appl Physiol.* 1953;5:510.)

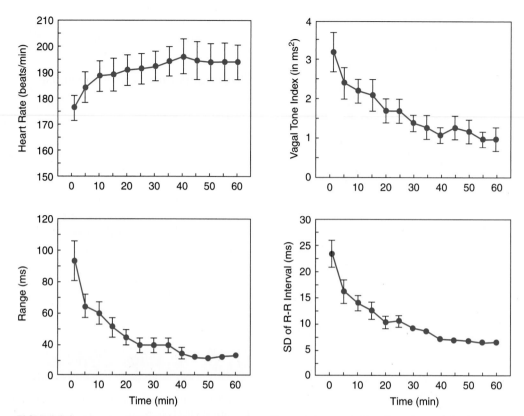

FIGURE 7.6 Heart rate and three measures of cardiac vagal tone during 60 minutes of sub-maximal treadmill running (6.4 kpm at a 10% grade) in 13 dogs. The upward drift in heart rate is associated with reductions in cardiac vagal tone during the initial 40 minutes of exercise, and both responses plateau over the last 20 minutes. These observations support the idea that cardiac vagal withdrawal plays an important role in mediating the heart rate drift during prolonged submaximal exercise. (From Kukielka M, Seals DR, Billman GE. Cardiac vagal modulation of heart rate during prolonged submaximal exercise in animals with healed myocardial infarctions: effects of training. *Am J Physiol Heart Circ Physiol.* 2006;290:H1680–H1685.)

Sympathoadrenal Response

Onset of exercise

The integrative response of the efferent SNS at the onset of conventional large-muscle dynamic exercise is unclear based on the available experimental evidence. Specifically, there is evidence for selective regional (tissue or organ specific), but not diffuse (systemic) SNS activation with the initiation of exercise. In experimental animals, renal (32,33) and cardiac (34) SNS activity increase at the onset of exercise. In human subjects, skin SNS activity, at least SNS sudomotor (sweat gland) activity, increases with the onset of isometric handgrip exercise in humans (35), but there are no direct (microneurographic) recordings of skin sympathetic nerve activity at the onset of conventional large-muscle dynamic exercise. In contrast, results of experiments employing direct recordings of SNS activity to inactive skeletal muscle demonstrate a reduction in SNS activity from baseline resting levels during preparation for and early during dynamic exercise (36,37) (Fig. 7.7).

In human subjects, SNS β-adrenergic blockade does not affect the increase in heart rate at the onset of upright leg-cycling exercise (29), indicating no physiologically relevant increase in cardiac sympathetic nerve activity (at least to the sinoatrial node), with the initiation of conventional dynamic exercise (Fig. 7.2). Due to technical limitations, it is unknown whether an SNS-mediated increase in epinephrine secretion from the adrenal medulla occurs at the onset of exercise. If so, this likely occurs only in response to heavy submaximal or maximal intensities of exercise and/or during sudden movement associated with a fight-or-flight response.

The lack of a consistent or uniform SNS response at the onset of exercise could be physiologic; that is, tissue-or organ-selective SNS activation may be evoked in order to meet specific needs aimed at preserving homeostasis. For example, increases in SNS outflow to the heart would stimulate heart rate and increase cardiac output, and renal SNS activation would produce vasoconstriction in the kidney, which would allow the increased cardiac output to be preferentially distributed to active muscle. Inhibition of SNS activity to muscle would acutely decrease vasoconstrictor tone, thus reducing opposition to locally mediated vasodilation in active muscle. On the other hand, the

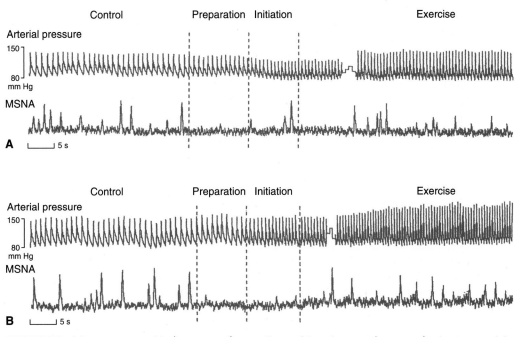

FIGURE 7.7 Microneurographic (intraneural) recordings of inactive muscle sympathetic nerve activity (MSNA) from the radial nerve in the arm during resting control, preparation for, and initiation of light (**A**) and moderate (**B**) intensity leg-cycling exercise in a healthy young subject. Note the marked inhibition of MSNA during preparation for and initiation of exercise compared with resting control. During the early (first minute) exercise period, MSNA remained suppressed during light intensity exercise, but it returned toward resting control levels at the higher exercise intensity. (Modified from Callister R, Ng AV, Seals DR. Arm sympathetic nerve activity during preparation for and initiation of leg-cycling exercise in humans. *J Appl Physiol.* 1994;77:1406.)

increase in cardiac SNS activity observed at the onset of treadmill exercise in conscious cats (34) is at odds with the fact that β-adrenergic blockade does not affect the heart rate response to the onset of large-muscle dynamic exercise in humans (29). The information needed to clarify these issues is not likely to be acquired in the foreseeable future because technical limitations restrict our ability to directly assess internal organ sympathetic (heart, kidney, gut) and adrenal medullary (epinephrine secretion) adjustments at the onset of large-muscle dynamic exercise in humans.

Exercise intensity

In general, in humans, SNS activation is initiated at exercise intensities ranging from about 25% to 50% of maximum work capacity (1,6,25); that is, at exercise intensities associated with heart rates above 100 beats per minute (6,22). The increase in SNS activity during these intensities of exercise appears to be widespread, including active and inactive skeletal muscle, the kidneys, the splanchnic region, the heart, the spleen, and the skin (6,19,38). Epinephrine secretion from the adrenal medulla is also increased during moderate to heavy exercise (typically 50% of maximal oxygen consumption or above) (21,26,39). Sympathoadrenal activation becomes progressively greater as exercise intensity increases from threshold

levels up to maximum. The overall evidence supporting sympathoadrenal system activation in response to moderate to heavy submaximal intensities of dynamic exercise includes the following:

- Progressively greater increases in PNE (*e.g.*, from 1.4 nmol/L at rest to 20 nmol/L at maximum) and PE (*e.g.*, from 0.25 nmol/L at rest to 2 nmol/L at maximum) with increasing exercise intensities up to maximum in humans (40–42) (Figs. 7.8 and 7.9)
- Increases in total (whole body) PNE (24,38,43) and PE (26) spillover rates from rest to exercise in humans that become greater with increasing exercise intensity (Fig. 7.10)
- Increases in directly recorded SNS activity to inactive skeletal muscle (muscle sympathetic nerve activity [MSNA]) from rest with increasing intensities of exercise in humans (36,44–47) (Fig. 7.11)
- Intensity-dependent increases in PNE arteriovenous difference and/or spillover to active and inactive skeletal muscle (46,48) (Fig. 7.12), the kidneys (24,38,49) (Fig. 7.9), the hepatomesenteric region (liver and gut) (49), and/or the heart (38,49) from rest to exercise in humans
- Intensity-dependent increases in renal SNS activity (32,33,48) and increases in liver NE spillover (50) with treadmill running in experimental animals,

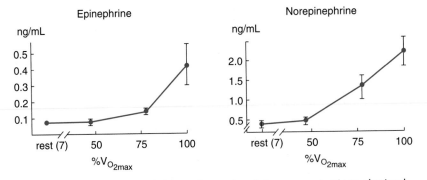

FIGURE 7.8 Plasma epinephrine and norepinephrine concentrations obtained from antecubital venous blood samples on healthy young adults at rest and during incremental treadmill running. Note the progressive increases in the concentrations of these catecholamines with increasing exercise intensity. (Modified from Galbo H. *Hormonal and Metabolic Adaptation to Exercise.* Stuttgart, New York: Thieme-Stratton; 1983:7. Based on data from Galbo H, Holst JJ, Christensen NJ. Glucagon and plasma catecholamine responses to graded and prolonged exercise in man. *J Appl Physiol.* 1975;38:70–76.)

and progressive inactive limb, renal, and splanchnic vasoconstriction and increases in plasma renin activity and angiotensin II concentrations from rest with increasing exercise intensities in humans and experimental animals (22,24) (Figs. 7.9 and 7.13)

- Increases in plasma concentrations of NPY from rest in response to heavy submaximal and maximal intensities of exercise in humans (23,24) (Fig. 7.9).

It is important to appreciate that the active limbs are a major target of the increase in SNS vasoconstrictor activity and a major source of the increase in PNE spillover during moderate and higher intensity dynamic exercise in humans (6,19,49) (Fig. 7.12). Indeed, Esler and associates (19) have estimated, based on measurements of total and regional PNE kinetics, that the skeletal muscle circulation accounts for about 60% of NE released from sympathetic nerve endings during submaximal large-muscle dynamic exercise. It is believed that this is an essential ANS adjustment to exercise because it counteracts locally mediated active muscle vasodilation (22,50). If unchecked by SNS-evoked vasoconstriction, the increases in active muscle and total vascular conductance would reduce arterial blood pressure (i.e., vital organ perfusion pressure for the brain and heart), threatening overall homeostasis.

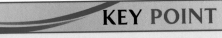

KEY POINT

Increased SNS activity to arterioles in active muscle is critical for proper cardiovascular regulation during exercise.

Prolonged submaximal exercise

Insight regarding the sympathoadrenal system adjustments to prolonged large-muscle dynamic exercise is largely limited to investigations assessing the changes in PNE and PE from rest during fixed moderate submaximal exercise (41,52,53). PNE increases progressively during sustained submaximal dynamic exercise (5,41,52,53) (Fig. 7.14), supporting the idea of increasing SNS activation during prolonged exercise. In healthy young adults, the rise in PNE above baseline control levels has been observed as early as 10 minutes after the onset of exercise and there is a clearly significant increase in PNE by 20 minutes (51). Continuous increases in PE also are observed during prolonged submaximal exercise (41,53), indicating time-dependent increases in epinephrine secretion from the adrenal medulla under these conditions (note that epinephrine release also can be triggered by hypoglycemia associated with prolonged large muscle dynamic exercise). Plasma concentrations of NPY appear to increase with exercise duration during moderate to heavy exercise intensities (23).

A limited amount of data from measurements of PNE kinetics and/or MSNA (inactive limbs) during submaximal exercise supports the observations on PNE. During sustained mild- or moderate-intensity cycling, the increase in PNE is either solely or primarily mediated by increases in total PNE spillover because total PNE clearance is either unchanged or only slightly reduced from levels at rest (Fig. 7.10). These findings indicate that changes in PNE during prolonged exercise reflect increases in SNS activity as estimated by changes in total PNE spillover. One target of the increase in overall SNS outflow during prolonged submaximal exercise appears to be nonactive skeletal muscle, as indicated by significant increases in arm MSNA during 30 minutes of light to moderate leg cycling exercise (53). Taken together, these findings support the idea of progressive, time-dependent sympathoadrenal system activation during prolonged submaximal exercise. The results also indicate that the greater the submaximal intensity, the greater the sympathoadrenal activation that occurs from early on to the end of the exercise period.

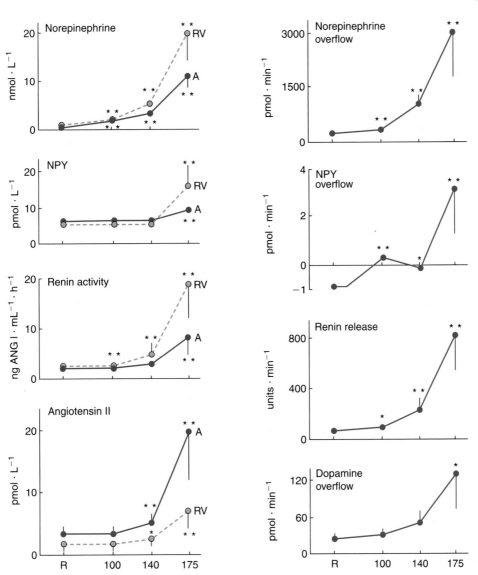

Heart Rate (beats/min)

FIGURE 7.9 *Left.* Arterial (A; *solid lines, closed symbols*) and renal vein (RV; *broken lines, open symbols*) plasma concentrations of norepinephrine, neuropeptide Y (NPY), renin activity, and angiotensin II. *Right.* Renal overflows of norepinephrine, NPY, renin, and dopamine, at rest (R) and during leg-cycling exercise at increasing levels of heart rate equivalent to 30%, 60%, and 80% to 90% of maximum workload in healthy young men. With increasing exercise intensity there are progressive increases in (a) total norepinephrine overflow, reflecting increasing net whole body sympathetic activation; (b) renal norepinephrine and dopamine overflow and renin release, reflecting increasing renal sympathetic nerve activation; and (c) increasing systemic and renal NPY overflow at the highest exercise intensity reflecting very high net whole body and renal sympathetic activation, respectively, during heavy sub-maximal to nearly maximal exercise intensities. (Reprinted with permission from Rowell LB, O'Leary DS, Kellogg DL. Integration of cardiovascular control systems in dynamic exercise. In: Rowell LB, Shepherd JT, eds. *Handbook of Physiology, Section 12: Exercise: Regulation and Integration of Multiple Systems.* New York: Oxford University; 1996:783. Based on data from Tidgren B, Hjemdahl P, Theodorsson E, et al. Renal neurohormonal and vascular responses to dynamic exercise in humans. *J Appl Physiol.* 1991;70:2279–2286.)

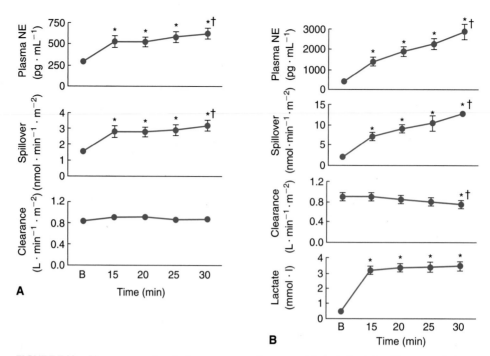

FIGURE 7.10 Plasma norepinephrine concentrations, total (whole body) spillover, and clearance in healthy young adults at rest and during 30 minutes of leg cycling performed at (**A**) a light (25% of maximum workload) and (**B**) a moderate (65% of maximum workload) exercise intensity. During light exercise, plasma norepinephrine concentrations are increased modestly (about 100% above rest) by 15 minutes of exercise mediated by an increase in norepinephrine spillover, reflecting an increase in net systemic sympathetic nervous system activation, which plateaus during the remainder of the exercise period. In contrast, moderate exercise results in a much more marked (about tenfold above rest) and progressive increase in sympathetic activation throughout the 30-minute exercise period. This progressive sympathetic activation is dissociated from the corresponding increase in plasma lactate concentration, a byproduct and marker of glycolytic metabolism. (Modified with permission from Leuenberger U, Sinoway L, Gubin S, et al. Effects of exercise intensity and duration on norepinephrine spillover and clearance in humans. *J Appl Physiol.* 1993;75:670–671.)

TEST YOURSELF

What is the likely sympathoadrenal system response to the types of exercise that you or someone you know typically perform, from weight lifting to endurance exercise?

Relation to plasma lactate response

There is a body of experimental evidence supporting the view that the increases in PNE and PE during incremental submaximal exercise are strongly related to the corresponding increases in plasma lactate concentrations (41,54). These findings suggest a physiologic connection between sympathoadrenal system activation and glycolytic metabolism during exercise. One explanation for this association is that sympathoadrenal activation, particularly increases in PE, stimulates β-adrenergic activation of phosphorylase, which, in turn, stimulates glycogenolysis in skeletal muscle and perhaps the kidneys, resulting in enhanced glycolytic flux and consequent formation of lactate (55). In contrast,

it has been noted that SNS activation occurs at exercise intensities associated with heart rates of about 100 beats per minute (*i.e.*, as low as 25%–40% of peak exercise capacity), whereas significant increases in plasma lactate concentrations typically are not observed until higher exercise intensities (*e.g.*, heart rates of about 140–150 beats per minute) (6,22,43) (Figs. 7.10 and 7.13). Moreover, during 30 minutes of moderate intensity leg cycling, both PNE and total PNE spillover increases progressively with time, whereas plasma lactate concentrations are increased above baseline early in exercise and remain at that level throughout exercise (43). These seemingly disparate observations may be explained by the fact that muscle lactate turnover increases even at mild exercise intensities, which is not immediately reflected by changes in plasma concentrations. Finally, there is evidence that lactate may actually suppress the catecholamine response to exercise, possibly via feedback inhibition (55).

Sympatholysis

The term *sympatholysis*, or functional sympatholysis, refers to the idea that the ability of the SNS to cause vasoconstriction

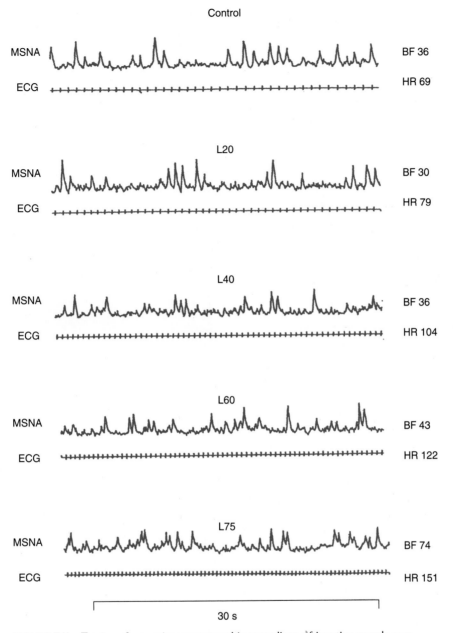

FIGURE 7.11 Tracings from microneurographic recordings of inactive muscle sympathetic nerve activity (MSNA) in the median nerve of the arm (*top to bottom*) during resting control conditions and increasing intensities of leg cycling exercise (20%–75% of maximum workload) in one subject. Compared with rest, MSNA is slightly reduced during light exercise, increasing progressively thereafter with increases in exercise intensity. BF, MSNA bursts frequency in bursts · min⁻¹. ECG, electrocardiogram; BF, burst frequency; HR, heart rate. (Modified from Saito M, Tsukanaka A, Yanagihara D, et al. Muscle sympathetic nerve responses to graded leg cycling. *J Appl Physiol.* 1993;75:664.)

of skeletal muscle arterioles is reduced in active muscle, either because of inhibition of NE release from sympathetic nerve endings or attenuation of the effects of NE release on postjunctional α-adrenergic receptors (22,50,57,58). The physiologic context in which this issue has received the most interest is during exercise when local changes in the production and accumulation of muscle metabolites (*e.g.*, potassium and hydrogen ions, hyperosmolarity) promote vasodilation in part by limiting SNS vasoconstriction of

arterioles in active muscle. As emphasized by Joyner and Thomas (57), this idea is attractive because it provides an additional regulatory mechanism by which the increase in cardiac output generated during exercise can be preferentially distributed to the active skeletal muscles and away from regions not requiring augmented flow in the face of widespread SNS activation. That is, functional sympatholysis would provide active muscle a powerful local mechanism for more precisely regulating blood flow to

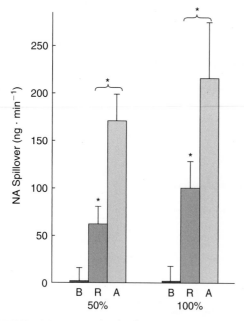

FIGURE 7.12 Noradrenaline (NA), or norepinephrine, spillover rates during one-legged knee extension exercise performed for 10 minutes at each of two intensities (50% and 100% of maximum workload) in healthy young men. Measurements were made under basal control conditions before exercise in the pooled (average of both) legs (B), in the resting leg during contralateral leg exercise (R), and in the active leg during exercise (A). NA spillover was progressively greater from rest to light-to-maximal intensities, reflecting incremental sympathetic activation to the legs across these conditions. Importantly, at both intensities sympathetic activation to the active (exercising) leg was much greater than that to the resting leg. (Modified from Savard G, Strange S, Kiens B, et al. Noradrenaline spillover during exercise in active versus resting skeletal muscle in man. *Acta Physiol Scand.* 1987;131:512.)

meet its metabolic demands. The potential disadvantage of such a mechanism would be the inability to produce sufficient SNS-mediated vasoconstriction in active muscle to limit the increase in systemic vascular conductance that can threaten arterial blood pressure and vital organ perfusion during whole body dynamic exercise (56,57). Under these conditions, the CNS must be able to produce effective SNS vasoconstriction in active muscle.

The concept of sympatholysis, which is discussed in depth elsewhere (22,51,57,58), has been controversial, with evidence that has been interpreted as both supporting and refuting the hypothesis. Although methodology issues affect the interpretation of data in this area (*e.g.*, the use of vascular conductance vs. vascular resistance) (22,58), it is well established that high local concentrations of vasodilatory metabolites, as produced during moderate to strenuous exercise of small muscle masses, can markedly reduce SNS-adrenergic vasoconstriction in active muscle (22). However, it is also clear that SNS-mediated vasoconstriction is not abolished in active muscle (*i.e.*, sympatholysis is not absolute) (22). Sympatholysis is most pronounced in the smaller, distal arterioles controlled

mainly by α_2-adrenergic receptors, which are highly susceptible to metabolic inhibition (22,50,57,58). In contrast, sympatholysis is less predominant in the larger proximal arterioles and feed arteries controlled mainly by α_1-adrenergic receptors. This differential expression of sympatholysis in the smaller and larger muscle arterioles results in a proximal shift in resistance from downstream to upstream vessels that optimizes blood flow distribution in the active muscles and maintains the ability to limit total systemic vascular conductance (57,58). As a consequence, SNS vasoconstriction is markedly reduced in the smaller arterioles in contracting muscle, whereas SNS vasoconstriction is largely preserved in the more proximal arterioles and feed arteries (57). This scheme provides an overall regulatory model by which functional sympatholysis can operate to ensure proper control of active muscle blood flow without threatening systemic cardiovascular homeostasis during large-muscle dynamic exercise (57).

TEST **YOURSELF**

Given the competing demands of active muscle blood flow, temperature regulation, and maintaining arterial blood pressure, would the physiologic influence of sympatholysis on active muscle blood flow differ at 5 versus 60 minutes of sustained endurance exercise performed under warm ambient conditions?

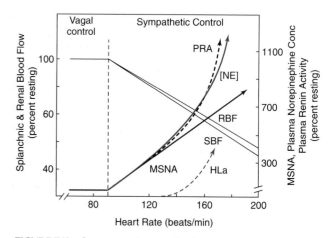

FIGURE 7.13 Summary of sympathetic responses to large-muscle dynamic exercise of increasing intensity. Diffuse sympathetic activation begins at moderate exercise intensities associated with heart rates above 100 beats per minute and increases exponentially up to maximal exercise intensities, as indicated by reductions in splanchnic (SBF) and renal (RBF) blood flow and corresponding increases in plasma renin activity (PRA), norepinephrine (NE), and muscle sympathetic nerve activity (MSNA). The increase in lactic acid (HLa) occurs at a higher intensity (associated with heart rates of 130–140 beats per minute) than sympathetic activation. (Modified from Rowell LB, O'Leary DS, Kellogg DL. Integration of cardiovascular control systems in dynamic exercise. In: Rowell LB, Shepherd JT, eds. *Handbook of Physiology, Section 12: Exercise: Regulation and Integration of Multiple Systems.* New York: Oxford University; 1996:782.)

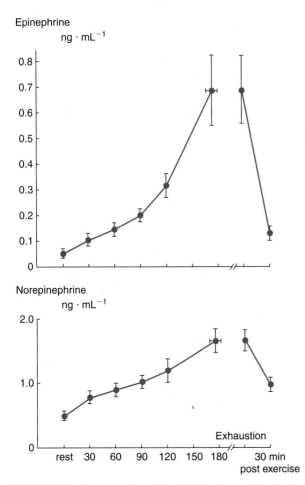

Epinephrine ng · mL^{-1}

Norepinephrine ng · mL^{-1}

Exhaustion

rest 30 60 90 120 150 180   30 min post exercise

FIGURE 7.14 Plasma epinephrine (*top*) and norepinephrine (*bottom*) concentrations at rest and during 3 hours of continuous treadmill running at an intensity associated with 60% of maximal oxygen consumption in healthy young adults. Note the progressive increases in the plasma concentrations of these catecholamines, reflecting progressively increasing sympathoadrenal system activation during prolonged moderate submaximal exercise. (Modified from Galbo H. *Hormonal and Metabolic Adaptation to Exercise*. Stuttgart, New York: Thieme-Stratton; 1983:7. Based on data from Galbo H, Holst JJ, Christensen NJ. Glucagon and plasma catecholamine responses to graded and prolonged exercise in man. *J Appl Physiol.* 1975;38:70–76.)

Modulatory Factors

Several factors or conditions can modify the ANS adjustments to acute exercise.

Absolute versus relative exercise intensities

Comparing individual subjects at the same absolute submaximal exercise intensity or level of maximal oxygen consumption results in marked variability among individuals in the ANS responses to exercise. This has been most thoroughly documented with regard to the plasma catecholamine responses to incremental exercise. In general, expressing these responses as a function of the percent of maximal oxygen consumption of the subject markedly reduces this variability (1,26,42), supporting the concept that the magnitude of the ANS adjustments to submaximal exercise is primarily determined by the relative (percent of maximum) rather than the absolute intensity (5,26,42). The absolute work rate or level of maximal oxygen consumption, however, does appear to contribute to the ANS response to exercise. One line of evidence supporting this idea is that during different types of dynamic exercise performed at the same percent of maximum, the increase in PNE is greater when the absolute workload or maximal oxygen consumption is greater (59). As such, it is likely that both the relative and the absolute workload determine the ANS response to submaximal dynamic exercise, with the former having the stronger influence.

Sex of individual

Plasma catecholamine responses to dynamic exercise may differ in men and women. PNE and PE may be higher in men than in women at various intensities of large-muscle dynamic exercise (60), including at the same relative workloads (60), although this is not a consistent finding (1). When observed, the greater PNE and PE in men may be explained by their higher maximal aerobic exercise capacity such that the same relative workload represents a much greater absolute exercise stimulus in men. Thus, women may undergo less sympathoadrenal system activation than men during large-muscle dynamic exercise performed at the same percent of maximal aerobic capacity.

Size of the active muscle mass

The sympathoadrenal response to dynamic exercise is influenced by the size of the active muscle mass. Specifically, the increases in PNE and PE are greater when the same absolute workload is performed by a smaller compared with a larger muscle mass (1,51,59). Thus, the greater amount of work performed and energy demand per unit of active muscle mass, the greater the activation of the sympathoadrenal system. Alternatively, when dynamic exercise is performed with different sized muscle masses (*e.g.*, one-arm vs. one-leg vs. two-leg cycling) at the same relative intensity (*i.e.*, the same percent of maximum for each respective mode of exercise), the magnitude of the increases in plasma catecholamine concentrations from rest to exercise are progressively greater with increasing size of the active muscle mass (59). Under these conditions, the larger muscle mass exercise is associated with a greater absolute workload and level of maximal oxygen consumption. The augmented SNS activation with the larger muscle mass exercise likely is necessary to produce vasoconstriction to counteract the greater active muscle vasodilation and consequent challenge to arterial blood pressure maintenance.

Ambient temperature and internal body temperature

ANS adjustments to dynamic exercise are influenced by both ambient and internal body temperature. With regard to the parasympathetic nervous system, HRV is lower during exercise performed in the heat than in thermoneutral control conditions (16). Indeed, there is an inverse relation between the high-frequency power of the HRV and rectal temperature during exercise (16). Thus, cardiac vagal modulation of heart rate is lower during exercise performed in warm ambient temperatures (with higher internal body temperature) than exercise under cool conditions. Both temperature extremes appear to influence the sympathoadrenal response to dynamic exercise in that the plasma catecholamine responses to exercise are augmented in temperature extremes compared to thermoneutral control conditions (5,16,61). The increased sympathoadrenal activation during exercise in warm conditions may be driven by the need to maintain arterial blood pressure in the face of marked cutaneous vasodilation produced for thermoregulatory needs. In particular, this requires a strong SNS-mediated vasoconstriction in the splanchnic and renal circulations (6,22). Increases in body temperature and the consequent cutaneous vasodilation and effects on arterial blood pressure also may act to stimulate SNS vasoconstrictor nerve activity during prolonged submaximal dynamic exercise performed in thermoneutral ambient conditions (52,54). The augmented sympathoadrenal activation during exercise performed in the cold likely is the result of an increase in baseline activity associated with the independent effects of cold. The increase in SNS activity during exercise in the cold is directed in part to the peripheral arterial blood vessels to maintain a high level of peripheral vasoconstriction to preserve internal body temperature by limiting access of the warm core blood to the cool body surface.

Body position and state of hydration

The increase in PNE is greater during dynamic exercise performed upright than supine (1,61,62). This augmented SNS response to exercise in the upright position likely is mediated, in part, by a greater baseline SNS activity as the result of reduced baroreflex inhibition of SNS outflow (baroreflex unloading). Greater SNS-mediated peripheral vasoconstriction is required to maintain arterial blood pressure in the upright body position (6). Body posture also modifies the SNS response to mild dynamic leg exercise (37), possibly via interactions with cardiopulmonary baroreceptors (discussed later). Exercise performed in the dehydrated state is also associated with an augmented PNE response over that of a hydrated state (1,5). This greater level of SNS activity likely is required to produce the elevated vasoconstrictor state necessary to maintain arterial blood pressure in the face of a reduced intravascular volume.

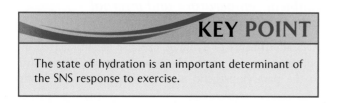

KEY POINT

The state of hydration is an important determinant of the SNS response to exercise.

Diet, plasma glucose, and caffeine ingestion

The ANS response to exercise also appears to be influenced by the composition of energy intake and circulating plasma glucose concentrations. For example, the increase in PE is greater when exercise is performed in a state of reduced circulating glucose (1,5). This augmented sympathoadrenal response to exercise with reduced availability of carbohydrate is likely mediated, in part, by the independent effects of hypoglycemia (1,5). Finally, caffeine ingestion appears to augment the PNE and/or PE responses to large-muscle dynamic exercise (63).

Hypoxia and hyperoxia

The ANS responses to exercise are modified by the level of inspired oxygen. Specifically, cardiac vagal modulation of heart rate is reduced and the increase in plasma catecholamine concentrations is augmented during exercise in low inspired oxygen (hypoxia or hypoxemia) conditions, and the reverse is true in hyperoxic states (6,64). See also Chapter 24 on hypoxia.

Small-Muscle Dynamic and Isometric Exercise

Dynamic exercise performed with a small muscle mass (*e.g.*, rhythmic handgrip exercise) or isometric exercise has been used frequently to study the regulation of ANS-mediated physiologic function during exercise (25,51,59). However, these types of exercise are not performed commonly in daily life. Therefore, only a brief description of the ANS adjustments is warranted here.

Many of the adjustments that occur during more conventional forms of dynamic exercise apply to small-muscle dynamic and isometric exercise. Cardiac vagal modulation of heart rate is reduced at the onset of these types of exercise and is responsible for the associated tachycardia (3,13,51). When these forms of exercise are sustained, eventually SNS activity and possibly PE will increase and stimulate heart rate via the β-adrenergic signaling pathway (3). Thus, as with more conventional forms of dynamic exercise, both withdrawal of cardiac vagal modulation and an increase in sympathoadrenal–β-adrenergic activation are responsible for the tachycardia associated with small-muscle dynamic and isometric exercise.

With regard to the sympathoadrenal system, in general, little or no activation is observed during mild (nonfatiguing) intensities and durations of small-muscle dynamic and isometric exercise or early on during contractions that eventually result in active muscle fatigue (1,25,26). However, total PNE spillover, cardiac NE spillover, nonactive limb MSNA (Fig. 7.15), skin sudomotor SNS activity, and epinephrine secretion from the adrenal medulla all are stimulated at intensities and durations associated with muscle fatigue (25,35,65), consistent with widespread sympathoadrenal system activation. During such sustained submaximal contractions, the increase in MSNA to the inactive limb parallels increases in active muscle electromyographic activity (66) (Fig. 7.16) and perceived

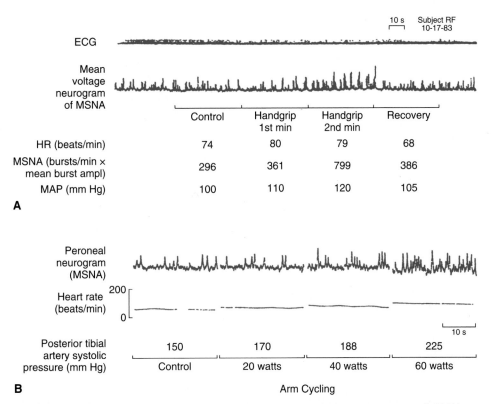

ECG

Mean voltage neurogram of MSNA

10 s Subject RF
10-17-83

	Control	Handgrip 1st min	Handgrip 2nd min	Recovery
HR (beats/min)	74	80	79	68
MSNA (bursts/min × mean burst ampl)	296	361	799	386
MAP (mm Hg)	100	110	120	105

A

Peroneal neurogram (MSNA)

Heart rate (beats/min)

200

0

10 s

Posterior tibial artery systolic pressure (mm Hg)	150	170	188	225
	Control	20 watts	40 watts	60 watts

B Arm Cycling

FIGURE 7.15 A. Peroneal neurogram of inactive leg muscle sympathetic nerve activity (MSNA) in a healthy young subject at rest (control), during 2 minutes of an isometric handgrip muscle contraction sustained at 30% of maximal voluntary contraction and during 2 minutes of relaxation (recovery) with corresponding mean values for heart rate (HR), MSNA, and mean arterial pressure (MAP). MSNA does not increase during the initial portion of the contraction period but becomes progressively stimulated during the second minute of the contraction. (Reprinted with permission from Mark AL, Victor RG, Nerhed C, et al. Neurographic studies of the mechanisms of sympathetic nerve responses to static exercise in humans. *Circ Res.* 1985;57:463. Subsequently published by Seals DR, Victor RG. Regulation of MSNA during exercise in humans. *Exerc Sport Sci Rev.* 1991;19:313–349.) **B.** Peroneal neurogram of inactive leg MSNA in a healthy young subject at rest (control) and during the final 30 s of two-arm cycling performed for 2 minutes each at 20, 40, and 60 watts (about 20%, 35%, and 50% of maximum workload). MSNA does not increase above control levels during light intensity submaximal arm cycling but increases progressively during the two higher submaximal workloads. (From Victor RG, Seals DR, Mark AL. Differential control of heart rate and sympathetic nerve activity during dynamic exercise: insight from direct intraneural recordings in humans. *J Clin Invest.* 1987;79:508–516. Modified with permission from Seals DR, Victor RG. Regulation of muscle sympathetic nerve activity during exercise in humans. *Exerc Sport Sci Rev.* 1991;19:319.)

sensations of fatigue (67), indicating a physiologic coupling between SNS activation and muscle fatigue (see Chapter 6). Renal SNS activity appears to increase immediately before or at the onset of brief voluntary isometric contractions in conscious cats (68). The increases in PNE, PE, and the spillover rates of the major catecholamines are relatively small compared with those produced by conventional whole body dynamic exercise (1,51,59), likely due to the absence of extensive active muscle vasodilation and, therefore, lack of need to counteract that vasodilation in exercises that involve a small muscle mass (22,51). Generally, the greater the active muscle mass involved in isometric contractions, the greater the magnitude of the increase in SNS activity produced (25).

These ANS adjustments to small-muscle dynamic and isometric exercise are critical for mediating the well-

established cardiovascular responses to these types of exercise, including increases in heart rate, cardiac output, and a marked elevation in arterial blood pressure. Indeed, these cardiovascular responses are eliminated when the sympathoadrenal–adrenergic signaling pathways are blocked by adrenergic receptor antagonists (3,13).

TEST YOURSELF

Which of these modulatory factors are influencing the SNS responses to the types of exercise that you typically perform? When you are performing a particular type of exercise with a friend of the opposite sex, how do your SNS responses likely differ?

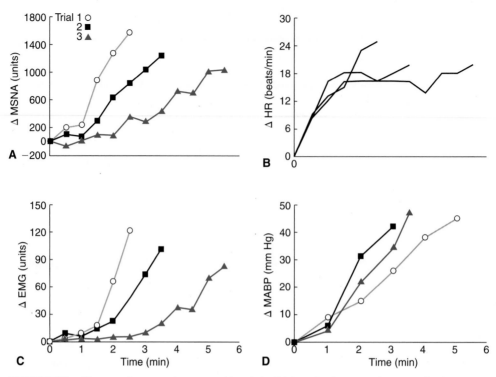

FIGURE 7.16   Changes from resting control levels in (**A**) inactive leg muscle sympathetic nerve activity (MSNA), (**B**) heart rate (HR), (**C**) contracting forearm muscle electromyographic (EMG) activity, and (**D**) mean arterial blood pressure (MABP) during three successive trials of isometric handgrip sustained at 30% of maximal voluntary contraction, each performed to exhaustion in one young healthy adult. Note the tight temporal coupling between MSNA and EMG within and among the trials, suggesting a physiologic link between the onset and development of local muscle fatigue and activation of the sympathetic nervous system during small-muscle mass exercise. In contrast, changes in EMG were not consistently associated with increases in HR or MABP. (Modified with permission from Seals DR, Enoka RM. Sympathetic activation associated with increases in EMG during fatiguing exercise. *J Appl Physiol.* 1989;66:90.)

Mechanisms Controlling the Autonomic Nervous System Adjustments to Acute Exercise

Brain regions and neuromodulators involved in autonomic nervous system control during exercise

The anatomical areas of the brain involved in mediating the ANS adjustments to acute exercise are discussed in detail elsewhere (69–71). This issue has been studied in both anesthetized animals during electrical stimulation of muscle contractions and in conscious animals during exercise (*e.g.*, treadmill running). Brain sites activated by exercise have been identified using several experimental approaches, including the following (69–71):

- Comparing ANS responses to exercise (*e.g.*, actual exercise, electrically stimulated muscle contractions, local arterial injections of reflex-activating metabolites into the skeletal muscle circulation) with and without anatomical or pharmacologic lesioning of selected areas of the brain, including the use of electrolytic and chemical lesions,

synaptic blocking agents, and various agonists or antagonists (in some cases, specific receptor antagonists were used to produce exercise responses)
- Recordings of single neuronal activity in various sites in the brain during electrically induced muscle contractions
- Global metabolic labeling of brain sites (*e.g.*, with 2-deoxyglucose or using c-fos immunocytochemistry) during exercise or electrically stimulated contractions compared with resting conditions
- Functional brain imaging in humans

There are limitations in interpreting these data, including (a) the ability to generalize results obtained from electrically induced muscle contractions to actual exercise and the nonspecific stress responses associated with forced treadmill running in experimental animals to the responses to voluntary exercise in humans and (b) the inability to determine whether the activated neurons are inhibitory or excitatory for ANS responses when using brain labeling techniques during actual exercise. Nevertheless, these technically challenging studies have provided substantial insight into the nature of the CNS nuclei that determine

ANS outflow to the periphery during exercise, either by generating excitatory or inhibitory action potentials or by processing sensory feedback from receptors in the peripheral nervous system. Based on evidence obtained from these experimental models, specific areas of the brain activated during exercise that appear to be linked to the stimulation of exercise-associated ANS-cardiorespiratory responses include the following (Fig. 7.17)

Insular cortex: This telencephalic area is considered a principal site of CNS regulation of peripheral ANS activity during exercise based on functional imaging studies in humans (72) and studies in experimental animals (73).

Diencephalon: Areas of the ventromedial caudal hypothalamus involved in classic defense reactions as well as hypothalamic locomotor regions (posterior and lateral hypothalamus), possibly activated via inhibition of GABAergic cells (69). Neurons in the caudal hypothalamus are stimulated by feedback from contracting hind limb muscles (discussed later) and therefore appear to be activated by those neural inputs (69,71).

Midbrain and pons: The periaqueductal gray matter appears to be among the most activated areas in the midbrain region during exercise (69,74). Both the medial and lateral aspects of the cuneiform nucleus, that is, the so-called mesencephalic locomotor region that evokes locomotion upon stimulation (69,71), demonstrates significant activation during exercise (69). The lateral parabrachial neurons in this area also appear to be stimulated by exercise (69).

Medulla: Several areas of the medulla appear to be activated during exercise:

- The dorsal column nuclei, particularly in the nucleus gracilis (69).
- The medial aspect of the nucleus of the tractus solitaries (69,75,76), possibly linked to stimulation of baroreceptor and/or chemoreceptor feedback (discussed later), as well as contraction-sensitive cells.
- The rostral and caudal ventrolateral medulla. These areas have direct projections to the spinal cord intermediolateral cell column and have been implicated as a major region involved in the stimulation of preganglionic sympathetic neurons and the regulation of SNS outflow to the periphery under a number of conditions. Activation of cells in the caudal ventrolateral medulla as well as the sympathoexcitatory parapyramidal region also occurs with exercise (69).
- The raphe nuclei and ventromedial medulla are activated during exercise, possibly via the stimulation of reflexes produced by muscle contraction (69).

Thus, as summarized elsewhere (69,72), ANS-mediated cardiorespiratory adjustments to exercise appear to be controlled by selected nuclei in several areas of the brain (Fig. 7.17). However, the separate and interactive roles of these specific regions of the brain in producing the ANS responses to exercise are incompletely understood.

There is relatively little information available as to the receptor–neurochemical signaling pathways involved in the transduction of neural information generated or received by these regions of the brain into ANS outflow during exercise. Evidence obtained from studies in experimental animals during real or simulated (*e.g.*, electrically induced muscle contractions) exercise supports a role for several of the prominent CNS neurotransmitter systems including nor adrenergic (77–79), dopaminergic (77), serotonergic (77), and GABAergic (80,81) in the regulation of the ANS responses to exercise.

Central and peripheral neural mechanisms mediating the autonomic nervous system adjustments to exercise

The central and peripheral neural mechanisms involved in the control of the ANS adjustments to exercise are summarized next. This topic has been reviewed extensively (50,70–72) and also is discussed in Chapter 9.

CENTRAL COMMAND Central command, as initially envisioned by Krogh and Lindhard as discussed by Rowell (6), refers to a CNS-generated signal that is believed to be a primary stimulus mediating the ANS adjustments to exercise (25,51,71,72). Central command is thought to originate in the nuclei in the brain (*e.g.*, primary motor cortex) involved in producing the neural excitation leading to activation of motor nerves and muscle contraction. These areas include nuclei in the cerebral cortex (primary motor cortex); diencephalon (hypothalamic and subthalamic locomotor regions); mesencephalon (mesencephalic locomotor region); and selected portions of the pons, medulla (pontomedullary locomotor strip), and possibly, the amygdala (71). A detailed review of the functional neuroanatomy of central command based on neuroimaging studies in humans is available elsewhere (72), as well as recent data from direct recordings of brain nuclei in patients implicating the periaqueductal gray area (74).

The basic concept is that this descending central motor command signal is generated in response to the intent to exercise and not only results in appropriate activation of spinal motor units and muscle, but also causes stimulation of areas of the brain involved in the regulation of ANS outflow to the periphery (Fig. 7.18). As such, the central command signal is believed to produce the initial motor and ANS effector responses to the initiation of exercise. This signal could then be adjusted as exercise is sustained and also could be complemented by various sources of sensory feedback to achieve the appropriate overall set of physiologic responses in a particular exercise state. This is an attractive regulatory control hypothesis for at least three reasons:

- It provides a means by which the CNS can play an active role in the maintenance of overall physiologic homeostasis during the stress of exercise.
- It provides a feed-forward neural mechanism by which the necessary ANS adjustments can be produced at the initiation of exercise.

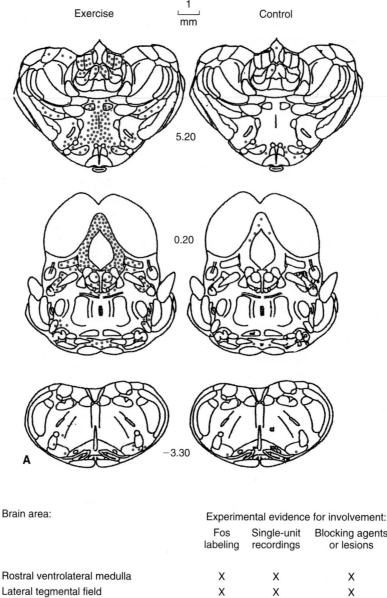

Brain area:	Experimental evidence for involvement:		
	Fos labeling	Single-unit recordings	Blocking agents or lesions
Rostral ventrolateral medulla	X	X	X
Lateral tegmental field	X	X	X
Raphe nuclei	X	X	
Caudal hypothalamus and locomotor region	X	X	X
	X		
Mesencephalic locomotor region	X	X	X
Periaqueductal gray matter	X	X	X
Nucleus of the solitary tract	X		

B

FIGURE 7.17 **A.** Representative Fos data of selected standard rat brain stereotactic planes in separate animals either in response to a single bout of treadmill running or during resting control: 5.20 is the level of the caudal hypothalamus, 0.28 is midbrain, and −3.30 is rostral medulla. Each dot signifies two cells. The control animal showed little or no Fos immunoreactivity labeling compared with the exercised animal in the following areas: rostral ventrolateral medulla; lateral tegmental field area just lateral to Gi; raphe nuclei; caudal hypothalamus, including locomotor region (ventromedial part of 5.2 level); mesencephalic locomotor region (cuneiform); and periaqueductal gray matter (dorsomedial part of 0.28 level surrounding cerebral aqueduct). At these levels the lateral tegmental field, raphe nuclei, and medial nucleus of the solitary tract (a sensory relay) were not labeled but were at other levels and in other animals. (Stereotactic figures and other abbreviations are adapted from Paxinos G, Watson C. *The Rat Brain in Stereotaxic Coordinates*, 2nd ed. Orlando: Academic Press; 1986. Modified with permission from Iwamoto GA, Wappel SM, Fox GM, et al. Identification of diencephalic and brainstem cardiorespiratory areas activated during exercise. *Brain Res.* 1996;726:113, 115–116.) **B.** Summary of brain sites for which there is evidence for activation during acute exercise that could contribute to control of ANS activity to the periphery. (Unpublished table courtesy of Professor Gary Iwamoto of the University of Illinois.)

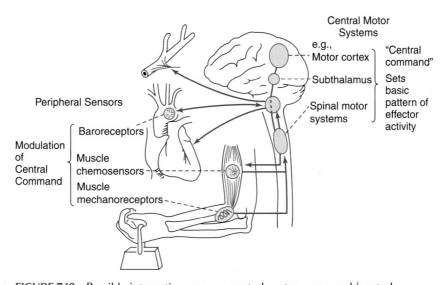

FIGURE 7.18   Possible interactions among central motor command (central command), arterial baroreflexes, and active muscle chemoreflexes and mechanoreflexes in controlling autonomic nervous system (ANS) efferent activity during exercise. In this scheme, central command would be responsible for the feed-forward stimulation of ANS changes at initiation of and during exercise. In contrast, the arterial baroreflexes and active muscle reflexes would provide fine-tuning feedback from the periphery that would modify the effects of central command to produce the most appropriate combination of ANS responses for maintaining overall physiologic homeostasis. (Modified with permission from Rowell LB. *Human Cardiovascular Control.* New York: Oxford University; 1993:442.)

- It provides a control system in which the magnitude of the ANS adjustments can be graded to the exercise stimulus and, therefore, better meet the specific physiologic demands imposed by the nature of the exercise being performed.

> # KEY POINT
>
> Central command is an important mechanism triggering ANS responses at the onset of exercise.

Central command also may function as a feedback system by which the effort or exertion associated with exercise is sensed by the CNS, providing further information that can be used to adjust ANS outflow to the periphery (72).

There is considerable experimental evidence that central command can influence the ANS responses to voluntary exercise and/or muscle contraction. Central command is a/the key mechanism responsible for the reduction in cardiac vagal modulation of heart rate with exercise, which contributes importantly to increases in cardiac output, particularly in the early period of exercise and at mild to moderate intensities (22,25,51). In contrast, there is much less evidence for a broad role of central command in the stimulation of sympathoadrenal system activity during exercise (22,25,51).

The experimental findings supporting a significant modulatory effect of central command on the ANS during exercise include the following:

- Exercise-like responses to intended muscle activity; that is, muscle contraction is prevented by administration of neuromuscular blocking agents, so that no feedback from active muscle is possible, which isolates the effects of central command. Under these conditions, a normal increase in heart rate is observed during attempted handgrip exercise (13,81) (Fig. 7.19). The increase in heart rate is abolished by pretreatment with atropine, but unaffected by β-adrenergic receptor antagonists (13,82), indicating that withdrawal of cardiac vagal modulation of heart rate is the key mechanism by which central command produces tachycardia during exercise.
- Augmented ANS responses with increases in voluntary effort (central command) during performance of a constant muscle force contraction (*i.e.,* manipulation of central command with fixed muscle afferent feedback) using partial neuromuscular blockade. Partial neuromuscular blockade, which requires increased voluntary effort to achieve and maintain a particular submaximal force, is associated with an augmented arterial blood pressure response to isometric exercise in humans (6,51); this increased blood pressure response is mediated primarily by greater increases in heart rate and cardiac output.

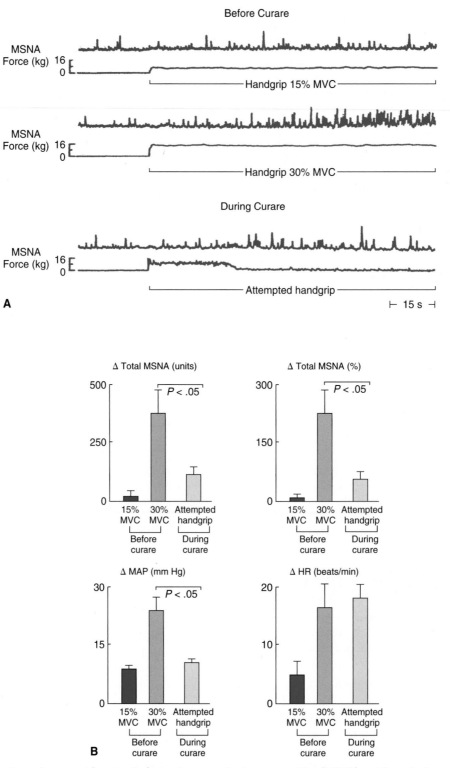

FIGURE 7.19 **A.** Tracings of peroneal (inactive leg) muscle sympathetic nerve activity (MSNA) and force before and during isometric handgrip contractions performed at 15% (*top*) and 30% (*middle*) of maximal voluntary contraction (MVC) prior to curare infusion (partial neuromuscular blockade), and attempted handgrip during curare infusion (*bottom*) in one subject. MSNA increased during handgrip at 30% MVC but not at 15% MVC. During partial neuromuscular blockade, which eliminated the ability to produce even the normal 15% of MVC handgrip force (removing active muscle reflex feedback and isolating the influence of central command), MSNA increased only slightly despite maximal effort (intent to perform the contraction), suggesting that even maximal levels of central command have little effect on MSNA. **B.** Mean changes in MSNA, mean arterial blood pressure (MAP), and heart rate (HR) in response to the same conditions. Although attempted handgrip contraction had little effect on MSNA, it produced normal increases in HR (abolished with atropine), indicating a primary influence of central command in producing cardiac vagal withdrawal-mediated tachycardia during exercise. (Modified with permission from Victor RG, SL Pryor, NH Secher, et al. Effects of partial neuromuscular blockade on sympathetic nerve responses to static exercise in humans. *Circ Res.* 1989;65:471–472.)

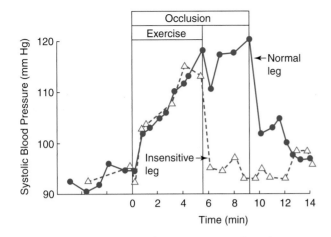

FIGURE 7.20 Systolic blood pressure responses to leg exercise and postexercise leg ischemia performed with a normal leg (intact central command and active muscle reflex feedback) and a leg without functional sensory afferent feedback (intact central command without active muscle reflex feedback). Note the normal blood pressure response to exercise of the leg with sensory loss, suggesting that central command alone can produce this autonomically mediated cardiovascular response to exercise. Also note the importance of sensory afferent feedback in maintaining blood pressure elevations during postexercise ischemia via the muscle chemoreflex. (Modified from Rowell LB. *Human Circulation Regulation During Physical Stress*. New York: Oxford University; 1986:213–416. Adapted from Alam M, Smirk FH. Unilateral loss of a blood pressure raising, pulse accelerating, reflex from voluntary muscle due to a lesion of the spinal cord. *Clin Sci.* 1938;3:297.)

- Normal ANS and cardiovascular responses to exercise performed by limbs without intact sensory feedback, which demonstrates the ability of central command to evoke the necessary adjustments to exercise without feedback from active muscle (83) (Fig. 7.20).
- Both imagined exercise (central command in the absence of muscle activity) (84) and perceived increases in effort during constant submaximal-intensity leg cycling exercise while under hypnosis (increased central command with fixed active muscle feedback) (85) increase heart rate, blood pressure, and blood flow to cortical regions of the brain thought to be involved in mediating the effects of central command.
- In experimental animals, electrical stimulation of the CNS sites (*e.g.*, subthalamus) thought to be involved in central command–induced ANS physiologic adjustments produce exercise-like motor, cardiorespiratory, neuroendocrine, and metabolic responses (69,71).

Experimental evidence supporting the view that central command has little if any role in the stimulation of sympathoadrenal system activity during exercise includes these points:

- Even maximal levels of central command (*i.e.*, maximal voluntary effort to perform handgrip exercise with total neuromuscular blockade) have a relatively small effect on MSNA (82) (Fig. 7.19).

- No increase in MSNA takes place during the initiation of exercise or during mild intensities of exercise despite physiologically significant central command–evoked cardiac vagal withdrawal–mediated increases in heart rate (82) (Figs. 7.11, 7.15, and 7.19).

As described earlier, renal SNS activity may increase soon after the initiation of exercise, at least in experimental animals (32,33). It could be argued that this is mediated by central command, although muscle mechanoreflexes and/or baroreflexes (discussed later) also could produce this response. There is also evidence that central command can stimulate SNS activity to skin during voluntary and electrically stimulated isometric muscle contractions and "intended" exercise models (35,86).

ACTIVE MUSCLE REFLEXES   As reviewed in detail previously (25,51,70), there is extensive experimental evidence that feedback from active skeletal muscles can influence the ANS-physiologic adjustments to exercise and therefore serve as the other primary CNS exercise signal along with central command. The peripheral neural substrate providing this feedback is group III and IV sensory nerves, which are stimulated by chemical, mechanical, and/or thermal stimuli produced by active muscle (25,51,70). The feedback is reflex in origin: Excitatory action potentials from muscle sensory afferents project to the brain via synaptic transmissions in the dorsal root of the spinal cord. This exerts effects on specific nuclei in the brain (primarily caudal and rostral aspects of the ventrolateral medulla) (70), which, in turn, inhibit vagal and/or stimulate sympathetic preganglionic neurons, thus producing selective efferent ANS responses to target tissues in the periphery (*e.g.*, heart and arterial vasculature).

This type of exercise-evoked CNS signal is attractive from a control system perspective because it would theoretically provide information from active muscle as to the appropriateness of the central command (feed-forward controller) produced ANS-physiologic adjustments to exercise. In this way, the initial, grosser ANS-physiologic activation generated by central command could be fine-tuned by information from the active muscle fibers (Fig. 7.18). Feedback indicating, for example, a mismatch between active muscle oxygen demand and delivery could produce the necessary ANS-cardiovascular adjustments to augment active muscle perfusion. Thus, active muscle feedback would complement the central command signal, providing more precise regulatory control for maintaining active muscle homeostasis during the changing metabolic demands imposed by the exercise state.

Two primary classifications of these reflexes have been identified: (a) those activated by chemical stimuli produced as a consequence of active muscle metabolism and (b) mechanical stimuli generated by the contracting muscle fibers (Fig. 7.18). The possible involvement of these reflexes, as well as active muscle thermoreflexes, in ANS control during exercise has been discussed in detail elsewhere (25,51,70).

Muscle chemoreflexes (muscle metaboreflexes) Muscle chemoreflexes appear to be activated when the metabolic state of the active muscle fibers changes during exercise in a manner that reflects an adverse (unwanted) internal metabolic environment posing a potential challenge to the maintenance of homeostasis. Under these conditions, the metabolism of the active muscle fibers will shift from oxidative to more glycolysis-driven adenosine triphosphate production, and the metabolic milieu both within the muscle cell and in the interstitial fluid surrounding those muscle fibers will change accordingly. The altered chemical composition of the interstitium stimulates the endings of group III and IV sensory neurons in the extracellular space surrounding these muscle fibers, increasing their discharge rates and initiating a reflex modulation of efferent ANS activity. The basic idea is that this reflex provides a local sensor to monitor the biochemical state of the active muscle fibers and transduce to the CNS information concerning the functional status of those cells. Thus, if inadequate oxygen delivery results in shifts in intracellular metabolism and corresponding changes in the interstitial fluid reflecting a mismatch with oxygen demand, the reflex would attempt to correct this error by stimulating ANS-cardiovascular adjustments resulting in increased perfusion of the active muscle fibers.

The specific biochemical changes that occur in the interstitium to activate chemically sensitive group III and IV nerve endings and engage this reflex have been discussed (22,25,69). These putative changes include increases in interstitial concentrations of carbon dioxide, hydrogen ion, lactic acid, arachidonic acid, potassium, phosphate, cyclooxygenase products, bradykinin, and prostaglandins (22,70), whereas changes in adenosine do not appear to be involved (86). Increases in potassium concentrations likely have only transient, if any, effects in stimulating these sensory afferents (22). Although a reduction in pH appears to be a key step in activating this reflex, hydrogen ion itself may not actually stimulate chemically sensitive afferents during exercise, but rather the conversion of monoprotonated phosphate to its diprotonated form (H_2PO_4) (22,70,88). At this time, the individual chemical triggers and/or interactions that result in muscle chemoreflex activation in vivo during exercise remain only partially understood.

The specific ANS effects of muscle chemoreflex activation appear to involve primarily increases in SNS activity including β-adrenergic stimulation of tachycardia, but with no obvious effect on cardiac vagal modulation of heart rate (22,25,51,70). Experimental evidence supporting the ability of muscle chemoreflexes to influence the SNS adjustments to exercise includes the following:

- During small-muscle dynamic and isometric exercise (45,66,67) (Figs. 7.15, 7.16, and 7.19A) (a) the absence of any increase in MSNA during the initial period of exercise that precedes accumulation of muscle chemoreflex activating metabolites and (b) a progressive and marked increase in MSNA thereafter as exercise is sustained, coinciding with the development of muscle fatigue and perceptions of muscle discomfort consistent with buildup of glycolytic metabolites. This temporal pattern of the MSNA response is consistent with the correspondingly delayed pattern of activation of chemically sensitive muscle afferents when stimulated by isometric contractions in anesthetized cats (51,70).

- Augmentation of the MSNA (inactive limb vasoconstrictor) and/or arterial blood pressure responses during exercise performed with compared to without partial or complete occlusion of blood flow to the active limbs (26,51,89); the occlusion of blood flow both increases the production and traps the buildup of muscle chemoreflex–activating metabolites in the active muscles.

- Maintenance of the exercise-induced elevation in MSNA, inactive limb vasoconstriction, and arterial blood pressure during a period of postexercise occlusion of blood flow to the previously active limb (i.e., as compared with a non–blood flow occluded recovery period postexercise) (25,83,89) (Fig. 7.20). During postexercise occlusion, the muscle chemoreflex remains activated in the absence of central command or other exercise-dependent CNS stimuli (i.e., muscle mechanoreflex input, discussed later).

- During isometric and dynamic handgrip exercise, increases in MSNA and inactive limb vascular resistance are consistently related to the intracellular hydrogen ion accumulation and pH (i.e., chemoreflex activating stimuli) of the active forearm muscles (90,91). In contrast, in patients with muscle phosphorylase deficiency (McArdle's disease), who cannot break down glycogen, produce lactic acid, or therefore increase hydrogen ion (reduce pH) during exercise (i.e., cannot activate the muscle chemoreflex), there is no increase in MSNA during the same handgrip exercise stimulus that results in a doubling of MSNA in normal subjects (92).

- In dogs, activation of muscle chemoreflexes (via occlusion of the terminal aorta) during treadmill running produces cardiac SNS–mediated coronary artery vasoconstriction (93), as well as increases in arterial blood pressure and systematic vascular resistance (22).

The concept that acidotic active skeletal muscle could trigger a reflex that would stimulate SNS vasoconstriction and augment arterial perfusion pressure is attractive from a control theory perspective when considered together with functional sympatholysis. That is, the SNS activation evoked by the reflex would produce widespread vasoconstriction except in tissues under increased metabolic demand, such as active skeletal muscle. In the latter, functional sympatholysis would secure increased blood flow for the most metabolically active tissues.

Despite a substantial body of experimental evidence demonstrating that activation of muscle chemoreflexes affects the ANS-cardiovascular responses to exercise, we still lack a clear understanding of the role, if any, these reflexes play in cardiovascular control during conventional large-muscle dynamic exercise. It is well established that these reflexes stimulate SNS activity in experimental animals and/or humans during these events:

- Fatiguing levels of isometric exercise, that is, exercise in which the sustained contractions mechanically compress arteries, resulting in a natural restriction in blood flow (Figs. 7.15A, 7.16, and 7.19)
- Fatiguing levels of dynamic exercise performed with small muscle groups (*e.g.*, handgrip and arm cycling), that is, exercise in which the demand for energy production per active muscle fiber is great and, therefore, glycolytic flux and intracellular acid production and accumulation are high within the active muscles (Fig. 7.15B)
- Large-muscle dynamic exercise performed under conditions of mild to severe occlusion of active muscle blood flow (22,51)

However, although muscle chemoreflexes can influence the ANS responses to exercise, that does not necessarily mean that they actually contribute to ANS-cardiovascular regulation during conventional forms of dynamic exercise performed without artificial occlusion of active muscle blood flow. At present, we have no direct or convincing evidence that the muscle chemoreflex is normally engaged during the submaximal levels of large-muscle dynamic exercise typi-

---

KEY POINT

Additional research is needed to determine the role of active muscle chemoreflexes in mediating the ANS adjustments to conventional forms of submaximal aerobic exercise.

---

cally performed by humans for health and fitness purposes. These forms of exercise are not obviously associated with restricted active muscle perfusion or with excessive accumulation of glycolytic metabolites or reductions in pH. If the muscle chemoreflex were activated during normal (free flow) large-muscle dynamic exercise, this likely would be limited to heavy submaximal and/or maximal intensities of work.

Muscle mechanoreflexes   The possible involvement of active muscle mechanoreflexes in ANS-cardiovascular control during exercise has been discussed previously (22,51,70). These reflexes are stimulated by mechanical stimuli (stretch and/or compression) in the active muscle fibers that activate mechanically sensitive group III and IV afferents. Evidence that these reflexes can modulate ANS adjustments to exercise includes:

- Stimulation of mechanically sensitive group III and IV sensory afferents produces a reflex increase

in systolic arterial blood pressure (presumably mediated by the ANS) in experimental animals (22,51,70); compression or increases in the intravascular volume of the active forearm muscles during exercise augments MSNA in humans (22,94).
- The onset of electrically induced muscle contraction in humans (*i.e.*, in the absence of central command and before the possible activation of muscle chemoreflexes) is associated with an increase in heart rate (22,25,51), a response shown to be mediated by cardiac vagal withdrawal (13) and an increase in skin (sudomotor) SNS activity (35).
- Brief muscle contractions are associated with corresponding bursts of cardiac SNS activity in cats, which is positively related to the muscle tension produced (22,51,70).

As with muscle chemoreflexes, the actual involvement of muscle mechanoreflexes in ANS-cardiovascular control during conventional forms of dynamic exercise is unknown. Mechanically sensitive muscle afferents appear to be active only at the onset of exercise, with their discharge rates returning rapidly to resting control levels (22,51,70). Therefore, any involvement of these potential signals would likely be confined to the initiation of exercise, severely limiting the possible scope of this mechanism in contributing to ANS control during sustained exercise.

Muscle thermoreflexes   In addition to responding to chemical and/or mechanical stimuli, many group III and IV sensory afferents are thermosensitive (22,70). Because active muscle temperatures can increase significantly during sustained moderate to heavy submaximal exercise, it is possible that these afferents could be stimulated and provide feedback to the CNS regarding the thermal status of the active muscle fibers (22). Although this remains a possibility, experimental findings are insufficient to determine the role of this mechanism in ANS-cardiovascular control during exercise.

ARTERIAL BAROREFLEXES   Arterial baroreflexes evoke beat-to-beat changes in cardiac vagal modulation of heart rate as well as SNS activity to the heart and vasculature in response to changes in arterial blood pressure (6,22,51). Specifically, increases in arterial blood pressure would deform the walls of the aortic arch and carotid sinus in which these mechanically sensitive receptors are located, stimulating their afferent nerve endings and signaling the CNS to increase cardiac vagal modulation of heart rate and decrease SNS activity to the heart and vasculature. These reflex ANS adjustments would act to reduce cardiac output (by decreasing heart rate and left ventricular contractility) and systemic vascular resistance (by dilating arterial resistance vessels), thus lowering arterial blood pressure. The opposite ANS-cardiovascular adjustments are induced in response to reductions in arterial blood pressure, which deactivates the arterial baroreflex.

The role of the arterial baroreflex in ANS-cardiovascular control during exercise (Fig. 7.18) has been reviewed in

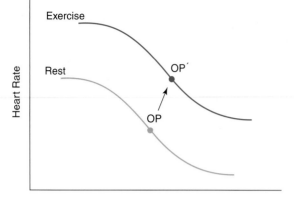

FIGURE 7.21 Resetting of the arterial baroreflex operating point (OP) for control of heart rate upward and to the right with acute exercise. (Modified with permission from O'Leary D. Heart rate control during exercise by baroreceptors and skeletal muscle afferents. *Med Sci Sports Exerc.* 1996;28:212.)

baroreflex is simply reset to regulate arterial blood pressure at a higher operating point during exercise (6,22,51,95,96) (Fig. 7.21). Indeed, it has been established that not only does the arterial baroreflex operate normally during exercise, but also that an intact arterial baroreflex is essential for producing the necessary ANS-cardiovascular adjustments. The primary experimental evidence for this conclusion comes from studies on animals in which arterial blood pressure falls markedly with the onset of large-muscle dynamic exercise following denervation of the sinoaortic and cardiopulmonary baroreceptors (22,51,95–97) (Fig. 7.22). Although blood pressure returns toward normal levels during moderate to heavy submaximal exercise in these animals, during light exercise blood pressure remains below control levels and demonstrates unusual instability (22,51,97). The key concept advanced is that the arterial baroreflex is essential for maintaining arterial blood pressure at the onset of large-muscle dynamic exercise and throughout at least lower intensity dynamic exercise. This is because the arterial baroreflex counteracts the extensive active muscle vasodilation and increase in total vascular conductance produced during exercise by evoking reflex decreases in cardiac vagal modulation of heart rate and increases in SNS vasoconstriction (6,22,51). With the onset of exercise the arterial baroreflex is reset, likely by central command (discussed later), to a higher operating pressure, resulting in the prevailing blood pressure being perceived as inappropriately low (i.e., as hypotension) and

detail elsewhere (6,22,51,95,96). Because systolic and arterial pulse pressures increase during conventional forms of large-muscle dynamic exercise and because both systolic and diastolic blood pressure increase during small-muscle dynamic and isometric contractions, originally it was believed that the arterial baroreflex was inhibited during exercise. However, it is now understood that the arterial

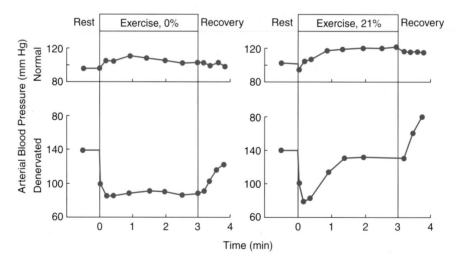

FIGURE 7.22 Arterial blood pressure at rest (left of 0 time points) and in response to light (0% grade, *left*) and heavier (21% grade, *right*) submaximal treadmill exercise (5.5 km · hr⁻¹) in healthy dogs with either intact (*top*) or denervated (*bottom*) baroreflexes. Note the immediate fall in blood pressure at the onset of both intensities of exercise in the barodenervated state. Blood pressure remains below resting control levels throughout light exercise but returns toward resting levels after the initial minute of heavier exercise, probably as a result of increased central command and/or muscle chemoreflex activation arising from the effect of low arterial blood pressure on active muscle blood flow. (Modified with permission from Rowell LB. Human circulation regulation during physical stress. New York: Oxford University; 1986:320. Adapted from Melcher A, Donald DE. Maintained ability of carotid baroreflex to regulate arterial pressure during exercise. *Am J Physiol.* 1981;241:H838–H849.)

evoking ANS-cardiovascular responses aimed at raising arterial pressure. Activation of reflexes from active skeletal muscles and feedback from cardiopulmonary baroreceptors (see next) also can contribute to arterial baroreflex resetting during exercise (96). Therefore, the contemporary view is that the arterial baroreflex does not oppose the ANS-cardiovascular adjustments by which arterial blood pressure is increased during exercise, but rather actually supports ANS-cardiovascular evoked increases in arterial pressure with exercise. More recent evidence indicates that the resetting of the arterial baroreflex is a dynamic process with increasing intensity and duration of exercise (98,99).

CARDIOPULMONARY BAROREFLEXES Cardiopulmonary baroreflexes monitor cardiopulmonary blood volume by sensing changes in the filling pressure (distension) of the chambers of the heart and pulmonary arteries and veins, as well as cardiac contractility and afterload (6,22,97). Increases in these stimuli activate mechanically sensitive receptors in these structures, stimulating vagal afferent fibers that signal the CNS to inhibit SNS activity. The latter results in systemic vasodilation and a reduction in systemic vascular resistance. This, in turn, increases the compliance of the arterial circulation and reduces the normal displacement of blood to the venous circulation and its return to the heart and pulmonary circulation, thus reducing cardiopulmonary blood volume. The release of extracellular fluid–regulating hormones also is modulated by this reflex in a manner that would act to facilitate water and sodium excretion under these conditions of hypervolemia. The opposite set of responses would be evoked in response to reductions in cardiopulmonary blood volume. These reflexes operate in an integrative fashion with arterial baroreflexes, generally one reflex opposing the effects of the other.

The possible involvement of these homeostatic reflexes in ANS-cardiovascular control during exercise has been reviewed previously (6,8,22,50). Because of active skeletal muscle pump–evoked increases in cardiac filling (preload) and contractility during conventional forms of upright dynamic exercise in humans, it might reasonably be assumed that these reflexes actively inhibit SNS outflow under these conditions. The possible modulatory effects of cardiopulmonary baroreflexes on the ANS-cardiovascular adjustments to exercise have been studied in both humans and experimental animals. The results of these studies are equivocal, with evidence both supporting and refuting a physiologically significant effect of cardiopulmonary baroreflexes in ANS control during exercise (6,22,51). The most compelling evidence for the involvement of this reflex in modulating ANS function during exercise in humans comes from observations of inhibition of nonactive limb MSNA during the onset and early phase of upright dynamic exercise (22,36,37). The theory advanced is that the activation of the muscle pump with the initiation of dynamic exercise would augment cardiac filling and central blood volume, stimulating these mechanoreceptors and producing reflex SNS inhibition. However, such a muscle pump–produced increase in blood volume in the central circulation at the onset of dynamic exercise also increases cardiac output and systolic blood pressure and, therefore, likely causes distension of the aortic arch and carotid sinus regions, possibly activating the arterial baroreflex and producing sympathoinhibition via that mechanism (22). More recent evidence suggests that cardiopulmonary baroreflexes may be reset during exercise to an operating point consistent with the associated increase in cardiac filling volume (100).

CENTRAL THERMOREFLEXES The role of central thermoreflexes in ANS-cardiovascular control during exercise has been reviewed elsewhere (6,22). These reflexes modulate neural vasoconstrictor and vasodilator outflow to the cutaneous circulation to ensure optimal circulatory conditions for heat dissipation during exercise, particularly that performed in warm ambient conditions. In performing these regulatory functions, central thermoreflexes interact with arterial and cardiopulmonary baroreflexes and other neural inputs to the CNS during exercise to maintain internal homeostasis. During sustained submaximal exercise in warm ambient conditions, cutaneous vasomotor outflow is adjusted to allow increased blood flow and volume to the skin circulation (6,22). If sufficiently great, this redistribution of the cardiac output to the skin can restrict active muscle blood flow, producing competition between exercise signals (central command and active muscle reflexes) aimed at ensuring perfusion of the contracting muscle fibers and thermal inputs charged with maintaining core temperature within the appropriate range. Moreover, the increased cutaneous vascular conductance during exercise in the heat acts to lower systemic vascular resistance, threatening arterial blood pressure, particularly in the face of marked active muscle vasodilation. Thus, under these conditions, a robust interaction occurs among exercise-specific and exercise-nonspecific neural inputs to the CNS, each attempting to produce ANS-cardiovascular responses to meet their particular homeostatic needs. The CNS must interpret these competing signals and generate efferent ANS outflow that attempts to support these diverse demands on the systemic circulation. In general, it appears that the top regulatory priority of the CNS is the maintenance of arterial blood pressure to ensure perfusion of vital organs followed in order by maintenance of internal body temperature and support of active locomotor muscle blood flow. Thus, the ability to sustain exercise is sacrificed first, for example, via SNS vasoconstriction of active muscle blood flow in order to maintain systemic vascular resistance and arterial blood pressure and to provide flow to the cutaneous circulation for thermoregulation. If necessary, the skin will undergo vasoconstriction to protect systemic arterial pressure, but vital organ perfusion will be protected at all costs.

ARTERIAL CHEMOREFLEXES Arterial chemoreflexes monitor and help maintain arterial oxygen and carbon dioxide levels and pH within their respective homeostatic ranges via effects on pulmonary ventilation and arterial blood acid–base balance (6,67). Stimulation of arterial chemoreflexes also has pronounced effects on the ANS, a key feature of which appears to be SNS activation by hypoxia, hypercapnia, and/or acidosis (6,70). Because exercise normally is associated with maintenance of Pa_{O_2}, normal or reduced arterial carbon dioxide, and maintenance of blood pH within acceptable ranges, the role of the arterial chemoreflexes in ANS control during conventional submaximal exercise at sea level or mild elevations in altitude is incompletely understood. Arterial chemoreflexes may be activated during exercise performed upon acute exposure to higher altitudes in normal subjects (*i.e.*, before compensatory adaptations), during exercise in patients with lung disease demonstrating arterial hypoxemia and/or hypercapnia, and/or during heavy submaximal and maximal exercise in endurance-trained athletes who demonstrate hypoxemia under these conditions. Moreover, experimentally induced acidosis augments the PNE response (101), and experimentally produced alkalosis can attenuate the PNE and PE responses (102) to exercise in humans, consistent with the concept that arterial chemoreflexes can influence sympathoadrenal responses to exercise under conditions of altered systemic acid–base balance.

LUNG INFLATION REFLEXES AND RESPIRATORY METABO-REFLEXES   In anesthetized animals, lung inflation stimulates vagal afferent nerves projecting to the CNS, producing a reflex inhibition of efferent SNS activity (6,70). Similarly, in humans MSNA is inhibited during inspiration and stimulated during expiration under resting conditions (103). Breathing (6) also influences cardiac vagal modulation of heart rate. Because breathing frequency, tidal volume, and minute ventilation all increase during exercise, it is possible that reflexes activated by lung inflation participate in ANS control during exercise. There is little information providing insight into this possibility. In healthy humans, simulated exercise hyperpnea (*i.e.*, isocapnic high frequency elevated tidal volume breathing) has no obvious influence on mean levels of MSNA at rest or during muscle metaboreflex activation produced by either isometric handgrip exercise or ischemia of the previously active forearm post handgrip (103). Thus, at present, there is no clear evidence that stimulation of lung inflation reflexes modulates SNS activity during exercise. However, given the limited information available, this possibility cannot be ruled out.

The work of Dempsey and colleagues (104) is consistent with the existence of a "respiratory muscle chemoreflex" (respiratory metaboreflex). The concept is that such a reflex can be activated during heavy submaximal and/or maximal exercise that is associated with a sustained elevation in work of breathing and development of respiratory muscle fatigue (105) (Fig. 7.23). Under these conditions, glycolytic metabolites may stimulate group III and IV phrenic afferents, increasing their discharge to the CNS and evoking a reflex excitation of efferent SNS activity to peripheral tissues, including the active locomotor muscles. The latter would produce active muscle vasoconstriction and a reduction in blood flow with a consequent reduction in exercise performance. This vasoconstriction would act to redistribute car-

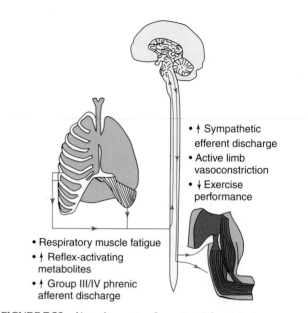

• ↑ Sympathetic efferent discharge
• Active limb vasoconstriction
• ↓ Exercise performance

• Respiratory muscle fatigue
• ↑ Reflex-activating metabolites
• ↑ Group III/IV phrenic afferent discharge

FIGURE 7.23   Key elements of a potential respiratory muscle metaboreflex. The concept is that sustained high-volume ventilation during exercise, particularly during high resistance to flow, could produce respiratory muscle fatigue with an associated increase in glycolytic metabolism, increased production, release and accumulation of reflex-activating (glycolytic) metabolites, and consequent activation of chemically sensitive group III/IV respiratory muscle sensory afferents. The latter would project to the CNS, producing a reflex increase in efferent sympathetic activity evoking peripheral vasoconstriction, including in arterioles perfusing the active locomotor muscles. This vasoconstriction would reduce active locomotor muscle blood flow, potentially providing increased flow and oxygen delivery to the respiratory muscles to maintain ventilation and, therefore, arterial blood gases and acid–base balance within ranges consistent with homeostasis. (Modified from Seals DR. Robin Hood for the lungs? A respiratory metaboreflex that "steals" blood flow from locomotor muscles. *J Physiol [Lond].* 2001;537:2.)

diac output to the respiratory muscles, increasing their blood flow in an attempt to address the "flow error" via a classic muscle chemoreflex response. Teleologically, this respiratory muscle metaboreflex could have as its primary regulatory aim the preservation of respiratory muscle perfusion during physiologic states in which there is competition for cardiac output with locomotor muscles. Because the respiratory muscles are essential for producing pulmonary ventilation at the necessary levels to maintain arterial blood gases and pH, the proper perfusion of the respiratory muscles should be a high priority for maintaining organismic homeostasis. Under these conditions, it could be argued that blood flow to the locomotor muscles and support of locomotion would constitute a far less important regulatory goal.

INTEGRATIVE CONTROL OF THE ANS ADJUSTMENTS TO EXERCISE   How do these CNS inputs control ANS function during exercise? Which of these signals actually contribute to integrative ANS-cardiovascular regulation during conventional forms of large-muscle dynamic exercise?

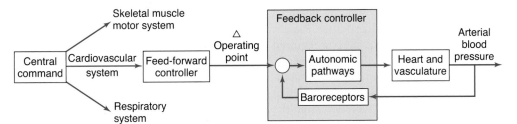

FIGURE 7.24 Hypothesized effect of central command in stimulating autonomic nervous system (ANS) adjustments to exercise via both direct effects on ANS controllers in the central nervous system (CNS) and indirectly by eliciting a resetting of the arterial baroreflex operating point, which, in turn, influences ANS adjustments during exercise. (Modified with permission from Rowell LB. *Human Cardiovascular Control*. New York: Oxford University; 1993:463.)

Which signals are not actively involved, perhaps participating only under specific or unusual exercise conditions? At this time, we only have pieces of the answers to these questions. However, Rowell (51) has advanced an overall model as to how the ANS adjustments to large-muscle dynamic exercise may be mediated. This hypothesis represents an integrative scheme attempting to explain the primary signals involved and how those signals may interact to produce these ANS adjustments to exercise.

In this theory, the central command (feed-forward) signal generated with the onset of exercise would cause the arterial baroreflex to be reset to a higher operating pressure (Fig. 7.24). Under these conditions, the prevailing arterial blood pressure would be interpreted by the CNS as hypotension, and reflex ANS adjustments would be evoked to increase blood pressure to the new operating point to correct the presumed blood pressure error (Fig. 7.25). Because cardiac vagal modulation of heart rate is the fastest ANS adjustment available to the arterial baroreflex for correcting blood pressure errors, the hypothesis is that cardiac vagal withdrawal–mediated increases in heart rate and cardiac output are produced initially to raise arterial blood pressure to the new exercise operating point (there is also evidence that central command can directly stimulate cardiac vagal withdrawal with the initiation of exercise independent of arterial baroreflex resetting) (22). Based on data from studies in experimental animals (32–34), an increase in cardiac and/or renal SNS activity also may be part of this initial ANS response to resetting of the arterial baroreflex operating pressure with the initiation of exercise (22). In any case, the key concept is that vagally mediated tachycardia and an increase in cardiac output would be the primary mechanism by which blood pressure would increase at the onset of exercise via central command–evoked arterial baroreflex resetting. The augmentation of cardiac output would also increase blood flow to active muscle, thus initiating a necessary increase in oxygen delivery to meet the increased metabolic demands of muscle activity.

Rowell's model (51) (Fig. 7.25) also predicts that if the exercise intensity is within the range in which the increases in heart rate required to raise cardiac output and arterial blood pressure could be met solely by cardiac vagal withdrawal (i.e., up to about 100 beats per minute), little or no sympathoadrenal system activation would be required. Additional increases in exercise

intensity would require further increases in the central motor command signal, producing further resetting of the arterial baroreflex to progressively higher operating pressures. At these greater intensities of exercise, the required increases in arterial blood pressure

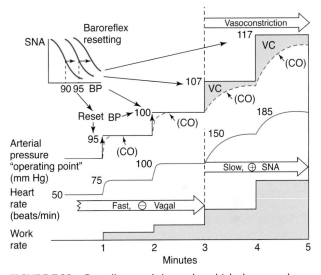

FIGURE 7.25 Overall control theory by which the central nervous system (CNS) mediates autonomic nervous system (ANS) adjustments to exercise via the available neural inputs. In this model, arterial baroreflex resetting by central command with the initiation of exercise causes a shift in the arterial blood pressure (BP) operating point to a higher pressure and results in a perceived pressure error (hypotension). At the onset of exercise and during transitions from light to light-moderate intensity of exercise, this error is eliminated (i.e., the new higher operating blood pressure is achieved) via rapid cardiac vagal withdrawal–mediated increases in heart rate and cardiac output (CO). During transitions to higher exercise intensities associated with heart rates above 100 beats per minute—that is, beyond the range in which the necessary blood pressure increases can be met solely by cardiac vagal withdrawal—sympathetic activation to the heart (to further increase heart rate and cardiac output) and arterioles (to produce vasoconstriction [VC] and increases in vascular resistance) is required to raise blood pressure and eliminate the pressure error produced by the exercise intensity–dependent arterial baroreflex resetting. SNA, sympathetic nerve activity. (Modified with permission from Rowell LB. *Human Cardiovascular Control*. New York: Oxford University; 1993:469.)

cannot be met by cardiac vagal withdrawal–mediated tachycardia-induced increases in cardiac output. Rather, increases in SNS activity to the heart would be required to further augment cardiac output via β-adrenergic stimulation of heart rate and left ventricular contractility. At heavy submaximal to maximal exercise intensities, SNS stimulation of epinephrine secretion from the adrenal medulla would also occur. This would increase circulating concentrations of this hormone, which binds to β-adrenergic receptors in the sinoatrial node and left ventricular muscle, providing a mechanism for further stimulation of heart rate and left ventricular contractility. Moreover, at these exercise intensities, increases in SNS vasoconstrictor activity to the resistance vessels in the arterial circulation, including active muscle, will be necessary to counteract active muscle vasodilation, hence to maintain systemic vascular conductance at levels necessary to achieve the higher arterial blood pressure set point. The overall increase in sympathoadrenal activity would be progressively greater up to maximal intensities of exercise to meet the cardiovascular demands of the intensity-dependent upward resetting of the arterial baroreflex operating pressure. Thus, in this theory, the arterial baroreflex is the primary mechanism by which the ANS adjustments to large-muscle dynamic exercise are mediated. Central command also plays a critical role in ANS control by stimulating exercise intensity–specific arterial baroreflex resetting and possibly exerting a direct effect on cardiac vagal modulation of heart rate.

KEY POINT

Central command–evoked resetting of the arterial baroreflex is an important signal mediating the ANS adjustments to exercise.

However, in this model, the involvement of active muscle reflexes are not required to explain the ANS responses to exercise, although these reflexes can contribute to arterial baroreflex resetting during exercise (96). A major strength of the model is that it accounts for the key ANS adjustments observed:

- Cardiac vagal withdrawal with the onset of exercise, increasing with exercise intensity
- The lack of need for an immediate increase in sympathoadrenal activity at the onset of exercise and during mild exercise (because the necessary increases in arterial blood pressure can be achieved under these conditions solely via cardiac vagal withdrawal–mediated increases in heart rate and cardiac output)
- Progressive increases in sympathoadrenal system activity from moderate submaximal to maximal intensities of exercise, as indicated by progressive increases in PNE and PE with increasing exercise intensity over this range

Moreover, this regulatory model also explains (a) why arterial blood pressure falls at the onset of exercise (instead of increasing) in experimental animals without intact baroreflexes (6,97) and (b) how SNS activation can occur at intensities of large-muscle dynamic exercise below that which produces a metabolic state consistent with muscle chemoreflex stimulation.

Acceptance of this control theory does not preclude the involvement of other signals under these or other exercise conditions. For example, as mentioned earlier in this chapter, it is possible that cardiopulmonary baroreflex stimulation in response to activation of the locomotor muscle pump and increased cardiac filling could contribute to or even explain the sympathoinhibition observed in inactive muscle at the onset of upright dynamic exercise in humans (22,36,37). It is also possible that during heavy submaximal and maximal large-muscle dynamic exercise in humans, active locomotor (and, possibly, respiratory) muscles attain a biochemical state in which the concentrations of glycolytic metabolites and other putative agents are sufficiently great to activate muscle chemoreflexes that contribute to sympathoadrenal system stimulation. The general homeostatic reflexes described earlier presumably operate in their normal roles during exercise, that is, as sensors actively monitoring their respective stimuli and transducing any perceived errors (potential threats) into corrective efferent ANS responses aimed at maintaining homeostasis. For example, thermoreflexes that would not be expected to have much, if any, active involvement in ANS control at the onset of dynamic exercise or during mild exercise performed under cool ambient conditions presumably play a more active role during prolonged moderate to heavy submaximal exercise, particularly in the heat. As mentioned earlier, the ANS adjustments to exercise upon acute sojourn to high altitude likely are modulated by arterial chemoreflexes responding to arterial hypoxemia and so on (see Chapter 24). It is also important to understand that the various neural inputs during exercise interact with and modify (enhance or inhibit) each other in producing the ANS and cardiovascular responses to exercise (106,107).

Finally, because isometric and small-muscle dynamic exercise pose such a different challenge to the maintenance of homeostasis from that of conventional forms of large-muscle dynamic exercise, the mechanisms controlling ANS responses to these types of exercise also likely differ (22,51). It appears that during large-muscle dynamic exercise, maintenance of arterial blood pressure in the face of marked active muscle vasodilation constitutes the primary threat to homeostasis (i.e., the need to prevent or correct pressure errors). Under these conditions, it follows that arterial baroreflexes would play a prominent role in ANS control, working interactively with exercise-specific signals (e.g., central motor command). In contrast, isometric and small-muscle dynamic exercise does not produce widespread active muscle vasodilation. Rather, the high intramuscular pressures associated with these forms of exercise result in mechanical compression of the conduit (feed) arteries, producing local occlusions of blood flow and limiting perfusion of the active muscle fibers (25,45,51). Under these conditions, there will be (a) a shift in energy production to greater dependence on glycolysis and a consequent increased rate of production of glycolytic metabolites and (b) natural occlusion of venous outflow and trapping of glycolytic metabolites in the active muscles. These two events together result in increases in the concentrations of these metabolites in the extracellular space surrounding the active muscle fibers, stimulation of chemically sensitive group III and IV sensory afferents, activation of muscle chemoreflexes, and a strong chemoreflex-mediated efferent SNS response (51,70). On the other hand, isometric, small-muscle dynamic, and large-muscle dynamic exercise all require tachycardia-mediated increases in cardiac output to increase arterial blood pressure and blood flow to active muscle with the initiation of exercise. Accordingly, under both exercise conditions central command–evoked cardiac vagal withdrawal appears to be used for most economically achieving this particular regulatory need (22,51). The key point is that the specific challenges to homeostasis imposed by the overall exercise conditions (including factors such as the ambient temperature, state of hydration, and fitness of the subject) determine the regulatory mechanisms that mediate the necessary ANS adjustments.

Summary

A reduction in cardiac vagal activity produces an increase in heart rate and cardiac output at the onset of exercise to increase active muscle blood flow and support arterial blood pressure (in the face of active muscle dilation). With increasing intensity of exercise, cardiac vagal withdrawal becomes greater and the sympathoadrenal system is activated. The latter stimulates heart rate and left ventricular contractility (further increasing cardiac output), causes vasoconstriction in selective regional circulations in order to redistribute blood flow to active muscle, and limits active muscle vasodilation such that systemic vascular conductance and arterial pressure are properly maintained. The temporal patterns and magnitudes of these adjustments are influenced by numerous factors. Finally, the ANS adjustments to acute exercise are controlled by a variety of neural inputs (central command, feedback from active muscle, cardiovascular reflexes, etc.) to regions of the brain that translate these multiple signals into ANS outflow to peripheral tissues and organs with the goal of maintaining physiologic homeostasis.

TEST YOURSELF

Which of these signals are influencing the ANS adjustments to the types of exercise that you typically perform? Which are exerting the greatest influence?

Autonomic Nervous System Adaptations to Chronic Exercise

As with many physiologic systems, the ANS undergoes specific adaptations in cardiac vagal and sympathoadrenal system function in response to repeated bouts of whole body dynamic exercise. Such adaptations may be observed, at rest but are particularly evident during exercise performed at the same submaximal intensity after compared with before exercise training. These ANS adaptations, in turn, help mediate exercise training–induced cardiovascular, metabolic, and thermoregulatory adaptations observed at rest and during acute exercise. Although it is important to remember the specific ANS adaptations to chronic exercise and the corresponding effects these changes produce in other physiologic systems, it is even more important to understand why the body produces these changes. What is the organism attempting to accomplish by producing such adaptations? What advantages (benefits) does the adaptation confer to a body repeatedly exposed to exercise?

In this context, it is helpful to consider acute exercise as a form of physiologic stress. Depending on the intensity of the exercise involved and other factors (*e.g.*, ambient temperature), this stress can induce physiologic systems, including the ANS, to sustain function at the extreme portion of their respective operating ranges (*i.e.*, at levels associated with little or no physiologic reserve). Doing so represents a challenge to homeostasis: the greater the stress imposed by the exercise training stimulus, the greater the challenge (acute threat) to overall organismic homeostasis each time that stimulus is applied (each exercise training session). The adaptations that the body undergoes in response to frequent exposure to such an exercise stress are intended to reduce the acute challenge to homeostasis. In other words, the improvements allow the acute exercise to be performed at a lower level of the operating range, that is, with greater functional reserve than before training. This can be achieved by either of the following:

1. Being able to perform the exercise at a lower absolute level of the original (unchanged) operating range for the function in question (*e.g.*, after endurance training, performing the same absolute submaximal dynamic exercise at a lower absolute level of heart rate than before training, with little or no change in resting or maximal heart rate)
2. Being able to perform exercise at the same absolute level of an increased operating range for the function in question (*e.g.*, after exercise training that produced increases in maximal cardiac output and maximal oxygen consumption—again, a common scenario— performing the same absolute submaximal dynamic exercise at the same absolute levels of maximal oxygen consumption and cardiac output as before training)

In this way, exercise training produces a physiologic state that is more resistant to the loss of homeostasis in response to the application of that particular stress than it was before the initiation of training. This is the intrinsic wisdom of the body as it relates to exercise training (or adaptation to the repeated exposure of any form of stress). Understanding the teleology of this process allows the physiologist to understand and predict the adaptations that are required to defend homeostasis while allowing the sustained performance of exercise.

The ANS adaptations to exercise training and information concerning the underlying mechanisms are discussed in the following sections. Unless otherwise stated, *exercise training* will refer to the chronic performance of sustained large-muscle dynamic exercise, that is, aerobic or endurance exercise. The term *exercise-trained state* refers either to the physiologic state after a period of regular exercise within a particular individual or group (*i.e.*, after vs. before an exercise intervention) or to the physiologic state of exercise-trained adults compared with sedentary age- and sex-matched peers (*i.e.*, cross-sectional comparison of exercise-trained and sedentary subjects). Findings supporting the conclusions are based on research involving both experimental animals and human subjects, generally healthy young and middle-aged adults. The reader is referred to selective previous reviews of this topic for additional information (1,6,17).

Cardiac Vagal Modulation of Heart Rate

At rest

Cardiac vagal modulation of heart rate appears to be increased under tonic (resting) conditions after a period of exercise training in some experimental animals and human subjects. The experimental evidence supporting such an adaptation includes the following:

- Greater increases in heart rate in response to acute intravenous administration of atropine at rest in the exercise-trained than in the sedentary state (17,108,109).
- Greater HRV at rest (17,110,111) and over the entire day (112) in the exercise-trained than in the sedentary state.
- Higher cardiac acetylcholine concentrations in the exercise-trained than in the sedentary state (113).

However, there is a significant body of evidence that does not support enhanced cardiac vagal tone in the endurance-trained state, including observations of similar heart rate increases in response to atropine in the trained and untrained states (17,114). The reasons for the lack of consistent findings likely include at least two factors (17):

- Between-study differences in the strength of the exercise training stimulus (*i.e.*, differences in the duration, intensity, frequency, and/or length of exercise training); a milder exercise stress may produce no adaptation or possibly only a small adaptation that could be missed because of normal measurement error and variability among subjects.

- Law of initial baseline; that is, subjects with low cardiac vagal modulatory tone at baseline (before the initiation of exercise training) would have the most potential for adaptation (increase in vagal tone with training), and vice versa.

Accordingly, the greatest possibility of an increase in cardiac vagal modulation of heart rate would be under these conditions:

- Subjects with very low baseline levels (*e.g.*, older adults or patients with cardiovascular diseases) undergoing vigorous and prolonged exercise training
- Comparing highly endurance exercise–trained with very sedentary adults

Thus, the role of increased cardiac vagal modulation of heart rate in the so-called training bradycardia (lower resting heart rate in the exercise-trained state) is not uniformly clear. The available evidence supports the view that this mechanism could contribute to the resting bradycardia in some endurance-trained subjects, but not necessarily in all. In the absence of such an effect, current evidence supports an important role for a reduction in the intrinsic heart rate (*i.e.*, heart rate in the absence of extrinsic [autonomic-adrenergic] influences) in mediating the training bradycardia (108,114,115).

> **KEY POINT**
>
> Reductions in intrinsic heart rate likely play a major role in mediating training bradycardia.

Also, recent findings (116) provide compelling support for the likelihood that intense and sustained endurance training, so-called overtraining, in athletes results in reduced HRV and, therefore, reduced cardiac vagal modulation of heart rate and an associated increase in resting heart rate. Thus, excessive exercise training may produce at least a temporary state of *adverse* physiologic stress characterized by reduced cardiac vagal tone and a shift in cardiac ANS balance toward an increased cardiac SNS predominance.

During acute exercise

A physiologist might reasonably speculate that cardiac vagal modulation of heart rate (greater vagal tone) would be greater during performance of the same absolute submaximal workload in the exercise-trained compared with the sedentary state. At the same relative submaximal workload (same percent of maximal exercise capacity), one would predict that cardiac vagal modulation of heart rate would be similar in the exercise-trained and untrained states. This speculation is consistent with the following facts:

- Heart rate is lower and unchanged, respectively, during submaximal dynamic exercise performed at the same absolute and relative work rates in the endurance trained than in the sedentary state (6,22).

- HRV at the offset of acute submaximal exercise is higher after than before exercise training (17,111).

Although there are no data concerning this issue in humans, findings in dogs support this idea (31). During 60 minutes of treadmill running at the same submaximal work rate as before training, after endurance training dogs exercised at a lower heart rate and HRV, suggesting maintenance of higher cardiac vagal activity in the trained state

Sympathoadrenal System Activity at Rest and throughout a Day

At rest

Although there is a widespread belief that sympathoadrenal system and/or SNS activity is lower in the exercise-trained than in the sedentary state under resting conditions, the experimental data on this issue are highly inconsistent. With regard to the SNS, PNE has been reported to be either unchanged (117,118) (Fig. 7.26) or lower (39,103) in the

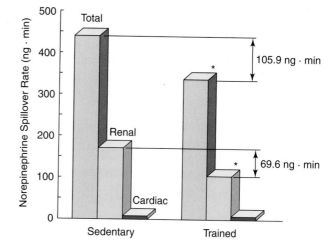

FIGURE 7.27 Total, renal, and cardiac norepinephrine spillover rates determined during resting conditions before and after endurance exercise training in healthy young and middle-aged men. Total norepinephrine spillover rate was lower after training, mediated largely by a corresponding reduction in renal norepinephrine spillover rate, indicating training-associated reductions in average whole body and kidney sympathetic activity at rest. In contrast, cardiac norepinephrine spillover rate, which was already low in the sedentary state, was not further reduced after exercise training, suggesting no effect of regular endurance exercise on cardiac sympathetic activity in healthy men of this age. (Modified with permission from Meredith TT, Friberg P, Jennings GL, et al. Exercise training lowers resting renal but not cardiac sympathetic activity in humans. *Hypertension.* 1991;18:579.)

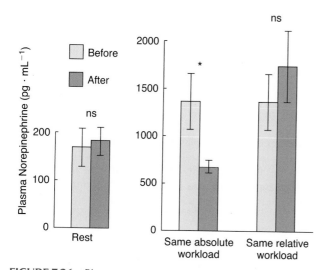

FIGURE 7.26 Plasma norepinephrine concentrations determined under resting conditions (*left*) and during submaximal leg cycling exercise (*right*) performed at the same absolute and relative (percent of maximum) intensities before and after endurance exercise training in 10 healthy young and middle-aged men. Plasma norepinephrine concentrations were not different under resting conditions or during exercise performed at the same relative workload before and after exercise training, indicating unchanged sympathetic activity with endurance training under these conditions. In contrast, plasma norepinephrine concentrations were lower at the same absolute submaximal workload after compared with before exercise training, indicating a markedly lower sympathetic activity after training under this condition. (Modified with permission from Peronnet F, Cleroux J, Perrault H, et al. Plasma norepinephrine response to exercise before and after training in humans. *J Appl Physiol.* 1981;51:813.)

exercise-trained than in the sedentary state. There are few data on total PNE spillover rate, a more precise measure of average whole-body SNS activity than PNE, comparing the exercise-trained and sedentary states. In young adults, a reduction in total PNE spillover rate at rest has been reported after a period of daily exercise training (119), but findings are inconsistent as to the effects of less frequent (3 days a week) training (115,119) (Fig. 7.27). In contrast, in older adults total PNE spillover rate at rest has been found to be either elevated (120) or not different (121) in the exercise-trained compared with the untrained state.

With reference to possible changes in regional SNS activity under resting conditions, a reduction in renal PNE spillover rate has been reported in young adult males after endurance exercise training compared with a period of sedentary living (115); the decrease in renal PNE spillover accounted for about two-thirds of the reduction in total PNE spillover rate after training (Fig. 7.27). MSNA generally has been found not to be different in the exercise-trained and sedentary states in young adult human subjects (122,123) or in middle-aged and older men (117,124), and is increased in exercise-trained postmenopausal women (117). In experimental animals, NE content and/or turnover has been found to be elevated in the brain (125), not different in the liver (21,126), and lower in the spleen (125) in the endurance-trained state.

Findings concerning the effects of exercise training on SNS activity to the heart also are inconsistent. Observations of (a) a smaller reduction in heart rate in response to acute β-adrenergic receptor blockade in the exercise-trained than in sedentary states (108) and (b) reduced NE content (127) and turnover (125) in whole-heart preparations and in right atrial β-adrenergic receptor density and affinity (128) in exercise-trained compared with untrained experimental animals are consistent with a reduction in cardiac SNS tone after endurance exercise training. However, findings of (a) no difference in heart rate in response to β-adrenergic receptor blockade (114), (b) no change in cardiac PNE spillover rate (115), and (c) no difference (21,126) or increased (125) NE content of the heart in the exercise-trained compared with sedentary states do not support an exercise training–associated reduction in cardiac SNS tone. Thus, the role of reduced sympathoadrenal β-adrenergic modulation of heart rate in contributing to the training bradycardia observed in the exercise-trained state is not clear. This mechanism could play some role, but the available experimental evidence is more consistent for enhanced cardiac vagal modulation and, particularly, a reduction in intrinsic heart rate in mediating the training bradycardia observed at rest.

Under resting conditions, epinephrine secretion from the adrenal medulla appears to be either unchanged or augmented in the endurance exercise–trained compared with the sedentary state. PE generally has been found to be not different in the trained and untrained states (42,115,119), nor is tissue epinephrine content in the adrenal medulla different in exercise-trained compared with sedentary rats under resting conditions (21). In contrast, there is evidence supporting enhanced epinephrine secretion rate from the adrenal medulla in the endurance-trained state (26), including elevated PE and increased epinephrine secretion, with unchanged epinephrine clearance.

PNE and PE over an entire 24-hour period in endurance exercise–trained and untrained young males have been established using serial blood sampling (129). Normal daily exercise training sessions were included in the analysis. Peak plasma concentrations of the catecholamines were much greater in the trained males as a result of their exercise training session. Mean 24-hour PNE and PE were twice as great in the trained as in the untrained men (Fig. 7.28), despite similar mean levels of heart rate. These unique data support the possibility that average daily sympathoadrenal system activity actually is greater in the endurance exercise–trained than in the sedentary state. This could be the result of greater tonic SNS stimulation associated with a state of chronically elevated "energy flux" as discussed later.

During acute exercise

The most consistently observed sympathoadrenal system adaptation to aerobic endurance exercise training is lower PNE and PE during performance of the same absolute

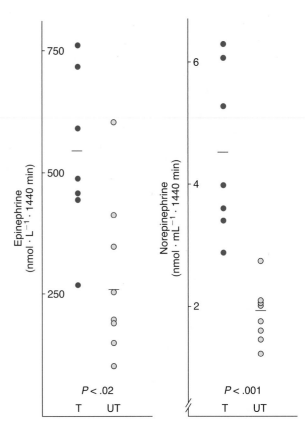

FIGURE 7.28   Mean 24-hour plasma epinephrine (*left*) and norepinephrine (*right*) concentrations in groups of endurance exercise–trained (T) and untrained (UT) healthy young men. The average 24-hour concentrations of these catecholamines were much higher in the endurance-trained than in the untrained men, suggesting that trained men have greater daily sympathoadrenal system activity and consequent circulating plasma epinephrine and norepinephrine levels than untrained men. (Modified from Dela F, Mikines KJ, von Linstow M, et al. Heart rate and plasma catecholamines during 24 h of everyday life in trained and untrained men. *J Appl Physiol.* 1992;73:2392.)

submaximal exercise condition in the trained than in the untrained state (40,118,130) (Fig. 7.26). This adaptation is observed at moderate to heavy submaximal exercise intensities that evoke significant sympathoadrenal system activation in the untrained state. The temporal pattern of this adaptation has not been extensively studied, but reductions in PNE and PE have been observed to be complete by the third week of a 7-week intensive endurance training program (130) (Fig. 7.29). These training-induced reductions in PNE and PE during submaximal exercise are abolished after a period of no exercise training (131). PE actually may be augmented in endurance-trained compared with untrained subjects during *prolonged* submaximal exercise performed to exhaustion (26), consistent with the concept of an increased capacity for adrenal medullary secretion of epinephrine under stressful conditions (*e.g.*, threat of hypoglycemia) in the exercise-trained state.

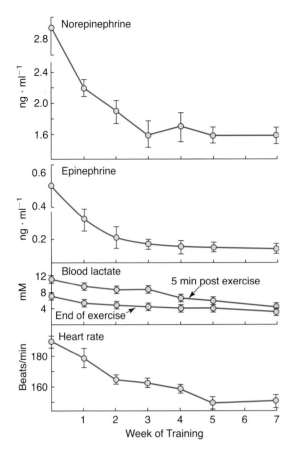

FIGURE 7.29   Changes in plasma norepinephrine and epinephrine, blood lactate, and heart rate during leg-cycling exercise performed at the same absolute submaximal workload before (far-left vertical axis points) and weekly throughout an intense 7-week exercise training program in healthy young men. Plasma norepinephrine and epinephrine concentrations during exercise decreased significantly throughout the initial 3 weeks of training and remained unchanged thereafter, indicating that this sympathoadrenal system adaptation was complete by the third week of exercise training. In contrast, exercise heart rate continued to decrease until the fifth week of training, suggesting that nonsympathetic mechanisms contribute to reductions in heart rate after the third week of training. (Modified from Winder WW, Hagberg JM, Hickson RC, et al. Time course of sympathoadrenal adaptation to endurance exercise training in man. *J Appl Physiol.* 1978;45:372.)

KEY POINT

Sympathoadrenal system activation during performance of the same absolute level of submaximal exercise is lower after aerobic exercise training.

PNE and PE usually are not different during exercise performed at the same relative submaximal workload (percent of maximal exercise capacity) (Fig. 7.26) or at maximum in the exercise-trained and sedentary states (40,42,118), although greater levels of PNE and/or PE also have been observed under these conditions (26,132).

Greater PNE at the same relative submaximal exercise intensity and/or at maximum following endurance training may be linked to the greater absolute work rates and VO_2, and a consequent greater active muscle mass compared with the untrained state (132). This would, in turn, require greater active muscle blood flow and vascular conductance, producing a greater threat to the maintenance of arterial blood pressure in the trained state. To maintain total vascular conductance and arterial blood pressure in the face of greater active muscle vasodilation, the arterial baroreflex would allow a correspondingly greater increase in SNS vasoconstrictor activity, which accounts for the higher PNE values in the trained state under these conditions.

The effects of these sympathoadrenal system adaptations to exercise training on cardiovascular function during acute exercise include the following (6,8):

- Less nonactive muscle and internal organ (renal, splanchnic) vasoconstriction during the same absolute submaximal workload in the trained state as a consequence of the reduced SNS activity
- Similar (or slightly greater) nonactive muscle and internal organ (renal, splanchnic) vasoconstriction during the same relative workload in the trained state as a consequence of the similar (or slightly greater) SNS activity
- The slope of the line relating renal and splanchnic blood flow to percent of maximal oxygen consumption is unchanged with exercise training; thus, a greater absolute workload can be performed with the same increase in SNS activity and associated renal and splanchnic vasoconstriction (6,22)
- Sympathoadrenal system activation occurs at a higher absolute submaximal workload after endurance training, although the heart rate–SNS activity relation is not altered in the exercise-trained state (6,22)

TEST YOURSELF

During the types of acute exercise that you perform, how would your ANS responses differ from a friend of the same size and sex, but who does not exercise regularly?

Role of the sympathoadrenal system in mediating physiologic adaptations to exercise training

The role of an intact sympathoadrenal system in mediating the physiologic adaptations to aerobic endurance exercise training is controversial (8), as limited evidence supports the need for an intact SNS in producing the bradycardia and other cardiovascular adaptations associated with endurance training (133,134). This information is obtained by comparing the physiologic responses to exercise training in experimental animals or humans with either an intact sympathoadrenal system or the absence of a functional sympathoadrenal system produced by SNS denervation, adrenalectomy, or adrenergic receptor blockade. The observation that chronic infusion of dobutamine, a β-adrenergic receptor agonist, can produce exercise training–like cardiovascular adaptations also is consistent with the idea that sympathoadrenal system stimulation of the β-adrenergic signaling pathways in the heart and other key peripheral tissues is an important mechanism in mediating the cardiovascular adaptations to exercise training (135). However, there is alternative experimental support for the position that the physiologic adaptations to exercise training, including increases in maximal aerobic capacity, can be produced without an intact sympathoadrenal system, including in the absence of β-adrenergic system signaling (8,11). Thus, at present, this issue remains controversial.

Influence of resistance exercise training on sympathoadrenal system function

There is a limited amount of information on the effects of resistance exercise training on sympathoadrenal activity. With regard to whole body measures of sympathoadrenal activity, PNE and PE concentrations at rest are not different in the resistance exercise–trained compared with the untrained state (136,137). PNE and PE during the same absolute submaximal workloads of large muscle dynamic exercise also are the same before and after resistance exercise training (137). Concerning regional SNS activity, MSNA determined under resting conditions is unchanged after resistance exercise training in young adults (138). Thus, based on the available experimental evidence, resistance exercise training does not appear to influence sympathoadrenal system activity under resting conditions or during conventional submaximal dynamic exercise. Sympathoadrenal system activation could be reduced during acute submaximal resistance exercise in the resistance exercise–trained state. However, this remains to be established experimentally.

Central and Peripheral Neural Mechanisms Mediating the Autonomic Nervous System Adaptations to Large-Muscle Dynamic Exercise Training

Any changes in efferent ANS activity in the exercise-trained compared with the untrained state must be mediated by corresponding changes in the peripheral nervous system and/or CNS mechanisms that control that activity under the specific set of physiologic conditions in which the ANS adaptation is observed. As such, exercise training–related changes in ANS activity observed under resting conditions would be mediated by changes in CNS nuclei involved in automatic rhythm generation of ANS activity (i.e., vagal and SNS preganglionic nerve activity) and/or sensory afferent feedback from tonic homeostatic reflexes (e.g., baroreflexes, arterial chemoreflexes). Of course, indirect cardiovascular measures of ANS activity, such as HRV, also are subject to nonneural peripheral adaptations

(e.g., changes in muscarinic receptor density or sensitivity). Exercise training–associated changes in ANS activity during acute exercise could be mediated by changes in these tonic control mechanisms, but also are affected by changes in neural signals specific to physical exercise (i.e., central command and feedback from active muscle reflexes).

Autonomic nervous system adaptations observed under resting conditions

It is difficult to speculate about the mechanisms that may mediate ANS adaptations to exercise training observed under resting conditions for at least two reasons. First, as noted earlier, these adaptations have not been observed consistently, particularly in human subjects. Second, unlike adaptations observed under conditions of submaximal exercise, there are not one or two specific signals that are believed to dominant ANS control under resting conditions but rather an integration of basic CNS outflow tonically modulated by feedback input from a number of homeostatic reflexes. When observed, increased HRV and reduced PNE may be mediated, in part, by increased vagal and reduced SNS activity from hypothalamic, medullary, and possibly other regions of the subcortical brain known to control tonic ANS outflow (139). However, increased cardiac vagal modulation of heart rate could also be mediated, in part, by peripheral adaptations in acetylcholine release from the vagus nerve and/or muscarinic receptor density and affinity for and sensitivity to acetylcholine. Similarly, reduced PNE could be mediated, in part, by training-associated changes in presynaptic modulation of NE release from sympathetic nerve endings (i.e., reduced NE release per unit sympathetic nerve discharge).

Possible changes in baroreflex control of heart rate and SNS activity at rest in the exercise-trained and untrained states have been studied extensively in both human subjects and experimental animals. As discussed in detail recently (140), the results of studies in humans indicate that baroreflex control of ANS-cardiovascular function (i.e., heart rate, MSNA, and/or arterial blood pressure) is increased (141), unchanged (124,140), or reduced (142) in the exercise-trained versus sedentary state. Findings from investigations in experimental animals are much more consistent, indicating impaired baroreflex control of the circulation in the endurance exercise–trained condition (143). However, the potential mechanistic role of changes in baroreflex function (when observed) in mediating the ANS-cardiovascular adaptations to endurance exercise training under resting conditions (when observed) has not been established.

Finally, inconsistency in ANS activity, particularly SNS activity, under resting conditions in the exercise-trained and untrained conditions could be mediated, in part, by changes in the state of energy flux. Energy flux refers to the absolute levels of energy intake and energy expenditure during a period of energy balance. A state of high-energy flux would be associated with high daily energy expenditure (e.g., as a result of daily endurance exercise training) and correspondingly high-energy intake required to maintain energy balance, and vice versa. High-energy flux states involving regular large-muscle dynamic exercise are associated with correspondingly greater levels of SNS activity (based on PNE values) and resting metabolic rate compared with a low energy flux state involving sedentary energy-balanced conditions (144). Accordingly, this poorly appreciated influence on the ANS should be considered in attempts to interpret findings related especially to the effects of endurance training on resting SNS activity.

Autonomic nervous system adaptations observed during submaximal exercise

As emphasized earlier, the most consistently evident ANS adaptations to exercise training are the (presumed) higher levels of cardiac vagal modulation of heart rate and the well-established lower overall sympathoadrenal system activity at the same absolute submaximal workload in the exercise-trained compared with the untrained state. Because central motor command, feedback from active muscle reflexes, and feedback from arterial baroreflexes are believed to be the three major neural signals mediating the ANS adjustments to acute exercise (51,70,71), most of the related experimental results to date concern the possible involvement of these mechanisms.

CENTRAL COMMAND   During exercise central command is believed to (22,51):

- Directly or indirectly (via baroreflex resetting) stimulate a reduction in cardiac vagal activity, with a resulting increase in heart rate
- Indirectly (via baroreflex resetting) stimulate increases sympathoadrenal activity, with resulting increases in heart rate and region-specific vasoconstriction

Therefore, one might reasonably hypothesize that a reduced level of central command is a key mechanism underlying the lower heart rate, PNE, renal and splanchnic vasoconstriction, and PE observed during the same absolute submaximal exercise load in the endurance-trained compared with the sedentary state. Three primary lines of experimental evidence support such an idea:

1. Reduced heart rate and blood pressure responses to the same absolute submaximal bout of dynamic cycling exercise performed with the untrained leg after compared with before one-leg exercise training (145). The interpretation of such results is that because the untrained leg has not undergone metabolic or other adaptations that occur in the trained leg, the feedback from the active muscles of the untrained leg during acute exercise should be the same before and after the period of exercise training. As such, the mechanism mediating the lower ANS-evoked cardiovascular adjustments to acute exercise with the untrained leg after contralateral leg training must involve a CNS-based adaptation, presumably a lower central motor command mediated by some type of crossover effect on the untrained limb.

2. Reduced heart rate and diastolic blood pressure responses to voluntary, but not electrically stimulated (involuntary) submaximal isometric exercise in the untrained limb after compared with before exercise training of the contralateral trained limb (146). The fact that the attenuated heart rate and diastolic blood pressure responses in the untrained limb after contralateral limb training was not observed during involuntary exercise (i.e., when only feedback from active muscle reflexes were stimulating ANS responses) implicates a lower level of central command in mediating the adaptations observed during voluntary exercise of the untrained limb post training.

3. Lower active muscle electromyographic (EMG) activity during performance of the same submaximal muscle activity in the endurance-trained compared with the untrained state (147). Active muscle EMG activity has been used as an indirect measure of central command; thus, a lower level of EMG during exercise is interpreted as representing a lower level of central command in the exercise-trained state.

KEY POINT

Reduced central command likely contributes to altered ANS responses during performance of the absolute level of submaximal exercise following aerobic exercise training.

FEEDBACK FROM ACTIVE MUSCLE REFLEXES   Feedback from active muscle reflexes, particularly from muscle chemoreflex activation, can stimulate SNS outflow to the heart (raising heart rate) and to the arterial blood vessels (producing vasoconstriction in nonactive muscle, the kidney, and the splanchnic circulations), although the contributions of these mechanisms during conventional large-muscle dynamic exercise are not clear (discussed earlier). Thus, it is possible that reduced SNS-mediated responses to acute exercise in the endurance-trained compared with the untrained state could be the result of reduced feedback from active muscle reflexes. Experimental evidence supporting this possibility includes these findings:

1. Greater reductions in heart rate and arterial blood pressure during the same absolute level of submaximal leg cycling exercise performed with the trained limb versus the untrained limb after compared with before one-leg endurance training (148). The idea is that because of CNS crossover effects produced by training, central command should be similarly reduced during performance of acute exercise with the trained and untrained limbs following exercise training. Therefore, any differences observed in ANS-mediated responses can be attributed to less feedback from active muscle reflexes.

2. Reductions in muscle lactate concentrations during acute submaximal large-muscle dynamic exercise as well as less hyperemia postexercise in the active muscles following exercise training (148,149). Because muscle chemoreflex activation during exercise is related to the extent of glycolytic metabolism and the production and accumulation of glycolytic metabolites, as well as to mismatches between oxygen demand and delivery, these observations suggest a metabolic state in the active muscles following training consistent with less muscle chemoreflex activation.

3. Reduced MSNA response to small-muscle dynamic exercise after training (150) associated with evidence for reduced active muscle chemoreflex (e.g., reduced accumulation of reflex-activating metabolites) (151) and possibly mechanoreflex (150) activation.

Based on the discussion of the involvement in these reflexes in ANS control during acute exercise presented earlier in this chapter, changes in these mechanisms likely play a more important role in mediating ANS adaptations to small-muscle and perhaps very high-intensity large-muscle exercise training than the adaptations observed in response to conventional intensities and durations of large-muscle endurance training.

BAROREFLEXES   As discussed previously, the resetting of the arterial baroreflex to a higher operating pressure from rest may be a key mechanism by which the ANS adjustments, particularly increases in SNS activity, to acute large-muscle dynamic exercise are mediated. Thus, changes in baroreflex function could contribute to or even explain the ANS adaptations observed during the same absolute intensity of submaximal exercise in the endurance-trained compared with the sedentary state. Unfortunately, direct experimental evidence is not available either to support or to refute this possibility, because studies to date have investigated baroreflex function in the trained and untrained states only under resting conditions (discussed earlier).

INTEGRATIVE MODEL EXPLAINING TRAINING-ASSOCIATED ANS ADAPTATIONS DURING SUBMAXIMAL DYNAMIC EXERCISE   A key question, therefore, remains unanswered: how are the smaller withdrawal of cardiac vagal nerve activity and sympathoadrenal system activation observed during the same absolute submaximal level of large-muscle dynamic exercise in the endurance-trained state mediated? This is unknown, but based on previous discussion we can construct a working model that attempts to explain how these adaptations may be produced.

In the regulatory scheme advanced by Rowell (51) (Fig. 7.25), the increase in heart rate during exercise requiring levels below 100 beats per minute is mediated by central command–stimulated cardiac vagal withdrawal. Exercise requiring greater increases in heart rate also necessitates activation of the SNS, which produces further increases

in heart rate and cardiac output along with vasoconstriction in the nonactive skeletal muscle, renal, and splanchnic circulations. At least the SNS activation appears to involve a resetting of the arterial baroreflex to a higher operating pressure. Given this scenario, it seems reasonable to postulate that the ANS adaptations to endurance training that are expressed during the performance of submaximal exercise are mediated by changes to these two key control mechanisms: central command and arterial baroreflex resetting. For example, a lower central motor command in the trained state would presumably cause less CNS-mediated cardiac vagal withdrawal and, therefore, result in the lower heart rate observed during submaximal exercise. In addition, the lower central command would cause less resetting of the arterial baroreflex and, therefore, the operating point for arterial blood pressure would be lower during submaximal exercise in the endurance-trained than in the sedentary state. During submaximal exercise performed at heart rates below 100 beats per minute (in the untrained state), less withdrawal of cardiac vagal activity and a smaller increase in heart rate would be required in the endurance-trained state to achieve the lower exercise-associated operating pressure. This would explain the lower heart rate and arterial blood pressure in the endurance-trained versus untrained state during mild to moderate submaximal exercise. During higher intensities of exercise requiring SNS activation, the smaller central command–mediated arterial baroreflex resetting would explain not only greater cardiac vagal tone in the endurance-trained state, but also the accompanying smaller increases in SNS activity to the heart and peripheral arterial vessels. That is, compared with the untrained state, less SNS activation (less NE release from sympathetic nerve endings and less epinephrine secretion from the adrenal medulla) would be needed because less of an increase in heart rate and regional vasoconstriction would be required to attain the lower operating pressure in the exercise-trained state. This would explain the smaller sympathoadrenal–β-adrenergic stimulation of heart rate, SNS-mediated α-adrenergic reductions in regional blood flow and vascular conductance (i.e., increases in vascular resistance), and increases in PNE and PE during moderate to heavy submaximal exercise observed in the endurance-trained state. Thus, in this regulatory scheme, the key mechanism involved in producing the ANS adaptations observed during submaximal large-muscle dynamic exercise in the trained state is a smaller central motor command.

ROLE OF REDUCED CNS NEURONAL ACTIVATION AND REMODELING IN ANS ADAPTATIONS OBSERVED DURING SUBMAXIMAL EXERCISE   Regardless of the exact mechanisms that contribute to the ANS adaptations to training observed during submaximal exercise, one would hypothesize that neuronal activity in selective regions of the brain involved in ANS-cardiorespiratory control during exercise would be different in the endurance-trained compared with the sedentary state. In particular, it might be postulated that areas of the brain implicated in stimulating

SNS outflow to the heart and arterial blood vessels during exercise would demonstrate less activation during submaximal exercise in the trained state. Iwamoto and colleagues (139) provide experimental evidence for this concept. Fos-like (c-Fos) immunocytochemistry was used to establish neuronal activation in specific regions of the brain thought to be involved in ANS-cardiorespiratory control during exercise. Rats who underwent spontaneous (voluntary) wheel running training were compared with sedentary controls during wheel running at the same submaximal running velocity. Submaximal exercise resulted in less neuronal activation in the posterior (caudal) hypothalamus, periaqueductal gray, nucleus of the tractus solitarius, rostral ventrolateral medulla, and cuneiform nucleus in the exercise-trained compared with the sedentary rats (Fig. 7.30). Thus, based on these results, neuronal activation in selective sites at all levels of the CNS appears to be lower during submaximal dynamic exercise in the endurance-trained than in the sedentary state. This altered state of CNS activation likely is mediated by some combination of reduced central command, less arterial baroreflex resetting, and possibly reduced excitatory feedback from the active muscles.

More recent data from Iwamoto and colleagues (152,153) provide evidence for a possible role of neuronal remodeling in the reduced CNS neuronal activity associated with performance of submaximal exercise in the exercise-trained state. Specifically, structural changes consisting of reductions in the dendritic fields of neurons located in the cardiorespiratory and locomotor control sites described previously were found in animals who had undergone up to 4 months of voluntary wheel running compared with sedentary animals (Fig. 7.30). These changes were reversed after a period of cessation of wheel running (detraining). The findings support the idea that chronic exercise causes "remodeling" of neurons in the brain activated by exercise, which may cause or contribute to reduced neuronal activation during submaximal exercise, which, in turn, results in altered ANS outflow to the periphery (i.e., increased vagal activity to the heart and/or reduced SNS activity). The altered peripheral ANS activity would cause or contribute to the changes in physiologic function observed during submaximal exercise in the trained state. Work from Mueller and colleagues (154) provide strong support for the idea that habitual exercise evokes adaptations in neuroplasticity in the rostral ventrolateral medulla and other areas of the brain that, in turn, influence sympathetic outflow.

KEY POINT

Habitual exercise influences neuroplasticity in the brain, which changes central ANS outflow to peripheral tissues.

TEST YOURSELF

Which of these signals likely have been altered by the type of physical activity that you (or a friend) regularly perform and, thus, contribute to your present ANS activity at rest and during acute submaximal exercise?

Endurance Training and Tissue Responsiveness to Adrenergic Stimulation

There is extensive experimental literature concerning the effects of endurance exercise training on tissue responsiveness to adrenergic receptor stimulation. Unfortunately, overall the results of this research are highly inconsistent.

Endurance training and vascular responsiveness to α-adrenergic stimulation

The influence of the endurance exercise–trained state on vascular responsiveness to α-adrenergic stimulation has been studied by examining the vasoconstrictor response of isolated arterial blood vessels, specific regional circulations, or the overall (systemic) circulation to specific α-adrenergic agonists (typically phenylephrine) or to NE, a nonspecific adrenergic agonist. The advantage of agonists such as phenylephrine is greater specificity for the α-adrenergic receptor (i.e., the associated vasoconstrictor response is presumed to be largely or solely mediated by this receptor signaling system); the disadvantage is some potential nonspecific β-adrenergic agonist effects and the fact that phenylephrine is not a natural endogenous (physiologic) agonist but rather a pharmacologic stimulus. The advantage of NE is that it is the primary neurotransmitter released from postganglionic sympathetic nerve endings that binds to α-adrenergic receptors and evokes physiologic vasoconstriction, although the actions of exogenously administrated NE are thought to be somewhat different from those of neuronally released NE. (This can be avoided by administering drugs that stimulate endogenous NE release from sympathetic nerve endings such as hexamethonium.) The major disadvantage of NE as an α-adrenergic receptor agonist is that it is also an agonist for β-adrenergic receptors. Because of this, the vasoconstrictor effects of NE mediated by stimulation of α-adrenergic receptors cannot be isolated because of the potential for concomitant stimulation of vasodilation via β_2-adrenergic receptors.

Vasoconstrictor responsiveness to phenylephrine has been found to be reduced (155), not different (140,143,156), or enhanced (26,157) in the endurance-trained compared with the untrained state. Similarly, vasoconstrictor responsiveness to NE has been reported to be impaired (158), not different (143), or increased (159) in the exercise-trained state. When exercise training–associated reductions in vasoconstrictor responsiveness to α-adrenergic receptor stimulation are observed,

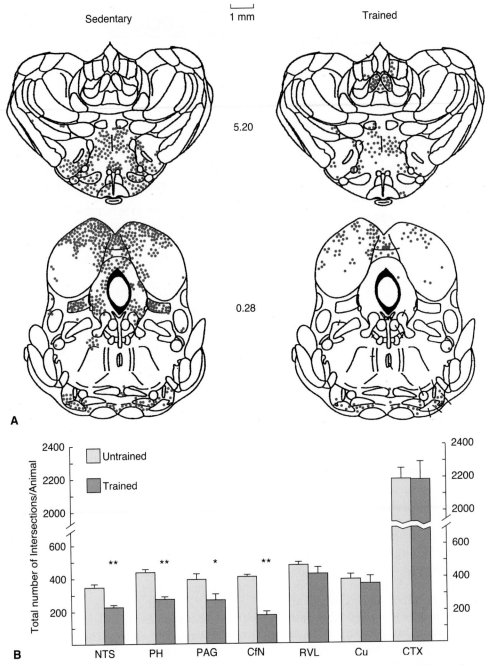

FIGURE 7.30   A. Representative Fos data contrasting a single bout of exercise wheel activity at a fixed submaximal speed in an endurance exercise–trained and an untrained rat in selected standard rat brain stereotaxic planes: 5.20 is the level of the caudal hypothalamus and 0.28 is midbrain. Each dot signifies three cells. Other areas in the medulla were studied, but are not depicted. Each of the following areas showed a statistically significant reduction in Fos immunoreactivity in the trained versus the seden-tary animals in response to the exercise bout: rostral ventrolateral medulla; caudal hypothalamus and locomotor region (ventro-medial part of 5.2 level); mesencephalic locomotor region (cuneiform); periaqueductal gray matter (dorsal medial part of 0.28 level surrounding cerebral aqueduct); and medial nucleus of the tractus solitarius. Areas showing large reductions in activity that did not quite reach levels of statistical significance included the lateral hypothalamus and cuneiform nucleus (mesencephalic loco-motor region). (Stereotaxic figures adapted from Paxinos G, Watson C. *The Rat Brain in Stereotaxic Coordinates.* 2nd ed. Orlando, FL: Academic Press; 1986. Modified with permission from Ichiyama RM, Gilbert AB, Waldrop TG, et al. Changes in the exercise activation of diencephalic and brainstem cardiorespiratory areas after training. *Brain Res.* 2002;947:230.). **B.** Summary data from a Sholl analysis depicting the number of dendrites at fixed distances from the soma ("intersections"), a direct reflection of the size of the dendritic field, in exercise-trained and untrained (sedentary) animals in response to acute exercise. Note that in critical car-diovascular control areas the number of intersections and, hence, the size of the dendritic arborization is reduced with training indicating structural remodeling of neurons. NTS, nucleus of the tractus solitarius; PH, posterior hypothalamus; PAG, periaq-ueductal gray; CfN, cuneiform nucleus; RVL, rostral ventrolateral medulla; Cu, nucleus cuneatus; CTX, cerebral cortex (motor areas); * $P < 0.05$; ** $P < 0.01$ vs. sedentary. (From Nelson AJ, Juraska JM, Musch TI, et al. Neuroplastic adaptations to exercise: neuronal remodeling in cardiorespiratory and locomotor areas. *J Appl Physiol.* 2005;99:2312–2322.)

there is evidence that the reductions are mediated by increased nitric oxide–dependent endothelial vasodilatory tone (155). However, the overall results concerning the relation between endurance exercise training and vascular responsiveness to α-adrenergic receptor stimulation are equivocal.

Endurance training and tissue responsiveness to β-adrenergic stimulation

The effects of endurance exercise training on tissue responsiveness to β-adrenergic receptor stimulation has been studied by measuring cardiac (heart rate, ventricular contractility) and/or vascular (vasodilation in arterial blood vessels or the overall arterial circulation) responses to infusion of β-adrenergic receptor agonists such as isoproterenol or dobutamine. Cardiac responses are mediated by both β_1- (primarily) and β_2-adrenergic receptors, whereas peripheral vasodilation is mediated by β_2-adrenergic receptors. Most often the nonselective β-adrenergic receptor agonist isoproterenol has been used to determine both cardiac and peripheral vascular responsiveness.

Using these methods, cardiac and vascular responsiveness to β-adrenergic receptor stimulation has been found to be reduced (128,157,160), not different (161,162), or augmented (163,164) in the exercise-trained versus sedentary state. Similarly, β-adrenergic receptor density and affinity have been reported to be decreased (160), not different (157,162), or increased (165). Thus, as with vasoconstrictor responsiveness to α-adrenergic receptor stimulation, the results of investigations concerning the effects of the endurance-trained state on cardiac and vascular responsiveness to β-adrenergic receptor stimulation, as well as on β-adrenergic receptor properties, are equivocal.

Sources of variability in data concerning endurance training and tissue responsiveness to adrenergic stimulation

Because tissue responsiveness to SNS adrenergic stimulation plays such a key role in the ANS-mediated physiologic adaptations to exercise training, it is important to understand the potential sources of the variability in the experimental results just described. These sources include the following:

- Use of various experimental animal models and human subjects (species differences).
- Local versus systemic arterial administration of adrenergic receptor agonists.
- Systemic infusion of adrenergic agonists with intact versus absent baroreflexes; intact baroreflexes will actively counter-regulate agonist-induced changes in arterial blood pressure by evoking ANS adjustments, which in turn confound interpretation of the results (140,156,166).

- Use of selective (*e.g.*, specific β_1-adrenergic) versus nonselective (*e.g.*, nonspecific β_1- and β_2-adrenergic) agonists causes stimulation of different receptor populations.
- Use of cross-sectional compared with intervention study designs.
- Comparisons of responses between different cardiovascular tissues (*e.g.*, heart vs. peripheral arterial blood vessels) or different functions within the same organ (*e.g.*, heart rate vs. left ventricular contractile response).
- Differences in baseline adrenergic responsiveness in the untrained subject groups among studies as a result of differences in age, degree of sedentary lifestyle (deconditioning), and so on.
- Differences in fiber type of the muscles in which blood flow measurements are made in animal studies (167).

CHAPTER SUMMARY

The ANS plays an important role in mediating the cardiovascular, thermoregulatory, and metabolic adjustments required to maintain internal homeostasis during acute physical exercise. These ANS-mediated physiologic adjustments are necessary to achieve one's true maximal aerobic capacity and submaximal endurance exercise performance.

A variety of experimental approaches, each with its own strengths and limitations, have been used to study the ANS at rest and during acute exercise. Using these methods, experimental evidence has established that cardiac vagal activity is reduced at the onset of even mild exercise, which produces an immediate increase in heart rate and cardiac output, providing blood flow to active muscle while supporting arterial blood pressure in the face of active muscle vasodilation–associated increases in total vascular conductance. Activation of the sympathoadrenal system occurs at moderate to heavy submaximal exercise intensities, further increasing cardiac output via stimulation of heart rate and left ventricular contractility. This sympathoadrenal activation also produces vasoconstriction of arterioles that (a) redistributes the increased cardiac output away from certain regional circulations (kidney, gut, inactive muscle) to active muscle and (b) restricts active muscle vasodilation to maintain systemic vascular resistance and most important, arterial blood pressure at levels required for proper perfusion of vital organs. The temporal pattern and magnitude of these ANS adjustments during acute exercise are determined by a number of modulatory influences including the intensity and duration of the exercise, sex of the individual or group, type of exercise, size of the active muscle mass, ambient temperature, and body position, among others. The ANS adjustments

The Milestone of Discovery experiment on the autonomic nervous system and exercise actually is two novel complementary experiments, both conducted by Professor Ron Victor and colleagues at Southwestern Medical School in Dallas. The studies addressed a critical but unanswered question at the time: the nature of the intracellular biochemical events that are responsible for activation of active muscle chemoreflexes during exercise in humans. These investigations were chosen for their use of novel experimental approaches, how well they complement each other, and the influence of the results on our understanding of the physiology of these events and on future research in this area.

Both investigations focus on the association between isometric exercise–induced increases in glycolysis, consequent generation of hydrogen ion and reductions in pH, and the increases in efferent sympathetic nervous system (SNS) activity (inactive muscle sympathetic nerve activity [MSNA]). In the first study, published in 1988, Dr. Victor and his colleagues performed simultaneous measurements of phosphorus nuclear magnetic resonance spectroscopy (^{31}P-NMR) in the active forearm muscle and MSNA in the peroneal nerve of an inactive leg during sustained submaximal isometric and rhythmic handgrip exercise in healthy young adult humans. During both types of exercise, increases in MSNA

coincided with intracellular accumulation of hydrogen ion and reductions in pH in the active forearm muscles. During sustained exercise, MSNA correlated strongly with reductions in intracellular pH (Fig. 7.31). Their primary conclusion was that stimulation of SNS outflow during exercise-evoked muscle chemoreflex activation is coupled to intracellular accumulation of hydrogen ions.

In the second study, published in 1990, Dr. Victor and his colleagues used an "experiment of nature" to independently confirm these initial observations. Specifically, they studied the physiologic responses to isometric handgrip exercise in groups of normal subjects and in patients with muscle phosphorylase deficiency. This disorder, McArdle's disease, is an inborn enzymatic defect of skeletal muscle that prevents glycolysis and, therefore, hydrogen ion accumulation and reductions in pH during exercise. Normal subjects demonstrated exercise-induced reductions in active forearm muscle pH and corresponding increases in peroneal MSNA in an inactive leg. In contrast, during exercise, the patients with McArdle's disease did not produce a reduction in active forearm muscle pH nor did they demonstrate increases in peroneal MSNA (Fig. 7.32). These findings confirmed that muscle chemoreflex–evoked stimulation of MSNA depends on augmentation of intracellular glycolysis and reduction in pH in the active muscles.

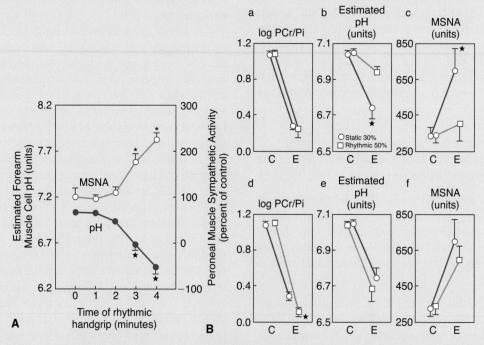

FIGURE 7.31 **A.** Active forearm muscle pH and peroneal (inactive leg) muscle sympathetic nerve activity (MSNA) during 4 minutes of rhythmic handgrip exercise (2 minutes at 30% maximal voluntary contraction [MVC] followed by 2 minutes at 50% MVC) performed by healthy young subjects. Note the tight association between the exercise-induced reductions in pH and increases in MSNA. **B.** MSNA changes from resting control levels in response to handgrip exercise with (*a–c*) comparable reductions in [PCr]/[Pi] or with (*d–f*) comparable reductions in pH. The MSNA responses were consistently associated with changes in pH but not with changes in [PCr]/[Pi]. (Modified from Victor RG, Bertocci LA, Pryor SL, et al. Sympathetic nerve discharge is coupled to muscle cell pH during exercise in humans. *J Clin Invest.* 1988;82:1301–1305, as published by Seals DR, Victor RG. Regulation of sympathetic nerve activity during exercise in humans. *Exerc Sport Sci Rev.* 1991;19:336.)

A **MILESTONE** OF DISCOVERY

The key conclusion from these studies, which were confirmed and subsequently extended and refined by the elegant work of MacLean and colleagues (87) and Sinoway and associates (87,89), was that intracellular biochemical events linked to the stimulation of active muscle glycolysis are important mechanisms underlying activation of muscle chemoreflexes and the increase in MSNA during small-muscle exercise in humans.

Victor RG, Bertocci LA, Pryor SL, et al. Sympathetic nerve discharge is coupled to muscle cell pH during exercise in humans. J Clin Invest. 1988;82:1301–1305.

Pryor SL, Lewis SF, Haller RG, et al. Impairment of sympathetic activation during static exercise in patients with muscle phosphorylase deficiency (McArdle's disease). J Clin Invest. 1990;85:1444–1449.

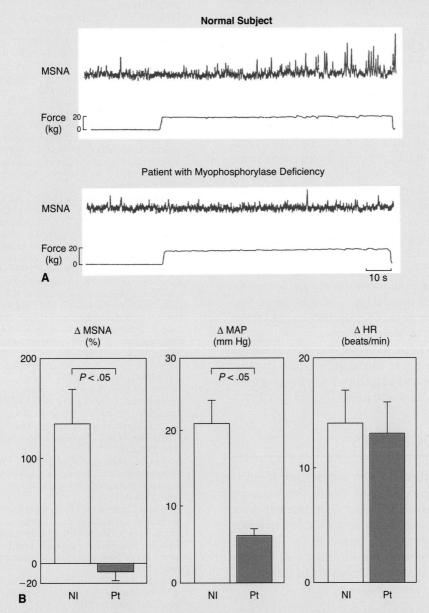

FIGURE 7.32   A. Peroneal muscle sympathetic nerve activity (MSNA) and handgrip force before and during 90 seconds of isometric handgrip exercise at 30% of maximal voluntary contraction (MVC) in a normal subject (*top*) and a patient with myophosphorylase deficiency (*below*). The MSNA increased during handgrip exercise in the normal subject but not in the patient. **B.** Increases above resting control levels of MSNA, mean arterial blood pressure (MAP), and heart rate (HR) during isometric handgrip exercise in groups of normal subjects (NI) and patients (Pt). In contrast to the normal subjects, the patients failed to evoke any increase in MSNA, produced an attenuated MAP response, but demonstrated normal tachycardia during handgrip exercise. (Modified from Pryor SL, Lewis SF, Haller RG, et al. Impairment of sympathetic activation during static exercise in patients with muscle phosphorylase deficiency [McArdle's disease]. *J Clin Invest.* 1990;85:1444–1449 as published by Seals DR, Victor RG. Regulation of muscle sympathetic nerve activity during exercise in humans. *Exerc Sport Sci Rev.* 1991;19:339.)

to acute exercise are stimulated by central command signals generated as part of neuromuscular activation; these central command signals are modulated by several sources of sensory afferent feedback from the periphery to the CNS, including active muscle reflexes and arterial baroreflexes. The key interaction may involve central command–induced resetting of the arterial baroreflex operating pressure. These collective CNS inputs modify the neuronal activity of various regions of the brain involved in ANS-cardiorespiratory control to produce the appropriate efferent (peripheral) ANS adjustments during acute exercise.

Repeated performance of large-muscle dynamic exercise results in specific ANS adaptations that are intended to accommodate the demands of the exercise and allow the exercise to be sustained while reducing tissue stress, thus increasing the resistance of the body to loss of homeostasis. Such ANS adaptations are most consistently evident during submaximal exercise performed at the same absolute intensity and duration in the exercise-trained and the sedentary states. Under these exercise conditions, there is less of a reduction in cardiac vagal modulation of heart rate and less sympathoadrenal activation in the endurance-trained state. These reduced ANS adjustments to submaximal exercise in the trained state are associated with correspondingly reduced neuronal activation in regions of the brain involved in the control of ANS outflow to the periphery, perhaps as a result of dendritic remodeling in nuclei involved in cardiorespiratory and locomotor control. This reduced neuronal activation in the trained state is most likely mediated by a smaller level of central command and arterial baroreflex resetting during the same submaximal exercise condition. The role of changes in tissue responsiveness to adrenergic receptor stimulation in mediating the ANS adaptations to endurance exercise training has not been established.

ACKNOWLEDGMENTS

For this revision, I thank Kristen Jablonski for identifying the new experimental literature, Dorincy Mariathas for administrative assistance, Professor Gary Iwamoto from the University of Illinois for his important contributions related to the sections on CNS control of the ANS with acute and chronic exercise, and Professor Gail Thomas from the Cedars Sinai Medical Center in Los Angeles for editing the section on sympatholysis.

REFERENCES

1. Christensen NJ, Galbo H. Sympathetic nervous activity during exercise. *Annu Rev Physiol.* 1983;45:139–153.
2. Epstein S, Robinson BF, Kahler RL, et al. Effects of beta-adrenergic blockade on the cardiac response to maximal and submaximal exercise in man. *J Clin Invest.* 1965;44:1745–1753.
3. Martin CE, Shaver JA, Leon DF, et al. Autonomic mechanisms in hemodynamic responses to isometric exercise. *J Clin Invest.* 1974;54:104–115.
4. Robinson BF, Epstein SE, Beiser GD, et al. Control of heart rate by the autonomic nervous system. Studies in man on the interrelation between baroreceptor mechanisms and exercise. *Circ Res.* 1966;19:400–411.
5. Galbo H. *Hormonal and Metabolic Adaptation to Exercise.* Stuttgart, New York: Thieme-Stratton; 1983.
6. Rowell LB. *Human Circulation Regulation During Physical Stress.* New York: Oxford University; 1986.
7. Nonogaki K. New insights into sympathetic regulation of glucose and fat metabolism. *Diabetologia.* 2000;43:533–549.
8. Tipton CM. *The Autonomic Nervous System.* New York: Oxford University; 2003.
9. Robinson S, Pearcy M, Brueckman FR, et al. Effects of atropine on heart rate and oxygen intake in working man. *J Appl Physiol.* 1953;5:508–512.
10. Ekblom B, Goldbarg AN, Kilbom A, et al. Effects of atropine and propranolol on the oxygen transport system during exercise in man. *Scand J Clin Lab Invest.* 1972;30:35–42.
11. Wilmore JH, Ewy GA, Freund BJ, et al. Cardiorespiratory alterations consequent to endurance exercise training during chronic beta-adrenergic blockade with atenolol and propranolol. *Am J Cardiol.* 1985;55:142D–148D.
12. Joyner MJ, Freund BJ, Jilka SM, et al. Effects of beta-blockade on exercise capacity of trained and untrained men: a hemodynamic comparison. *J Appl Physiol.* 1986;60:1429–1434.
13. Freyschuss U. Elicitation of heart rate and blood pressure increase on muscle contraction. *J Appl Physiol.* 1970;28:758–761.
14. Billman GE, Dujardin JP. Dynamic changes in cardiac vagal tone as measured by time-series analysis. *Am J Physiol.* 1990;258:H896–H902.
15. O'Leary DS, Rossi NF, Churchill PC. Substantial cardiac parasympathetic activity exists during heavy dynamic exercise in dogs. *Am J Physiol.* 1997;273:H2135–H2140.
16. Brenner IK, Thomas S, Shephard RJ. Autonomic regulation of the circulation during exercise and heat exposure: inferences from heart rate variability. *Sports Med.* 1998;26:85–99.
17. Carter JB, Banister EW, Blaber AP. Effect of endurance exercise on autonomic control of heart rate. *Sports Med.* 2003;33:33–46.
18. Casadei B, Cochrane S, Johnston J, et al. Pitfalls in the interpretation of spectral analysis of the heart rate variability during exercise in humans. *Acta Physiol Scand.* 1995;153:125–131.
19. Esler M, Jennings G, Lambert G, et al. Overflow of catecholamine neurotransmitters to the circulation: source, fate, and functions. *Physiol Rev.* 1990;70:963–985.
20. Grassi G, Esler M. How to assess sympathetic activity in humans. *J Hypertens.* 1999;17:719–734.
21. Mazzeo RS. Catecholamine responses to acute and chronic exercise. *Med Sci Sports Exerc.* 1991;23:839–845.
22. Rowell LB, O'Leary DS, Kellogg DL. Integration of cardiovascular control systems in dynamic exercise. In: Rowell LB, Sheperd JT, eds. *Handbook of Physiology.* New York: Oxford University; 1996:770–838.
23. Pernow J, Lundberg JM, Kaijser L, et al. Plasma neuropeptide Y-like immunoreactivity and catecholamines during various degrees of sympathetic activation in man. *Clin Physiol.* 1986;6:561–578.
24. Tidgren B, Hjemdahl P, Theodorsson E, et al. Renal neurohormonal and vascular responses to dynamic exercise in humans. *J Appl Physiol.* 1991;70:2279–2286.
25. Seals DR, Victor RG. Regulation of muscle sympathetic nerve activity during exercise in humans. *Exerc Sport Sci Rev.* 1991;19:313–349.
26. Kjaer M. Epinephrine and some other hormonal responses to exercise in man: with special reference to physical training. *Int J Sports Med.* 1989;10:2–15.
27. Bachman ES, Dhillon H, Zhang CY, et al. betaAR signaling required for diet-induced thermogenesis and obesity resistance. *Science.* 2002;297:843–845.
28. Arai Y, Saul JP, Albrecht P, et al. Modulation of cardiac autonomic activity during and immediately after exercise. *Am J Physiol.* 1989;256:H132–H141.
29. Fagraeus L, Linnarsson D. Autonomic origin of heart rate fluctuations at the onset of muscular exercise. *J Appl Physiol.* 1976;40:679–682.
30. Yamamoto Y, Hughson RL, Peterson JC. Autonomic control of heart rate during exercise studied by heart rate variability spectral analysis. *J Appl Physiol.* 1991;71:1136–1142.

31. Kukielka M, Seals DR, Billman GE. Cardiac vagal modulation of heart rate during prolonged submaximal exercise in animals with healed myocardial infarctions: effects of training. *Am J Physiol Heart Circ Physiol*. 2006;290:H1680–H1685.

32. DiCarlo SE, Bishop VS. Onset of exercise shifts operating point of arterial baroreflex to higher pressures. *Am J Physiol*. 1992;262:H303–H307.

33. O'Hagan KP, Bell LB, Mittelstadt SW, et al. Effect of dynamic exercise on renal sympathetic nerve activity in conscious rabbits. *J Appl Physiol*. 1993;74:2099–2104.

34. Tsuchimochi H, Matsukawa K, Komine H, et al. Direct measurement of cardiac sympathetic efferent nerve activity during dynamic exercise. *Am J Physiol Heart Circ Physiol*. 2002;283:H1896–H1906.

35. Saito M, Naito M, Mano T. Different responses in skin and muscle sympathetic nerve activity to static muscle contraction. *J Appl Physiol*. 1990;69:2085–2090.

36. Callister R, Ng AV, Seals DR. Arm muscle sympathetic nerve activity during preparation for and initiation of leg-cycling exercise in humans. *J Appl Physiol*. 1994;77:1403–1410.

37. Ray CA, Rea RF, Clary MP, et al. Muscle sympathetic nerve responses to dynamic one-legged exercise: effect of body posture. *Am J Physiol*. 1993;264:H1–H7.

38. Hasking GJ, Esler MD, Jennings GL, et al. Norepinephrine spillover to plasma during steady-state supine bicycle exercise: comparison of patients with congestive heart failure and normal subjects. *Circulation*. 1988;78:516–521.

39. Esler M, Kaye D, Thompson J, et al. Effects of aging on epinephrine secretion and regional release of epinephrine from the human heart. *J Clin Endocrinol Metab*. 1995;80:435–442.

40. Bloom SR, Johnson RH, Park DM, et al. Differences in the metabolic and hormonal response to exercise between racing cyclists and untrained individuals. *J Physiol*. 1976;258:1–18.

41. Galbo H, Holst JJ, Christensen NJ. Glucagon and plasma catecholamine responses to graded and prolonged exercise in man. *J Appl Physiol*. 1975;38:70–76.

42. Lehmann M, Keul J, Huber G, et al. Plasma catecholamines in trained and untrained volunteers during graduated exercise. *Int J Sports Med*. 1981;2:143–147.

43. Leuenberger U, Sinoway L, Gubin S, et al. Effects of exercise intensity and duration on norepinephrine spillover and clearance in humans. *J Appl Physiol*. 1993;75:668–674.

44. Saito M, Tsukanaka A, Yanagihara D, et al. Muscle sympathetic nerve responses to graded leg cycling. *J Appl Physiol*. 1993;75:663–667.

45. Victor RG, Seals DR, Mark AL. Differential control of heart rate and sympathetic nerve activity during dynamic exercise: insight from intraneural recordings in humans. *J Clin Invest*. 1987;79:508–516.

46. Savard G, Strange S, Kiens B, et al. Noradrenaline spillover during exercise in active versus resting skeletal muscle in man. *Acta Physiol Scand*. 1987;131:507–515.

47. Mazzeo RS, Rajkumar C, Jennings G, et al. Norepinephrine spillover at rest and during submaximal exercise in young and old subjects. *J Appl Physiol*. 1997;82:1869–1874.

48. Ichinose M, Saito M, Fujii N, et al. Modulation of the control of muscle sympathetic nerve activity during incremental leg cycling. *J Physiol*. 2008;586:2753–2766.

49. Manhem P, Lecerof H, Hokfelt B. Plasma catecholamine levels in the coronary sinus, the left renal vein and peripheral vessels in healthy males at rest and during exercise. *Acta Physiol Scand*. 1978;104:364–369.

50. Coker RH, Krishna MG, Zinker BA, et al. Sympathetic drive to liver and nonhepatic splanchnic tissue during prolonged exercise is increased in diabetes. *Metabolism*. 1997;46:1327–1332.

51. Rowell LB. *Human Cardiovascular Control*. New York: Oxford University; 1993.

52. Davy KP, Johnson DG, Seals DR. Cardiovascular, plasma norepinephrine, and thermal adjustments to prolonged exercise in young and older healthy humans. *Clin Physiol*. 1995;15:169–181.

53. Hagberg JM, Seals DR, Yerg JE, et al. Metabolic responses to exercise in young and older athletes and sedentary men. *J Appl Physiol*. 1988;65:900–908.

54. Saito M, Sone R, Ikeda M, et al. Sympathetic outflow to the skeletal muscle in humans increases during prolonged light exercise. *J Appl Physiol*. 1997;82:1237–1243.

55. Mazzeo RS, Marshall P. Influence of plasma catecholamines on the lactate threshold during graded exercise. *J Appl Physiol*. 1989;67:1319–1322.

56. Fattor JA, Miller BF, Jacobs KA, et al. Catecholamine response is attenuated during moderate-intensity exercise in response to the "lactate clamp." *Am J Physiol Endocrinol Metab*. 2005;288:E143–E147.

57. Joyner MJ, Thomas GD. Having it both ways? Vasoconstriction in contracting muscles. *J Physiol*. 2003;550:333.

58. Thomas GD, Segal SS. Neural control of muscle blood flow during exercise. *J Appl Physiol*. 2004;97:731–738.

59. Blomqvist CG, Lewis SF, Taylor WF, et al. Similarity of the hemodynamic responses to static and dynamic exercise of small muscle groups. *Circ Res*. 1981;48:187–192.

60. McMurray RG, Forsythe WA, Mar MH, et al. Exercise intensity-related responses of beta-endorphin and catecholamines. *Med Sci Sports Exerc*. 1987;19:570–574.

61. Galbo H, Houston ME, Christensen NJ, et al. The effect of water temperature on the hormonal response to prolonged swimming. *Acta Physiol Scand*. 1979;105:326–337.

62. Watson RD, Hamilton CA, Jones DH, et al. Sequential changes in plasma noradrenaline during bicycle exercise. *Clin Sci (Lond)*. 1980;58:37–43.

63. Anderson DE, Hickey MS. Effects of caffeine on the metabolic and catecholamine responses to exercise in 5 and 28 degrees C. *Med Sci Sports Exerc*. 1994;26:453–458.

64. Escourrou P, Johnson DG, Rowell LB. Hypoxemia increases plasma catecholamine concentrations in exercising humans. *J Appl Physiol*. 1984;57:1507–1511.

65. Esler MD, Thompson JM, Kaye DM, et al. Effects of aging on the responsiveness of the human cardiac sympathetic nerves to stressors. *Circulation*. 1995;91:351–358.

66. Seals DR, Enoka RM. Sympathetic activation is associated with increases in EMG during fatiguing exercise. *J Appl Physiol*. 1989;66:88–95.

67. Saito M, Mano T, Iwase S. Sympathetic nerve activity related to local fatigue sensation during static contraction. *J Appl Physiol*. 1989;67:980–984.

68. Matsukawa K, Mitchell JH, Wall PT, et al. The effect of static exercise on renal sympathetic nerve activity in conscious cats. *J Physiol*. 1991;434:453–467.

69. Iwamoto GA, Wappel SM, Fox GM, et al. Identification of diencephalic and brainstem cardiorespiratory areas activated during exercise. *Brain Res*. 1996;726:109–122.

70. Kaufman MP, Forster H. *Reflexes Controlling Circulatory, Ventilatory and Airway Responses to Exercise*. New York: Oxford University; 1996.

71. Waldrop T, Eldridge FL, Iwamoto GA, et al. *Central Neural Control of Respiration and Circulation During Exercise*. New York: Oxford University; 1996.

72. Williamson JW, Fadel PJ, Mitchell JH. New insights into central cardiovascular control during exercise in humans: a central command update. *Exp Physiol*. 2006;91:51–58.

73. Ichiyama RM, Waldrop TG, Iwamoto GA. Neurons in and near insular cortex are responsive to muscular contraction and have sympathetic and/or cardiac-related discharge. *Brain Res*. 2004;1008:273–277.

74. Green AL, Wang S, Purvis S, et al. Identifying cardiorespiratory neurocircuitry involved in central command during exercise in humans. *J Physiol*. 2007;578:605–612.

75. Potts JT, Waldrop TG. Discharge patterns of somatosensitive neurons in the nucleus tractus solitarius of the cat. *Neuroscience*. 2005;132:1123–1134.

76. Potts JT, Fong AY, Anguelov PI, et al. Targeted deletion of neurokinin-1 receptor expressing nucleus tractus solitarii neurons precludes somatosensory depression of arterial baroreceptor-heart rate reflex. *Neuroscience*. 2007;145:1168–1181.

77. Elam M, Svensson TH, Thoren P. Brain monoamine metabolism is altered in rats following spontaneous, long-distance running. *Acta Physiol Scand*. 1987;130:313–316.

78. Pagliari R, Peyrin L. Norepinephrine release in the rat frontal cortex under treadmill exercise: a study with microdialysis. *J Appl Physiol*. 1995;78:2121–2130.

79. Scheurink AJ, Steffens AB, Gaykema RP. Hypothalamic adrenoceptors mediate sympathoadrenal activity in exercising rats. *Am J Physiol*. 1990;259:R470–R477.

80. Overton JM, Redding MW, Yancey SL, et al. Hypothalamic GABAergic influences on treadmill exercise responses in rats. *Brain Res Bull*. 1994;33:517–522.

81. Potts JT. Exercise and sensory integration: role of the nucleus tractus solitarius. *Ann N Y Acad Sci.* 2001;940:221–236.
82. Victor RG, Pryor SL, Secher NH, et al. Effects of partial neuromuscular blockade on sympathetic nerve responses to static exercise in humans. *Circ Res.* 1989;65:468–476.
83. Alam M, Smirk FH. Unilateral loss of a blood pressure raising, pulse accelerating, reflex from voluntary muscle due to a lesion of the spinal cord. *Clin Sci.* 1938;3:247–252.
84. Williamson JW, McColl R, Mathews D, et al. Brain activation by central command during actual and imagined handgrip under hypnosis. *J Appl Physiol.* 2002;92:1317–1324.
85. Williamson JW, McColl R, Mathews D, et al. Hypnotic manipulation of effort sense during dynamic exercise: cardiovascular responses and brain activation. *J Appl Physiol.* 2001;90:1392–1399.
86. Vissing SF, Hjortso EM. Central motor command activates sympathetic outflow to the cutaneous circulation in humans. *J Physiol.* 1996;492 (pt 3):931–939.
87. MacLean DA, Vickery LM, Sinoway LI. Elevated interstitial adenosine concentrations do not activate the muscle reflex. *Am J Physiol Heart Circ Physiol.* 2001;280:H546–H553.
88. Sinoway LI, Smith MB, Enders B, et al. Role of diprotonated phosphate in evoking muscle reflex responses in cats and humans. *Am J Physiol.* 1994;267:H770–H778.
89. Alam M, Smirk FH. Observations in man upon a blood pressure raising reflex arising from the voluntary muscles. *J Physiol (London).* 1937;89:372–383.
90. Sinoway L, Prophet S, Gorman I, et al. Muscle acidosis during static exercise is associated with calf vasoconstriction. *J Appl Physiol.* 1989;66:429–436.
91. Victor RG, Bertocci LA, Pryor SL, et al. Sympathetic nerve discharge is coupled to muscle cell pH during exercise in humans. *J Clin Invest.* 1988;82:1301–1305.
92. Pryor SL, Lewis SF, Haller RG, et al. Impairment of sympathetic activation during static exercise in patients with muscle phosphorylase deficiency (McArdle's disease). *J Clin Invest.* 1990;85:1444–1449.
93. Ansorge EJ, Shah SH, Augustyniak RA, et al. Muscle metaboreflex control of coronary blood flow. *Am J Physiol Heart Circ Physiol.* 2002;283:H526–H532.
94. Herr MD, Imadojemu V, Kunselman AR, et al. Characteristics of the muscle mechanoreflex during quadriceps contractions in humans. *J Appl Physiol.* 1999;86:767–772.
95. Joyner MJ. Baroreceptor function during exercise: resetting the record. *Exp Physiol.* 2006;91:27–36.
96. Raven PB, Fadel PJ, Ogoh S. Arterial baroreflex resetting during exercise: a current perspective. *Exp Physiol.* 2006;91:37–49.
97. Melcher A, Donald DE. Maintained ability of carotid baroreflex to regulate arterial pressure during exercise. *Am J Physiol.* 1981;241:H838–H849.
98. Ichinose M, Saito M, Kondo N, et al. Time-dependent modulation of arterial baroreflex control of muscle sympathetic nerve activity during isometric exercise in humans. *Am J Physiol Heart Circ Physiol.* 2006;290:H1419–H1426.
99. Ogoh S, Fisher JP, Raven PB, et al. Arterial baroreflex control of muscle sympathetic nerve activity in the transition from rest to steady-state dynamic exercise in humans. *Am J Physiol Heart Circ Physiol.* 2007;293:H2202–H2209.
100. Ogoh S, Brothers RM, Barnes Q, et al. Cardiopulmonary baroreflex is reset during dynamic exercise. *J Appl Physiol.* 2006;100:51–59.
101. Goldsmith SR, Iber C, McArthur CD, et al. Influence of acid-base status on plasma catecholamines during exercise in normal humans. *Am J Physiol.* 1990;258:R1411–R1416.
102. Bouissou P, Defer G, Guezennec CY, et al. Metabolic and blood catecholamine responses to exercise during alkalosis. *Med Sci Sports Exerc.* 1988;20:228–232.
103. Seals DR, Suwarno NO, Dempsey JA. Influence of lung volume on sympathetic nerve discharge in normal humans. *Circ Res.* 1990;67:130–141.
104. Rodman JR, Henderson KS, Smith CA, et al. Cardiovascular effects of the respiratory muscle metaboreflexes in dogs: rest and exercise. *J Appl Physiol.* 2003;95:1159–1169.
105. Seals DR. Robin Hood for the lungs? A respiratory metaboreflex that "steals" blood flow from locomotor muscles. *J Physiol.* 2001;537:2.
106. Sala-Mercado JA, Ichinose M, Hammond RL, et al. Muscle metaboreflex attenuates spontaneous heart rate baroreflex sensitivity during dynamic exercise. *Am J Physiol Heart Circ Physiol.* 2007;292:H2867–H2873.
107. Kim JK, Sala-Mercado JA, Rodriguez J, et al. Arterial baroreflex alters strength and mechanisms of muscle metaboreflex during dynamic exercise. *Am J Physiol Heart Circ Physiol.* 2005;288:H1374–H1380.
108. Ekblom B, Kilbom A, Soltysiak J. Physical training, bradycardia, and autonomic nervous system. *Scand J Clin Lab Invest.* 1973;32:251–256.
109. Frick MH, Elovainio RO, Somer T. The mechanism of bradycardia evoked by physical training. *Cardiologia.* 1967;51:46–54.
110. Kenney WL. Parasympathetic control of resting heart rate: relationship to aerobic power. *Med Sci Sports Exerc.* 1985;17:451–455.
111. Yamamoto K, Miyachi M, Saitoh T, et al. Effects of endurance training on resting and post-exercise cardiac autonomic control. *Med Sci Sports Exerc.* 2001;33:1496–1502.
112. Goldsmith RL, Bigger JT Jr, Steinman RC, et al. Comparison of 24-hour parasympathetic activity in endurance-trained and untrained young men. *J Am Coll Cardiol.* 1992;20:552–558.
113. Herrlich HC, Raab W, Gigee W. Influence of muscular training and of catecholamines on cardiac acetylcholine and cholinesterase. *Arch Int Pharmacodyn Ther.* 1960;129:201–215.
114. Katona PG, McLean M, Dighton DH, et al. Sympathetic and parasympathetic cardiac control in athletes and nonathletes at rest. *J Appl Physiol.* 1982;52:1652–1657.
115. Meredith IT, Friberg P, Jennings GL, et al. Exercise training lowers resting renal but not cardiac sympathetic activity in humans. *Hypertension.* 1991;18:575–582.
116. Iellamo F, Legramante JM, Pigozzi F, et al. Conversion from vagal to sympathetic predominance with strenuous training in high-performance world class athletes. *Circulation.* 2002;105:2719–2724.
117. Ng AV, Callister R, Johnson DG, et al. Endurance exercise training is associated with elevated basal sympathetic nerve activity in healthy older humans. *J Appl Physiol.* 1994;77:1366–1374.
118. Peronnet F, Cleroux J, Perrault H, et al. Plasma norepinephrine response to exercise before and after training in humans. *J Appl Physiol.* 1981;51:812–815.
119. Jennings G, Nelson L, Nestel P, et al. The effects of changes in physical activity on major cardiovascular risk factors, hemodynamics, sympathetic function, and glucose utilization in man: a controlled study of four levels of activity. *Circulation.* 1986;73:30–40.
120. Poehlman ET, Danforth E Jr. Endurance training increases metabolic rate and norepinephrine appearance rate in older individuals. *Am J Physiol.* 1991;261:E233–E239.
121. Marker JC, Cryer PE, Clutter WE. Simplified measurement of norepinephrine kinetics: application to studies of aging and exercise training. *Am J Physiol.* 1994;267:E380–E387.
122. Seals DR. Sympathetic neural adjustments to stress in physically trained and untrained humans. *Hypertension.* 1991;17:36–43.
123. Svedenhag J, Wallin BG, Sundlof G, et al. Skeletal muscle sympathetic activity at rest in trained and untrained subjects. *Acta Physiol Scand.* 1984;120:499–504.
124. Sheldahl LM, Ebert TJ, Cox B, et al. Effect of aerobic training on baroreflex regulation of cardiac and sympathetic function. *J Appl Physiol.* 1994;76:158–165.
125. Ostman-Smith I. Adaptive changes in the sympathetic nervous system and some effector organs of the rat following long term exercise or cold acclimation and the role of cardiac sympathetic nerves in the genesis of compensatory cardiac hypertrophy. *Acta Physiol Scand Suppl.* 1979;477:1–118.
126. Mazzeo RS, Grantham PA. Norepinephrine turnover in various tissues at rest and during exercise: evidence for a training effect. *Metabolism.* 1989;38:479–483.
127. DeSchryver C, DeHerdt P, Lammerant J. Effect of physical training on cardiac catecholamine concentrations. *Nature.* 1967;214:907–908.
128. Hammond HK, White FC, Brunton LL, et al. Association of decreased myocardial beta-receptors and chronotropic response to isoproterenol and exercise in pigs following chronic dynamic exercise. *Circ Res.* 1987;60:720–726.
129. Dela F, Mikines KJ, von Linstow M, et al. Heart rate and plasma catecholamines during 24 h of everyday life in trained and untrained men. *J Appl Physiol.* 1992;73:2389–2395.

‌
‌
‌

130. Winder WW, Hagberg JM, Hickson RC, et al. Time course of sympathoadrenal adaptation to endurance exercise training in man. *J Appl Physiol.* 1978;45:370–374.
131. Hagberg JM, Hickson RC, McLane JA, et al. Disappearance of norepinephrine from the circulation following strenuous exercise. *J Appl Physiol.* 1979;47:1311–1314.
132. Greiwe JS, Hickner RC, Shah SD, et al. Norepinephrine response to exercise at the same relative intensity before and after endurance exercise training. *J Appl Physiol.* 1999;86:531–535.
133. Ordway GA, Charles JB, Randall DC, et al. Heart rate adaptation to exercise training in cardiac-denervated dogs. *J Appl Physiol.* 1982;52:1586–1590.
134. Wolfel EE, Hiatt WR, Brammell HL, et al. Effects of selective and nonselective beta-adrenergic blockade on mechanisms of exercise conditioning. *Circulation.* 1986;74:664–674.
135. Liang C, Tuttle RR, Hood WB Jr, et al. Conditioning effects of chronic infusions of dobutamine: comparison with exercise training. *J Clin Invest.* 1979;64:613–619.
136. Fry AC, Kraemer WJ, van Borselen F, et al. Catecholamine responses to short-term high-intensity resistance exercise overtraining. *J Appl Physiol.* 1994;77:941–946.
137. Peronnet F, Thibault G, Perrault H, et al. Sympathetic response to maximal bicycle exercise before and after leg strength training. *Eur J Appl Physiol Occup Physiol.* 1986;55:1–4.
138. Carter JR, Ray CA, Downs EM, et al. Strength training reduces arterial blood pressure but not sympathetic neural activity in young normotensive subjects. *J Appl Physiol.* 2003;94:2212–2216.
139. Ichiyama RM, Gilbert AB, Waldrop TG, et al. Changes in the exercise activation of diencephalic and brainstem cardiorespiratory areas after training. *Brain Res.* 2002;947:225–233.
140. Christou DD, Jones PP, Seals DR. Baroreflex buffering in sedentary and endurance exercise-trained healthy men. *Hypertension.* 2003;41:1219–1222.
141. Grassi G, Seravalle G, Calhoun DA, et al. Physical training and baroreceptor control of sympathetic nerve activity in humans. *Hypertension.* 1994;23:294–301.
142. Smith SA, Querry RG, Fadel PJ, et al. Differential baroreflex control of heart rate in sedentary and aerobically fit individuals. *Med Sci Sports Exerc.* 2000;32:1419–1430.
143. Bedford TG, Tipton CM. Exercise training and the arterial baroreflex. *J Appl Physiol.* 1987;63:1926–1932.
144. Bullough RC, Gillette CA, Harris MA, et al. Interaction of acute changes in exercise energy expenditure and energy intake on resting metabolic rate. *Am J Clin Nutr.* 1995;61:473–481.
145. Clausen JP, Klausen K, Rasmussen B, et al. Central and peripheral circulatory changes after training of the arms or legs. *Am J Physiol.* 1973;225:675–682.
146. Fisher WJ, White MJ. Training-induced adaptations in the central command and peripheral reflex components of the pressor response to isometric exercise of the human triceps surae. *J Physiol.* 1999;520(Pt 2):621–628.
147. Hakkinen K, Komi PV. Electromyographic changes during strength training and detraining. *Med Sci Sports Exerc.* 1983;15:455–460.
148. Saltin B, Nazar K, Costill DL, et al. The nature of the training response: peripheral and central adaptations of one-legged exercise. *Acta Physiol Scand.* 1976;96:289–305.
149. Elsner R, Carlson L. Post exercise hyperemia in trained and untrained subjects. *J Appl Physiol.* 1962;17:436–440.
150. Sinoway L, Shenberger J, Leaman G, et al. Forearm training attenuates sympathetic responses to prolonged rhythmic forearm exercise. *J Appl Physiol.* 1996;81:1778–1784.
151. Mostoufi-Moab S, Widmaier EJ, Cornett JA, et al. Forearm training reduces the exercise pressor reflex during ischemic rhythmic handgrip. *J Appl Physiol.* 1998;84:277–283.
152. Nelson AJ, Juraska JM, Musch TI, et al. Neuroplastic adaptations to exercise: neuronal remodeling in cardiorespiratory and locomotor areas. *J Appl Physiol.* 2005;99:2312–2322.
153. Nelson AJ, Iwamoto GA. Reversibility of exercise-induced dendritic attenuation in brain cardiorespiratory and locomotor areas following exercise detraining. *J Appl Physiol.* 2006;101:1243–1251.
154. Mueller, PJ. Physical (in)activity-dependent alterations at the rostral ventrolateral medulla: influence on sympathetic nervous system regulation. *Am J Physiol Regul Integr Comp Physiol.* 2010;298:R1468–R1474.
155. Delp MD, McAllister RM, Laughlin MH. Exercise training alters endothelium-dependent vasoreactivity of rat abdominal aorta. *J Appl Physiol.* 1993;75:1354–1363.
156. Jones PP, Shapiro LF, Keisling GA, et al. Is autonomic support of arterial blood pressure related to habitual exercise status in healthy men? *J Physiol.* 2002;540:701–706.
157. Svedenhag J, Martinsson A, Ekblom B, et al. Altered cardiovascular responsiveness to adrenoceptor agonists in endurance-trained men. *J Appl Physiol.* 1991;70:531–538.
158. Wiegman DL, Harris PD, Joshua IG, et al. Decreased vascular sensitivity to norepinephrine following exercise training. *J Appl Physiol.* 1981;51:282–287.
159. LeBlanc J, Boulay M, Dulac S, et al. Metabolic and cardiovascular responses to norepinephrine in trained and nontrained human subjects. *J Appl Physiol.* 1977;42:166–173.
160. Sylvestre-Gervais L, Nadeau A, Nguyen MH, et al. Effects of physical training on beta-adrenergic receptors in rat myocardial tissue. *Cardiovasc Res.* 1982;16:530–534.
161. Stratton JR, Cerqueira MD, Schwartz RS, et al. Differences in cardiovascular responses to isoproterenol in relation to age and exercise training in healthy men. *Circulation.* 1992;86:504–512.
162. Williams RS, Schaible TF, Bishop T, et al. Effects of endurance training on cholinergic and adrenergic receptors of rat heart. *J Mol Cell Cardiol.* 1984;16:395–403.
163. Hopkins MG, Spina RJ, Ehsani AA. Enhanced beta-adrenergic-mediated cardiovascular responses in endurance athletes. *J Appl Physiol.* 1996;80:516–521.
164. Lash JM. Exercise training enhances adrenergic constriction and dilation in the rat spinotrapezius muscle. *J Appl Physiol.* 1998;85:168–174.
165. Lehmann M, Dickhuth HH, Schmid P, et al. Plasma catecholamines, beta-adrenergic receptors, and isoproterenol sensitivity in endurance trained and non-endurance trained volunteers. *Eur J Appl Physiol Occup Physiol.* 1984;52:362–369.
166. Evans YM, Funk JN, Charles JB, et al. Endurance training in dogs increases vascular responsiveness to an alpha 1-agonist. *J Appl Physiol.* 1988;65:625–632.
167. Plourde G, Rousseau-Migneron S, Nadeau A. Effect of endurance training on beta-adrenergic system in three different skeletal muscles. *J Appl Physiol.* 1993;74:1641–1646.

CHAPTER 8

The Respiratory System

Lee M. Romer, A. William Sheel,
and Craig A. Harms

Abbreviations

$A\text{-}aD_{O_2}$	Alveolar to arterial oxygen partial pressure difference	$P_{A_{O_2}}$	Alveolar oxygen partial pressure
Ca_{O_2}	Arterial oxygen content	Pa_{O_2}	Arterial oxygen partial pressure
CNS	Central nervous system	P_{di}	Transdiaphragmatic pressure
COPD	Chronic obstructive pulmonary disease	P_{ga}	Gastric pressure
$C\bar{v}_{CO_2}$	Carbon dioxide content in mixed venous blood	P_{it}	Intrathoracic pressure
		P_{lung}	Lung surface pressure
$C\bar{v}_{O_2}$	Oxygen content in mixed venous blood	P_{pl}	Pleural pressure
EELV	End-expiratory lung volume	$\dot{Q}$	Pulmonary blood flow
EILV	End-inspiratory lung volume	Sa_{O_2}	Arterial oxyhemoglobin saturation
f_R	Respiratory frequency	TLC	Total lung capacity
FRC	Functional residual capacity	$\dot{V}_A$	Alveolar ventilation
NTS	Nucleus of the solitary tract	$\dot{V}_E$	Minute ventilation
P_{ab}	Abdominal pressure	$\dot{V}_{O_2}$	Oxygen uptake
P_{CO_2}	Carbon dioxide partial pressure	$\dot{V}_{O_{2max}}$	Maximum oxygen uptake
Pa_{CO_2}	Alveolar carbon dioxide partial pressure	$\dot{V}_{CO_2}$	Carbon dioxide production
Pa_{CO_2}	Arterial carbon dioxide partial pressure	V_D	Dead space volume
P_{O_2}	Oxygen partial pressure	V_T	Tidal volume

Introduction

The respiratory system is responsible for the first two steps in oxygen transport from inspired air to muscle mitochondria: the bulk transport of oxygen from atmospheric air to alveoli and the transfer of oxygen from alveolar gas to pulmonary capillaries. The respiratory system is also responsible for regulating carbon dioxide levels in the body and for much of the regulation of pH. Importantly, arterial blood gas homeostasis should be maintained at a minimum energy expense to the organism. In addition, pulmonary vascular resistance and vascular pressures must remain low to limit the load on the right heart and prevent trauma to the delicate alveolar–capillary interface.

From rest to moderate exercise, these goals are readily met in the healthy humans with use of only a small portion of the structural and functional capabilities of the respiratory system. However, during high-intensity exercise, the respiratory system may present a significant limitation to systemic oxygen delivery and exercise performance due to an exercise-induced reduction in oxygen content (hypoxemia) and/or a decrease in limb blood flow in response to the considerable ventilatory requirements needed at high metabolic rates. This chapter examines how the normal human respiratory system is structured and how it is regulated by the nervous system to meet these exercise requirements. Emphasis is on the respiratory physiology of the healthy young adult exercising at sea level. We also consider the special needs and adaptations of the respiratory system that accompany development, aging and physical training, and the special circumstances that determine the balance (or imbalance) between metabolic demand and respiratory system capacity in both normal and highly trained subjects.

Control of Breathing

In healthy humans, breathing in all physiologic states (including wakefulness, sleep, and exercise) is remarkably well controlled. Consider that although the partial pressure of oxygen (PO_2) and partial pressure of carbon dioxide (PCO_2) within the alveoli are regulated precisely within a few millimeters of mercury, we are rarely aware of taking a breath and we effortlessly speak, cough, chew, swallow, and breathe, all through the same airway and using many of the same muscles. The control system that allows this multitasking to occur with such precision and efficiency consists of three highly integrative, overlapping levels of control:

- The central controller (or driver) of respiratory rhythm and pattern
- Distribution and synchronization of respiratory motor output to the appropriate respiratory muscles
- Sensory inputs to the central pattern generator

A schematic of most known components of the control system coupled with an outline of the primary motor and sensory pathways is shown in Figure 8.1. We briefly describe each of these components and their interactions before attempting to put them together to consider the complex mechanisms of exercise hyperpnea.

Central Controller

Nearly a century of research using neural lesioning and intracellular and extracellular neural recordings in mammalian preparations has begun to unmask a significant portion of the complex mystery surrounding the morphology and physiology of the central respiratory pattern generator. Eupneic breathing rhythm seems to reflect the output of a pontomedullary neuronal circuit. Within the ventral lateral medulla, a tiny area labeled the pre-Bötzinger complex and an even smaller adjacent area contain a combination of pacemaker-like neurons linked to a neural network. Together, this hybrid pacemaker and network system is capable of generating an oscillatory, respiratory-like rhythm (1). The rostral area of the pons is also capable of generating a respiratory rhythm (2). Ablation of either of these areas greatly disrupts the normal eupneic rhythm and it seems likely that the entire pontomedullary network is required for central generation of the respiratory rhythm.

The underlying rhythm from this network is relayed to larger adjacent networks of respiratory premotor medullary neurons called the ventral respiratory group and the ventral lateral nucleus of the solitary tract (NTS). Within these neuronal networks, the respiratory pattern is further sculpted in response to several types of sensory inputs, which are added to the basic rhythm (discussed later). This rhythmic

pattern is passed on via the spinal cord to the phrenic, intercostal, and abdominal motor nerves, which, in turn, drive the respiratory pump muscles to generate the appropriate level of intrathoracic pressure (P_{it}) for a breath. In addition, this same pattern of respiratory output is directed in parallel to cranial motor neurons, which lie primarily in the nucleus ambiguus and project out of cranial nerves IX to XII to innervate skeletal muscles of the upper airway, tongue, and smooth involuntary muscles of the trachea and bronchi.

Respiratory Motor Output

Although the breathing rhythm is conceptually simple (good air in, bad air out), the pattern of respiratory motor output from premotor neurons in the medulla must be much more than a simple sine wave. Indeed, a carefully sculpted, patterned output containing essential features such as precise timing and amplitude of pump muscle contractions and carefully controlled coordination of activation of the rib cage and the diaphragm musculature is necessary. Equally important, the motor control of the skeletal muscles regulating the extrathoracic (upper) airway that run from the tip of the nares (alae nasae) to the larynx (posterior cricoarytenoid) must be synchronized precisely with the chest wall pump muscles. This coordination ensures that the upper airway is prepared (via dilation and stiffening) for the subatmospheric (P_{it}) generated by the pump muscles with each inspiration.

This precise coordination of motor output requires not only several different types of premotor neurons in the medullary pattern generator but also a means for these neurons to know precisely what each other is doing throughout every millisecond of the breath. Six types of neurons within the central pattern generator have been identified with some, but incomplete, certainty: three for inspiration and three for expiration (Fig. 8.2A). Inspiratory and expiratory premotor neurons do not discharge simultaneously, but rather one set of neurons is silent while the other is active (Fig. 8.2B). Furthermore, the onset of inspiratory activity in cranial nerves innervating the muscles of the upper airway precedes that of the phrenic nerves (Fig. 8.2C). The coordination among neuronal activities is critically dependent on the principle of reciprocal inhibition among neurons such that the discharge of the inspiratory neuronal activity inhibits all expiratory neuronal activity and vice versa.

Summary

The past decade has brought significant advances in our understanding of the neuroanatomical basis for respiratory rhythm generation. Nevertheless, there is much controversy in the field and huge gaps in our knowledge still exist, even on such fundamental questions as the minimal pontomedullary structures required for the eupneic rhythm. We also have no information on the principles governing exactly how these neuronal networks integrate the underlying rhythm with the multitude of demands

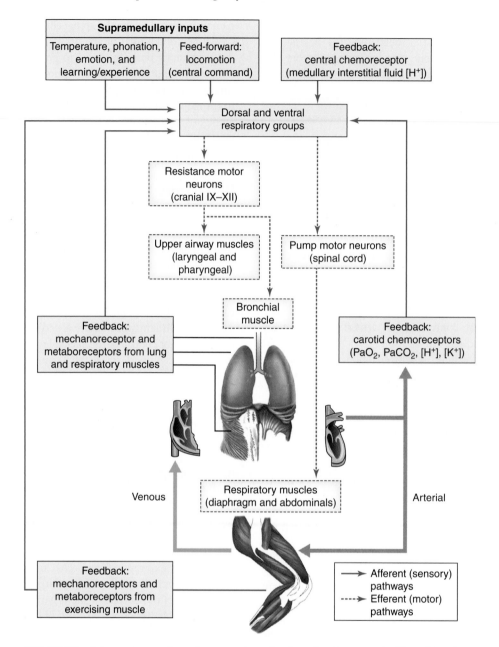

FIGURE 8.1   Schematic overview of proposed mechanisms for the control of breathing during exercise. Efferent (motor) pathways: motor output carried in cranial and spinal nerves and innervating muscles of the upper airway, bronchial muscle, and respiratory muscles. Afferent (sensory) pathways: inputs to the dorsal and ventral respiratory groups (medulla oblongata) originating from central (supramedullary regions, central chemoreceptors) and peripheral sites (working muscles, lung, respiratory muscles, carotid chemoreceptors). (Redrawn from Stickland MK, Amann M, Katayama K, et al. Pulmonary responses to exercise and limitations to human performance. In: Taylor NA, Groeller H, eds. *Physiological Bases of Human Performance during Work and Exercise*. New York: Churchill Livingstone; 2008:31, with permission.)

imposed by the many and varied sensory inputs to produce the desired breath. A major problem is that although in vitro and in situ preparations offer great advantages in terms of increased feasibility of intracellular recordings and expanded possibilities for precise ablation and experimental manipulation, these reduced preparations are unphysiologic. For example, in vitro brainstem–spinal cord preparations have no blood supply and are therefore anoxic at their inner core. Furthermore, these preparations are extremely limited in the extent to which they can mimic the ever-changing respiratory behaviors of the in vivo state, such as those that occur with hyperpnea. Perhaps even the specific types of neurons (Fig. 8.2A) may take on different roles as total respiratory drive is

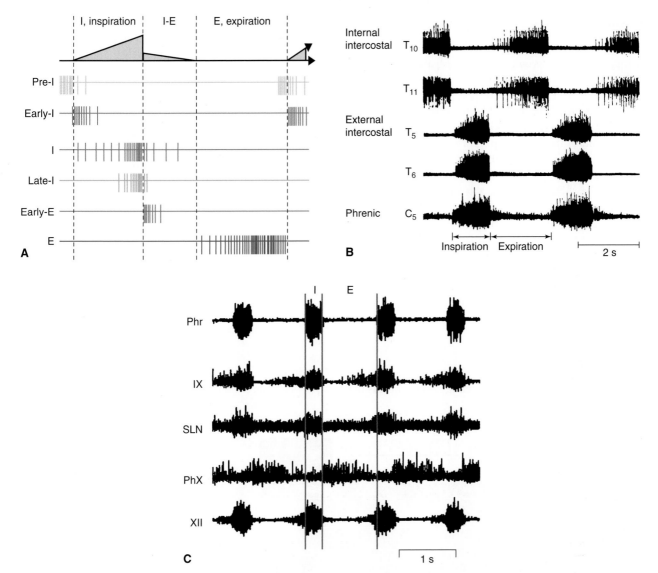

FIGURE 8.2 **A.** Patterns of discharge of the phrenic nerve (blue shaded area) and of brainstem respiratory neurons (traces at bottom) are shown to distinguish three stages in the respiratory cycle—namely, inspiration, inspiration–expiration transitions, and expiration—along with six types of respiratory neurons, three during inspiration and three during different phases of expiration. (Redrawn from Hilaire G, Pasaro R. Genesis and control of the respiratory rhythm in adult mammals. *News Physiol Sci.* 2003;18:26, with permission.) **B.** Spinal respiratory motor nerve activities to the expiratory intercostals (T_{10} and T_{11}), the inspiratory intercostals (T_5 and T_6), and the phrenic nerve to the diaphragm (C_5). Note the apparent reciprocal inhibition of expiratory nerve activity by inspiratory nerve activity and vice versa. Also note the continued phrenic nerve activity into early expiration, commonly called postinspiratory activity of the diaphragm; this activity is abruptly inhibited when ventilation is increased during exercise. (Redrawn from Hlastala MP, Berger AJ. *Physiology of Respiration.* New York: Oxford University Press; 1996:173, with permission.) **C.** Patterns of spontaneous respiratory activity on selected cranial and phrenic (Phr) nerves. Vertical lines indicate phase transitions between inspiration (I) and expiration (E). Note that the onset of inspiratory activity on cranial nerves to the muscles of the upper airway precedes that on Phr to the diaphragm. IX, glossopharyngeal nerve innervating muscles of the pharynx and tongue; SLN, superior laryngeal nerve innervating muscles of the larynx and constrictor muscles of the pharynx; PhX, pharyngeal branch of the vagus nerve; XII, hypoglossal nerve innervating intrinsic muscles of the tongue and neighboring pharyngeal muscles. (Redrawn from Hayashi F, McCrimmon DR. Respiratory motor responses to cranial nerve afferent stimulation in rats. *Am J Physiol.* 1996;271:R1055, with permission.)

changed, and each neuronal type may contribute to more than one phase of activity during the respiratory cycle. Almost all in vivo preparations used to study rhythm generation require anesthesia or decerebration, procedures which greatly blunt the sensitivity and stability of

the neuronal networks under study. A few chronically instrumented unanesthetized preparations are available, and these have provided valuable albeit limited data thus far on the genesis of respiratory rhythm in waking and sleeping states (3).

Sensory Inputs

Sensory inputs to the medulla originating in the periphery, the higher central nervous system (CNS), and the medulla itself are essential for the organism to breathe and for respiratory rhythm and pattern to respond appropriately to all physiologic states. It is claimed by scientists working with in vitro preparations that sensory afferents are not required for formation of the basic respiratory pattern because the respiratory-like rhythm from the phrenic nerve was shown to persist when the preparation was fully deafferented (4). However, the rhythm of the in vitro preparation is absolutely dependent on the addition of a significant concentration of carbon dioxide in the bathing medium; hence, at least one type of sensory input is required for rhythmic respiratory motor output.

We now describe two types of sensory inputs—chemical and mechanical—and leave consideration of sensory inputs related to locomotion to our later discussion of exercise hyperpnea.

Chemoreceptor feedback

Mammals have two types of chemoreceptors. One set is in the periphery and is exposed to arterial blood, whereas the other is central in the medulla and bathed by brain interstitial fluid. Traditionally, these receptors were viewed as independent entities responding solely to the oxygen partial pressure (P_{O_2}), P_{CO_2}, and pH in their environments. Newer evidence, however, has shown that these two types of receptors are not functionally separate, but rather they are dependent on one another such that the sensitivity of the medullary chemoreceptors is critically determined by input from the peripheral chemoreceptors and vice versa (5,6).

The carotid chemoreceptors are small (1-mm diameter) organs located bilaterally near the bifurcations of the common carotid arteries (Fig. 8.3A) and that respond quickly to changes in P_{O_2}, P_{CO_2}, and pH of the arterial blood on the way to the brain. Sensory activity is carried via the carotid sinus nerve, a branch of the glossopharyngeal nerve (cranial nerve IX), to stimulate the brainstem medullary respiratory neurons and influence motor nerve activity to the respiratory muscles. These organs receive the highest blood flow per gram of tissue of any organ and are especially important because they are the only receptors responsible for rapidly stimulating ventilation when oxygen availability is low. There are neurons in the ventral medulla that can sense low levels of oxygen, but it is not yet established what role they play in regulating breathing

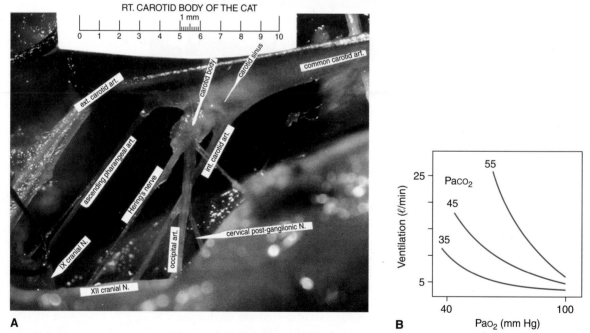

A   **B**

FIGURE 8.3   A. The intact carotid chemoreceptor of the cat. Head is to the left and heart to the right. Note the highly vascularized carotid body at the bifurcation of the common carotid artery. The sensory carotid sinus nerve, labeled here as its older designation, Hering's nerve, projects to the ninth nerve (glossopharyngeal), which, in turn, projects to the petrosal ganglion and then to the nucleus of the solitary tract. (Courtesy of Dr. E. H. Vidruk of the University of Wisconsin-Madison.) **B.** Effects of hypoxia and carbon dioxide on minute ventilation in the normal human. As arterial oxygen partial pressure (P_{aO_2}) is reduced (by gradually reducing inspired oxygen partial pressure), ventilation increases in a hyperbolic fashion. This effect of hypoxia on ventilation is enhanced by increasing arterial carbon dioxide partial pressure (P_{aCO_2}). Thus in the lowest response curve, P_{aCO_2} is maintained at 35 mm Hg and in the highest response curve at 55 mm Hg. These differences in P_{aCO_2} are achieved by adding carbon dioxide to the inspired gas as the P_{aO_2} is reduced. Note the strong interactive (greater than additive) effect of carbon dioxide on the hypoxic ventilatory response.

in the intact awake animal when both the central chemoreceptors and the brain are hypoxic.

Figure 8.3B shows the curvilinear response of ventilation to reductions in Pa_{O_2}. Normally, Pa_{CO_2} would be reduced when alveolar ventilation ($\dot{V}_A$) was stimulated, but in this case, Pa_{CO_2} was held constant by adding carbon dioxide to the inspired air so as to demonstrate the full strength of the hypoxic stimulus. The ventilatory response to hypoxia is curvilinear; under isocapnic conditions the response becomes brisk at 60 mm Hg Pa_{O_2}. This Pa_{O_2} corresponds to the shoulder of the oxyhemoglobin dissociation curve, below which oxyhemoglobin saturation drops severely and tissue hypoxia probably occurs. Reduced Pa_{O_2} and increased Pa_{CO_2} both stimulate ventilation via the carotid body and, when applied together, that is, during asphyxia, they have powerful synergistic effects on ventilatory output (7). The carotid chemoreceptors also respond briskly to ionic changes in the arterial blood, especially metabolically induced changes in pH, that is, metabolic acidosis or alkalosis. Furthermore, with acute changes in metabolic acid-base status, the carotid chemoreceptors are solely responsible for the ventilatory response. Carotid chemoreceptors respond to reduced Pa_{O_2} but do not respond to reduced arterial oxygen content (Ca_{O_2}) per se when it is caused by decreased hemoglobin concentration.

How chemoreception occurs within the carotid bodies is not entirely clear. The microscopic anatomy of this remarkable sensor reveals two types of cells, with the peripheral nerve endings terminating in the glomus, or type I cells. There is general consensus that an important step in the chemoreceptor response to decreased Pa_{O_2} is closure of potassium channels in type I cells, leading to cell depolarization and opening of voltage-gated calcium channels, calcium entry into the cell, release of various neurotransmitters, and transduction of the signal from the carotid body cells to the sensory nerve fiber. Possible sites for the oxygen sensors in type I cells include complexes of the mitochondrial electron transport chain, an extra-mitochondrial rotenone-sensitive protein, and a plasma membrane-associated heme oxygenase-2. Stimulation of the chemoreceptors by an increased Pa_{CO_2} is dependent on carbonic anhydrase (present in the type I cell) and there is therefore the possibility of both raised P_{CO_2} and decreased arterial pH acting through an increase in intracellular $[H^+]$.

Some of the medullary chemoreceptors have yet to be isolated anatomically, although several locations near the ventrolateral surface of the medulla are very sensitive to changes in interstitial brain fluid pH, especially when pH is changed by an increase or decrease in P_{CO_2} (8) (Fig. 8.3B). The cerebral fluid environment of these medullary chemoreceptors has a closely regulated ionic composition because of the selective permeability of the capillary endothelium of cerebral blood vessels, that is, the so-called blood–brain barrier. Thus, metabolic acids and bases in the plasma enter the brain interstitial fluid very slowly, whereas carbon dioxide crosses readily and changes the pH of the medullary interstitial fluid very quickly and substantially.

On balance, the ventilatory response to increased carbon dioxide in the arterial blood and the brain is a result of both peripheral carotid chemoreceptor and central medullary chemoreceptor stimulation. In the steady state, after several minutes of raised arterial carbon dioxide partial pressure (Pa_{CO_2}), the medullary chemoreceptors are the major contributors to the increased ventilation. However, the carotid chemoreceptors still respond strongly to small increases and decreases in Pa_{CO_2}. Furthermore, when Pa_{CO_2} is changing dynamically, the carotid chemoreceptors are the sole initiators of the ventilatory response.

The ventilatory response to inhaled carbon dioxide is much more linear than to hypoxia. This likely reflects the fact that even small changes in carbon dioxide will change plasma and tissue pH, and that the sensitive ventilatory response to acute changes in carbon dioxide is designed to defend pH. On the other hand, when arterial oxygen partial pressure (Pa_{O_2}) is reduced, the high affinity of hemoglobin for oxygen at Pa_{O_2} levels greater than 70 mm Hg prevents appreciable reductions in oxyhemoglobin saturation and systemic oxygen transport until Pa_{O_2} is greatly reduced. Thus, the ventilatory response to "pure" hypoxemia is more linearly related to the percentage of oxyhemoglobin saturation.

Chemoreceptors perform classical negative feedback control of breathing and, as such, are intimately involved as error detectors every time breathing is changed. For example, if for any reason $\dot{V}_A$ is increased or reduced out of proportion to tissue carbon dioxide production (V_{CO_2}) or oxygen consumption, alveolar and arterial P_{CO_2} and P_{O_2} will rise or fall, respectively. Within the circulation time from the alveoli to the carotid chemoreceptor (<10 seconds) the carotid chemoreceptors will react by changing phrenic nerve output and ventilation in a direction that restores the P_{CO_2} to its normal range. Roughly 15 to 20 seconds later, the medullary chemoreceptors will follow suit and respond to the lingering changes in P_{CO_2}. Accordingly, these chemoreceptors are the vigilant guardians of their own chemical environment and—as we shall see—are important to the regulation of exercise ventilation.

Mechanoreceptor feedback

To maintain precise and mechanically efficient control of breathing, it is crucial that the pattern generating neurons in the medulla are constantly made aware of the mechanical state of the lung and the mechanical and metabolic state of the respiratory muscles. Accordingly, the lung and airways are richly innervated by vagal afferents serving several types of receptors and afferent fibers. The slowly adapting fibers in the lung respond to lung stretch by providing feedback to the medulla via the vagus nerves to inhibit inspiration. This inhibitory effect limits end-inspiratory lung volume (EILV), usually to the linear portion of the lung's compliance curve, thereby avoiding the increased stiffness of the lung at high lung volumes. Input from the pontine respiratory neurons to the medullary pattern generator provides an additional source of inhibition to inspiration. Lung stretch receptors also provide an excitatory input to the medullary respiratory neurons in response to lung deflation; thus, they may be responsible for activating augmented inspirations (or sighs), which occur periodically to prevent excessive airway narrowing at low lung volumes. Additional vagally mediated receptors in the lung parenchyma include unmyelinated C-fiber endings, which respond to changes in lung interstitial fluid pressure and have marked effects on ventilatory drive and frequency. Finally, many other receptors in the intrathoracic airways are sensitive to pressure deformation of the mucosal wall, particulate matter, temperature, and so on, most of which cause coughing or changes in bronchial smooth muscle tone to protect the lung from injury and foreign matter.

Respiratory muscles, including the diaphragm and abdominal muscles, have receptors that are classified as type III (primarily mechanical) and type IV (primarily metabolic) (9). These receptors send feedback to the medulla via afferent fibers within the major motor nerves, such as the phrenic which innervates the diaphragm. Feedback from these receptors exerts significant effects on the control of both ventilation and circulation (discussed later in the section *Cardiorespiratory Interactions during Exercise*). Afferent feedback from upper airway skeletal muscles, responding to pressure and airway wall deformation, is also important for the activation of cranial nerve motor activity directed at stiffening and abducting the pharyngeal and laryngeal musculature for purposes of protecting upper airway patency.

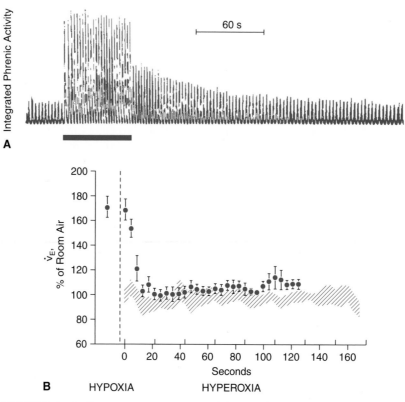

FIGURE 8.4 **A.** Short-term potentiation of the ventilatory response to carotid chemoreceptor stimulation. Electrical stimulation of the carotid sinus nerve was used to suddenly increase carotid sinus nerve activity and to suddenly withdraw that activity in the anesthetized cat. Phrenic nerve activity increased during carotid sinus nerve stimulation and then slowly dissipated to return to control several seconds following the sudden cessation of carotid sinus nerve stimulation. (Redrawn from Eldridge FL, Gill-Kumar P. Lack of effect of vagal afferent input on central neural respiratory afterdischarge. *J Appl Physiol.* 1978;45:341, with permission.) **B.** Similar short-term potentiation effects have been shown in sleeping humans using brief periods of isocapnic hypoxia to stimulate ventilation and then hyperoxia to achieve sudden cessation of carotid chemoreceptor stimulation. Note that 45 seconds of isocapnic hypoxia increased ventilation ($\dot{V}_E$) to 170% of baseline $\dot{V}_E$. Then, after the third breath of hyperoxia, $\dot{V}_E$ remained more than 20% greater than control (hatched area) and did not return to control until the ninth hyperoxic recovery breath following hypoxia. (Redrawn from Badr MS, Skatrud JB, Dempsey JA. Determinants of poststimulus potentiation in humans during NREM sleep. *J Appl Physiol.* 1992;73:1962, with permission.)

Significant influences from these types of mechanoreceptor feedback on the control of breathing are well established for laboratory mammals, including rats, cats, dogs, and others. Vagal feedback from lung stretch has also been shown to be very powerful in the newborn human. However, the role of these mechanoreceptor feedback mechanisms in adult humans is less well established. Studies that have used mechanical ventilators to alter tidal volumes (V_T) in sleeping humans (to avoid behavioral responses to lung inflation) or in patients with denervated transplanted lungs have suggested that the pulmonary stretch reflex does play a role in inhibiting inspiratory ventilatory drive in adult humans, but the sensitivity to changes in lung volume seems to be significantly less than in most mammals (10).

Short-term Potentiation

The full effect of any given ventilatory stimulus on respiratory motor output lasts beyond the time of application of the stimulus. Examples of this memory response are shown during and following electrical stimulation of the carotid sinus nerve in the anesthetized animal (*i.e.*, mimicking carotid body stimulation) and after brief hypoxic ventilatory stimulation in the sleeping human (11) (Fig. 8.4). These aftereffects on respiratory motor output also occur in response to a wide variety of sensory stimuli, including those from central chemoreceptors or skeletal muscle (excitatory), or from vagal or superior laryngeal nerves (inhibitory). Thus, just as activation of a synapse and the firing of any neuron leaves behind an altered state of the neuron, or a memory of the preceding excitatory events, the network of neurons in the respiratory pattern generator also displays an intrinsic afterdischarge, or short-term potentiation, in response to its own neuronal activity. These lingering aftereffects are attributed to changes in the presynaptic membrane because repetitive neuronal firing causes gradual accumulation of calcium ions and increased neurotransmitter release, whereas the slow exponential decline in neural discharge is attributable to a slow removal of calcium ions from nerve terminals.

The implications of short-term potentiation for understanding the control of breathing are many, including the realization that the full ventilatory response to a given stimulus does not occur immediately and that short-term potentiation serves as a self-amplifying effect to boost the ventilatory output. Short-term potentiation also serves to smooth or stabilize the ventilatory response to prevent overshoots and undershoots during ventilatory transitions.

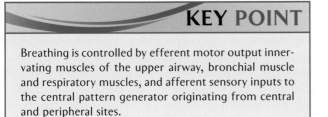

KEY POINT

Breathing is controlled by efferent motor output innervating muscles of the upper airway, bronchial muscle and respiratory muscles, and afferent sensory inputs to the central pattern generator originating from central and peripheral sites.

Exercise Hyperpnea

Requisites for Hyperpnea

The extra ventilation generated during exercise must accomplish two aims. First, increased $\dot{V}_A$ must be proportional to the increase in $\dot{V}_{CO_2}$ and oxygen uptake ($\dot{V}_{O_2}$) demanded by the muscular work according to the strict rules of the alveolar gas equations. These relationships are also shown graphically in Figure 8.5.

$$P_{ACO_2} = [\dot{V}_{CO_2} \div \dot{V}_A]\,K$$
$$P_{ACO_2} = P_{IO_2} - [\dot{V}_{O_2} \div \dot{V}_A]\,K \qquad [1]$$

where P_{ACO_2} and P_{AO_2} are alveolar carbon dioxide and oxygen partial pressures (it is assumed $P_{ACO_2} \approx$ arterial P_{CO_2}); $\dot{V}_{CO_2}$ and $\dot{V}_{O_2}$ are volumes of carbon dioxide expired and oxygen consumed; $\dot{V}_A$ is alveolar ventilation; P_{IO_2} is inspired partial pressure of oxygen; and K is constant (0.863).

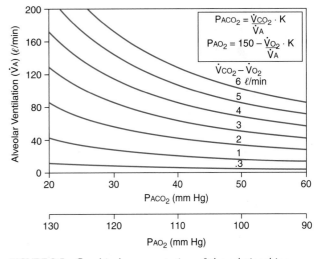

FIGURE 8.5 Graphical representation of the relationships between alveolar ventilation $\dot{V}_A$ and alveolar carbon dioxide partial pressure (P_{ACO_2}) at varying oxygen uptake and between $\dot{V}_A$ and P_{ACO_2} at varying carbon dioxide production ($\dot{V}_{CO_2}$). All P_{ACO_2} values are for breathing room air near sea level. To estimate total ventilation during exercise from the $\dot{V}_A$, multiply the $\dot{V}_A$ by 1.15. This assumes an average dead space to tidal volume ratio (V_D/V_T) of 0.15 throughout exercise. Because of the hyperbolic relationship between $\dot{V}_A$ and arterial carbon dioxide partial pressure (P_{aCO_2}), note the following circumstances. In a normal untrained subject at a $\dot{V}_{CO_2}$ of 3.5 L · min⁻¹ at maximum exercise, the requirement for $\dot{V}_A$ is about 80 L · min⁻¹ to maintain P_{ACO_2} constant at resting value, that is, 40 mm Hg. To achieve an average degree of hyperventilation at maximum exercise, which would drive P_{aCO_2} down to about 30 mm Hg, an $\dot{V}_A$ of about 95 to 100 L · min⁻¹ is required (and a total minute ventilation of 100–115 L · min⁻¹). Contrast this ventilatory requirement to that in a highly trained individual of similar body mass to the untrained but with a $\dot{V}_{CO_2}$ of 6 L · min⁻¹. To achieve the same amount of alveolar hyperventilation (P_{aCO_2} = 30 mm Hg and P_{AO_2} = 120 mm Hg) the highly trained subject would require an $\dot{V}_A$ of 180 L · min⁻¹, or slightly over 200 L · min⁻¹ total ventilation.

Alveolar gases may be calculated from these equations if $\dot{V}CO_2$ and $\dot{V}O_2$ are expressed in milliliters per minute and $\dot{V}_A$ is expressed in liters per minute. For example, if P_IO_2 is 150 mm Hg, $\dot{V}O_2$ is 240 mL $\cdot$ min^{-1} STPD (standard temperature pressure dry), and $\dot{V}_A$ is 4.0 L $\cdot$ min^{-1} BTPS (body temperature pressure saturated), then PAO_2 is 98 mm Hg. The same applies to the calculation of $PACO_2$, only this is simplified because carbon dioxide is almost absent in the inspired air.

TEST YOURSELF

Use Equation 8.1 and an inspired PO_2 of 150 mm Hg to calculate what would happen to $PACO_2$ and PAO_2 if, for example, you exercise at a moderate intensity requiring a fourfold increase from rest in $\dot{V}CO_2$ and $\dot{V}O_2$ (e.g., $\dot{V}CO_2$ and $\dot{V}O_2$ = 0.25 L $\cdot$ min^{-1} at rest and 1.0 L $\cdot$ min^{-1} during exercise) but failed to increase your $\dot{V}_A$ above a resting level of 4.0 L $\cdot$ min^{-1}. Furthermore, determine how much you would have to increase $\dot{V}_A$ during this same level of exercise to maintain $PACO_2$ and PAO_2 at resting levels.

Clearly then, to protect the alveolar gases, that is, the first line of defense in the oxygen transport system, you must increase your $\dot{V}_A$ quickly and precisely in tune with the metabolic requirement. Picture the alveolar gas as a compartment of gas that resides between the conducting airways (source of fresh inspired air and dead space air) and the pulmonary capillaries (source of metabolic carbon dioxide brought to the lung in the venous blood and oxygen taken up from the lung). If the alveolar gases are not protected, PaO_2 and $PACO_2$ will quickly deteriorate, and oxygen transport to tissue and elimination of carbon dioxide and tissue acid-base status will be severely compromised. Also, recall that total ventilation ($\dot{V}_E = f_R \times V_T$, where $\dot{V}_E$ is minute ventilation, f_R is respiratory frequency, and V_T is tidal volume) does not fully aerate the alveoli; rather, about one-third of each breath in the resting subject is dead space gas (V_D), defined as gas low in oxygen and high in carbon dioxide that remains in the conducting airways at end-expiration and must be inhaled into the alveoli on each subsequent inspiration. Thus, the higher the f_R, the greater the contribution of V_D to total ventilation.

$$\dot{V}_A \text{ (L} \cdot \text{min}^{-1}) = f_R \times \dot{V}_T \times (1 - \dot{V}_D/\dot{V}_T). \qquad [2]$$

Fortunately, the proportion of each breath occupied by dead space gas is reduced during exercise at a time when the demand for $\dot{V}_A$ is high.

The second requisite for the exercise hyperpnea is that the work and metabolic cost of the increased ventilation are minimized. We simply cannot expend a great deal of energy and devote an excessive portion of our cardiac output to our respiratory muscles during exercise, when the blood flow and $\dot{V}O_2$ of locomotor muscles must be a top priority. Furthermore, we cannot afford to be made aware of our breathing effort to the point of even mild distraction from the locomotor task at hand.

Optimal Response Strategy

Given the aforementioned requisites, the ideal hyperpneic response to increasing exercise intensities would contain the following features. First, $\dot{V}_A$ must increase in proportion to metabolic requirements so that alveolar gases are maintained or improved. The increase in $\dot{V}_A$ must not be too much (energetically wasteful, creating hypocapnia and alkalosis) or too little (causing hypercapnia, acidosis, and hypoxemia), and the speed of the response must be neither too slow nor too fast. Second, the control system must be sensitive to and capable of responding to any special needs for extra $\dot{V}_A$ beyond the basic metabolic requirements of a rising tissue $\dot{V}CO_2$. Third, a carefully selected combination of increased frequency and V_T must be achieved, taking into account the need for minimizing dead space ventilation (V_D) (i.e., the increase in respiratory frequency [f_R] should not be excessive). At the same time, this combination protects against an excessive increase in V_T, which would require excessive generation of subatmospheric P_{it} and, therefore, large amounts of work by the inspiratory muscles (discussed later). Fourth, the work of breathing must be shared and carefully coordinated among all inspiratory, expiratory, and airway muscles. Furthermore, respiratory muscle length must be carefully guarded and optimized so that force production is maximized for a given motor command. Finally, underlying a precise neural control system for regulating ventilation and breathing pattern must be adequate structural capacities of the respiratory muscles. These muscles must be capable of producing and sustaining the large forces necessary for changing P_{it} as required across the continuum of demands for ventilation with increasing exercise intensity. Similarly, lung and airway structural capacities must be capable of responding to the pressure changes and producing the appropriate volumes and flow rates.

This combination of a highly sensitive multifaceted control system with an adequately structured lung and chest wall exists in normal subjects across most of the lifespan. The result is—with few exceptions—a nearly perfect and highly efficient ventilatory response to exercise. We now describe this response and examine in detail some of the proposed underlying mechanisms.

Primary Stimulus for Exercise Hyperpnea

Figure 8.6 and Table 8.1 show the well-established hallmarks of the ventilatory response to light and moderate exercise requiring less than 60% maximum oxygen uptake ($\dot{V}O_{2max}$). Ventilation increases abruptly from resting levels at the onset of exercise and then increases more gradually over time until a steady state is achieved at each work rate. The steady state ventilatory response is almost directly in proportion to the increase in $\dot{V}CO_2$. Accordingly, throughout light to moderate exercise, alveolar PO_2 is controlled within 5% to 10% of resting levels and

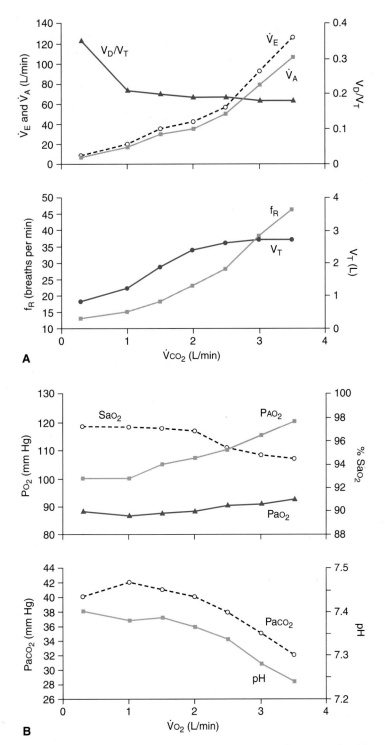

FIGURE 8.6   A. Ventilatory responses to progressive steady state increases in work rate in a healthy recreationally active young man ($\dot{V}_{O_{2max}}$ = 45 mL · kg⁻¹ · min⁻¹). $\dot{V}_E$, total minute ventilation; $\dot{V}_A$, alveolar ventilation; V_D/V_T, dead space to tidal volume ratio; f_R, respiratory frequency; V_T, tidal volume; $\dot{V}_{CO_2}$, CO_2 production. **B.** Arterial blood gases and acid-base status during progressive steady state increases in work rate. Sa_{O_2}, percent arterial oxyhemoglobin saturation; PA_{O_2}, alveolar P_{O_2}; Pa_{O_2}, arterial P_{O_2}; Pa_{CO_2}, arterial P_{CO_2}; pH, arterial pH. The fall in pH at the two highest work rates was caused by a rise in the concentration of lactic acid and a reduction in plasma bicarbonate in arterial blood. Pa_{CO_2} is fairly constant over the first four work rates but falls commensurately with the metabolic acidosis at the two heaviest work rates. Thus, the arterial blood acid–base status at the final two work rates is primary metabolic acidosis partially compensated by hyperventilation (and hypocapnia).

TABLE 8.1   Representative Values for Ventilation, Pulmonary Gas Exchange, and Pulmonary Circulation at Rest and during Maximal Incremental (Ramp) Exercise in Healthy, Untrained Young Adults (body mass 70 kg; $\dot{V}o_{2max}$ 40–45 mL · kg^{-1} · min^{-1}) and Peak Exercise Values for Two Highly Trained Young Adults (body mass 70 kg; $\dot{V}o_{2max}$ 75 mL · kg^{-1} · min^{-1})

		Untrained				Trained A	Trained B
		Exercise intensity (% maximum oxygen uptake)					
	Rest	30	60	90	100	100	100
$\dot{V}o_2$ (L · min^{-1})	0.24	0.90	1.80	2.70	3.00	5.25	5.25
$\dot{V}co_2$ (L · min^{-1})	0.19	0.77	1.71	2.85	3.30	6.04	6.04
$\dot{V}_E$ (L · min^{-1})	6	22	51	89	113	183	168
$\dot{V}_A$ (L · min^{-1})	4	18	41	74	93	150	138
V_T (L)	0.6	1.2	2.2	2.7	2.7	3.1	2.9
f_R (breaths · min^{-1})	10	18	23	33	42	59	58
V_D/V_T	0.35	0.21	0.19	0.18	0.18	0.18	0.18
EELV (% TLC)	0.50	0.46	0.44	0.42	0.42	0.48	0.48
Gas exchange							
Pao_2 (mm Hg)	91	93	92	92	92	85	70
PAo_2 (mm Hg)	96	101	107	114	117	115	112
$Paco_2$ (mm Hg)	39	38	36	33	31	35	38
A-aDo_2 (mm Hg)	5	8	15	22	25	30	42
pH	7.40	7.38	7.34	7.29	7.28	7.27	7.27
Sao_2 (%)	97	97	97	96	95	95	88
$\dot{V}_A/\dot{Q}$	0.8	2.0	2.9	3.7	4.4	4.4	4.1
Cao_2 (mL O_2 · 100 mL^{-1})	20.5	20.5	20.4	20.2	20.1	20.1	18.6
$C\bar{v}o_2$ (mL O_2 · 100 mL^{-1})	16.0	9.5	7.4	5.1	4.1	3.1	1.6
Pulmonary circulation							
$\dot{Q}$ (L · min^{-1})	5	9	14	20	21	34	34
PCBV (mL)	83	107	137	173	180	220–260	220–260
Transit time (s)	1.00	0.71	0.59	0.52	0.51	0.39–0.45	0.39–0.45
P_{pa} (mm Hg)	12	16	21	27	28	41	41
PVR (mm Hg · L · min^{-1})	2.40	1.76	1.49	1.35	1.33	1.21	1.21

$\dot{V}o_2$, oxygen uptake; $\dot{V}co_2$, carbon dioxide production; $\dot{V}_E$, minute ventilation; $\dot{V}_A$, alveolar ventilation; V_T, tidal volume; f_R, respiratory frequency; V_D/V_T, dead space to tidal volume ratio; EELV (% TLC), end-expiratory lung volume as a percentage of total lung capacity; Pao_2, partial pressure of arterial oxygen; PAo_2, partial pressure of alveolar oxygen; $Paco_2$, partial pressure of arterial carbon dioxide; A-aDo_2, alveolar to arterial oxygen partial pressure difference; Sao_2, oxyhemoglobin saturation; $\dot{V}_A/\dot{Q}$, global alveolar ventilation to perfusion ratio; Cao_2, arterial oxygen content; $C\bar{v}o_2$, mixed venous oxygen content; $\dot{Q}$, pulmonary blood flow; PCBV, pulmonary capillary blood volume; transit time, mean pulmonary capillary transit time; P_{pa}, mean pulmonary artery pressure; P_{paw}, pulmonary artery wedge pressure; PVR, pulmonary vascular resistance.

Cardiac output calculated from Rowell L. *Human Cardiovascular Control*. New York: Oxford University; 1993:162–203.

Pulmonary capillary blood volume calculated from Hsia CC, McBrayer DG, Ramanathan M. Reference values of pulmonary diffusing capacity during exercise by a rebreathing technique. *Am J Respir Crit Care Med*. 1995;152:658–665.

Mean pulmonary artery pressure and pulmonary vascular resistance calculated from Reeves JT, Dempsey JA, Grover RF. Pulmonary circulation during exercise. In: Weir EK, Reeves JT, eds. *Pulmonary Vascular Physiology and Pathophysiology*. New York: Marcel Dekker; 1989:107–133.

All other data compiled from authors' laboratory.

$Paco_2$, Pao_2, and pH are also tightly regulated. This direct relationship between $\dot{V}_A$ and $\dot{V}co_2$ holds for all types of large-muscle exercise, such as cycling, walking, and running. However, a tendency for a mild hyperventilatory response to exercise is fairly common during running (rather than walking) and during exercise with smaller muscle groups, such as with the arms in humans. The time course of the ventilatory response to exercise onset (from a baseline of rest) is very fast, usually faster than the concomitant rate of rise of cardiac output and $\dot{V}co_2$, resulting in transient levels of mild hypocapnia. However, if an increase in exercise intensity is initiated from moderate exercise (rather than rest) the increase in $\dot{V}_A$ is in closer proportion to the increase in $\dot{V}co_2$, and $Paco_2$ changes very little. This difference between ventilatory changes from the resting and the exercise baseline suggests that some extra behavioral response may be causing the transient hyperventilation often noted in the transition from rest to exercise.

For more than 130 years physiologists have been fascinated with the power and precision of this hyperpneic response to exercise and many have asked the same question, namely: what mechanism will stimulate ventilation in direct proportion to the increasing production of carbon dioxide by the working muscles?

Several candidate stimuli have emerged based on ingenious experiments performed using human and animal models. The primary candidates include:

- Carbon dioxide flow ($\dot{Q} \cdot C\bar{v}co_2$; where $\dot{Q}$ is pulmonary blood flow in $L \cdot min^{-1}$ and $C\bar{v}co_2$ is CO_2 content in the mixed venous blood in mL CO_2/100 mL blood) sensed by afferents located within the lung, or in the circulation on either the right or left side of the lung.
- Locomotor muscle mechanoreceptors and metaboreceptors sensitive to the muscle's work rate, muscle metabolite accumulation, and/or blood vessel distension.
- Central locomotor command proportional to the work rate of the locomotor muscles.

Of course, all of these potential mechanisms occur simultaneously during exercise. The experimental approach to teasing out a role for each of these stimuli has been to isolate the specific stimulus and determine whether it alone will produce a physiologic, hyperpneic, exercise-like response.

Carbon dioxide flow to the lung

This humoral mechanism is extremely attractive because of the nearly perfect correlation of increases in $\dot{V}_A$ to $\dot{V}co_2$ with steady state exercise and because the proposed primary driver to increasing $\dot{V}_A$ (i.e., carbon dioxide) is also the controlled variable. Now, how can one isolate this humoral stimulus and yet be sure that any change in carbon dioxide is not seen on the arterial (as well as the venous) side of

the circulation by the carotid chemoreceptors? Remember, $Paco_2$ remains very constant during exercise, and therefore any significant changes in $Paco_2$ (or Pao_2 or arterial pH) would not mimic the exercise response and would activate additional chemoreceptors that would not ordinarily be brought into play. The approach has been to use an extracorporeal gas exchanger in resting experimental animals (dogs or sheep) attached to the inferior vena cava, so that mixed venous carbon dioxide and/or blood flow can be raised or lowered over a limited range. When carbon dioxide flow to the lung ($\dot{Q} \cdot C\bar{v}co_2$) was changed in either the resting awake or anesthetized animal, $\dot{V}_A$ changed in proportion to the change in $\dot{V}co_2$. Amazingly, in one study using docile, awake sheep, as carbon dioxide was scrubbed from the venous return, $\dot{V}_A$ fell until prolonged apneas ensued (12). Other investigators argued that very small changes in $Paco_2$ occurred during venous loading and unloading, and that these changes were sufficient to explain much or all of the observed ventilatory response. One answer to this controversy was to use two extracorporeal gas exchangers in the anesthetized animal—one to change $\dot{Q} \cdot C\bar{v}co_2$ and the other to control carotid arterial blood gases to be absolutely sure that the $Paco_2$ was maintained constant at baseline values. Even with these stringent controls, significant ventilatory responses to changes in pulmonary $\dot{Q} \cdot C\bar{v}co_2$, per se, were still obtained (13).

Other approaches used to examine the carbon dioxide flow hypothesis in resting humans have demonstrated a proportional sensitivity of ventilation to small changes in carbon dioxide flow, including the following:

- An increased isocapnic ventilatory response to increases in $\dot{V}co_2$ and respiratory quotient induced by augmenting the proportion of carbohydrate in the diet.
- A reduction in ventilation (and unstable breathing) produced in renal dialysis patients produced by lowering the carbon dioxide in the dialysate (and therefore in the venous return).
- An increase in ventilation occurring in proportion to the coincident increase in $\dot{V}co_2$ caused by electrically stimulating the lower limb muscles to contract in patients with complete spinal cord lesions. Carbon dioxide flow would be the main mechanism for the hyperpnea in the absence of functional afferent neural pathways from contracting limbs to medulla and with no apparent central command (also discussed later).

There is little doubt, then, that carbon dioxide flow per se (i.e., without accompanying locomotion) does influence ventilation, but how? Several possible mechanisms have been investigated. For example, vagally mediated feedback receptors on both the right and left sides of the pulmonary circulation mediate increases in ventilation in response to infused acid solutions and to changes in vascular pressures. Furthermore, the phasic ventilation of the lung causes intrabreath fluctuations in alveolar and also in systemic $PaCO_2$ and PaO_2, and these fluctuations are sensed by and can influence the sensory output from the carotid chemoreceptors. These PCO_2 fluctuations are augmented around a constant mean value as carbon dioxide returning to the lungs increases during exercise.

To summarize, both correlational data linking $\dot{V}CO_2$ to $\dot{V}_A$ during dynamic exercise and the logical appeal of self-regulation of carbon dioxide as the dependent variable are excellent points in support of carbon dioxide flow–linked mechanisms of exercise hyperpnea. Furthermore, as outlined previously, isolated studies in the resting (and usually anesthetized) animal show that feedback receptors on both the right and left side of the circulation do exist and are ideally situated to influence ventilation quickly in response to each of the components of carbon dioxide flow. This broaches the next question: is the sensitivity of these receptors sufficient to produce the 10- to 12-fold increases in steady state ventilation above resting levels that accompany light to moderate exercise?

The bulk of evidence speaks against such a major role in exercise hyperpnea for these carbon dioxide flow feedback receptors (13). For example, artificially controlling stroke volume, cardiac output, and therefore carbon dioxide flow in exercising animals did not produce concomitant or proportional changes in $\dot{V}_A$ (14). Also, the extracorporeal gas exchange studies in awake animals (as cited earlier) were conducted over narrow ranges of increasing $\dot{V}CO_2$ in which even small changes in $PaCO_2$ (i.e., within the measurement error) could have explained the entire observed ventilatory response. Furthermore, enhanced fluctuations in $PaCO_2$ and arterial pH were shown *to modulate but not to stimulate* ventilation to a significant extent. Finally, these chemoreceptors (or flow measurement receptors) are not required for the normal hyperpnea, as shown by the normal isocapnic ventilatory responses to steady state exercise obtained in human heart or heart–lung transplant recipients, in humans with denervated carotid bodies studied following surgery, or an animal model studied both before and after vagal or carotid body denervations.

Collectively, we think the findings in animal models and humans point to an essential role for carbon dioxide flow ($\dot{V}CO_2$), possibly mediated via right-sided feedback receptors, in the very sensitive regulation of breathing near resting eupneic levels. This metabolic rate effect on normal eupnea may be viewed as forming the essential underpinning to the control of breathing. This metabolic rate effect also remains an important determinant of ventilatory output, even in the presence of other strong stimuli such as hypoxia, which has the dual effect of simultaneously increasing chemoreceptor stimulation and reducing whole-body metabolic rate (15). However, the control of exercise hyperpnea clearly requires additional more powerful stimuli that are engaged by the act of locomotion. At first glance, it may appear as though these mostly nonmetabolic locomotor-linked stimuli do not fit with the arterial blood gas homeostatic role for hyperpnea (as was clearly

the case for carbon dioxide flow). Indeed, it is logical that the controlled variable (PCO_2) should also have a major say in its means of control (i.e., $\dot{V}_A$). On the other hand, with dynamic exercise, there is a highly predictable and linear relationship between increasing work rate and metabolic rate. Accordingly, the tight relationship of increasing $\dot{V}_A$ to $\dot{V}CO_2$ may be attributed more to strictly locomotor-related rather than to metabolic or cardiovascular linked ventilatory control mechanisms. We now examine these locomotor-linked mechanisms.

Feedback from locomotor muscles

It is well established that various types of receptors in limb skeletal muscle and tendons are sensitive to mechanical events (stretch, pressure, tension), to metabolic changes produced by muscle contraction (lactic acid and bradykinin), and to venous vascular distention caused by increasing muscle blood flow (16). The most important nerve fibers sensing these perturbations in muscle are those that are very thinly myelinated or unmyelinated, classified as type III (primarily mechanical) and type IV (primarily metabolic), respectively. These skeletal muscle afferents synapse in the laminae of the dorsal horn of the spinal cord and project to the medulla, including the NST relay area, which also receives other cardiorespiratory afferents carried in the vagus and glossopharyngeal nerves. When these afferent fibers are stimulated (electrically, pharmacologically, or via perfusion of acid or other metabolites into the arterial blood supply), phrenic nerve activity and f_R increase, as do sympathetic nerve activity, systemic vascular resistance, and blood pressure. These cardiorespiratory responses are prevented by ganglionic blockade or by lesioning of the sensory nervous pathways. Furthermore, when muscle contraction is caused by direct electrical stimulation and the venous effluent blood from the working muscle is directed to another animal via cross circulation anastomosis—thereby eliminating the carbon dioxide flow stimulus—hyperpnea is readily achieved. There is also limited evidence in humans supporting a significant role for peripheral muscle feedback in exercise hyperpnea, including the hyperpneic responses to electrical stimulation of muscle and to muscle ischemia.

The aforementioned evidence shows that ventilatory and especially circulatory responses to stimuli originating in the locomotor muscle do occur; but what are these stimuli and how effective are they during dynamic exercise? First, it seems as though a sensitive and potent stimulus for activating the type III and IV sensory afferents is simply rhythmic muscle contraction. This was demonstrated by stimulating motor areas of the higher CNS in the decorticate cat and observing activation of type III and IV afferents in the biceps femoris muscle during evoked rhythmic contractions, even of mild intensity (17). Increasing the force of limb muscle contraction per se has little effect on ventilatory output, whereas frequency of limb movement and changes in the distention of veins within the muscle and/or intramuscular pressure appear to have marked effects on sensory afferent input to the medulla and increasing ventilation. The proposed relationship of muscle venous distention and muscle blood flow to sensory output and ventilatory drive is teleologically attractive because it links muscle blood flow to the hyperpnea, and blood flow is a critical variable in determining carbon dioxide flow to the lung. Furthermore, many of the type III and IV fibers terminate within the adventitia of the venous vasculature of the muscle and respond to the mechanical changes associated with venous distention (18).

Summary

When rhythmic muscle contraction is viewed as an isolated stimulus it appears to provide sufficient sensory feedback stimulation to increase ventilation. This feedback mechanism also has appeal simply because there are extremely vast numbers of afferent receptors throughout the large mass of skeletal muscle tissue that are available for substantial sensory input during muscle contraction. The relatively recent evidence linking local muscle blood flow and muscle receptors to exercise hyperpnea is especially worthy of further investigation because it incorporates a powerful feedback effect—relative to previously proposed carbon dioxide flow mechanisms operating in the central circulation or at the carotid chemoreceptors (see previous section)—to explain the $\dot{V}_A$ - $\dot{V}CO_2$ relationship. As to the relative role of this mechanism in the total scheme of exercise hyperpnea, we speculate that it contributes a significant portion to both the immediate increase in ventilation at exercise onset and the sustained hyperpnea in the steady state. This proposed feedback role for hyperpnea, although significant, contrasts with the more critical dependence of sympathetic vasoconstrictor outflow on these feedback influences from metabolite accumulation in contracting muscle.

Central command

The third proposal for a major locomotor-induced primary stimulus to exercise hyperpnea is the *feed-forward* pathway (as opposed to the feedback pathways provided by the carbon dioxide flow and muscle mechanoreceptors and metaboreceptors). This stimulus is called *central command,* denoting the cardiorespiratory responses caused by direct action of the supramedullary locomotor center neurons on respiratory pattern–generating medullary neurons, whose output, in turn, regulates respiratory motor output to the airway and chest wall muscles (as well as parasympathetic and sympathetic efferent output to the heart and blood vessels). Thus, central command involves a parallel simultaneous excitation of the neuronal circuits containing locomotor and cardiorespiratory neurons. Anatomically, several motor areas involved in this response have been identified in multilabel nerve tracing studies. These motor areas are located principally in discrete regions of the hypothalamus, in the diencephalon of the midbrain, and in the premotor cortex; they project to the medullary cardiorespiratory neurons and also directly to cervical and lumbar spinal motor neurons.

As with the two hypotheses discussed earlier, to determine a role for central command in exercise hyperpnea requires isolation of the specific stimulus. The concept of a central command over cardiorespiratory function was first suggested prior to the last century (19) and named cortical irradiation. It was not until the past two decades that researchers devised methods using first electrical and then pharmacologic stimulation of these specific CNS locomotor regions in unanesthetized, decorticate cats to cause rhythmic locomotion of the limbs similar to that produced voluntarily (20). When locomotion was initiated via this type of hypothalamic stimulation, phrenic nerve activity and cardiac output increased, and blood flow was redistributed from inactive to active tissues. Most important, these exercise-like cardiorespiratory changes occurred even when limb muscles were paralyzed (*i.e.*, so-called fictive locomotion), thereby providing strong evidence that central command was capable—by itself—of producing normal exercise hyperpnea (see Milestone of Discovery at the end of this chapter). These impressive findings were confirmed in several laboratories using the decorticate-animal central command model. However, skepticism continues, especially concerning how precisely this model mimics actual physiologic exercise.

In humans, there is circumstantial evidence favoring a significant role for central command in exercise hyperpnea. Most often cited are the very fast ventilatory responses at exercise onset and cessation, which appear to be almost anticipatory of these exercise transitions and apparently, occur faster than any feedback mechanism could operate (19). Exercise following partial muscle paralysis caused a fast-onset hyperventilatory response, attributed to the additional central command required to recruit more muscle motor units in an attempt to produce a given amount of force in the compromised muscle (21). Other studies have used hypnotic suggestion of exercise in resting humans to uncouple feedback from central command. Merely the suggestion of exercise in a resting subject, or of heavier exercise in the lightly exercising subject, caused exercise-like tachycardia and hyperventilation (22). Furthermore, neuroimaging techniques measuring brain blood flow distribution have shown that several motor cortical areas activated with purely volitional hyperpnea are also activated using imagined exercise (23). Whether these are the same higher CNS areas activated by the true central command during normal physiologic exercise is a question that must be answered before these types of findings can be applied with confidence to the exercise hyperpnea question.

TEST YOURSELF

A healthy person is running at a moderate intensity on a treadmill. If the inspired fraction of oxygen is abruptly changed from 0.21 to 0.12, there is a corresponding fall in the PaO_2 and SaO_2 and a rise in $\dot{V}_E$. Explain all of the steps that lead to the increase in ventilation.

Hyperventilation during Heavy Exercise

As exercise intensity increases beyond ~60% of $\dot{V}O_{2max}$ in untrained subjects, ventilation first increases out of proportion to $\dot{V}O_2$ (causing alveolar PO_2 to rise) and then, at a slightly higher workload, disproportionately more with respect to $\dot{V}CO_2$ (causing arterial PCO_2 to fall). The degree of hyperventilation can be substantial, sufficient at maximal exercise to drive $PaCO_2$ 8 to 15 mm Hg below resting values. What causes this extra drive to breathe? The popular choice for the past 60 years or so has been metabolic acidosis as arterial plasma lactic acid and hydrogen ions begin to rise with the onset of the hyperventilatory response. Reasonably, the hyperventilation is viewed as a ventilatory compensation (i.e., reduced $PaCO_2$) for a primary metabolic acidosis. The carotid chemoreceptors are exposed to the metabolic acidosis and are, therefore, the logical choice as the main transducer of the hyperventilatory response. Support for this hypothesis stems from clinical evidence showing that neither the mildly asthmatic patient with denervated carotid bodies (24) nor the rare patient with normal lungs but a demonstrated absence of ventilatory response to chemoreceptor stimuli (carbon dioxide or hypoxia) shows a hyperventilatory response to heavy exercise, even though they both have a normal isocapnic hyperpnea in moderate exercise. Accordingly, unlike the dilemma of hyperpnea of moderate-intensity exercise, the hyperventilation of heavy exercise would at first glance appear to have a clearly defined stimulus and reflex receptor site.

Unfortunately, several lines of evidence preclude such a clear-cut conclusion. When dietary-induced glycogen depletion is used to prevent almost all of the exercise-induced increase in lactic acid, a normal hyperventilatory response persists (25). Patients with McArdle's syndrome are incapable of producing lactic acid, but hyperventilation occurs during heavy exercise (26). When exercising animals are studied before and after carotid body denervation, the ventilatory response to heavy exercise is, if anything, slightly greater after the carotid body denervation, despite similar levels of metabolic acidosis (9). Furthermore, infusion of dopamine to reduce the tonic activity and responsiveness of the carotid chemoreceptors diminishes the hypoxic ventilatory response but has no effect on the ventilatory response during heavy exercise (27). Collectively, these findings suggest that neither metabolic acidosis nor the carotid bodies is *required* for the hyperventilation during heavy exercise.

What can we conclude from these conflicting results? Given the well-described ventilatory response of the carotid chemoreceptors to circulating hydrogen ions, it is safe to say that the carotid chemoreceptors are involved to a significant extent in the ventilatory response to heavy exercise. However, carotid chemoreceptor feedback is unlikely to be a sufficiently strong stimulus to explain the 20% to 30% extra increase in ventilation (20–40 L · min^{-1} in normal young subjects) observed during heavy exercise. Additional carotid body stimuli, such as increasing concentrations of norepinephrine and potassium, occur in heavy exercise. Other powerful locomotor-linked nonchemoreceptor stimuli might also cause hyperventilation. For example, as limb locomotor muscle fatigue occurs in heavy exercise, more central command must be generated to maintain locomotor muscle force, and this would be expected to have a coincident augmenting effect on respiratory motor output. There is no direct evidence to support this suggestion, but electromyographic activity of limb muscle has been shown to increase markedly (suggesting an increase in central command) coincident with the onset of both heavy exercise and hyperventilation (28). Furthermore, heavy exercise causes substantial activation of limb muscle metaboreceptors and/or mechanoreceptors that may contribute to the extra ventilatory response. Support for this idea stems from recent work showing substantial hypoventilation across a wide range of exercise intensities in response to partial blockade of muscle afferent feedback (29).

In summary, the hyperventilation of heavy exercise presents as many or perhaps even more opportunities for known feed-forward and feedback sensory inputs to influence ventilation than the isocapnic hyperpnea of moderate exercise. The major obvious difference is that in heavy exercise there are large changes in additional known chemoreceptor stimuli in arterial blood that surely contribute to some extent to the hyperventilatory response. However, the available evidence also points to the additional (and perhaps interactive) strong ascending influences of augmented feedback from fatiguing locomotor muscles and descending influences from central command. Logically, this central command influence may also rely critically on stored information from past memorable experiences of heavy exercise (discussed later).

Finally, sustaining constant work-rate exercise at heavy intensities beyond about 5 to 10 minutes causes a time-dependent tachypneic (i.e., increased f_R) hyperventilatory response. An important difference between short- and long-term heavy exercise is that arterial hydrogen ion concentration may actually be falling in the long term as opposed to rising in short-term heavy exercise. The reason is that net release of lactic acid from the working muscle may actually fall over time at constant work rates, and the level of hypocapnia resulting from hyperventilation becomes the dominant determinant of arterial hydrogen ion concentration (30). Nevertheless, carotid chemoreceptor stimuli in the form of time dependent increases in circulating norepinephrine and potassium continue to be present in long-term exercise, in addition to the potentially augmented central command influences associated with locomotor limb fatigue. An additional consideration here is the time-dependent rise in core and blood temperature, which in humans elicits a predominant tachypneic rather than V_T response. In this regard, preventing most of this temperature increase via skin cooling was shown to reduce some of the time-dependent tachypneic hyperventilation in long-term exercise (31). Exactly where the increase in temperature might be acting to cause hyperventilation is uncertain. Perhaps this tachypneic response is stimulated by increased hypothalamic temperature and serves as a thermoregulatory response for selective brain cooling (32), analogous to that commonly experienced in the fur-bearing, panting animal.

Interim Summary and Future Considerations

After more than a century of investigation, does the mechanism of exercise hyperpnea remain a true dilemma and an ultra secret—as expressed two decades ago by the late Frederick Grodins (1915–1989), one of the pioneering modelers of the ventilatory control system? Not completely! On the positive side, we clearly have two candidates in the locomotor-linked stimuli, namely central command (feedforward) and muscle receptors (feedback). When studied in isolation, each is capable of producing fast and significant increases in respiratory motor output and ventilation. The finding that hypothalamic locomotor centers received sensory input from skeletal muscle receptors also shows the presence of the neural circuitry for providing interaction between these two main drives to breathe (33). Thus, we propose that these two major stimuli act together to provide the primary stimulus to exercise hyperpnea, perhaps with backup error detection by carotid chemoreceptors to provide fine tuning of the ventilatory response to ensure sufficient and precise normocapnic hyperpnea. This combination of stimuli provides an explanation for the first (fast) phase of increased ventilation at exercise onset and the final normocapnic steady state ventilation achieved at a given exercise intensity. The memory or self-amplifying effect of short-term potentiation would account for the gradual time-dependent increase in ventilation between exercise onset and steady state, and also explain the lack of large transient overshoots and undershoots in ventilation in transitional phases at exercise onset, on achievement of the steady state, and during recovery from exercise.

We propose this control scheme for hyperpnea as an interim working hypothesis. Future research should also consider the following findings. When either of the two primary mechanisms is removed, via lesioning of the spinal cord (in the case of feedback) or destruction of hypothalamic locomotor center neurons (in the case of central command), the ventilatory response to exercise remains near normal (34). Apparently, then, *neither input is required* for normal exercise hyperpnea. Perhaps we can explain

this finding by the concept of redundant biologic mechanisms or the multifaceted effects of lesioning. At the same time, it is difficult to accept any given mechanism as the *primary* driver of such a substantial physiologic response when it is not also an *obligatory* mechanism!

> # KEY POINT
>
> There is an unfortunate drawback to denervation experiments. They provide very important understanding to the relative importance of certain sensory pathways. However, negative results allow only the conclusion that these receptors are not required and do not rule out a significant role for these receptors in the intact subject. The key problem with such preparations is that removal of these sensory inputs is not the only significant change in the neural control system as a result of the denervations. To the contrary, sensory pathways such as those contained in vagal or carotid sinus nerves contain important tonic inputs to the medulla under normal intact conditions; accordingly, when they are denervated and this input is removed, adaptive changes are likely to occur either at the level of the neurons that generate central integrative respiratory patterns or by upregulation of other sensory receptors. For example, carotid body denervation was shown by histologic studies to have marked detrimental effects on the metabolic integrity (and therefore the neuronal function) of the medullary rhythm-generating neurons in the pre-Bötzinger complex (35) and over time to cause sensitization of the other sites of peripheral chemoreception in aortic chemoreceptors (36).

Attempts have been made to test how these two powerful locomotor-linked ventilatory stimuli might interact during exercise. This was accomplished by activation of each of the mechanisms separately and then together in anesthetized animals (37). Surprisingly, the sum of the response of each of the mechanisms acting alone was always greater than the two acting simultaneously. Strong interactive effects of combined ventilatory stimuli do commonly occur, for example, with all carotid chemoreceptor stimuli. However, there is as yet no direct evidence that this synergistic effect on ventilation occurs between the two locomotor-linked ventilatory stimuli.

An emerging concept is based on the capability of the organism to make accurate ventilatory responses to locomotion without guidance from identifiable error signals (see lesioning studies earlier in the chapter). This concept proposes that the brain—in our case, the medullary respiratory controller—is unlikely to solve complex differential equations in response to the many sensory inputs it receives from the higher CNS motor areas, muscular contraction, chemoreceptors, and short-term potentiation during exercise. Rather, the brain learns to make accurate ventilatory responses by trial and error, correcting them time after time during maturation. That is, the CNS anticipates present and future needs based on experience (38).

The identified sensory inputs for hyperpnea would certainly be important, especially during the learning-maturation phase, for the CNS to have knowledge of its errors. However, it is also proposed that the brain must rely on stored or learned information to achieve error-free regulation (38,39). This idea of learning the appropriate exercise hyperpneic response has been named *adaptive feed-forward control*. As implied from the cardiorespiratory responses and neuroimaging findings obtained during exercise suggested under hypnosis (discussed previously), the prefrontal cortex may be a critical area for encoding a respiratory motor program that evolves as motor tasks are learned in development (22). Further tests of these intriguing but still highly theoretical hypotheses will occur as our knowledge of the neurophysiology of learning and memory evolves.

KEY POINT

Two major stimuli act together to provide the primary stimulus to exercise hyperpnea, namely descending output from central command (feed-forward) and ascending input from muscle receptors (feedback).

Mechanics of Breathing

The lungs are inflated by negative pressure ventilation, whereby intrapleural and then alveolar pressure is reduced below atmospheric pressure by the expanding action of the inspiratory muscles on the chest wall. When the inspiratory muscles contract, they must provide sufficient force to overcome two mechanical impedances in the lung, namely, (a) resistance to flow through the airways, and (b) the lung's elastic recoil forces, which—when unopposed by the outward recoil of the chest wall—will cause the lung to collapse to its smallest volume. A balance between lung inward recoil and chest wall outward recoil occurs at functional residual capacity (FRC); that is, the lung volume averaging 45% to 50% of total lung capacity (TLC) and from which under quiet resting conditions each inspiration is initiated. This elastic characteristic for any given lung volume is defined by the lung compliance, which is calculated as the change in volume divided by a given change in pleural pressure (P_{pl}) (Δ volume/Δ pressure). The compliance of the lung decreases exponentially above a certain lung volume such that the lung is stiff at high lung volumes. The resistance to flow through the airways is expressed in centimeters of water per liter per second and is determined primarily by the radius of the airway according to Poiseuille's law, which governs flow through rigid tubes. As lung volume increases, there is a linear increase in airway caliber and a decrease in flow resistance.

Given the huge demands of exercise for increases in V_T and flow rate, it is extremely important that the elastic and resistive characteristics are regulated to minimize the magnitude of intrapleural pressure changes and, hence, prevent excessive amounts of work by the respiratory muscles. For the most part, these goals are met during exercise because the lungs, airways, and parenchymal tissue are anatomically suited to the increased ventilatory demands and also because the nervous control of breathing pattern and airway caliber is nearly optimal. We now address each of these anatomical and physiologic characteristics in detail.

Control of Airway Caliber

Even though airflow increases as much as five- to sixfold during moderate-intensity exercise, and up to 10-fold during high-intensity exercise whereupon airflow turbulence increases, the total resistance to airflow remains fairly constant. Thus, when airway resistance is compared at identical flow rates between rest and exercise, airway resistance is markedly lower during exercise. This reduced resistance to airflow reflects a major effect of exercise on both the stiffening (*i.e.*, the airway is less collapsible) and dilating of the upper and lower airways.

Extrathoracic airways

The upper airways consist of the nose, mouth, pharynx, and larynx. The diameters of these structures are regulated by more than 20 pairs of skeletal muscles innervated by the cranial nerves. This complex upper airway structure is responsible for phonation, swallowing, coughing, and mastication, in addition to providing a critical conduit for airflow. It also offers a tortuous and potentially high-resistance breathing route. However, several key mechanisms activated during exercise ensure that resistance to airflow is minimized. The route of airflow switches from predominantly nasal at rest to oral during light exercise requiring about 25 to 50 L · min⁻¹ V_E. This switch largely bypasses the nasal cavity, which has the smallest cross-sectional area in the upper airway. Cessation of nasal airflow is accomplished by activation of pharyngeal muscles which bring the soft pallet into contact with the posterior pharyngeal wall. The diameter of the oral pharynx is increased primarily via activation of the genioglossus muscle (which controls tongue position), as well as other palatal and pharyngeal muscles. The pharyngeal muscles are activated slightly before the inspiratory pump muscles (Fig. 8.2C), thereby stiffening the upper airway and preventing airway narrowing or collapse in the face of the highly subatmospheric P_{it} generated by the inspiratory muscles during exercise.

Finally, the cartilaginous larynx connects the pharynx with the trachea. The valve-like regulation of the laryngeal vocal folds, principally by the posterior cricoarytenoid and the thyroarytenoid muscles, is a key

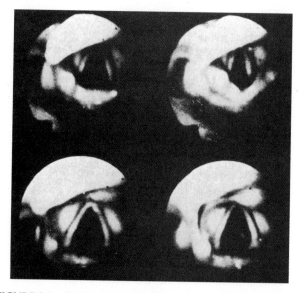

FIGURE 8.7 Position of the human vocal cords, as viewed through a laryngoscope, during mid inspiration (*left side*) and mid expiration (*right side*) from typical breaths at rest (eupneic breathing; *top panel*) and during moderate exercise (hyperpnea; *bottom panel*). The vocal cords are much more abducted during exercise than during rest. The major effect of hyperpnea on the position of the vocal cords occurred during expiration: they markedly narrowed at rest during expiration but underwent only minor narrowing during exercise. (Reprinted from England SJ, Bartlett D Jr. Changes in respiratory movements of the human vocal cords during hyperpnea. *J Appl Physiol.* 1982;52:782, with permission.)

determinant of upper airway resistance. At rest, the glottal laryngeal opening widens on inspiration and narrows on expiration, providing a slight brake on expiratory airflow—presumably to prevent EELV from dropping below FRC. During exercise, with increased f_R and shortened inspiratory and expiratory times, the glottal opening is widened and there is little or no narrowing on expiration (Fig. 8.7).

There are multiple levels of control of the diameter and compliance of the upper airway during exercise. First, activation of the nasal, pharyngeal, and laryngeal skeletal muscles is under similar feed-forward and feedback control (via the cranial nerves) as explained in detail earlier for the respiratory pump muscles during exercise. Output from the medullary respiratory pattern generator is the primary determinant of the timing and magnitude of the contractions of all the respiratory muscles, including those of the upper airway and chest wall (Fig. 8.1). Sympathetic activation during exercise also causes vasoconstriction of the nasal mucosa, thereby increasing nasal airway diameter and reducing nasal resistance. Finally, purely mechanical forces associated with increased contraction of the inspiratory chest wall muscles increase laryngeal diameter by caudal traction on the trachea (*i.e.*, the so-called "tracheal tug").

Intrathoracic airways

Intrathoracic airway caliber is under the involuntary control of smooth muscle. A powerful dilation of the bronchi occurs during exercise, as evidenced by the increase in the maximal amount of air forced out of the lungs during 1 second (FEV_1) immediately after exercise in both normal and asthmatic subjects. Several mechanisms contribute to this exercise-induced bronchodilation. The most important is the immediate and sustained withdrawal of vagal parasympathetic tone to the airways, which occurs primarily reflexively via neural feedback from limb locomotor muscle mechanoreceptor activation at exercise onset (9). This mechanism is also responsible, in part, for the reduced vagal efferent output to the heart during exercise resulting in increased heart rate. Mechanical influences may also play a substantial role in increasing airway caliber. Because the airways are tethered open by the lung parenchyma, increasing EILV during exercise will increase airway diameter. In addition, evidence from airway smooth muscle strip preparations in vitro has shown that even small amounts of airway stretch result in reductions in bronchial smooth muscle crossbridge formation by disturbing the bronchiolar smooth muscle latch state, and that these reductions decrease smooth muscle stiffness and promote bronchial smooth muscle relaxation (40). Local release of chemical mediators from airway resident and nonresident cells might also increase airway caliber during exercise.

Although major changes in airway caliber and resistance do occur during exercise, the elastic characteristics of the lung and chest wall are essentially unaltered. Thus, respiratory system compliance and, therefore, TLC are unchanged during and after exercise. However, the elastic work performed by the respiratory muscles on the lungs and chest wall is also critically dependent on the operating lung volume. If hyperinflation occurs secondary to expiratory flow limitation, lung compliance will be reduced during tidal breathing and the elastic work of breathing markedly increased. In addition, reductions in vital capacity following maximum short-term and long-term exercise may occur because maximum expiratory flow rates are reduced at low lung volumes consequent to small-airway narrowing (also discussed later).

Breathing Pattern

In addition to the total amount of ventilation required and the mechanical characteristics of the lung and airways, precisely how the timing and amplitude of *each* breath is sculpted during exercise is a critical determinant of the amount of mechanical work done by the respiratory muscles. The important variables requiring control under these conditions include tidal, EILV and EELV, inspiratory and expiratory flow rates, f_R, and duty cycle.

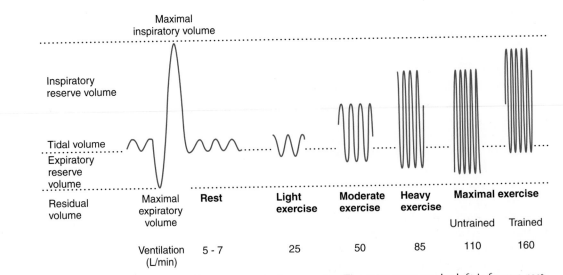

FIGURE 8.8 Changes in breathing pattern during exercise. The spirogram on the left is from a rest-ing subject showing normal tidal volume, maximal expiration to residual volume, then maximal inspi-ration to total lung capacity. With light to heavy exercise (in untrained and highly trained subjects) the increase in ventilation is achieved by increasing respiratory frequency and tidal volume. Tidal volume increases by encroaching on the expiratory and inspiratory reserve volumes. The reduced end-expiratory lung volume is maintained at maximal exercise in the untrained subject ($\dot{V}O_{2max}$ 45 mL · kg^{-1} · min^{-1}). In the trained subject ($\dot{V}O_{2max}$ 75 mL · kg^{-1} · min^{-1}), ventilation, respiratory frequency and tidal volume are all higher, and at maximal exercise end-expiratory lung volume is increased to near resting values due to expiratory flow limitation.

During light to moderate exercise, the increase in ventilation is achieved by increases in both respiratory frequency and tidal volume ($\dot{V}_E = f_R \cdot V_T$), whereas at higher intensities V_T tends to level off and an increase in frequency accounts for all of the further increase in venti-lation (Figs. 8.6 and 8.8). This tachypneic breathing pat-tern also occurs over time during submaximal endurance exercise. Increases in f_R are brought about by reductions in inspiratory and expiratory times. The respiratory duty cycle, defined as inspiratory time relative to total breath time, increases slightly, but most of the total breath time remains in expiration and the T_I is usually maintained at less than 50% of the total breath time. Finally, the increase in V_T is achieved by a reduction in EELV below FRC and an increase in EILV (Fig. 8.8).

These changes in breathing pattern are important for ensuring optimal mechanics of breathing during exercise. By increasing V_T rather than simply increas-ing f_R ensures that V_D is minimized and effective $\dot{V}_A$ is maximized ($\dot{V}_A = f_R \cdot [V_T - \dot{V}_D]$). This breathing pat-tern also minimizes flow rate and, hence, the flow-resis-tive work of breathing. The increase in V_T is limited to 70% of vital capacity during heavy exercise and EELV is reduced below resting levels (Fig. 8.8); these adjust-ments are important in minimizing the elastic work of breathing.

Why are these changes in breathing pattern and lung volumes such important determinants of both the work and the perception of breathing? First, by increas-ing tidal volume on the linear (and therefore most

compliant) portion of the respiratory system pressure–volume relationship (or compliance curve), the least amount of negative P_{it} has to be generated by the inspira-tory muscles for a given increase in volume. Second, the reduced EELV, achieved via activation of the abdominal expiratory muscles, means that intra-abdominal pres-sure (P_{ab}) is elevated and the diaphragm is lengthened at end-expiration enabling this muscle to operate near its optimal length for force generation. Third, the reduced EELV below relaxation volume (FRC) allows for the stor-age of elastic energy in the chest and abdominal walls during expiration; this energy can be used to produce a significant portion of the work required during the ensuing inspiration, thereby potentially sparing the inspiratory muscles. Fourth, it is important that inspira-tory time remains less than one-half the total breath time as forceful diaphragmatic contractions increase P_{ab}, compress the vessels supplying the diaphragm, and reduce its blood flow. Thus, the shorter the inspiration, the lesser the reduction in diaphragmatic blood flow and the less likelihood of diaphragmatic fatigue (also dis-cussed later).

TEST **YOURSELF**

Why is it important, especially during exercise, that we begin each inspiration from a lung volume that is at or below our resting FRC?

Flow–Volume Relationships

The maximum volitional flow–volume envelope is commonly used to quantify the maximum limits of the lungs and respiratory muscles for these variables (Fig. 8.9). Inspiratory flow is primarily limited by the ability of the inspiratory muscles to generate negative P_{it}, which is the key determinant of the pressure gradient for airflow between the atmosphere and the alveoli. Thus, as inspiratory effort and the magnitude of the subatmospheric P_{it} increases, flow rate increases at any given lung volume. In contrast, expiratory flow is dependent on the force of expiratory muscle effort, only very early in expiration (*i.e.*, near peak flow rate at high lung volume). Over most of the ensuing forced expiration, flow rate at any given lung volume is determined by the pressure difference across the airway. This so-called transmural pressure is the difference between the intra-airway pressure (determined by lung elastic recoil) and the collapsing positive P_{it} outside the airway (determined by compressive forces produced by expiratory muscles). Thus, in contrast to inspiration, maximum expiratory flow at any given lung volume is reached when expiratory muscle pressure is only a small portion of the maximum achievable pressure. The lowest expiratory pressure that generates

maximum expiratory flow is termed maximum effective pressure; any extra expiratory muscle effort beyond this point will cause airway narrowing or collapse and will not increase flow further.

In Figure 8.9, inspiratory and expiratory flow rates increase progressively during incremental exercise, whereas end-expiratory and EILVs gradually decrease and increase, respectively (41). The maximum pressures at any given flow rate and lung volume are also shown for inspiration and expiration (detailed explanation in the legend). For young healthy adults with normal $\dot{V}O_{2max}$ and maximum $\dot{V}_E$ of about 110 to 120 L · min^{-1}, the maximum mechanical limits of the flow–volume envelope are not reached, even during maximal exercise. EELV remains below resting levels and EILV is 70% to 80% of TLC. Clearly then, the maximum mechanical capability of the inspiratory muscles to produce maximum flow substantially exceeds the ventilatory requirements normally observed during exercise—at least in untrained subjects. In highly trained subjects, $\dot{V}O_{2max}$ and $\dot{V}_E$ increase further, but the maximum flow–volume envelope is unchanged from that of the untrained subjects. Accordingly, the expiratory flow during tidal breathing now commonly intersects with the maximum flow–volume envelope. EELV is now forced upward,

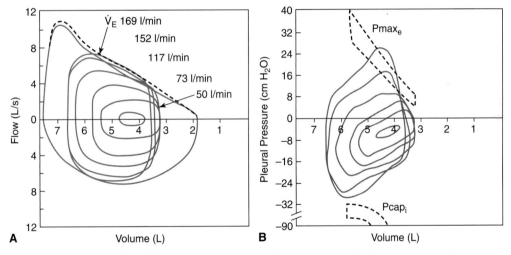

FIGURE 8.9   Flow–volume (**A**) and pressure–volume (**B**) relationships for healthy young adults at rest and during progressive exercise. Tidal flow–volume loops are shown plotted within flow constraints set by pre- (*solid line*) and postexercise (*dashed line*) maximum volitional flow–volume loops. Tidal pressure–volume loops are shown within constraints for effective pressure generation on expiration (Pmax$_e$) and within capacity for pressure generation on inspiration (Pcap$_i$). Up to a minute ventilation ($\dot{V}_E$) of ~115 L · min^{-1}, approximating peak exercise in an untrained adult, the inspiratory and expiratory flow–volume limits are not reached, and the pressures produced by the inspiratory muscles are only 40% to 60% of maximum dynamic capacity. In more highly trained subjects exercising at high metabolic rates and with ventilations in excess of 150 L · min^{-1} the tidal flow–volume loop encroaches on the maximum flow–volume envelope, end-expiratory lung volume rises, and peak inspiratory muscle pressures approach 90% of capacity or greater. The dashed area on the expiratory side of **B** indicates an expiratory pressure for any given lung volume, beyond which extra expiratory muscle effort will not produce a higher flow. In almost all instances up to 150 L · min^{-1} $\dot{V}_E$, this critical expiratory pressure is not exceeded, but it is exceeded slightly in the highly trained athlete at maximum exercise. (Redrawn from Johnson BD, Saupe KW, Dempsey JA. Mechanical constraints on exercise hyperpnea in endurance athletes. *J Appl Physiol.* 1992;73:878, with permission.)

so that there will be room within the maximum flow–volume envelope to increase flow rate further. However, this increase in flow is accomplished at the expense of lung hyperinflation. At high lung volumes the lung is stiffer (less compliant) and the diaphragm is shorter such that its capacity to generate pressure is impaired. Lung hyperinflation also impairs the pressure-generating capacity of the inspiratory chest wall muscles, but in contrast to the diaphragm, this effect is largely related to the orientation and motion of the ribs rather than the ability of the muscles to generate force.

TEST YOURSELF

To appreciate the importance of changes in lung volume, try this experiment on yourself. Voluntarily increase your V_T about three times above your resting level for five or six breaths. Do this starting at three different EELV: (a) from your relaxed EELV (FRC), (b) from your residual lung volume, and (c) from an EELV well above your FRC, about halfway between FRC and TLC. Accomplish this latter EELV by first breathing in to well above FRC, and then hold your breath for a second or two before you start breathing at the high V_T. Now you should be able to appreciate how much more effort it takes to accomplish the same V_T starting in a hyperinflated state versus starting with a normal or a deflated lung volume.

The most common approach to measuring expiratory flow limitation is to position spontaneous tidal flow–volume loops within a maximum volitional flow–volume envelope according to a measured inspiratory capacity at the end of a tidal expiration (Fig. 8.9). This approach provides an excellent visual representation of the breathing strategy used during exercise, the inspiratory and expiratory flow reserves, as well as the magnitude of expiratory flow limitation (42). The magnitude of expiratory flow limitation is quantified by calculating the percent overlap of the tidal expiratory flow–volume loop with the maximum flow–volume envelope, and the resultant value is used as a measure of the degree of ventilatory constraint during exercise. Although this approach is used widely, there are some methodologic errors that can influence the degree of expiratory flow limitation (43). First, the thoracic gas compression artifact of the maximum flow–volume envelope may underestimate the true capacity for flow generation. Second, differences in the volume and time history that precede tidal and forced expiratory maneuvers may lead to a false detection of expiratory flow limitation. Although gas compression can be corrected by measuring the maximum flow–volume envelope with a volume displacement plethysmograph, or so-called body box, this technique is rarely implemented because it requires subjects to exercise in a confined space. A more practical approach to correct

for gas compression is to perform three to five expiratory maneuvers at different efforts from TLC to residual volume and take the highest flow obtained at each lung volume (44). Another consideration when measuring expiratory flow limitation is the increase in maximal flows due to exercise-induced bronchodilation with the consequence that flows measured during exercise could exceed the maximum flow–volume envelope measured before exercise. Therefore, a maximum flow–volume loop obtained immediately after exercise may provide the simplest and most accurate estimate of maximal available flow and volume during the exercise. An alternative method of detecting expiratory flow limitation during exercise is to apply a negative expiratory pressure (NEP) at the mouth and to compare the flow–volume curve during the ensuing expiration with that of the preceding breath (45). Unlike the traditional approach of placing the exercise tidal flow–volume loop within the maximum flow–volume envelope, the NEP method does not require forced expiratory efforts or correction for gas compression. However, the NEP may cause upper airway collapse, resulting in a false comparison with spontaneous expirations. Other limitations include an inability to detect changes in EELV and the "all or none" quantification of expiratory flow limitation, both of which provide little information regarding the degree of ventilatory constraint.

TEST YOURSELF

Why is the expiratory half of the maximum flow–volume envelope a different shape than the inspiratory half?

Respiratory Pump Muscles in Exercise

Ventilatory requirements are directly served by several groups of skeletal muscles, namely upper airway dilators and stiffeners (as described earlier), and muscles of the respiratory pump comprising the inspiratory and expiratory muscles. The diaphragm is the most important inspiratory muscle in humans and accounts for around 70% of ventilation in healthy adults. The other inspiratory muscles are the scalenes and parasternal intercostals, which are usually active during quiet breathing, and the sternocleidomastoids, which become active when respiratory effort increases. The primary expiratory muscles, namely the rectus abdominis, external obliques, internal obliques, transversus abdominis, and triangularis sterni, are inactive in normal subjects when supine because expiration in that situation is a passive process, but they are readily recruited if $\dot{V}_E$ is increased for any reason or indeed in many cases on adopting the upright position.

Structurally, respiratory muscles are similar to skeletal muscle elsewhere in the body, such as the quadriceps, and therefore exhibit similar physiologic properties. In healthy humans, the diaphragm contains approximately 50% type I and 50% type II fibers, which, in turn, are a mix of type IIa and type IIx. The fatigue resistance of the diaphragm derives from its relatively high oxidative capacity and to the short capillary-to-mitochondrial diffusion distances for oxygen achieved by the very low muscle fiber cross-sectional area.

Respiratory muscle recruitment patterns

To provide mechanically efficient increases in V_T and f_R during exercise requires the following:

- Force output and velocity of shortening of the pump muscles must increase.
- Volumes of the rib cage and the abdominal compartments must increase.
- Respiratory muscle fibers must be regulated at close to optimal lengths.
- Respiratory system compliance (Δ volume/Δ pressure) must remain high so that minimal amounts of pressure are needed for changes in V_T.

The combined and highly coordinated actions of the respiratory pump muscles accomplish all of these required responses to exercise. It is impossible to measure actual length changes or force production of the respiratory muscles in humans. Nevertheless, balloon-catheter systems do provide estimates of the mechanical properties of the respiratory system. P_{pl} is measured by means of esophageal pressure relative to body surface pressure. Abdominal pressure (P_{ab}) is the pressure within the abdominal cavity and is usually measured by means of gastric pressure (P_{ga}). The difference between P_{ab} and P_{pl} is termed transdiaphragmatic pressure (P_{di}). Accurate measurements of rib cage and abdominal volume changes are extremely difficult, especially during exercise. The most accurate estimates to date have been made through the use of three-dimensional video tracking of reflective markers placed at many locations over the upper and lower rib cage and abdomen (46).

At rest, motor command from the medulla activates the phrenic motor neurons and, in turn, shortens the diaphragm, whose descent expands the thoracic cavity and causes a more negative P_{pl}. As the diaphragm shortens and descends toward the abdominal cavity during inspiration, P_{ab} and P_{di} increase. Thus, at rest the diaphragm is the major force generator, the rib cage muscles are a minor force generator, and the expiratory muscles are inactive because expiration is passive. With increasing exercise intensity, motor command is distributed to all three sets of respiratory pump muscles, but now the diaphragm is no longer the only major force developer. Although the work performed by the diaphragm increases more than tenfold during exercise, it now serves as the major flow producer by increasing its velocity of shortening (discussed later), whereas the inspiratory rib cage muscles now become the major force producers to expand rib cage volume and reduce P_{pl} during inspiration. Furthermore, the expiratory abdominal muscles now become major force producers to reduce abdominal and rib cage volumes and to increase P_{ab}

during active expiration. We now address how the active expiration achieved by the abdominal muscles influences diaphragm function during exercise.

The abdominal expiratory muscles are important in many ways to diaphragmatic function during exercise. Active expiration begins even with light exercise, causing P_{ab} to move in an increasingly positive direction and abdominal compartment volume to be reduced during expiration. At the end of the active expiration, the expiratory muscles relax rapidly and the abdominal wall recoils outward. Thus, during inspiration P_{ab} initially falls as abdominal volume increases, and this occurs in parallel with the falling P_{pl}. Thus, the contracting, descending diaphragm is not faced with an increasing P_{ab} and is, therefore, unloaded during inspiration and capable of generating a high velocity of shortening. In addition, as mentioned earlier, the phasic activation of the abdominal muscles during expiration reduces EELV and aids the diaphragm during exercise in two other important ways: (a) with increasing P_{ab} and stretching of the diaphragm on expiration, diaphragmatic descent at the onset of the ensuing inspiration will occur purely passively, that is, prior to the initiation of active diaphragmatic contraction; and (b) diaphragm length is optimized in preparation for active force generation during the ensuing inspiration. During weight-supported locomotion, such as jogging or running, the abdominal muscles are tonically activated, and mean levels of P_{ab} increase. Thus, the abdominal cavity acts as a shock absorber during exercise, thereby substantially lessening the concussive forces transmitted to the vertebral column and cranium from the impact of each foot plant.

TEST YOURSELF

Because expiratory flow is effort independent at most lung volumes, why even have expiratory muscles?

Oxygen cost of the work of breathing

The muscles of the diaphragm, rib cage, and abdomen perform both elastic work to produce lung expansion during inspiration and resistive work to produce increases in inspiratory and expiratory flow, the latter increasing nonlinearly at very high exercise intensities as flow becomes fully turbulent. Accordingly, total respiratory muscle work increases several fold from rest to high-intensity exercise. Estimates of the oxygen cost of this increase in ventilatory work (Fig. 8.10) averaged 1.8 mL $\dot{V}_{O_2} \cdot L^{-1} \dot{V}_E \cdot min^{-1}$ during moderate exercise. Thereafter, the oxygen cost of breathing rose out of proportion to the increasing $\dot{V}_E$ and averaged 2.9 mL $\dot{V}_{O_2} \cdot L^{-1} \cdot \dot{V}_E \cdot min^{-1}$ at maximal exercise. As a fraction of total body $\dot{V}_{O_2}$, the oxygen cost of exercise hyperpnea averaged 3% to 5% during moderate exercise and 8% to 10% at $\dot{V}_{O_{2max}}$ in untrained young adults (40–50 mL $\cdot$ kg$^{-1} \cdot$ min^{-1}). The values for respiratory muscle $\dot{V}_{O_2}$ during

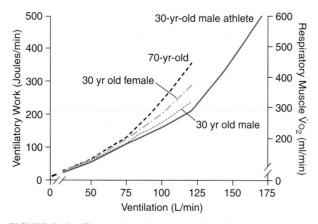

FIGURE 8.10 The work and oxygen cost of breathing at different levels of steady state ventilation during exercise in four different types of subjects. In the 30-year-old untrained male at maximum oxygen uptake ($\dot{V}O_{2max}$)the oxygen cost of breathing approximates 10% of $\dot{V}O_{2max}$, whereas in the highly trained 70-year-old male and 30-year-old female (at comparable $\dot{V}O_{2max}$ as the young untrained male) the work and oxygen cost of breathing are significantly higher. In the young highly trained endurance athlete working at much higher $\dot{V}O_{2max}$ (75 mL · kg^{-1} · min^{-1}) and at much higher minute ventilation the oxygen cost of breathing approaches 15% to 16% of $\dot{V}O_{2max}$.

maximal exercise were variable among subjects, with some trained subjects ($\dot{V}O_{2max} > 60$ mL · kg^{-1} · min^{-1}) requiring 13% to 16% of the total $\dot{V}O_{2max}$ (47).

Respiratory muscle blood flow

Skeletal muscle blood flow increases during exercise with increasing metabolic requirements. The magnitude of this increase is dependent on the net influences of the specific muscle's arteriolar smooth muscle response to local vasodilators (such as nitric oxide and muscle metabolites) and to sympathetic vasoconstrictor activity. Both of these opposing influences increase with exercise intensity (48). The network of vessels supplying blood flow to the diaphragm is extensive, including tributaries from the phrenic, lobar, and mammary arteries.

In experimental animals, data on respiratory muscle blood flow and $\dot{V}O_2$ during exercise are derived using radiolabeled microspheres to determine local blood flow and cannulation of the phrenic vein to obtain arteriovenous oxygen difference across the diaphragm. In this way, diaphragm $\dot{V}O_2$ may be obtained ($\dot{V}O_2$ = blood flow · a-$\bar{v}DO_2$). Although exercise effects vary greatly *among* species and *within* species, it is clear that vascular conductance and blood flow (per 100 g of tissue) to the inspiratory and expiratory muscles increase substantially, probably to a similar extent as to limb locomotor muscles. Diaphragm $\dot{V}O_2$ also increases many times above resting values as a result of both increased blood flow and increased oxygen extraction. In total, during maximal exercise, blood flow to the inspiratory and expiratory muscles approximates 15% to 16% of the total cardiac output.

The fraction of cardiac output devoted to respiratory muscles in running equines as measured with microspheres (49) is similar to that estimated indirectly in humans from measuring the reduction in cardiac output and $\dot{V}O_2$ after unloading the respiratory muscles with a mechanical ventilator during maximum exercise (Fig. 8.11) (50). Furthermore, the fraction of the total $\dot{V}O_2$ devoted to breathing agrees closely with that obtained by measuring the increase in $\dot{V}O_2$ when the work of breathing during exercise was mimicked voluntarily by resting subjects (Fig. 8.10). Certainly none of these methods is without some error in estimating the total blood flow devoted to breathing during exercise. For example, the blood flow measured in the des-

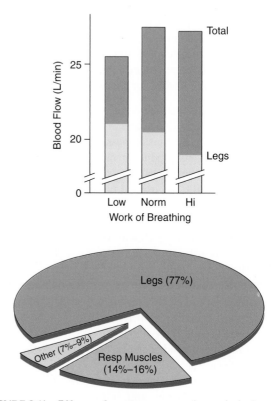

FIGURE 8.11 Effects of respiratory muscle work during exercise on cardiac output and its distribution in endurance-trained male subjects cycling at $\dot{V}O_{2max}$ ($\dot{V}O_2$ = 65 mL · kg^{-1} · min^{-1}; cardiac output = 28 L · min^{-1}). The estimated distribution of blood flow to the limb locomotor and respiratory muscles is shown in the pie chart. These estimates come from three sources: (a) the oxygen cost of breathing at maximum exercise (47), (b) measurements based on microsphere distribution to the respiratory muscles during maximum exercise in the pony (49), and (c) the change in cardiac output and limb muscle blood flow in response to unloading the respiratory muscles during maximum exercise (50,104). These effects of respiratory muscle unloading at maximum exercise on limb blood flow and on total cardiac output are shown in the insert. With reduced respiratory muscle work, that is, unloading, the total cardiac output falls and the limb muscle blood flow rises, whereas with respiratory muscle loading and increased work of breathing at maximum exercise, the maximum cardiac output remains unchanged but the limb blood flow is reduced.

ignated respiratory muscles of the abdomen and rib cage in the exercising quadruped is likely devoted in large part to trunk stabilization and locomotion. Furthermore, a portion of the reductions in stroke volume and cardiac output achieved via mechanical unloading of the respiratory muscles in the human was likely due to reductions in the negativity of P_{it} (see section *Cardiorespiratory Interactions during Exercise*). For now we can only conclude that a substantial portion of the total cardiac output and total $\dot{V}O_2$, probably in the range of 10% to 16% (depending on the maximum metabolic and ventilatory requirements of the individual), is devoted to inspiratory and expiratory muscle work during maximum exercise.

Recent studies have provided some promise that blood flow to the respiratory muscles can be determined in humans under exercising conditions. The method is based on the Fick principle and requires the measurement of indocyanine green dye concentration in the tissue microcirculation using near infrared spectroscopy and in the arterial blood using photodensitometry. Using this technique, Guenette et al. (51) found that respiratory muscle blood flow in the region of the seventh intercostal space increased progressively with voluntary increases in ventilation (from rest to $120\,L \cdot min^{-1}$). As ventilation rose, respiratory muscle blood flow correlated with cardiac output and work of breathing. A limitation of the method is that it is impossible to determine the relative blood flow contributions of the various muscles located within the field of view of the optodes over the seventh intercostal space. Nonetheless, the technique does have the potential to provide insight into human respiratory muscle blood flow during exercise.

Respiratory muscle fatigue

Muscle fatigue is universally defined as a reduction in force output and/or velocity of shortening in response to muscle activity that recovers with rest. The most objective method of assessing respiratory muscle fatigue is to estimate the force output of the muscle in question by measuring the P_{it} response to motor nerve stimulation. For the diaphragm, force development across the muscle (P_{di}) is estimated by measuring the difference between P_{ga} and esophageal pressure induced by electrical or magnetic stimulation of both phrenic nerves at one or more stimulation frequency (52). For the abdominal muscles, force output is estimated by measuring the P_{ga} response to magnetic stimulation of the thoracic nerve roots (53).

These nerve stimulation techniques have been used to show that under certain conditions, dynamic exercise can induce contractile fatigue of the diaphragm (54) and abdominal muscles (55). After short-term, progressive exercise to exhaustion in untrained or trained subjects, stimulated P_{di} was not reduced below pre-exercise values. Similarly, stimulated P_{di} was unaffected by constant-load exhaustive exercise at intensities less than 80% of $\dot{V}O_{2max}$. However, after sustained exercise continued to exhaustion at intensities greater than 80% to 85% of $\dot{V}O_{2max}$, stimulated P_{di} was reduced by

15% to 30% and did not return to near pre-exercise values until 1 to 2 hours after the exercise (54). When hypoxic gas mixtures were breathed during exercise, diaphragmatic fatigue occurred with shorter exercise times, and stimulated P_{di} took longer to recover (56). More recent studies have reported postexercise declines of about 15% to 25% in the P_{ga} response to magnetic stimulation of the thoracic nerves at work rates eliciting >90% of $\dot{V}O_{2max}$ (55), indicating that like the diaphragm the abdominal muscles are also susceptible to fatigue with sustained, high-intensity exercise.

What factors contribute to exercise-induced respiratory muscle fatigue? The ventilatory parameters that lead to diaphragmatic fatigue have been determined for subjects at rest who voluntarily control their breath timing and respiratory muscle force production. The key variables include the f_R, the ratio of force developed with tidal breathing to maximum force available (as determined by the maximum P_{di} developed via maximum inspiratory effort against a closed airway), and the inspiratory duty cycle. The product of these latter two variables is the so-called tension–time index (57). Combinations of these variables produced voluntarily in normal subjects at rest while breathing against resistance can certainly cause diaphragm fatigue. At rest, however, diaphragm fatigue does not occur until the forces developed by the diaphragm are substantially greater than those present with tidal breathing during whole body exercise at intensities that caused exercise-induced diaphragmatic fatigue (58).

Why is the fatigue threshold of force production for the diaphragm so much lower during whole body exercise than at rest? The probable explanation is that at rest, the volitional increases in diaphragmatic work mean large shares of the total cardiac output are devoted to the diaphragm, whereas during exercise the diaphragm and locomotor muscles must compete for a share of the available cardiac output. The less the blood flow to the diaphragm, the less the oxygen delivery and carbon dioxide removal, the greater the likelihood of fatigue.

The physiologic consequences of exercise-induced respiratory muscle fatigue are not entirely clear. It is important to clarify that significant *fatigue* of the respiratory muscles does not mean *task failure* in terms of compromised ventilatory response to exercise. Nevertheless, two consequences of respiratory muscle fatigue that do occur during sustained heavy exercise are: (a) a decrease in the relative contribution of the diaphragm to total ventilation over time as accessory inspiratory and expiratory muscles are recruited to deliver a progressive hyperventilatory response; and (b) a tachypneic breathing pattern characterized by an increase in f_R. Both of these effects would be expected to reduce the mechanical efficiency of breathing. Exercise-induced respiratory muscle fatigue may also influence systemic blood flow distribution, with implications for exercise performance limitation (see *Respiratory Limitations to Exercise*).

Exercise-induced transient abdominal pain, or the so-called abdominal stitch, is commonly felt during sustained heavy exercise and may be associated with some aspect of diaphragmatic contraction and/or fatigue during exercise. This sharp, stabbing pain occurs in the lumbar region of the abdomen and may also involve shoulder tip pain. It occurs commonly in exercise involving repetitive torso movements, is exacerbated by fluid ingestion and distention of the stomach, and is relieved by physical measures that reduce abdominal volume (such as abdominal strapping). Diaphragm ischemia has been cited as a possible cause, but this seems unlikely. More likely causes include irritation of the ligaments extending from the diaphragm to the abdominal viscera that may be provoked by repeated diaphragm shortening, and irritation of the abdominal portion of the parietal peritoneum caused by increased P_{ab} and stomach distention (59).

KEY POINT

Diaphragm and abdominal muscles are susceptible to fatigue under conditions of sustained, high-intensity endurance exercise.

Neural Regulation of Breathing Pattern and Respiratory Muscle Recruitment

What mechanisms within the ventilatory control system are responsible for the timing of the respiratory pattern and the actions of the inspiratory and expiratory muscles? Vagally mediated feedback from lung stretch and airway receptors (Fig. 8.1) has been studied in exercising animals whose vagus nerves were isolated, placed in a skin flap in the neck, and blocked quickly and reversibly by external cooling. In humans, patients with transplanted denervated lungs have been studied, and topical airway anesthesia has also been used to block feedback from the lung in normal intact humans. Data from such studies show that blockade of vagal feedback causes frequency to slow and V_T to increase via increases in EILV, thereby demonstrating that vagal feedback was critical to limiting the increase in V_T, at least during moderate exercise. Furthermore, phasic expiratory abdominal muscle activity was enabled and rib cage expiratory muscle activity inhibited by vagal feedback during exercise. Because active expiration begins even during very light exercise, these findings suggest that vagal feedback control of active expiration via the expiratory abdominal muscles is highly sensitive to even small changes in lung stretch in both humans and dogs. Feed-forward activation of expiratory abdominal muscles, originating from locomotor areas of the higher CNS commensurate with the onset of locomotion, may also account for some of this early increase in expiratory muscle activity.

The control of breathing pattern appears to be more complex at higher exercise intensities, especially when expiratory flow limitation first appears as shown by the intersection of the tidal flow–volume loop with the maximum volitional loop (Fig. 8.9). Key questions here include the following: What constrains the expiratory muscles from developing excessive pressures beyond those effective in increasing expiratory flow rate? Is there neural feedback control over the hyperinflation that occurs as airways narrow during expiration (i.e., avoiding impending flow limitation), or does this hyperinflation occur simply because of mechanical constraint on expiratory flow rate imposed by the narrowed airways (i.e., forcing lung volume upward)? With high exercise intensities the chemoreceptor and locomotor-linked drives to breathe become intense, producing hyperventilation. However, the responsiveness of V_T and frequency to these stimuli is mechanically constrained in many subjects with a greater than average $\dot{V}O_{2max}$. This constraint has been demonstrated by showing that the slope of the V_T and ventilatory responses to added inspired carbon dioxide is reduced during heavy exercise versus that in light or moderate exercise; and that this ventilatory response to carbon dioxide during heavy exercise is enhanced if the maximum flow–volume envelope is enlarged and flow limitation is relieved by breathing HeO_2, a low-density gas mixture (60).

What about feedback from the inspiratory and expiratory muscles themselves to control breathing pattern and/or respiratory muscle recruitment? As with any negative feedback system, it makes sense that the best source of feedback should be from the structures that are the most affected by the efferent motor output, in this case, the respiratory muscles. As for limb skeletal muscles, there are high densities of sensory nerve endings in the inspiratory and expiratory muscles. Evidence in anesthetized preparations shows that type IV receptors are activated by diaphragm fatigue (61), and accumulation of lactic acid in the diaphragm muscle may actually inhibit phrenic nerve activity (62). Perhaps this inhibitory feedback from a fatiguing diaphragm may be an attempt to spare this crucial inspiratory muscle from further fatigue (or even damage). So the potential for significant feedback reflex effects from the respiratory muscles themselves on cardiorespiratory control is clearly present. These feedback influences from the diaphragm appear to be similar but probably less effective—at least over the control of ventilation—than the feedback from similar receptors in working limb skeletal muscle.

Locomotor–Respiratory Coupling

Just as there is a dual role for respiratory abdominal and rib cage muscles in assisting locomotion, it has also been claimed that locomotion affects breathing pattern and ventilation. There are certain examples of clear entrainment of f_R with stride frequency. In bipedal humans, such entrainment occurs on occasion—but is not observed consistently. The entrainment seems to occur most often in running (vs. cycling) and at high intensities in experienced (vs. novice) athletes. In quadrupeds, 1:1 locomotor-respiratory coupling is observed consistently only in galloping animals, such as horses. In the canine such strict entrainment is rare, as the high respiratory frequencies associated with panting (2–5 Hz) are common for purposes of thermal regulation.

Contribution of locomotor forces during running to the generation of airflow is commonly claimed in both humans and quadrupeds, based on the concept that the to-and-fro movements of the liver act as a visceral piston against the diaphragm. However, extensive electromyographic evidence in exercising dogs shows that each inspiration, regardless of f_R, is accompanied by diaphragmatic electrical activity and active shortening of the diaphragm (63). Furthermore, in running humans, airflow associated with the foot plant was shown to contribute less than 2% of the total V_T generated during active inspiration. So, although there are certainly important mechanical links between locomotion and respiratory muscle function, exercise hyperpnea and breathing pattern during bipedal exercise are not commonly determined by the mechanical consequences of locomotor activity. Thus, neural control mechanisms are clearly required for this coupling between locomotion and ventilation. Again, the usual suspects invoked to explain this coupling are central locomotor command and peripheral feedback. By using an in vitro brainstem–spinal cord preparation and electrical stimulation of sensory afferent pathways to simulate the effects of muscle contraction, sensory feedback from the legs during walking was shown to play a key role in providing timing information for the respiratory system to couple the breathing frequency to the locomotor rhythm (64).

This neuroanatomical linkage originating in proprioceptor afferents from the lumbar spinal cord, with sensory input to the medullary respiratory network and motor output to phrenic motor neurons and diaphragm, may provide the basis for locomotor-respiratory coupling in many mammals. These types of findings represent an important advance in understanding because of the unique capability of these preparations to isolate and separate specific mechanisms. However, whether the demonstrated dominance of peripheral over central locomotor input on respiratory rhythm will hold during actual dynamic exercise in the intact animal remains untested.

Perception of Breathlessness

In our discussions of the control of breathing and exercise hyperpnea, we have emphasized the brainstem as the sole depository of afferent inputs from reflex receptors in the periphery and from higher locomotor centers. However, common experience tells us that the cerebral cortex must also receive information related to the effort to breathe. For example, we commonly express an awareness of an increased effort to breathe during moderate exercise. With further increases in exercise intensity, most healthy persons will eventually express an unpleasant sensation commonly called shortness of breath, breathlessness, or dyspnea. This dyspneic sensation assumes great significance to daily living in many patients with pulmonary or cardiac disease, who often have debilitating and truly painful levels of dyspnea during even light exercise. Such symptoms become a major limitation to exercise tolerance and likely play a role in the conscious decision on

the part of these patients whether to engage in exercise in their daily living. It is also likely that these cortical perceptions of breathing effort play some significant role in determining f_R and V_T in an attempt to minimize breathing discomfort. It is now relatively common in routine exercise testing to assess subjective perceptions of dyspnea (in addition to those of limb discomfort) using various rating scales (e.g., Borg, visual analogue).

There is a sound anatomical and neurophysiologic basis for the CNS to be made aware of excessive sensory input associated with breathing efforts and ventilatory stimuli. Sensory input received by the medullary pattern generator, in addition to providing motor output to stimulate the respiratory muscles, also gives rise to neural information that is relayed to and perceived by higher (supramedullary) nervous system structures as an unpleasant sensation emanating from increased respiratory effort. Evidence that neural pathways from the medulla to higher centers exist stems from the finding that peripheral chemostimulation elicits rhythmic neuronal activity in mesencephalic and thalamic neurons (65).

The mechanisms underlying the perception of breathlessness remain a mystery. Is dyspnea due only to the magnitude of sensory input? What types of input are important? What is the role of efferent motor output to the respiratory pump muscles in the perception of respiratory effort, and how does one distinguish the effect of a high motor output from that due to the summation of massive sensory inputs alone to the higher CNS? Because only humans can provide feedback concerning their perception of effort, remarkable experiments have been conducted in such models as patients with high cervical spinal cord lesions, experimental respiratory muscle paralysis in normal subjects, and patients with heart–lung transplants (66). Most evidence supports an important role for mechanoreceptor afferent feedback from respiratory muscles, rib cage, and lung volume accompanying the hyperpnea of exercise. Furthermore, a long-held concept is that sensations of dyspnea are most likely to occur when there is a marked discrepancy between the magnitude of the central neural drive and/or the neuromuscular effort exerted by the respiratory muscles on the one hand and the ventilation (volume and flow) achieved on the other. This discrepancy and the ensuing unpleasant and often even painful perception of breathing has been aptly described as "unsatisfied inspiration." This combination of factors is most commonly encountered in patients with lung, chest wall, or cardiac diseases because of mechanical impedances to lung expansion (decreased compliance) or airflow (higher resistance) especially when the drives to breathe and the ventilatory requirements are augmented during exercise. However, the discrepancy between neural input and ventilatory output also occurs in healthy subjects during heavy exercise, especially when dynamic lung hyperinflation occurs in the face of expiratory flow limitation. Heavy exercise in the hypoxia of high altitudes often elicits extreme dyspneic sensations, probably owing to the extremely high sensory inputs emanating from hypoxemic and acidotic carotid chemoreceptors in combination with the markedly increased levels of respiratory muscle work.

Pulmonary Gas Exchange

Demands Imposed on the Lung by Exercise

Exercise places huge demands on the lung. First, the lung is faced with large changes in oxygenation ($P\bar{v}O_2$ declining to <20 mm Hg) and carbon dioxide ($P\bar{v}CO_2$ rising to >75 mm Hg), as the locomotor muscles use oxygen and produce carbon dioxide (Table 8.1). Second, because of a rising $\dot{Q}$, the lung has a greatly reduced time to equilibrate the deoxygenated mixed venous blood with the alveolar gas in order to maintain PaO_2 (and $PaCO_2$) near resting levels. Third, the lung is the only organ that receives all of the blood pumped from the heart and, thus, must accommodate the entire increase in cardiac output during exercise. This huge increase in blood flow has the potential to substantially increase pulmonary vascular pressures, thereby increasing the load placed on the right ventricle

and presenting a large hydrostatic pressure gradient that could force plasma water out of the vasculature and into the alveoli. The exudation of even small amounts of fluid into the alveoli would substantially reduce the diffusion of oxygen into the pulmonary capillaries, resulting in severe arterial hypoxemia.

We know that these dire events do not usually occur in the normal lung even during heavy exercise, as PaO_2 is (with some exceptions) maintained near resting levels and the increase in pulmonary capillary pressure is limited to less than double its resting value. Pulmonary vascular resistance falls dramatically as cardiac output rises. The alveoli remain dry. To appreciate this remarkable homeostatic response, it is necessary to understand the unique microstructure of the gas–blood interface.

Lung Structure Suits Function

The structure of the pulmonary circulation is aimed at preserving a low vascular resistance and providing the maximum alveolar–capillary surface area for diffusion (Fig. 8.12). To this end, vessels in the lung are thin-walled,

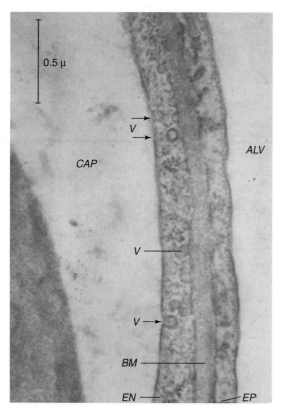

A

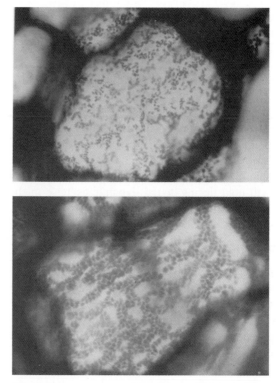

B

FIGURE 8.12   A. The alveolar–capillary blood gas barrier and the alveolar-to-capillary diffusion pathway. In the capillary, the clear area is plasma and the darker area in the left bottom corner is a red blood cell. Between the alveolar epithelium and the capillary endothelium lies the interstitial fluid space, which is important to lymphatic drainage of extravascular lung water. ALV, alveolar gas; EP, alveolar epithelium; BM, basement membrane; EN, capillary endothelium; CAP, capillary. **B.** Single alveolar walls face on to show the extent of filling of the capillary network. *Top.* Capillaries relatively empty of erythrocytes in a midgravitational zone of the lung in the resting human. *Bottom.* Alveoli under higher flow conditions (such as with exercise) in which the capillary network is fully recruited and distended; the capillary network around each alveolus forms a nearly continuous sheet of blood when all capillaries are recruited.

highly compliant, and contain relatively little smooth muscle. At rest, the average resistance to blood flow in the pulmonary vasculature is only about one-tenth that in the systemic circulation.

The pulmonary arterioles at the entrance to the lung's gas exchange area contain smooth muscle and respond vigorously to local alveolar hypoxia or carbon dioxide accumulation. While this smooth muscle is innervated by motor nerves from the sympathetic branch of the autonomic nervous system, pulmonary arterioles do not constrict vigorously with reflex sympathetic activation. This lack of sympathetic vasoconstriction is important to maintaining a low resistance in the pulmonary vasculature during exercise.

The pulmonary circulation includes an extensive interdigitating capillary network within the alveolar walls (Fig. 8.12B). This capillary network has been likened more to sheets of blood than to individual channels, with its huge surface area of many square meters containing only 70 to 90 mL of blood (about 2% of the total circulating blood volume) under resting conditions. This blood volume in the pulmonary capillaries can expand more than threefold with only very small changes in perfusion pressure, as $\dot{Q}$ rises linearly with increasing work rate.

It is important for gas exchange that the alveoli are kept dry. To this end, capillary perfusion pressures are maintained relatively low during exercise. At rest there is a small outward flow of plasma fluid (about 10–20 mL · h⁻¹) from the capillaries into the interstitial space of the alveolar wall that passes into the perivascular and peribronchiolar spaces of the lung (Fig. 8.12A). In turn, the lymphatic system transports fluid from the interstitial spaces out of the lung to the hilar lymph nodes. The flow of lymph increases substantially with increasing cardiac output as hydrostatic pressure rises in the capillaries and the alveolar–capillary surface expands. This lymphatic storm sewer is vitally important to preventing exudation of fluid into the alveoli during exercise (67).

The alveolar–capillary barrier must be both *extremely thin,* so that diffusion distance is kept to a minimum, and *very strong,* so that it does not break down when capillary pressures are raised with increases in blood flow through the lung. This barrier is indeed extremely thin, less than a fraction of the thickness of a human hair, and its strength is maintained by an extremely thin layer of collagen tissue (68).

Pulmonary Vascular Response to Exercise and the Blood–Gas Barrier

The net driving force for blood flow through the lung is the pressure difference between the pulmonary artery (P_{pa}) and the pulmonary capillary (P_{cap}). The P_{pa} is measured directly via right heart catheterization. The P_{cap} is estimated from the so-called wedge pressure, obtained using a balloon-tipped catheter advanced into a lobar branch of the pulmonary artery. Changes in wedge pressure with exercise closely approximate those in left ventricular end-diastolic pressure. With the onset of moderate exercise, there is a parallel rise in both pulmonary arterial and wedge pressure with no change in the driving pressure ($P_{pa} - P_{cap}$) across the lung (Fig. 8.13). Nevertheless, $\dot{Q}$ increases, indicating an abrupt fall in pulmonary vascular resistance. This reduced resistance reflects an increase in cross-sectional area of the pulmonary vasculature as more capillaries are recruited, especially in the lung apices, and as already recruited capillaries become

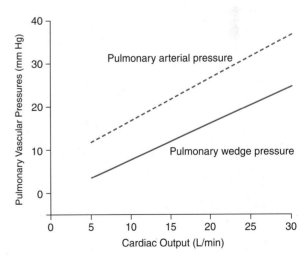

FIGURE 8.13 Pressures in the pulmonary artery and pulmonary capillaries (wedge pressures) plotted against cardiac output during progressive steady state exercise. The relationships between the increasing pulmonary blood flow and the increasing vascular pressures were such that pulmonary vascular resistance fell from rest to moderate exercise and remained low through heavy exercise. (Modified from Reeves JT, Dempsey JA, Grover RF. Pulmonary circulation during exercise. In: Weir EK, Reeves JT, eds. *Pulmonary Vascular Physiology and Pathophysiology.* New York: Marcel Dekker; 1989:107–133.)

distended (Fig. 8.12B). As exercise intensity increases further, the linear increase in blood flow through the lung is achieved with only minor further reductions in pulmonary vascular resistance, principally by increasing the driving pressure within the pulmonary vasculature.

With progressive increases in exercise intensity, the purely mechanical effects of a rising left atrial filling pressure and pulmonary capillary pressure secondary to the increase in $\dot{Q}$ exert the dominant effect on recruitment and distension of the delicate, thin-walled, highly compliant lung capillaries. This rise in left atrial pressure accounts for almost all of the upstream increase in P_{pa}.

Increased shear stress on the pulmonary vasculature induces release of potent vasodilators, such as nitric oxide, from the vascular endothelium. However, these humoral vasodilators are of only minor importance in regulating pulmonary hemodynamics during progressive exercise. During prolonged constant-load exercise, pulmonary vascular resistance falls over time, and this may involve active vasodilatation secondary to the release of vasodilators from the endothelium.

Fluid homeostasis within the lung microcirculation is governed by Starling forces, which include the hydrostatic pressure gradient from the vessel lumen to the interstitial fluid space, the oncotic pressures governing reabsorption into the capillary, and the permeability of the blood–gas barrier. Heavy exercise places significant stress on the integrity of the blood–gas barrier. First, pulmonary capillary wedge pressures during maximal exercise often exceed 20 mm Hg in untrained subjects (at cardiac outputs of about 25 L · min^{-1}) and 30 to 35 mm Hg in highly trained subjects (at cardiac outputs of 30 to 35 L · min^{-1}). These elevated capillary wedge pressures are approaching those shown to cause fluid accumulation in isolated lung lobes. Second, lungs stretched to extreme volumes (as may occur with dynamic hyperinflation in high-intensity exercise) will narrow capillaries, increase pulmonary vascular resistance, and increase the permeability of the pulmonary capillaries by increasing longitudinal tension in the alveolar walls. In addition, the alveolar–capillary surface area increases substantially with capillary recruitment during exercise, thereby promoting increased fluid flux across the blood–gas barrier.

Fluid filtration in the lungs can be determined using the following equation:

$$Q_{vc} = L_p A[(P_c - P_{ti,f}) - \sigma(\pi_c - \pi_{ti})]$$

where Q_{vc} is fluid filtration; L_p is filtration constant per unit area (index of permeability); A is membrane area available for filtration; P_c is hydrostatic pressure within the lumen; $P_{ti,f}$ is hydrostatic pressure of the interstitial fluid surrounding the vessel; σ is reflection coefficient for proteins; π_c is plasma oncotic pressure; and π_{ti} is tissue fluid oncotic pressure.

What are the consequences of these changes in extravascular fluid flux and high capillary pressures in the lung? When extravascular fluid does accumulate, it appears first as interstitial fluid cuffs surrounding larger vessels and airways outside the alveolar–capillary region. With further transvascular fluid flux, alveolar flooding may occur. It seems unlikely that exercise causes substantial fluid accumulation because fluid reabsorption from the interstitial space is enhanced by an increased capillary osmotic pressure gradient, and the thoracic lymph flow rises several orders of magnitude in proportion to the increased $\dot{Q}$. The lymphatic system is vitally important in keeping the lung dry during exercise (67). In spite of these mechanisms, there is some evidence that high-intensity, sustained exercise of maximum or near maximum effort might induce an accumulation of extravascular fluid, as demonstrated by a postexercise increase in lung density measured using noninvasive imaging techniques. In contrast, however, several other studies using similar methods have not shown an increase in lung density after exercise. The discrepancy could be attributable to differences in exercise duration and/or intensity, imaging procedure, subject fitness, or timing of postexercise imaging. For now, we must recognize that exercise-induced accumulation of extravascular fluid in humans remains a physiologic possibility but that the evidence is less than certain (69).

An extreme point on the continuum of the lung's response to stress is pulmonary capillary stress failure (Fig. 8.14). During maximal, sustained exercise in highly trained athletes there is evidence for an increased permeability of the blood–gas barrier, allowing the transport of red blood cells and plasma proteins to the alveolar spaces (70). In the thoroughbred horse, even submaximal exercise routinely causes widespread alveolar hemorrhage. In this equine athlete, the enormous cardiac output (>750 L · min^{-1} at a $\dot{V}O_{2max}$ >160 mL · kg^{-1} · min^{-1}) relative to the morphometric dimensions of the pulmonary vasculature results in left atrial pressures above 70 mm Hg, P_{pa} above 120 mm Hg, and P_{pc} approximating 100 mm Hg—these values exceed by several fold those in humans (see Fig. 8.13 and Table 8.1). The capillary stress failure occurs because of intracellular disruptions in endothelial and epithelial cells. Once the capillary pressures are reduced to normal after exercise, the intracellular disruptions close rapidly.

Regulation of A-aDo$_2$ and Pao$_2$ during Exercise

Determinants of A-aDo$_2$

The alveolar to arterial Po$_2$ difference (A-aDo$_2$) is a measure of the efficiency of pulmonary gas exchange. Its magnitude is determined primarily by the uniformity with which V_A is distributed relative to $\dot{Q}$ throughout the 300 million alveolar capillary gas exchange units in the lung. The $\dot{V}_A/\dot{Q}$

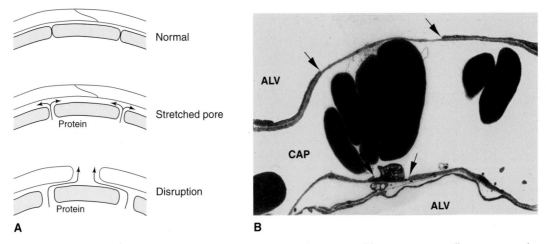

FIGURE 8.14   A. Three hypothetical stages of pulmonary edema caused by increasing capillary transmural pressure. *Top.* Normal morphology, with low protein hydrostatic edema when capillary pressure is raised. *Middle.* Pore stretching, with increased permeability of endothelium and leakage of protein into interstitium; epithelium remains intact. *Bottom.* Endothelial and epithelial disruption caused by stress failure and consequent movement of protein into alveolar space. (Redrawn from West JB, Tsukimoto K, Mathieu-Costello O, et al. Stress failure in pulmonary capillaries. *J Appl Physiol.* 1991;70:1740, with permission.) **B.** Stress failure in pulmonary capillaries (CAP) in response to very high capillary transmural pressures caused by experimentally increasing perfusion pressure in an in situ rabbit lung preparation. Both the alveolar (ALV) epithelial layer (*top*) and capillary endothelial layer (*bottom*) are disrupted (disrupted areas shown by *arrows*), with a platelet close to the basement membrane (*bottom*). (Reprinted from West JB, Tsukimoto K, Mathieu-Costello O, et al. Stress failure in pulmonary capillaries. *J Appl Physiol.* 1991;70:1733, with permission.)

distribution cannot be quantified accurately in humans, but it can be estimated in two ways. First, lung imaging of inhaled and infused radioactive tracers yields useful information on topographical gravity-dependent distribution of $\dot{V}_A/\dot{Q}$. However, this approach lacks resolution because of the large tissue volumes that must be averaged. A second approach uses intravenously infused inert gases of varying solubility in blood to provide a near-continuous measurement of $\dot{V}_A/\dot{Q}$ distribution throughout the lung. This multiple inert gas elimination technique is based on the principle that the excretion and retention of each of the inert gases by the lung depends on the magnitude of the $\dot{V}_A/\dot{Q}$ ratio and the solubility of the gas (71).

The A-aDO_2 is also determined by the extrapulmonary shunting of deoxygenated mixed venous blood that bypasses the pulmonary circulation entirely. To date, the only significant extrapulmonary shunt of deoxygenated venous blood known for sure to be present in healthy humans is that of the Thebesian venous drainage, originating in the coronary vasculature and emptying into the left ventricle. This shunt is estimated to constitute 1% to 2% of the resting cardiac output. Estimating the exact amount of shunt is usually done by determining the effects of breathing 100% oxygen on PaO_2 and A-aDO_2 and is based on the premise that increases in alveolar PO_2 to more than 600 mm Hg will readily correct any contributions to the A-aDO_2 of simply low (but > 0) $\dot{V}_A/\dot{Q}$ regions or deficient diffusion capacity (discussed later). Due to the difficulty encountered in measuring very high levels of PO_2 in blood and several of the assumptions that must be made, this

technique is of questionable value in quantifying shunts less than 10% of cardiac output.

The final determinant of the A-aDO_2 is the diffusion equilibrium of alveolar gas with end-pulmonary capillary blood, as determined by the alveolar–capillary surface area, the diffusion gradient from alveolar to capillary PO_2, and the time available for equilibration in the pulmonary capillary (Fig. 8.15). The available diffusion surface area in the lung can be estimated by inspiring small concentrations of carbon monoxide and measuring its rate of disappearance from the lung because carbon monoxide uptake is dependent on the rate of diffusion from alveolar gas to capillary blood. Diffusion disequilibrium has been quantified using the multiple inert gas elimination technique, based on the A-aDO_2 not accounted for by $\dot{V}_A/\dot{Q}$ maldistribution.

At rest, the A-aDO_2 averages 5 to 15 mm Hg in normal, healthy nonsmoking young adults and rises another 5 to 10 mm Hg or so by age 70. It is truly amazing that the A-aDO_2 is this narrow, given the marked topographical heterogeneity from lung apex to base in the distribution of $\dot{V}_A$ (four- to fivefold difference), $\dot{Q}$ (ninefold difference), and $\dot{V}_A/\dot{Q}$ (3–4 at the apex vs. 0.8 at the lung bases). Furthermore, even in the normal lung there is structural heterogeneity in vessels and airways that gives rise to nongravitational maldistribution of $\dot{V}_A$ and $\dot{Q}$ within any lung region (72). Nonetheless, the inert gas measurements show that functional $\dot{V}_A/\dot{Q}$ distribution is narrow in the normal lung at rest, with an average $\dot{V}_A/\dot{Q}$ ratio of ~0.8 to 0.9 and a variation about this mean from ~0.4 to

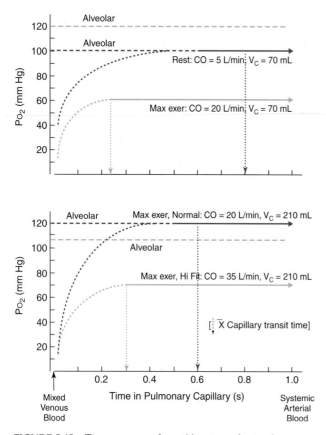

FIGURE 8.15 Time course of equilibration of mixed venous blood with alveolar gas in the pulmonary capillary at varying cardiac outputs, pulmonary capillary blood volumes (V_C), and degrees of alveolar hyperventilation (and alveolar Po_2.) *Top.* Untrained subject at rest and at maximum exercise, with normal increases in cardiac output, alveolar ventilation, and alveolar Po_2 but assuming a pulmonary capillary blood volume fixed at resting levels. The mean capillary transit time is greatly reduced from rest to exercise because cardiac output increased without a corresponding increase in pulmonary capillary blood volume. This theoretical example emphasizes the importance of the normal pulmonary capillary expansion to gas exchange during exercise. *Bottom.* Contrast between a normal untrained subject and a fit highly trained subject at maximum oxygen uptake ($\dot{V}o_{2max}$). Pulmonary capillary blood volumes are assumed to be similar in the two subjects, but maximum cardiac output and, therefore, $\dot{V}o_{2max}$ are substantially greater in the trained subject. In addition, the trained subject has not hyperventilated to the same extent as the untrained subject. Note the slower rate of equilibration of mixed venous blood with alveolar oxygen in the pulmonary capillary and the markedly shortened mean transit time in the pulmonary capillary; this is due to a cardiac output that increased out of proportion to the pulmonary capillary blood volume. Arterial hypoxemia occurs because pulmonary capillary blood reached the end of the pulmonary capillary before it reached equilibration with alveolar gas. This scenario represents one theoretical explanation for arterial hypoxemia in heavy exercise in highly trained subjects.

1.3. This distribution of $\dot{V}_A/\dot{Q}$ could account for about half of the resting A-aDo_2; the remainder is likely due to the small anatomical shunt, with no portion of the A-aDo_2 attributable to diffusion disequilibrium (Fig. 8.16).

Increased A-aDo$_2$ during exercise

A-aDo_2 begins to rise with light exercise and continues to widen to about 20 to 30 mm Hg at maximal exercise in the untrained subject and by as much as 35 to 50 mm Hg in many, but not all, endurance-trained subjects. In most subjects the increased A-aDo_2 is due to a rise in PAo_2 only because $\dot{V}_A$ increases out of proportion to $\dot{V}o_2$ resulting in the maintenance of Pao_2 near resting levels. In extreme cases of A-aDo_2 widening, arterial hypoxemia can occur (*i.e.*, Pao_2 20 to 30 mm Hg below resting levels and arterial oxyhemoglobin saturation [Sao_2] <94%). This exercise-induced arterial hypoxemia is often exacerbated by an inadequate compensatory hyperventilation (and therefore minimal rise in PAo_2) due to mechanical constraint of airflow (see *Flow–Volume Relationships*) and/or a deficiency in sensitivity to ventilatory stimuli.

We can now examine the three major mechanisms of A-aDo_2 (discussed earlier) to determine why pulmonary gas exchange becomes more inefficient as exercise intensity increases (Fig. 8.16). First, a small but significant increase, about 20% to 30% as determined via the inert gas method, occurs in the overall nonuniformity of $\dot{V}_A/\dot{Q}$ distribution throughout the lung with moderate to heavy exercise. Interestingly, topographic (or gravity dependent) $\dot{V}_A/\dot{Q}$ distribution becomes much more uniform during exercise, as perfusion to lung apices is greatly improved by an increased pulmonary arterial pressure coincident with the increase in cardiac output (Fig. 8.13). Accordingly, we presume that the increased heterogeneity in overall $\dot{V}_A/\dot{Q}$ distribution must derive from greater maldistribution within *isogravitational* lung regions. The reasons for this small increase in $\dot{V}_A/\dot{Q}$ maldistribution are unknown, but the possibilities range from release of inflammatory mediators in the airways and/or vasculature that would increase local resistances to airflow or blood flow, cuffing of airways, to accumulation of plasma water around small vessels. The most likely explanation is simply the normal anatomical heterogeneity of vessel and airway diameters and compliances within specific isogravitational lung regions. The effect of even small increases in $\dot{V}_A/\dot{Q}$ maldistribution on A-aDo_2 is magnified during exercise by the progressively reduced mixed venous oxygen content (C$\bar{v}o_2$) resulting from the increased extraction of oxygen by the working muscles (Table 8.1).

Although these combined effects of $\dot{V}_A/\dot{Q}$ maldistribution and reduced C$\bar{v}o_2$ would tend to widen A-aDo_2 and reduce Pao_2 during exercise, these effects are opposed by the disproportionate increase in total $\dot{V}_A$ relative to cardiac output. This means that average $\dot{V}_A/\dot{Q}$ increases from <1 at rest to 4 to 5 during heavy exercise. Accordingly, even the lowest $\dot{V}_A/\dot{Q}$ regions of the lung during exercise are greater in magnitude (and therefore well ventilated with high

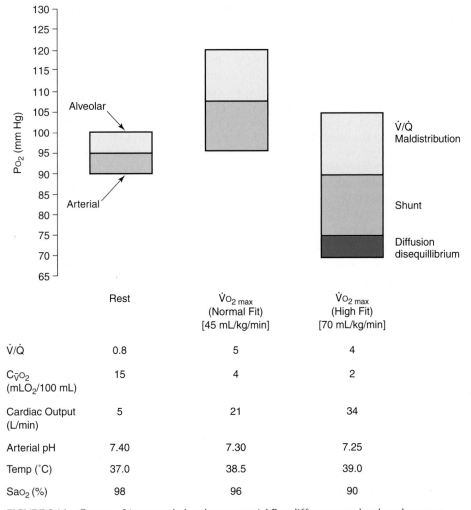

	Rest	$\dot{V}o_{2\,max}$ (Normal Fit) [45 mL/kg/min]	$\dot{V}o_{2\,max}$ (High Fit) [70 mL/kg/min]
$\dot{V}/\dot{Q}$	0.8	5	4
$C_{\bar{v}}o_2$ (mLO$_2$/100 mL)	15	4	2
Cardiac Output (L/min)	5	21	34
Arterial pH	7.40	7.30	7.25
Temp (°C)	37.0	38.5	39.0
Sao$_2$ (%)	98	96	90

FIGURE 8.16   Causes of increased alveolar to arterial Po_2 difference and reduced percent oxyhemoglobin saturation during maximum exercise in a normally fit subject and in a highly fit subject with exercise-induced arterial hypoxemia. In the normally fit subject, the A-aDo$_2$ at maximum exercise is due to approximately equal contributions from $\dot{V}_A/\dot{Q}$ maldistribution and a small anatomical shunt of mixed venous blood. Both contributions to the A-aDo$_2$ from these sources are magnified because of the exercise-induced reductions in mixed venous oxygen content ($C\bar{v}o_2$). In the highly fit subject, most of the A-aDo$_2$ at maximum exercise is caused by $\dot{V}_A/\dot{Q}$ maldistribution and shunt. In addition, it has been proposed that alveolar capillary diffusion disequilibrium is present, perhaps because of a shortened red cell transit time. The reduced Pao$_2$ in the highly fit subject is also due to blunted hyperventilation (note the lower alveolar Po_2). The reduced Sao$_2$ is due almost equally to the reduced Pao$_2$ and to a rightward shift in the hemoglobin-oxygen dissociation curve in arterial blood because of reduced arterial pH and increased core temperature.

alveolar Po_2) than the highest $\dot{V}_A/\dot{Q}$ regions at rest. Thus, the ventilatory response to exercise is a key protector of pulmonary gas exchange and arterial Po_2 during exercise.

Although $\dot{V}_A/\dot{Q}$ maldistribution accounts for about half of the increase in A-aDo$_2$ during exercise, what accounts for the remainder of the increase? Two popular postulates are shunting and diffusion disequilibrium. There is no definitive way to partition these potential contributions to the A-aDo$_2$. Extrapulmonary shunting must be a significant contributor to the increased A-aDo$_2$, because we know that venous drainage from the coronary sinuses to the left ventricle via the Thebesian veins does exist in the human. Furthermore, as myocardial $\dot{V}o_2$ increases during exercise,

the oxygen content of coronary sinus effluent blood must fall and the absolute flow of shunted blood increase. Other potential conduits for shunting mixed venous blood may open up during exercise, as cardiac output and pulmonary arterial pressure increase. Intracardiac shunts from patent foramen ovale (PFO) are thought to be present in more than 30% of the normal population, and significant intracardiac shunts have been reported during exercise in hypoxic environments (73). Recent work suggests that large-diameter intrapulmonary arteriovenous shunt vessels are recruited during exercise (74–76), but it is not yet clear whether these shunts contribute significantly to the widening of A-aDo$_2$ during exercise (77,78).

Can alveolar–capillary diffusion disequilibrium occur during exercise and explain a portion of the widened A-aDO$_2$? This will depend on the rate of equilibration of mixed venous blood with alveolar PO$_2$ (*i.e.*, diffusion capacity) and the time available in the pulmonary capillary for this equilibrium to occur (Fig. 8.15). The transit time of the red blood cell in the pulmonary capillary depends critically on how closely changes in pulmonary capillary blood volume match those in cardiac output during exercise.

Mean transit time of the pulmonary capillaries (s) = pulmonary capillary blood volume (mL) ÷ pulmonary blood flow (mL · s^{-1})

For example, at rest:
$$\text{Transit time} = 70 \text{ mL} \div 5000 \text{ mL} \cdot \text{min}^{-1}$$

Thus,
$$\text{Transit time} = 70 \text{ mL} \div 83 \text{ mL} \cdot \text{s}^{-1} = 0.8 \text{ s}$$

If one exercises at high intensity, so that cardiac output increases to 20 L · min^{-1} and pulmonary capillary blood volume does not change from resting levels, the mean transit time would fall to about 0.2 seconds and there is an excellent chance that diffusion disequilibrium of capillary blood with alveolar gas would occur. However, four important adaptations during exercise counteract this potential diffusion disequilibrium in the pulmonary capillary. First, alveolar–capillary surface area increases, which greatly increases the *diffusion capacity* of the lung (*i.e.*, oxygen diffused and taken up by the capillary blood per millimeter of mercury of diffusion gradient). Second, the extremely short alveolar–capillary diffusion distance is preserved by preventing plasma fluid from entering the alveoli via reductions in pulmonary vascular resistance combined with high lymphatic drainage of the lung interstitium (discussed previously). Third, alveolar PO$_2$ increases (via hyperventilation) as the venous PO$_2$ falls (via muscle oxygen extraction), increasing the diffusion gradient of alveolar to capillary PO$_2$. Finally, pulmonary capillary blood volume gradually expands, as capillaries are recruited with increased cardiac output, and reaches values of 200 to 250 mL in normal-sized adults (or about three times resting values). This expanded pulmonary capillary volume probably approaches the maximum morphologic capacity of the entire pulmonary capillary vasculature during maximal exercise; that is, all capillaries are recruited and maximally distended (Fig. 8.12B). Thus, at 20 L · min^{-1} cardiac output, mean transit time is 0.5 to 0.6 seconds and diffusion equilibrium is readily achieved in the pulmonary capillaries. Estimates of the influence of these changes on the rate of and the time for equilibration of oxygen in the pulmonary capillaries are shown schematically in Figure 8.15.

To summarize, the A-aDO$_2$ of 20 to 25 mm Hg achieved in most normal, untrained subjects at $\dot{V}O_{2max}$ is attributable primarily to $\dot{V}_A/\dot{Q}$ maldistribution and reduced $C\bar{v}O_2$, plus some significant (but still unquantified) contribution from anatomical shunts (Fig. 8.16). Diffusion disequilibrium is unlikely to play a significant role in these subjects.

However, in some endurance-trained subjects who widen A-aDO$_2$ to more than 30 mm Hg at higher $\dot{V}O_{2max}$ there is a greater probability that diffusion equilibrium is incomplete, due in part to the extremely short capillary transit times. This may occur in these subjects because maximum cardiac output is higher than in the untrained while maximum pulmonary capillary blood volume may only approximate that in the untrained subject (see *Training Effects and Plasticity in the Respiratory System*). In addition, many trained subjects have little or no hyperventilatory response to heavy exercise such that alveolar PO$_2$ and the alveolar-to-capillary diffusion gradient are less than normal.

Finally, the ratio of pulmonary capillary volume to blood flow is likely to be distributed heterogeneously throughout the lung. Accordingly, the distribution of red cell transit times will also be heterogeneous. In turn, during heavy exercise when calculated mean transit time is barely sufficient to ensure diffusion equilibrium it is likely that at least a small, but significant, portion of capillary blood flow will perfuse gas exchange areas with a low pulmonary capillary volume and, therefore, markedly shorten transit time. In these areas of the lung, diffusion equilibrium may not occur. In the face of a falling $C\bar{v}O_2$, these small areas of the lung with very short transit times would be expected to contribute significantly to the overall widening of A-aDO$_2$.

> ## KEY POINT
>
> Impairment of pulmonary gas exchange with exercise is caused by ventilation-perfusion maldistribution, extrapulmonary shunting, intracardiac and intrapulmonary shunting, diffusion limitations, and mechanical ventilatory constraints.

> ## TEST YOURSELF
>
> The pulmonary system faces several "challenges" with exercise. Increased muscle metabolism at high exercise intensities causes a fall in mixed venous O$_2$ content and a rise in mixed venous PCO$_2$. However, even during heavy exercise arterial PO$_2$ and PCO$_2$ usually remain close to resting values. What are the anatomic/functional aspects of the pulmonary system and the physiologic adjustments that enable this to occur? Consider your answer from (a) rest to (b) light exercise to (c) near-maximal exercise.

Cardiorespiratory Interactions during Exercise

It makes sense that the functions of the cardiovascular and respiratory systems should be tightly linked and that their neural control systems communicate, simply because both organ systems acting together are the major determinants of oxygen and carbon dioxide transport (oxygen transport is the product of CaO_2 and blood flow). It would serve no useful purpose to activate one system at the onset of exercise, for example, an increase in $\dot{V}O_2$ and cardiac output, without increasing ventilation to maintain CaO_2. Accordingly, there is ample evidence to show that the two primary mechanisms proposed for exercise hyperpnea also have major cardiovascular influences during exercise. First, central locomotor command has parallel neural pathways to medullary neural networks, which in turn affect increases in both ventilation and cardiac output. Second, activation of type III and IV afferents in contracting limb skeletal muscle reflexively increases both ventilation and sympathetic efferent vasoconstrictor activities. Furthermore, one important trigger for these afferents is the venous distention in muscle that is secondary to increased muscle blood flow (16). There are many other such examples of cardiorespiratory interactions operating during dynamic exercise. We briefly address two fundamental interactions: One is an important determinant of venous return and cardiac output via mechanical heart-lung interdependencies, and the other may influence sympathetic vasoconstrictor outflow and blood flow distribution during exercise via mechanoreflexes and metaboreflexes from the respiratory muscles. Chapter 9 discusses several of these cardiac regulators and our intention here is to show how those regulators are impacted by respiration.

Mechanical Interactions between the Respiratory and Circulatory Systems

The performance of the right and left ventricles is in large part determined by the influence of end-diastolic volume (i.e., preload) and systolic wall stress (i.e., afterload). Perhaps the greatest challenge to understanding cardiorespiratory interactions is forcing oneself to think in terms of *transmural* pressures (inside pressure minus outside pressure). The heart, situated within the intrathoracic space, is unavoidably exposed to excursions in P_{it}, and its juxtaposition to the lungs in the cardiac fossa provides an additional mechanical interface. At any given point in the respiratory cycle, cardiac preload and afterload will be a function of not only intracardiac pressure but also P_{it} and lung surface–cardiac fossa pressure (P_{lung}). Similar relationships hold true for the transmural wall stress across the blood vessels within the abdominal compartment or rib cage, which can also be influenced by P_{it}, P_{lung}, or P_{ab}. To facilitate the understanding of the basic mechanical interactions between the pulmonary and circulatory systems, the effects of inspiratory and expiratory pressure production are first discussed in the resting human (see also Fig. 8.17).

Mechanical effects of P_{it} and P_{lung} on cardiac preload and afterload at rest

During inspiration, the negative pressure generated in the intrathoracic space widens the pressure gradient across the walls of the heart. Such a widened transmural pressure is thought to improve ventricular filling by lowering the pressures within the heart's chambers and augmenting cardiac preload. Of particular importance are the reductions in right atrial pressure during inspiration that widen the pressure gradient for venous return from the limbs and splanchnic vasculature and increase the return of blood to the heart. However, the increases in ventricular preload during inspiration due to a reduced P_{it} can be limited by increases in lung surface pressure (P_{lung}) as the cardiac fossa becomes less compliant with increasing lung volumes (79). These increases in P_{lung} usually become significant only at higher lung volumes (e.g., >75% TLC), and the transmural pressure across the walls of the heart is predominantly influenced by changes in P_{it}. During the ensuing expiration, ventricular filling is impeded by a narrowing of the transmural pressure gradient due to a positive shift in P_{it}, which also reduces the pressure gradient for venous return.

During systole, the reductions in P_{it} during inspiration widen the transmural pressure gradient across the walls of the heart and actually *hinder* ventricular emptying. Conversely, during expiration, the positive shift in P_{it} can actually *aid* the emptying of the ventricle by the narrowing of the transmural pressure gradient (i.e., the positive P_{it} pushes inward on the ventricle as it contracts inward). Although increases in P_{it} during expiration may increase stroke volume very transiently (e.g., modulation over the course of a breath), the volume of blood ejected from the heart with each contraction is largely dependent on ventricular preload, and reductions in cardiac preload will usually predominate over reductions in transmural wall stress because of the dependence of stroke volume on the Frank-Starling mechanism in normal humans.

Mechanical effects of diaphragm contraction and intra-abdominal pressure on venous return at rest

Although the previous section implies that reductions in P_{it} always increase venous return to the heart, increases in inferior vena caval blood flow are not always observed during inspiration at rest. This is primarily because increases in P_{ab} due to diaphragmatic descent can compress the abdominal inferior vena cava and impede venous return from the lower limb (80). Further, complicating matters is the observation that diaphragmatic contraction decreases venous return from the splanchnic circulation via compression of the liver, with this phenomenon occurring independently of changes in P_{ab} (81). A third and final consideration in the prediction of the effects of breathing on venous return is the blood volume status of the inferior vena cava. If abdominal vena caval blood volume is high (e.g., immediately preceding an inspiration at rest), increases in P_{ab} will translocate a relatively large volume of blood up toward the heart during inspiration as a

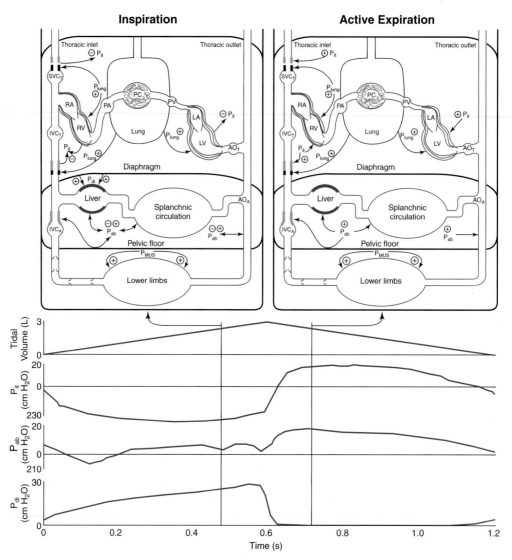

FIGURE 8.17 The cardiovascular effects of respiratory muscle pressure production during high-intensity exercise ($>90\%$ $\dot{V}O_{2max}$, $f_R = 50$ breaths $\cdot$ min^{-1}) at the same lung volume during inspiration and expiration. During inspiration, intrathoracic pressure (P_{it}) can decrease to less than -30 cm H$_2$O, resulting in a substantial widening of the pressure gradient across the walls of the heart (denoted by a negative sign). During expiration, P_{it} becomes positive, decreasing the transmural pressure across the walls of the heart (denoted by a positive sign). These shifts in P_{it} also result in significant changes in the transmural pressure across the thoracic inferior and superior venae cavae (IVC$_T$ and SVC$_T$, respectively), which can markedly alter the resistance to venous return via changing vessel cross-sectional area. Lung surface pressure (P_{lung}) increases exponentially with increases in lung volume and will have a compressive effect on the heart and great vessels. However, its magnitude is likely to be far less than that of P_{it} except in cases of severe dynamic hyperinflation. The contraction of the abdominal muscles shifts intra-abdominal pressure (P_{ab}) positive during expiration, resulting in compression of the vasculature within the abdominal compartment and driving of end-expiratory lung volume below functional residual capacity. This contributes to the biphasic P_{ab} pattern observed during inspiration, as the relaxation of the abdominal muscles during early inspiration results in a rapid outward recoiling of the abdominal wall and a reduction in P_{ab}. This occurs in spite of contraction of the diaphragm (increasing P_{di}), as its descent lags behind the outward movement of the abdominal wall until later during inspiration, when further increases in P_{di} elicit roughly proportional increases in P_{ab}. Although increases in P_{di} consistently reduce blood flow through the liver via compression of the hepatic sinusoids, the dynamics of P_{ab} result in distention of the abdominal inferior vena cava (IVC$_A$) during early inspiration (when P_{ab} is decreased), followed by moderate compression of the IVC$_A$ during the last half of inspiration (when P_{ab} is increasing). P_{ab} is smaller at all time points during inspiration than at expiration, resulting in a *relative* distention of the IVC$_A$ throughout inspiration. The modulatory effects of P_{it} and P_{ab} on venous return from the lower limbs are lower than during rest because of the powerful rhythmic contraction of the locomotor muscles that compresses the veins within them and forces blood toward the heart.

result of the compression of the abdominal vena cava (with the venous valves preventing retrograde flow), resulting in increases in venous return. However, if blood volume is low (*e.g.*, at end-inspiration at rest), a relatively small volume of blood will be translocated upward, and venous return will decrease during inspiration as a result of a decreased blood flow *through* the inferior vena cava (82).

So, predicting the effect of inspiration or expiration on cardiac filling and emptying requires knowledge not only of the magnitude and directionality of P_{it} and P_{lung}, but also of P_{ab} and P_{di}. Reductions in P_{it} cannot increase venous return from the lower limbs and splanchnic vasculature without permissive changes in P_{ab} and P_{di} (83). The role of blood volume in the cardiovascular response to changes in P_{it}, P_{ab}, and P_{di} is only beginning to be understood but is likely to play a significant role as well.

Mechanical effects of respiratory muscle pressure production on cardiovascular function during exercise

To facilitate understanding of the principles of mechanical cardiorespiratory interactions, all of the preceding discussion has focused on the effects of respiratory muscle pressure on cardiovascular function at rest. When considering these interactions during exercise, one must account for the mechanical effects of the phasic contraction of the locomotor muscles that push blood back to the heart. This is frequently referred to as the skeletal muscle pump, and it is thought to be critical in the maintenance of venous return during upright exercise. Indeed, the rhythmic contraction of the lower limb locomotor muscles alone can empty more than 25% of the blood volume contained in the lower limb vasculature. With such a powerful force pushing blood back to the heart, are the negative pressures produced during inspiration actually *required* for normal venous return and cardiac output during exercise? An idealistic approach to answering this question involves the analysis of both within-breath and steady state cardiac function.

The examination of within-breath modulation of cardiovascular function is useful because the marked modulation of venous return and cardiac output implies that the cardiovascular system is susceptible to manipulation by respiratory pressure. Unfortunately, technical limitations have resulted in few data regarding the within-breath effects of breathing on cardiovascular function during whole body exercise. Although early measures of inferior vena cava blood *velocity* implied a profound modulatory effect of ventilation on venous return during cycling exercise (84), it is difficult to translate these measures into blood *flow*, given the high compliance of the veins and relatively large changes in venous cross-sectional area that occur over the course of a breath. Nonetheless, this observation suggests that experimentally altering respiratory muscle pressure production could have significant effects on cardiac function in the steady state.

There are few data on the effects of respiratory muscle pressure on steady state cardiac output (*i.e.*, blood flow). Perhaps the most insightful intervention has been the application of positive pressure mechanical ventilation during inspiration, which makes P_{it} less negative during inspiration by forcing air into the lungs. Under these conditions, significant decreases in stroke volume and cardiac output have been observed in the steady state of moderate and heavy exercise (50,85), likely because a less negative P_{it} limits cardiac preload. These data provide strong support to the hypothesis that the pressures produced by the respiratory muscles during inspiration can contribute significantly to the normal cardiac output and stroke volume responses to dynamic exercise.

You may wonder how the negative P_{it} during inspiration can facilitate venous return from the exercising limbs if P_{ab} increases with diaphragmatic contraction. The answer lies in the mechanics used to minimize the work of breathing during exercise. Even at the onset of light exercise, expiration becomes active, P_{ab} becomes positive, and the contraction of the abdominal muscles forces EELV below FRC. Now, when the abdominal muscles relax, the abdominal wall quickly moves outward, and P_{ab} actually *decreases* during inspiration. This occurs despite the contraction of the diaphragm, as the outward movement of the abdominal wall is faster than the descent of the diaphragm. During very heavy exercise, P_{ab} can actually become *negative* (Fig. 8.17), which would widen the transmural pressure gradient across the inferior vena cava, preventing its collapse and allowing the reductions in P_{it} (which in turn reduce right atrial pressure) to facilitate the return of blood to the heart from the locomotor limbs.

Although there are few data concerning the effects of respiratory pressure production during active expiration on cardiac function, it is likely that the excessively high positive expiratory pressures produced during maximal exercise in athletes with expiratory flow limitation and in patients with chronic obstructive pulmonary disease (COPD) present a substantial limitation on cardiac function. Positive P_{it} during expiration reduces ventricular transmural pressure, thereby decreasing the rate of ventricular filling during diastole and reducing stroke volume and cardiac output (86,87). In addition, active expiration against positive resistance impedes femoral venous return, even in the face of an active muscle pump (88).

Ventricular interdependence and the matching of right and left ventricular stroke volumes

Although breathing can have a profound modulatory effect on cardiac preload by changing the transmural pressure across the right and left ventricular free walls, the effects of inspiration and expiration on ventricular filling are limited by an intrinsic autoregulatory cardiac mechanism termed *ventricular interdependence*; that is, the preload of one ventricle affects the other. Simply put, the filling of one ventricle shifts their common wall—the interventricular septum—toward the opposite ventricle, which limits filling. The magnitude of the septal shift depends in large part on septal compliance, in addition to the individual elastances of the right and left ventricular free walls, and will also be markedly affected by the extent to which the pericardium constrains the heart (89). For example, with high levels of pericardial constraint (which may occur during maximal exercise), the only way the right ventricle can increase its filling is by shifting the septal wall leftward, which, in turn, impedes left ventricular filling. However, when pericardial constraint is low, it is more likely that the right ventricular free wall will move outward to accommodate the increased end-diastolic volume, and left ventricular filling is not likely to be substantially compromised. In any event, this reciprocal relationship between right and left ventricular filling serves to equalize stroke volumes over time, as reductions in the output of one ventricle will inevitably reduce the filling of the other, and vice versa.

Although this section highlights some of the most common direct mechanical effects of respiratory pressure production on cardiovascular function, it is by no means comprehensive. A nearly endless number of permutations exists for each variable we have discussed, all yielding slightly different cardiovascular effects both over the course of a breath and over time. However, our understanding of most of these effects is poor, as data on whole body exercise in humans are limited. For detailed discussions of many of these topics in reduced animal preparations, see Scharf and associates (90). In the next section, we discuss an equally important component of ventricular afterload that may be affected by respiratory influences on autonomic function— the resistance of the skeletal muscle vascular beds.

Respiratory-Induced Autonomic Effects on Cardiovascular Function

Breathing has significant influences over sympathetic vasoconstrictor outflow and heart rate, which are manifested in two ways. First, a modulatory influence on sympathetic nerve activity and heart rate occurs within each respiratory cycle; second, overall levels of sympathetic nerve activity are increased and systemic vasoconstriction occurs when respiratory muscles undergo fatiguing contractions.

Within-breath cardiovascular modulation

In humans, muscle sympathetic nerve activity to a resting limb as measured via microneurography is markedly depressed throughout the latter half of inspiration and early expiration, and rises and peaks during mid to late expiration. The modulatory effect of ventilation on muscle sympathetic nerve activity is critically dependent on lung volume, with both V_T and the lung volume from which inspiration begins being important determinants of the extent of modulation (91). However, the magnitude of central respiratory motor output does not affect the modulation

of muscle sympathetic nerve activity over the course of a breath (91). These observations demonstrate that lung stretch is important to sympathetic inhibition during inspiration and to its modulation over the course of a breath. The neural pathway controlling this feedback modulation originates in the pulmonary stretch receptors in the lung parenchyma, travels through the vagus nerves to the NTS, and eventually meets a common pool of cardiorespiratory interneurons in the medulla. These interneurons, in turn, affect output from the NTS and contribute to the control of the spinal preganglionic neurons that regulate systemic vascular sympathetic tone. The most important influence of lung stretch on sympathetic nerve activity is probably through its effectiveness in modulating the sympathetic responses to baroreceptor input to the NTS, which is markedly depressed during inspiration and augmented during expiration (92).

A second well-known respiratory influence is the parasympathetically mediated within-breath variation in heart rate, by which the RR interval on an electrocardiogram in shortened during inspiration and lengthened during expiration. This so-called respiratory sinus arrhythmia is markedly dependent on V_T and requires intact feedback from pulmonary stretch receptors in the human, as demonstrated by the lack of response in lung-denervated transplant patients (93). Unlike the respiratory modulation of sympathetic activity, however, central respiratory motor output has a significant influence on respiratory sinus arrhythmia by way of direct modulation of the cardiac vagal preganglionic neurons. Collectively, these examples of within-breath modulation clearly demonstrate a strong respiratory influence on both parasympathetic and sympathetically mediated cardiovascular function in the human.

Metabochemoreceptor effects on sympathetic vasoconstrictor outflow and blood flow distribution

As detailed in the chapter on autonomic control (48), mechanoreceptors and metaboreceptors in the working skeletal muscle, together with central command from locomotor areas of the higher CNS, are important determinants of sympathetic vasoconstrictor outflow to the cardiac and systemic vasculature during exercise of all intensities, especially during high-intensity exercise. These are the same feed-forward and feedback mechanisms we previously discussed in detail as potential primary determinants of exercise hyperpnea. It is believed that augmentation of sympathetic outflow during dynamic exercise occurs in part by the integration of feedback (from muscle) and feedforward (from higher CNS locomotor centers) signals at the level of the NTS in the lateral medulla, which, in turn, results in the resetting of the baroreceptor set point (94). However, intact baroreceptors are not *required* for an exercise-induced increase of sympathetic nerve activity (95).

Evidence from animal models has shown, not surprisingly, that mechanoreceptors and metaboreceptors are also present in great quantities in the diaphragm and other inspiratory and expiratory muscles, just as they are in limb skeletal muscles (Fig. 8.18). Furthermore, diaphragm metaboreceptor activity relayed via afferent fibers in the phrenic nerves to the NTS is increased when diaphragm fatigue is produced in the anesthetized animal (62). In turn, when these metaboreceptors in the diaphragm or abdominal muscles are stimulated pharmacologically or with local lactic acid injections, increases occur in mean arterial pressure and in vascular resistance in several systemic vascular beds, including those in the limb muscle, renal, and mesenteric vasculatures (96,97). In addition, when humans fatigue their inspiratory or expiratory muscles by voluntarily breathing against resistance at a high level of respiratory motor output, muscle sympathetic nerve activity in the resting limb increases and vascular conductance and blood flow fall in a time-dependent fashion (98–100). These findings with high-intensity contractions of the respiratory muscles are similar to the increased muscle sympathetic nerve activity in resting limbs that occurs secondary to rhythmic fatiguing contractions of the forearm musculature (48).

Certainly, the mechanisms are present for respiratory muscle afferent stimulation to contribute to the general increase in efferent sympathetic vasoconstrictor activity that occurs with exercise, so long as the exercise is sufficiently intense to activate respiratory muscle metaboreceptors. This activation may begin to occur during moderate exercise (17) but is much more likely to occur during sustained heavy exercise, when diaphragm fatigue is known to be present.

Central respiratory motor output is also high during exercise, but in contrast to the excitatory effects of high central *locomotor* command on sympathetic efferent activity, there is no evidence that central *respiratory* motor output is excitatory in this regard. Even at very high (voluntary) inspiratory efforts, muscle sympathetic nerve activity is *reduced during inspiration,* apparently because of the dominant inhibitory effect of increased lung volume over augmented respiratory motor output on sympathetic efferent activity (91) (also discussed previously in the section *Within-Breath Cardiovascular Modulation*).

Another respiratory-related source of sympathetic activation in heavy exercise that is not often considered is the carotid chemoreceptors. Stimulation of these sensors by a variety of circulating hormonal stimuli with exercise elicits significant increases in sympathetic vasoconstrictor activity (see *Hyperventilation of Heavy Exercise*). In addition to mediating a reflex increase in ventilation, these receptors are an important source of sympathetic vasoconstrictor activity and their sensitivity is enhanced with exercise (101,102). It is generally assumed that the increased sympathetic nervous activity with exercise is due to feed-forward mechanisms such as central command, feedback from muscle metaboreceptors and mechanoreceptors, and/or a resetting of systemic baroreceptors (103).

We now address what respiratory-related activations of sympathetic nerve activity may have to do with systemic blood flow distribution during dynamic exercise. Recall that the locomotor muscles receive about 80% of the cardiac output during exercise. The magnitude of any increase in muscle blood flow depends on the opposing effects of strong local vasodilators on the one hand versus the braking effects (and blood pressure–sparing effects) of sympathetic vasoconstrictor activity, both of which increase with increasing exercise intensity (48). This broaches the question whether the sympathetic excitation originating from respiratory muscle metaboreceptors and/or carotid chemoreceptors can

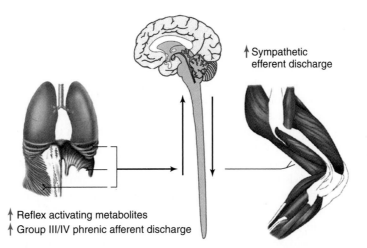

↑ Sympathetic efferent discharge

↑ Reflex activating metabolites
↑ Group III/IV phrenic afferent discharge

FIGURE 8.18   The diaphragm metaboreflex based on data in the resting human (98), the exercising dog (97), the anesthetized dog (96), and the anesthetized rat (61). Collectively, these data show that either fatiguing contractions of the diaphragm or local infusion of lactic acid into the phrenic artery increase the activity of type III/IV afferents in the diaphragm and trigger a supraspinal reflex that increases sympathetic nerve activity to the resting limb muscle vasculature and causes decreased vascular conductance and blood flow to the limb both at rest and during light exercise.

overcome the regional vasodilator effects present in locomotor muscles and redistribute a portion of flow to the respiratory muscle vasculature.

Preceding sections have provided strong evidence that the respiratory muscles:

1. Demand a significant amount of blood flow during dynamic exercise
2. Are richly innervated with afferent fibers that detect force and metabolite production and project to autonomic control centers in the medulla
3. Can elicit sympathetic activation in response to high, sustained levels of respiratory muscle work
4. Can reduce vascular conductance and blood flow to resting limb muscle

Collectively, these observations suggest that the respiratory muscles are well designed to compete for a significant fraction of cardiac output during maximal dynamic exercise, and there is a growing body of evidence that this may be so. Certainly, the 10% to 16% of total cardiac output devoted to the respiratory muscles must come from somewhere, and the locomotor muscles with their high levels of blood flow would seem to be the logical source.

The first observation that respiratory muscles could steal blood flow from the limbs came from studies using a mechanical ventilator to unload the respiratory muscles during exercise (104). When the work of breathing was reduced by about 50% during maximal exercise in fit humans, limb locomotor muscle blood flow and vascular conductance increased 7% to 10% and in proportion to decreases in norepinephrine spillover, an index of local sympathetic activity (Fig. 8.11). Furthermore, data in dogs exercising at moderate intensity (97) showed that activation of the respiratory muscle metaboreflex from the diaphragm or abdominal muscles (invoked via local lactic acidosis) caused vasoconstriction in exercising hind limb muscle and reduced blood flow a small but significant amount despite increases in systemic blood pressure.

However, phrenic afferent stimulation has been shown to increase sympathetic activity to *several* vascular beds (96), suggesting that sympathetic activity increases globally. How can blood flow be redistributed to the respiratory muscles via global sympathetic activation? This redistribution may be facilitated by regional differences in adrenergic receptor sensitivity. In vitro studies of isolated vessels have shown that α-adrenergic receptors in the diaphragm vasculature are less responsive to changes in catecholamines than in limb locomotor vasculature (105). Thus, at least theoretically, a global increase in sympathetic activity would result in greater vasoconstriction in the locomotor than respiratory muscle vasculature and, in turn, redirect blood flow to the respiratory muscles. However, technical limitations have precluded rigorous testing of these hypotheses during high-intensity dynamic exercise in vivo, a requisite for these concepts to progress beyond speculation from in vitro preparations.

As discussed previously, the carotid chemoreceptors are an important source of sympathetic vasoconstrictor activity and are sensitized with exercise. What are the effects of an enhanced carotid chemosensitivity with exercise on systemic blood flow distribution during exercise? Specific inhibition of the carotid chemoreceptors in exercising dogs caused peripheral vasodilatation, as demonstrated by increases in hind limb flow and conductance. In addition, the vasodilatation after carotid chemoreceptor inhibition was abolished with α-adrenergic blockade, suggesting that vasodilatation was due to a reduction in sympathetic outflow. By comparing both responses, the carotid chemoreceptors were shown to account for about one-third of the total increase in sympathetic nerve activity with exercise (102).

> ## KEY POINT
>
> Two fundamental cardiorespiratory interactions occur during exercise, namely mechanical heart–lung effects on venous return and cardiac output, and metabochemoreceptor effects on sympathetic vasoconstrictor outflow and blood flow distribution.

Respiratory System Across the Lifespan

The pulmonary system undergoes changes from childhood through normal healthy aging. The ventilatory response of children is altered in a variety of ways based on growth and maturation-related development. Compared to adults, children ventilate more relative to metabolic demand (106) and have smaller airways as a function of lung size (107). Even when controlled for body size, ventilation at rest and during submaximal exercise is elevated in prepubescent children. The explanation for the exaggerated ventilatory response for a given metabolic demand is not entirely clear, but may be due to a greater neural respiratory drive (108) and/or greater sensitivity of the respiratory centers to carbon dioxide in the blood (109). The increased ventilation occurs via more rapid and shallow breathing, which tends to increase V_D and decrease breathing efficiency. This breathing strategy may cause children to reach ventilatory constraints during maximal exercise at a lower relative $\dot{V}O_2$ than in adults (110). As a result, the work of breathing is likely to be elevated in children more than in adults. However, maximal respiratory pressures are surprisingly well preserved in children compared to adults (111). This may be due to the small radius of curvature of the rib cage, diaphragm, and abdomen, which, according to the Laplace relationship, converts small tensions into relatively high pressures. Nevertheless, children are unable to sustain a given percentage of their maximal pressure for as long as adults (112).

Normal healthy aging causes progressive deterioration in the structure and function of the respiratory system (113). Most of these changes begin in the mid 20s, with disproportionate changes in the fifth to sixth decades of life. In the lung, the major structural changes with aging include: (a) increased lung compliance, reflecting loss of elastic recoil of the lung due to loosening in the spatial arrangement and cross linking of the elastin collagen fiber network; and (b) reduced surface area for diffusion, due to loss of alveoli and an enlargement of the alveolar airspaces. Functionally, the loss of elastic recoil combined with a decreased tethering of small airways results in excessive airway narrowing during forced expiration. Thus, older airways tend to close at higher lung volumes (Fig. 8.19A). Accordingly, distribution of inspired air and $\dot{V}_A/\dot{Q}$ become significantly more heterogeneous with aging. The aforementioned increase in lung compliance is paralleled by a decrease in chest wall compliance, reflecting stiffening of the chest wall due to calcification of the costal cartilages and/or progressive osteoporosis-induced changes in the shape and configuration of the thorax. The strength and endurance of the respiratory muscles is also markedly reduced with age, due in part to a loss of muscle mass.

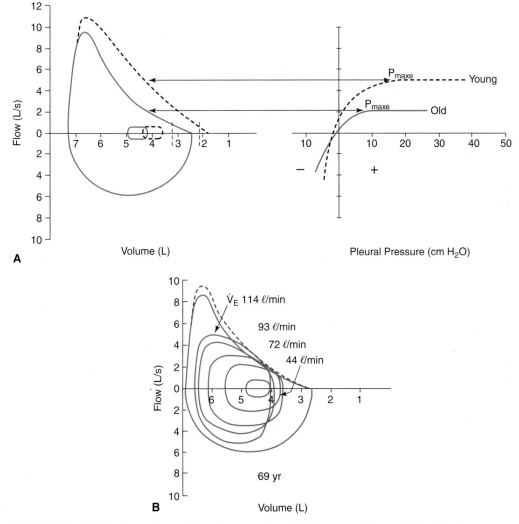

FIGURE 8.19   A. Maximum flow–volume loops and isovolume pressure-flow relationships for a 30-year-old and a 70-year-old nonsmoking man. *Left.* In the older subject the scooping in the expiratory limb of the maximum flow–volume loop indicates that airways are narrowing, thereby reducing flow rate at any given lung volume during most of forced expiration. The end-expiratory lung volume is higher in the older subject, as is the airway closing volume (vertical dashed line). *Right.* Expiratory flow increases with increasing expiratory effort up to a critical closing pressure (P_{maxe}); at which point, despite additional expiratory effort, airways narrow and close and flow no longer increases (note the much lower P_{maxe} in the older subject). These changes to the flow–volume loop, airway closing volume, and critical closing airway pressure occur with aging because of reduced lung elastic recoil. **B.** Tidal flow–volume loops at increasing levels of ventilation during steady state exercise plotted within the maximum flow–volume loop for endurance-trained 70-year-old subjects. Contrast these loops with those for young adult subjects in Figure 8.9. For the older subjects significant expiratory flow limitation begins at exercise ventilations (<70 L · min⁻¹) that are much lower than in the younger subjects (>100 L · min⁻¹). With the intersection of the tidal expiratory flow–volume loop with the maximum flow-volume envelope, end-expiratory lung volume increases to and even exceeds resting levels. (Redrawn from Johnson BD, Reddan WG, Seow KC, et al. Mechanical constraints on exercise hyperpnea in a fit aging population. *Am Rev Respir Dis.* 1991;143:968–977, with permission.)

These changes in the lung and chest wall have significant implications for the magnitude and efficiency of the respiratory system's response to exercise. In contrast to the fairly uniform respiratory responses in young adults (discussed previously), the marked variability in the effects of aging on organ system function means that the response to exercise also varies widely among individuals. Nonetheless, some generalizations regarding healthy aging effects on the acute response to exercise can be drawn.

Compared with young adults, the overall ventilatory response to exercise is higher in the elderly due to a progressive increase in V_D; thus, for a given metabolic rate, V_A is only slightly elevated. In the young adult V_D/V_T averages 0.30 to 0.35 at rest and 0.15 to 0.20 during exercise, whereas in the healthy, nonsmoking 70-year-old V_D/V_T averages 0.40 to 0.50 at rest and 0.25 to 0.30 during exercise. The high V_D/V_T likely reflects heterogeneous airway narrowing leading to a maldistribution of ventilation in the elderly. Age-related declines in vital capacity (due to an increase in residual lung volume via the loss of lung elastic recoil) limit V_T during exercise. Thus, at any given ventilation, f_R is higher and V_T lower, thereby increasing V_D. The end result is that the total ventilatory response (alveolar plus V_D) in the aged is excessive and therefore inefficient.

Figure 8.19B shows average values for the flow–volume relationship at rest and during exercise for healthy elderly subjects. The most striking contrast with younger subjects is that the elderly begin to exhibit significant expiratory flow limitation even during mild-to-moderate exercise at relatively low ventilations ($60–70 \; L \cdot min^{-1}$), and this flow limitation worsens as exercise intensity and ventilation increase further in fit elderly subjects (114). These responses are in sharp contrast to the typical young adult subject, who does not begin to show any flow limitation until ventilation exceeds $\sim130 \; L \cdot min^{-1}$ (Fig. 8.9). The exercise-induced flow limitation in the elderly results from the increased ventilatory requirements of exercise (due to augmented dead space) and the relatively reduced maximal ventilatory reserve (due to reduced lung elastic recoil).

At any given ventilation during exercise the work of breathing is higher in the elderly subject compared to control. Expiratory flow limitation accounts for much of this increase, because it not only increases expiratory resistance but, more importantly, causes hyperinflation and therefore increases elastic work during inspiration. Consequently, the older flow-limited subject must breathe along the upper, stiffer portion of the pressure–volume relationship of the lung. The lower compliance of the chest wall in the aged adult also contributes to increased ventilatory work during exercise. It is presumed that this elevated ventilatory work during exercise will require greater oxygen consumption and blood flow by the respiratory muscles. Furthermore, the increased work of breathing likely contributes to the age-related increase in exertional dyspnea (66). Lastly, respiratory muscle efficiency is reduced because of the expiratory

flow limitation and the associated lung hyperinflation. When exercising in the hyperinflated state, the diaphragm and other inspiratory muscles will be shortened and maximum force-generating capacity reduced. Accordingly, during heavy exercise the inspiratory muscles of elderly subjects operate in excess of 80% of dynamic capacity. In contrast, younger subjects at comparable $\dot{V}O_{2max}$ and $\dot{V}E_{max}$ typically operate at only 40% to 60% of maximum dynamic capacity for pressure generation (Fig. 8.9).

The aforementioned changes in pulmonary structure and function could have a negative impact on exercise gas exchange. The normally fit older adult widens the A-aDO_2 to a similar extent during maximal exercise as the young athlete at an equivalent metabolic rate, and PaO_2 during maximal exercise remains within $\sim5 \; mm \; Hg$ of resting values (114). However, some highly active and fit elderly subjects with a $\dot{V}O_{2max}$ 1.5 to 2 times that of age-matched controls (and about equal to untrained 30 year olds) do exhibit substantially widened A-aDO_2 ($\sim35 \; mm \; Hg$), limited hyperventilation ($PaCO_2$ 35–41 mm Hg), and arterial hypoxemia (PaO_2 <75 mm Hg, SaO_2 85%–94%) (114,115). Thus, fit elderly subjects encounter arterial hypoxemia for the same reasons as a subpopulation of highly trained younger subjects: widened A-aDO_2 and limited hyperventilation due to mechanical constraints. However, the arterial hypoxemia occurs in fit elderly subjects with a relatively low $\dot{V}O_{2max}$ ($40–55 \; mL \cdot kg^{-1} \cdot min^{-1}$), whereas in young adult subjects much higher levels of $\dot{V}O_{2max}$ are required before hypoxemia is observed.

Given the deleterious effects of aging on airway closure, ventilation distribution, and alveolar diffusion surface, it is surprising that a much higher prevalence of arterial hypoxemia is not observed in healthy fit elderly subjects. It appears that a reduction in maximal metabolic demand ($\dot{V}O_{2max}$) occurs with age at a rate equal to or greater than that of respiratory system deterioration. Accordingly, the maximal *demands* for ventilation and alveolar-to-arterial oxygen transport relative to the *capacity* for maximum airflow and alveolar capillary diffusion are usually no greater in young than in healthy elderly subjects. There remain, however, exceptionally active, highly fit elderly individuals whose $\dot{V}O_{2max}$ (demand) declines substantially less than normal with age but whose age-dependent decline in structural capacities of the lung and airways is normal and unaffected by their lifelong physical training regimen (114,115). Mechanical ventilatory constraint, arterial hypoxemia, and thus exercise limitation are most likely to occur in this population.

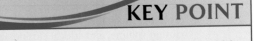

KEY POINT

Reductions in lung elastic recoil, vital capacity, diffusion surface area, and chest wall compliance are a normal consequence of aging that may result in an excessive/inefficient ventilatory response and limit endurance exercise performance via mechanical ventilatory constraint and arterial hypoxemia.

Sex Differences in Respiratory Function

The human response to exercise has traditionally been studied in male rather than female subjects. Male–female differences have been documented for many of the major determinants of exercise performance, such as substrate metabolism, fatigability of skeletal muscle, and autonomic control of the cardiovascular system. Sex differences in pulmonary function have received much less attention. There are at least two differences between men and women that may influence the integrated response to exercise.

Gas Exchange

The total number of alveoli is present by the age of 2 years with little or no subsequent alveolar multiplication. Rather, with normal lung growth, it is the alveolar size that increases. Studies using morphometric techniques applied to autopsied lungs show that for a given stature and age, boys have more alveoli and a larger surface area than girls (116). Women have significantly smaller lung volumes and a lower resting diffusion capacity than men, even when corrected for body size and hemoglobin concentration. Sex differences in lung diffusion capacity can be explained by fewer alveoli and smaller airway diameters relative to lung size in women, and these differences probably become significant late in the growth period of the lung. Given the pulmonary structural differences that exist between men and women, it is reasonable to predict that pulmonary gas exchange disturbances and hypoxemia would be more likely in women than in men. Support for this assertion stems from a recent literature review which showed that females had a greater A-aDo$_2$ and a lower Pao$_2$ at the same relative $\dot{V}o_2$ (117).

Dysanapsis

There is direct anatomical evidence that the pattern of airway-parenchymal growth is different for boys and girls (116). Postmortem lungs obtained from children showed that boys had larger lungs than girls starting at approximately 2 years. Even when lung volume was corrected for differences in body length, boys continued to have larger lungs per unit of stature. If there is perfectly proportional growth of the airways and lung parenchyma, then the ratio of airway area to lung volume should be constant and independent of lung volume. By extension, any deviation would reflect unequal growth or *dysanapsis*. In this regard, it has been shown that women have airways that are smaller relative to lung size than men (107,118). However, previous studies have been limited by the use of indirect estimates of airway size or by the assessment of airways above the tracheal carina. A more recent study using high-resolution computed tomography in a group of elderly men and women showed that women have smaller luminal areas of the large and central airways (trachea,

generation 0 through lobar generation 2, and many of the segmental airways) that are not accounted for by differences in lung size (Fig. 8.20). Based on the principles that govern airflow (see *Mechanics of Breathing*), it is reasonable to predict that a woman with the same size lungs as a man would have higher airway resistance and more turbulent airflow during exercise. Indeed, there is now evidence that these differences in airway size manifest themselves during exercise in three ways (119,120). First, women are more likely to develop expiratory flow limitation because the demand for high expiratory flows encroaches on the maximum flow–volume envelope. Second, as maximal exercise is approached, women increase EELV back toward resting values in response to the expiratory flow limitation. In addition, EILV is higher at maximal exercise in women and, hence, there is an increased elastic load on the inspiratory muscles. Third, the flow-resistive work of breathing is higher in women compared to men at increasing exercise intensities and $\dot{V}_E$ (see also Fig. 8.10). Although the aforementioned sex differences might be expected to increase the likelihood of developing exercise-induced diaphragmatic fatigue in women, recent evidence suggests that the prevalence and severity of exercise-induced diaphragmatic fatigue is *lower* in women versus men (121). These findings are in line with previous studies showing greater fatigue resistance of limb locomotor muscles in women versus men. Commonly cited mechanisms associated with greater fatigue resistance in women include differences in muscle mass/morphology, substrate utilization, and neuromuscular activation (122).

KEY POINT

Women have smaller diameter airways, lung volumes, and diffusion surfaces relative to men of the same height.

Training Effects and Plasticity in the Respiratory System

Lung, Airway, and Vascular Structures

There is clear evidence that the cardiovascular and skeletal muscular systems adapt quickly and substantially to chronic exercise training (48,123,124). On the other hand, endurance training has minimal or no positive effects on lung, airway, and pulmonary vascular structures. A striking example of the disparity among organ systems in their relative adaptabilities to increased metabolic demand was demonstrated in a series of studies comparing athletic and sedentary mammalian species of similar body size but with up to threefold difference in $\dot{V}o_{2max}$ (*e.g.*, horse vs. cow; dog vs. goat). The higher $\dot{V}o_{2max}$ was accompanied by comparable increases in heart and limb muscle mitochondrial volume and capillary density in the athletic versus the

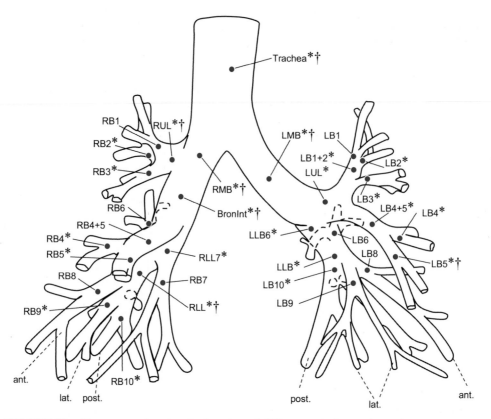

FIGURE 8.20 Airway tree showing the location of differences in luminal area between men and women. The large and central airways in women were significantly smaller than those of men even after controlling for lung size. Labels refer to segments but are assigned to terminating branchpoint of respective segment. LMB, left main bronchus; LUL, left upper lobe; LB, left bronchus; LLB, left lower lobe; RMB, right main bronchus; RUL, right upper lobe; RB, right bronchus; Bronint, intermediate bronchus; RLL, right lower lobe; post, posterior; lat, lateral; ant, anterior. *Significant difference between men and women of varying body size ($P < 0.05$). †Significant difference between subjects matched for lung size ($P < 0.05$). (Reprinted from Sheel AW, Guenette JA, Yuan R, et al. Evidence for dysanapsis using computed tomographic imaging of the airways in older ex-smokers. *J Appl Physiol.* 2009;107:1625, with permission.)

sedentary animal, but only 20% to 30% differences in the lung's alveolar–capillary surface area (125). Further evidence that lung structure is mostly independent of habitual physical activity stems from studies that report nonsignificant changes in lung diffusion surface, airways, and pulmonary vasculature after chronic heavy exercise training in the maturing lung of rodents.

In humans, lung diffusion capacity and pulmonary capillary blood volume are not substantially different between endurance trained and normal untrained subjects, either at rest or during exercise. Furthermore, static lung volumes and maximum flow–volume loops of endurance-trained subjects are not different from those of untrained individuals. There is evidence from in vitro studies in pigs to suggest that short-term training enhances vasorelaxation of the pulmonary artery via an increase in endothelial nitric oxide protein in the smooth muscle (126). In vivo studies are required to determine the implications of these findings in isolated vessels to changes in pulmonary vascular resistance during exercise.

Swimmers may be an exception to the assertion that physical activity has minimal influence on pulmonary structure and function. Swimmers tend to have larger lungs than the normal population. However, cross-sectional studies suffer from selection bias. That is, swimmers may have a strong genetic predisposition for large lungs. Nevertheless, longitudinal data from already fit adult subjects suggest that competitive swim training promotes slight but significant increases in static lung volumes (127). The mechanism responsible for these improvements in lung function is unclear, but swimmers during training inspire repeatedly to TLC, which may result in an increased ability to contract inspiratory muscles to shorter lengths. Daily bouts of either voluntary hyperpnea or flow resistive loading directed specifically at the inspiratory muscles have been shown to promote small but significant increases in both static and dynamic pulmonary function over several weeks (128).

Despite only limited evidence of a positive training effect on the lung, recent evidence suggests that physical training may improve airway function. Well-trained athletes exhibit lower airway responsiveness to inhaled methacholine than individuals who do not exercise vigorously in their daily life (129). Moreover, short-term (5–10 weeks) aerobic exercise substantially reduces the bronchoconstrictive effect of inhaled methacholine in normal subjects (130). Whether these findings in healthy subjects extend to patients with obstructive pulmonary disease is not entirely clear. However, repeated bouts of aerobic exercise have been shown to attenuate airway hyperresponsiveness in children with mild stable asthma (131) and to reduce airway inflammation in adult patients with moderate-to-severe persistent asthma (132). Physical training could influence airway function through the repeated stretch associated with increased ventilation during exercise causing a modification of the contractile mechanism of airway smooth muscle (133) or via a remodeling of the airway smooth muscle (134).

Evidence in children suggests that physical training prepuberty may accelerate lung growth as an adaptive response to the exercise. Maximal flow–volume loops tend to be larger in endurance trained than untrained prepubescent children (135). Moreover, there is evidence that prepubescent children may increase lung volumes and expiratory flow rates with long-term endurance training (136,137). Several studies have attempted to determine whether exercise training protects against the normal age-dependent deterioration in lung function. Cross-sectional comparisons of subjects with normal versus high $\dot{V}O_{2max}$ suggest that highly active elderly subjects have higher maximum expiratory flow rates and higher lung diffusion capacities than do less fit or sedentary subjects (138). At first glance, these findings suggest that age-dependent rates of decline in the lung elastic recoil and diffusion surface area are curtailed with habitual physical activity. In contrast, a longitudinal study of competitive distance runners in their sixth and seventh decades showed that chronic dynamic exercise training ensured high aerobic fitness but did not modify either the normal deterioration in resting lung function or the increased levels of ventilatory work during exercise that occur with normal healthy aging (139). Thus, the enhanced lung function of habitually active elderly subjects noted in cross-sectional studies was most likely *brought to,* rather than *resulted from,* their active lifestyle. The absence of a true training effect on the aging lung contrasts sharply with the beneficial effects of habitual exercise on cardiac function, systemic vasculature, limb skeletal muscle oxidative capacity and strength, and $\dot{V}O_{2max}$ (140).

Because the lungs and airways do not change appreciably with exercise training, it is reasonable to question whether these structures adapt to other types of external stimuli. Humans native to high altitude, and to lesser extent lowlanders who reside for many years at high altitude, have higher lung diffusion capacities and pulmonary capillary blood volumes than their sea-level contemporaries (141). This enhanced diffusion capacity translated into a reduced A-aDo$_2$ and a more efficient gas exchange

during exercise in hypoxia. Another stimulus to which the lungs adapt is calorie restriction. Studies on rodents show that calorie restriction increases the distance between alveolar walls and decreases alveolar surface area. Furthermore, these negative effects of calorie restriction are reversed with refeeding (142). Adaptation also occurs when a portion of lung is removed surgically (pneumonectomy). Compensatory growth of the remaining lung occurs in response to this procedure in the form of an increased alveolar–capillary surface area (143). Finally, there are striking examples of genetic adaptation of the lung in some mammalian species with extremely high aerobic capacity. For example, in the pronghorn antelope (with a $\dot{V}O_{2max}$ >300 mL $\cdot$ kg^{-1} $\cdot$ min^{-1}), the alveolar–capillary surface area, like cardiovascular and muscle adaptations, is enlarged in proportion to the elevated $\dot{V}O_{2max}$.

If the lung is indeed malleable to specific chronic stimuli, why does exercise training not elicit these kinds of adaptations? An obvious explanation is that dynamic exercise is not sufficiently stressful to warrant a positive adaptive response. However, there is ample evidence that the limits of lung function and structure are being challenged, at least during heavy exercise in the highly trained human, as shown by the occasional development of arterial hypoxemia, expiratory flow limitation, stress failure of the blood–gas barrier, and significant release of inflammatory mediators in the airways and pulmonary vasculature. In superhuman athletes, like the thoroughbred horse, the lung parenchyma actually hemorrhages at multiple sites during exercise. One can imagine a significant scarring and stiffening of the lung parenchyma because of the repeated insults in these animals.

Limited evidence in human athletes suggests that instead of a positive adaptation to intense physical training, a pulmonary maladaptation may actually occur in some susceptible athletes, especially when the training is carried out in the presence of cold, dry air or urban pollutants and at high, sustained intensities. Lung biopsy studies in cross-country skiers show increased collagen deposition and remodeling in the bronchiolar airway walls (144). Perhaps repeated release of inflammatory mediators in the airways may be, in part, responsible for these structural changes. One wonders whether the high prevalence of asthma-like symptoms in endurance athletes may be attributed in part to these training-induced structural changes. Pulmonary maladaptations are also implied by the excessively widened A-aDo$_2$ and hypoxemia in some highly trained athletes even during submaximal exercise. It is certainly reasonable to suspect that the acute injuries to or fractures of the alveolar–capillary interface, or profound shear stresses at high flow rates acting on the pulmonary vascular endothelium produce permanent structural alterations in the diffusion pathway.

Collectively, these observations suggest that with exercise training not only does the lung lag behind the adaptations made by the cardiovascular system and the locomotor muscles but also the key elements of lung structure may be compromised or remodeled to the point where this interferes significantly with airway reactivity, ventilation and perfusion distribution, and gas exchange, even at submaximal requirements for oxygen transport. Confirmation of this postulate requires much more detailed longitudinal study of the lung and airways throughout training.

Respiratory Muscles

It is now clear that respiratory muscles are both metabolically and structurally plastic and respond to the regular contractile activity associated with chronic physical training (145). Evidence in rodents shows that heavy dynamic exercise training promotes 20% to 30% increases in mitochondrial enzyme activity within the costal diaphragm, as well as in specific accessory inspiratory (parasternal and external intercostals) and expiratory muscles (rectus abdominis and external oblique). The magnitude of these training-induced changes in oxidative capacity in the respiratory muscles are substantially less than those reported for limb locomotor muscles with fiber type composition similar to that of the diaphragm (e.g., plantaris). The differences in adaptation are likely attributable to differences in the work performed by diaphragm versus limbs during dynamic exercise training. In contrast to the changes in oxidative capacity, endurance training has little effect on most respiratory muscle glycolytic enzymes. However, training does elicit increases in the activities of key antioxidant enzymes within the diaphragm of rodents. This increased antioxidant capacity will improve the diaphragm's ability to scavenge reactive oxygen species and protect against the effects of exercise-induced oxidative stress, such as reductions in maximal tension and rate of force development, and early onset of fatigue. Endurance exercise training also promotes phenotypic adaptations in the diaphragm, as shown in a shift of type IIx to IIa in the fast myosin heavy chain isoforms. Furthermore, decreases occur in the cross-sectional area of costal diaphragm fibers, resulting in a reduced distance from capillary to mitochondria for diffusion of gases, metabolites, and/or substrates in the diaphragm. Studies in rodents also show that the respiratory dilator muscles of the upper airway adapt to chronic exercise as shown by a fast-to-slow shift in the myosin heavy chain isoform phenotype, together with an increase in oxidative and antioxidant capacities in the digastric and sternohyoid muscles (146).

Biopsy studies in humans attest to the plasticity of the diaphragm in response to chronic overload. Patients with COPD who underwent specific inspiratory muscle training via loaded breathing showed significant increases in the proportion of type I fibers and the size of type II fibers in the external intercostals (147). Furthermore, cross-sectional comparisons of diaphragm muscle biopsies in either chronic heart failure or severe COPD patients showed substantial increases in the proportion of type I fibers and the concentration of mitochondrial oxidative enzymes in the costal diaphragm, apparently resulting from the progressive increase in load placed on the respiratory muscles over several years

or decades (148). Indirect evidence also suggests that the respiratory muscles undergo a training effect after a dynamic exercise training regimen in normal humans. The endurance-trained athlete will, like his or her sedentary counterparts, show significant diaphragm fatigue in response to heavy exercise continued to exhaustion. However, the endurance-trained athlete has diaphragm fatigue only at levels of total ventilation and respiratory muscle work that are far greater than in sedentary individuals (149).

Although much attention has been paid to the diaphragmatic adaptations to chronic overload, little is known about the effects of detraining on diaphragmatic structure and function. Hemidiaphragmatic inactivity (induced by unilateral chemical blockade of phrenic nerve conduction or sectioning of the phrenic nerve) results in significant reductions in peak diaphragmatic force production and type II muscle fiber cross-sectional area in the inactive hemidiaphragm within 2 weeks (150). However, pure diaphragmatic quiescence (i.e., complete bilateral absence of diaphragmatic electrical activity) induced by mechanical ventilation for as little as 18 hours results in marked atrophy of both type I and type II fibers in the diaphragm (151). Thus, removal of the normal phasic activation of the diaphragm has a substantial effect in a relatively short time, with the period required for recovery remaining unclear.

An impressive diaphragmatic adaptation in an animal model of COPD is the loss of sarcomeres in series with elastase-induced emphysema. As lung elastic recoil decreases and more air is trapped in the lungs (i.e., FRC increases), the diaphragm is forced to operate at shorter lengths and in a flatter geometric configuration. In an attempt to optimize sarcomere length and force production under these conditions, sarcomeres in series are progressively lost from the diaphragmatic myofibrils (152). In this regard, the remaining sarcomeres are able to operate closer to their optimal length and the length–tension relationship of the diaphragm is shifted to the left, with the magnitude of sarcomere loss inversely proportional to the increase in FRC (153). Similar structural adaptations appear to occur in the expiratory musculature, as evidenced by the loss of sarcomeres in series in the transversus abdominis of animals with experimental emphysema (154). After lung volume reduction surgery, and the resulting reduction in FRC and lengthening of the diaphragm, diaphragmatic sarcomeres are added back in series (155), and the length–tension relationship of the diaphragm is shifted rightward (156).

Control of Breathing

Exercise training has been shown to reduce the ventilatory response to moderate and heavy exercise. This reduced ventilatory response is likely due to a decrease in circulating stimuli (including hydrogen ions, potassium, and norepinephrine), temperature, and a decrease in central motor command as limb fatigue is delayed to higher work rates in the trained subject. Second, the ventilatory response to hypoxia and inhaled carbon dioxide is known to be markedly heterogeneous in the normal human population. Many endurance-trained athletes have lower than average ventilatory responsiveness to these chemoreceptor stimuli, although this is not a universal finding. However, in athletes who do show reduced ventilatory chemoresponsiveness, this characteristic may have practical implications for gas exchange during exercise and perhaps even exercise performance. Specifically, a reduced hyperventilatory response in the presence of an excessive A-aDO$_2$ is responsible for arterial hypoxemia in some highly trained subjects. A portion of this inadequate hyperventilatory response is due to a mechanical constraint on exercise ventilation, primarily due to expiratory flow limitation (Fig. 8.9). However, purely mechanical constraint of ventilation does not account for all of the blunted hyperventilation during heavy exercise in these subjects with arterial hypoxemia. In some subjects, failure to achieve sufficient hyperventilation occurs even when they are ventilating well within the maximal capacities defined by the envelope of their maximum flow–volume loop and when the pressures generated by their inspiratory muscles are substantially less than their capacity. Therefore, their failure to increase ventilation further may be due, in part, to their relative insensitivity to prevailing ventilatory stimuli, especially humoral stimuli, which are known to influence the carotid chemoreceptors.

KEY POINT

Intense endurance training stimulates the development of high oxidative, fatigue-resistant respiratory muscles, but the structures of the lung and airways appear resistant to training and may even be negatively impacted by the repeated shear stresses and inflammatory mediatory release accompanying high-intensity exercise.

Respiratory Limitations to Exercise

It is generally agreed that $\dot{V}O_{2max}$ is in large part determined by systemic oxygen transport, that is, the product of maximal cardiac output ($\dot{Q}$) and CaO_2, at least in normal adults with $\dot{V}O_{2max}$ in the range of 35 to 85 mL · kg^{-1} · min^{-1} (157,158). Support for this premise stems from findings showing a strong positive correlation between $CaO_2 · \dot{Q}_{max}$ and $\dot{V}O_{2max}$ in subjects of widely varying fitness (157). In addition, experimental evidence in animals and humans shows that as CaO_2 varies (via changing the fractional oxygen concentration of inspired air or the hemoglobin concentration) or V_{max} is raised (via changing circulating blood volume or pericardectomy), $\dot{V}O_{2max}$ is also altered in accordance with the change in $CaO_2 · \dot{Q}$.

Of the two components of systemic oxygen transport, it is generally believed that maximum stroke volume, and therefore cardiac output, is the key limiter to maximum oxygen delivery in most untrained young adults with a $\dot{V}O_{2max}$ in the normal range. As detailed throughout this chapter, the maintenance of CaO_2 is usually not a problem in health because in general the lungs, airways, and respiratory muscles are structurally overbuilt with respect to maximum metabolic requirements for gas transport. Thus, a large diffusion surface area and a short alveolar–capillary diffusion distance, coupled with a substantial capacity for flow rate, volume, and ventilation, ensures that at $\dot{V}O_{2max}$: (a) the A-aDO$_2$ widens only two to three times resting levels, and (b) alveolar hyperventilation raises alveolar PO_2 sufficiently to compensate for the widened A-aDO$_2$, and arterial PO_2 and oxyhemoglobin saturation are maintained near resting levels.

On the other hand, evidence has accumulated to show that as aerobic capacity increases because of training or in already highly fit individuals, the normal pulmonary system in some humans and some other mammals may not be so overbuilt with respect to metabolic requirements. As detailed in the section *Training Effects and Plasticity in the Respiratory System* earlier in the chapter, the lung diffusion surface and airways and even the respiratory muscles do not adapt to the training stimulus nearly to the same extent as do other links in the oxygen transport system. The result is that the respiratory system in many highly trained subjects is relatively underbuilt with respect to the extraordinarily high metabolic requirements and may contribute significantly to limiting exercise performance. Two specific types of respiratory system limitation to exercise have been identified to date, namely, arterial hypoxemia and high levels of respiratory muscle work.

Exercise-Induced Arterial Hypoxemia

Arterial oxyhemoglobin desaturation ranging from 5% to 15% below resting levels occurs during high-intensity endurance exercise in many, but not all, athletes capable of high aerobic work. Arterial hypoxemia has been reported most frequently in young endurance-trained men. However, recent studies of smaller numbers of trained women and older trained men also reported a high prevalence of arterial hypoxemia, even though the $\dot{V}O_{2max}$ of these subjects was substantially lower than in the young trained men with arterial hypoxemia. The thoroughbred horse, with a $\dot{V}O_{2max}$ twice that of even the most highly trained human, has a substantially underbuilt lung relative to its extraordinary metabolic requirements. Accordingly, all such horses studied to date demonstrate severe arterial hypoxemia, as well as marked CO_2 retention at moderate to severe exercise intensities (159).

Arterial oxygen desaturation during endurance exercise occurs most commonly due to a rightward shift in the oxyhemoglobin dissociation curve, mediated by increases in core temperature and arterial acidity. Additional desaturation occurs in a minority of subjects due to a fall below resting levels in PaO_2 secondary to excessive widening of A-aDO$_2$. This widening of A-aDO$_2$ has been attributed to a combination of $\dot{V}_A/\dot{Q}$ maldistribution, extrapulmonary and intrapulmonary shunt, and diffusion disequilibrium. Arterial oxygen desaturation can be explained to a less consistent extent by an inadequate compensatory hyperventilation due to a mechanical constraint on airflow and/or insensitivity to the ventilatory stimuli associated with heavy exercise (see *Pulmonary Gas Exchange*).

The effect of arterial hypoxemia on $\dot{V}O_{2max}$ has been determined by preventing the desaturation via a mildly hyperoxic inspirate to maintain SaO_2 at resting levels (Fig. 8.21). Using this approach, arterial hypoxemia was shown to impact negatively on $\dot{V}O_{2max}$ when the oxyhemoglobin desaturation exceeded 3% below resting levels, with the effect approximating a 1.5% to 2% decrement in $\dot{V}O_{2max}$ for each 1% reduction in SaO_2 (160). The most commonly encountered levels of arterial hypoxemia among fit males, females, and older subjects are usually modest and will cause less than a 10% reduction in $\dot{V}O_{2max}$. A small, but significant, number of endurance athletes have greater levels of arterial hypoxemia during maximal exercise, and the resulting decrement in $\dot{V}O_{2max}$ ranges from 8% to 15%. In the thoroughbred horse, whose arterial oxyhemoglobin desaturates to almost 20% below resting levels at maximum exercise, $\dot{V}O_{2max}$ is reduced by 30% below levels achieved when arterial hypoxemia is prevented. In athletes with high $\dot{V}O_{2max}$, exercising at even modest elevations in altitude (~1000–1500 meters) exacerbates the severity of

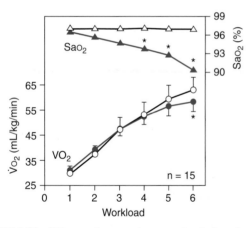

FIGURE 8.21 Effects of preventing exercise-induced arterial hypoxemia via an inspired O_2 fraction of 0.26 on SaO_2 and $\dot{V}O_2$ in 15 fit female subjects during treadmill running. Treadmill grade increased 2% every 2.5 min while treadmill speed was maintained (6–10 mph). Note the gradual reduction in SaO_2 with progressive increases in workload in normoxia (*blue triangles*). At submaximal workloads, preventing oxygen desaturation (*white triangles*) had no effect on $\dot{V}O_2$ (*blue circles*) whereas at peak workloads $\dot{V}O_2$ was significantly increased (*white circles*). *Significant difference at the same workload ($P < 0.05$). (Data from Harms CA, McClaran SR, Nickele GA, et al. Effect of exercise-induced arterial O_2 desaturation on $\dot{V}O_{2max}$ in women. *Med Sci Sports Exerc.* 2000;32:1101–1108; and Harms CA, McClaran SR, Nickele GA, et al. Exercise-induced arterial hypoxaemia in healthy young women. *J Physiol [Lond].* 1998;507(pt 2):619–628.)

arterial hypoxemia and further limits $\dot{V}O_{2max}$ (160–162). The reason arterial hypoxemia causes a reduction in $\dot{V}O_{2max}$ is likely found in the Fick equation. That is, reduced CaO_2 decreases oxygen transport to the working locomotor muscles, thereby reducing the maximal attainable arterial to mixed venous oxygen partial pressure difference across the working muscle. More recent studies using supplemental inspired oxygen to prevent arterial hypoxemia have shown that it contributes significantly to the development of exercise-induced locomotor muscle fatigue and impacts negatively on high-intensity endurance exercise performance (163,164). This effect of oxygen transport on exercise performance becomes progressively more important as SaO_2 is further reduced at high altitudes (165).

Respiratory Muscle Work

We have previously documented that heavy dynamic exercise causes substantial increases in the work of the inspiratory and expiratory muscles, both in untrained human subjects and especially in the highly trained. These high levels of work require 10% to 16% of the $\dot{V}O_{2max}$ and cardiac output. The diaphragm and abdominal muscles fatigue in response to heavy sustained exercise. Furthermore, experimentally relieving the work of the respiratory muscles (via mechanical ventilation) during heavy exercise reduces cardiac output and $\dot{V}O_2$, and increases vascular conductance and blood flow to the limb locomotor muscles. Finally, maintaining the required levels of ventilation and the associated respiratory muscle work leads to intense perceptions of breathing effort, that is, exertional dyspnea.

One approach used to determine whether respiratory muscle work/fatigue and/or dyspnea affect exercise performance has been to partially unload the respiratory muscles during the exercise using a mechanical ventilator (Fig. 8.22). Using this approach, exercise-induced diaphragm fatigue was prevented, exercise time to exhaustion was increased by a mean of 14%, and the rates of rise in $\dot{V}O_2$ and perceptions of dyspnea and limb discomfort throughout the exercise were reduced (166). The significant effect of respiratory muscle unloading on exercise performance is consistent with the deleterious effect on subsequent exercise performance of prefatiguing the respiratory muscles (167,168).

Of course, such studies do not tell us *why* high levels of respiratory work might affect endurance performance. Exercise-induced respiratory muscle fatigue does not limit the hyperventilatory response during exercise (54,55). However, it does trigger a metaboreflex from the fatiguing respiratory muscles, which, in turn, causes sympathoexcitation and vasoconstriction of the vasculature of the exercising limb, resulting in reduced limb blood flow and oxygen transport (169). When a mechanical ventilator was used to partially unload the inspiratory muscles during heavy exercise, a significant portion of the exercise-induced quadriceps muscle fatigue was prevented (170). This effect was likely related to preventing the respiratory muscle

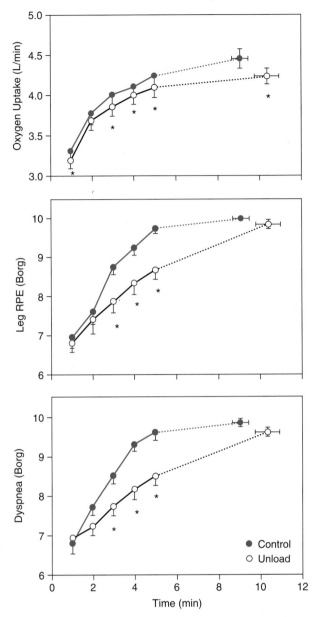

FIGURE 8.22 Effects of respiratory muscle unloading via mechanical ventilation on endurance exercise performance at a work rate requiring ~90% of $\dot{V}O_{2max}$ in endurance-trained cyclists (n = 7). Group mean data are shown for minutes 1 to 5 of exercise and at exhaustion. Absolute time to exhaustion under control conditions averaged 9.1 ± 2.6 min (mean ± SD). Reducing the normal work of breathing by 50% from control increased time to exhaustion in 76% of trials by 1.3 ± 0.4 min (14 ± 5%). Unloading caused reductions in oxygen uptake ($\dot{V}O_2$; top) and the rate of rise in perceptions of limb discomfort (leg ratings of perceived exertion [RPE]; middle) and respiratory discomfort (dyspnea; bottom) throughout the duration of exercise. *Significantly different from control (P < 0.05). (Redrawn from Harms CA, Wetter TJ, St Croix CM, et al. Effects of respiratory muscle work on exercise performance. *J Appl Physiol.* 2000;89:131–138, with permission.)

metaboreflex effect on reducing limb blood flow. Exercise in hypoxia increases the hyperventilatory response, the work of breathing, and diaphragm fatigue. Accordingly, the work of the respiratory muscles is likely to have an even more prominent influence on the development of peripheral locomotor muscle fatigue and exercise performance at high altitudes (171).

> ## KEY POINT
>
> Exercise-induced arterial hypoxemia and fatiguing levels of respiratory muscle work compromise oxygen delivery to locomotor muscles and limit endurance performance.

Overcoming the Respiratory System Limitations to Exercise

We are not permitted to provide supplemental oxygen during competitive endurance events, and we are unable to store previously inhaled hyperoxic gases within our body. Neither can one conceive of transporting a mechanical ventilator or breathing low-density gas mixtures to relieve the work of breathing during competition. Thus, although these ergogenic aids may be of substantial benefit to the supervised rehabilitation of patients with heart failure or COPD, the healthy athlete must seek alternative ways of overcoming the proposed pulmonary limitations.

In the case of exercise-induced arterial hypoxemia, the most practical advice to be gained by its measurement is its predictive capabilities. That is, endurance athletes who tend to desaturate even marginally at sea level will in all likelihood desaturate substantially with even mild increases in altitude (160–162). Accordingly, when such athletes compete or train at altitude they will be at a substantial disadvantage and should probably avoid such practices.

We know of no antidote to exercise-induced arterial hypoxemia in susceptible subjects, although some attempts have been made by intravenously infusing alkalinizing agents, such as sodium bicarbonate (172). This will overcome a significant amount of the arterial oxyhemoglobin desaturation, that is, what is due to metabolic acidosis, but this might also interfere with offloading of oxygen at the muscle capillary or reduce respiratory drive and $\dot{V}_A$. Anti-inflammatory medications have not been shown to reduce A-aDO$_2$ and prevent arterial hypoxemia in young nonasthmatic subjects (173), but have been shown to be effective in improving gas exchange abnormalities in older master athletes (174) and habitually active asthmatics (175) (Fig. 8.23). Of course, adding hemoglobin (and oxygen-carrying capacity) by intermittent hypoxic exposures or via the illegal practices of blood doping or exogenous erythropoietin would readily negate any reduction in CaO$_2$ secondary to arterial hypoxemia.

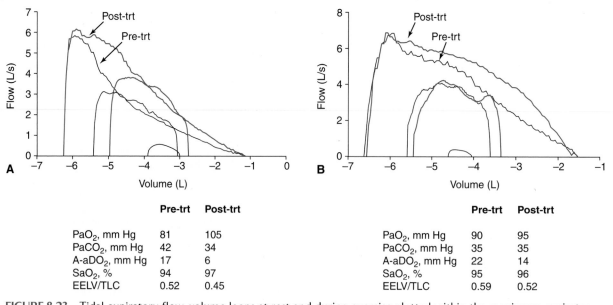

	Pre-trt	Post-trt
PaO_2, mm Hg	81	105
$PaCO_2$, mm Hg	42	34
$A\text{-}aDO_2$, mm Hg	17	6
SaO_2, %	94	97
EELV/TLC	0.52	0.45

	Pre-trt	Post-trt
PaO_2, mm Hg	90	95
$PaCO_2$, mm Hg	35	35
$A\text{-}aDO_2$, mm Hg	22	14
SaO_2, %	95	96
EELV/TLC	0.59	0.52

FIGURE 8.23 Tidal expiratory flow–volume loops at rest and during exercise plotted within the maximum expiratory flow–volume loop before and after 6 weeks of treatment with inhaled corticosteroid in a single habitually active subject with mild-to-moderate asthma. Also shown are the pre- and posttreatment exercise responses for PaO_2, $PaCO_2$, $A\text{-}aDO_2$, SaO_2, and EELV/TLC ratio. *Pre-treatment*: note the severe expiratory flow limitation (at a $\dot{V}_E$ of only 47 L · min^{-1}) and the ensuing dynamic hyperinflation; also note the arterial hypoxemia, alveolar hypoventilation ($PaCO_2$ >40 mm Hg), and decreased SaO_2 during exercise. *Posttreatment*: note the increased size of the maximum flow–volume loop and increased exercise peak expiratory flow rate. Also note that PaO_2 and SaO_2 were increased whereas $A\text{-}aDO_2$ and $PaCO2$ were decreased relative to pretreatment; EELV was maintained at less than FRC. Despite the increased ventilatory capacity, the subject still reached expiratory flow limitation during the exercise but at much higher expiratory flow rates and $\dot{V}E$ than pretreatment. Thus, the treatment of airway inflammation improved arterial blood oxygenation during exercise (and increased exercise capacity by 74%) due to increased alveolar ventilation secondary to an increased maximal flow-volume envelope, and improved pulmonary gas exchange efficiency (*i.e.*, decreased $A\text{-}aDO_2$). (Redrawn from Haverkamp HC, Dempsey JA, Pegelow DF. Treatment of airway inflammation improves exercise pulmonary gas exchange and performance in asthmatic subjects. *J Allergy Clin Immunol.* 2007;120:45, with permission.)

Many have tested the hypothesis that specific training of the respiratory pump muscles will enhance exercise performance (176). The two principal methods are resistance training using imposed external loads at the mouth and endurance training using voluntary hyperpnea. Early studies produced contradictory findings, primarily because of poor research designs and inappropriate outcome measures. Several recent studies using a placebo-controlled experimental design have shown that aerobic exercise performance improves when resistance training is directed specifically at the inspiratory muscles. Several controlled trials of respiratory muscle endurance training have also shown improvements in aerobic exercise performance. In addition to the potential ergogenic effect of respiratory muscle training on aerobic exercise performance, several controlled studies of resistance inspiratory muscle training have demonstrated improvements in repetitive sprint performance.

The underlying mechanisms for the potential ergogenic effect of respiratory muscle training on aerobic exercise performance are unlikely through increases in $\dot{V}O_{2max}$ or maximal lactate steady state (177,178). The ergogenic effect could be due to relief of respiratory muscle fatigue (179,180) or limb muscle fatigue (181), perhaps by increasing the threshold for activation of the respiratory muscle metaboreflex (182) (see *Cardiorespiratory Interactions during Exercise*). However, the perceptual benefit obtained by relieving the discomfort associated with high levels of respiratory muscle work or fatigue may also be responsible for at least some of the improvements in exercise performance (183).

CHAPTER SUMMARY

It is important for the student of exercise physiology to appreciate that much of this field of study is relatively new. Accordingly, our understanding of many fundamental problems concerning exercise and the respiratory system is incomplete. Furthermore, we are several steps away from applying much of our knowledge of basic physiology to improving the performance of the competitive athlete. We conclude this chapter by addressing a few of the more pressing needs in this field.

- *Regulation of exercise hyperpnea.* Two major locomotor-linked mechanisms appear to account for much of the steady state hyperpnea during exercise, but the key

A MILESTONE OF DISCOVERY

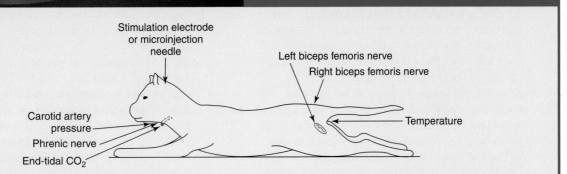

FIGURE 8.24   Decorticate, paralyzed, ventilated cat preparation used to study the cardiorespiratory effects of fictive locomotion. (Redrawn from Eldridge FL, Millhorn DE, Waldrop TG. Exercise hyperpnea and locomotion: parallel activation from the hypothalamus. *Science.* 1981;211:845, with permission.)

The question was whether central command of locomotion originating in the hypothalamic locomotor regions of the CNS also caused parallel activation of ventilation and circulation. By the end of the 1970s, neurochemical feedback from the periphery was the most popularly purported primary stimulus for exercise hyperpnea. However, Fred Eldridge, a Stanford-trained physician and professor of physiology at the University of North Carolina–Chapel Hill, believed strongly in the Krogh hypothesis of cortical irradiation as an explanation for exercise hyperpnea. Teaming with his research fellows, Tony Waldrop and David Millhorn, Eldridge expanded significantly on the original central command experiments conducted by Rushmer in anesthetized animals some 20 years earlier. The Eldridge model was the unanesthetized decorticate cat (similar to a preparation described in the Russian literature), in which they used either electrical or pharmacologic stimulation of the hypothalamic locomotor region to produce rhythmic limb contractions sufficient to cause revolutions of a treadmill belt. This caused immediate increases in ventilation, cardiac output and blood pressure, analogous to the normal exercise response. Then, to completely isolate the central command stimulus, they paralyzed all skeletal muscles so that hypothalamic stimulation caused fictive locomotion (Fig. 8.24). Amazingly, cardiorespiratory responses were identical to those obtained in the intact animal, that is, when both feed-forward and feedback stimulation were present (Fig. 8.25).

These findings formally established central command as a significant player in exercise hyperpnea and served to stimulate the conduct of many subsequent studies throughout the 1980s and 1990s, which showed the following:

1. Stimulation of other CNS areas, such as the mesencephalic locomotor areas and the amygdala, produced cardiorespiratory responses that were similar to those caused by stimulation of the hypothalamic areas.
2. Hypothalamic stimulation also engaged the parasympathetic and sympathetic nervous systems, leading to increases in cardiac output and a redistribution of systemic blood flow similar to that caused by exercise.
3. Descending projections were discovered linking the caudal hypothalamus to the cardiorespiratory medullary neurons.
4. Hypothalamic locomotor centers were shown to receive sensory input from skeletal muscle receptor afferents.

Nevertheless, lesioning of the hypothalamic locomotor areas did not prevent a normal cardiorespiratory response to exercise in the awake animal. It is likely, then, that these powerful central feed-forward and peripheral feedback mechanisms, which occur simultaneously during exercise, are somewhat redundant in their functional influences on exercise hyperpnea.

Eldridge FL, Millhorn DE, Waldrop TG. Exercise hyperpnea and locomotion: parallel activation from the hypothalamus. Science. 1981;211:844–846.

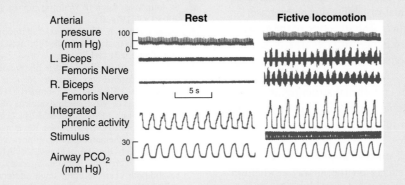

FIGURE 8.25   Example of cardiovascular and respiratory responses during fictive locomotion induced by stimulation of the hypothalamic locomotor region. (Redrawn from Eldridge FL, Millhorn DE, Waldrop TG. Exercise hyperpnea and locomotion: parallel activation from the hypothalamus. *Science.* 1981;211:845, with permission.)

questions of how these inputs interact with one another and with other fine-tuning mechanisms remain unanswered. The influence of prior learning and the role of nervous system plasticity also are complex important questions concerning the mechanisms of hyperpnea. Innovative approaches employing unanesthetized, nervously intact preparations with control system sensitivities in the physiologic range are needed.

- *Breathing mechanics.* Reflexes from the lung, airways, and chest wall have been shown to have important influences on breath timing and respiratory muscle recruitment. Experimental evidence in the exercising state is needed to determine the specific role of these reflexes on breathing pattern, the recruitment of accessory respiratory muscles as diaphragm and abdominal muscle fatigue develops in heavy sustained exercise, and the regulation of operating lung volumes as expiratory flow limitation is approached.

- *Cardiorespiratory interactions.* Large cyclical fluctuations in intrathoracic and P_{ab} occur throughout the respiratory cycle during exercise, especially when expiratory flow limitation is present and expiratory time is prolonged. Future exploration in the exercising human is needed to determine how these respiratory-induced changes in pressure influence left-ventricular output. We also know that respiratory muscle metaboreceptors and carotid chemoreceptors are capable of reflexively increasing sympathetic vasoconstrictor outflow. What is unclear is how these feedback receptors are activated during exercise, and what their net influence is on blood flow distribution to respiratory and locomotor muscles.

- *Gas exchange.* It is surprising how little we understand of the structure of the pulmonary circulation in the face of an increase in cardiac output during dynamic exercise. If we could measure both red cell transit time distribution and extravascular fluid accumulation, and if we could image arteriovenous shunt pathways potentially capable of carrying deoxygenated mixed venous blood, perhaps we could explain the causes of gas exchange inefficiency and its marked individual variability during exercise.

- *Exercise training effects.* The structure of the airways and of the gas exchange surface area is usually viewed as unresponsive to the stimulus of exercise training. However, little attention has been paid to training effects on endothelial structure and reactivity in the pulmonary arterioles or in vessels regulating blood flow to the diaphragm and accessory respiratory muscles. Furthermore, recent evidence demonstrates that intense physical training may have deleterious effects on the airway epithelium and even on pulmonary gas exchange. The excellent animal models available to explore training effects on locomotor muscles and the systemic

vasculature should be applied to these questions concerning training-induced structural changes in the lung, airways, and respiratory muscles.

- *Respiratory limitations.* Exercise-induced arterial hypoxemia and fatiguing levels of respiratory muscle work have been shown to compromise oxygen transport to working limbs—the former by reducing CaO_2, and the latter by triggering vasoconstriction and reducing limb blood flow. What needs to be determined, however, is whether exercise limitation is a direct effect of peripheral locomotor muscle fatigue, or if significant local fatigue (of both respiratory and limb locomotor muscles) impacts via neural feedback effects on effort perception causing reduced central motor output to the working limbs. We also need to explore whether the significant effects of changes in intrathoracic and P_{ab} during breathing on venous return and left ventricular output impact on exercise performance.

These are some of the key problems concerning the respiratory system biology of exercise. Equally fascinating and even more challenging is the need to address similar questions in subpopulations (*e.g.*, children, elderly, women, patients with pulmonary disease) and during exercise in extreme environments (*e.g.*, high and low altitudes, heat and cold).

ACKNOWLEDGMENTS

Portions of this chapter are adapted from the first edition of ACSM's *Advanced Exercise Physiology*. Therefore, the previous efforts of Professor Jerome Dempsey and Dr. Jordan Miller are gratefully acknowledged.

REFERENCES

1. Smith JC, Ellenberger HH, Ballanyi K, et al. Pre-Botzinger complex: a brainstem region that may generate respiratory rhythm in mammals. *Science.* 1991;254(5032):726–729.
2. St -John WM, Paton JF. Defining eupnea. *Respir Physiol Neurobiol.* 2003;139(1):97–103.
3. Orem J, Netick A. Characteristics of midbrain respiratory neurons in sleep and wakefulness in the cat. *Brain Res.* 1982;244(2):231–241.
4. Feldman JL, Mitchell GS, Nattie EE. Breathing: rhythmicity, plasticity, chemosensitivity. *Annu Rev Neurosci.* 2003;26:239–266.
5. Takakura AC, Moreira TS, Colombari E, et al. Peripheral chemoreceptor inputs to retrotrapezoid nucleus (RTN) CO2-sensitive neurons in rats. *J Physiol.* 2006;572(pt 2):503–523.
6. Blain GM, Smith CA, Henderson KS, et al. Contribution of the carotid body chemoreceptors to eupneic ventilation in the intact, unanesthetized dog. *J Appl Physiol.* 2009;106(5):1564–1573.
7. Lahiri S, DeLaney RG. Stimulus interaction in the responses of carotid body chemoreceptor single afferent fibers. *Respir Physiol.* 1975;24(3):249–266.
8. Nattie E, Li A. Central chemoreception is a complex system function that involves multiple brain stem sites. *J Appl Physiol.* 2009;106(4):1464–1466.

9. Kaufman MP, Forster HV. Reflexes controlling ventilatory and airway responses to exercise. In: Rowell L, Shephard RJ, eds. *Handbook of Physiology: Exercise.* New York: Oxford Press; 1996:381–447.

10. Rice AJ, Nakayama HC, Haverkamp HC, et al. Controlled versus assisted mechanical ventilation effects on respiratory motor output in sleeping humans. *Am J Respir Crit Care Med.* 2003;168(1):92–101.

11. Badr MS, Skatrud JB, Dempsey JA. Determinants of poststimulus potentiation in humans during NREM sleep. *J Appl Physiol.* 1992;73(5):1958–1971.

12. Phillipson EA, Duffin J, Cooper JD. Critical dependence of respiratory rhythmicity on metabolic CO2 load. *J Appl Physiol.* 1981;50(1):45–54.

13. Dempsey JA, Vidruk EH, Mitchell GS. Pulmonary control systems in exercise: update. *Fed Proc.* 1985;44(7):2260–2270.

14. Huszczuk A, Whipp BJ, Adams TD, et al. Ventilatory control during exercise in calves with artificial hearts. *J Appl Physiol.* 1990;68(6):2604–2611.

15. Olson EB Jr, Dempsey JA. Rat as a model for humanlike ventilatory adaptation to chronic hypoxia. *J Appl Physiol.* 1978;44(5):763–769.

16. Haouzi P, Hill JM, Lewis BK, et al. Responses of group III and IV muscle afferents to distension of the peripheral vascular bed. *J Appl Physiol.* 1999;87(2):545–553.

17. Pickar JG, Hill JM, Kaufman MP. Dynamic exercise stimulates group III muscle afferents. *J Neurophysiol.* 1994;71(2):753–760.

18. Haouzi P, Chenuel B, Huszczuk A. Sensing vascular distension in skeletal muscle by slow conducting afferent fibers: neurophysiological basis and implication for respiratory control. *J Appl Physiol.* 2004;96(2):407–418.

19. Krogh A, Lindhard J. The regulation of respiration and circulation during the initial stages of muscular work. *J Physiol.* 1913;47(1–2):112–136.

20. Eldridge FL, Millhorn DE, Waldrop TG. Exercise hyperpnea and locomotion: parallel activation from the hypothalamus. *Science.* 1981;211(4484):844–846.

21. Innes JA, De Cort SC, Evans PJ, et al. Central command influences cardiorespiratory response to dynamic exercise in humans with unilateral weakness. *J Physiol.* 1992;448:551–563.

22. Thornton JM, Guz A, Murphy K, et al. Identification of higher brain centres that may encode the cardiorespiratory response to exercise in humans. *J Physiol.* 2001;533(pt 3):823–836.

23. Williamson JW, McColl R, Mathews D, et al. Brain activation by central command during actual and imagined handgrip under hypnosis. *J Appl Physiol.* 2002;92(3):1317–1324.

24. Wasserman K, Whipp BJ, Koyal SN, et al. Effect of carotid body resection on ventilatory and acid-base control during exercise. *J Appl Physiol.* 1975;39(3):354–358.

25. Busse MW, Maassen N, Konrad H. Relation between plasma K+ and ventilation during incremental exercise after glycogen depletion and repletion in man. *J Physiol.* 1991;443:469–476.

26. Hagberg JM, Coyle EF, Carroll JE, et al. Exercise hyperventilation in patients with McArdle's disease. *J Appl Physiol.* 1982;52(4):991–994.

27. Henson LC, Ward DS, Whipp BJ. Effect of dopamine on ventilatory response to incremental exercise in man. *Respir Physiol.* 1992;89(2):209–224.

28. Mateika JH, Duffin J. Coincidental changes in ventilation and electromyographic activity during consecutive incremental exercise tests. *Eur J Appl Physiol Occup Physiol.* 1994;68(1):54–61.

29. Amann M, Blain GM, Proctor LT, et al. Group III and IV muscle afferents contribute to ventilatory and cardiovascular response to rhythmic exercise in humans. *J Appl Physiol.* 2010;109:947–948.

30. Hanson P, Claremont A, Dempsey J, et al. Determinants and consequences of ventilatory responses to competitive endurance running. *J Appl Physiol.* 1982;52(3):615–623.

31. MacDougall JD, Reddan WG, Layton CR, et al. Effects of metabolic hyperthermia on performance during heavy prolonged exercise. *J Appl Physiol.* 1974;36(5):538–544.

32. White MD. Components and mechanisms of thermal hyperpnea. *J Appl Physiol.* 2006;101(2):655–663.

33. Waldrop TG, Mullins DC, Millhorn DE. Control of respiration by the hypothalamus and feedback from contracting muscles in cats. *Respir Physiol.* 1986;64(3):317–328.

34. Waldrop TG, Mullins DC, Henderson MC. Effects of hypothalamic lesions on the cardiorespiratory responses to muscular contraction. *Respir Physiol.* 1986;66(2):215–224.

35. Liu Q, Kim J, Cinotte J, et al. Carotid body denervation effect on cytochrome oxidase activity in pre-Botzinger complex of developing rats. *J Appl Physiol.* 2003;94(3):1115–1121.

36. Serra A, Brozoski D, Hodges M, et al. Effects of carotid and aortic chemoreceptor denervation in newborn piglets. *J Appl Physiol.* 2002;92(3):893–900.

37. Waldrop TG, Eldridge FL, Iwamoto G. Central neural control of respiration and circulation during exercise. In: Rowell LB, Shepherd JT, eds. *Handbook of Physiology.* New York: Oxford University; 1996:333–380.

38. Somjen GG. The missing error signal: regulation beyond negative feedback. *News Physiol Sci.* 1992;7:15–19.

39. Houk JC. Control strategies in physiological systems. *Faseb J.* 1988;2(2):97–107.

40. Fredberg JJ, Inouye D, Miller B, et al. Airway smooth muscle, tidal stretches, and dynamically determined contractile states. *Am J Respir Crit Care Med.* 1997;156(6):1752–1759.

41. Johnson BD, Saupe KW, Dempsey JA. Mechanical constraints on exercise hyperpnea in endurance athletes. *J Appl Physiol.* 1992;73(3):874–886.

42. Johnson BD, Weisman IM, Zeballos RJ, et al. Emerging concepts in the evaluation of ventilatory limitation during exercise: the exercise tidal flow-volume loop. *Chest.* 1999;116(2):488–503.

43. Guenette JA, Dominelli PB, Reeve SS, et al. Effect of thoracic gas compression and bronchodilation on the assessment of expiratory flow limitation during exercise in healthy humans. *Respir Physiol Neurobiol.* 2010;170(3):279–286.

44. Olafsson S, Hyatt RE. Ventilatory mechanics and expiratory flow limitation during exercise in normal subjects. *J Clin Invest.* 1969;48(3):564–573.

45. Koulouris NG, Dimopoulou I, Valta P, et al. Detection of expiratory flow limitation during exercise in COPD patients. *J Appl Physiol.* 1997;82(3):723–731.

46. Aliverti A, Cala SJ, Duranti R, et al. Human respiratory muscle actions and control during exercise. *J Appl Physiol.* 1997;83(4):1256–1269.

47. Aaron EA, Seow KC, Johnson BD, et al. Oxygen cost of exercise hyperpnea: implications for performance. *J Appl Physiol.* 1992;72(5):1818–1825.

48. Seals DR. The autonomic nervous system. In: Farrell PA, Joyner MJ, Caiozzo VJ, eds. *ACSM's Advanced Exercise Physiology* (2nd ed.). Baltimore: Lippincott Williams & Wilkins; 2011.

49. Manohar M. Blood flow to the respiratory and limb muscles and to abdominal organs during maximal exertion in ponies. *J Physiol.* 1986;377:25–35.

50. Harms CA, Wetter TJ, McClaran SR, et al. Effects of respiratory muscle work on cardiac output and its distribution during maximal exercise. *J Appl Physiol.* 1998;85(2):609–618.

51. Guenette JA, Vogiatzis I, Zakynthinos S, et al. Human respiratory muscle blood flow measured by near-infrared spectroscopy and indocyanine green. *J Appl Physiol.* 2008;104(4):1202–1210.

52. Aubier M, Farkas G, De Troyer A, et al. Detection of diaphragmatic fatigue in man by phrenic stimulation. *J Appl Physiol.* 1981;50(3):538–544.

53. Kyroussis D, Mills GH, Polkey MI, et al. Abdominal muscle fatigue after maximal ventilation in humans. *J Appl Physiol.* 1996;81(4):1477–1483.

54. Johnson BD, Babcock MA, Suman OE, et al. Exercise-induced diaphragmatic fatigue in healthy humans. *J Physiol.* 1993;460:385–405.

55. Taylor BJ, How SC, Romer LM. Exercise-induced abdominal muscle fatigue in healthy humans. *J Appl Physiol.* 2006;100(5):1554–1562.

56. Babcock MA, Johnson BD, Pegelow DF, et al. Hypoxic effects on exercise-induced diaphragmatic fatigue in normal healthy humans. *J Appl Physiol.* 1995;78(1):82–92.

57. Bellemare F, Grassino A. Effect of pressure and timing of contraction on human diaphragm fatigue. *J Appl Physiol.* 1982;53(5):1190–1195.

58. Babcock MA, Pegelow DF, McClaran SR, et al. Contribution of diaphragmatic power output to exercise-induced diaphragm fatigue. *J Appl Physiol.* 1995;78(5):1710–1719.

59. Morton DP, Callister R. Characteristics and etiology of exercise-related transient abdominal pain. *Med Sci Sports Exerc.* 2000;32(2):432–438.

60. McClaran SR, Wetter TJ, Pegelow DF, et al. Role of expiratory flow limitation in determining lung volumes and ventilation during exercise. *J Appl Physiol.* 1999;86(4):1357–1366.

61. Hill JM. Discharge of group IV phrenic afferent fibers increases during diaphragmatic fatigue. *Brain Res.* 2000;856(1–2):240–244.

62. Jammes Y, Balzamo E. Changes in afferent and efferent phrenic activities with electrically induced diaphragmatic fatigue. *J Appl Physiol.* 1992;73(3):894–902.

63. Ainsworth DM, Smith CA, Henderson KS, et al. Breathing during exercise in dogs—passive or active? *J Appl Physiol.* 1996;81(2):586–595.

64. Morin D, Viala D. Coordinations of locomotor and respiratory rhythms in vitro are critically dependent on hindlimb sensory inputs. *J Neurosci.* 2002;22(11):4756–4765.

65. Chen Z, Eldridge FL, Wagner PG. Respiratory-associated rhythmic firing of midbrain neurones in cats: relation to level of respiratory drive. *J Physiol.* 1991;437:305–325.

66. Jensen D, Ofir D, O'Donnell DE. Effects of pregnancy, obesity and aging on the intensity of perceived breathlessness during exercise in healthy humans. *Respir Physiol Neurobiol.* 2009;167(1):87–100.

67. Coates G, O'Brodovich H, Jefferies AL, et al. Effects of exercise on lung lymph flow in sheep and goats during normoxia and hypoxia. *J Clin Invest.* 1984;74(1):133–141.

68. West JB. Invited review: pulmonary capillary stress failure. *J Appl Physiol.* 2000;89(6):2483–2489;discussion 97.

69. Hopkins SR, Sheel AW, McKenzie DC. Point: pulmonary edema does/does not occur in human athletes performing heavy sea-level exercise. *J Appl Physiol.* 2010;109:1270–1272.

70. Hopkins SR, Schoene RB, Henderson WR, et al. Intense exercise impairs the integrity of the pulmonary blood-gas barrier in elite athletes. *Am J Respir Crit Care Med.* 1997;155(3):1090–1094.

71. Wagner PD, Gale GE, Moon RE, et al. Pulmonary gas exchange in humans exercising at sea level and simulated altitude. *J Appl Physiol.* 1986;61(1):260–270.

72. Sinclair SE, McKinney S, Glenny RW, et al. Exercise alters fractal dimension and spatial correlation of pulmonary blood flow in the horse. *J Appl Physiol.* 2000;88(6):2269–2278.

73. Allemann Y, Hutter D, Lipp E, et al. Patent foramen ovale and high-altitude pulmonary edema. *JAMA.* 2006;296(24):2954–2958.

74. Stickland MK, Welsh RC, Haykowsky MJ, et al. Intra-pulmonary shunt and pulmonary gas exchange during exercise in humans. *J Physiol.* 2004;561(pt 1):321–329.

75. Lovering AT, Haverkamp HC, Romer LM, et al. Transpulmonary passage of 99mTc macroaggregated albumin in healthy humans at rest and during maximal exercise. *J Appl Physiol.* 2009;106(6):1986–1992.

76. Eldridge MW, Dempsey JA, Haverkamp HC, et al. Exercise-induced intrapulmonary arteriovenous shunting in healthy humans. *J Appl Physiol.* 2004;97(3):797–805.

77. Lovering AT, Eldridge MW, Stickland MK. Counterpoint: exercise-induced intrapulmonary shunting is real. *J Appl Physiol.* 2009;107(3):994–997.

78. Hopkins SR, Olfert IM, Wagner PD. Point: exercise-induced intrapulmonary shunting is imaginary. *J Appl Physiol.* 2009;107(3):993–994.

79. Lloyd TC Jr. Respiratory system compliance as seen from the cardiac fossa. *J Appl Physiol.* 1982;53(1):57–62.

80. Willeput R, Rondeux C, De Troyer A. Breathing affects venous return from legs in humans. *J Appl Physiol.* 1984;57(4):971–976.

81. Moreno AH, Katz AI, Gold LD. An integrated approach to the study of the venous system with steps toward a detailed model of the dynamics of venous return to the right heart. *IEEE Trans Biomed Eng.* 1969;16(4):308–324.

82. Takata M, Wise RA, Robotham JL. Effects of abdominal pressure on venous return: abdominal vascular zone conditions. *J Appl Physiol.* 1990;69(6):1961–1972.

83. Miller JD, Pegelow DF, Jacques AJ, et al. Skeletal muscle pump versus respiratory muscle pump: modulation of venous return from the locomotor limb in humans. *J Physiol.* 2005;563(pt 3):925–943.

84. Wexler L, Bergel DH, Gabe IT, et al. Velocity of blood flow in normal human venae cavae. *Circ Res.* 1968;23(3):349–359.

85. Miller JD, Smith CA, Hemauer SJ, et al. The effects of inspiratory intrathoracic pressure production on the cardiovascular response to submaximal exercise in health and chronic heart failure. *Am J Physiol Heart Circ Physiol.* 2007;292(1):H580–H592.

86. Miller JD, Hemauer SJ, Smith CA, et al. Expiratory threshold loading impairs cardiovascular function in health and chronic heart failure during submaximal exercise. *J Appl Physiol.* 2006;101(1):213–227.

87. Stark-Leyva KN, Beck KC, Johnson BD. Influence of expiratory loading and hyperinflation on cardiac output during exercise. *J Appl Physiol.* 2004;96(5):1920–1927.

88. Miller JD, Pegelow DF, Jacques AJ, et al. Effects of augmented respiratory muscle pressure production on locomotor limb venous return during calf contraction exercise. *J Appl Physiol.* 2005;99(5):1802–1815.

89. Belenkie I, Smith ER, Tyberg JV. Ventricular interaction: from bench to bedside. *Ann Med.* 2001;33(4):236–241.

90. Scharf SM, Pinsky MR, Magder S, et al. *Respiratory-Circulatory Interactions in Health and Disease.* New York: Marcel Dekker; 2001.

91. St Croix CM, Satoh M, Morgan BJ, et al. Role of respiratory motor output in within-breath modulation of muscle sympathetic nerve activity in humans. *Circ Res.* 1999;85(5):457–469.

92. Eckberg DL, Kifle YT, Roberts VL. Phase relationship between normal human respiration and baroreflex responsiveness. *J Physiol.* 1980;304:489–502.

93. Taha BH, Simon PM, Dempsey JA, et al. Respiratory sinus arrhythmia in humans: an obligatory role for vagal feedback from the lungs. *J Appl Physiol.* 1995;78(2):638–645.

94. Potts JT, Paton JF, Mitchell JH, et al. Contraction-sensitive skeletal muscle afferents inhibit arterial baroreceptor signalling in the nucleus of the solitary tract: role of intrinsic GABA interneurons. *Neuroscience.* 2003;119(1):201–214.

95. Hajduczok G, Hade JS, Mark AL, et al. Central command increases sympathetic nerve activity during spontaneous locomotion in cats. *Circ Res.* 1991;69(1):66–75.

96. Hussain SN, Chatillon A, Comtois A, et al. Chemical activation of thin-fiber phrenic afferents. 2. Cardiovascular responses. *J Appl Physiol.* 1991;70(1):77–86.

97. Rodman JR, Henderson KS, Smith CA, et al. Cardiovascular effects of the respiratory muscle metaboreflexes in dogs: rest and exercise. *J Appl Physiol.* 2003;95(3):1159–1169.

98. St Croix CM, Morgan BJ, Wetter TJ, et al. Fatiguing inspiratory muscle work causes reflex sympathetic activation in humans. *J Physiol.* 2000;529(pt 2):493–504.

99. Sheel AW, Derchak PA, Morgan BJ, et al. Fatiguing inspiratory muscle work causes reflex reduction in resting leg blood flow in humans. *J Physiol.* 2001;537:277–289.

100. Derchak PA, Sheel AW, Morgan BJ, et al. Effects of expiratory muscle work on muscle sympathetic nerve activity. *J Appl Physiol.* 2002;92(4):1539–1552.

101. Stickland MK, Morgan BJ, Dempsey JA. Carotid chemoreceptor modulation of sympathetic vasoconstrictor outflow during exercise in healthy humans. *J Physiol.* 2008;586(6):1743–1754.

102. Stickland MK, Miller JD, Smith CA, et al. Carotid chemoreceptor modulation of regional blood flow distribution during exercise in health and chronic heart failure. *Circ Res.* 2007;100(9):1371–1378.

103. Rowell LB, O'Leary DS. Reflex control of the circulation during exercise: chemoreflexes and mechanoreflexes. *J Appl Physiol.* 1990;69(2):407–418.

104. Harms CA, Babcock MA, McClaran SR, et al. Respiratory muscle work compromises leg blood flow during maximal exercise. *J Appl Physiol.* 1997;82(5):1573–1583.

105. Aaker A, Laughlin MH. Diaphragm arterioles are less responsive to alpha(1)- adrenergic constriction than gastrocnemius arterioles. *J Appl Physiol.* 2002;92(5):1808–1816.

106. Cooper DM, Kaplan MR, Baumgarten L, et al. Coupling of ventilation and CO2 production during exercise in children. *Pediatr Res.* 1987;21(6):568–572.

107. Mead J. Dysanapsis in normal lungs assessed by the relationship between maximal flow, static recoil, and vital capacity. *Am Rev Respir Dis.* 1980;121(2):339–342.

108. Gaultier C, Perret L, Boule M, et al. Occlusion pressure and breathing pattern in healthy children. *Respir Physiol.* 1981;46(1):71–80.

109. Rowland TW, Cunningham LN. Development of ventilatory responses to exercise in normal white children: a longitudinal study. *Chest.* 1997;111(2):327–332.

110. Nourry C, Deruelle F, Fabre C, et al. Evidence of ventilatory constraints in healthy exercising prepubescent children. *Pediatr Pulmonol.* 2006;41(2):133–140.

111. Cook CD, Mead J, Orzalesi MM. Static volume-pressure characteristics of the respiratory system during maximal efforts. *J Appl Physiol.* 1964;19:1016–1022.

112. Koechlin C, Matecki S, Jaber S, et al. Changes in respiratory muscle endurance during puberty. *Pediatr Pulmonol.* 2005;40(3):197–204.

113. Janssens JP. Aging of the respiratory system: impact on pulmonary function tests and adaptation to exertion. *Clin Chest Med.* 2005;26(3):469–484, vi–vii.

114. Johnson BD, Reddan WG, Seow KC, et al. Mechanical constraints on exercise hyperpnea in a fit aging population. *Am Rev Respir Dis.* 1991;143(5 Pt 1):968–977.

115. Prefaut C, Anselme F, Caillaud C, et al. Exercise-induced hypoxemia in older athletes. *J Appl Physiol.* 1994;76(1):120–126.

116. Thurlbeck WM. Postnatal human lung growth. *Thorax.* 1982;37(8):564–571.

117. Hopkins SR, Harms CA. Gender and pulmonary gas exchange during exercise. *Exerc Sport Sci Rev.* 2004;32(2):50–56.

118. Martin TR, Castile RG, Fredberg JJ, et al. Airway size is related to sex but not lung size in normal adults. *J Appl Physiol.* 1987;63(5):2042–2047.

119. McClaran SR, Harms CA, Pegelow DF, et al. Smaller lungs in women affect exercise hyperpnea. *J Appl Physiol.* 1998;84(6):1872–1881.

120. Guenette JA, Witt JD, McKenzie DC, et al. Respiratory mechanics during exercise in endurance-trained men and women. *J Physiol.* 2007;581(pt 3):1309–1322.

121. Guenette JA, Romer LM, Querido JS, et al. Sex differences in exercise-induced diaphragmatic fatigue in endurance-trained athletes. *J Appl Physiol.* 2010;109(1):35–46.

122. Hicks AL, Kent-Braun J, Ditor DS. Sex differences in human skeletal muscle fatigue. *Exerc Sport Sci Rev.* 2001;29(3):109–112.

123. Moore RL. The cardiovascular system: cardiac function. In: Farrell PA, Joyner MJ, Caiozzo VJ, eds. *ACSM's Advanced Exercise Physiology.* 2nd ed. Baltimore: Lippincott Williams & Wilkins; 2011.

124. Caiozzo VJ. The muscular system: structural and functional plasticity. In: Farrell PA, Joyner MJ, Caiozzo VJ, eds. *ACSM's Advanced Exercise Physiology* (2nd ed.). Baltimore: Lippincott Williams & Wilkins; 2011.

125. Weibel ER, Taylor CR, Hoppeler H. Variations in function and design: testing symmorphosis in the respiratory system. *Respir Physiol.* 1992;87(3):325–348.

126. Johnson LR, Rush JW, Turk JR, et al. Short-term exercise training increases ACh-induced relaxation and eNOS protein in porcine pulmonary arteries. *J Appl Physiol.* 2001;90(3):1102–1110.

127. Clanton TL, Dixon GF, Drake J, et al. Effects of swim training on lung volumes and inspiratory muscle conditioning. *J Appl Physiol.* 1987;62(1):39–46.

128. Leith DE, Bradley M. Ventilatory muscle strength and endurance training. *J Appl Physiol.* 1976;41(4):508–516.

129. Scichilone N, Morici G, Marchese R, et al. Reduced airway responsiveness in nonelite runners. *Med Sci Sports Exerc.* 2005;37(12):2019–2025.

130. Scichilone N, Morici G, Zangla D, et al. Effects of exercise training on airway responsiveness and airway cells in healthy subjects. *J Appl Physiol.* 2010;109(2):288–294.

131. Bonsignore MR, La Grutta S, Cibella F, et al. Effects of exercise training and montelukast in children with mild asthma. *Med Sci Sports Exerc.* 2008;40(3):405–412.

132. Mendes FA, Almeida FM, Cukier A, et al. Effects of aerobic training on airway inflammation in asthmatic patients. *Med Sci Sports Exerc.* 2011;43:197–203.

133. Scichilone N, Togias A. The role of lung inflation in airway hyperresponsiveness and in asthma. *Curr Allergy Asthma Rep.* 2004;4(2):166–174.

134. Hewitt M, Estell K, Davis IC, et al. Repeated bouts of moderate-intensity aerobic exercise reduce airway reactivity in a murine asthma model. *Am J Respir Cell Mol Biol.* 2010;42(2):243–249.

135. Nourry C, Deruelle F, Fabre C, et al. Exercise flow-volume loops in prepubescent aerobically trained children. *J Appl Physiol.* 2005;99(5):1912–1921.

136. Courteix D, Obert P, Lecoq AM, et al. Effect of intensive swimming training on lung volumes, airway resistance and on the maximal expiratory flow-volume relationship in prepubertal girls. *Eur J Appl Physiol Occup Physiol.* 1997;76(3):264–269.

137. Nourry C, Deruelle F, Guinhouya C, et al. High-intensity intermittent running training improves pulmonary function and alters exercise breathing pattern in children. *Eur J Appl Physiol.* 2005;94(4):415–423.

138. Hagberg JM, Yerg JE 2nd, Seals DR. Pulmonary function in young and older athletes and untrained men. *J Appl Physiol.* 1988;65(1):101–105.

139. McClaran SR, Babcock MA, Pegelow DF, et al. Longitudinal effects of aging on lung function at rest and exercise in healthy active fit elderly adults. *J Apply Physiol.* 1995;78(5):1957–1968.

140. Seals DR, Walker AE, Pierce GL, et al. Habitual exercise and vascular ageing. *J Physiol.* 2009;587(pt 23):5541–5549.

141. Dempsey JA, Reddan WG, Birnbaum ML, et al. Effects of acute through life-long hypoxic exposure on exercise pulmonary gas exchange. *Respir Physiol.* 1971;13(1):62–89.

142. Massaro D, Massaro GD, Baras A, et al. Calorie-related rapid onset of alveolar loss, regeneration, and changes in mouse lung gene expression. *Am J Physiol Lung Cell Mol Physiol.* 2004;286(5):L896–L906.

143. Hsia CC, Fryder-Doffey F, Stalder-Nayarro V, et al. Structural changes underlying compensatory increase of diffusing capacity after left pneumonectomy in adult dogs. *J Clin Invest.* 1993;92(2):758–764.

144. Karjalainen EM, Laitinen A, Sue-Chu M, et al. Evidence of airway inflammation and remodeling in ski athletes with and without bronchial hyperresponsiveness to methacholine. *Am J Respir Crit Care Med.* 2000;161(6):2086–2091.

145. Powers S, Shanley R. Exercise-induced changes in diaphragmatic bioenergetic and antioxidant capacity. *Exerc Sport Sci Rev.* 2002;30(2):69–74.

146. Vincent HK, Shanely RA, Stewart DJ, et al. Adaptation of upper airway muscles to chronic endurance exercise. *Am J Respir Crit Care Med.* 2002;166(3):287–293.

147. Ramirez-Sarmiento A, Orozco-Levi M, Guell R, et al. Inspiratory muscle training in patients with chronic obstructive pulmonary disease: structural adaptation and physiologic outcomes. *Am J Respir Crit Care Med.* 2002;166(11):1491–1497.

148. Levine S, Nguyen T, Shrager J, et al. Diaphragm adaptations elicited by severe chronic obstructive pulmonary disease: lessons for sports science. *Exerc Sport Sci Rev.* 2001;29(2):71–75.

149. Babcock MA, Pegelow DF, Johnson BD, et al. Aerobic fitness effects on exercise-induced low-frequency diaphragm fatigue. *J Appl Physiol.* 1996;81(5):2156–2164.

150. Zhan WZ, Sieck GC. Adaptations of diaphragm and medial gastrocnemius muscles to inactivity. *J Appl Physiol.* 1992;72(4):1445–1453.

151. Levine S, Nguyen T, Taylor N, et al. Rapid disuse atrophy of diaphragm fibers in mechanically ventilated humans. *N Engl J Med.* 2008;358(13):1327–1335.

152. Farkas GA, Roussos C. Adaptability of the hamster diaphragm to exercise and/or emphysema. *J Appl Physiol.* 1982;53(5):1263–1272.

153. Farkas GA, Roussos C. Diaphragm in emphysematous hamsters: sarcomere adaptability. *J Appl Physiol.* 1983;54(6):1635–1640.

154. Arnold JS, Thomas AJ, Kelsen SG. Length-tension relationship of abdominal expiratory muscles: effect of emphysema. *J Appl Physiol.* 1987;62(2):739–745.

155. Shrager JB, Kim DK, Hashmi YJ, et al. Sarcomeres are added in series to emphysematous rat diaphragm after lung volume reduction surgery. *Chest.* 2002;121(1):210–215.

156. Shrager JB, Kim DK, Hashmi YJ, et al. Lung volume reduction surgery restores the normal diaphragmatic length-tension relationship in emphysematous rats. *J Thorac Cardiovasc Surg.* 2001;121(2):217–224.

157. Saltin B, Calbet JA. Point: in health and in a normoxic environment, VO2 max is limited primarily by cardiac output and locomotor muscle blood flow. *J Appl Physiol.* 2006;100(2):744–745.

158. Wagner PD. Counterpoint: in health and in normoxic environment VO2max is limited primarily by cardiac output and locomotor muscle blood flow. *J Appl Physiol.* 2006;100(2):745–747; discussion 7–8.

159. Bayly WM, Hodgson DR, Schulz DA, et al. Exercise-induced hypercapnia in the horse. *J Appl Physiol.* 1989;67(5):1958–1966.

160. Dempsey JA, Hanson PG, Henderson KS. Exercise-induced arterial hypoxaemia in healthy human subjects at sea level. *J Physiol.* 1984;355:161–175.

161. Gore CJ, Little SC, Hahn AG, et al. Reduced performance of male and female athletes at 580 m altitude. *Eur J Appl Physiol Occup Physiol.* 1997;75(2):136–143.

162. Lawler J, Powers SK, Thompson D. Linear relationship between VO2max and VO2max decrement during exposure to acute hypoxia. *J Appl Physiol.* 1988;64(4):1486–1492.

163. Romer LM, Haverkamp HC, Lovering AT, et al. Effect of exercise-induced arterial hypoxemia on quadriceps muscle fatigue in healthy humans. *Am J Physiol Regul Integr Comp Physiol.* 2006;290(2):R365–R375.

164. Amann M, Eldridge MW, Lovering AT, et al. Arterial oxygenation influences central motor output and exercise performance via effects on peripheral locomotor muscle fatigue. *J Physiol.* 2006;575:937–952.

165. Amann M, Calbet JA. Convective oxygen transport and fatigue. *J Appl Physiol.* 2008;104(3):861–870.

166. Harms CA, Wetter TJ, St. Croix CM, et al. Effects of respiratory muscle work on exercise performance. *J Appl Physiol.* 2000;89(1):131–138.

167. Mador MJ, Acevedo FA. Effect of respiratory muscle fatigue on subsequent exercise performance. *J Appl Physiol.* 1991;70:2059–2065.

168. Taylor BJ, Romer LM. Effect of expiratory muscle fatigue on exercise tolerance and locomotor muscle fatigue in healthy humans. *J Appl Physiol.* 2008;104(5):1442–1451.

169. Romer LM, Polkey MI. Exercise-induced respiratory muscle fatigue: implications for performance. *J Appl Physiol.* 2008;104(3):879–888.

170. Romer LM, Lovering AT, Haverkamp HC, et al. Effect of inspiratory muscle work on peripheral fatigue of locomotor muscles in healthy humans. *J Physiol.* 2006;571(pt 2):425–439.

171. Amann M, Pegelow DF, Jacques AJ, et al. Inspiratory muscle work in acute hypoxia influences locomotor muscle fatigue and exercise performance of healthy humans. *Am J Physiol Regul Integr Comp Physiol.* 2007;293(5):R2036–R2045.

172. Nielsen HB, Bredmose PP, Stromstad M, et al. Bicarbonate attenuates arterial desaturation during maximal exercise in humans. *J Appl Physiol.* 2002;93(2):724–731.

173. Wetter TJ, Xiang Z, Sonetti DA, et al. Role of lung inflammatory mediators as a cause of exercise-induced arterial hypoxemia in young athletes. *J Appl Physiol.* 2002;93(1):116–126.

174. Prefaut C, Anselme-Poujol F, Caillaud C. Inhibition of histamine release by nedocromil sodium reduces exercise-induced hypoxemia in master athletes. *Med Sci Sports Exerc.* 1997;29(1):10–16.

175. Haverkamp HC, Dempsey JA, Pegelow DF, et al. Treatment of airway inflammation improves exercise pulmonary gas exchange and performance in asthmatic subjects. *J Allergy Clin Immunol.* 2007;120(1):39–47.

176. McConnell AK, Romer LM. Respiratory muscle training in healthy humans: resolving the controversy. *Int J Sports Med.* 2004;25(4):284–293.

177. Johnson MA, Sharpe GR, Brown PI. Inspiratory muscle training improves cycling time-trial performance and anaerobic work capacity but not critical power. *Eur J Appl Physiol.* 2007;101(6):761–770.

178. McConnell AK, Sharpe GR. The effect of inspiratory muscle training upon maximum lactate steady-state and blood lactate concentration. *Eur J Appl Physiol.* 2005;94(3):277–284.

179. Romer LM, McConnell AK, Jones DA. Inspiratory muscle fatigue in trained cyclists: effects of inspiratory muscle training. *Med Sci Sports Exerc.* 2002;34(5):785–792.

180. Verges S, Lenherr O, Haner AC, et al. Increased fatigue resistance of respiratory muscles during exercise after respiratory muscle endurance training. *Am J Physiol Regul Integr Comp Physiol.* 2007;292(3):R1246–R1253.

181. McConnell AK, Lomax M. The influence of inspiratory muscle work history and specific inspiratory muscle training upon human limb muscle fatigue. *J Physiol.* 2006;577(pt 1):445–457.

182. Witt JD, Guenette JA, Rupert JL, et al. Inspiratory muscle training attenuates the human respiratory muscle metaboreflex. *J Physiol.* 2007;584(pt 3):1019–1028.

183. McConnell AK, Romer LM. Dyspnoea in health and obstructive pulmonary disease: the role of respiratory muscle function and training. *Sports Med.* 2004;34(2):117–132.

CHAPTER 9

The Cardiovascular System: Design and Control

Donal S. O'Leary, Patrick J. Mueller, and Javier A. Sala-Mercado

Abbreviations

bpm	Beats per minute	NE	norepinephrine
CO	Cardiac output	NO	Nitric oxide
dP/dt	rate of change in pressure within the left ventricle	R-R interval	Period between successive R waves of the electrocardiogram, period between heart beats, inverse of HR
E_{max}	Maximal ventricular elastance		
HR	Heart rate	SV	Stroke volume

Introduction

Strenuous dynamic exercise presents one of the greatest challenges to cardiovascular control. In response to increasing work rates and oxygen consumption (*e.g.*, treadmill running, bicycling), heart rate (HR) increases progressively toward maximal values. This tachycardia coupled with sustained or modestly increased stroke volume (SV) (amount of blood pumped by the heart with each heartbeat) causes large (fourfold to fivefold) increases in blood flow to the systemic circulation (termed *cardiac output* [CO]). Marked vasodilation occurs in the active skeletal muscles, such that virtually all of this increase in CO is directed to the active muscles, although skin blood flow may also rise if internal temperature increases sufficiently. Blood flow to inactive areas (*e.g.*, splanchnic, renal circulations) decreases as a result of substantial activation of the sympathetic nervous system and this flow is redistributed to the active skeletal muscle as well. With the marked changes in autonomic nervous activity, increases in CO, and vasoconstriction in inactive vascular beds, arterial pressure rises. With strenuous static muscle contraction, increases in HR and CO also occur, as does vasoconstriction in inactive beds, but vasodilation within the active muscle becomes mechanically restricted due to physical compression of blood vessels by the large increases in muscle tissue pressure and arterial systolic blood pressures may increase to extreme levels (>300 mm Hg).

The mechanisms mediating these substantial cardiovascular and autonomic responses to exercise are not completely understood, but they involve the action and likely interaction between at least three systems: central command, the arterial baroreflex, and activation of afferents within the active skeletal muscle (both mechanically sensitive and chemically sensitive receptors) (Fig. 9.1). This chapter focuses on what cardiovascular parameters are controlled during dynamic and resistance exercise and the mechanisms by which they are controlled. Given the limited space for this chapter, see other reviews for more detailed discussion (1,2).

Design: What Is Controlled?

The Pump: Control of Cardiac Output

CO is the amount of blood pumped by the heart into the systemic circulation per unit of time, most often expressed as liters per minute. CO can be calculated as the product of SV and HR—that is, the amount of blood pumped per

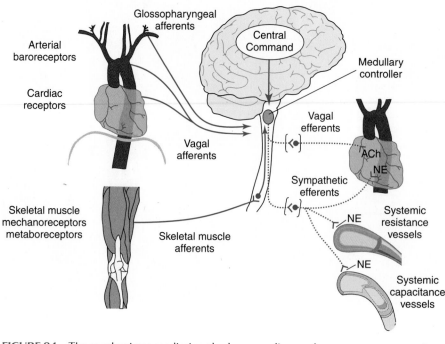

FIGURE 9.1   The mechanisms mediating the large cardiovascular responses to exercise. Activation of central command, skeletal muscle afferents, and resetting of the arterial and perhaps cardiopulmonary baroreflexes together affect central areas that control sympathetic and parasympathetic activity to the heart and peripheral blood vessels. ACh, acetylcholine; NE, norepinephrine.

heartbeat (stroke volume) times the number of times the heart contracts per unit of time (usually expressed as beats per minute [bpm]):

$$CO = SV \times HR$$

where CO is cardiac output and HR is heart rate.

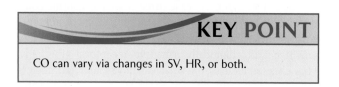

KEY POINT

CO can vary via changes in SV, HR, or both.

Control of Heart Rate

HR is controlled primarily via changes in parasympathetic and sympathetic activity to the pacemaker area of the heart, the sinoatrial node. Increases in parasympathetic activity decrease HR, and increases in sympathetic activity increase HR. With no activity of either sympathetic or parasympathetic nerves to the heart (*e.g.,* cardiac transplant patients), HR is ~100 to 110 bpm. Resting HR in normal humans is ~60 to 70 bpm, so tonic restraint of HR exists via sustained moderate levels of parasympathetic tone. A small amount of functional sympathetic activity to the heart also exists at rest. Thus, in response to exercise, HR can increase via reductions in parasympathetic activity and via increases in sympathetic activity.

Control of Stroke Volume

As HR changes, SV can vary as a result of the changes in the time for filling of the ventricles. Figure 9.2 shows the results of an experiment wherein HR was varied from about 40 to about 220 bpm via a pacemaker in conscious dogs with atrioventricular block (3). As HR increased from 40 to about 100 bpm, a fairly linear increase in CO occurred. CO increased because SV was well maintained. However, from about 110 to about 180 bpm little further increase in CO occurred, because of the concomitant fall in SV as the filling time for the ventricles lessened. Above 180 bpm, further increases in HR actually caused decreases in CO because of the severe fall in SV as filling time decreased markedly. This can happen in patients with ventricular tachycardia, even more so if atrial contraction does not contribute to ventricular filling (as was the case in the study cited above which only used ventricular stimulation) (3). These are important considerations in understanding cardiac control mechanisms during exercise. Changes in HR per se may be of little consequence in the steady state control of CO, unless other mechanisms are engaged to maintain or increase SV despite marked reductions in ventricular filling time. In contrast to the effects of HR per se on CO, the broken line in Figure 9.2 shows the changes in CO as a function of HR in conscious dogs during treadmill exercise. As HR increased from about 120 bpm to the maximal level of about 280 bpm, substantial increases in CO occurred. In this setting, the increases in HR are accompanied by increases in ventricular performance, left ventricular filling pressure, and end diastolic volume, which together act to maintain or even increase SV, despite

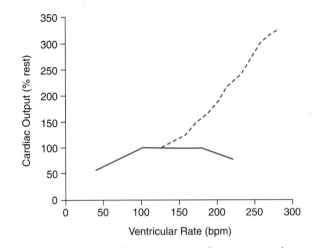

FIGURE 9.2 Relationship between cardiac output and ventricular rate when ventricular rate is altered via a pacemaker (*solid line*) versus during treadmill exercise to maximal exercise intensities in dogs. For the *solid line*, heart rate was varied via a pacemaker in conscious dogs with atrioventricular block (so that very low heart rates could be produced). As heart rate increases, initially increases in cardiac output occur, however above about 110 bpm, little further increase in cardiac output occurs because of substantial decreases in stroke volume. Above 180 bpm, further increases in heart rate actually decrease cardiac output because of severe reductions in stroke volume that result from limitations in ventricular filling time. (Data from White S, Higgins CB, Vatner SF, et al. Effects of altering ventricular rate on blood flow distribution in conscious dogs. *Am J Physiol.* 1971;221:H1402–H1407). In contrast, during normal dynamic exercise (*broken line*), substantial increases in cardiac output occur with the normal tachycardia because of sustained or increased stroke volume with increases in heart rate. (Data with permission from Musch TI, Friedman DB, Pitetti KH, et al. Regional distribution of blood flow of dogs during graded dynamic exercise. *J Appl Physiol.* 1987;63:2269–2277.)

the markedly reduced ventricular filling time (from more than 0.5 seconds at rest to <0.1 seconds at maximal exercise). Similar results are observed during strong static muscle contractions (resistive exercise). HR and CO increase while SV remains essentially constant or increases modestly.

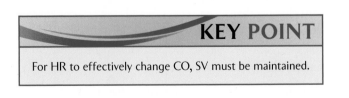

KEY POINT

For HR to effectively change CO, SV must be maintained.

Role of preload, afterload, and ventricular contractility

As HR increases and ventricular filling time decreases, there can be less filling of the ventricles, less tension developed, and thus less ability to eject blood into the arterial circulation. This relationship between SV and ventricular preload (ventricular volume immediately prior to contraction) can

be modified via activation of the sympathetic nerves to the heart. With the release of norepinephrine and stimulation of β-adrenergic receptors on the ventricular myocardium, the strength of each individual contraction increases and the relationship between SV and ventricular preload is improved, in that a larger SV will occur at a given preload. This represents an increase in ventricular contractility, also termed an increased inotropic state of the heart (see Chapter 10).

With each ventricular contraction, pressure inside the left ventricle must exceed pressure in the aorta before the aortic valve opens and blood can be expelled (often termed the afterload on the ventricle, a term borrowed from skeletal muscle mechanics and is the load lifted by a muscle—the cardiac muscle does not lift a load but rather expels blood against resistance which creates pressure, but both are work performed by the muscle). Thus, changes in arterial pressure can also affect SV. At high arterial pressures, it takes longer to generate enough pressure to open the aortic valve, and the valve closes sooner. Therefore, the time during which ejection of blood can occur is lessened, and SV falls. This relationship between SV and afterload can also be modified by changes in ventricular contractility. With stimulation of sympathetic nerves to the heart and an increase in ventricular contractility, the heart becomes less sensitive to changes in ventricular afterload, allowing the left ventricle to maintain SV over a wider range of arterial pressures.

Ventricular contractility is exceedingly difficult to measure (perhaps because there is no universally accepted rigorous definition—generally, we consider changes in contractility to reflect changes in ventricular function independent of changes in preload and afterload). Nearly all indirect indices—such as SV, the rate of change in pressure within the left ventricle (dP/dt), how fast the ventricle contracts, and what fraction of the blood is ejected—can all vary with changes in preload and afterload, as well as inotropic state. Studies using more invasive measurements are often performed in an anesthetized animal model and general anesthetics agents and acute surgical trauma may profoundly alter the central nervous system regulation of circulatory responses, affect the baseline sympathetic and parasympathetic activity, and therefore baseline HR and contractility as well as response to neural interventions (4–6).

One technique to measure contractility pioneered by Sagawa and colleagues (7) is analysis of ventricular contractions in the pressure–volume relationship. As the heart contracts and develops tension, it becomes more stiff. This maximal stiffness (termed *maximal elastance*; E_{max}) varies in direct proportion to the contractility and is relatively insensitive to changes in ventricular preload and afterload. One caveat is that most of these studies were made in isolated hearts or during acute experiments in animals when the chest was opened. However, with the fairly recent advent of indirect techniques to measure ventricular volume and pressure in subjects during exercise, some insight into regulation of ventricular contractility during exercise has been possible (8,9).

The Peripheral Vasculature

Arterial resistance

Control of the arterial resistance occurs primarily at the level of the arterioles. These are thick-walled vessels capable of marked changes in diameter. Inasmuch as the resistance to flow is inversely proportional to the radius of the blood vessel raised to the fourth power, even small changes in radius can yield large changes in resistance and therefore in blood flow. This relationship between flow and resistance is governed by a hydraulic analog of Ohm's law:

$$\text{perfusion pressure} = \text{flow} \times \text{resistance}$$

Changes in the level of activity of the vascular smooth muscle in the arterioles can vary as a result of changes in sympathetic activity to the arterioles (see Chapter 11). Sympathetic nerves innervate the peripheral blood vessels and release NE as the primary neurotransmitter. NE acts on α-receptors and elicits increased activity of the vascular smooth muscle, causing vasoconstriction, which decreases the radius of the arteriole. As described earlier, even small changes in radius can yield large changes in resistance and therefore blood flow (assuming a constant perfusion pressure, discussed in more depth later in the chapter).

Changes in the interstitial concentration of chemical substances released from cells can also modulate resistance. These metabolic vasodilators include bradykinin, prostaglandins, adenosine, K^+, carbon dioxide, and lactate, among others. Decreases in local PO_2 can also elicit release of adenosine triphosphate from hemoglobin, which can activate purinergic receptors on the vascular smooth muscle, causing vasodilation. Furthermore, the endothelium lining the interior of the arterioles can also release a variety of substances that can affect vasomotor tone. Most notable is nitric oxide (NO). In response to increases in the shear stress, NO is released and causes vasodilation of the arterioles. Sheriff and associates (10) demonstrated that NO may contribute to the vasodilation in skeletal muscle accompanying mild to moderate treadmill exercise. The role of other endothelial factors, such as endothelin and endothelium-derived hyperpolarizing factor, in the regulation of skeletal muscle blood flow during exercise is unclear. Many if not all of the vasodilator substances described earlier likely contribute to the rapid vasodilation that occurs in skeletal muscle with the onset of dynamic exercise. With static muscle contractions, the production of metabolites also increases, but the vasodilation may be prevented mechanically by the increased muscle tissue pressure physically compressing the blood vessels.

Venous capacitance

Approximately 70% of blood volume resides on the venous side of the circulation. Increased sympathetic activity to the veins causes venous smooth muscle contraction resulting in mobilization of blood volume from the periphery to the central veins, which can aid in the increase of ventricular filling pressure, preload, and therefore SV. In addition, with locomotion, the repetitive dynamic contractions of the skeletal muscle act to squeeze the veins and pump the blood back toward the heart (this pumping, of course, occurs only once with static contractions). The "muscle pump" likely aids in maintaining or even increasing ventricular filling pressure, preload, and thereby SV during dynamic exercise.

Feed-Forward and Feedback Reflex Cardiovascular Control during Exercise

The autonomic and neurohormonal responses to exercise are the result of the action and likely interaction among at least three systems: central command, the arterial baroreflex, and activation of skeletal muscle afferents (Fig. 9.1).

Central Command

Central command is the concept that the volition to exercise can elicit cardiovascular responses. This is a feed-forward system that, by its very nature, is difficult to study. The theory is that with activation of the motor cortex, there is a parallel activation of pathways that descend into the brainstem areas controlling sympathetic and parasympathetic activities.

Victor and colleagues (12) performed an insightful series of experiments that strongly support the concept that central command can cause substantial inhibition of parasympathetic activity; the role of central command in the control of sympathetic activity remains less certain. These investigators had subjects perform static forearm contractions before and after treatment with a neuromuscular blocker. In the control setting, the static contraction raised arterial pressure, HR, and sympathetic nerve activity to resting skeletal muscle. After neuromuscular blockade, the subjects attempted the contraction but were able to generate little, if any, force despite near maximal effort. In this setting of high levels of attempted effort and presumed high central command, the increase in arterial pressure and muscle sympathetic nerve activity were much smaller than in the control experiment; however, a similar increase in HR occurred. This rise in HR with attempted contractions could be blocked by an antagonist to the parasympathetic nerves and was unaffected by an antagonist to the cardiac sympathetic nerves. Thus, the increase in HR with strong activation of central command occurred via inhibition of tonic parasympathetic tone to the heart. Strong increases in central command can also elicit some increase in sympathetic tone (13). In animal models, electrical or chemical stimulation of certain central sites will elicit locomotor responses, as well as large increases in sympathetic activity (14,15). To what extent this reflects "central command" seen in normal volitional exercise is unknown. Matsukawa et al. (16) did observe small increases (less than 25%) in renal sympathetic activity immediately before the start of static exercise in cats trained to perform static forelimb contractions. Because no contraction had occurred yet, this is likely due to activation of central command.

KEY POINT

The initial rapid increase in HR at the initiation of exercise may stem from activation of central command causing rapid decreases in parasympathetic activity that will elicit very fast increases in HR.

Whereas activation of central command can elicit rapid parasympathetic withdrawal and increased CO due to a rise in HR, no studies to our knowledge have investigated whether central command can directly increase the inotropic state of the heart. As previously mentioned, it is controversial whether central command modulates sympathetic nerve activity, but it is clear that central command modulates parasympathetic activity to the heart and it is mainly responsible of the initial tachycardia observed at the onset of exercise. The physiologic significance of the parasympathetic control of ventricular inotropicity has been less established than for the sympathetic nervous system (see Chapter 10). In conscious dogs, blockade of parasympathetic nerves at rest caused a significant tachycardia with no concomitant change in left ventricular dP/dt suggesting that, although (at rest) there is a substantial atrial parasympathetic tone

modulating HR, there is little or no parasympathetic influence on ventricular contractility (17). Supporting this study would be the fact that choline esters alone produce little or no reduction on ventricular contractility and that histochemical studies have shown dense cholinergic innervation of the atria and conducting system, however sparse innervation along the ventricular myocardium (18,19). In addition, although Xenopoulos and Applegate (20) observed negative inotropism (decreased left ventricular E_{max}) with vagal stimulation in anesthetized dogs, Matsuura et al. (21) showed in sympathectomized rabbits that vagal stimulation hardly affects ventricular contractility (E_{max}) as long as HR is kept constant. As a result, central command through altering parasympathetic nerve activity to the heart is important in modulating HR but it has little if any role in direct modulation of ventricular contractility.

TEST YOURSELF

Describe the evidence that supports a role for "central command" in controlling parasympathetic withdrawal at the onset of exercise.

Baroreflexes

Within the walls of the carotid sinus and aortic arch are receptors that sense the level of arterial pressure, termed the arterial baroreceptors. In response to changes in arterial pressure (mean pressure as well as pulse pressure), the baroreceptors change their level of activity. For example, as pressure rises, the activity of the baroreceptors increases. This information is relayed to the brainstem via cranial nerves IX and X (for carotid and aortic arch baroreceptors, respectively) and a reflex increase in parasympathetic and decrease in sympathetic activity occurs. This causes HR and CO to decrease and peripheral vasodilation of resistance and capacitance vessels, which decreases pressure. Opposite responses occur with decreases in blood pressure from the normal levels. Thus, the arterial baroreflex is the primary short-term controller of arterial pressure on a beat-to-beat basis. Removal of the arterial baroreceptors results in marked variability of arterial pressure at rest and during mild exercise.

For many years, it was thought that because both HR and arterial pressure rise during exercise, the arterial baroreflex must be inhibited; otherwise, the rise in arterial pressure would elicit a baroreflex reduction in HR. Much of the support for this concept came from a series of studies wherein the chronotropic responses to rapid increases in arterial pressure were observed in humans at rest and during dynamic exercise of various intensities (22). These studies concluded that the strength of the baroreflex was progressively lessened, as exercise intensity increased. However, two factors can markedly affect the conclusions from these experiments: (a) arterial pressure was raised rapidly via bolus intravenous infusion of a vasoconstrictor and

(b) the chronotropic response was quantified as the change in interbeat interval (electrocardiographic R-R interval, the time between heart beats). With the bolus method, the changes in arterial pressure are so rapid that mainly only the parasympathetic component of the chronotropic response is observed because the speed of the sympathetic responses is much slower than the fast parasympathetic responses. Second, although R-R interval and HR are reciprocally related, they are often thought to be interchangeable. However, a reciprocal relationship is highly nonlinear. Figure 9.3 shows the relationship between R-R interval and HR. The problem in the analysis comes when a large change in baseline HR occurs, as between rest and exercise. For example, assume that at rest HR is 60 bpm (R-R interval of 1000 ms) and that arterial pressure is raised by 10 mm Hg, causing a 10-bpm baroreflex bradycardia. Baroreflex sensitivity would be 1 bpm per mm Hg, or 20.0 ms per mm Hg. If in response to exercise HR increases to 165 bpm (R-R interval of 363.6 ms) and the same 10-mm Hg increase in arterial pressure causes the same 10-bpm baroreflex bradycardia, then in terms of HR, baroreflex strength is undiminished (again, 1 bpm per mm Hg). But, when analyzed in terms of R-R interval, baroreflex sensitivity is reduced nearly to one-tenth—to 2.3 ms per mm Hg. Thus, the same data yield completely different conclusions when analyzed in terms of HR versus R-R interval. Indeed, in a similar study Bevegard and Shepherd (23) observed similar baroreflex HR responses at rest and during exercise (note these authors used HR for analysis, rather than R-R interval). Which is correct? An important consideration is that HR is not the variable sensed and controlled by the arterial baroreflex; rather, that variable is arterial pressure.

In a classic study, Melcher and Donald (24) vascularly isolated the carotid sinus baroreceptors such that the pressure exposed to the carotid baroreceptors could be controlled in conscious animals at rest and during graded treadmill exercise. Thus, these investigators could change the pressure at the baroreceptors and observe the changes in systemic arterial pressure and HR. They found that the strength of the baroreflex was not reduced during exercise; rather, the reflex was reset to a higher pressure (see the Milestone of Discovery at the end of this chapter). These conclusions have been confirmed by several other investigators in other species, including humans (15,25–27). Thus, rather than being turned off by exercise, the arterial baroreflex is reset to a higher pressure and now defends this higher pressure. Therefore, a portion of the rise in sympathetic activity and decrease in parasympathetic activity with exercise could be due to the resetting of the baroreflex; that is, rather than opposing the rise in pressure, the arterial baroreflex reinforces this increase. The factors that cause this resetting are unknown. However, recent studies implicate both central command (discussed previously) as well as activation of skeletal muscle afferents (discussed later) in mediating resetting of the arterial baroreflex during exercise (15,28).

There is controversy whether the strength or gain of the baroreflex decreases somewhat, as exercise intensity approaches maximal levels. In a series of studies, Raven and colleagues (25,26) investigated carotid baroreflex control of HR and arterial pressure by manipulating the transmural pressure at the carotid sinuses by applying pressure or suction around the neck. They showed that as exercise intensity increased, the operating point (prevailing point on the stimulus–response relationship; point at which the reflex is operating) of the baroreflex moved away from the center of the carotid sinus pressure–HR relationship and toward the threshold for the baroreflex (Fig. 9.4). Thus, as exercise intensity increased, the operating point moved from a high-gain portion of the curve (in the center) to a low-gain portion of the curve. Both the operating range (range of pressures over which the reflex is operating) and the response range (range of the HR response; maximal HR minus minimal HR) decreased at higher exercise intensities; however, the maximal gain (maximal slope of the curve; centering point) did not change, but the operating point became progressively displaced from the centering point, as exercise intensity increased. Similar results were obtained by Sala-Mercado and associates (30) who observed the chronotropic responses to small spontaneous changes in arterial pressure and found that the responses became smaller as exercise intensity increased. Theoretically, as HR approaches maximal levels, the operating point for the HR responses must move closer to the baroreflex threshold, inasmuch as further tachycardia becomes limited as the subject approaches maximal HR. Interestingly, the same large shift in the operating point with dynamic exercise was significantly less for the relationship between carotid sinus pressure and arterial pressure, and no changes in the operating or response ranges

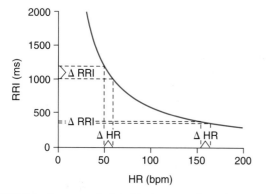

FIGURE 9.3 Inverse relationship between heartbeat interval (RRI) and heart rate (HR) *(solid line)*. The line of identity between the two indices *(broken lines)*. When HR is low, a 10 bpm change in HR will yield a large change in RRI, whereas when the baseline level of HR is elevated, the same 10 bpm change in HR will be calculated as a very small change in RRI. (Reprinted with permission from O'Leary DS. Heart rate control during exercise by baroreceptors and skeletal muscle afferents. *Med Sci Sports Exerc.* 1995;28:210–217.)

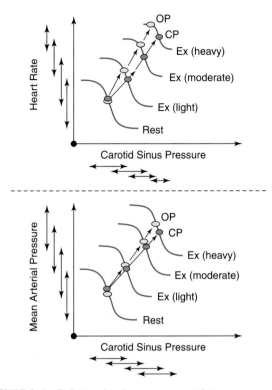

FIGURE 9.4 Relationship between carotid sinus pressure and heart rate (*top*) and carotid sinus pressure and mean arterial pressure (*bottom*) at rest and during graded exercise. At rest for both relationships, the operating point (OP) is at the high-gain portion of the curve near the center of the relationship (centering point, or CP). As exercise intensity rises, the OP for the heart rate responses moves away from the CP toward a lower gain portion of the curve. Less movement of the OP for the mean arterial pressure responses occurs. For the heart rate responses, both the range of the responses (*arrows on y-axis*) and the operating range (*arrows on x-axis*) decreases as exercise intensity rises, although no change in maximal gain was observed. Little change in either the response or operating ranges for the arterial pressure responses occurred. (Fig. 9.4 redrawn from unpublished figure courtesy of Dr. Peter B. Raven based on several recent studies from his laboratory, located at the University of North Texas Health Science Center in Fort Worth, Texas. Figure is based on investigation conducted in Raven's laboratory or in colleague's laboratories where he was a coinvestigator.)

occurred (the arterial pressure response was shown to be virtually entirely due to changes in vasomotor tone, not CO [26]). In this setting, effective baroreflex buffering of a hypotensive response could occur only via peripheral vasoconstriction (discussed later in the chapter).

KEY POINT

The arterial baroreflex effectively regulates arterial pressure from at rest and mild through strenuous work rates.

Exercise Alters Baroreflex Mechanisms

With the large changes in CO, HR, and regional blood flow accompanying exercise, the mechanisms mediating baroreflex responses can change between rest and exercise.

Heart rate

In humans and other species such as dogs, resting HR is primarily under parasympathetic control. Thus, baroreflex-mediated reductions in HR occur mainly if not solely via increases in the tonic parasympathetic activity, inasmuch as little, if any, sympathetic activity exists to be withdrawn, but baroreflex-mediated tachycardia can occur via both inhibition of the high tonic parasympathetic activity and increases in sympathetic tone. In contrast, during moderate to heavy exercise, the baseline levels of autonomic activity to the heart have shifted. In this setting, parasympathetic activity is less (although not totally inhibited), and sympathetic activity is elevated. Thus, both baroreflex-mediated tachycardia and bradycardia can occur via changes in both sympathetic and parasympathetic activity in response to both decreases and increases in arterial pressure, respectively (31). One possible contributing factor to conclusions regarding baroreflex control of HR during exercise is the method used to manipulate baroreceptor activity. The initial, rapid chronotropic responses to changes in arterial pressure are virtually entirely due to rapid changes in parasympathetic tone, which has an exceedingly short time lag for full expression of its effects on HR. Full expression of the HR responses to changes in sympathetic tone take much longer to develop (31). Therefore, if the change in baroreceptor activity is transient, such as when utilizing the spontaneous oscillations in arterial pressure or rapid changes in pressure induced by bolus infusion of vasoactive drugs, the observed HR responses are likely only due to changes in parasympathetic activity. As exercise intensity increases, parasympathetic activity decreases. Thus, the reduction in baroreflex control over rapid changes in HR with exercise seen in some studies may reflect the limited remaining parasympathetic tone, as well as limitations in the methods used to study the baroreflex.

The arterial baroreflex effect on ventricular inotropicity is not as pronounced as its influence on HR and the peripheral vasculature. In conscious, chronically instrumented dogs, there is no significant decrease in left ventricular dP/dt after carotid sinus nerve stimulation (32). This observation corresponds with the concept that in conscious normal dogs and humans under physiologic conditions at rest there is low sympathetic tone and, as a result, it cannot be further withdrawn. In addition, also at rest, unloading of the arterial baroreceptors in conscious dogs (intravenous nitroglycerine; bilateral carotid occlusion) has shown to elicit a small yet significant increase left ventricular dP/dt (32). The carotid sinus reflex through modifying sympathetic discharge to the adrenal glands has been shown to alter catecholamines secretion. However, the importance of circulating catecholamines in regulating the contractile state of the heart during dynamic exercise is controversial. Shimizu et al. (33) have shown in anesthetized cats that vagotomy and cardiac sympathectomy attenuated but did not abolish the dP/dt responses to carotid sinus pressure alteration and concluded that induced adrenal gland secretion of catecholamines plays a significant role in the reflex control of cardiac contractility. On the other hand, infusions of catecholamines in conscious chronically instrumented dogs yield no significant increase in left ventricular dP/dt until plasma catecholamines reach 1000 pg · mL^{-1} (34). In normal dogs, plasma catecholamines do not reach such high levels during moderate to heavy dynamic exercise (35), whereas left ventricular dP/dt nearly doubles, and E$_{max}$ significantly increases (36). Thus, moderate dynamic exercise in normal dogs is associated with a relatively small rise in circulating catecholamines with large increases in ventricular inotropicity. Human studies performed at rest and during dynamic exercise have shown that SV is not significantly altered during carotid baroreflex stimulation (acute changes in carotid transmural pressure) (26,29). However, because SV is dependent on factors in addition to ventricular contractility (e.g., preload and afterload), these results should be viewed with caution. Therefore, whereas substantial baroreflex-induced changes in HR occur even during heavy exercise, only limited (at most) baroreflex changes in inotropic state have been observed using relatively indirect methods to assess ventricular contractility.

Even substantial baroreflex-induced increases in ventricular contractility would have limited ability to cause sustained increases in CO without some mechanism(s) to increase central blood volume mobilization. This is due to the inverse relationship between CO and ventricular preload. As CO increases, blood volume is transferred from the central veins to the systemic circulation, thereby lowering central venous pressure. Baroreflex activation via carotid sinus hypotension is capable of increasing central venous pressure modestly (37), which would thereby support some sustained increase in CO via the concomitant reflex tachycardia and increase in contractility.

Peripheral vasculature

The most important component of the arterial baroreflex compensatory responses to a hypotensive challenge is peripheral vasoconstriction. In response to decreases in arterial pressure, vasoconstriction occurs in virtually all vascular beds except the brain. The ability of vasoconstriction within a given vascular bed to affect arterial pressure depends on the extent of the vasoconstriction and on the fraction of the CO directed to that vascular bed. This is an important consideration because, during dynamic exercise, a greater and greater fraction of the CO is directed to the active skeletal muscle as exercise intensity increases, such that (at heavy exercise intensities) active muscles receives more than 80% of CO. Theoretically, in this setting, effective arterial pressure control can occur only via modulation of vascular tone within the active skeletal muscle. Yet, this idea remains somewhat controversial because, in 1962, Remensnyder and associates (38) concluded that the ability of skeletal muscle to vasoconstrict in response to sympathetic activation was depressed during exercise, termed *functional sympatholysis*. To some extent, however, this conclusion regarding the existence of sympatholysis may also depend on the method of data analysis (39).

Blood flow can be affected by changes in both perfusion pressure and vasomotor tone, so an appropriate index quantifying vasoconstriction or dilation must reflect only changes in vasomotor tone. The two indices used are either vascular resistance (perfusion pressure divided by blood flow) or conductance (blood flow divided by perfusion pressure). As with the relationship between HR and R-R interval, discussed earlier, the reciprocal relationship between resistance and conductance is highly nonlinear. Thus, when marked changes in the baseline level of vasomotor tone occur (as within skeletal muscle between rest and exercise), opposite conclusions can be drawn regarding the magnitude of a vasomotor response when quantified according to the changes in resistance versus conductance. This apparent dichotomy is demonstrated in Figure 9.5. For simplicity we assume that arterial pressure remains constant. At both a low-flow (rest) and a high-flow (exercise) state, a 50% decrease in blood flow occurs in response to sympathetic activation. As can be seen, in terms of resistance, a much larger change occurs during rest, whereas in terms of conductance, a much greater change occurs during exercise. Which is correct? To make matters even more confusing, quantified as percent changes, the responses are exactly the same between the low- and high-flow states. Between rest and exercise, how can a vasomotor response be larger (Δ conductance), smaller (Δ resistance), and exactly the same (% Δ)? Clearly, the conclusions depend on the definition of the term *vasoconstriction*. To resolve this apparent discrepancy, O'Leary (39) proposed that when large changes in blood flow occur between states, vascular conductance is the most appropriate index of vasomotor responses because, at constant pressure, changes in conductance are linearly related to changes in flow. Furthermore, the effect of a given change in regional conductance on arterial pressure is much less dependent on the baseline level than that for resistance. Using a similar approach, Collins et al. (40) directly quantified the contribution of vasoconstriction within skeletal muscle to the rise in arterial pressure with unloading of carotid baroreceptors at rest and during exercise. Because both total flow (CO) and blood flow to the hind limb skeletal muscles were measured, they could directly calculate what fraction of the carotid baroreflex pressor responses could be directly attributed to vasoconstriction in the hind limb skeletal muscles. They concluded that as exercise intensity increased, vasoconstriction within the active skeletal muscle became progressively more important in mediating the rise in arterial pressure with unloading of the carotid baroreceptors. Importantly, these conclusions are independent of whether resistance or conductance, absolute values,

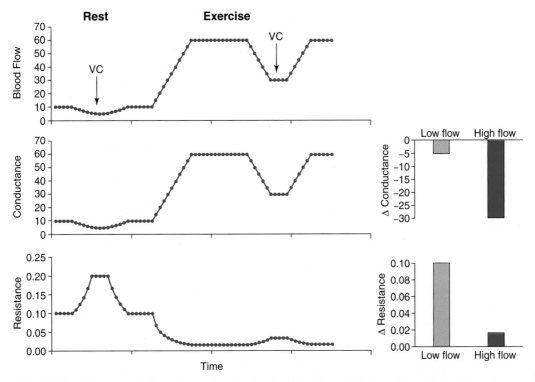

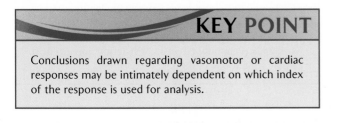

FIGURE 9.5 Theoretical effect of a 50% reduction in blood flow *(VC at arrows)* to skeletal muscle at rest and during exercise on the calculated changes in resistance and conductance. Opposite conclusions would be drawn using each index of the vasomotor response.

or percent changes are used for the calculations; that is, we are no longer trying to measure vasoconstriction but are evaluating the importance of the response in the regulation of arterial pressure. What is not known is whether this greater pressor effect of muscle vasoconstriction seen during exercise is produced by similar increases in sympathetic activity as seen at rest (*e.g.*, little sympatholysis) or whether during dynamic exercise, this greater pressor effect requires a much greater rise in sympathetic activity to overcome substantial sympatholysis.

> # KEY POINT
>
> Conclusions drawn regarding vasomotor or cardiac responses may be intimately dependent on which index of the response is used for analysis.

Skeletal Muscle Afferents

Skeletal muscle is extensively supplied with afferents that sense both the mechanical and metabolic environment. These afferents are lightly myelinated (group III) and unmyelinated (group IV) fibers. In general, the group III fibers tend to be more mechanosensitive and the group IV fibers more sensitive to changes in the chemical environment (termed *chemoreceptors* or *metaboreceptors*). The larger group I and II fibers have no role in cardiovascular control (1).

Muscle metaboreceptors

The cardiovascular effects of the skeletal muscle afferents were first discovered in 1937 by Alam and Smirk (41). They observed in humans that if blood flow to the active skeletal muscles was occluded at the cessation of exercise, arterial pressure remained elevated for as long as the occlusion was maintained. This technique of circulatory occlusion postexercise has been widely used to investigate the role of the muscle metaboreceptors, with the theory being that during the circulatory occlusion, metabolites responsible for activating the receptors (lactate, H^+, phosphate, bradykinin, and prostaglandins, among others) are entrapped within the formerly active muscle and maintain metaboreceptor activation. Activation of the muscle metaboreflex, especially with a large muscle mass, is capable of eliciting profound increases in sympathetic activity and arterial pressure. This rise in arterial pressure is buffered by arterial and cardiopulmonary reflexes. Left unbuffered by the arterial baroreflex, this reflex rivals that from cerebral ischemia in the ability to increase arterial pressure (42). Metaboreflex activation increases CO, HR, ventricular performance, peripheral vasoconstriction, and central blood volume mobilization, which raises arterial pressure, presumably in an attempt to increase blood flow to the ischemic muscles (43,44). The existence of circulatory occlusion responses to moderate-to-intense static muscle contractions postexercise provides compelling evidence that this reflex becomes activated in these settings.

To what extent the muscle metaboreflex is normally activated during dynamic exercise is not well understood. Reductions in skeletal muscle blood flow during mild exercise do not cause metaboreflex responses until blood flow is reduced below a critical threshold level, which indicates that during mild exercise this reflex is not tonically active (2). However, as exercise intensity increases, the threshold level of skeletal muscle blood flow required to elicit reflex responses moves closer and closer to the normal level of flow, such that at moderate exercise intensities often no threshold is apparent—even small reductions in the normal level of flow elicit reflex cardiovascular responses. At even higher exercise intensities no threshold is detected (45). This indicates that either the reflex is indeed tonically active or that the reflex sits just at the blood flow threshold and any reduction in flow triggers metaboreflex responses. In pathophysiologic states, such as peripheral claudication or heart failure, wherein the normal level of skeletal muscle blood flow is reduced, the muscle metaboreflex likely contributes to the exaggerated sympathetic activation observed during exercise (46,47).

One quandary in this area is that with sustained metaboreceptor activation during circulatory occlusion postexercise, whereas arterial pressure remains elevated, most often HR recovers toward resting values with a time course similar to that during the normal recovery from exercise (48). These results have led several investigators to conclude that the muscle metaboreflex has little control over HR. In contrast, when blood flow to active muscle is reduced during sustained dynamic exercise, decreasing oxygen delivery and increasing metabolite production due to partial ischemia, substantial increases in HR and CO and sympathetic nerve activity are observed (45,49–51). One resolution of the discrepancy is that if postexercise occlusion is performed after blockade of the parasympathetic nerves, then, like blood pressure, HR remains elevated for the duration of the occlusion (52,53), indicating that sympathetic activity to the heart as well as to the peripheral vasculature remains elevated. The repeated observation of a fairly normal recovery of HR during circulatory occlusion postexercise likely stems from increases in parasympathetic activity, which can overwhelm the effects of sustained increases in sympathetic activity. The mechanisms mediating the rise in parasympathetic activity in this setting are not known, but may stem from the loss of central command with the cessation of exercise. (As discussed earlier, activation of central command inhibits parasympathetic tone, so the reduction in central command would be expected to increase parasympathetic activity.) Or it may be due to the arterial baroreflex in an attempt to return arterial pressure to normal levels. This remains to be investigated.

The mechanisms mediating the often substantial increases in arterial pressure by the muscle metaboreflex during dynamic exercise appear dependent on the ability of the heart to increase CO (46,47). During submaximal exercise in normal subjects, the primary mechanism is to raise CO. Thus, this can be thought of as a flow sensitive, flow raising reflex that is initiated by underperfused skeletal muscle and acts to increase the total blood flow available for perfusion (*e.g.*, CO). This substantial increase in CO occurs via the tachycardia, marked central blood volume mobilization (greater than three times that from the arterial baroreflex), and substantial increases in ventricular contractility as indicated by substantial increases in dP/dt_{max}, E_{max}, and preload-recruitable stroke work (a reflection of the ability of the heart to increase the amount of work performed with increases in ventricular preload) (9,36,54). Whether these reflexes exert direct control over cardiac lusitropic function (ability of the heart to relax) is still uncertain.

In settings wherein increases in CO are limited such as at maximal exercise or in pathophysiologic situations such as congestive heart failure, the metaboreflex now elicits pronounced vasoconstriction. This may be self-limiting because during dynamic exercise, most of the total vascular conductance is active skeletal muscle and, therefore, a substantial increase in arterial pressure can only occur via vasoconstriction of this vascular bed. Whether the metaboreflex preferentially shifts blood flow from relatively well-perfused skeletal muscle toward that more ischemic is one possibility. Sympathetic vasoconstriction within the heart accomplishes much the same by preferentially protecting the interior layers of the ventricle, which are more susceptible to ischemia.

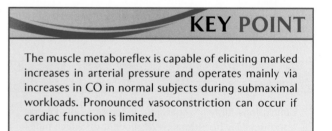

Muscle mechanoreceptors

Less is known about the normal role of mechanoreceptors in mediating the cardiovascular responses to dynamic and resistance exercise. Static muscle contraction likely activates both mechanoreceptors and metaboreceptors, although the time course of activation may be different, inasmuch as more time is required for generation of metabolites for metaboreflex activation (1). In addition, some mechanosensitive afferents increase their activity with ischemia (55). However, via tendon stretch, tension in the muscle can be increased without contraction and this maneuver does elicit increases in sympathetic activity, HR, ventilation, and arterial pressure. To investigate differentiation between the roles of mechanoreceptors and metaboreceptors in mediating the responses to static muscle contraction, Hayes and Kaufman (56) observed the responses before and after infusion of gadolinium, which blocks mechanosensitive channels. Gadolinium significantly attenuated the rise in arterial pressure and HR in response to both static muscle contraction and tendon stretch, indicating that a portion of the cardiovascular response to static muscle contraction may be mediated via activation of the mechanoreceptors.

Interaction between Central Command, Arterial Baroreflexes, and Skeletal Muscle Afferents

The reflex cardiovascular responses to exercise are likely the result of the action of and interaction between central command, the arterial baroreflex, and the activation of skeletal muscle afferents. With the transition from rest to mild dynamic exercise, the immediate rapid tachycardia is the result of rapid partial withdrawal of parasympathetic activity, which is likely due to activation of central command, rapid resetting of the arterial baroreflex, or activation of skeletal muscle mechanoreceptors. As exercise intensity progresses, marked sympathetic activation is not seen until moderate exercise intensities (although this can vary widely with species). This may be due to the ability to raise CO via parasympathetic withdrawal in combination with the increased central blood volume mobilization arising from the skeletal muscle pump, which thereby maintains or increases ventricular filling pressure, allowing SV to be sustained despite the reduced filling time (2). If parasympathetic withdrawal increases CO sufficiently to supply the active skeletal muscles with enough oxygen to prevent marked accumulation of ischemic metabolites, then the muscle metaboreflex is likely not strongly engaged. In addition, if the increase in CO is large enough to raise arterial pressure toward the reset baroreflex set point, then the baroreflex is likely also not strongly engaged. Thus, little afferent signals would exist for substantial sympathetic activation via either the muscle metaboreflex or arterial baroreflex. (Whether muscle mechanoreflexes or central command could raise sympathetic activity in this setting is not well established.) With further increases in exercise intensity sympathetic activation is clearly evident. This increase in sympathetic tone could come about via further increases in central command, activation of skeletal muscle afferents, and/or resetting of the arterial baroreflex to a higher set point. With heavy or maximal exercise intensities, parasympathetic activity is reduced to very low levels and sympathetic activity is greatly elevated. The relative roles for central command, skeletal muscle afferents, and the arterial baroreflex in this setting are not well understood, but it is likely that all are strongly activated and participate in the autonomic adjustments both to increase the delivery of oxygen to the active skeletal muscles and to maintain arterial pressure in the face of large peripheral vasodilation.

These reflexes also likely interact. Recent studies strongly support the concept that both activation of skeletal muscle afferents and central command can reset the arterial baroreflex (15,57). Furthermore, with strong stimulation of skeletal muscle afferents, the sympathetic activation is buffered by the arterial baroreflex: much larger pressor responses are observed after baroreceptor denervation (42,58). Indeed, one recent idea is that the arterial baroreflex buffers the muscle metaboreflex primarily via limiting the ability of the metaboreflex to cause peripheral vasoconstriction. In settings such as heart failure, baroreflex strength is diminished, thereby lessening the opposition and allowing more pronounced vasoconstrictor responses. That is, the arterial baroreflex may act to protect skeletal muscle from being vasoconstricted by the muscle metaboreflex (59). Thus, situations can exist when these reflexes are exerting changes in sympathetic activity in opposite directions. For example, during dynamic exercise in subjects with peripheral claudication or during intense static muscle contractions, the sympathetic activation due to strong metaboreflex activation may raise pressure above the baroreflex set point and, thus, this increase in sympathetic activity would be partially suppressed by the baroreflex. It is likely that more often, these reflexes are eliciting changes in autonomic outflow in the same direction, as with the responses to graded exercise described earlier. In pathophysiologic settings, such as heart failure, enormous increases in sympathetic activity can occur during exercise (35). In this setting, both arterial pressure (especially pulse pressure) and skeletal muscle blood flow are below normal levels. This likely results in strong activation of both the arterial baroreflex and the muscle metaboreflex to increase sympathetic activity, which can cause profound vasoconstriction in inactive vascular beds and even within the active skeletal muscle itself. This restraint of skeletal muscle vasodilation could exacerbate the situation, although it is possible that redistribution of flow within the muscles between motor units, which may be activated to different degrees, may occur to optimize the distribution of the restricted delivery of oxygen to areas most underperfused.

Physical Activity and Inactivity

Traditionally termed "exercise training," regular vigorous physical activity can result in increased functional capacity of the cardiovascular system (e.g., increased $\dot{V}O_{2max}$). Conversely, a period following exercise training in which there is little or no regular physical activity is termed "detraining" and implies a return to the original (albeit reduced) functional capacity of the cardiovascular system. Although still valid, these more traditional exercise physiology terms are now being reviewed in light of the recent trends in our society toward a more sedentary lifestyle.

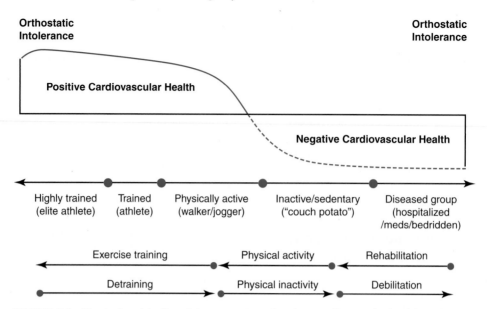

FIGURE 9.6 Physical activity/inactivity spectrum related to cardiovascular health and disease. (Modified from Booth FW, Lees SJ. Physically active subjects should be the control group. *Med Sci Sports Exerc.* 2006;38:405–406.)

Indeed, physical inactivity is listed by the American Heart Association as a major risk factor for cardiovascular disease and has been viewed by many as one of the major public health concerns of this century (60). With this in mind, it is important to recognize that the propensity toward cardiovascular (and other) disease states may be viewed on a physiologic spectrum related to both increased physical activity, as well as decreased physical activity (see Fig. 9.6). However, direct relationship between the amount of activity and cardiovascular health is complex. Based on studies from the Cooper Institute (61,62), the population that appears to derive the biggest increase in benefit from an increased level of physical activity are those in the lowest quartile of activity or fitness. This relationship is represented by the steep slope in cardiovascular health when transitioning from inactive to physically active. Although cardiovascular benefits are believed to increase with greater and greater levels of activity, the phenomenon of overtraining does appear to exist. Dysregulation of the cardiovascular system can be manifested in the form of orthostatic intolerance observed in highly fit athletes (63). Interestingly, orthostatic intolerance is also observed at the other end of the physical activity spectrum, especially in individuals with extremely low levels of activity (i.e., bedrest patients) or individuals subjected to the microgravity of space (i.e., astronauts) (64,65).

Although it has been long known that regular exercise positively affects the cardiovascular system, the idea that a sedentary lifestyle may engage mechanisms that produce cardiovascular disease has only recently been examined (66–68). This important concept applies directly to the human species, as we have become more and more sedentary despite a set of genes that has evolved to "expect" physical activity based on the evolution of the hunter/gatherer phenotype (66). In addition, it has been speculated that the mechanisms by which a sedentary lifestyle may elicit detrimental cardiovascular effects (*dotted line* in Fig. 9.6) may not simply be a reversal of the same mechanisms by which regular physical activity produces cardiovascular benefits (68). Therefore, the study of "inactivity" physiology is gaining momentum and has implications not only in the study of cardiovascular physiology but also endocrinology, metabolism, and other fields (*e.g.*, insulin signaling, triglyceride metabolism, adipose regulation).

It is well established that individuals with existing cardiovascular risk factors (*i.e.*, hypertension) or frank cardiovascular disease (*i.e.*, heart failure, etc.) can benefit from exercise therapies, if performed at appropriate levels. For example, mild-to-moderate exercise intensities (typically 60%–70% of $\dot{V}_{O_{2max}}$) appear to be beneficial in lowering blood pressure in hypertensive animals (69,70) and, indeed, in humans with borderline hypertension, a moderate exercise program can lower blood pressure to normal levels (71). In addition, exercise decreases blood clotting, stroke risk, incidence of myocardial infarction (first and recurrent events), and lowers blood vessel inflammation and damage induced by stress hormones. Exercise can lower overactivity of the sympathetic nervous system in congestive heart failure patients (72) and animal models (73). In contrast, higher intensity exercise may offset or

KEY POINT

Alterations of the cardiovascular system likely occur along the physical activity/inactivity spectrum with functionally overt dysregulation occurring at both high and low ends of the spectrum.

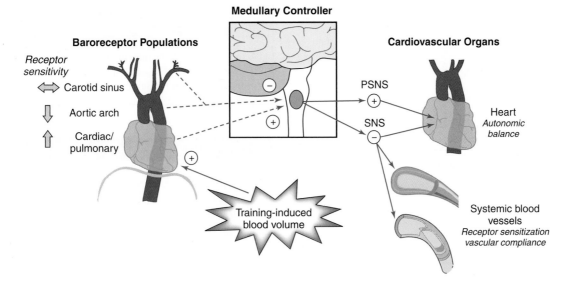

FIGURE 9.7   Physical activity–induced changes in baroreceptor reflexes. The important adaptive changes brought about by increases and decreases in physical activity that alter reflex regulation of the cardiovascular system. Dynamic exercise training attenuates arterial (aortic) baroreflex responses and sensitizes cardiopulmonary afferents. This is accompanied by resting bradycardia, reduced sympathetic activity, and blunted cardiovascular responses to exercise. Mechanisms possibly contributing to training-induced changes in cardiovascular reflexes include altered baroreflex function, structural and/or autonomic changes to the heart and blood vessels, and altered hemodynamic responses during exercise. Conversely, physical inactivity may produce opposite changes and in extreme cases may also lead to orthostatic intolerance that is observed in highly fit individuals. PSNS, parasympathetic nervous system; SNS, sympathetic nervous system.

even worsen cardiovascular risk factors including hypertension (70,74). Therefore, it is important that patients with existing cardiovascular disease work closely with their physicians when using exercise in conjunction with other beneficial therapies.

Figure 9.7 summarizes the effects of physical activity and inactivity on reflex control of the cardiovascular system. The major components include expansion of blood volume, structural changes in the heart and blood vessels, as well as changes in the major cardiovascular reflexes discussed previously. Likewise, the alterations in SV, along with altered sympathetic-parasympathetic balance, likely contribute to the changes in HR at rest and during acute bouts of exercise. The cellular mechanisms underlying changes in reflex function remain to be elucidated. In addition, the contribution of the neurohumoral axis, which was not discussed here, must also be considered for complete understanding of the physiologic adaptations that result from chronic physical activity and inactivity.

The effects of physical activity and inactivity on baroreflex control of sympathetic outflow can be related to current trends in our society toward a more inactive lifestyle and the prevalence of cardiovascular disease in sedentary individuals. For example, although somewhat controversial in the human literature, work from DiCarlo and Bishop (75) and Negrao and coworkers (76) clearly demonstrated in conscious rabbits and rats, respectively, that chronic treadmill exercise reduces baroreflex-mediated sympathoexcitation. These results are represented in Figure 9.8A and, along with other studies, have been interpreted as an effect of exercise training to lower resting and baroreflex-mediated sympathetic outflow. Because these changes are expressed in relative terms (exercise vs. sedentary), an alternate (or additional) interpretation of these data can be reached if the experimental groups are relabeled as in Figure 9.8B. We and other have suggested that the physically active group might be better identified as the control or "healthy" group (77,78) based on the aforementioned premise that our genes and physiologic systems (including the cardiovascular system) have evolved to "expect" physical activity as the norm. With this perspective, one could conclude that sympathoexcitation is actually exacerbated under sedentary conditions at least on a relative basis. This idea is supported by the fact that inactivity-related diseases, such as hypertension, obesity, and diabetes, are associated with overactivity of the sympathetic nervous system (79–82) and that excess sympathetic nervous system activity is strong predictor of cardiovascular disease/mortality (83,84).

TEST YOURSELF

The chapter provides several examples concerning how the expression of data can alter the interpretation of results. Which of the examples provided in the chapter do you feel is the most important example? Defend your choice.

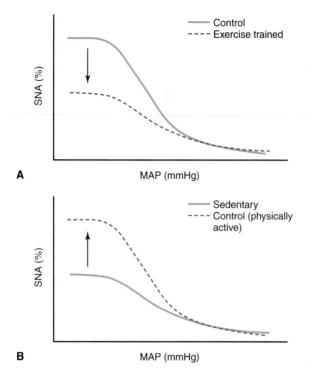

FIGURE 9.8 Generalized results from DiCarlo and Bishop (85) and Negrao and coworkers (76) in which alterations in physical activity influences baroreflex-mediated sympatho-excitation. In **A**, experimental groups are labeled with traditional terms of control and exercise trained, whereas in **B**, groups are relabeled "sedentary" and "control" to represent the paradigm shift that addresses the more recent trend toward sedentary living in our society. SNA, symphatetic nerve activity; MAP, mean arterial pressure.

KEY POINT

A sedentary lifestyle may be an important contributor to cardiovascular disease, at least in part, due to elevations in sympathetic nervous system activity.

CHAPTER SUMMARY

Whole body dynamic exercise presents one of the greatest challenges to cardiovascular control. CO must increase to meet the markedly increased metabolic demands, as well as maintain blood pressure in the face of massive peripheral vasodilation in the active skeletal muscle. These challenges are met via the combined action of the feed-forward role of central command and the feedback action of baroreflexes and reflexes arising from activation of skeletal muscle afferents. These reflexes act to control parasympathetic and sympathetic activity to increase HR, ventricular contractility, and central blood volume mobilization to raise CO and vasoconstrict inactive vascular beds, as well as limit skeletal muscle vasodilation to prevent a large fall in arterial pressure. With the initiation of exercise, there is an immediate rapid increase in HR due to rapid withdrawal of parasympathetic activity. This is likely due to activation of central command with possible contribution of resetting of the arterial baroreflex and activation of skeletal muscle mechanoreceptors. As work rate progresses, parasympathetic activity progressively declines and sympathetic activity rises. At moderate

A MILESTONE OF DISCOVERY

As discussed in the section on baroreflexes, for many years it was thought that the arterial baroreflex was functionally inhibited (turned off) during exercise. This idea stemmed from two observations: (a) both arterial pressure and HR increase during exercise, therefore the baroreflex should inhibit any rise in HR with the increase in arterial pressure; and (b) the increases in R-R interval (bradycardia) with rapid increases in arterial pressure became smaller and smaller as exercise intensity increased (22). The latter observation had been challenged, inasmuch as baroreflex-mediated HR responses were undiminished (Fig. 9.3). However, HR is neither sensed nor controlled by the arterial baroreflex; rather, arterial pressure is sensed and is controlled via changes in CO and vasomotor tone.

In their study, Melcher and Donald (24) used the innovative and technically demanding surgical approach of reversibly isolating the carotid sinuses to test the hypothesis that the carotid baroreflex remains functional during dynamic exercise. This technique allowed the vascular isolation of the carotid sinuses and, thus, pressure at the carotid baroreceptors to be controlled and the reflex changes in arterial pressure and HR observed. This was the first study to explore the entire range of baroreflex response at rest and during exercise.

Importantly, this nearly heroic surgery allowed observations in a conscious animal running on a treadmill; thus, the detrimental effects of anesthesia and acute surgical trauma were avoided. Melcher and Donald (24) found that baroreflex control of arterial pressure was reset upward to a higher pressure (later studies also showed a rightward shift in the curves, per Fig. 9.4). Importantly, they showed that the strength of the reflex (reflex gain) was undiminished from rest to heavy exercise. They also described how the baroreflex mediated changes in HR were time dependent—again, reinforcing the problems of using HR for baroreflex analysis. Thus, these investigators conclusively demonstrated that the arterial baroreflex is not inhibited during exercise but rather the reflex is reset to a higher pressure in proportion to the exercise intensity. These observations, along with the innovative surgical techniques, have led many investigative teams to use similar approaches over the past 20 years or more to investigate the baroreflex, its action, and interaction with other reflexes at rest, during exercise, and in pathophysiologic conditions.

Melcher A, Donald DE. Maintained ability of carotid baroreflex to regulate arterial pressure during exercise. Am J Physiol. 1981;241:H838–H849.

workloads, the skeletal muscle metaboreflex may also be engaged. As work rate rises to maximal levels, parasympathetic activity to the heart is very low and sympathetic activity to the heart and peripheral vasculature is high resulting in maximal CO, vasoconstriction of inactive vascular beds such as the kidney and splanchnic vasculatures, and even active skeletal muscle, as well as the coronary circulation are restrained from maximal vasodilation. Chronic physical activity and inactivity can have marked consequences on both the ability of the cardiovascular system to respond to dynamic exercise, as well as the ability to exercise per se. The relative roles of these cardiovascular reflexes in normal and especially pathophysiologic states such as heart failure (a setting wherein often severe activation of the sympathetic nervous system during exercise often occurs) are not well understood but clearly substantial interaction between these reflexes likely occurs presenting a classical example of integrative physiologic function.

REFERENCES

1. Mitchell JH, Schmidt RF. Cardiovascular reflex control by afferent fibers from skeletal muscle receptors. In: *Handbook of Physiology*. Bethesda, MD: American Physiological Society; 1983:623–658.
2. Rowell LB, O'Leary DS, Kellogg DL. *Integration of Cardiovascular Control Systems in Dynamic Exercise*. New York: Oxford Press; 1996:770–838.
3. White S, Patrick T, Higgins CB, et al. Effects of altering ventricular rate on blood flow distribution in conscious dogs. *Am J Physiol*. 1971;221:1402–1407.
4. Manders WT, Vatner SF. Effects of sodium pentobarbital anesthesia on left ventricular function and distribution of cardiac output in dogs, with particular reference to the mechanism for tachycardia. *Circ Res*. 1976;39:512–517.
5. Vatner SF, Smith NT. Effects of halothane on left ventricular function and distribution of regional blood flow in dogs and primates. *Circ Res*. 1974;34:155–167.
6. Vatner SF, Braunwald E. Cardiovascular control mechanisms in the conscious state. *N Engl J Med*. 1975;293(19):970–976.
7. Sagawa K, Maughan L, Suga H, et al. *Cardiac Contraction and the Pressure–Volume Relationship*. New York: Oxford University Press Inc.; 1988.
8. Cheng CP, Igarashi Y, Little WC. Mechanism of augmented rate of left ventricular filling during exercise. *Circ Res*. 1992;70:9–19.
9. Sala-Mercado JA, Hammond RL, Kim JK, et al. Heart failure attenuates muscle metaboreflex control of ventricular contractility during dynamic exercise. *Am J Physiol Heart Circ Physiol*. 2006;292(5):H2159–H2166.
10. Sheriff DD, Nelson CD, Sundermann RK. Does autonomic blockade reveal a potent contribution of nitric oxide to locomotion-induced vasodilation? *Am J Physiol Heart Circ Physiol*. 2000;279:H726–H732.
11. Sheriff DD, Van BR. Flow-generating capability of the isolated skeletal muscle pump. *Am J Physiol*. 1998;274:H1502–H1508.
12. Victor RG, Pryor SL, Secher NH, et al. Effects of partial neuromuscular blockade on sympathetic nerve responses to static exercise in humans. *Circ Res*. 1989;65:468–476.
13. Victor RG, Secher NH, Lyson T, et al. Central command increases muscle sympathetic nerve activity during intense intermittent isometric exercise in humans. *Circ Res*. 1995;76:127–131.
14. Hayes SG, Kaufman MP. MLR stimulation and exercise pressor reflex activate different renal sympathetic fibers in decerebrate cats. *J Appl Physiol*. 2002;92:1628–1634.
15. McIlveen SA, Hayes, SG, Kaufman MP. Both central command and exercise pressor reflex reset carotid sinus baroreflex. *Am J Physiol*. 2001;280:H1454–H1463.
16. Matsukawa K, Mitchell JH, Wall PT, et al. The effect of static exercise on renal sympathetic nerve activity in conscious cats. *J Physiol*. 1991;434:453–467.
17. Vatner SF, Rutherford JD, Ochs HR. Baroreflex and vagal mechanisms modulating left ventricular contractile responses to sympathomimetic amines in conscious dogs. *Circ Res*. 1979;44:195–207.
18. Blukoo-Allotey JA, Vincent NH, Ellis S. Interactions of acetylcholine and epinephrine on contractility, glycogen and phosphorylase activity of isolated mammalian hearts. *J Pharmacol Exp Ther*. 1969;170:27–36.
19. Jacobowitz DAV, Cooper THE, Barner HB. Histochemical and chemical studies of the localization of adrenergic and cholinergic nerves in normal and denervated cat hearts. *Circ Res*. 1967;20:289–298.
20. Xenopoulos NP, Applegate RJ. The effect of vagal stimulation on left ventricular systolic and diastolic performance. *Am J Physiol Heart Circ Physiol*. 1994;266:H2167–H2173.
21. Matsuura W, Sugimachi M, Kawada T, et al. Vagal stimulation decreases left ventricular contractility mainly through negative chronotropic effect. *Am J Physiol Heart Circ Physiol*. 1997;273:H534–H539.
22. Bristow JD, Brown EB Jr, Cunningham DJC, et al. Effect of bicycling on the baroreflex regulation of pulse interval. *Circ Res*. 1971;28:582–592.
23. Bevegard BS, Shepherd JT. Circulatory effects of stimulating the carotid arterial stretch receptors in man at rest and during exercise. *J Clin Invest*. 1966;45:132–142.
24. Melcher A, Donald DE. Maintained ability of carotid baroreflex to regulate arterial pressure during exercise. *Am J Physiol*. 1981;241:H838–H849.
25. Potts JT, Shi XR, Raven PB. Carotid baroreflex responsiveness during dynamic exercise in humans. *Am J Physiol*. 1993;265:H1928–H1938.
26. Ogoh S, Fadel PJ, Nissen P, et al. Baroreflex-mediated changes in cardiac output and vascular conductance in response to alterations in carotid sinus pressure during exercise in humans. *J Physiol (Lond)*. 2003;550:317–324.
27. O'Leary DS, Seamans DP. Effect of exercise on autonomic mechanisms of baroreflex control of heart rate. *J Appl Physiol*. 1993;75:2251–2257.
28. Potts JT, Li J. Interaction between carotid baroreflex and exercise pressor reflex depends on baroreceptor afferent input. *Am J Physiol*. 1998;274:H1841–H1847.
29. Ogoh S, Fadel PJ, Monteiro F, et al. Haemodynamic changes during neck pressure and suction in seated and supine positions. *J Physiol (Lond)*. 2002;540(Pt 2):707–716.
30. Sala-Mercado JA, Ichinose M, Hammond RL, et al. Muscle metaboreflex attenuates spontaneous heart rate baroreflex sensitivity during dynamic exercise. *Am J Physiol Heart Circ Physiol*. 2007;292(6):H2867–H2873.
31. O'Leary DS, Seamans DP. Effect of exercise on autonomic mechanisms of baroreflex control of heart rate. *J Appl Physiol*. 1993;75:2251–2257.
32. Vatner SF, Higgins CB, Franklin D, et al. Extent of carotid sinus regulation of the myocardial contractile state in conscious dogs. *J Clin Invest*. 1972;51(4):995–1008.
33. Shimizu T, Bishop VS. Mechanism of reflex control of cardiac contractility by carotid sinus baroreceptors. *Am J Physiol Heart Circ Physiol*. 1980;239:H65–H72.
34. Young MA, Hintze TH, Vatner SF. Correlation between cardiac performance and plasma catecholamine levels in conscious dogs. *Am J Physiol Heart Circ Physiol*. 1985;248:H82–H88.
35. Hammond RL, Augustyniak RA, Rossi NF, et al. Alteration of humoral and peripheral vascular responses during graded exercise in heart failure. *J Appl Physiol*. 2001;90:55–61.
36. Sala-Mercado JA, Hammond RL, Kim JK, et al. Muscle metaboreflex control of ventricular contractility during dynamic exercise. *Am J Physiol Heart Circ Physiol*. 2006;290:H751–H757.
37. Bennett TD, Wyss CR, Scher AM. Changes in vascular capacity in awake dogs in response to carotid sinus occlusion and administration of catecholamines. *Circ Res*. 1984;55:440–453.
38. Remensnyder JP, Mitchell JH, Sarnoff SJ. Functional sympatholysis during muscular activity. Observations on influence of carotid sinus on oxygen uptake. *Circ Res*. 1962;11:370–380.
39. O'Leary DS. Regional vascular resistance vs. conductance: which index for baroreflex responses? *Am J Physiol*. 1991;260:H632–H637.
40. Collins HL, Augustyniak RA, Ansorge EJ, et al. Carotid baroreflex pressor responses at rest and during exercise: cardiac output vs. regional vasoconstriction. *Am J Physiol Heart Circ Physiol*. 2001;280:H642–H648.

41. Alam M, Smirk FH. Observations in man upon a blood pressure raising reflex arising from the voluntary muscles. *J Physiol*. 1937;89:372–383.

42. Sheriff DD, O'Leary DS, Scher AM, et al. Baroreflex attenuates pressor response to graded muscle ischemia in exercising dogs. *Am J Physiol*. 190;258:H305–H310.

43. Sheriff DD, Augustyniak RA, O'Leary DS. Muscle chemoreflex-induced increases in right atrial pressure. *Am J Physiol*. 1998;275:H767–H775.

44. O'Leary DS, Sheriff DD. Is the muscle metaboreflex important in control of blood flow to ischemic active skeletal muscle in dogs? *Am J Physiol*. 1995;268:H980–H986.

45. Augustyniak RA, Collins HL, Ansorge EJ, et al. Severe exercise alters the strength and mechanisms of the muscle metaboreflex. *Am J Physiol Heart Circ Physiol*. 2001;280:H1645–H1652.

46. Hammond RL, Augustyniak RA, Rossi NF, et al. Heart failure alters the strength and mechanisms of the muscle metaboreflex. *Am J Physiol*. 2000;278:H818–H828.

47. Crisafulli A, Salis E, Tocco F, et al. Impaired central hemodynamic response and exaggerated vasoconstriction during muscle metaboreflex activation in heart failure patients. *Am J Physiol Heart Circ Physiol*. 2007;292:H2988–H2996.

48. Wallin BG, Victor RG, Mark AL. Sympathetic outflow to resting muscles during static handgrip and postcontraction muscle ischemia. *Am J Physiol*. 1989;256:H105–H110.

49. Wyss CR, Ardell JL, Scher AM, et al. Cardiovascular responses to graded reductions in hindlimb perfusion in exercising dogs. *Am J Physiol*. 1983;245:H481–H486.

50. Sheriff DD, Wyss CR, Rowell LB, et al. Does inadequate oxygen delivery trigger pressor response to muscle hypoperfusion during exercise? *Am J Physiol*. 1987;253:H1199–H1207.

51. O'Hagan KP, Casey SP, Clifford PS. Muscle chemoreflex increases renal sympathetic nerve activity. *J Appl Physiol*. 1997;82:1818–1825.

52. O'Leary DS. Autonomic mechanisms of muscle metaboreflex control of heart rate. *J Appl Physiol*. 1993;74:1748–1754.

53. Fisher JP, Seifert T, Hartwich D, et al. Autonomic control of heart rate by metabolically sensitive skeletal muscle afferents in humans. *J Physiol*. 2010;588:1117–1127.

54. Crisafulli A, Salis E, Pittau G, et al. Modulation of cardiac contractility by muscle metaboreflex following efforts of different intensities in humans. *Am J Physiol Heart Circ Physiol*. 2006;291(6):H3035–H3042.

55. Kaufman MP, Rybicki KJ, Waldrop TG, et al. Effect of ischemia on responses of group III and IV afferents to contraction. *J Appl Physiol*. 1984;57:644–650.

56. Hayes SG, Kaufman MP. Gadolinium attenuates exercise pressor reflex in cats. *Am J Physiol Heart Circ Physiol*. 2001;280:H2153–H2161.

57. Potts JT, Mitchell JH. Rapid resetting of carotid baroreceptor reflex by afferent input from skeletal muscle receptors. *Am J Physiol Heart Circ Physiol*. 1998;44:H2000–H2008.

58. Kim JK, Sala-Mercado JA, Rodriguez J, et al. The arterial baroreflex alters the strength and mechanisms of the muscle metaboreflex pressor response during dynamic exercise. *Am J Physiol Heart Circ Physiol*. 2005;288:H1374–H1380.

59. Kim JK, Sala-Mercado JA, Hammond RL, et al. Attenuated arterial baroreflex buffering of muscle metaboreflex in heart failure. *Am J Physiol Heart Circ Physiol* 2005;289:H2416–H2423.

60. Blair SN. Physical inactivity: the biggest public health problem of the 21st century. *Br J Sports Med*. 2009;43:1–2.

61. Blair SN, Morris JN. Healthy hearts—and the universal benefits of being physically active: physical activity and health. *Ann Epidemiol*. 2009;19:253–256.

62. Sui X, LaMonte MJ, Laditka JN, et al. Cardiorespiratory fitness and adiposity as mortality predictors in older adults. *JAMA*. 2007;298:2507–2516.

63. Raven PB, Pawelczyk JA. Chronic endurance exercise training: a condition of inadequate blood pressure regulation and reduced tolerance to LBNP. *Med Sci Sports Exerc*. 1993;25:713–721.

64. Watenpaugh DE, Hargens AR. The cardiovascular system in microgravity. In: Fregly MJ, Blatteis CM, eds. *Handbook of Physiology*. New York: Oxford University Press; 1996:631–674.

65. Pavy-Le TA, Heer M, Narici MV, et al. From space to Earth: advances in human physiology from 20 years of bed rest studies (1986–2006). *Eur J Appl Physiol*. 2007;101:143–194.

66. Booth FW, Lees SJ. Physically active subjects should be the control group. *Med Sci Sports Exerc*. 2006;38:405–406.

67. Hamilton MT, Hamilton DG, Zderic TW. Exercise physiology versus inactivity physiology: an essential concept for understanding lipoprotein lipase regulation. *Exerc Sport Sci Rev*. 2004;32:161–166.

68. Hamilton MT, Hamilton DG, Zderic TW. Role of low energy expenditure and sitting in obesity, metabolic syndrome, type 2 diabetes, and cardiovascular disease. *Diabetes*. 2007;56:2655–2667.

69. Bertagnolli M, Schenkel PC, Campos C, et al. Exercise training reduces sympathetic modulation on cardiovascular system and cardiac oxidative stress in spontaneously hypertensive rats. *Am J Hypertens*. 2008;21:1188–1193.

70. Tipton CM, Matthes RD, Marcus KD, et al. Influences of exercise intensity, age, and medication on resting systolic blood pressure of SHR populations. *J Appl Physiol*. 1983;55:1305–1310.

71. Kenney MJ, Seals DR. Postexercise hypotension: key features, mechanisms, and clinical significance. *Hypertension*. 1993;22:653–664.

72. Roveda F, Middlekauff HR, Rondon MU, et al. The effects of exercise training on sympathetic neural activation in advanced heart failure: a randomized controlled trial. *J Am Coll Cardiol*. 2003;42:854–860.

73. Zucker IH. Novel mechanisms of sympathetic regulation in chronic heart failure. *Hypertension*. 2006;48:1005–1011.

74. Veras-Silva AS, Mattos KC, Gava NS, et al. Low-intensity exercise training decreases cardiac output and hypertension in spontaneously hypertensive rats. *Am J Physiol*. 1997;273:H2627–H2631.

75. Dicarlo SE, Bishop VS. Exercise training attenuates baroreflex regulation of nerve activity in rabbits. *Am J Physiol*. 1988;255:H974–H979.

76. Negrao CE, Irigoyen MC, Moreira ED, et al. Effect of exercise training on RSNA, baroreflex control, and blood pressure responsiveness. *Am J Physiol*. 1993;265:R365–R370.

77. Lees SJ, Booth FW. Sedentary death syndrome. *Can J Appl Physiol*. 2004;29:447–460.

78. Mueller PJ. Exercise training and sympathetic nervous system activity: evidence for physical activity dependent neural plasticity. *Clin Exp Pharmacol Physiol*. 2007;34:377–384.

79. Schlaich MP, Lambert E, Kaye DM, et al. Sympathetic augmentation in hypertension: role of nerve firing, norepinephrine reuptake, and Angiotensin neuromodulation. *Hypertension*. 2004;43:169–175.

80. Straznicky NE, Lambert EA, Lambert GW, et al. Effects of dietary weight loss on sympathetic activity and cardiac risk factors associated with the metabolic syndrome. *J Clin Endocrinol Metab*. 2005;90:5998–6005.

81. Julius S, Valentini M. Consequences of the increased autonomic nervous drive in hypertension, heart failure and diabetes. *Blood Press Suppl*. 1998;3:5–13.

82. Esler M, Rumantir M, Kaye D, et al. Sympathetic nerve biology in essential hypertension. *Clin Exp Pharmacol Physiol*. 2001;28:986–989.

83. Benedict CR, Shelton B, Johnstone DE, et al. Prognostic significance of plasma norepinephrine in patients with asymptomatic left ventricular dysfunction. SOLVD Investigators. *Circulation*. 1996;94:690–697.

84. Zoccali C, Mallamaci F, Parlongo S, et al. Plasma norepinephrine predicts survival and incident cardiovascular events in patients with end-stage renal disease. *Circulation*. 2002;105:1354–1359.

85. Dicarlo SE, Bishop VS. Exercise training attenuates baroreflex regulation of nerve activity in rabbits. *Am J Physiol*. 1988;255:H974–H979.

CHAPTER 10

The Cardiovascular System: Cardiac Function

Russell L. Moore and David A. Brown

Abbreviations

ACh	Acetylcholine	$G_s\alpha$	Stimulatory g-protein
AdC	Aadenylate cyclase activity	HR	Heart rate
ADP	Adenosine diphosphate	LV	Left ventricle
ANS	Autonomic nervous system	NCX	Sodium-calcium exchanger
ATP	Adenosine triphosphate	PKA	Protein kinase A
ATPase	Adenosine triphosphatase	PLB	Phospholamban
cAMP	Cyclic adenosine monophosphate	RyR	Ryanodine receptor
CE	Contractile element	SAN	Sinoatrial node
CICR	Calcium-induced calcium release	SERCA	Sarco(endo)plasmic reticulum calcium ATPase
CO	Cardiac output		
EC	Excitation-contraction	SR	Sarcoplasmic reticulum
EDV	End-diastolic volume	SV	Stroke volume
ESV	End-systolic volume	TCA	Tricarboxylic acid cycle
$\Delta G_{ATP,synthesis}$	Phosphorylation potential (energy required to synthesize ATP)	TnI	Troponin I
		$\dot{V}O_2$	Rate of oxygen consumption

Introduction

Physical activity represents a large portion of a continuum of normal physiologic states in humans. To successfully exist in this continuum, significant alterations must occur in cardiac output (CO) and central cardiac function to accommodate the systemic demands imposed on an organism by physical activity. The autonomic nervous system (ANS) is primarily responsible for the integrated control of the cardiovascular system and is of central importance in enabling an organism to match O_2 supply with the metabolic demands that occur during physical activity (see Chapter 9). Although the ANS is critical to the integrated control of the cardiovascular system and its responses to physical activity, there are significant elements regulating pump function that are intrinsic to the heart. These intrinsic control elements are absolutely critical to the overall systemic response of an organism to acute exercise, and some respond adaptively to exercise training. Training-induced improvements in maximal and submaximal work capacity are accompanied by several central cardiovascular adaptations that are regarded as "signatures" of the trained state. These fundamental adaptive changes, which have been documented in humans and all mammalian species examined, include a resting and submaximal exercise bradycardia, increased maximal stroke volume, an increase in left ventricular end-diastolic dimension, improved myocardial contractile function, and subtle to moderate increases in myocardial mass.

General Cardiovascular Adjustments to Acute Exercise

During exercise, systemic oxygen consumption ($\dot{V}O_2$) increases in response to the increase in metabolic demand of active muscle. The cardiovascular system is responsible for increasing the delivery of blood and O_2 to working

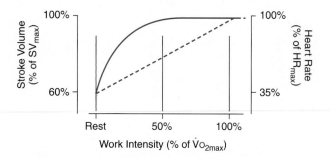

FIGURE 10.1 The relationship between work intensity, heart rate (HR), and stroke volume (SV). In general, between the resting state and $\dot{V}O_{2max}$, HR increases approximately linearly as a function of work intensity. The adjustment in stroke volume across the same continuum is curvilinear, with most of the increase occurring at the lower work intensities ($<50\%$ $\dot{V}O_{2max}$).

skeletal muscle and the pulmonary vasculature. The attendant increase in CO is accomplished via increases in heart rate (HR), stroke volume (SV), systolic blood pressure, myocardial contractile activity, a general reduction in systemic vascular resistance, and only small changes in mean arterial and diastolic blood pressure (1–3). In quantitative terms, the increased demands for oxygen consumption that occur during physical exercise are met according to the following relationship: $\dot{V}O_2 = HR \times SV \times$ arteriovenous O_2 content difference ($\Delta a - vO_2$). Two components of the product describing $\dot{V}O_2$, (i.e., HR and SV) are directly attributable to the performance of the heart. As the demands for systemic blood flow increase, both HR and SV increase (Fig. 10.1). Over the continuum of dynamic aerobic work intensity, the adjustment in SV occurs early on and is virtually complete at 40% to 50% $\dot{V}O_{2max}$ whereas HR increases continuously from rest until $\dot{V}O_{2max}$ is achieved. With the onset of exercise, key events that occur at the level of the heart that contribute to augmented HR, SV, and pump function include an increase in sympathetic drive, venous return, and, as the work bout proceeds, changes in the ion composition of the extracellular milieu (4). The overall consequence is that cardiac contractile activity increases concomitantly with the demand that is placed on the processes that are involved in excitation and contraction.

Myocardial Mechanisms for Heart Rate Control

$$\dot{V}O_2 = HR \times SV \times \Delta a - vO_2$$

Under normal circumstances, HR is governed in large part by the cardio-depressant and cardio-accelerator influences of the parasympathetic and sympathetic nervous systems, respectively. Across the continuum from rest to $\dot{V}O_{2max}$, adjustments in HR occur as a result of alterations in the relative magnitudes of parasympathetic and sympathetic input into the heart (see Chapter 7). Specifically, the ANS controls HR by modulating the intrinsic pacemaker activity of the heart. To understand the cellular basis for this type of *chronotropic* modulation, the ionic basis for intrinsic pacemaker activity of the heart, and how these ionic events are influenced by the ANS, must be reviewed.

HR is controlled via the primary pacemaker activity of cardiocytes in the sinoatrial node (SAN). The spontaneous cyclic depolarization of primary pacemaker cells in the SAN that establish intrinsic HR arises from the unique time-dependent characteristics of a variety of depolarizing and hyperpolarizing currents. Over the last ~5 to 10 years, the number of candidate currents (and intracellular mechanisms) that contribute to the primary pacemaker activity of SAN myocytes has markedly increased, as have the theoretical descriptions of the mechanisms by which cardiac pacemaker activity occurs (5–8). The classical description of the ionic basis of SAN pacemaker activity is that action potential configuration is determined by two outward hyperpolarizing K^+ currents, I_K and I_{K1}, and two depolarizing inward currents, I_{Ca} and I_f, that are carried primarily by Ca^{2+} and Na^+, respectively. During diastole, the membrane potential of SAN pacemaker cells exhibits a depolarizing drift until such time as a threshold potential is achieved. The gradual membrane depolarization that precedes the threshold activation of an action potential has been attributed to an overall decline in the net conductance of hyperpolarizing K^+ currents and a prominent increase in I_f in the latter diastolic phase of the pacemaker potential. Once a threshold potential is reached, I_{Ca} (an L-type current) markedly increases and the rapid upstroke phase of the action potential ensues. Action potential repolarization occurs as a result of the net increase in the magnitudes of the hyperpolarizing K^+ currents.

One version of an emerging and more contemporary view (simplified) of SAN pacemaker activity is that, in addition to the diminution in hyperpolarizing K^+ currents and the increase in I_f, the slow membrane depolarization that leads to the triggered action potential is due to an increase in a transient (T-type) inward Ca^{2+} current ($I_{Ca,T}$), a progressive filling of the sarcoplasmic reticulum (SR) with Ca^{2+} during diastole that leads to an increase in the magnitude of leak of Ca^{2+} from the SR into a confined space in close proximity to the sarcolemma, and an increase in a forward sodium-calcium exchange current (I_{NaCa}) (Fig. 10.2A and B). During the earliest phase of the diastolic pacemaker potential, slow membrane depolarization begins to occur as a result of a reduction in the magnitude of hyperpolarizing K^+ currents and an increase in the magnitude of I_f. This initial depolarization leads to the activation of $I_{Ca,T}$, a depolarizing current, that leads to further membrane depolarization and activation of $I_{Ca,T}$ during the latter depolarization phase. During diastole, several other key events occur that also contribute to late phase membrane depolarization. The progressive increase in $I_{Ca,T}$ not only has a depolarizing effect on the membrane, but there is also evidence to support the idea that the inward Ca^{2+} current is also sufficient to increase the occurrence of small focal Ca^{2+} releases from the SR (Ca^{2+} sparks). The frequency of Ca^{2+} sparks increases during the latter phase of the diastolic depolarization and results in increased $[Ca^{2+}]$ in a confined space between the SR and the sarcolemma. This increase in subsarcolemmal $[Ca^{2+}]$ ($[Ca^{2+}]_{ss}$) elicits the activation of forward sodium-calcium

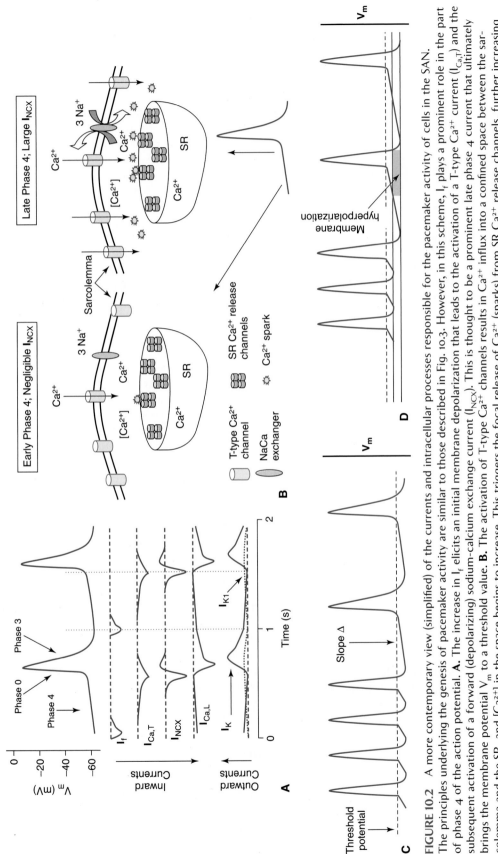

FIGURE 10.2   A more contemporary view (simplified) of the currents and intracellular processes responsible for the pacemaker activity of cells in the SAN. The principles underlying the genesis of pacemaker activity are similar to those described in Fig. 10.3. However, in this scheme, I_f plays a prominent role in the part of phase 4 of the action potential. **A.** The increase in I_f elicits an initial membrane depolarization that leads to the activation of a T-type Ca^{2+} current ($I_{Ca,T}$) and the subsequent activation of a forward (depolarizing) sodium-calcium exchange current (I_{NCX}). This is thought to be a prominent late phase 4 current that ultimately brings the membrane potential V_m to a threshold value. **B.** The activation of T-type Ca^{2+} channels results in Ca^{2+} influx into a confined space between the sarcolemma and the SR, and $[Ca^{2+}]$ in the space begins to increase. This triggers the focal release of Ca^{2+} (sparks) from SR Ca^{2+} release channels, further increasing $[Ca^{2+}]$ in the space. This in turn leads to the activation of I_{NCX} and further membrane depolarization toward a threshold potential. Increased vagal stimulation slows the pacemaker activity of the SAN. **C.** At lower levels of vagal input, depolarizing currents (e.g., I_f) are suppressed. This leads to a decrease in the slope of phase 4 of the action potential, an increase in the time required to reach threshold, and a slowing of heart rate. **D.** When vagal input is more robust, ACh-sensitive K^+ channels are activated, and this leads to membrane hyperpolarization. This effect, in combination with the effect described in **C**, contributes to a further slowing of heart rate.

exchange that mediates a "Ca^{2+} out/Na^+ in" exchange in an attempt to normalize $[Ca^{2+}]_{ss}$. Because the stoichiometry of the exchange is 3 Na^+ for 1 Ca^{2+}, the exchange is electrogenic and mediates a net inward current, I_{NaCa}, that leads to further depolarization of the cell membrane. The interrelated actions of $I_{Ca,T}$, SR Ca^{2+} sparks, and I_{NaCa} creates a positive feedback loop that culminates in a progressive membrane depolarization to a threshold potential. Once threshold is achieved, there is a rapid activation of an L-type current and an action potential is triggered.

KEY POINT

In the healthy heart, HR is determined by the spontaneous depolarization of pacemaker cell membrane potential, mediated by a combination of potassium, sodium, and calcium currents. During exercise, the increased HR is due to (a) increasing the rate of spontaneous depolarization of SAN cells, and (b) repolarizing to a less negative membrane potential that is closer to threshold.

The intrinsic pacemaker activity of cardiocytes in the SAN is powerfully modulated by the actions of the ANS. HR across the physiologic range is determined by the combined influences of the sympathetic and parasympathetic nervous systems. Increased vagal (parasympathetic) input into the SAN decreases the frequency at which pacemaker cells spontaneously depolarize (Fig. 10.2C and D). Classically, this is thought to occur via combinations of three different mechanisms that include:

1. A reduction in the rate of diastolic depolarization
2. Action potential hyperpolarization
3. An upward shift in action potential threshold potential

Of these three mechanisms, the first two are probably the most prominent. The events that give rise to the slowing of pacemaker activity with vagal stimulation are quite complex (6). These events can be simplified in concept by describing them as being modifications of depolarizing and hyperpolarizing currents, particularly during the diastolic phase of the action potential. Vagal stimulation results in the release of acetylcholine (ACh) from nerve endings at the SA node. Released ACh binds to muscarinic receptors (M_2) on SAN myocytes, which results in the activation or modulation of several important processes. First, ACh can directly activate a specific class of K^+ channels (K_{ACh}) in SAN myocytes. Activation of K_{ACh} channels in the SAN produces a hyperpolarizing current that opposes the effects of depolarizing currents during the diastolic phase of the action potential. Second, several depolarizing diastolic currents are suppressed by ACh. The latter mechanism is thought to occur at lower levels of vagal activation and can provide a conceptual explanation for a reduction in the rate of dia-

stolic depolarization without prominent membrane hyperpolarization (Fig. 10.2C). The former mechanism is more prominent at higher levels of vagal activation, and provides an explanation of ACh-mediated action potential hyperpolarization (Fig. 10.2D). The net effect of both mechanisms is to prolong the time required for diastolic depolarization to proceed to an action potential threshold level.

The release of ACh onto SAN myocytes can also slow HR by suppressing membrane bound adenylate cyclase activity (AdC) via a G protein coupled M_2-AdC mechanism. This mechanism is relevant to more contemporary theories of intrinsic SAN pacemaker activity where processes that are involved in diastolic membrane depolarization are strongly influenced by cyclic adenosine monophosphate (cAMP)-dependent protein kinases. For example, both inward Ca^{2+} current activity and SR Ca^{2+} spark frequency can be increased by cAMP-dependent processes. These contribute the acceleration of diastolic membrane depolarization via the actions of I_{NaCa} whereas suppression of these processes would result in a reduction in the rate of membrane depolarization.

Sympathetic stimulation accelerates the pacemaker activity of SAN myocytes. This is manifested as a marked increase in the rate of diastolic depolarization and an increase in the amplitude of the pacemaker action potential (Fig. 10.3). The increase in the rate of diastolic depolarization results from an increase in the magnitude of I_f as well as a cAMP-mediated increase in SR Ca^{2+} spark frequency. The latter occurs as a result of a phosphorylation-induced increase in the "open probability" of the SR Ca^{2+} release channel (direct) and to an increase in SR Ca^{2+} pump activity and Ca^{2+} load (indirect). The net effect would be that $[Ca^{2+}]_{ss}$ would increase more rapidly which would in turn lead to an augmentation of I_{NaCa} and further membrane depolarization to an action potential threshold. Once the threshold is achieved, the amplitude of the ensuing action potential is augmented. Explanations for this phenomenon include cAMP-mediated increases in the open probability of L-type Ca^{2+} channels and an augmentation in I_{Ca}, as well as an augmentation in I_{NaCa} that occurs secondary to a greater release of Ca^{2+} from SR with greater Ca^{2+} loads.

Overall, in the transition from rest to exercise of increasing intensity, HR initially increases as a result of withdrawal of vagal input to the SAN. As work intensity increases, further increases in HR are produced via the continued withdrawal of parasympathetic drive and increased sympathetic drive to the pacemaker cells in the SAN.

Summary

With the onset of exercise, increased HR is accomplished by a reduction in parasympathetic *and* an increase in sympathetic drive to the pacemaker cells of the SAN. These changes result in a decrease in K^+ conductance and an increase in I_f (carried primarily by sodium), which brings the SAN membrane potential to threshold more quickly, resulting in an increased HR.

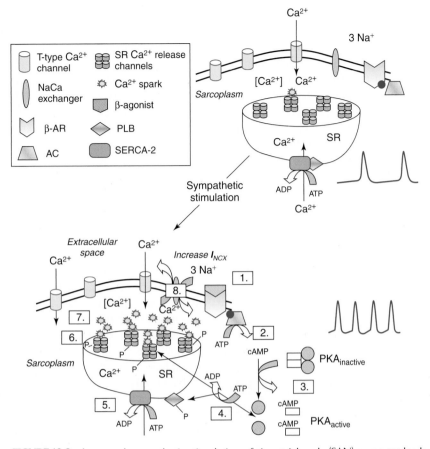

FIGURE 10.3   Increased sympathetic stimulation of sinoatrial node (SAN) myocytes leads to an increase in heart rate via a variety of mechanisms. Part of the effect of β-agonist on SAN pacemaker activity is thought to be secondary to modulation of intracellular Ca^{2+} handling. The binding of β-agonist to β-adrenergic receptors (β-AR) (*1*) leads to the G protein–mediated activation of a membrane-bound adenylate cyclase (AC), the formation of cyclic adenosine monophosphate (cAMP) (*2*), and subsequent activation of a cAMP-dependent protein kinase (PKA) (*3*). The active catalytic subunits of PKA are thought to lead to the phosphorylation of a variety of proteins that include phospholamban (PLB) and sarcoplasmic reticulum (SR) Ca^{2+} release channels (*4*). This elicits an increase in SR Ca^{2+} pump (SERCA-2) activity (*5*) and SR Ca^{2+} loading as well as the Ca^{2+} spark frequency (*6*). These events culminate in a faster increase in $[Ca^{2+}]$ in the confined space between the SR and sarcolemma (*7*) and a more robust activation of a depolarizing sodium-calcium exchange current (I_{NCX}) (*8*). The acceleration of processes *6* to *8* results in a shortening of phase 4 of the pacemaker action potential and an increase in heart rate.

Myocardial Mechanisms for Heart Rate Control: Adaptations to Training

A hallmark of the exercise trained state is resting and submaximal exercise bradycardia. Based on the observation that resting bradycardia persists under conditions of sympathetic and parasympathetic blockade in both humans and animals (4,9), it appears that the intrinsic pacemaker activity of the heart is altered by training. However, no data are currently available regarding if and how the various pacemaker currents (or associated processes) respond adaptively to training. Finally, it is likely that training-induced alterations in the autonomic control of the cells in the SAN play a more pronounced role in the bradycardia that occurs during submaximal exercise. This issue is addressed in detail in Chapter 9.

Some work, however, has been devoted to determining whether or not training bradycardia is a result of intrinsic changes in atrial adrenergic and cholinergic muscarinic receptor systems. Hammond et al. (9) found that chronic exercise elicited a decrease in β-adrenergic receptor number and no changes in muscarinic cholinergic receptor number in right atrial membranes isolated from endurance trained pigs. In this porcine model of training, it was also found that the HR response to adrenergic stimulation was attenuated in trained animals. These data strongly implicate a training-induced down-regulation of the right atrial β-adrenergic system as being a contributing factor to training bradycardia in the porcine model of exercise training. In a subsequent study, Hammond et al. (10) found that the training-induced reduction in right atrial β-adrenergic receptor number was accompanied by an increase in stimulatory G-protein ($G_{s\alpha}$) content. The increase in $G_{s\alpha}$ was associated with a training-induced reduction in the dose of isoproterenol required to elicit 50% of a maximal HR response even though training elicited a marked reduction in the maximal isoproterenol-stimulated HR response (10). In addition to the effect of training on HR and the right atrial β-adrenergic receptor system, it was also demonstrated that intrinsic HR in the presence of β-adrenergic and muscarinic cholinergic blockade was reduced (10). Schaefer et al. (11) clearly demonstrated in the running rat model of exercise training that intrinsic atrial firing frequency was reduced by training and that this atrial bradycardia was due to factors other than those associated with receptor-mediated signal transduction mechanisms. The idea that training bradycardia is also due, at least in part, to intrinsic atrial adaptations independent of sympathetic and parasympathetic mechanisms is also supported by other work in rat and human models of endurance training (4). Brown et al. (12) found that the resting HR from chronically trained rats was ~10% lower than sedentary counterparts, although a mechanism underlying this bradycardia was not investigated in their study and represents an area for future research.

TEST YOURSELF

Based on your knowledge of ionic currents in the SAN, how might the magnitude of I_f and I_K be altered at rest in the heart of an exercise trained individual?

Myocardial Mechanisms Influencing Stroke Volume during Exercise

$$\dot{V}O_2 = HR \times SV \times \Delta a - vO_2$$

Left ventricular stroke volume is the amount of blood that is ejected from the left ventricle (LV) during a single cardiac cycle and is described as the difference between LV end-diastolic volume (EDV) and end-systolic volume (ESV). Although somewhat variable as a function of sex, body size, and a variety of other factors, a reasonable approximation of SV is ~70 mL in a normal healthy adult. Maximal SV values range from ~100 to 200 mL, variable as a function of a person's maximal CO and aerobic capacity. Factors that influence LV-EDV include the size of the heart, LV filling pressure, and the compliance of the LV during the diastolic filling phase of the cardiac cycle. Factors that influence ESV include afterload and LV myocardial contractile force. As exercise intensity increases, both LV-EDV and LV-ESV contribute to the increase in SV: LV-EDV increases and LV-ESV decreases (1,13). The increase in LV-EDV with the onset of exercise has been associated with increases in venous return and LV filling pressure. The progressive decrease in LV-ESV with increasing exercise intensity is attributable to augmented myocardial contractile function. Increased pumping by the heart results from

increased sympathetic drive to the heart and second messenger–mediated modulation of contractile function, as well as from intrinsic mechanisms. These intrinsic mechanisms can be length dependent (heterometric) or length independent (homeometric), and are described in detail later in this chapter. During exercise, all of these mechanisms work in concert to optimize LV diastolic and systolic function. An appreciation of the elegant integration of these processes requires a basic understanding of the cellular processes that are involved in myocardial excitation, contraction, and relaxation (see Bers [14] for review).

In the heart, an action potential that originates in the SAN is propagated through the atria and into both ventricles of the heart. This membrane depolarization is the triggering event in the excitation-contraction (EC) coupling process (Fig. 10.4). Action potential conduction into the T-tubular system elicits the voltage-dependent opening of L-type Ca^{2+} channels and the generation of a small inward Ca^{2+} current (I_{Ca}). Many of the L-type Ca^{2+} channels in the T-tubular membrane are found to be in a highly ordered association with and in close proximity to large conductance SR Ca^{2+} release channels in the terminal cisternal face of the SR. These SR Ca^{2+} release channels act as highly specific receptors for the plant alkaloid, ryanodine. Ryanodine alters SR Ca^{2+} channel function and at high μM concentrations it suppresses SR Ca^{2+} release. Accordingly, SR Ca^{2+} release channels are often referred to as ryanodine receptors, or RyRs. Different SR Ca^{2+} release channel/RyR isoforms exist in cardiac, skeletal, and smooth muscle; the cardiac isoform is RyR2.

A very small confined space exists between the T-tubular membrane (containing L-type channels) and the terminal cisternal face of the SR membrane (containing RyRs). This is significant because when a small I_{Ca} is triggered by an action potential, the Ca^{2+} entering the small confined space produces an increase $[Ca^{2+}]$ in the space to the extent that Ca^{2+} can bind to specific Ca^{2+} binding sites on RyRs. The binding of Ca^{2+} to RyRs promotes the opening of these channels and facilitates the focal release of Ca^{2+} from small, spatially organized clusters of RyRs. Initially, SR Ca^{2+} release appears as discrete, spatiotemporally organized Ca^{2+} release, or Ca^{2+} "sparks." Although it was once thought that a single "spark" represented the release of Ca^{2+} from a single RyR, it is now known that a "spark" is the result of the simultaneous release of Ca^{2+} from clusters (about 10–20) or RyRs. With the occurrence of multiple Ca^{2+} "sparks," $[Ca^{2+}]$ in the confined space and around other RyRs elicits a rapid and explosive opening of more RyRs and a massive release of Ca^{2+} from the SR ensues. This general process of I_{Ca}-triggered release of Ca^{2+} from the SR is referred to as Ca^{2+}-induced Ca^{2+} release (CICR). Once CICR is initiated, Ca^{2+} rapidly diffuses from the confined space into the myofibrillar space of each sarcomere. The subsequent elevation in $[Ca^{2+}]$ around the contractile apparatus elicits Ca^{2+} binding to troponin C, the release of the steric inhibition of actin-myosin interactions by the troponin-tropomyosin complex, and the activation of crossbridge cycling and cardiac muscle contraction. These are the events of EC coupling (14–17).

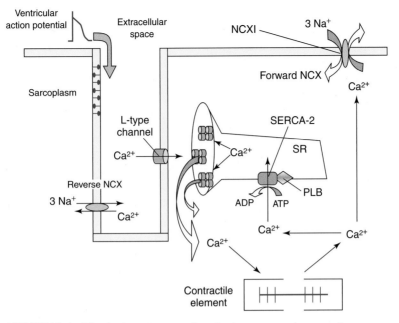

FIGURE 10.4   The basic processes of excitation-contraction coupling in ventricular myocardium. NXC, sodium-calcium exchanger; SERCA-2, sarco(endo)plasmic reticulum Ca^{2+} pump; SR, sarcoplasmic reticulum; ADP, adenosine diphosphate; ATP, adenosine triphosphate; PLB, phospholamban.

The relaxation phase of the cardiac cycle occurs when $[Ca^{2+}]$ around the contractile apparatus is reduced. This reduction occurs primarily via the actions of the 2A isoform of the sarco(endo)plasmic reticulum Ca^{2+} ATPase (SERCA 2A) and the cardiac sarcolemmal sodium-calcium exchanger (NCX1). On a beat-to-beat basis, Ca^{2+} removal by the SR is quantitatively the most important and, depending on animal species, accounts for about 70% to 85% of the reduction in sarcoplasmic $[Ca^{2+}]$. Although NCX1-mediated Ca^{2+} extrusion from the cell is quantitatively less important in the beat-to-beat regulation of sarcoplasmic $[Ca^{2+}]$, it does play a critical role in providing a mechanism to regulate cardiocyte Ca^{2+} content by quantitatively balancing the Ca^{2+} influx into the cell that occurs via I_{Ca}. Transient imbalances between cardiocyte Ca^{2+} influx and efflux over several beats can markedly influence cellular Ca^{2+} content, SR Ca^{2+} load, and the amount of Ca^{2+} that is released from the SR during a single EC coupling cycle. The NCX1 is an electrogenic exchanger (3 Na^+ for 1 Ca^{2+}) and under physiologic conditions, operation in the forward (Ca^{2+} out $-$ Na^+ in) mode is favored at membrane potentials more negative than about -35 mV. This will be relevant to a discussion of rate-dependent modulation of cardiac contractile force that follows.

TEST YOURSELF

The concentration of what ion is most important in mediating cardiac relaxation? Name two extrusion pathways responsible for lowering the cytosolic concentration of this ion. Which of these two pathways is quantitatively more important?

Sarcomere Length–Tension Relationship

With the onset of exercise, the increase in LV-EDV and decrease in LV-ESV are not independent phenomena. Starling's law of the heart states that myocardial contractile force increases in proportion to increases in myocardial muscle fiber length, such as would occur with increases in LV-EDV. Functionally, this provides for quantitative homeostatic control of venous return and CO to ensure that the blood presented to the LV is pumped from the LV. Several cellular mechanisms contribute to Starling's law of the heart. The effect of myocardial fiber length on myocardial contractile force can be explained, in part, in the context of the sliding filament theory where maximal muscle contractile force is directly proportional to the degree of thin–thick filament overlap in the sarcomere (18). This is manifest as the classic length–tension relationship that is exhibited in all striated muscle (Fig. 10.5A). In the heart, the physiologically operational sarcomere length range is between 1.85 and 2.20 μ, and in this range there is a very steep length–tension relationship (19). With the onset of exercise, an increase in LV-EDV would force average sarcomere lengths toward the apex of the length–tension relationship and optimize myocardial contractile force during systole and result in an increase in stroke volume.

$[Ca^{2+}]$–Tension Relationship

Myocardial contractile force varies as a function of the amount of Ca^{2+} that is presented to the contractile element (20) (Fig. 10.5B). In normal myocardium, sarcoplasmic diastolic $[Ca^{2+}]$ is in the 100 to 200 nM range, and during contraction, it approaches μM concentrations.

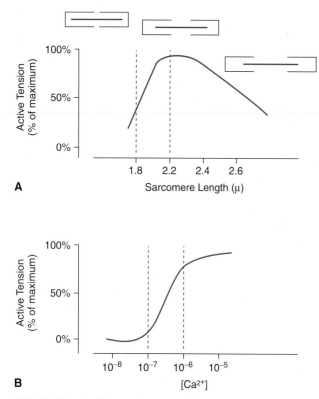

A

B

FIGURE 10.5 **A.** The cardiac muscle length–tension relationship. Note the very steep increase in tension between sarcomere lengths of 1.8 and 2.2 μ (the ascending limb). The decline in tension on the descending limb of the relationship is more gradual. The descending limb is rarely encountered physiologically except in severely pathologic conditions. **B.** A representation of the cardiac muscle [Ca²⁺]–tension relationship. The vertical broken lines denote the theoretical intracellular [Ca²⁺] boundaries between diastole (*left*) and systole (*right*). The relationship is presented in a semilogarithmic fashion.

The sensitivity of the myocardial contractile element to activation by Ca^{2+} is greater than that observed in skeletal muscle. Factors that influence the amount of Ca^{2+} released by the SR during EC coupling have a direct effect on the extent of thin filament–mediated contractile element activation and, therefore, of myocardial contractile force. In addition, the [Ca²⁺]–tension relationship is not static. Rather, it is subject to regulation by several factors. The [Ca²⁺]–tension relationship varies as a function of muscle (sarcomere) length (Fig. 10.6A and B). Increasing muscle length within the physiologically relevant range of sarcomere lengths causes a leftward shift in the [Ca²⁺]–tension relationship (21,22). This results in a sensitization of the contractile element (CE) to activation by Ca^{2+}. The molecular basis for the length dependence of the pCa versus tension relationship is thought to involve simple alterations in the geometry of the sarcomere. If one considers the sarcomere to be a constant volume entity, then as length increases, cross-sectional dimension must decrease. The consequence of the latter is that thick filaments are in closer proximity to thin filaments, thus increasing the probability of force generating actin-myosin encounters when myosin-binding domains

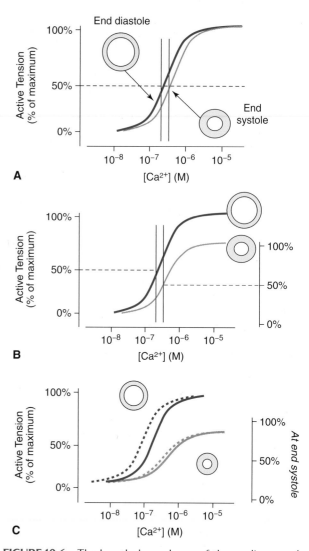

A

B

C

FIGURE 10.6 The length dependence of the cardiac muscle [Ca²⁺]–tension relationship. **A.** During end diastole, when chamber volume is large and muscle length is long, the [Ca²⁺]–tension relationship lies to the left of that occurring during end systole, when chamber volume is small and muscle length is short. Maximal forces occurring at long and short sarcomere lengths are scaled to illustrate the length-dependent shift in sensitivity of the contractile element to activation by Ca²⁺. **B.** In reality, at shorter sarcomere lengths, not only is there a rightward shift in the [Ca²⁺]–tension relationship, but maximal force-generating capabilities are diminished as a result of a movement to the left on the length–tension relationship (compare part **A**). Both phenomena optimize the system for relaxation. **C.** Training alters the length dependence of the [Ca²⁺]–tension relationship. Diffee and Nagle (47) found that the sensitivity of the cardiac contractile element to activation by Ca²⁺ was altered by training only at long (*e.g.*, end-diastolic) sarcomere lengths. The hypothetical consequences of this type of adaptation are illustrated here. At long sarcomere lengths, during end diastole (*black lines*), the sensitivity of the myocardial contractile element to activation by Ca²⁺ is greater in myocardium from the trained (*broken lines*) than in the sedentary (*solid lines*) state. Contractile force development is favored in the trained state under these conditions. However, during end systole (*gray lines*), when sarcomere lengths are short, relaxation is favored similarly in both the trained and sedentary states.

on actin become exposed. Conversely, the pCa versus tension relationship moves rightward when sarcomere length is decreased. This property of the $[Ca^{2+}]$–tension relationship makes good sense in that at long sarcomere lengths, such as those that occur during end diastole, the CE is sensitized to activation by Ca^{2+}. This sensitization would provide for a more forceful contraction at the beginning of systole. As blood is ejected from the heart, sarcomere length decreases and the $[Ca^{2+}]$–tension relationship moves back to the right rendering the CE less sensitive to activation by Ca^{2+}. Desensitization of the CE at the end of the ejection phase of the cardiac cycle also makes good sense because it would favor myocardial relaxation and filling of the ventricle with blood during diastole. The dynamic length-dependent modulation of the $[Ca^{2+}]$–tension relationship provides another mechanism that contributes to Starling's law of the heart.

A third length-dependent mechanism has been identified that may also contribute to Starling's law of the heart. There is evidence that the amount of Ca^{2+} released from the SR during an EC coupling cycle is proportional to myocardial segment length (23,24). This may be a result of an augmentation in the magnitude of I_{Ca}, SR Ca^{2+} load, and release of Ca^{2+} from the SR. Collectively, the increase in myocardial segment length that occurs during the filling phase of the cardiac cycle sets up conditions that are ideal for the generation of myocardial contractile force: the degree of thick–thin filament overlap is optimized, the sensitivity of the contractile element to activation by Ca^{2+} is increased as is the amount of Ca^{2+} that is delivered to the contractile element.

TEST YOURSELF

At which part of the cardiac phase are the myofilaments the most sensitive to calcium? At which phase are the myofilaments the least sensitive to calcium? How does this benefit the pumping function of the heart?

Summary

The onset of exercise leads to increased LV-EDV, which increases the amount of force that the myofilaments generate (Frank-Starling mechanism), resulting in increased SV. The length–tension relationship in the heart is believed to be due to three factors: (a) increased proximity of the actin-myosin binding sites; (b) higher sensitivity of the CE to Ca^{2+} at longer resting sarcomere lengths; and (c) enhanced Ca^{2+} release from the SR at longer sarcomere lengths.

Rate-dependent Regulation of Myocardial Contraction

For more than 100 years (25,26), it has been well known that an increase in HR is accompanied by a progressive increase in contractile force of the myocardium, or the "staircase" phenomenon (25) (Fig. 10.7). There is good evidence to indicate that this rate-dependent augmentation in cardiac contractile force results from a progressive increase in Ca^{2+} content of the SR, and in the amount of SR

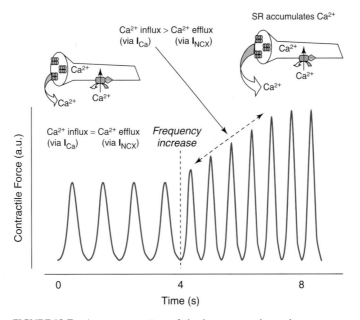

FIGURE 10.7 A representation of the heart rate–dependent increase in cardiac contractile force development, or the staircase (or treppe) phenomenon. As heart rate increases, muscle contractile force increases to a new steady-state plateau. The increase in force is secondary to a transient imbalance in cellular Ca^{2+} influx and efflux (favoring influx), an increase in sarcoplasmic reticulum (SR) Ca^{2+} content, and a larger SR Ca^{2+} release during each excitation-contraction coupling cycle. I_{NCX}, sodium-calcium exchange current.

Ca^{2+} released on a beat-to-beat basis (14). The progressive increase in SR Ca^{2+} content with an increase in contraction frequency is thought to be due to a transient imbalance that is created between Ca^{2+} influx via I_{Ca} and Ca^{2+} efflux via sodium-calcium exchange (NaCa exchange). As mentioned earlier, NaCa exchange is electrogenic and its operation in the forward "Ca^{2+} out/Na^+ in" mode is favored at hyperpolarized membrane potentials, whereas during membrane depolarization (*i.e.*, the action potential), reverse "Ca^{2+} in/Na^+ out" exchange is favored. A simple explanation for the HR-dependent increase in SR Ca^{2+} load is as follows. In any given window of time, when HR is increased, the frequency of I_{Ca} increases and this contributes to an increase in Ca^{2+} influx into the cell. In addition, the time between EC coupling events is decreased resulting in less time for Ca^{2+} extrusion from the cell. In combination with the increase in Ca^{2+} influx, an increase in the amount of Ca^{2+} that is taken up by the SR during diastole occurs. Finally, when HR is increased, a greater fraction of time in the cardiac cycle is occupied by conditions where the myocardial membrane is depolarized, a condition that is not conducive to forward NaCa exchange. The net effect is that when HR is increased, the delicate and dynamic equilibrium that exists between cellular Ca^{2+} influx and efflux is transiently shifted in favor of influx and the excess Ca^{2+} is retained by and subsequently released from the SR. (Note: An exception to the general observation that myocardial contractile force increases in direct proportion to HR is seen in hearts from smaller rodents [rat, mouse]. In these species, a "negative staircase" is typically observed, and related to a rate-dependent depletion of Ca^{2+} from the SR [14]. Species-dependent differences in the relative durations of the cardiac action potential and the intracellular $[Ca^{2+}]$ transient are thought to contribute to this species difference.)

β-adrenergic Modulation of Myocardial Contraction

The increase in sympathetic drive that occurs with the onset of exercise not only affects HR via effects on pacemaker cells in the SAN, it also affects myocardial contractile force (Fig. 10.8A). Hallmark alterations in cardiac contractile function resulting from β-adrenergic stimulation include a marked increased in peak contractile force generation, and an acceleration in myocardial relaxation. Overall, this culminates in a contraction that is larger in magnitude, but shorter in duration. This adaptation is ideal to accommodate the generation of large stroke volumes at high frequencies (*e.g.*, HRs). The cellular basis for the effects of β-adrenergic agonists on the characteristics of cardiac contractile force has been well characterized.

In cardiocytes of the ventricular myocardium, the binding of agonists (epinephrine, norepinephrine) to β_1-adrenergic receptors (β-AR) results in the G-protein mediated activation of adenylate cyclase, the formation of cAMP and subsequent activation of cAMP-dependent pro-

tein kinase (PKA) (Fig. 10.8B). Although the active catalytic subunit of PKA has numerous intracellular targets, there are at least four that are thought to contribute to augmented myocardial pump function during exercise (14–17). Myocardial contractile force is known to be modulated by the PKA-mediated phosphorylation of the L-type Ca^{2+} channel, the SR proteins phospholamban (PLB) and RyR2, and the thin filament protein troponin I (TnI). Phosphorylation of TnI produces a rightward shift in the $[Ca^{2+}]$–tension relationship. This desensitization of the CE to activation by Ca^{2+} would promote myocardial relaxation. Phospholamban acts to suppress the activity of the SR Ca^{2+} pump. Phosphorylation of PLB by PKA acts to release the inhibitory effects of PLB on SR Ca^{2+} pump activity, and this increases in the rate of Ca^{2+} clearance from the sarcoplasm by the SR and promotes relaxation. With respect to the PKA-mediated mechanisms that augment myocardial relaxation, the PLB phosphorylation is probably of greater quantitative significance than the TnI phosphorylation. Phosphorylation of L-type Ca^{2+} channels by PKA increases L-type channel open probability and open time, and the physiologic consequence is that I_{Ca} is markedly increased. There is also evidence I_{Ca} can be increased by β-adrenergic agonists via a more direct β-AR/G protein mediated process (27). Because I_{Ca} is the "trigger" for CICR, one consequence of an increase in I_{Ca} would be that the magnitude of Ca^{2+} release from the SR would increase (28).

In addition, β-adrenergic stimulation creates a situation where the amount of Ca^{2+} available to be released from the SR is increased (Fig. 10.8B). The augmentation in SR Ca^{2+} load occurs via two mechanisms. First, the increase in I_{Ca} magnitude that occurs on a beat-to-beat basis creates a situation where the influx of Ca^{2+} into the cell is increased. Because NaCa exchange is not directly influenced by β-adrenergic stimulation, a transient imbalance between cellular Ca^{2+} influx and efflux would occur and the Ca^{2+} retained by the cell would be taken up into the SR. Second, because β-adrenergic stimulation markedly increases SR Ca^{2+} pump activity, a greater fraction of the Ca^{2+} that is removed from the sarcoplasm by the combined actions of SR pump activity and NaCa exchange would be removed via the SR mechanism. In other words, the sarcoplasmic Ca^{2+} clearance pathway that favors cellular Ca^{2+} retention (*e.g.*, the SR Ca^{2+} pump activity) competes more effectively with the NaCa exchange, the Ca^{2+} extrusion pathway. Again, the net effect is that SR Ca^{2+} load increases and more Ca^{2+} is available for release when CICR is "triggered" by I_{Ca}. An increase in SR Ca^{2+} load also has the powerful effect of increasing the sensitivity of SR Ca^{2+} release from the SR by I_{Ca}.

Finally, under the influence of β-adrenergic stimulation, the sensitivity of the cardiac SR Ca^{2+} release mechanism to the "triggering" effects of I_{Ca} is increased via two mechanisms. First, the sensitivity of the SR Ca^{2+} release channel to opening by I_{Ca} is powerfully (~geometrically) influenced by SR Ca^{2+} load. Very small increases in SR Ca^{2+} load produce very large changes in SR Ca^{2+} release channel open probability. The link between SR Ca^{2+} load

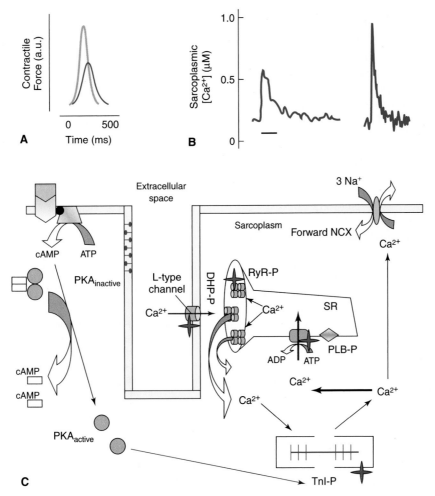

FIGURE 10.8   β-Adrenergic stimulation increases cardiac contractile force and accelerates myocardial relaxation. **A.** With β-adrenergic stimulation, cardiac contractile force markedly increases (*light blue tracing*). In addition, the duration of the force transient is abbreviated. The former effect favors more powerful systolic ejection, whereas the latter effect favors diastolic filling, as would be required at high heart rates. **B.** The mechanical effects depicted in **A** are associated with similar alterations in the magnitude and duration of the intracellular [Ca²⁺] transient. [Ca²⁺] transients occur in the same cell prior to (*left*) and after (*right*) exposure to β-agonist. (Representative data acquired from our laboratory for purposes of illustration only.) **C.** The effects of β-agonist on the intracellular [Ca²⁺] transient and myocardial contractile force are secondary to the effects of protein kinase A (PKA)-mediated phosphorylations of phospholamban (PLB-P), ryanodine receptor (RyR), troponin I (TnI-P), and the L-type of Ca²⁺ channels. The scheme and symbols used in this panel are consistent with those in Figs. 10.3 and 10.4.

and SR Ca²⁺ release channel open probability occurs via a physical coupling of RyRs with the intraluminal SR protein, calsequestrin (via the proteins junctin and triadin). Calsequestrin is a high capacity Ca²⁺ binding protein and increased Ca²⁺ binding to calsequestrin (*i.e.*, when SR Ca²⁺ load increases) exerts a strong influence on SR Ca²⁺ release channel sensitivity to "triggered" opening by I_Ca. Second, RyRs exist as complex multimeric protein complexes that include both the catalytic and regulatory subunits of PKA. Under the influence of β-adrenergic stimulation, RyRs are directly phosphorylated by PKA and this phosphorylation elicits a direct increase in the sensitivity of the SR Ca²⁺ release mechanism to the "triggering" effects of I_Ca.

Summary

Overall, β-adrenergic stimulation enhances both contraction and relaxation. β-adrenergic stimulation promotes myocardial relaxation and diastolic filling via the phosphorylations of PLB and TnI. Once the heart fills with blood, systolic function is increased via augmented SR Ca²⁺ release. The enhanced SR Ca²⁺ release occurs both *directly* from the phosphorylations of L-type Ca²⁺ channels increasing RyR release, and *indirectly* from augmented SR Ca²⁺ loading due to higher PLB activity.

Integration of Mechanisms to Improve Cardiac Contractile Function during Exercise

With the onset of exercise, parasympathetic drive is reduced and sympathetic drive increases to augment CO. At the level of the SAN, this results in an increase in the frequency of pacemaker activity and a subsequent increase in HR. Because CO = HR × SV, the impact of this adjustment in pacemaker activity on CO is obvious. In addition, independent of the direct effects of sympathetic input on the ventricular myocardium, the rate-dependent augmentation in SR Ca^{2+} may also act to increase myocardial contractile force and have an impact on stroke volume.

At the level of the ventricular myocardium, the onset of exercise brings about several important changes. An increase in venous return, significantly augmented by the skeletal muscle pump, to the heart elicits an increase in LV-EDV and an increase in end-diastolic sarcomere length. In addition, increased sympathetic β-adrenergic stimulation acts on processes that improve both the *lusitropic* and *inotropic* function of the heart (Fig. 10.9). During EC coupling, the magnitude of SR Ca^{2+} release is markedly increased by β-adrenergic stimulation. The resulting increase in sarcoplasmic $[Ca^{2+}]$ that occurs during EC coupling is easily sufficient to overcome any desensitization of the CE that occurs via TnI phosphorylation. In addition, bear in mind that in a normal cardiac cycle, EC coupling is initiated when diastolic volume is maximal and sarcomere lengths are near the apex of the length–tension curve. This not only optimizes the degree of thick-thin filament overlap at the beginning of systole, but this length increase also acts to sensitize the CE to activation by Ca^{2+} by eliciting a leftward shift in the $[Ca^{2+}]$–tension relationship, thus opposing any desensitization caused by TnI phosphorylation. The net result is that all of these processes act to optimize contractile force upon the initiation of systole. This is the basis for the observation that ESV decreases in the transition from rest to exercise.

After the ejection phase of the cardiac cycle, myocardial relaxation and ventricular filling are required to sustain effective myocardial pump function. This is particularly important during exercise where elevated HRs are achieved primarily via the abbreviation of diastole as opposed to systole. Two primary mechanisms contribute

Myocardial Relaxation Optimized
- Ca^{2+} desensitized contractile element length, TnI phosphorylation
- on ascending limb of length–tension relationship
- increased SR Ca^{2+} pump activity (PLB phosphorylation)

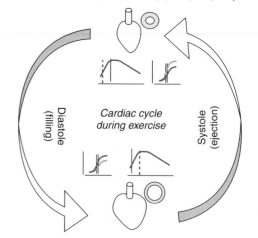

Contractile Force Development Optimized
- Resensitization of contractile element to activation by Ca^{2+}
  Length effect
- Near apex of length–tension relationship
- Increased SR Ca^{2+} release
  increased I_{Ca}
  • L-type Ca^{2+} channel phosphorylation
  Increased SR Ca^{2+} load
  • Heart rate
  • Increase SR Ca^{2+} pump activity (PLB phosphorylation)

FIGURE 10.9 The mechanisms activated to improve cardiac function during exercise. The processes that favor both systole and diastole are listed in the context of the cardiac cycle.

to improved relaxation during the abbreviated diastolic filling period during exercise. First, the marked acceleration in sarcoplasmic Ca^{2+} clearance by the SR that occurs secondary to PLB phosphorylation profoundly accelerates the relaxation of the heart. Second, relaxation is further facilitated via the length-dependent rightward shift that occurs in the $[Ca^{2+}]$–tension relationship when LV-ESV is small and sarcomere lengths are short. The net result of these processes is that myocardial relaxation and ventricular filling can occur rapidly and optimal LV-EDVs can be achieved prior to the onset of another EC coupling event, even when exercise HRs are high. It should be noted that these lusitropic processes begin to fail to compensate for the extreme shortening in diastolic filling times that occur at extremely high HRs (*e.g.*, approximately >200 bpm). This failure is manifest as a reduction in LV-EDV at extremely high HRs.

Bioenergetics of the Exercised Heart

Maintenance of Myocardial ATP Levels during Exercise

As CO increases during the onset of exercise, the oxygen consumption by the heart *itself* also increases three to four times higher than resting levels. Oxygen is delivered to the myocardium via the coronary arteries, and most perfusion of the heart occurs during diastole, when wall pressure decreases. Increased oxygen delivery to the heart during exercise can be accomplished by either increasing the amount of oxygen extracted from the blood, or by increasing the coronary flow rate. In heart, the amount of oxygen that the heart extracts from the blood is already ~80% of maximal at rest, so during exercise there is not a large increase in the amount of extracted oxygen (in stark contrast to skeletal muscle, see Chapter 11). In the heart, the increased oxygen delivery during exercise is mostly accomplished by increasing the coronary flow rate, with the exercise-induced vasodilation driven primarily by local metabolic factors.

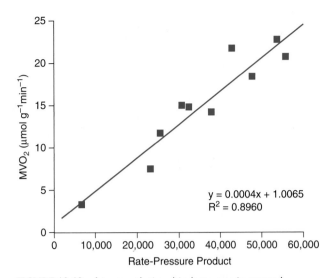

FIGURE 10.10   Linear relationship between increased cardiac work and oxygen consumption. Cardiac function is expressed as the rate-pressure product (rate-pressure product = heart rate × peak systolic pressure). Oxygen consumption was measured in isolated guinea pig hearts and is expressed as μmol O_2 per gram of heart dry weight per minute (DA Brown, unpublished observations).

> ## KEY POINT
>
> Increased oxygen delivery to the heart during exercise is accomplished primarily by increasing coronary flow rates. Oxygen extraction by the heart is near maximal even at rest.

There is a direct linear relationship between increased cardiac work and oxygen consumption by the heart (Fig. 10.10; unpublished observation by Brown). During exercise, heightened cardiac work translates to increased hydrolysis of ATP due to increases in:

1. Number and frequency of actin/myosin cross-bridge cycling (accounting for ~70% of all myocardial ATP hydrolysis)
2. Calcium reuptake by the SR (accounting for ~25% of all myocardial ATP hydrolysis)
3. Restoration of ion gradients across the sarcolemmal membrane by the Na^+/K^+ ATPase and the sarcolemmal Ca^{2+} pump (accounting for ~5% of all myocardial ATP hydrolysis)

Given the increase in myocardial ATP breakdown following the onset of exercise, there is a very brief buffering of ATP by phosphocreatine (29). Over the course of exercise, the heart relies primarily on the aerobic breakdown of carbohydrates and fat by mitochondria to increase ATP supply to match heightened demand. Heart tissue is well suited to tolerate increasing workloads, as approximately 30% of mammalian heart cell volume is comprised by mitochondria (30,31). Although this represents one of the highest densities of mitochondria of any tissue in the body, the mechanisms through which cardiac mitochondria enhance ATP production during exercise have not been fully characterized.

Supply and demand matching in the heart

A common observation in all types of striated muscle is that muscle ATP content is not altered immediately following the onset of exercise. Clearly, both heart and skeletal muscle are well adapted to compensate for higher amounts of ATP hydrolysis after exercise begins. What is less clear, however, is *how* this ability to buffer ATP is accomplished within each muscle cell. As described in detail in Chapter 13, the compensatory increase ATP production in skeletal muscle during extensive exercise is largely attributed to a decreased ATP/ADP ratio (due to elevated ADP). This elevated ADP lowers the phosphorylation potential ($\Delta G_{ATP,synthesis}$) at the level of the F_1F_O-ATPase (Complex V) of the respiratory chain. A reduction in $\Delta G_{ATP,synthesis}$ allows for increased proton flux into the mitochondrial matrix, which provides more energy to phosphorylate ADP. As proton flux into the matrix increases, electron flow down the respiratory chain is augmented, and more oxygen is consumed (as oxygen is the terminal acceptor of electrons). In this paradigm, the increased products of ATP hydrolysis (namely, ADP and Pi) are said to "pull" electrons down the respiratory chain by lowering the $\Delta G_{ATP,synthesis}$.

Unlike skeletal muscle, discernible changes in adenine nucleotide concentrations are not typically observed in heart tissue during exercise. The reason for this discrepancy between heart and skeletal muscle is because, unlike skeletal muscle, the heart is a muscle that is never at rest (when skeletal muscle is chronically paced and then workload is increased, there is no longer an observable change in the level of ATP hydrolysis products with increases in work [32]). In heart, the observation that increased cardiac work does not lead to altered levels of high-energy phosphate compounds was first noted in the 1950s (33) and has since been supported by a number of studies (34). Although absence of changes in ATP hydrolysis products in the heart could be due to compartmentation, this has been disputed and is an area of ongoing investigation.

The importance of Ca^{2+} in cardiac muscle contraction has been known since the early experiments of Sydney Ringer more than 125 years ago (35). More recently, Ca^{2+} appears to have a role in regulating respiration via a process known as "parallel activation." In this mechanism of matching supply with demand, Ca^{2+} bears the responsibility of simultaneously stimulating contraction of the myofilaments and increasing the production of ATP. By stimulating the activity of dehydrogenases (α-ketoglutarate dehydrogenase, pyruvate dehydrogenase, and isocitrate dehydrogenase) in the TCA cycle, Ca^{2+} mediates increased production of reducing equivalents that feed into the respiratory chain. Through this pathway, Ca^{2+} is thought to "push" electrons down the respiratory chain (contrasted with the "pull" mechanism as described previously). If Ca^{2+} influx into the matrix is inhibited, heart mitochondria are not able to effectively match ATP supply with demand (29). Although the feed-forward and feedback mechanisms have been discussed previously as two potential regulators of heart respiration, these two pathways are not mutually exclusive. For example, in addition to stimulating enzymes in the TCA cycle, Ca^{2+} has also been shown to increase the rate at which complex V synthesizes ATP, leading to an increased rate of respiration (36). In the intact heart, there is likely a combination of compartmentalized changes in phosphorylation potential and parallel activation by Ca^{2+} that translates to a rapid matching of energy supply with the ATP demand exerted by exercise.

Summary

Increased CO during exercise leads to higher amounts of ATP hydrolysis by the heart itself, and cardiac mitochondria match ATP demand with an increased supply. Under physiologic conditions, there are no discernible changes in ATP or ADP in the heart upon the onset of exercise. Activation of TCA and electron transport chain enzymes by calcium mediate the increased supply of ATP. Compartmentalized changes in myocardial nucleotide content may occur with increased work, but have been difficult to measure to date.

The Effect of Training on Myocardial Energy Metabolism

In general, it can be stated that, unlike skeletal muscle where endurance training can produce dramatic increases in oxidative metabolic potential, the adaptive response of myocardial energy metabolism to exercise training is at best subtle. The observation that the activities of the key oxidative enzymes in rat heart are two to four times higher than those seen in skeletal muscle (41) suggest that the pathways of oxidative metabolism are already well adapted to support the energy demands imposed by daily bouts of exercise. This is not surprising in view of the fact that, even at rest, the heart exhibits chronic mechanical activity around the clock, whereas skeletal muscle is largely quiescent. This is not to say, however, that the heart does not exhibit the potential for metabolic adaptations. Experimentally, it is known that the activities of key enzymes of myocardial oxidative energy metabolism can be increased in response to sustained increases in HR and mechanical work that are brought about by electrical pacing (4,39). It is also clear, however, that the stimulus imposed by intermittent and relatively brief (~1–2 h) daily bouts of exercise is not sufficient to elicit significant changes in these enzymatic markers of myocardial energy production (42). A significant and complex body of literature exists on the adaptive effects of exercise training on myocardial energy metabolism and in-depth reviews on the subject can be found elsewhere (4,39).

Although the expression of glycolytic and oxidative enzymes does not change in response to exercise training, there have been noted differences in the oxidant scavenging ability of the heart. Upregulated antioxidant enzymes, such as glutathione, catalase, and manganese superoxide dismutase, have been observed in hearts from trained animals (43–45). It seems plausible that these changes in antioxidant potential in hearts may be a very important adaptation to exercise that can protect the heart in the face of severe metabolic deficit (such as ischemia, discussed later).

Summary

Overall, the normal healthy heart is well adapted to meet the metabolic demands that are placed on it on a daily basis and the metabolic potential of the heart is not markedly influenced by training.

Adaptations of the Heart to Chronic Exercise Training

Training-induced Adaptations to Stroke Volume during Submaximal and Maximal Exercise

Among the most fundamental systemic characteristics of the endurance-trained state include (a) an increase organismic maximal oxygen consumption ($\dot{V}O_{2max}$) where $\dot{V}O_{2max} = HR_{max} \times$ maximal stroke volume (SV_{max}) $\times$ maximal arteriovenous O_2 content difference ($\Delta a - vO_{2max}$) and (b) a resting and submaximal exercise bradycardia. Adaptations in HR_{max} do not contribute to training-induced increases in $\dot{V}O_{2max}$. As a general rule, $\geq 50\%$ of the training-induced increase in $\dot{V}O_{2max}$ can be attributed to an increase in SV_{max} and the remainder to an increase in $\Delta a - vO_{2max}$ (2,37,38). It can generally be stated that training-induced increases in SV_{max} are virtually always associated with increases in LV-EDV, whereas the contribution of augmented myocardial contractile function (and a decrease in LV-ESV) to SV_{max} is variable (2,37,38). Training-induced increases in maximal LV end-diastolic volume (LV-EDV$_{max}$) might be achieved by a variety of mechanisms that include (a) an increase in the intrinsic compliance of the myocardium, (b) an increase in end-diastolic filling pressure, and/or (c) an increase in LV chamber dimension secondary to myocyte growth.

Augmentation of LV-EDV with training

The effect of training on the intrinsic compliance of normal, healthy myocardium has not been unambiguously identified. In the normal heart, training has been found to increase or leave unaltered myocardial compliance in diastole (4,39). These discrepant findings may be due in part to the different techniques used, as well as interpretive assumptions associated with making compliance determinations in a dynamic system. Diastolic compliance of the heart is determined by both passive and active tissue properties. In certain disease states (or with aging), the decreased compliance of the heart is associated with changes in the amount and composition of interstitial connective elements, which have a marked effect on the passive compliance of the myocardial material. In a dynamically contracting and relaxing system, active properties certainly affect the compliance of the heart and influence its ability to relax and fill during diastole. An example of an active property that affects diastolic compliance is sarcoplasmic Ca^{2+} handling. In animal models of advanced age and diabetes mellitus, diminished sarcoplasmic Ca^{2+} clearance and alterations in the sensitivity of the CE to activation by Ca^{2+} have been shown to contribute to increased diastolic stiffness (40). It has been clearly demonstrated that in pathologic settings, exercise training can increase the compliance of the heart during diastole. Furthermore, this type of improvement in diastolic compliance has been clearly shown to be associated with active, rather than passive properties of the heart. Blood and plasma volume expansion occurring as a result of exercise training could also contribute to increases in LV-EDV$_{max}$. In normal healthy subjects, such a phenomenon has been observed and provides an attractive mechanism for improved diastolic filling during maximal exercise (1).

An important mechanism for training-induced augmentation of LV-EDV$_{max}$ is myocardial growth that produces an intrinsic increase in the LV chamber dimension. Exercise training has been shown to elicit small to modest increases in the mass of the heart (0%–25%). If cardiac myocytes are assumed to be terminally differentiated, training-induced increases in myocardial mass must be accomplished via hypertrophy of individual myocytes. In a variety of animal models of exercise training, increases in mean myocyte dimension can account for all of the increase in ventricular mass that is produced by training. Myocyte growth in both

the longitudinal and cross-sectional dimensions have been shown to occur (4,39). Importantly, with exercise training longitudinal myocyte growth occurs in the absence of intrinsic alterations in sarcomere length. This increase in cell length without changing sarcomere length is accomplished by adding sarcomeres "in series" with existing sarcomeres and is termed eccentric hypertrophy. With eccentric hypertrophy, the increase in cell size is primarily due to an increase in myocyte length. Eccentric hypertrophy is often seen in states where there is volume overload, such as with endurance training or in late-stage heart failure (although the latter is also accompanied by thinning of the ventricular wall). In contrast, hypertrophic myocyte growth in early heart failure or hypertension is accomplished by adding sarcomeres "in parallel" with other sarcomeres, leading to increased myocyte cross-sectional area). This is referred to as concentric hypertrophy and is classically observed in pressure-overloaded hearts.

The cardiocyte hypertrophy that is observed in the endurance-trained state has several very important consequences for the LV. Because LV dimension can be approximated as a surface of revolution around a longitudinal axis, a 5% increase in mean LV myocyte length would produce a 5% increase in mean circumferential dimension as well as a ~5% increase in the length of the axis of revolution. The net result would be that longitudinal myocyte growth of 5% would elicit a ~16% increase in LV chamber volume. In addition, according to La Place's Law of the heart, this type of increase in chamber volume would only elicit a small (≤5%) increase in ventricular wall stress which is likely offset by a commensurate increase in myocyte cross-sectional dimension with training.

Increases in intrinsic LV chamber volume would have several important functional consequences. First, an increase in stroke volume would be expected to occur even if the contractility and fractional shortening of myocytes in the LV myocardium were unaltered by training. Second, an increase in LV-EDV resulting purely from longitudinal myocyte growth would produce a situation where EDV could be increased independent of increases in mean sarcomere length. Such an elegantly simple mechanism would leave the Frank-Starling mechanism intact to further improve cardiac function via an optimization of the "sarcomere length vs. tension" relationship and other length-dependent mechanisms. This mechanism also provides a simple cellular basis to explain the observation that a training-induced increase in LV-EDV produces a rightward but parallel shift in the ventricular "pressure vs. volume" relationship (4,39).

Finally, a relative bradycardia during rest and submaximal exercise is a classic marker of the trained state. Because the relationship between EDV, systemic oxygen consumption, and the absolute amount of external work performed within a species is highly invariant, it follows that stroke volume at rest and during fixed, absolute submaximal workloads is augmented by training. The mechanisms identified in the preceding paragraphs to explain the effect of training on SV_{max} are also applicable when explaining the effect of training on submaximal stroke volume.

In addition, however, it is probable that increased diastolic filling time secondary to a training-induced bradycardia contribute to augmented SV during rest and submaximal work in the trained state.

Summary

Exercise training-induced increases in SV_{max} are virtually always associated with increases in LV-EDV. The latter almost certainly results from intrinsic alterations in LV chamber geometry that result from cardiac hypertrophy that is accompanied by longitudinal myocyte growth. There is also evidence that increased LV-EDV with training may be partly due to increased LV filling pressures that result from training-induced plasma volume expansion. Although training has been clearly shown to normalize (increase) the compliance of the heart in pathologic settings, this adaptation to training has not been clearly confirmed in normal, healthy myocardium.

Intrinsic Alterations in Contractile Function with Training

The body of evidence supportive of the concept that chronic aerobic exercise can invoke adaptive changes in intrinsic myocardial contractile function is substantial (4,37,39). Interestingly, attempts to elucidate the cellular mechanisms that underlie these functional changes have not yet produced clear and unified ideas about what systems respond adaptively to training, and how these adaptations actually contribute to training-induced improvements in the contractile performance of the heart. Over the last 30 years, much effort has been focused on determining how training influences (a) contractile element composition and intrinsic function, (b) the complex events that are involved in sarcoplasmic $[Ca^{2+}]$ regulation during the cardiac cycle, (c) the metabolic processes that are responsible for defending the tight coupling between ATP supply and demand that must be maintained in support of normal contractile activity, and (d) on systems that can modulate cardiocyte energy metabolism and mechanical function.

The effect of training on the myocardial contractile element

Considerable attention has been devoted to characterizing the effects of chronic exercise on contractile element protein composition. In small rodents, training elicits compositional change in myosin that is reflected as a shift in myosin isoform composition toward the native V_1 form (an isoform possessing a higher ATPase activity). However, it is now clear that changes in ventricular myosin ATPase activity and/or isoform composition are not obligatory for improved ventricular performance secondary to chronic exercise.

There is some evidence from animal models that training may increase the sensitivity of the contractile element to activation by Ca^{2+}. This idea is supported by the observation that paced myocytes isolated from trained and sedentary rats shortened to the same extent even though the cytosolic $[Ca^{2+}]$ achieved during contraction was lower in the myocytes from the trained animals (39). In addition, it has been recently demonstrated that in chemically "skinned" cardiocytes that were subject to strict sarcomere length control that endurance training produced a leftward shift in the $[Ca^{2+}]$–tension relationship (46). In addition, it was also demonstrated that this training-induced sensitization of the CE to activation by Ca^{2+} was only apparent at long (e.g., diastolic) sarcomere lengths but not at short (e.g., systolic) sarcomere lengths (47). This is also consistent with the recent observation in intact cardiocytes that the steepness of the length–tension relationship is increased by training (48) (Fig. 10.6C). Such an adaptation would provide for a training-induced optimization of contractile element activation at the beginning of the ejection phase of the cardiac cycle, whereas the effect would be lost at short sarcomere lengths and would not contribute to impaired myocardial relaxation when chamber filling is initiated. It should be noted that this adaptation has not been confirmed in species other than the rat and whether or not this type of adaptation occurs in larger mammals is not known.

The effect of training on EC coupling and sarcoplasmic $[Ca^{2+}]$ regulation

Because myocardial contractile force is governed in large part by the amount of Ca^{2+} presented to the contractile element, it is not surprising that considerable effort has been spent on determining whether or not training alters cardiocyte EC coupling and/or Ca^{2+} regulation. Critical examination of the extensive literature in the field (4,39) reveals two safe conclusions in this regard. First, in normal healthy myocardium, training does not appear to elicit striking effects on EC coupling and/or cellular Ca^{2+} regulation. In this regard, it must be recognized that cardiocyte Ca^{2+} homeostasis and control during EC coupling is delicately balanced by myriad processes. It is unlikely that profound alterations in any of these processes would be conducive to the fine control of myocardial contractile force. In addition, seemingly subtle alterations in points of Ca^{2+} control may, in fact, elicit physiologic significant adjustments in control that contribute to improved cardiac function in the trained state. Second, in pathologic settings where aberrant Ca^{2+} regulation can be readily detected, training has been shown to be effective in normalizing cardiocyte Ca^{2+} regulation. For example, age- and diabetes-related deficits in myocardial relaxation have been attributed to slowed sarcoplasmic Ca^{2+} clearance by the SR, and training has been shown to be particularly effective in ameliorating these deficits.

The effect of training on β-adrenergic signaling in the heart

A significant number of processes involved in the control of cardiac function can be modulated by β-adrenergic receptor agonists via the actions of PKA. The effects of aerobic exercise training on various aspects of the β-adrenergic system have been examined in a variety of training models. One clear characteristic of the trained state is that at a given absolute submaximal work load sympathetic drive, as reflected by circulating catecholamine levels, is attenuated relative to that observed in untrained subjects (see Chapter 7). At the level of the heart, however, the issue of whether or not training influences the inotropic sensitivity of the heart to β-agonists is not clear. Following training, the contractile responsiveness of the heart to catecholamines has been reported to increase, decrease, or remain unchanged (4,39). The adaptive responsiveness of key elements of the β-adrenergic signaling cascade to exercise training also has been examined in considerable detail and a clear consensus has not been reached. However, at present, it would appear that training-induced alterations in β-adrenergic signaling in ventricular myocardium are minimal whereas at the level of the right atrium, β-adrenergic receptor number is probably down-regulated, perhaps contributing to the bradycardia that occurs following exercise training (9).

The Effect of Training on the Coronary Vasculature

The regulation of cardiac function cannot be fully appreciated without acknowledging the important contribution of coronary vasculature in matching O_2 delivery with myocardial O_2 demand (as discussed previously). Training-induced alterations in cardiocyte dimension produce significant consequences with respect to the coronary vasculature and its ability to properly service the working myocardium. For example, if training-induced cardiocyte growth was not accompanied by angiogenesis and/or adaptations in the mechanisms regulating myocardial perfusion, then the heart may be exposed to energetic risk during periods of increased mechanical activity. Clearly, cardiocyte growth without parallel adaptations in the coronary vasculature is maladaptive. In most circumstances, exercise training-induced cardiocyte growth is accompanied by parallel (at least) growth of the coronary vasculature (39,49,50). Exercise training has been shown to elicit structural changes in the vasculature of the heart, including growth of the larger, proximal coronary arteries such that arterial size increases are commensurate with or greater than the relative increase in myocardial mass that is produced by training. Overall, training usually elicits adaptation in the coronary vasculature such that, at a minimum, microvasculature development occurs in parallel with the modest myocyte hypertrophy that is often observed in response to exercise training (4). It should be noted that in more severe models of training, cardiac hypertrophy is not accompanied by sufficient growth and restructuring of the coronary microvasculature; normalization of capillary-to-midmyocyte diffusion distances does not appear to occur (4). An analogous mismatch in microvascular growth is observed in pressure overload models of ventricular hypertrophy where myocyte cross-sectional area is increased dramatically and capillarity is decreased. Finally, training elicits robust effects on the reactivity of the coronary vasculature to humoral and mechanical stimuli. In a variety of animal models of exercise training, both the coronary smooth muscle and vascular endothelium appear to respond adaptively to training and in most cases, these adaptations are vasodilatory in nature (49–55). These types of adaptations likely represent physiologic mechanisms to preserve adequate regional coronary blood flow during periods of increased cardiac work.

Summary

Growth of the cardiac coronary vasculature, along with increased vasodilatory responsiveness, occur in response to chronic exercise training and enhance the ability of the heart to deliver blood to working muscle.

Beneficial Effect of Chronic Exercise in the Context of Heart Disease

Ischemic heart disease remains the leading cause of death in the industrialized world. Humans who exercise regularly are more likely to survive a myocardial infarction (56), and there appear to be several contributing factors leading to improved outcomes. First, exercise is very well known to decrease risk factors associated with heart disease, including obesity, hypertension, hyperglycemia, and hyperinsulinemia. Second, in animal models exposed to experimental ischemia/reperfusion, the pumping function of the heart is better maintained in the face of an ischemic event (45,57). Third, the amount of tissue injury after infarction (infarct size) is much smaller in exercise trained versus sedentary hearts. This adaptation has been observed in a variety of animals and is particularly important in promoting long-term survival after an infarction (58). Fourth, exercise training has been shown to reduce the incidence of arrhythmia during ischemia (59). Finally, beneficial adaptations in coronary reactivity (as described previously) enhance the hyperemic response and quickly restore coronary flow after a myocardial infarction. Exercise clearly represents one of the most robust nonpharmacologic interventions that promotes both short- and long-term health benefits for the heart.

TEST YOURSELF

Of all the information provided in this chapter, what do you consider the most important fact or facts about cardiac adaptations to regular exercise, which explains a reduced death rate in people who are physcially active?

A MILESTONE OF DISCOVERY

With the disclaimer that singling out specific "milestones of discovery" is a contrivance that risks doing disservice to the many giant contributions to the field of muscle physiology, we provide a point of view on two works that have added significantly to our understanding of how cardiac contractile force is dynamically regulated in the cardiac cycle.

The cellular basis for Starling's law of the heart is often described in the context of the classic work of Gordon and Huxley (18) where they elegantly demonstrated that in frog skeletal muscle, the length–tension relationship could be attributed to the degree of thin–thick filament overlap in the sarcomere. However, in cardiac muscle, although the same principles of sarcomere geometry certainly apply, Allen et al. (19) observed that the steepness of the ascending limb of the length–tension relationship of cardiac muscle was much greater than that observed in skeletal muscle. This observation defied explanation solely by the principles of the sliding filament theory, and it was proposed that activation processes of some sort contributed to this difference. Subsequent to this key observation, Hibberd and Jewell (21) demonstrated a marked length dependence in the cardiac $[Ca^{2+}]$–tension relationship. Specifically, at longer (e.g., end-diastolic) sarcomere lengths, the sensitivity of the contractile element to activation by Ca^{2+} was significantly greater than that occurring at shorter (e.g., end-systolic) sarcomere lengths. In addition, Allen and

Kurihara (24) conducted experiments demonstrating that in the physiologic sarcomere length range, there was a direct relationship between the magnitude of the intracellular $[Ca^{2+}]$ transient and sarcomere length.

Collectively, these observations were important for several key reasons. First, it is now clear that across sarcomere lengths that occur physiologically (i.e., between end systole and end diastole), only part (approximately <50%) of the length-dependent regulation of cardiac contractile force can be explained in the context of the sliding filament theory. Second, the marked length dependencies of Ca^{2+} release to the contractile element and the sensitivity of the contractile element to activation by Ca^{2+}, provide viable explanations for the steepness of the ascending limb of the cardiac muscle length–tension relationship. Third, and most importantly, this also provides for an elegant and powerful scheme of regulation, whereby cardiac contractile force development is optimized once the heart fills with blood, and the processes favoring relaxation are optimized after blood has been ejected.

Allen DG, Kurihara S. The effects of muscle length on intracellular calcium transients in mammalian cardiac muscle. J Physiol. 1982;327:79–94.

Hibberd MB, Jewell BR. Calcium- and length-dependent force production in rat ventricular muscle. J Physiol. 1982;329:527–40.

CHAPTER SUMMARY

In this chapter we described the effect of exercise on cardiac function. Adaptations in HR and SV are discussed as mediating increased CO during exercise. Further, several distinct adaptations are found in hearts from animals that have been chronically exercise trained, resulting in enhanced SV and improved CO. Although the benefits of exercise on the intact heart function have been well characterized, much work needs to be done to identify cellular and subcellular adaptations that contribute to training-induced adaptations in HR and SV.

ACKNOWLEDGMENTS

We would like to express thanks to Drs. Douglas R. Seals and Robert Mazzeo for their useful and insightful discussions. We would also like to acknowledge Ruben C. Sloan III and Chad R. Frasier for valuable editorial contributions.

REFERENCES

1. Rowell LB. *Human Cardiovascular Control.* New York: Oxford University Press; 1993:162–479.
2. Saltin B, Blomqvist G, Mitchell JH, et al. Response to exercise after bed rest and after training: a longitudinal study of adaptive changes in oxygen transport and body composition. *Circulation.* 1968;38:1–78.
3. Saltin B, Rowell LB. Functional adaptations to physical activity and inactivity. *Fed Proc.* 1980;39:1506–1513.
4. Moore R, Korzick D. Cellular adaptations of the myocardium to chronic exercise. *Prog Cardiovasc Dis.* 1995;37(6):371–396.
5. Katz AM. *Physiology of the Heart.* 2nd ed. New York: Raven Press; 1992:687.
6. Demir SS, Clark JW, Giles WR. Parasympathetic modulation of sinoatrial node pacemaker activity in rabbit heart: a unifying model. *Am J Physiol.* 1999;276(45):H2221–H2244.
7. Lipsius SL, Huser J, Blatter LA. Intracellular Ca^{2+} release sparks atrial pacemaker activity. *News Physiol Sci.* 2001;16:101–106.
8. Trautwein W. Cellular pacemakers. In: Carpenter D, ed. *I. Mechanisms and Pacemaker Generation.* New York: Wiley; 1981:127–160.
9. Hammond HK, White FC, Brunton LL, et al. Association of decreased myocardial β-receptors and chronotropic response to isoproterenol and exercise in pigs following chronic dynamic exercise. *Circ Res.* 1987;60(5):720–726.
10. Hammond HK, Ransas LA, Insel PA. Noncoordinate regulation of cardiac G_s protein and β-adrenergic receptors by a physiological stimulus, chronic dynamic exercise. *J Clin Invest.* 1988;82:2168–2171.
11. Schaefer ME, Allert JA, Adams HR, et al. Adrenergic responsiveness and intrinsic sinoatrial automaticity of exercise-trained rats. *Med Sci Sports Exerc.* 1992;24(8):887–894.
12. Brown DA, Chicco AJ, Jew KN, et al. Cardioprotection afforded by chronic exercise is mediated by the sarcolemmal, and not the mitochondrial, isoform of the KATP channel in the rat. *J Physiol.* 2005;569:913–924.
13. Poliner LR, Dehmer GJ, Lewis SE, et al. Left ventricular performance in normal subjects: a comparison of the responses to exercise in the upright and supine positions. *Circulation.* 1980;62:528–534.

14. Bers DM. *Excitation-Contraction Coupling and Cardiac Contractile Force*. 2nd ed. Dordrecht, The Netherlands: Kluwer Academic Publishers; 2001:427.

15. Korzick DH. Regulation of cardiac excitation-contraction coupling: a cellular update. *Adv Physiol Educ*. 2003;27:192–200.

16. Marks AR. Cardiac intracellular calcium release channels: role in heart failure. *Circ Res*. 2000;87:8–11.

17. Bers DM. Cardiac excitation-contraction coupling. *Nature*. 2002;415:198–205.

18. Gordon AM, Huxley AF, Julian FJ. The variation in isometric tension with sarcomere length in vertebrate muscle fibres. *J Physiol*. 1966;184:170–192.

19. Allen DG, Jewell BR, Murray JW. The contribution of activation processes to the length tension relation in cardiac muscle. *Nature*. 1974;248:606–607.

20. Solaro RJ, Wise RM, Shiner JS, et al. Calcium requirement for cardiac myofibrillar activation. *Circ Res*. 1974;34:525–530.

21. Hibberd MG, Jewell BR. Calcium- and length-dependent force production in rat ventricular muscle. *J Physiol*. 1982;329:527–540.

22. Kentish JC, ter Keurs HE, Ricciardi L, et al. Comparison between the sarcomere length-force relations of intact and skinned trabeculae from rat right ventricle. *Circ Res*. 1986;58:755–768.

23. Fabiato A. Calcium release in skinned cardiac cells: variations with species, tissues, and development. *Fed Proc*. 1982;41:2238–2244.

24. Allen DG, Kurihara S. The effects of muscle length on intracellular calcium transients in mammalian cardiac muscle. *J Physiol*. 1982;327:79–94.

25. Woodworth RS. Maximal contraction, "staircase" contraction, refractory period, and compensatory pause of the heart. *Am J Physiol*. 1902;8:213–249.

26. Bowditch HP. Uber die eigenthumlichkeiten der reizbarkeit, welche die muskelfasem des herzens zeigen. *Ber Sachs Ges Wiss*. 1871;23:652–689.

27. Yatani A, Codina J, Imoto Y, et al. A G protein directly regulates mammalian cardiac calcium channels. *Science*. 1987;238:1288–1292.

28. Fabiato A. Stimulated calcium current can both cause calcium loading in and trigger calcium release from the sarcoplasmic reticulum of a skinned canine Purkinje cell. *J Gen Physiol*. 1985;85:291–320.

29. Unitt JF, McCormack JG, Reid D, et al. Direct evidence for a role of intramitochondrial Ca2+ in the regulation of oxidative phosphorylation in the stimulated rat heart. Studies using 31P n.m.r. and ruthenium red. *Biochem J*. 1989;262(1):293–301.

30. David H, Meyer R, Marx I, et al. Morphometric characterization of left ventricular myocardial cells of male rats during postnatal development. *J Mol Cell Cardiol*. 1979;11(7):631–638.

31. Schaper J, Meiser E, Stammler G. Ultrastructural morphometric analysis of myocardium from dogs, rats, hamsters, mice, and from human hearts. *Circ Res*. 1985;56(3):377–391.

32. Clark BJ III, Acker MA, McCully K, et al. In vivo 31P-NMR spectroscopy of chronically stimulated canine skeletal muscle. *Am J Physiol*. 1988;254(2 pt 1):C258–C266.

33. Wollenberger A. Relation between work and labile phosphate content in the isolated dog heart. *Circ Res*. 1957;5(2):175–178.

34. Balaban RS. Domestication of the cardiac mitochondrion for energy conversion. *J Mol Cell Cardiol*. 2009;46:832–841.

35. Ringer S. A further contribution regarding the influence of the different constituents of the blood on the contraction of the heart. *J Physiol*. 1883;4(1):29–42.3.

36. Territo PR, Mootha VK, French SA, et al. Ca(2+) activation of heart mitochondrial oxidative phosphorylation: role of the F(0)/F(1)-ATPase. *Am J Physiol Cell Physiol*. 2000;278(2):C423–C435.

37. Schaible TF, Scheuer J. Cardiac adaptations to chronic exercise. *Prog Cardiovasc Dis*. 1985;27(5):297–324.

38. Scheuer J, Tipton CM. Cardiovascular adaptations to physical training. *Annu Rev Physiol*. 1977;39:221–251.

39. Moore RL, Palmer BM. Exercise training and cellular adaptations of normal and diseased hearts. *Exerc Sport Sci Rev*. 1999;27:285–315.

40. Lakatta EG. Cardiovascular regulatory mechanisms in advanced age. *Physiol Rev*. 1993;73(2):413–467.

41. Baldwin KM, Cooke DA, Cheadle WG. Time course adaptations in cardiac and skeletal muscle to different running programs. *J Appl Physiol*. 1977;42(2):267–272.

42. Laughlin MH, Hale CC, Novela L, et al. Biochemical characterization of exercise-trained porcine myocardium. *J Appl Physiol*. 1991;71(1):229–235.

43. Liu J, Yeo HC, Overvik-Douki E, et al. Chronically and acutely exercised rats: biomarkers of oxidative stress and endogenous antioxidants. *J Appl Physiol*. 2000;89(1):21–28.

44. Starnes JW, Taylor RP, Park Y. Exercise improves postischemic function in aging hearts. *Am J Physiol Heart Circ Physiol*. 2003;285(1):H347–H351.

45. Brown DA, Jew KN, Sparagna GC, et al. Exercise training preserves coronary flow and reduces infarct size after ischemia-reperfusion in rat heart. *J Appl Physiol*. 2003;95(6):2510–2518.

46. Diffee GM, Seversen EA, Titus MM. Exercise training increases the Ca^{2+} sensitivity of tension in rat cardiac myocytes. *J Appl Physiol*. 2001;91:309–315.

47. Diffee GM, Nagle DF. Exercise training alters the length dependence of contractile properties in rat myocardium. *J Appl Physiol*. 2003;94:1137–1144.

48. Natali AJ, Wilson LA, Peckham M, et al. Different regional effects of voluntary exercise on the mechanical and electrical properties of rat ventricular myocytes. *J Physiol*. 2002;541:863–875.

49. Laughlin MH, Oltman CL, Bowles DK. Exercise training-induced adaptations in the coronary circulation. *Med Sci Sports Exerc*. 1998;30:352–360.

50. Laughlin MH, et al. Adaptation of coronary circulation to exercise training. In: Fletcher GF, ed. *Cardiovascular Response to Exercise*. Mount Kisco, NY: Futura Publishing Company, Inc; 1994:175–205.

51. Bowles DK, Woodman CR, Laughlin MH. Coronary smooth muscle and endothelial adaptations to exercise training. *Exerc Sport Sci Rev*. 2000;28:57–62.

52. Laughlin MH, Overholser KA, Bhatte MJ. Exercise training increases coronary transport reserve in miniature swine. *J Appl Physiol*. 1989;67(3):1140–1149.

53. Laughlin MH, Tomanek RJ. Myocardial capillarity and maximal capillary diffusion capacity in exercise-trained dogs. *J Appl Physiol*. 1987;63(4):1481–1486.

54. Laughlin MH, McAllister RM. Exercise training-induced coronary vascular adaptation. *J Appl Physiol*. 1992;73(6):2209–2225.

55. Laughlin MH, Rubin LJ, Rush JW, et al. Short-term training enhances endothelium-dependent dilation of coronary arteries, not arterioles. *J Appl Physiol*. 2003;94:234–244.

56. Morris JN, Everitt MG, Pollard R, et al. Vigorous exercise in leisure-time: protection against coronary heart disease. *Lancet*. 1980;2(8206):1207–1210.

57. Bowles DK, Farrar RP, Starnes JW. Exercise training improves cardiac function after ischemia in the isolated, working rat heart. *Am J Physiol*. 1992;263:H804–H809.

58. Brown DA, Moore RL. Perspectives in innate and acquired cardioprotection: cardioprotection acquired through exercise. *J Appl Physiol*. 2007;103(5):1894–1899.

59. Hamilton KL, Quindry JC, French JP, et al. MnSOD antisense treatment and exercise-induced protection against arrhythmias. *Free Radic Biol Med*. 2004;37(9):1360–1368.

CHAPTER 11

Organization and Control of Circulation to Skeletal Muscle

Steven S. Segal and Shawn E. Bearden

Abbreviations

ATP	Adenosine triphosphate	SNA	Sympathetic nerve activity
IP_3	Inositol trisphosphate	TA	Terminal arteriole
MVU	Microvascular unit	VOCCs	Voltage-operated Ca^{++} channels
RBCs	Red blood cells	$\dot{V}O_2$	Oxygen consumption

Introduction

Blood flow to skeletal muscle is dictated by the perfusion pressure across the vascular bed and the total resistance presented by vessel branches. With arterial and venous pressures maintained, changes in muscle blood flow are governed through changes in vascular resistance, which resides primarily in the precapillary vasculature (see *A Milestone of Discovery* at the end of this chapter). Through relaxation of vascular smooth muscle, the magnitude of blood flowing through skeletal muscle can increase from approximately 5 mL · min · 100 g^{-1} at rest to more than 250 mL · min · 100 g^{-1} during aerobic exercise. This functional, or exercise, hyperemia represents a dynamic range of 50-fold or more (1,2). The positive relationships among muscle contraction, oxygen consumption ($\dot{V}O_2$), and blood flow indicate that the convection and diffusion of oxygen from the vasculature are related intimately to energy expenditure. Moreover, the elevation of blood flow in response to contractile activity demonstrates the intrinsic coupling between skeletal muscle and its vascular supply.

Blood flow to skeletal muscle is also determined by the activity of the sympathetic nervous system and the need to maintain systemic blood pressure. Indeed, sympathetic vasoconstriction diverts flow from inactive tissues to redistribute (as well as enhance) cardiac output to active skeletal muscle (3). Considerable knowledge has been gained in understanding the regulation of muscle blood flow during exercise and its adaptations to physical training (2). The goal of this chapter is to illustrate the functional organization of the vascular supply to skeletal muscle and explore how muscle blood flow is controlled in light of the physical determinants of oxygen delivery to active muscle fibers during exercise.

Organization of the Vascular Supply

The Microcirculation is a Highly Branched Network

Understanding how the peripheral vasculature is organized anatomically is integral to understanding the nature of blood flow control to skeletal muscle. Upon leaving the heart, the convection of blood through large conduit vessels (*e.g.*, brachial and femoral arteries) rapidly conveys blood to peripheral tissues with minimal hemodynamic resistance. The vascular resistance to blood flow begins with the small muscular feed arteries that are external to skeletal muscles and arise from the larger conduit arteries. Feed arteries are positioned to control the total amount of blood entering the muscle and can present half of the total resistance to blood flow (4). When maximally dilated, the diameter of feed arteries ranges from 100 to several hundred micrometers in rodents and on the order of millimeters in muscles of humans and larger animals.

Because feed arteries are located external to the muscle, they are physically removed from vasoactive stimuli produced by skeletal muscle fibers.

Upon entering skeletal muscle, feed arteries give rise to arteriolar networks, which provide the major resistance to blood flow. The primary arterioles, which arise from feed arteries, typically branch into second- and third-order arterioles (Fig. 11.1). These intermediate branches distribute blood throughout the muscle and thereby control regional tissue perfusion. In some muscles, anastomoses between arteriolar branches provide alternative pathways for the delivery of blood. Arising from the distributing arterioles are the fourth-order arterioles and terminal arterioles (TA), which control the perfusion of capillaries with red blood cells (RBCs) (5). The effluent blood from capillaries drains into collecting venules, which converge into progressively larger branches that often course along arterioles as they carry blood back toward the heart (Fig. 11.1). The maximal (dilated) diameter of arterioles declines with successive orders of branching, ranging from more than 100 μm in proximal (1A) branches to 10 to 15 μm in distal (TA) branches (6). The mechanisms and signaling pathways underlying the coordination of vasodilation along branches of arteriolar networks and their feed arteries are considered later in this chapter.

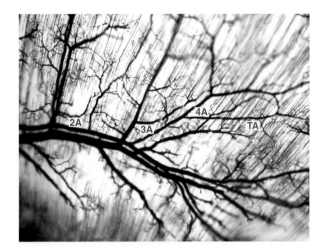

FIGURE 11.1 Arteriolar and venular networks are paired in skeletal muscle. A vascular cast of the mouse gluteus maximus muscle begins with the second-order arterioles (*2A*) to illustrate network branching into third-order (*3A*) and fourth-order (*4A*) arterioles. The primary arteriole and feed artery, which are proximal to *2A*, are not shown. Venules (not labeled) are often paired with arterioles, particularly in the larger proximal branches. Distal arterioles diverge from venules and form microvascular units (see Fig. 11.5). TA, terminal arteriole.

Because of their circumferential orientation, contraction of smooth muscle cells causes vasoconstriction, thereby reducing vessel diameter and increasing the resistance to blood flow. Conversely, relaxation of smooth muscle cells causes vasodilation, thereby increasing diameter and the conductance for blood flow (6). Resistance vessels assume a smooth and cylindrical shape when they are fully dilated. However, longitudinal ridges and folds form along the intima during smooth muscle cell shortening and vasoconstriction (7). This inward deformation

Resistance Vessels are Composed of Smooth Muscle Lined by Endothelium and Surrounded by Sympathetic Nerves

The primary physiologic mechanism for controlling blood flow is through changes in the diameter of resistance vessels, which is determined by the contractile status of vascular smooth muscle cells. The media of arterioles and feed arteries typically contains a single layer of smooth muscle cells. Adjacent smooth muscle cells form a continuous layer throughout much of the resistance network but can become discontinuous in distal arteriolar branches. Individual smooth muscle cells are about 5 μm in diameter and can exceed 100 μm in length when fully relaxed. Thus, a single smooth muscle cell can wrap completely around the lumen of smaller arterioles (Fig. 11.2) but do not completely circumscribe the larger proximal arterioles or feed arteries. As they encircle the vessel, each smooth muscle cell spans up to 20 adjacent endothelial cells.

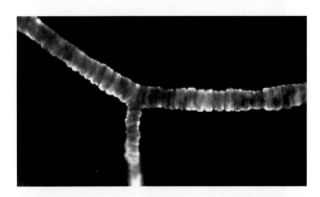

FIGURE 11.2 A continuous monolayer of arteriolar smooth muscle cells. A third-order arteriole (resting diameter, 20 μm) gives rise to a fourth-order daughter branch in the mouse gluteus maximus muscle. Smooth muscle cells are visualized by immunolabeling for α-actin. Note how each cell wraps completely around the vessel and abuts its neighbor to form a continuous monolayer surrounding the vessel lumen within.

of the vessel wall amplifies the reduction in vessel caliber during vasoconstriction.

As with all blood vessels, the intimal surface of the resistance vasculature is lined by a continuous monolayer of endothelial cells that are oriented along the vessel axis and in direct contact with blood flowing within the vessel lumen (Fig. 11.3). Individual endothelial cells of arterioles and feed arteries are 50 to 100 μm long, about 5 to 10 μm wide, and less than 1 μm thick. Each endothelial cell spans up to 20 smooth muscle cells along the vessel wall. Such spatial arrangements between respective cell layers are integral to blood flow control by coordinating vasodilator and vasoconstrictor responses through intercellular signaling. Although smooth muscle cells and endothelial cells are physically separated from each other by the internal elastic lamina, fenestrations in the internal elastic lamina enable projections from respective cells to form myoendothelial contacts (6) that enable the transfer of ions and second messenger molecules between cell layers.

Within the adventitia surrounding feed arteries and arterioles, a rich plexus of perivascular sympathetic nerve

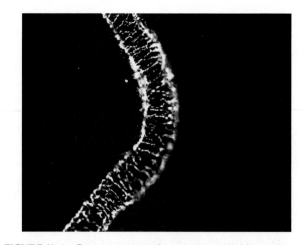

FIGURE 11.4 Resistance vessels are surrounded by sympathetic nerves. A feed artery (resting diameter, 75 μm) of the hamster retractor muscle is shown following histochemical staining for glyoxylic acid to reveal catecholamine-containing nerve fibers in the adventitia surrounding the smooth muscle cell layer. In skeletal muscle, this rich plexus of nerve fibers extends throughout the arteriolar network but not into capillaries or venules.

fibers courses over the smooth muscle cells (Fig. 11.4). During sympathetic nerve activity (SNA), norepinephrine is released (along with co-transmitters adenosine triphosphate [ATP] and neuropeptide Y; we focus here on norepinephrine) from varicosities along these nerve fibers and causes smooth muscle contraction. Capillaries are comprised of a single layer of endothelial cells, which minimizes the barrier for exchanging solutes between the blood and muscle fibers. Although individual capillaries are the smallest of all blood vessels, their total number and cross-sectional area far exceeds that of all other vessel branches. Thus, capillaries have the lowest total resistance and greatest surface area of the entire vascular tree. Beyond the capillaries, smooth muscle cells return in the venules. Although venules in skeletal muscle are not directly innervated, spillover of norepinephrine released around nearby arterioles or carried in the bloodstream can constrict venular smooth muscle cells, reducing capacitance and promoting venous return of blood to the heart (8). Capillaries and venules are also the primary loci for regulating vascular permeability and inflammation, which are not considered further here.

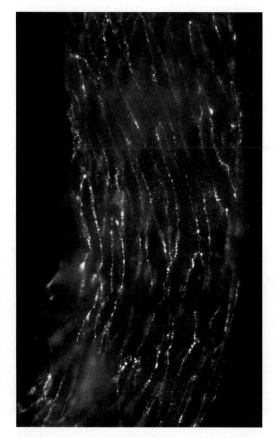

FIGURE 11.3 A continuous monolayer of endothelial cells lines the lumen of all blood vessels. Shown is a feed artery (resting diameter, 75 μm) of the hamster retractor muscle following immunolabeling for connexin-43, a protein that is integral to the formation of gap junction channels at the borders of endothelial cells in feed arteries and arterioles. Cell-to-cell coupling via gap junction channels enables electrical signals to travel rapidly along the vessel wall.

Summary

The control of blood flow in the microcirculation is dictated by the contraction and relaxation of vascular smooth muscle cells in arterioles and their feeding arteries. Under resting conditions, smooth muscle cells are partially contracted in a state of spontaneous vasomotor tone. From this resting baseline, smooth muscle cells can either relax to increase blood flow (vasodilation) or contract to reduce blood flow (vasoconstriction). The endothelial cells forming the intima are in contact with the flowing blood and promote vasodilation by signaling smooth muscle cells to relax. Sympathetic nerve fibers surrounding smooth muscle cells cause vasoconstriction when they are activated to release norepinephrine. Because of its essential role in blood flow control during exercise, the regulation of vasomotor tone is a central theme of this chapter. In venules, smooth muscle cell contraction reduces capacitance and promotes the return of effluent blood from capillaries back to the heart.

Capillaries are Organized into Microvascular Units

The functional unit of blood flow control can be defined as the smallest volume of tissue to which oxygen delivery can be independently controlled (9). In skeletal muscle, this functional entity is the microvascular unit (MVU), which consists of all of the capillaries arising from a common TA. The branching of a TA into a group of capillaries and the control of their perfusion by their parent TA is analogous to the branching of a single motor neuron to control a group of muscle fibers within a motor unit. TAs are typically oriented perpendicular to muscle fibers, giving rise to a group of about 20 capillaries that course between and along muscle fibers for a distance of about 1 mm in each direction (often with intercapillary anastomoses) and then empty into collecting venules (Fig. 11.5). The volume of muscle tissue within a MVU is about 0.1 mm^3, with average dimensions of 1 to 2 mm long, 0.5 mm wide, and 0.2 mm thick. These dimensions result in 10 to 20 MVUs per cubic millimeter (or milligram) of intact skeletal muscle. The volume of muscle supplied by each MVU contains segments of about 20 muscle fibers. However, because individual muscle fibers within a motor unit are dispersed throughout a larger cross-sectional area of the muscle, the adjacent muscle fibers within the tissue volume perfused by each MVU are typically derived from different motor units. As a result of these differences in their spatial organization, a particular capillary or MVU may have from one to several adjacent muscle fibers consuming oxygen at a given moment, according to respective patterns of MVU perfusion and motor unit recruitment (10).

The perfusion of capillaries with RBCs is not controlled at the level of individual capillaries. Instead, each TA serves as the functional equivalent of a precapillary sphincter by being the last branch of the arteriolar network with smooth muscle cells that actively control vessel diameter. Thus, constriction of a TA prevents the entire group of capillaries within an MVU from receiving blood flow, whereas dilation of a TA results in perfusion of the entire MVU (5). However, the distribution of RBCs within a MVU is not uniform among capillaries; it is determined passively by differences in the physical determinants of RBC entry into each capillary (11) and variations in the hemodynamic resistance of respective capillary segments, attributable to corresponding differences in their lengths and branching characteristics (12).

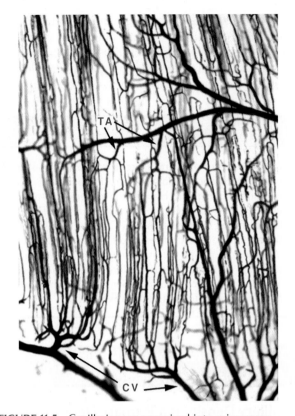

FIGURE 11.5   Capillaries are organized into microvascular units (MVUs) along skeletal muscle fibers. Microscopic examination of a vascular cast near a thin edge of the mouse gluteus maximus muscle shows terminal arterioles (TAs) giving rise to groups of capillaries that extend for about 1 mm and converge on collecting venules. A TA typically gives rise to capillaries in both directions along muscle fibers. Furthermore, collecting venules (CV) typically receive blood from capillaries that originate from more than one TA. As muscle thickness increases, MVUs stack on top of and next to each other, making it difficult to resolve capillaries associated with individual MVUs.

Each Muscle Fiber Spans Multiple Microvascular Units

Individual striated muscle fibers are typically several centimeters long, which contrasts with the 1- to 2-mm distance that is spanned by each MVU. Because metabolic demand increases along the entire length of an active muscle fiber, the perfusion of multiple MVUs is required to deliver oxygen and nutrients to each muscle fiber. In turn, because muscle fibers of each motor unit are dispersed through the muscle, the firing of a motor neuron will result in perfusion of far more capillaries than needed to supply only the active fibers, particularly at low levels of motor unit recruitment (10). This functional organization precludes any selective increase in blood flow to only those muscle fibers that are active. Within the muscle, individual MVUs are situated next to each other (5). This arrangement results in blood flow being concurrent between some capillaries (e.g., those arising in the same direction from TAs) while being countercurrent between capillaries arising in the opposite direction along muscle fibers. In turn, the proximity of adjacent MVUs promotes oxygen diffusion between neighboring capillaries that can offset local heterogeneities in oxygen delivery.

TEST YOURSELF

Blood flow control during exercise is dependent on the functional organization of the microcirculation as well as that of skeletal muscle. How do the anatomy and physiology of an MVU determine the spatial domain of capillary perfusion in skeletal muscle? Conversely, how does the anatomy of muscle fibers and distribution of motor units correspond to the architecture of their vascular supply? In light of this organization, what requirements are imposed on the microcirculation for increasing blood flow to active motor units during exercise?

Oxygen is Transported from Microvessels to Muscle Fibers

Capillary Density is a Primary Determinant of Oxygen Diffusion

Early in the twentieth century, August Krogh proposed that each capillary supplies oxygen to a cylindrical region of muscle fibers surrounding it (13). This Krogh cylinder model of oxygen diffusion has dominated much of the thinking about the supply and utilization of oxygen in skeletal muscle. Krogh based many of his conclusions on spatial relationships determined in muscle cross-sections, which remains a common practice today. Thus, the ability of the microcirculation to present oxygen to muscle fibers is typically evaluated in terms of capillary density (number of capillaries per square millimeter) or as the capillary-to-fiber ratio in cross-sections of whole muscles or muscle biopsies (14). Human skeletal muscle fibers typically have one or two capillaries in contact at each point along their length (14). Although it is well established that the capillary supply and vascular transport capacity of skeletal muscle are enhanced in response to physical training (14), it has not yet been resolved whether branches of the arteriolar network increase in proportion to capillarity. With respect to the control of capillary perfusion discussed previously, an important issue that still remains for future research is to resolve whether individual MVUs increase in size, total number, or both.

The capillary-to-fiber ratio can be remarkably consistent among muscles (or muscle regions) in the presence of large differences in capillary density. This property is explained by corresponding differences in the diameter of muscle fibers. For example, the distance between capillaries will be less for type I muscle fibers (slow oxidative), which have a small diameter, than for type IIB muscle fibers (fast glycolytic), which have a larger diameter (14). The capillary supply of skeletal

muscle considered in three dimensions is more accurately expressed in terms of volume density, that is, the total volume of capillaries per volume of muscle (15), because this estimate accounts for capillary anastomoses and tortuosity that are not apparent in individual tissue cross-sections.

KEY POINT

The capillary supply of skeletal muscle is described in several ways, the most common being capillary density and the capillary-to-fiber ratio. With no change in capillary supply, changes in muscle fiber diameter will have a reciprocal effect on capillary density.

An increase in metabolic rate will lower intracellular Po_2 in myocytes and increase the gradient for oxygen diffusion from the capillary to respiring mitochondria within muscle fibers. Once capillary Po_2 falls below a critical level, $\dot{V}o_2$ becomes limited by blood (i.e., RBC) flow through the capillary (16). The occurrence of flow-limited $\dot{V}o_2$ can be delayed by perfusing additional capillaries (i.e., dilating TAs that control MVUs) as metabolic demand increases. In response to physical conditioning, capillary proliferation further reduces the distance and increases the surface area for oxygen diffusion. As a result, capillary Po_2 can fall to lower levels and still maintain myocyte Po_2 above limiting values. This explains why an increase in capillary volume density enhances oxygen flux from blood to muscle fibers and supports the aerobic production of ATP through oxidative phosphorylation. Nevertheless, structural indices alone cannot fully describe the physiologic properties of capillary networks or the diffusion of oxygen from blood to muscle fibers.

TEST YOURSELF

Exercise training can increase the capillary-to-fiber ratio in the recruited skeletal muscles. In light of motor unit architecture, what are the structural adaptations in microvascular network organization that may account for this effect of training? How would such adaptations influence the control processes of blood flow to active (and inactive) motor units? What experiment(s) would you design to determine how such adaptation of the microcirculation actually occurs?

Red Blood Cell Transit Time in Capillaries is a Determinant of Oxygen Extraction

The duration that RBCs remain within the capillaries is known as the capillary transit time. It is proportional to the length of the path taken by a RBC from TA to collecting venule and inversely proportional to flow velocity (12). Intuitively, transit time affects the degree to which the oxygen content of the capillary blood can be lowered; that is, longer transit times should facilitate oxygen extraction. At any given level of blood flow, transit time is also influenced by the total number (volume) of capillaries perfused. Acutely, this can be altered through MVU recruitment by dilating TAs and over time by increasing the number of capillaries through physical training (14). Thus, increasing the total number (volume density) of perfused capillaries will prolong transit times as a result of the greater cross-sectional area in which RBCs are distributed. These adaptations allow skeletal muscle to take greater advantage of the other circulatory responses to exercise training (e.g., greater muscle blood flow with increased oxygen-carrying capacity per unit of blood).

Measurements of total muscle blood flow and the estimated capillary density per unit volume of biopsied tissue have led to calculated mean capillary transit times of several seconds at rest to less than 1 second during heavy exercise. However, the idea of a mean capillary transit time is misleading, because it treats the flow of RBCs through capillaries as homogeneous. Direct observations using intravital microscopy have revealed both temporal and spatial heterogeneity in the flow of RBCs through capillary networks. Indeed, actual flow path lengths taken by RBCs (e.g., through interconnecting capillary anastomoses) can be considerably greater than direct anatomical path lengths, resulting in a broad distribution of values for capillary transit time as well as for RBC flux (cells per second) and capillary flow path length (12). These dynamic rheologic properties of blood flow suggest that individual capillaries are not uniform in their ability to supply oxygen to the surrounding tissue, although such heterogeneity in capillary perfusion can be offset by the diffusional interactions within and among neighboring MVUs.

The RBC Content of Capillaries Increases during Hyperemia

The volume fraction of a capillary that is occupied by RBCs is referred to as "tube hematocrit" and varies with the vasomotor state of resistance vessels and with the metabolic demand of muscle fibers (16). Capillary tube hematocrit is calculated from the number of RBCs per unit of capillary length by accounting for the volume of individual RBCs relative to the total volume within the capillary lumen. Because RBCs are the source of oxygen in the bloodstream capillary tube hematocrit provides an index of capillary oxygen content at any given moment. Capillary tube hematocrit can be less than 20% of systemic hematocrit in resting muscle, but during hyperemia it increases rapidly to approximate that of the systemic circulation (16). Thus, the oxygen content of a capillary will increase with the number of RBCs it contains, which has the effect of maintaining a higher P_{O_2} along the capillary at a given level of tissue $\dot{V}_{O_2}$. Further, by reducing plasma gaps between RBCs, an increase in capillary hematocrit during high $\dot{V}_{O_2}$ can augment the effective capillary surface for oxygen diffusion to mitochondria

within the muscle fibers even with no change in the total number of capillaries perfused (16).

Changes in capillary tube hematocrit are explained by the presence of a glycocalyx on the luminal surface of the capillary endothelial cells that can change its thickness according to the rate of capillary blood flow. At rest (i.e., with low tube hematocrit), this glycocalyx results in a layer of stabilized plasma adjacent to the capillary wall that is nearly a micrometer thick and excludes RBCs. Remarkably, the thickness of this cell-free layer (i.e., of the glycocalyx) is diminished during hyperemia, when the flux of RBCs and capillary tube hematocrit increase during arteriolar dilation. In addition to enabling more of the capillary volume to fill with RBCs, the diffusion distance between RBCs and muscle fibers is reduced because the RBCs are closer to the capillary wall. Although capillary diameter is typically not considered to be a variable during exercise, this dynamic and reversible expansion of the capillary lumen can augment oxygen transport during exercise hyperemia. Thus, the ability of individual capillaries to deliver oxygen to muscle fibers is enhanced in response to an increase in metabolic demand.

TEST YOURSELF

The consumption of oxygen by muscle fibers increases with the intensity of aerobic exercise. What corresponding changes occur in the ability of individual capillaries to supply oxygen for surrounding muscle fibers? How can such behavior be explained in light of RBC hemodynamic responses, RBCs as determinants of oxygen diffusion from capillaries to tissue, and the role of RBCs in the local control of blood flow? Do adaptations to aerobic training affect any of these parameters and, if so, how?

Oxygen Diffuses Out of Arterioles and between Microvessels

Inherent to the idea that the capillary is the source of oxygen delivery to the tissue is the assumption that the oxygen content of blood decreases progressively along the capillary. However, studies of the living microcirculation reveal this to be an oversimplification (17). For example, countercurrent flow of RBCs in overlapping diffusion fields from adjacent MVUs may lead to mixing of capillary P_{O_2} rather than a progressive arterial-to-venous P_{O_2} gradient along each capillary. Indeed, mean P_{O_2} within individual capillaries, as well as arterioles and venules, can increase as well as decrease within 1 second, attributable to the gain and loss of oxygen to and from neighboring microvessels by diffusion. Further, RBCs can release substantive amounts of oxygen as they travel along arterioles before even reaching the capillaries (17). This should not be surprising because the single layer of smooth muscle cells surrounding the endothelial cells presents little barrier to the diffusion of oxygen across the arteriolar wall.

KEY POINT

Oxygen can diffuse freely between arterioles, capillaries, and venules according to their physical proximity to each other and local P_{O_2} gradients. The diffusion of oxygen between microvessels helps to buffer steep gradients in P_{O_2} within the tissue.

Although the P_{O_2} of venous blood reflects the extraction of oxygen within the muscle, it does not provide an accurate index of the local gradients driving oxygen diffusion from RBCs to mitochondria. For example, any variation in the flux of oxygen from individual capillaries (*e.g.*, due to changes in the velocity, flux, or spacing of RBCs) would be masked in a time-averaged blood sample. In turn, when capillaries supplied from different TAs empty into a common collecting venule, the returning blood from respective MVUs mixes and reaches some intermediate level of P_{O_2}. This homogenization is cumulative as venules converge and carry blood back toward the heart. Superimposed on the temporal and spatial mixing of postcapillary blood is the diffusion of oxygen from capillaries and arterioles in physical proximity to venules, which may set a lower limit on the amount of oxygen that can actually be extracted from the blood. Nevertheless, these diffusive interactions between microvessels help to offset local heterogeneities in oxygen content and tissue P_{O_2}.

Our focus on the control of blood flow through the peripheral circulation in terms of oxygen transport raises the question whether oxygen delivery or tissue P_{O_2} are actually regulated. In skeletal muscle, arteriolar diameter changes with ambient oxygen tension, constricting with an increase in P_{O_2} and dilating with a fall in P_{O_2}. This intrinsic response demonstrates that the resistance microvasculature is indeed sensitive to the balance between oxygen supply and demand. Remarkably, rather than changes in tissue P_{O_2} providing the vasoactive stimulus, the RBC itself may act as the oxygen sensor. Through this proposed mechanism, as RBCs enter a region of increased metabolic demand relative to supply and release oxygen, the fall in hemoglobin saturation evokes the release of a vasodilator substance (*e.g.*, ATP) to promote arteriolar dilation and thereby increase the local delivery of oxygen (18).

In contrast to being tightly regulated (*i.e.*, within a few Torr), tissue P_{O_2} in skeletal muscle has a broad distribution (19) that can shift according to local changes in oxygen supply and consumption. Within myocytes, particularly those adapted to endurance exercise (and those of diving mammals; see Chapter 25), the presence of myoglobin can help to buffer intracellular P_{O_2} above the level required to support mitochondrial respiration. Nevertheless, with respect to whether the peripheral circulation can support aerobic metabolism, the critical issue is whether (and, if so, how much of) the distribution of muscle P_{O_2} falls below that which supports the aerobic production of ATP.

Summary

The perfusion of capillaries with RBCs is not controlled at the level of individual capillaries in skeletal muscle. Instead, RBC perfusion into groups of about 20 capillaries is controlled by a TA with each group functioning as an MVU. Capillaries within each MVU can arise in either direction along muscle fibers from a common TA. Oxygen can diffuse between adjacent MVUs, and between arterioles and venules in close proximity. This intervessel diffusion helps to reduce local gradients in tissue P_{O_2}. Each MVU supplies a bundle of about 20 adjacent muscle fibers that originate from different motor units, but only along a short distance of 1 to 2 mm. In turn, each muscle fiber requires many MVUs to be perfused to deliver oxygen along its entire length. Capillary density describes the number of capillaries per muscle fiber. With greater capillary density, there is more surface area and shorter distances to for oxygen to diffuse from RBCs to mitochondria. As MVU perfusion increases during hyperemia, the spacing of RBCs within capillaries decreases because the thickness of the endothelial cell glycocalyx is diminished. This increased capillary hematocrit enhances the amount of oxygen that can be delivered per unit length of each capillary. When RBCs release oxygen in a region of low P_{O_2}, they can also release ATP that acts as a vasodilator to increase local blood flow and oxygen delivery.

Blood Flow is Controlled in Response to the Metabolic Demand of Skeletal Muscle Fibers

We now explore how blood flow is controlled in response to the metabolic demand of muscle fibers. These regulatory mechanisms are intrinsic to skeletal muscle and its vascular supply. We then consider how the sympathetic nervous system exerts extrinsic control over the vascular supply in the context of redistribution of cardiac output and maintenance of arterial blood pressure during exercise (3). Figure 11.6 illustrates the multiple dimensions of blood flow control at rest and during activity.

Muscle Blood Flow Increases with Oxidative Capacity

Blood flow to exercising muscle is proportional to the oxidative capacity of its constituent fibers. In rats, blood flow during exercise is highest in muscles and muscle regions that are composed primarily of oxidative fibers and

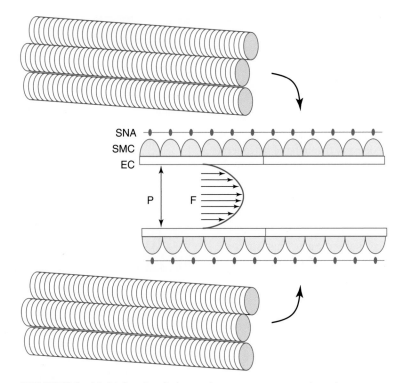

FIGURE 11.6 Multiple stimuli determine vasomotor tone in resistance vessels of skeletal muscle. Summary illustration depicts a segment of an arteriole embedded in muscle fibers (not to scale). The vessel is sectioned along its axis to show endothelial cells (EC) lining the lumen and circumscribed by smooth muscle cells (SMC), which are therefore in cross-section. In resting skeletal muscle, basal vasomotor tone reflects the interplay between two hemodynamic forces: transmural distending pressure (P), which promotes myogenic vasoconstriction, and blood flow (F) through the lumen, which exerts shear stress on the endothelium (indicated by parabolic flow profile; *arrows* indicate relative velocity) to stimulate the production of vasodilator autacoids (*e.g.*, prostacyclin and nitric oxide). Perivascular sympathetic nerve activity (SNA) increases vasomotor tone, whereas contraction of muscle fibers leads to the production of vasodilator stimuli (*curved arrows*) that reduce vasomotor tone.

lowest where fibers are primarily glycolytic (2). Differential control of blood flow in accord with muscle fiber type may be explained not only by the pattern of motor unit recruitment, but also by complementary adaptations in the architecture and reactivity of resistance vessels that supply muscles or muscle regions containing a predominance of a particular fiber type. Although human skeletal muscle characteristically lacks such regional differences in fiber type (14), this property does not preclude the ability of the vascular network to direct flow to particular muscles or muscle regions according to their capacity for oxidative metabolism and the organization of their vascular supply.

Motor Unit Recruitment Promotes Capillary Perfusion

The greater distances spanned by muscle fibers (several centimeters) as compared to MVUs (1–2 mm) implies that for capillary perfusion to increase along the fiber, a mechanism is required whereby the perfusion of multiple MVUs with RBCs is coordinated in some manner. Further, the dispersion of the individual muscle fibers belonging to each motor unit throughout a muscle implies that perfusion to regions of inactive muscle must increase in order to enhance the perfusion of capillaries associated with active fibers (10). Although it may seem wasteful to deliver RBCs to inactive muscle fibers, early perfusion of capillaries supplying inactive muscle fibers can provide a feed-forward mechanism of oxygen supply. Hence, upon the recruitment of additional motor units, the adjacent capillaries already contain RBCs, which would help to minimize any delay in elevating oxidative phosphorylation (20). Indeed, this relationship helps to explain how warm-up activity can facilitate a more rapid transition to aerobic energy production with an increase in energy expenditure. Further, rapidly increasing the functional capillary surface area facilitates the extraction of oxygen even before muscle blood flow increases significantly (1). We now consider how vasodilation is coordinated among branches of the resistance network.

Vasodilation Ascends the Resistance Network as Metabolic Demand Increases

The determinants of $\dot{V}o_2$ are expressed by the Fick relationship, which states that the oxygen consumed by a tissue is the product of its convective delivery through the peripheral circulation and its extraction through diffusion into muscle fibers. In resting skeletal muscle, the resistance vasculature maintains a high level of vasomotor tone and the extraction of oxygen from arterial blood is low relative to its oxygen content (1). With metabolic demand, the initial response is to increase the extraction of available oxygen. This is accomplished through a fall in myocyte Po_2, which increases the gradient for oxygen diffusion, along with the increase in capillary RBC perfusion upon dilation of TAs. These initial responses account for the large fall in venous Po_2 at the onset of exercise and during mild activity (1). However, greater total delivery of oxygen through the peripheral circulation is necessary to prevent a fall in tissue Po_2 below levels necessary to sustain oxidative metabolism.

Once a TA dilates and the capillaries within MVUs are perfused, the volume of blood delivered into capillaries is governed by dilation of the proximal vessel branches. Thus, as metabolic demand increases, vasodilation ascends progressively from the distal arterioles into larger arterioles and their feed arteries (21). Remember that these proximal branches govern the total amount of blood flowing into the muscle. The contributions of proximal and distal resistance vessels to the control of muscle blood flow can be represented using a simple model of resistance elements connected in series (see *A Milestone of Discovery*).

Summary

In the presence of high vasomotor tone throughout the resistance network, dilation of distal branches will increase blood flow through capillaries but hyperemia will be restricted by the resistance of proximal segments. The major increases in muscle blood flow occur when proximal vessels dilate in concert with distal vessels. The coordination of vasodilation between distal and proximal branches is intrinsic to the resistance vasculature and is essential to achieving maximal perfusion of skeletal muscle as the intensity of exercise increases. Consistent with this relationship, dilation of feed arteries as well as arterioles increases progressively with duty cycle and with motor unit recruitment (21). The integrated response of the resistance vasculature is reflected by the large increase in oxygen extraction at exercise onset and during light activity, leading to a progressive increase in total flow as workload increases (1).

TEST YOURSELF

The ability of skeletal muscle to consume oxygen can be limited by restricting the amount of oxygen delivered to the mitochondria within active muscle fibers. Under what conditions (*i.e.*, according to what criteria) would oxygen delivery from the microcirculation to muscle fibers be considered as being "flow-limited"? Is such limitation under physiologic control and, if so, how does this occur? Is there any way to alleviate such a limitation?

Multiple Signaling Pathways Govern Functional Hyperemia

Muscular activity produces a multitude of signals that contribute to functional hyperemia. No single stimulus or signaling pathway can explain the complex physiologic response of muscle blood flow to contracting muscle fibers. Instead, the initiation and maintenance of functional hyperemia reflects the integration of multiple stimuli that vary temporally as well as spatially through the resistance network. Furthermore, the effectiveness of a given stimulus can vary among vessel branches. These relationships are illustrated in Figure 11.7. The intent here is not to define the mechanism or site of action for each known stimulus but to use examples that illustrate how vascular resistance may be governed in response to a variety of signaling events. Therefore, in describing regulatory pathways, examples are intended to be conceptual rather than highly detailed.

Contraction and Relaxation of Vascular Smooth Muscle Controls Vascular Resistance

Blood flow control reflects changes in vessel diameter that result from the contraction or relaxation of smooth muscle cells comprising the media of arterioles and feed arteries. The contraction of smooth muscle typically results from an increase in the free (*i.e.*, unbound) concentration of intracellular Ca^{++}. The influx of Ca^{++} through the plasma membrane is controlled largely by voltage-operated (*e.g.*, L-type) Ca^{++} channels (VOCCs). The ionic conductance of these channels increases with depolarization and decreases with hyperpolarization. In turn, the entry of Ca^{++} through VOCCs is modulated largely through the activity of K^+ channels (Fig. 11.7). For example, as the ionic conductance of K^+ channels increases, the resulting hyperpolarization will close VOCCs and reduce intracellular Ca^{++} to promote smooth muscle cell relaxation (22).

Free intracellular Ca^{++} is also derived internally from the endoplasmic reticulum. The release of Ca^{++} from internal stores is largely independent of membrane potential and is affected via second messengers (*e.g.*, inositol-3-phosphate, IP_3) generated by receptor-mediated signaling events at the plasma membrane. Thus, events that suppress

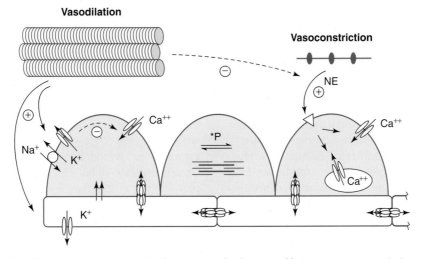

FIGURE 11.7   Multiple signaling pathways interact to determine whether vasodilation or vasoconstriction prevails during exercise. Summary illustration depicts the production of vasodilator stimuli from the contractile activity of muscle fibers and vasoconstriction through sympathetic nerve activity. Three smooth muscle cells are shown above a pair of adjacent endothelial cells (not to scale). On the left, vasodilation results from hyperpolarization of the smooth muscle cells through the activation of K^+ channels (*single arrow pointing up to left*) and/or stimulation of the Na^+/K^+ adenosine triphosphatase in their plasma membrane (*bidirectional arrows attached to circle*). Alternatively, activation of K^+ channels in endothelial cells (*vertical arrow pointing down*) can produce smooth muscle hyperpolarization by current flow through myoendothelial gap junction channels (*vertical bidirectional arrows*). Hyperpolarization of smooth muscle cells inhibits the influx of Ca^{++} across their plasma membrane through voltage-operated Ca^{++} channels (*broken arrow within smooth muscle cell at left*). Smooth muscle cell relaxation can also result from endothelial cell producing vasodilator autacoids (*double vertical arrow pointing up*). Cell-to-cell coupling between endothelial cells through gap junction channels (*horizontal bidirectional arrows*) enables hyperpolarization to travel rapidly along the vessel wall and thereby coordinate relaxation of smooth muscle cells within and between vessel branches. As shown on the right, sympathetic nerve activity releases norepinephrine (*curved arrow*) that diffuses to adrenoreceptors (*triangle*) on nearby smooth muscle cells to promote the opening of voltage-operated Ca^{++} channels in the plasma membrane and the release of Ca^{++} from internal stores to produce vasoconstriction. Sympathetic vasoconstriction is antagonized (*broken arrow at top*) by products of muscle fiber contraction. The middle smooth muscle cell indicates that contractile status can also be altered through modulation of regulatory kinase and phosphatase activities (**P*) to alter the sensitivity of the contractile machinery to intracellular Ca^{++}.

the production of IP_3 within smooth muscle cells also promote vasodilation. Unlike skeletal or cardiac muscle, vascular smooth muscle can also alter its contractile activity independent of changes in intracellular Ca^{++} through altering the phosphorylation state of regulatory proteins and the sensitivity of contractile proteins to Ca^{++}. Additionally, stimulation of endothelial cells can produce smooth muscle cell hyperpolarization through K^+ channel activation. For example, metabolites of arachidonic acid released by the endothelium stimulate calcium-activated K^+ channels in the smooth muscle membrane to produce hyperpolarization and relaxation (22). Alternatively, hyperpolarization can be initiated in the endothelium by vasoactive stimuli and then be transferred to smooth muscle cells through gap junction channels located at myoendothelial junctions (23).

> ## KEY POINT
>
> Vasodilator signals can act directly on smooth muscle cells or indirectly via endothelial cells. At each level of the resistance network, respective cell layers work in concert to govern muscle blood flow.

Transmural Pressure and Luminal Shear Stress Interact to Determine Vasomotor Tone

The vasculature is exposed continually to transmural pressure (*i.e.*, circumferential wall stress) and luminal shear stress. These mechanical forces give rise to myogenic (24) and flow-mediated (25) mechanisms of vasomotor control that are governed by smooth muscle cells and endothelial cells, respectively. In the absence of SNA, these regulatory processes interact to establish the resting contractile state (vasomotor tone) of vascular smooth muscle cells throughout the resistance network (Fig. 11.6). Resistance vessels supplying skeletal muscle typically rest at 50% to 70% of their maximal diameter (21). Thus, vasomotor tone establishes a baseline for regulatory "gain" in vasomotor control that, through dilating and constricting, encompasses a dynamic range in muscle blood flow of more than 50-fold.

Myogenic autoregulation is governed by smooth muscle cells

Smooth muscle cells of resistance vessels are inherently responsive to changes in transmural pressure. An increase in circumferential wall stress (proportional to the product of transmural pressure and lumen radius; inversely proportional to vessel wall thickness) stimulates smooth muscle contraction. This myogenic response is explained by mechanical transduction leading to depolarization and the activation of VOCC (24). Thus, with an increase in transmural pressure, the influx of Ca^{++} into smooth muscle cells produces vasoconstriction and thereby restores circumferential wall stress. In skeletal muscle, as observed in the cerebral and renal circulations, myogenic autoregulation of vasomotor tone acts dynamically to maintain the constancy of tissue blood flow throughout the physiologic range of perfusion pressures. During skeletal muscle contraction, the increase in tissue pressure can reduce transmural pressure throughout the arteriolar network and result in vasodilation. In this manner, myogenic vasodilation (along with the muscle pump, discussed later) can provide a transient increase in muscle blood flow immediately following skeletal muscle contraction (26).

Flow-mediated vasodilation is governed by endothelial cells

The flow of blood exerts shear stress (proportional to the product of blood flow velocity and blood viscosity, related inversely to internal vessel diameter) on the endothelial cells lining the vessel lumen (25). The endothelium responds by releasing autacoids (e.g., nitric oxide and metabolites of arachidonic acid) that induce relaxation of surrounding smooth muscle cells. Shear stress may also hyperpolarize endothelial cells by activating K^+ channels in the plasma membrane. As alluded to earlier, this electrical signal can be transmitted directly to smooth muscle through myoendothelial gap junction channels (Fig. 11.7). In turn, hyperpolarization of smooth muscle cells will inhibit VOCC and the fall in intracellular Ca^{++} will produce relaxation and vasodilation. An increase in perfusion pressure will produce myogenic vasoconstriction and increase luminal shear stress, which in turn stimulates the endothelium to promote smooth muscle relaxation and attenuate vasoconstriction. Conversely, with a fall in perfusion pressure, myogenic relaxation reduces shear stress and diminishes the production of autacoids by the endothelium, which reduces the stimulus for vasodilation. In this manner, flow-mediated vasodilation can provide negative feedback to both myogenic vasoconstriction and vasodilation.

Blood vessels remodel in response to sustained changes in pressure and flow

With chronic elevation of transmural pressure (days to weeks, such as occurs in hypertension), blood vessels remodel around a smaller lumen and with a thicker media to restore circumferential wall stress. When blood flow is consistently elevated over time, such as with regular endurance exercise, blood vessels can remodel to form an enlarged lumen through arteriogenesis, which continues until the prevailing shear stress returns to normal (27). This mechanism can increase the conductance of the supplying vessels and is especially important in the development of collateral circulation when the primary vascular supply is insufficient or interrupted. Signaling events underlying arteriogenesis include macrophage infiltration along with the release of growth factors and proteolytic enzymes essential to remodeling of the extracellular matrix. Complementary signaling events result in sprouting and proliferation of capillary endothelial cells (angiogenesis) in response to elevated shear stress as well as mechanical stretch (28). Taken together, these adaptations of the peripheral vasculature contribute to the enhanced vascular transport capacity of skeletal muscle in response to exercise conditioning (2,14).

Summary

Through physical forces exerted on vascular smooth muscle cells and endothelial cells, blood pressure and blood flow interact dynamically to establish the prevailing level of vasomotor tone. When maintained over time, changes in pressure and flow stimulate vascular remodeling to maintain circumferential wall stress and luminal shear stress. In such manner, hypertension causes thickening of the vessel wall, whereas chronic endurance exercise and the associated hyperemia promotes enlargement of the vessel lumen. Although the nature of signaling events varies between the acute and long-term regulation of vessel diameter, the end result is for the vascular supply to be able to meet the demands of its dependent cells and tissues.

TEST YOURSELF

Blood vessels are not simply passive tubes carrying blood, but are dynamically active both structurally and functionally. What is meant by "vasomotor tone" and how is it regulated? What role(s) do smooth muscle cells play and what are the key underlying signaling events effecting such regulation? What role(s) do endothelial cells play and what are the key underlying signaling events in mediating such action(s)?

Metabolic Vasodilators Initiate and Sustain Vasodilation

The metabolic theory of blood flow control (24) is based on the release of vasodilator substances from active muscle fibers in proportion to their energy expenditure (Fig. 11.6). These substances then diffuse to relax the arteriolar smooth muscle cells, producing vasodilation (29).

The ensuing increase in local blood flow removes vasoactive metabolites as they diffuse into capillaries and are carried away in the venous effluent. Thus, through negative feedback from vasodilator metabolites, hyperemia is maintained during activity at a level that is commensurate with the intensity of metabolic demand. Research into the regulation of the peripheral circulation has increasingly focused on the role of ion channels as sites of action for metabolic vasodilators (Fig. 11.7). For example, extracellular K^+ increases at the onset of muscle contraction. From a resting concentration of about 5 mM, an increase in extracellular K^+ to 10 mM will activate inward-rectifying K^+ channels to promote K^+ efflux and hyperpolarization (22). The elevation in extracellular K^+ can also stimulate Na^+/K^+ adenosine triphosphatase to hyperpolarize the smooth muscle cell membrane. However, the increase in extracellular K^+ from active skeletal muscle cells is transitory and it is unlikely that K^+ mediates sustained elevations in muscle blood flow.

Steady-state contractions are associated with a sustained reduction in P_{O_2} and corresponding elevation of P_{CO_2} in the venous blood. Both of these signals have long been implicated in the maintenance of functional hyperemia, and recent studies have shown both gases to modulate the activity of ion channels in vascular smooth muscle. For example, in addition to the effect of changing P_{O_2} on the metabolic production of vasodilators (e.g., adenosine), a more direct effect involves modulating the activation of VOCCs (e.g., depolarization and Ca^{++} influx with elevated P_{O_2}; hyperpolarization and relaxation as P_{O_2} falls). In a complementary manner, activation of ATP-sensitive K^+ channels with a fall in P_{O_2} (22) would promote vasodilation through hyperpolarization and inactivation of VOCCs (Fig. 11.7). As discussed earlier, local reductions in tissue P_{O_2} may act indirectly (e.g., via RBCs releasing ATP) to promote vasodilation, thereby increasing oxygen delivery according to increases in metabolic demand. Indeed, findings in human subjects are consistent with such a mechanism for governing exercise hyperemia, particularly during steady-state activity (30).

Venules also serve an important though often unrecognized role in the metabolic control of peripheral resistance. Adhesive junctions between endothelial cells of the venular wall are not as tight as those in arterioles or capillaries. This greater permeability of venular endothelium allows vasoactive metabolites carried in the effluent blood to pass readily into the interstitium. Thus, where venules run across or countercurrent to arterioles, metabolites can diffuse down their concentration gradients to influence the contractile status of arteriolar smooth muscle (31). Venular endothelial cells can also release dilator autacoids in response to chemical or physical stimuli. In such manner, vasodilator stimuli arising from venules provide concerted feedback for governing arteriolar diameter and local blood flow in accord with the metabolic status and $\dot{V}_{O_2}$ of dependent muscle fibers (31).

TEST YOURSELF

Muscle blood flow increases with the level of energy expenditure during exercise. How can vasodilation and the accompanying increase in blood flow be controlled by contractile activity of muscle fibers? Are the regulatory events that occur with the onset of exercise different from those that are manifested during steady-state aerobic performance? What are the key similarities and/or differences under respective conditions?

Conducted Vasodilation Coordinates Vasomotor Control

Up to this point, we have focused on vasomotor responses of vascular smooth muscle cells directly or indirectly (via endothelial cells) exposed to a stimulus. However, vascular resistance is distributed among proximal, as well as distal, branches of the precapillary network of arterioles and their feed arteries. We now consider how vasoactive signals initiated at distinct sites within a muscle can travel rapidly along resistance networks over considerable distances through cell to cell signaling (32). The conduction of vasodilation is enabled through gap junction channels in the vessel wall, particularly those expressed at the cell borders of endothelial cells (Fig. 11.3). The strong electrical coupling and the axial orientation of endothelial cells promote signal transmission along and between consecutive branches of arterioles and their feed arteries. Gap junction channels are also expressed between adjacent smooth muscle cells as well as at myoendothelial contacts between smooth muscle cells and endothelial cells. Analogous to the spread of electrical activity in the heart, electrical signals initiated in one location can thereby travel rapidly from cell to cell along the vessel wall. Indeed, conduction along the endothelium and into smooth muscle cells underlies the ability of feed arteries to dilate in concert with arterioles and thereby attain peak levels of muscle blood flow during contractile activity (33).

Conduction can also be initiated from capillaries and possibly venules (18), with vasoactive signals traveling upstream into corresponding TAs and their parent branches. Thus, conducted vasodilation provides an explanation of how MVU perfusion may be coordinated along (and among) active muscle fibers to increase the functional capillary surface area. Further, responses initiated in separate MVUs or arteriolar branches can be summed and integrated in their parent vessels. In this manner, vasomotor response of parent vessels reflects the integration of input from daughter branches along with vasoactive metabolites released in the vicinity of arteriolar smooth muscle cells (Fig. 11.7). The physiologic stimulus (or stimuli) for conducted vasodilation with muscle fiber contraction has yet to be established. Indeed, multiple signals could produce an electrical signal that can travel from cell to cell along the vessel wall (34). Under experimental conditions, the nature of conduction has been studied extensively using acetylcholine for its consistency in triggering conducted responses. In skeletal muscle, the end plate of somatic motor nerves is the apparent physiologic source of this neurotransmitter. Although it remains controversial whether spillover of acetylcholine from neuromuscular junctions can trigger conducted vasodilation on nearby capillary or arteriolar endothelial cells, growing evidence points to rapid onset dilation of arterioles and feed arteries that is initiated with muscle fiber recruitment (26). This rapid and coordinated response among distal and proximal vessel branches may well reflect intercellular electrical signaling (32) and can rapidly increase capillary RBC perfusion according to the local increase in metabolic demand.

TEST YOURSELF

Blood flow to skeletal muscle is controlled by the resistance vasculature. How do distal and proximal branches of resistance networks interact to control the distribution and magnitude of blood flow within exercising skeletal muscle? At what level is capillary perfusion regulated? Which vessel branches control the distribution of blood flow within the muscle? Which vessel branches control the maximum blood flow that a muscle can receive?

Summary

Vasodilation constrained to a single arteriole has little effect on local blood flow. In contrast, local blood flow increases significantly when vasodilation is conducted upstream into proximal arterioles and their feed arteries as the intensity of metabolic demand increases. Furthermore, vasodilation initiated in distal arterioles will increase blood flow through their parent arterioles and feed arteries upstream. In turn, this will elevate shear stress in these proximal vessels, where endothelium-dependent, flow-mediated vasodilation (25) can further promote and sustain functional hyperemia. Vasodilation in response to shear stress takes several seconds longer to occur when compared to the electrical signaling that underlies conducted vasodilation. Nevertheless, by working together in a coordinated fashion, conducted vasodilation initiated within the microcirculation arterioles ascends into the arterial supply where flow-mediated vasodilation further contributes to maintaining a sustained increase in muscle blood flow during exercise.

Sympathetic Vasoconstriction Interacts with Functional Vasodilation to Establish Peripheral Vascular Resistance

SNA increases with the mass of muscle recruited during exercise in accord with the intensity of muscular

contractions (3). In response to SNA, norepinephrine is released from perivascular nerve fibers and activates α-adrenoreceptors on vascular smooth muscle cells to produce vasoconstriction (Fig. 11.7). As discussed later, sympathetic vasoconstriction presents a dichotomy: It can restrict blood flow to exercising muscle and can be overridden by skeletal muscle contractions. Understanding the interaction between functional vasodilation and sympathetic vasoconstriction has long been a subject of intense study of the peripheral circulation.

Blood flow restriction through sympathetic vasoconstriction is particularly apparent when another large mass of muscle is active simultaneously and demands a substantial portion of cardiac output (3). The restriction of blood flow during SNA is most effective in feed arteries. Remarkably, during flow restriction the extraction of oxygen by active motor units is enhanced, indicating that muscle fibers become more effective in removing oxygen from the blood as flow becomes limiting. This adjustment occurs through the process of "functional sympatholysis" whereby sympathetic vasoconstriction is inhibited within contracting skeletal muscle (35). As discussed earlier, inhibiting arteriolar constriction promotes local vasodilation, thereby increasing capillary (MVU) perfusion with RBCs and providing greater surface area for oxygen diffusion to respiring mitochondria within active muscle fibers.

The inhibition of sympathetic vasoconstriction may occur presynaptically by preventing neurotransmitter release, as well as postsynaptically by interfering with intracellular signaling pathways activated by norepinephrine on vascular smooth muscle (35). Thus, as SNA increases, vasodilation prevails in distal arterioles to promote capillary perfusion and the extraction of oxygen, whereas the total increase of blood flow into the muscle is restricted progressively through constriction of feed arteries and primary arterioles (36). Indeed, the activation of α-adrenoreceptors can inhibit ascending vasodilation. Because feed arteries are external to the muscle, they are not directly exposed to the products of metabolism. In such manner, these vessels serve as a key site for maintaining total peripheral resistance and arterial pressure during peak demands on cardiac output and the corresponding increase in SNA (3,36).

In addition to the local inhibition of sympathetic neurotransmission, the conduction of vasodilation can attenuate sympathetic vasoconstriction, providing a complementary signaling pathway for antagonizing the effect of SNA on arteriolar resistance (35). A complementary mechanism for inhibiting the vasoconstrictor effect of SNA occurs as a result of increasing Ca^{++} in smooth muscle cells subsequent to the activation of α-adrenoreceptors. This response establishes a diffusion gradient for Ca^{++} into endothelial cells through myoendothelial gap junctions. As Ca^{++} enters the endothelium, it stimulates production of nitric oxide and activation of K^+ channels, both of which counter the vasoconstriction (35). Thus, multiple mechanisms can inhibit sympathetic vasoconstriction during muscular activity. Conversely, the activation of α-adrenoreceptors can inhibit conducted vasodilation (37).

It should be recognized that functional sympatholysis is integral to achieving high levels of blood flow to exercising skeletal muscle by promoting vasodilation where metabolic demand is high, at the same time, sympathetic vasoconstriction restricts blood flow to regions of the body with low metabolic demand. Moreover, the interaction between muscle contraction and SNA in controlling vessel diameter is graded with the intensity of respective stimuli and with the location of vessel branches within the resistance network (36). Indeed, recent findings illustrate that the recruitment of motor units within a defined muscle region can rapidly direct blood flow to the active muscle fibers by antagonizing the effects of SNA on arterioles and feed arteries supplying that muscle region (37).

Summary

There is interplay between SNA and conducted vasodilation in arterioles and feed arteries supplying exercising skeletal muscle. Thus, norepinephrine release can suppress the ability of vasodilation to ascend from arterioles into their feeding arteries, whereas conducted vasodilation can attenuate sympathetic vasoconstriction. The ability of respective constrictor and dilator signals to influence each other is graded with the level of SNA, the intensity of metabolic demand and the location of vessel branches in the resistance network. This interplay underscores the ability of active muscles to increase oxygen extraction at the same time total muscle flow is restricted to maintain arterial blood pressure.

TEST YOURSELF

The level of SNA increases with the intensity of exercise and active muscle mass. How does SNA influence vasomotor tone? Where in the vascular tree is this effect exerted in skeletal muscle? What about the gut and other regions of the body? If it is possible to override the effect of SNA during exercise, where in the vasculature does this occur, how does it happen, and what purpose does it serve?

The Muscle Pump Promotes Exercise Hyperemia

Muscle blood flow is typically evaluated as a mean value over time and is proportional to exercise intensity and the oxidative capacity of active muscle fibers (2). However, with each contraction, the rhythmic changes in muscle length and tension produce cyclic oscillations in intramuscular pressure. With venous valves preventing backflow, the squeezing and emptying of veins propels blood away from the muscle and back toward the heart. Thus, in the presence of constant arterial pressure, the reduction in venous pressure during relaxation between muscle contractions increases the effective pressure gradient for capillary perfusion. As vasodilation progresses from rest, the volume of blood within the muscle increases between contractions, analogous to the period of diastolic filling in the cardiac cycle. In such manner, the ejection of blood from active muscle during each contraction (analogous to cardiac systole) increases until a steady level of hyperemia is attained (38). In addition, this pumping action of skeletal muscle on the peripheral vasculature imparts substantial kinetic energy to the blood, thereby reducing stress on the heart.

KEY POINT

Nearly half of the total energy required for circulating the blood during exercise may be generated by the muscle pump and this kinetic energy is essential to achieving the high blood flows that accompany maximal aerobic exercise.

CHAPTER SUMMARY

This chapter describes the organization and control of peripheral circulation to skeletal muscle in the context of exercise hyperemia. We consider the functional anatomy of the resistance network, the cellular signaling pathways within and between smooth muscle and endothelium, how the activity of muscle fibers gives rise to vasomotor responses that encompass progressively greater portions of the resistance network, and how (as well as where) sympathetic innervation competes with functional vasodilation. It should now be apparent that the response of the peripheral circulation to the activity of skeletal muscle requires coordination among a diverse array of vasoactive signals and among multiple branches of the vascular tree.

Recent findings implicate novel mechanisms of vasomotor control that reflect physical coupling of arteriolar smooth muscle cells to elements of the extracellular matrix (39), the activation of particular K^+ channels together with specific connexin subunits of gap junction channels along the endothelium (34), and alternative mechanisms for tissue oxygen sensing through the endogenous production of hydrogen sulfide gas (40). At each level of the resistance network, vascular smooth muscle serves as an integrator of metabolic signals that arise from muscle fiber contraction, the mechanical effects of blood pressure (circumferential wall stress) and blood flow (shear stress on endothelial cells), the release of norepinephrine from perivascular sympathetic nerves, and the pumping actions of rhythmic muscle contractions.

At rest, in the absence of SNA, vasomotor tone and peripheral vascular resistance manifest the interaction between myogenic contraction of vascular smooth muscle cells and its modulation by the endothelium in response to luminal shear stress. Functional hyperemia has long been attributed to the production and release of vasodilator substances from active muscle fibers (29). However, metabolic vasodilation requires at least 5 to 6 seconds for substances to be produced by skeletal muscle fibers and diffuse to arteriolar smooth muscle cells in sufficient concentration to elicit vasodilation. Thus, metabolic vasodilation is too slow to account for the rapid onset (within 1 or 2 seconds) of functional hyperemia. Although the muscle pump effectively promotes venous return and increases the driving pressure for capillary perfusion, it is not fully effective until vasodilation and an increase in muscle blood volume have become established. Thus, the rapid onset of vasodilation, together with the coordinated increase in capillary perfusion, may best be explained by the initiation and conduction of vasodilation in conjunction with mechanical forces that are exerted coincident with motor unit recruitment. In turn, metabolic and flow-mediated vasodilation can effectively govern steady-state components of the hyperemic response, which is further enhanced by the muscle pump.

Vasodilation triggered by muscle fiber activation ascends from TAs into proximal arterioles and feed arteries as metabolic demand increases. Indeed, dilation of these proximal resistance vessels is essential to achieving peak levels of functional hyperemia. The location of feed arteries external to the muscle physically removes them from the direct influence of the vasoactive products of muscular activity. It is at this level of the peripheral circulation where sympathetic vasoconstriction effectively limits blood flow during exercise. Under such conditions, the volume of blood flow to active muscle (and thereby its $\dot{V}O_2$) is restricted while extraction is optimized by dilation of arterioles within the muscle.

Where and how is muscle blood flow actually controlled? Through the 1960s, it was recognized that different segments of the vasculature varied in their responses to vasoactive stimuli. In the mesenteric microcirculation, the sensitivity to humoral stimuli increased from proximal resistance vessels to the precapillary sphincters, yet these distal vessels appeared to be less responsive to sympathetic vasoconstriction. Others found that the functional capillary surface area of skeletal muscle remained high despite flow restriction during sympathetic nerve activity (SNA).

Folkow and coworkers tested the hypothesis that the site of flow restriction to skeletal muscle during SNA would vary over time and with metabolic demand. The nerve and vascular supply to calf muscles were isolated in anesthetized cats, and total blood flow into the muscle was measured with a flow meter. Blood pressure was measured at three key sites: upstream from the muscle in the femoral artery (Pa), downstream from the muscle in the femoral vein (Pv), and at an intermediate site (Pi) represented by the sural artery. The contributions of proximal resistance arteries (Rp) and distal precapillary arterioles (Rd) to total vascular resistance (Rt) were evaluated according to a model of resistive segments arranged in series, where Rt = Rp + Rd (Fig. 11.8). Relative to control conditions, an increase in Rd/Rt indicated that distal vessels had constricted more than proximal vessels. Conversely, a fall in Rd/Rt indicated that the proximal vessels were constricted more than distal vessels.

Blood flow decreased as Rt increased in resting muscle during SNA, whereas the ratio of Rd/Rt increased transiently and then declined as SNA was maintained. This behavior indicated that distal vessels were initially the primary site of constriction and then reversed to dilation over time, whereas constriction of the proximal vessels accounted for the sustained increase in Rt. In response to rhythmic muscle contractions, Rt decreased over time, with two characteristic components to the response: Rd fell rapidly over about the first 30 seconds and was attributed to the action of vasodilator metabolites on precapillary arterioles at the distal ends of resistance networks. This early decrease in Rd was succeeded by a decline in Rp over several minutes, indicating that vasodilation progressively ascended into the resistance arteries as exercise continued. When SNA was performed during steady-state muscle contractions, the increase in Rt was much lower than in resting muscle, and Rd/Rt declined. Thus, sympathetic vasoconstriction appeared to be inhibited in distal branches (which underwent dilation) but sustained in proximal branches.

These insightful experiments resolved distinct components of the integrated vasomotor response to SNA, to muscle contraction, and to the nature of interaction between these opposing stimuli at different levels of the resistance network. The predictions of vascular function that were made from the classic whole-organ experiments of Folkow and coworkers have been confirmed and extended using intravital microscopy. Complementary studies have demonstrated regional differences in the expression and inhibition of adrenore-

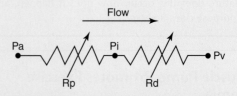

FIGURE 11.8 The contributions of proximal resistance arteries (Rp) and distal precapillary arterioles (Rd) to total vascular resistance (Rt) were evaluated according to a model of resistive segments arranged in series, where Rt = Rp + Rd. Pa, femoral artery; Pi, intermediate site; Pv, femoral vein.

A **MILESTONE** OF DISCOVERY

ceptor subtypes that mediate sympathetic vasoconstriction. The expression and regulation of ion channels and signaling pathways that govern and coordinate the contractile status of vascular smooth muscle cells are also now known to display regional variations in the peripheral vasculature. Furthering our understanding of the role of exercise in modifying the cellular, molecular, and genomic regulation of vascular smooth muscle and endothelium has broad implications for ameliorating such widespread diseases of the peripheral vasculature as atherosclerosis, diabetes, and hypertension.

Folkow B, Sonnenschein RR, Wright DL. Loci of neurogenic and metabolic effects on precapillary vessels of skeletal muscle. Acta Physiol Scand. 1971;81:459–471.

ACKNOWLEDGEMENT

Support for this work was provided by the National Institutes of Health, grants R37-HL041026, RO1-HL056786, and RO1- HL086483.

REFERENCES

1. Andersen P, Saltin B. Maximal perfusion of skeletal muscle in man. *J Physiol.* 1985;366:233–249.
2. Laughlin MH, Korthius RJ, Duncker DJ, et al. Control of blood flow to cardiac and skeletal muscle during exercise. In: Rowell LB, Shepherd JT, eds. *Handbook of Physiology, Section 12: Exercise: Regulation and Integration of Multiple Systems.* New York: Oxford University; 1996:705–769.
3. Rowell LB, O'Leary DS, Kellog DLJ. Integration of cardiovascular control systems in dynamic exercise. In: Rowell LB, Shepherd JT, eds. *Handbook of Physiology, Section 12: Exercise: Regulation and Integration of Multiple Systems.* New York: Oxford University; 1996:770–838.
4. Christensen KL, Mulvany MJ. Location of resistance arteries. *J Vasc Res.* 2001;38:1–12.
5. Delashaw JB, Duling BR. A study of the functional elements regulating capillary perfusion in striated muscle. *Microvasc Res.* 1988;36:162–171.
6. Rhodin JA. The ultrastructure of mammalian arterioles and precapillary sphincters. *J Ultrastruct Res.* 1967;18:181–223.
7. Greensmith JE, Duling BR. Morphology of the constricted arteriolar wall: physiological implications. *Am J Physiol.* 1984;247:H687–H698.
8. Marshall JM. The venous vessel within skeletal muscle. *NIPS.* 1991;6:11–15.
9. Bloch EH, Iberall AS. Toward a concept of the functional unit of mammalian skeletal muscle. *Am J Physiol.* 1982;242:R411–R420.
10. Fuglevand AJ, Segal SS. Simulation of motor unit recruitment and microvascular unit perfusion: spatial considerations. *J Appl Physiol.* 1997;83:1223–1234.
11. Klitzman B, Damon DN, Gorczynski RJ, et al. Augmented tissue oxygen supply during striated muscle contraction in the hamster: relative contributions of capillary recruitment, functional dilation, and reduced tissue Po_2. *Circ Res.* 1982;51:711–721.
12. Sarelius IH. Cell flow path influences transit time through striated muscle capillaries. *Am J Physiol.* 1986;250:H899–H907.
13. Krogh A. The number and distribution of capillaries in muscles with calculations of the oxygen pressure head necessary for supplying the tissue. *J Physiol.* 1918;52:409–415.
14. Saltin BG, Gollnick PD. Skeletal muscle adaptability: significance for metabolism and performance. In: Peachey LD, eds. *Handbook of Physiology, Section 10: Skeletal Muscle.* Bethesda, MD: American Physiological Society; 1983:555–631.
15. Weibel ER. Scaling of structural and functional variables in the respiratory system. *Annu Rev Physiol.* 1987;49:147–159.
16. Duling BR, Desjardins C. Capillary hematocrit: what does it mean? *NIPS.* 1987;2:66–69.
17. Tsai AG, Johnson PC, Intaglietta M. Oxygen gradients in the microcirculation. *Physiol Rev.* 2003;83:933–963.
18. Ellsworth ML, Ellis CG, Goldman D, et al. Erythrocytes: oxygen sensors and modulators of vascular tone. *Physiology.* 2009; 24:107–116.
19. Lund N, Jorfeldt L, Lewis DH. Skeletal muscle oxygen pressure fields in healthy human volunteers: a study of the normal state and the effects of different arterial oxygen pressures. *Acta Anaesth Scand.* 1980;24:272–278.
20. Bearden SE, Moffatt RJ. Vo_2 and heart rate kinetics in cycling: transitions from an elevated baseline. *J Appl Physiol.* 2001;90:2081–2087.
21. VanTeeffelen JW, Segal SS. Effect of motor unit recruitment on functional vasodilatation in hamster retractor muscle. *J Physiol.* 2000;524:267–278.
22. Jackson WF. Potassium channels in the peripheral microcirculation. *Microcirculation.* 2005;12:113–127.
23. Ledoux J, Werner ME, Brayden JE, et al. Calcium-activated potassium channels and the regulation of vascular tone. *Physiology.* 2006;21:69–78.
24. Davis MJ, Hill MA, Kuo L. Local control of microvascular perfusion. In: Tuma RF, Duran WN, Ley K, eds. *Handbook of Physiology, Microcirculation: Regulation of Microvascular Blood Flow.* 2nd ed. Amsterdam: Elsevier; 2008:161–284.
25. Davies PF. Flow-mediated endothelial mechanotransduction. *Physiol Rev.* 1995;75:519–560.
26. Clifford PS. Skeletal muscle vasodilatation at the onset of exercise. *J Physiol.* 2007;583:825–833.
27. Schaper W, Scholz D. Factors regulating arteriogenesis. *Arterioscler Thromb Vasc Biol.* 2003;23:1143–1151.
28. Haas TL. Molecular control of capillary growth in skeletal muscle. *Can J Appl Physiol.* 2002;27:491–515.
29. Haddy FJ, Scott JB. Metabolic factors in peripheral circulatory regulation. *Fed Proc.* 1975;34:2006–2011.
30. Gonzalez-Alonso J, Olsen DB, Saltin B. Erythrocyte and the regulation of human skeletal muscle blood flow and oxygen delivery: role of circulating ATP. *Circ Res.* 2002;91:1046–1055.
31. Hester RL, Hammer LW. Venular-arteriolar communication in the regulation of blood flow. *Am J Physiol.* 2002;282:R1280–R1285.
32. Bagher P, Segal SS. Regulation of blood flow in the microcirculation: role of conducted vasodilation. *Acta Physiol.* 2011;201:1–13.
33. Segal SS, Jacobs TL. Role for endothelial cell conduction in ascending vasodilatation and exercise hyperaemia in hamster skeletal muscle. *J Physiol.* 2001;536:937–946.
34. Milkau M, Köhler R, de Wit C. Crucial importance of the endothelial K^+ channel SK3 and connexin40 in arteriolar dilations during skeletal muscle contraction. *FASEB J.* 2010;24:3572–3579.
35. Thomas GD, Segal SS. Neural control of muscle blood flow during exercise. *J Appl Physiol.* 2004;97:731–738.
36. VanTeeffelen JW, Segal SS. Interaction between sympathetic nerve activation and muscle fibre contraction in resistance vessels of hamster retractor muscle. *J Physiol.* 2003;550:563–574.
37. Moore AW, Bearden SE, Segal SS. Regional activation of rapid onset vasodilatation in mouse skeletal muscle: regulation through α-adrenoreceptors. *J Physiol.* 2010;588:3321–3331.
38. Anrep GV, von Saalfeld E. The blood flow through the skeletal muscle in relation to its contraction. *J Physiol.* 1935;85:375–399.
39. Hocking DC, Titus PA, Sumagin R, et al. Extracellular matrix fibronectin mechanically couples skeletal muscle contraction with local vasodilation. *Circ Res.* 2008;102:372–379.
40. Olson KR, Whitfield NL. Hydrogen sulfide and oxygen sensing in the cardiovascular system. *Antioxid Redox Signal.* 2010;12:1219–1234.

CHAPTER 12

The Gastrointestinal System

G. Patrick Lambert, Xiaocai Shi, and Robert Murray

Abbreviations

DRTS	Disaccharidase-related transport system	$mOsm \cdot kg\ H_2O^{-1}$	Milliosmoles per kilogram water
GI	Gastrointestinal	NSAIDs	Nonsteroidal anti-inflammatory drugs
GLUT	Glucose transporter	SGLT1	Sodium-glucose cotransporter
kDa	KiloDalton	$\dot{V}O_{2max}$	Maximal oxygen uptake
$mEq \cdot L^{-1}$	Milliequivalents per liter	$\dot{V}O_{2peak}$	Peak oxygen uptake
mM	Millimolar		

Introduction

During strenuous and/or prolonged exercise in which dehydration, hyperthermia, and carbohydrate depletion can occur, proper gastrointestinal (GI) function is essential to maintain performance and safeguard health. Under such conditions, rapid gastric emptying and intestinal absorption of ingested fluid and solute (*e.g.*, carbohydrate, sodium) become imperative in supplying the water and substrate needed to sustain cardiovascular, thermoregulatory, and metabolic functions. On the other hand, GI dysfunction can negatively affect performance by causing problems such as fullness, nausea, and diarrhea.

Unfortunately, compared to most of the organ systems in the body, the GI system has received relatively little attention from exercise scientists. In fact, Gisolfi (1) emphasized that, in the past 150 years, few scientists have demonstrated more than just a passing interest in the effects of exercise on GI function. It was not until the 1970s and 1980s before exercise physiologists such as David Costill, Carl Gisolfi, and Ronald Maughan turned their attention to the subject of GI function during exercise. Currently, only a small portion of exercise-related research deals with the GI tract. Fortunately, much of that work is quite instructive, and this chapter relies on

that body of literature to address what we know, what we think we know, and what we do not know about GI function during exercise. In so doing, this chapter focuses on the effects of dynamic sustained exercise on GI function. Keep that in mind whenever the term exercise is used.

Basic Anatomy and Functions of the GI Tract

In essence, the GI tract is just a long tube (~9 m; ~30 ft) (2) designed to transport water and nutrients into the body. The transfer of nutrients into the body from the food and beverages we ingest is achieved by the processes of motility, secretion, digestion, and absorption. The effects of exercise on each of these functions are described in more detail as the chapter progresses. In addition to these basic GI functions, the GI mucosa (with associated secretions and immune cells) provides a defense against harmful substances found in the GI lumen. This defense mechanism is collectively known as the "GI barrier" or "gut barrier."

The processes of gastric emptying (a form of motility) and intestinal absorption receive the most emphasis in this chapter. This is because rapid emptying from the stomach and efficient absorption in the proximal small intestine will ultimately determine fluid and nutrient availability during exercise and thus will impact exercise-related performance and health.

Basic GI Regulation

To expedite the absorption of nutrients into the body and to minimize malabsorption and GI discomfort, GI processes must be regulated in a coordinated fashion. This is carried out through neural, hormonal, and local mechanisms. The GI system effectively has its own nervous system, the enteric nervous system, which extends from the esophagus to the anus. The enteric nervous system contains more than 100 million afferent and efferent neurons, roughly the same number as in the spinal cord (3), and, thus, it has sometimes been referred to as the "mini brain," "gut brain," or the "visceral brain." The primary purpose of the enteric nervous system is to ensure efficient absorption of water and solute by controlling muscular contraction, secretion, and blood flow. Interestingly, the GI system is endowed with a preponderance of afferent output that reflects the importance of regulatory signals from gut chemoreceptors, osmoreceptors, and mechanoreceptors to the brain and spinal cord.

The enteric nervous system has two primary plexuses, the myenteric plexus and the submucosal plexus; the activity of both plexuses can be modified by sympathetic and parasympathetic input. In general, parasympathetic fibers from the vagus nerve provide excitatory input for secretion and motility via acetylcholine release, whereas sympathetic fibers have an inhibitory effect via norepinephrine. Sympathetic activation causes vasoconstriction of intestinal blood vessels, inhibition of wall contractions, and decreased sphincter activity during the "fight-or-flight response," including the response to vigorous physical activity.

The smooth muscle of the GI system functions as a syncytium (*i.e.*, electrical signal generated in one cell is transmitted to adjacent cells) that allows action potentials to travel in all directions, helping facilitate the peristaltic contractions that churn and transport food and fluid in the gut. Ease of depolarization among smooth muscle cells occurs as a result of each cell having more than 200 gap-junction connections with adjacent cells (3). In resting humans, peristaltic contractions occur in the stomach at a rate of 1 to 2 per minute and the small intestine at a rate of 15 to 18 per minute (2). The type and strength of contractions change upon eating and drinking, such that stronger and more frequent contractions and peristaltic movements help empty the stomach and sweep the chyme along the small intestine.

The GI tract is also controlled by a number of regulatory agents, many of which it produces itself. These include hormones and peptides such as gastrin, cholecystokinin, secretin, motilin, gastric inhibitory peptide, and vasoactive intestinal peptide. These substances allow further regulation of GI motility, secretions, and blood flow. Interestingly, many gut peptides are also found in the brain, providing further credence to the notion of a "gut brain."

GI Blood Flow during Exercise

Blood flow to the GI tract is delivered via the splanchnic circulation. Within this circulation, branches of the celiac trunk serve the stomach and duodenum, whereas branches of the superior mesenteric artery provide blood to the small intestine and a good part of the large intestine. The inferior mesenteric artery also provides blood to the descending colon, sigmoid colon, and rectum. All blood exiting these organs passes to the liver via the hepatic portal vein.

Dynamic exercise has a profound effect on splanchnic blood flow. Rowell (4) notes that regional vasoconstrictor outflow is proportional to the severity of exercise, as reflected by the close relationship between heart rate and plasma norepinephrine at heart rates above 100 beats per minute; in brief, splanchnic blood flow decreases as heart rate increases. The decrease in splanchnic blood flow that occurs during exercise is a critical compensatory response to ensure the maintenance of adequate central blood volume and pressure, although how this affects blood flow to the intestinal mucosa via the superior and inferior mesenteric arteries is less clear. In theory, a substantial drop in mesenteric blood flow could impair absorption, because flowing blood removes water and solute and maintains the concentration gradient between the intestinal lumen and the intestinal epithelial cell (enterocyte). It has been found that when mesenteric blood flow declines to less than 50% of normal, both glucose absorption and oxygen uptake are reduced (5). In addition, should blood supply to the intestinal epithelium be severely compromised for a sufficient period, the resultant ischemia can alter barrier function and possibly cause epithelial necrosis. This can occur during prolonged dynamic exercise in the heat (6), when the combination of dehydration and hyperthermia can severely limit splanchnic blood flow. In fact, some endurance-trained athletes have developed such severe colonic ischemia during races that surgery was required to remove infarcted tissue (7).

KEY POINT

As exercise intensity increases, blood flow to the GI tract decreases. This is exacerbated by dehydration and heat stress.

Summary

GI blood flow declines with increasing levels of exercise intensity, heat stress, and dehydration. Depending on the severity of these factors, altered GI function can result.

Gastric Emptying during Exercise

General Concepts

The stomach is a semi-isolated holding tank for ingested food and fluid. With the exception of small amounts of alcohol and vitamin B_{12}, water and other nutrients are not absorbed from the stomach. For that reason, rapid gastric emptying is an essential prelude for rapid intestinal fluid and solute absorption required to sustain prolonged, vigorous exercise. For example, many athletes sweat at rates exceeding 2 L per hour, necessitating an aggressive fluid replacement regimen and unimpeded absorption if significant dehydration is to be avoided. Ingestion of beverages that are not optimally formulated will invariably result in delayed gastric emptying, as will ingestion of foods during exercise. Delayed gastric emptying reduces the rate at which ingested fluid can be absorbed across the epithelium of the small intestine, increasing the risk of gastric discomfort and slowing the rehydration process.

Measurement of Gastric Emptying Rate

Gastric emptying rate during rest and exercise is often assessed by means of a nasogastric tube that allows for measurements of the change in gastric volume based on changes in the concentration of a nonabsorbable marker such as phenol red (8,9). Other methods, such as magnetic resonance imaging, scintigraphy, electrical impedance, ultrasonography, and radiography, have also been used to study gastric emptying, but the nasogastric tube is often the method of choice because subjects can continue to exercise while gastric samples are collected, and the presence of the tube does not affect emptying rate (10).

Determinants of Gastric Emptying Rate

The stomach is the most distensible part of the GI system, and its unfilled volume is small, about 50 mL, yet it can quickly expand to 1000 mL without much change in intragastric pressure. In fact, the very act of swallowing causes reflex relaxation of the stomach, so that the initial intake of food or fluid does not result in a substantial rise in intragastric pressure (3).

Control of gastric motility occurs via afferent and efferent sympathetic and parasympathetic nerves, spinal feedback reflexes, and hormones released from the intestinal mucosa. Control of gastric activity is essential during both rest and dynamic exercise because unrestricted emptying of gastric contents into the duodenum and jejunum results in osmotic diarrhea and nutrient wasting. For this reason, gastric emptying is tightly controlled by neural, hormonal, and local factors to ensure that the intestine receives fluid and nutrients at rates that are less than its absorptive capacity and therefore compatible with efficient digestion and absorption. Vasoactive intestinal peptide, γ-amino-butyric acid, substance P, gastrin, cholecystokinin, serotonin, nitric oxide, gastric inhibitory polypeptide, and glucagon-like peptide are examples of hormones and neurotransmitters released by gastric and intestinal nerve and endocrine cells that influence gastric emptying, GI motility, and secretions from the pancreas and gallbladder in response to a meal.

Three layers of muscles surround the stomach, arrayed as an outer longitudinal layer, a middle circular layer, and an inner oblique layer. The frequency and strength of contractions of these muscles determines gastric emptying rate by altering the pressure in the antrum of the stomach (Fig. 12.1), the space closest to the pyloric sphincter. When pressure in the antrum exceeds the pressure in the duodenal bulb, the pylorus opens and stomach contents (chyme) enter the small intestine.

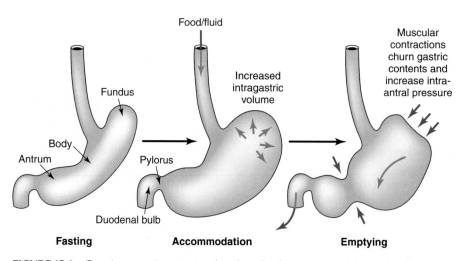

FIGURE 12.1 Gastric emptying rate is related to the frequency and strength of contractions of the gastric musculature. When pressure in the antrum exceeds that in the duodenal bulb, chyme passes through the pylorus. Increased gastric volume promotes rapid gastric emptying.

Gastric emptying rate varies widely among individuals; some people empty test solutions twice as rapidly as others. In general, the rate of gastric emptying follows an exponentially declining pattern regardless of the average rate of emptying. In other words, the most rapid gastric emptying rates occur in the first minutes after consumption, when gastric volume is high, and then the rate declines over time, reaching low values when most of the test meal or solution has left the stomach. Mean gastric emptying rates of 15 to more than 20 mL per minute are common during both rest and dynamic exercise when water or a dilute carbohydrate solution is ingested. Sustaining such rates is possible but requires repeated ingestion of such fluids to maintain the high gastric volume (11–14) that produces high antral pressure.

Based on the previous discussion, gastric volume appears to be the most important factor in promoting a high gastric emptying rate. The energy content of the ingested solution is the second most important factor (i.e., lower energy content promotes faster emptying). Other factors that can inhibit emptying are increased solution osmolality, increased solution temperature, reduced pH of the ingested solution, increased exercise intensity, dehydration, and increased heat stress (15).

KEY POINT

Gastric emptying rate is enhanced by maintenance of a relatively high gastric volume.

Most solutions consumed during exercise, other than water, contain carbohydrate as an energy source. It is well established that gastric emptying of carbohydrate solutions vary with the carbohydrate (energy) content, such that higher carbohydrate content results in slower gastric emptying (16). In general, the ingestion of a relatively dilute carbohydrate solution (e.g., 6% carbohydrate; 60 g/L) has been shown to result in a gastric emptying rate that is statistically indistinguishable from that of an equal volume of water (17). However, some investigators have reported delayed gastric emptying rates (compared to water) for carbohydrate solutions less than 6% (18), whereas others have found that gastric emptying is unimpeded even with solutions containing 10% carbohydrate (19,20). However, these inconsistent results are likely due to differences in the volume and frequency of fluid intake because research has shown that with repeated drinking, similar gastric emptying rates can be obtained among solutions with different carbohydrate content and/or osmolalities. Again, this appears to be the result of maintenance of a relatively high (~300–600 mL, depending on the solution) steady-state stomach volume (11,21–23). Therefore, all things considered, athletes with slow gastric emptying rates and those who sweat profusely can benefit from maintaining a large yet comfortable gastric volume, which will help maximize

gastric emptying rate. This can be achieved by drinking water or an appropriately formulated sports drink within 15 minutes before starting exercise and continuing to drink at frequent intervals (e.g., every 10–15 minutes) throughout exercise.

Effects of Acute Exercise on Gastric Emptying Rate

It appears that exercise below ~75% maximal oxygen uptake ($\dot{V}O_{2max}$) does not affect gastric emptying, and may actually enhance it (15). In addition, there does not appear to be a difference in gastric emptying between running and cycling (24). However, with prolonged exercise above 75% $\dot{V}O_{2max}$ or in sporting activities that require intermittent high-intensity efforts, such as in basketball and soccer, delayed gastric emptying is likely (25). Thus, during intermittent high-intensity sports, fluid ingestion during the low-intensity and rest periods should be encouraged, as this is when the opportunity for rapid gastric emptying can take place and drinking strategies should be adjusted to take advantage of such occasions.

Unfortunately, the mechanisms by which heavy exercise delays gastric emptying are unclear. Reduced GI blood flow, exacerbated by dehydration and/or hyperthermia, along with increased sympathetic discharge and catecholamine levels are all possible candidates (10,15).

Effects of Exercise Training on Gastric Emptying Rate

Chronic exercise training does not appear to influence gastric emptying rate (26); however, little has been done in this area and further research is needed. With regard to training, it has been recommended that athletes drink during training sessions to enhance tolerance to fluid ingestion during competition (10,27,28). This concept has been tested (29) and it was observed that repeated trials of drinking to match sweat rate (while running) result in improved stomach comfort during later trials. Thus, such results indicate that athletes can improve their tolerance to fluid ingestion during exercise. Interestingly, in that study, improved tolerance was not associated with improved gastric emptying.

Another area of research that requires more attention is how the athlete's overall diet and the "pre-game" meal may influence gastric emptying. The best that can currently be said is that individuals should avoid abrupt changes in diet prior to or during competition.

Effects of Dehydration and Hyperthermia on Gastric Emptying Rate during Exercise

Many individuals who engage in endurance training and competition have experienced the unfortunate chain of GI events that often begins with dehydration and hyperthermia. Such factors alone, or in combination, likely reduce gastric emptying rate (30,31), and problems such as bloating and GI discomfort can arise. The result is reduced voluntary fluid intake, greater dehydration, a higher body temperature, earlier fatigue, and an increased risk of heat injury. The only solution appears to be avoiding dehydration by limiting ingestion of foods and fluids that delay gastric emptying; that is, taking the steps necessary to maintain a high rate of gastric emptying.

The mechanisms by which dehydration and hyperthermia reduce gastric emptying are other areas of research that deserve further attention. At present, we can only speculate that, as with exercise itself, enhanced sympathetic discharge and/or reduced GI blood flow result in reduced gastric motility and/or reduced intestinal absorption, each of which can directly or indirectly influence gastric emptying.

KEY POINT

Gastric emptying rate can be reduced by high exercise intensity and exercise combined with dehydration and/or heat stress.

Summary

Gastric emptying rate may decline with high exercise intensity and exercise combined with dehydration and/or heat stress. In addition, ingestion of beverages that are too concentrated (*e.g.*, high glucose concentration) can reduce emptying rate. On the other hand, gastric emptying rate is enhanced by maintenance of a relatively high gastric volume that can be accomplished by repeated drinking during exercise.

TEST YOURSELF

What is the most likely mechanism for reduced gastric emptying rates during either high-intensity exercise or prolonged exercise combined with heat stress and/or dehydration?

Intestinal Absorption during Exercise

General Concepts

In the simplest characterization, the intestine functions as an absorbing surface for water and nutrients (solutes). In that regard, three fundamental concepts are worth remembering: (a) water absorption from hypoosmotic solutions can occur rapidly, especially in the duodenum, as a result of simple osmosis; (b) water absorption from isosmotic and hyperosmotic solutions is secondary to solute absorption because solute absorption establishes an

osmotic gradient that results in water absorption; and (c) alterations in the osmotic gradient across the intestinal epithelium can occur with the ingestion of inappropriate foods and fluids during exercise, resulting in net fluid secretion into the proximal gut.

From an anatomical standpoint, the small intestine is superbly designed for the absorption of water and solute. The first 25 to 30 cm (10–12 in) past the pylorus is the duodenum, an area characterized by a leaky epithelium. This characteristic allows for rapid osmotic equilibration of the gastric effluent because water freely flows across the duodenal epithelium in response to the prevailing osmotic gradient. As a result, a hypertonic effluent, such as a concentrated carbohydrate solution (*e.g.*, a regular soft drink or fruit juice), will provoke net secretion of water into the duodenum to reduce osmolality as a preface to net water absorption further down the small intestine. Hypotonic fluids such as water are quickly absorbed in the duodenum because water molecules are free to pass across the duodenal epithelium into the higher osmolality environment of the intracellular and extracellular fluid.

The next 100 cm (about 3 ft) of the small intestine is the jejunum (2), where microvilli-covered epithelial cells (*i.e.*, enterocytes) are rich in membrane-bound enzymes, transporters, and intercellular junctions that open and close in response to the prevailing luminal environment. Isotonic and hypertonic fluids containing substrates such as glucose and fructose will be absorbed more rapidly in this section of the small intestine compared to the duodenum. (The presence of mucosal folding and microvilli in the small intestine creates an absorptive surface area about the size of a doubles tennis court, 20 times the surface area of a smooth tube of like length.) The ileum is the final 200 cm (about 6–7) of the small intestine (2), but its function is not covered in this chapter because its role in water and solute absorption during exercise is usually minimal; among other functions, the ileum provides reserve absorptive capacity for water and solutes that escape absorption in the duodenum and jejunum.

Measurement of Water and Solute Absorption

Water and solute absorption and its transport mechanisms in the proximal small intestine can be studied using a variety of in vitro techniques (*e.g.*, Ussing chamber, tissue incubation, oocyte expression of transport proteins), tracer techniques (most often with deuterium oxide), and perfusion methods using double- and triple-lumen perfusion tubes. Among these methods, the triple-lumen perfusion technique, also called steady-state perfusion, is considered the gold standard for studying regional water and solute absorption in the resting or exercising human. One limitation of the perfusion technique is that it measures only the absorptive characteristics of the segment of intestine that is perfused, usually about 40 to 50 cm. However, this is an acceptable limitation for studying the absorption of water and carbohydrate and electrolyte beverages, because the majority of fluid absorption occurs within that length of the proximal small intestine (11,23). The perfusion technique requires a triple-lumen tube to be placed via the mouth into the subject's small intestine under fluoroscopic guidance. Once proper tube placement is verified, a test solution containing a nonabsorbable marker such as polyethylene glycol is ingested (14) or infused (32) into the small intestine and samples are collected from the proximal and distal ports of the other lumens for analysis of the nonabsorbable marker and solutes, such as carbohydrates and electrolytes. The change in the concentration of the nonabsorbable marker and solutes from the proximal and distal sampling sites allows calculation of the net flux of water and solutes, respectively.

Principles of Solute and Water Absorption

Solute absorption refers to the movement of nutrients, such as carbohydrates and amino acids, and minerals, such as sodium and potassium, from the intestinal lumen into the bloodstream either transcellularly (into the cell across the apical enterocyte membrane and out of the cell across the basolateral membrane) or paracellularly (between the enterocytes via the tight junctions). Water absorption, in general, is driven by solute absorption and follows the principle of osmosis.

Solute and water absorption are primarily linked by the activity of the sodium-glucose cotransporter (SGLT1), found in abundant quantities in the jejunal epithelium. Even prior to the identification of this protein, it was recognized that the combination of low concentrations of glucose and sodium in a solution enhanced water absorption from that solution. In fact, this has been the subject of considerable research attention for more than 50 years and such research has paved the way for the formulation of simple oral rehydration solutions that are used to save the lives of millions of people stricken with severe diarrheal disease. In the 1960s, the first sports drink was developed, based in part on the principle that water molecules quickly follow solute across the intestinal epithelium. An oral rehydration solution formulated to replace diarrheal fluid loss typically contains about 2% carbohydrate and high levels of sodium (45–75 mEq · L^{-1}) and potassium (20 mEq · L^{-1}), whereas sports drinks contain more carbohydrate (*e.g.*, 6%–7%) and less electrolytes (*e.g.*, 20–40 mEq · L^{-1} sodium; 3–5 mEq · L^{-1} potassium). The differences in formulation are due to differences in the intended benefits. Diarrheal electrolyte losses are usually considerably higher than electrolyte losses in sweat, so more electrolytes are needed in an oral rehydration solution to offset those losses. In terms of carbohydrate concentration, the 2% glucose concentration of an oral rehydration solution will stimulate rapid water absorption but will not provide the amount of exogenous carbohydrate required for improved exercise performance (16).

Carbohydrate digestion and absorption

Salivary amylases (secreted into the mouth) and pancreatic amylases (secreted into the duodenum) begin the process of starch digestion into limit dextrins, maltotriose, and maltose. At the brush border of the small intestine, lactase digests lactose, the primary carbohydrate in milk. (Lactose intolerance occurs when an individual fails to sufficiently produce this enzyme.) Sucrase digests sucrose into glucose and fructose. Isomaltase digests limit dextrins into glucose and maltose units, and maltase digests maltose and maltotriose into individual glucose monomers. These brush border enzymes are transcriptionally regulated, and their abundance in the cell membrane can be influenced by diet (33).

Glucose and galactose are absorbed across the brush border (apical) membrane by SGLT1 (Fig. 12.2). The concentration of SGLT1 in the membrane is primarily influenced by dietary carbohydrate content. For example, the presence of glucose and galactose in the gut can rapidly increase the trafficking of SGLT1 from intracellular storage sites to the brush border membrane (33). Such rapid response is an important functional characteristic of the small intestine because it ensures that the absorptive capacity of the intestine always exceeds nutrient intake, a critical balance if osmotic diarrhea is to be avoided. Interestingly, Kellett (34) has also proposed that glucose transporter type 2 (GLUT2) serves as a facilitated transporter of glucose and it is inserted into the apical membrane within minutes in response to SGLT1-initiated signaling events. Thus, it appears the plasticity of the small intestine is quite remarkable. Stevens (35) noted that reversible increases in absorptive capacity can occur within hours or days as a result of (a) mucosal hyperplasia and increased villus height, (b) increased number of solute transporters in response to the ingestion of specific solutes, and (c) local regulation of transporter kinetics.

The GLUT5 transporter shuttles fructose across the apical membrane into the intestinal epithelial cell (Fig. 12.2) by facilitated transport, a mechanism that allows for relatively faster absorption rates than that of passively absorbed carbohydrates, such as rhamnose, a nonmetabolizable monosaccharide, similar in size to glucose. However, GLUT5-facilitated transport of fructose is slower than that of actively transported carbohydrates, such as glucose and galactose, via SGLT1. Interestingly, the turnover of GLUT5 protein occurs in diurnal fashion in the rat, even in the absence of dietary fructose (33). Whether the same is true in humans is not yet known. Once inside the intestinal epithelial cell (enterocyte), glucose, galactose, and fructose exit the basolateral membrane of the intestinal epithelial cell into the portal blood via the GLUT2 transporter (33).

It is hypothesized but still unproven that the products of sucrose digestion (*i.e.*, glucose and fructose) are absorbed via a distinct transport system, the disaccharidase-related transport system (DRTS) (36). This transport mechanism appears to be associated with sucrose hydrolysis, but it is unclear whether the enzyme, sucrase, transfers the free glucose and fructose to DRTS or whether the carrier is an integral part of the enzyme itself (Fig. 12.2).

Another proposed solute transport mechanism is paracellular transport (37) (Fig. 12.2). SGLT1 solute transport

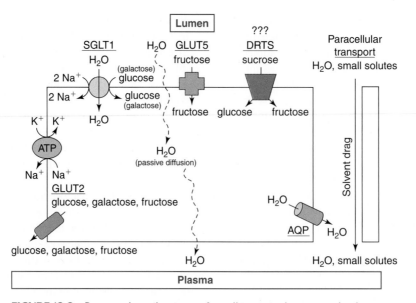

FIGURE 12.2 Proposed mechanisms of small intestinal water and solute absorption. Sodium and glucose cotransport by the SGLT1 transporter in the enterocyte apical membrane and extrusion of sodium and glucose across the basolateral membrane stimulate water and solute absorption through both transcellular and paracellular routes. The roles of glucose transporter (GLUT5), GLUT2, disaccharidase-related transport system (DRTS), Na⁺-K⁺ ATPase, and aquaporins (AQP) are also depicted. Following activation of SGLT1, water and solutes such as monosaccharides, minerals, and perhaps even small peptides and oligosaccharides can be absorbed via the paracellular pathway. ATP, adenosine triphosphate.

triggers contraction of perijunctional actomyosin to open tight junctions between enterocytes and thereby stimulates solvent drag (*i.e.*, solute transport as a result of water transport). For example, in addition to transport via GLUT5, fructose can be absorbed paracellularly, carried along by the solvent drag created by SGLT1 activation. This is also how glucose can be absorbed efficiently when luminal glucose concentrations are above and beyond the absorptive capacity of SGLT1.

In terms of the effects of exercise on carbohydrate absorption, the results are somewhat unclear. Fordtran and Saltin (38) found no effect of running at ~70% $\dot{V}O_{2max}$ on glucose absorption during small intestinal perfusion of a 13.3% glucose solution. In contrast, Lang et al. (39) found that running at 70% $\dot{V}O_{2max}$ resulted in reduced absorption of the glucose analogs, 3-O-methyl-D-glucose (actively absorbed), and D-xylose (passively absorbed), indicating reduced ability to absorb glucose. The discrepancy in results is likely due to methodologic differences and indicates a need for further research in this area.

Summary

Glucose is absorbed into enterocytes through the apical membrane by SGLT1, and possibly by GLUT2. Fructose is absorbed into enterocytes by GLUT5. Both exit the enterocyte at the basolateral membrane via GLUT2.

Absorptive capacity of glucose always exceeds glucose intake and this is regulated by changes in mucosal surface area, number of transporters, and transport kinetics. SGLT1-mediated tight junction opening also allows for paracellular absorption of glucose and fructose. Exercise at lower intensities does not likely affect carbohydrate absorption, however higher intensities may do so.

Amino acid absorption

There are a number of amino acid transporters in the gut (35). Some depend on cotransport of sodium, others do not. Some transporters are specific to cationic amino acids, others to anionic amino acids, yet others to dipolar amino acids. Even some dipeptides and tripeptides can be absorbed by enterocytes. The effect of dynamic exercise or exercise training on amino acid absorption has not been studied.

Because some amino acids are actively transported with sodium, and increased amino acid absorption alone would increase solute absorption, there has been interest in determining whether the addition of certain amino acids can augment water absorption from a carbohydrate–electrolyte beverage. To date, the results have been disappointing. For example, the amino acid glutamine is the preferred energy substrate for enterocytes (although they will also use glucose for energy when it is available in high concentrations), but there appears to be no absorption-related advantage of providing glutamine in a beverage formulated for consumption during exercise (40). This has also been shown for glycine (48) and L-arginine (unpublished findings). In fact, in high concentrations, L-arginine is known to promote fluid secretion (41).

Mineral absorption

There is no doubt that sodium is the mineral that plays the most pivotal role in water absorption in the small intestine. It is absorbed primarily by SGLT1, but can also be absorbed via the paracellular route (Fig. 12.2). Even in the fasted state, sodium is present in the intestinal lumen because the lumen is bathed in extracellular fluid. Luminal sodium is also supplied by food and drink, from sodium bicarbonate, and from bile salts. In the fasting human, sodium concentration in the duodenum (about 60 mEq $\cdot$ L^{-1}) is about half of that in the jejunum (about 140 mEq $\cdot$ L^{-1}). There is evidence that sodium absorption is influenced by the type of carbohydrate in the ingested beverage. For example, maltodextrin (glucose polymers) appear to produce a faster rate of sodium absorption than glucose and maltose; maltose is superior to glucose, and glucose and oligosaccharides are better than sucrose (42). Perfusion of a fructose solution initially results in sodium secretion and slower net sodium absorption than with a glucose solution (42). The practical ramifications of these differences have yet to be elucidated, but the principle is that rapid sodium absorption is an indispensable characteristic of an oral rehydration solution. Additional research is required to assess the effect of ingesting various blends of carbohydrates and electrolytes on sodium and water absorption; however, it is known that adding extra sodium to solutions of higher carbohydrate concentration does not enhance fluid absorption (22,43).

Chloride and potassium are largely transported by solvent drag through paracellular channels, whereas other minerals, such as calcium, iron, and zinc, rely on yet other solute-specific transport mechanisms. However, there is no evidence that water or solute absorption from an oral rehydration solution is augmented with the addition of common minerals other than sodium chloride.

The effect of dynamic exercise or exercise training on mineral absorption has not been well studied. One supposition is that because sodium absorption does not appear to be influenced by dynamic exercise (44), it is unlikely that the absorption of other minerals is affected.

Water absorption

Although the athlete's requirements for water, carbohydrate, and electrolytes during training and competition can be impressively high (*e.g.*, sweat rates above 2 L/hour, carbohydrate oxidation rates above 1 g/minute, and sodium losses above 1 g/L of sweat), those demands fall well below the capacity of the GI system to absorb water and solute. For example, the maximum rate of glucose and amino acid transport is estimated to exceed typical dietary intake by a factor of 2 (33). However, that is not to say that the small intestine has an unlimited capacity for water and solute absorption. That is clearly not the case and is one reason feedback inhibition

from intestinal osmoreceptors and chemoreceptors is needed to ensure that the gastric emptying rate does not exceed the absorptive capacity of the proximal small intestine.

Water molecules cross the enterocyte membrane via SGLT1 or by transcellular and paracellular diffusion driven by the osmotic gradient (Fig. 12.2). Considerable research and scientific debate have been devoted to quantifying the proportion of water absorption that occurs via paracellular versus transcellular transport. Suffice to say that, although the tide of evidence favors greater transcellular absorption, both mechanisms are critical in ensuring the water and solute absorption required during exercise.

SGLT1 is a 290-kDa molecule composed of four 73-kDa subunits (35). The activity of SGLT1 is driven by the transmembrane electrical potential that is maintained by active sodium-potassium transport in the basolateral membrane by the sodium-potassium pump and by facilitated transport of chloride from adjacent epithelial cells or from the intestinal lumen. The SGLT1 molecule is thought to function in the following way: When two sodium ions bind to the active site of SGLT1, a conformational change allows glucose to bind. Once glucose is bound, another conformational shift occurs, and the sodium ions and glucose molecule are transported across the membrane and released. SGLT1 then undergoes yet another conformational change back to its original position, ready to bind additional sodium and glucose.

In the absence of glucose or galactose, SGLT1 serves as a sodium uniporter and a passive water channel. An important feature of SGLT1 is that in its active state it also serves as a molecular pump for water, accounting for up to 70% of total daily water absorption in the jejunum. Each time that SGLT1 transports glucose and sodium into the enterocyte, approximately 260 water molecules follow (45). Assuming a rotation rate of 34 times per second (46), each SGLT1 molecule could be responsible for the absorption of 8840 water molecules per second. Scientifically formulated oral rehydration solutions and sports drinks take advantage of this fundamental concept to promote rapid solute and water absorption.

DETERMINANTS OF THE RATE OF WATER ABSORPTION A handful of factors influence the rate of water absorption in the proximal small intestine. Gastric emptying rate has an obvious influence on absorption; delayed gastric emptying results in delayed absorption. In addition to gastric emptying rate, the primary factors influencing the rate of water absorption are beverage osmolality, the concentration of carbohydrate, the type of carbohydrate, and the number of transportable solutes in the beverage. Solution temperature is not likely a factor because all solutions will be warmed to a similar temperature prior to absorption. The sheer number of interactions among the known influential variables, however, complicates the study of how beverage composition affects water absorption. Even so, a partial and instructive picture has emerged.

EFFECT OF BEVERAGE OSMOLALITY ON THE RATE OF WATER ABSORPTION The proximal small intestine, especially the duodenum, functions as an osmotic equilibrator that rapidly adjusts the osmolality of the gastric effluent toward iso-osmolality. For example, a hyperosmotic effluent will be diluted in the duodenum by water secretion, whereas a hypoosmotic effluent will promote solute secretion (primary sodium and chloride). As would be expected, the rate of water absorption in the proximal small intestine tends to be inversely related to the osmolality of the perfused solution (47,48), and certain hypotonic solutions have been shown to be absorbed more rapidly than isotonic solutions (49,50). However, this relationship may not always hold true. For example, in two studies, an isosmotic carbohydrate-electrolyte solution promoted greater water absorption than distilled water (51,52). In addition, Shi and associates (53) and Gisolfi and associates (23) reported no significant differences in water absorption at rest or during dynamic exercise, respectively, from carbohydrate-electrolyte beverages that varied in osmolality from hypoosmotic (186–197 mOsm · kg H_2O^{-1}), isosmotic (283–295 mOsm · kg H_2O^{-1}), to hyperosmotic (403–414 mOsm · kg H_2O^{-1}). Thus, it is likely the effect of beverage osmolality is modified by the concentration and types of carbohydrates in the beverage.

EFFECT OF CARBOHYDRATE CONCENTRATION ON THE RATE OF WATER ABSORPTION

The rate of water absorption is influenced by a solution's carbohydrate concentration, partly because carbohydrate concentration often determines the solution osmolality. Thus, an inverse relationship between carbohydrate concentration and water absorption is commonly observed in the literature (51,52). Generally speaking, carbohydrate concentrations above 7% to 8% reduce water absorption. For example, Ryan and colleagues (12) reported slower water absorption during exercise from 8% and 9% carbohydrate beverages than with water or from a 6% carbohydrate beverage. Similar results have been found in resting subjects (47). It is possible that beverages with more than 6% carbohydrate saturate the absorption process for glucose in the jejunum. In support of this possibility, Rolston and Mathan (54) estimated that the SGLT1 transporter process in the jejunum is saturated at approximately 200 mM glucose (about 35 g/L, the equivalent of a 3.5% glucose solution).

EFFECT OF CARBOHYDRATE TYPE ON THE RATE OF WATER ABSORPTION

There is little doubt that the type of carbohydrate can influence the rate of water absorption because of the differences in solution osmolality conferred by carbohydrate type (*e.g.*, equal concentrations of glucose, sucrose, and maltodextrins have widely varying osmolalities) and differences in the rates at which the carbohydrates are absorbed (*e.g.*, glucose more than fructose). For example, oral rehydration solutions typically contain 2% glucose (about 111 mM) because decades of studies have demonstrated that such solutions stimulate rapid water absorption and save lives. In contrast, carbohydrate-electrolyte beverages (*e.g.*, sports drinks) usually contain a blend of

carbohydrates at concentrations around 60 g · L^{-1} (*i.e.*, a 6% carbohydrate solution; about 333 mM). The higher amount of carbohydrate provides the palatability required for consumption during exercise and supplies enough exogenous substrate to improve performance (16). If such beverages are properly formulated, high rates of water absorption can be maintained. However, if the wrong blend of carbohydrate is used (*e.g.*, too much fructose), or if the carbohydrate concentration is too high (*e.g.*, more than 7%–8%), the rate of water absorption will likely be reduced.

A study by Shi and colleagues (48) (Fig. 12.3) demonstrated how water absorption in resting humans is influenced by the number of transportable substrates and solution osmolality. The effect of solution osmolality on water absorption was attenuated by enhanced solute absorption when more than one transportable carbohydrate was present in the solution. In other words, even slightly hyperosmotic beverages (*e.g.*, 300–400 mOsm · kg^{-1}) can be rapidly absorbed if more than one transportable substrate is present (23,53). Some evidence indicates that this may be the case with solutions of even higher osmolality (47). However, as Figure 12.3 illustrates, the obvious tendency is for lower osmolality solutions to be absorbed more rapidly.

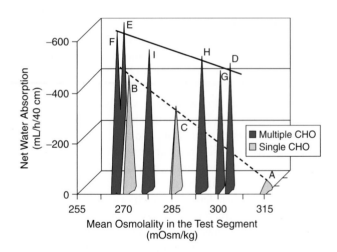

FIGURE 12.3 Relationship between water absorption and luminal osmolality for solutions containing single- and multiple-transportable carbohydrates. Negative values indicate net water absorption. Solution carbohydrate composition and test segment osmolality: A, 8% glucose, 314 mOsm · kg H_2O^{-1}; B, 6% maltodextrin, 271 mOsm · kg H_2O^{-1}; C, 8% maltodextrin, 286 mOsm · kg H_2O^{-1}; D, 4% glucose + 4% fructose, 304 mOsm · kg H_2O^{-1}; E, 4% sucrose + 2% glucose, 269 mOsm · kg H_2O^{-1}; F, 3% glucose + 2% sucrose + 1% maltodextrin, 268 mOsm · kg H_2O^{-1}; G, 3% glucose + 3% fructose + 2% sucrose, 300 mOsm · kg H_2O^{-1}; H, 8% sucrose, 296 mOsm · kg H_2O^{-1}; I, 4% sucrose + 2% glucose + 0.4% glycine, 276 mOsm · kg H_2O^{-1}. (Data from Shi X, Flanagan S, Summers RW, et al. Effects of carbohydrate type and concentration and solution osmolality on water absorption. *Med Sci Sports Exerc.* 1995;27:1607–1615.)

KEY POINT

Water absorption is enhanced by inclusion of two or more transportable substrates in a beverage.

EFFECT OF EXERCISE ON THE RATE OF WATER ABSORPTION
Does exercise affect the rate at which water is absorbed? Evidence on this important question is conflicting. In 1967, using the segmental perfusion technique, Fordtran and Saltin (38) reported no consistent effect of exercise on glucose, water, or electrolyte absorption during treadmill running for 1 hour at 64% to 78% $\dot{V}o_{2max}$. This finding was supported by Gisolfi and colleagues (44) during 1-hour bouts of cycle exercise at 30%, 50%, and 70% $\dot{V}o_{2max}$. Whether this finding is consistent remains to be determined. Part of the difficulty in quantifying the effects of intense exercise on water absorption is that very few subjects can sustain intense exercise long enough to allow for segmental perfusion measurements to be made.

EFFECTS OF DEHYDRATION AND HYPERTHERMIA ON THE RATE OF WATER ABSORPTION   Dehydration during exercise results in plasma hyperosmolality, reduced skin and splanchnic blood flow, decreased sweat rate, and an increased rate of rise in core body temperature. The combination of dehydration, hyperthermia, and heavy exercise has been linked to GI barrier dysfunction, ostensibly as a result of reduced GI blood flow and local ischemia. How these changes affect water and solute absorption is not well understood. Ryan and colleagues (12) investigated the effect of hypohydration (loss of 2.7% body mass prior to the commencement of exercise) on water absorption during 85 minutes of cycle exercise at 65% $\dot{V}o_{2max}$ in a cool environment. The results indicated that hypohydration did not affect absorption. Additional research is necessary to corroborate and extend these findings, to determine whether greater levels of dehydration affect absorption, and to investigate the interaction between dehydration and hyperthermia on water and solute absorption.

KEY POINT

Water absorption is not affected by moderate exercise intensity or low levels of dehydration.

EFFECT OF DIET ON THE RATE OF WATER ABSORPTION
Absorption of water in the small intestine follows the establishment of a favorable osmotic gradient due either to ingestion of a hypoosmotic beverage or secondary to the osmotic gradient established by solute absorption. In the latter regard, glucose is the solute that provokes the most robust stimulation of water absorption. The rate of carbohydrate absorption in the small intestine is related to the concentration and activity of SGLT1, GLUT5, and GLUT2 in the enterocyte membrane. Consequently, anything that affects the regulation of carbohydrate transporters may affect water absorption. Animal studies have shown that SGLT1 and GLUT5 transporter activity and site density are upregulated by consumption of a high-carbohydrate diet (33). In fact, within 4 hours of fructose exposure, GLUT5 mRNA protein levels rise (33). When animals are on a carbohydrate-free diet, levels of sucrase, isomaltase and SGLT1 decline (33).

Low sodium diets decrease glucose transport by decreasing the number of brush border GLUTs, whereas a high-sodium diet does not appear to effect SGLT1 trafficking. Aside from these findings, there is a dearth of evidence regarding the effects of changes in the macronutrient composition of the diet on water and solute absorption. Individuals in training typically ingest diets high in carbohydrate and sodium, providing the nutritional impetus for the maintenance of an ample quantity of membrane transporters. However, it would be useful to know more about how water absorption is influenced by short-term changes in diet.

EFFECT OF AGING ON THE RATE OF WATER ABSORPTION
The effect of aging on water absorption has not been extensively studied. However, carbohydrate malabsorption has been demonstrated in about one-third of healthy individuals older than age 65 (55), and altered carbohydrate absorption could retard water absorption. Impaired carbohydrate absorption with age may be due to a reduction in the effective absorptive surface of the small intestine and/or a reduction in splanchnic blood flow, but little is known about how dynamic exercise and exercise training affect water and solute absorption in older, physically active individuals. There is no reliable evidence that the intestine changes in length, weight, or permeability with aging.

Summary

Intestinal water absorption is not affected by moderate exercise intensity or low levels of dehydration, but can be enhanced by inclusion of two or more transportable substrates in a beverage and possibly by dietary manipulation.

TEST YOURSELF

How should a sports drink be formulated to maximize gastric emptying rate, water absorption, and solute absorption?

GI Transit, Motility, and Secretions during Exercise

The effect of exercise on GI transit and motility in humans has not received a great deal of attention. Of the available literature, it has been shown that mild exercise (*i.e.*, treadmill walking) increases mouth-to-cecum transit of a light, liquid meal in both healthy young men (56) and women (57). In contrast, it appears that during prolonged, strenuous cycling (90 minutes at 70% maximal workload) (58) or shorter, more intense cycling (59), mouth-to-cecum transit is unchanged. Gastric motility (assessed by gastric emptying of a solid meal consumed prior to exercise) does not appear to be affected by moderate intensity cycling (60). However, antroduodenal motility has been reported to increase during prolonged, strenuous exercise (180 minutes at 70% $\dot{V}_{O_{2peak}}$; run-bike-run protocol) when fluid is ingested, as has postprandial duodenojejunal motility in highly trained cyclists at higher intensities (80%–90% $\dot{V}_{O_{2max}}$) (59). Among well-trained subjects, it appears that colonic motility is increased during activity, especially among individuals who experience loose stools with exercise (61). However, in untrained subjects, motility was found to be decreased with increasing cycling intensity (25%, 50%, and 75% $\dot{V}_{O_{2max}}$) (62). Thus, factors such as exercise mode, exercise intensity, and level of training appear to play a role in the acute effects of exercise on GI transit and motility, but more research is needed.

In terms of the chronic effects of exercise, mouth-to-cecum transit has been found to be faster in men that are more physically active who have greater energy intakes. This indicates that intestinal adaptation allows for greater and more rapid nutrient absorption among individuals who require it (63). Furthermore, it has been reported (64) that regular physical activity may improve colonic transit time, which can be beneficial in reducing symptoms of constipation.

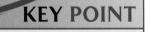

KEY POINT

GI transit and motility may be enhanced by acute and chronic exercise, but this could be related to exercise intensity and training status.

Little research has been conducted in humans examining the effect of acute or chronic exercise on digestive secretions. Based on the available literature (60,65), it does not appear that acute, moderate intensity exercise significantly affects gastric secretion. No studies, to our knowledge, have been conducted in humans to assess the effect of exercise on biliary or pancreatic secretions. In dogs, however, acute treadmill running has been shown to inhibit meal-induced gastric acid and pancreatic bicarbonate secretion, but not biliary bicarbonate secretion. In terms of chronic exercise, endurance training has been shown to increase pancreatic enzyme activity (66) and to improve pancreatic exocrine secretions (67) in rats.

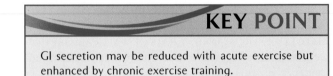

KEY POINT

GI secretion may be reduced with acute exercise but enhanced by chronic exercise training.

Summary

Research on GI transit, motility, and secretion is lacking. Of what is known, transit and motility appear to both be enhanced by acute and chronic exercise, but exercise intensity and training status also likely play important roles. In terms of GI secretion, acute exercise appears to reduce it, but chronic exercise enhances it.

GI Barrier Function during Exercise

The GI epithelium is only one cell thick, creating an enormous yet extremely thin interface between the body and the outside world. This epithelial layer is constantly exposed to a wide variety of undigested nutrients, antigens, hydrolytic enzymes, and microbes, any one of which could provoke an adverse reaction or inflammatory immune response. In addition to pathogens and foreign proteins ingested in foods and beverages, the GI system is home to more than 400 types of bacteria (68), so it should not be surprising that the gut has robust immune response capabilities. The healthy gut is endowed with effective barriers and a rich array of innate and adaptive immune response options that restrict or destroy harmful substances while allowing for the selective absorption of macronutrients, micronutrients, and water (69).

The "GI barrier" is formed by the surface mucus layer, the apical membrane of the enterocytes, the tight junctions between enterocytes, tissue macrophages, and the intestinal lymph nodes. Dysfunction of the barrier results in increased "GI permeability," defined as increased passage of large (>150 Da), normally restricted molecules from the GI lumen to the internal environment. Increased permeability can occur under a number of highly stressful conditions such as trauma/hemorrhage, severe hyperthermia, and severe psychological stress (70). Not surprisingly, the stress of prolonged, strenuous exercise in the heat (71), high-intensity aerobic exercise (72), and exercise combined with nonsteroidal anti-inflammatory drug (NSAID) use also increases GI permeability (73). The most obvious example of impaired gut barrier function during exercise is the intestinal bleeding sometimes seen in marathon runners (74,75). Heavy exercise has also been associated with mucosal lesions, such as hemorrhagic colitis (76), and increased permeability to large, normally restricted, molecules (77). One of the most immunogenic substances that can cross the GI barrier is endotoxin, derived from the walls of gram-negative bacteria. Thus, GI barrier dysfunction can result in endotoxemia and can produce an inflammatory response that is implicated in exertional heat stroke and organ damage.

Additional research is needed on potential interventions to reduce GI barrier dysfunction during prolonged exercise and/or heat stress. To date, there is evidence of improved gut barrier function with pre-exposure to exercise and/or heat stress (78). In addition, appropriate fluid consumption during exercise may reduce the effect of NSAIDs (79) and dehydration (80) on the GI barrier.

Summary

GI barrier dysfunction can occur with prolonged, strenuous exercise especially if heat stress and/or dehydration occur, or if NSAIDs are used.

TEST YOURSELF

What is a potential intervention that may attenuate GI barrier dysfunction during exercise-heat stress?

GI Symptoms during Exercise

GI discomfort is commonly observed before, during, and after prolonged, heavy exercise, primarily in long distance running, cycling, and triathlons. Research indicates that the GI symptoms occur in 20% to 50% of endurance athletes and can be as high as 83% in marathon participants. Symptoms include abdominal cramps, heartburn, nausea, vomiting, diarrhea, and bloody stools (74,75).

Many GI symptoms may be related to factors such as psychological stress; the mode, duration, and intensity of exercise; the type, amount, and timing of food and drink ingested before and during exercise; and the use of NSAIDs. In addition, endotoxemia, due to GI barrier dysfunction, is also believed to cause GI symptoms, such as nausea, vomiting, and diarrhea. These problems all can increase the risk of dehydration, heat exhaustion, and exertional heat stroke (6,78).

KEY POINT

GI symptoms and heat illness may be related to GI barrier dysfunction during exercise.

CHAPTER SUMMARY

Strenuous exercise can significantly reduce GI blood flow and, depending on factors such as exercise intensity, heat stress, and dehydration, can impair gastric emptying and GI barrier function. These effects can lead to GI symptoms, promote further dehydration and hyperthermia, increase the risk of heat-related illness, and reduce exercise performance (Fig. 12.4). To enhance gastric emptying and intestinal absorption of ingested fluids, a drinking strategy that maintains a constant, comfortable stomach volume should be employed and the beverages consumed should contain multiple transportable substrates, not exceeding 7% to

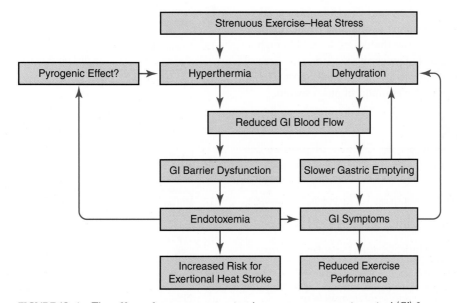

FIGURE 12.4 The effect of strenuous exercise–heat stress on gastrointestinal (GI) function and its relationship to reduced exercise performance and exertional heat stroke.

A MILESTONE OF DISCOVERY

Does heavy exercise affect gastrointestinal function? Specifically, does it interfere with the athlete's ability to replace sweat losses and replace energy during exercise? In the 1960s, there were only suggestions in the scientific literature that gut function might be adversely affected during exercise, and those suggestions were derived from studies on gastric emptying published in 1928 and 1934. A few studies in the early 1960s reported that exercise reduced blood flow to the gut, a further indication that water and solute absorption might be impaired. This led John Fordtran and Bengt Saltin to combine their scientific talents to conduct experiments measuring gastric emptying and intestinal absorption during treadmill exercise. They speculated that "were it possible to replace sweat losses and to maintain a sufficient supply of glucose during exercise, performance might be improved." They also noted that some elite cross-country skiers believed that drinking a glucose solution during competition was a key to improved performance. To address this, Fordtran and

Saltin designed a study in which subjects ran at 70% $\dot{V}O_{2max}$ while gastric emptying measurements were made on one day and absorption measurements on another. The test beverages were a 13.3% glucose solution, a 0.3% saline solution, and water. The results showed a clear negative effect of the concentrated glucose solution on gastric emptying rate but no effect of exercise itself on either gastric emptying or intestinal absorption. From these results, the authors surmised that it would be possible for active individuals to replace fluid loss and to supply carbohydrate and electrolytes "during heavy exercise, even in hot environments." This hallmark study not only set the stage for all future research along this line, but also established the scientific rationale for the subsequent formulation of effective sports drinks.

Fordtran JS, Saltin B. Gastric emptying and intestinal absorption during prolonged severe exercise. J Appl Physiol. 1967;23:331–335.

8% in total carbohydrate concentration. Further research on the effects of training, diet, dehydration, and hyperthermia is needed in this area. Also, research examining neural and hormonal regulation of the GI tract during exercise should be pursued. The value of such research may improve exercise performance, alleviate exercise-induced GI disorders, and reduce the risk of exertional heat injury and illness.

ACKNOWLEDGMENTS

We are grateful to the late Dr. Carl Gisolfi for his excellent mentorship and contributions to the area of GI function during exercise. Likewise, we thank Drs. Ronald Maughan and John Leiper for their pioneering work in this area of science. Finally, we acknowledge the Gatorade Sport Science Institute for their significant support of our research.

REFERENCES

1. Gisolfi CV. The gastrointestinal system. In: Tipton CM, ed. *Exercise Physiology: People and Ideas.* New York: Oxford University; 2003:475–495.
2. Van De Graaff KM. *Human Anatomy.* 6th ed. Boston: McGraw-Hill; 2002.
3. Davenport HW. *Physiology of the Digestive Tract.* Chicago: Year Book; 1982.
4. Rowell LB. *Human Circulation: Regulation During Physical Stress.* New York: Oxford University; 1986.
5. Gisolfi CV, Summers RW, Schedl HP. Intestinal absorption of fluids during rest and exercise. In: Gisolfi CV, Lamb DR, eds. *Perspectives in Exercise Science and Sports Medicine, 3: Fluid Homeostasis During Exercise.* Indianapolis: Benchmark; 1990:129–180.
6. Lambert GP. Role of gastrointestinal permeability in exertional heatstroke. *Exer Sport Sci Rev.* 2004;32(4):185–190.
7. Lucas W, Schroy PC. Reversible ischemic colitis in a high endurance athlete. *Am J Gastroenterology.* 1998;93:2231–2234.
8. Beckers EJ, Rehrer NJ, Brouns F, et al. Determination of total gastric volume, gastric secretion and residual meal using the double sampling technique of George. *Gut.* 1988;29(12):1725–1729.
9. George JD. New clinical method for measuring the rate of gastric emptying: the double sampling test meal. *Gut.* 1968;9:237–242.
10. Leiper JB. Gastric emptying and intestinal absorption of fluids, carbohydrates, and electrolytes. In: Maughan RJ, Murray R, eds. *Sports Drinks: Basic Science and Practical Aspects.* Boca Raton: CRC Press; 2001:89–128.
11. Lambert GP, Chang RT, Xia T, et al. Absorption from different intestinal segments during exercise. *J Appl Physiol.* 1997;83(1):204–212.
12. Ryan AJ, Lambert GP, Shi X, et al. Effect of hypohydration on gastric emptying and intestinal absorption during exercise. *J Appl Physiol.* 1998;84(5):1581–1588.
13. Mitchell JB, Voss KW. The influence of volume on gastric emptying and fluid balance during prolonged exercise. *Med Sci Sports Exerc.* 1991;23(3):314–319.
14. Lambert GP, Chang RT, Joensen D, et al. Simultaneous determination of gastric emptying and intestinal absorption during cycle exercise in humans. *Int J Sports Med.* 1996;17(1):48–55.
15. Costill DL. Gastric emptying of fluids during exercise. In: Gisolfi CV, Lamb DR, eds. *Perspectives in Exercise Science and Sports Medicine, 3: Fluid Homeostasis During Exercise.* Indianapolis: Benchmark Press; 1990:97–127.
16. Murray R. The effects of consuming carbohydrate-electrolyte beverages on gastric emptying and fluid absorption during and following exercise. *Sports Med.* 1987;4:322–351.
17. Murray R, Eddy DE, Bartoli WP, et al. Gastric emptying of water and isocaloric carbohydrate solutions consumed at rest. *Med Sci Sports Exerc.* 1994;26(6):725–732.
18. Vist GE, Maughan RJ. Gastric emptying of ingested solutions in man: effect of beverage glucose concentrations. *Med Sci Sports Exerc.* 1994;26:1269–1273.
19. Owen MD, Kregel KC, Wall PT, et al. Effects of ingesting carbohydrate beverages during exercise in the heat. *Med Sci Sports Exerc.* 1986;18(5):568–575.
20. Zachwieja JJ, Costill DL, Beard GC, et al. The effects of a carbonated carbohydrate drink on gastric emptying,

gastrointestinal distress, and exercise performance. *Int J Sport Nutr.* 1992;2:239–250.

21. Rogers J, Summers RW, Lambert GP. Gastric emptying and intestinal absorption of a low-carbohydrate sport drink during exercise. *Int J Sport Nutr Exerc Metab.* 2005;15:220–235.

22. Gisolfi CV, Lambert GP, Summers RW. Intestinal fluid absorption during exercise: role of sport drink osmolality and [Na+]. *Med Sci Sports Exerc.* 2001;33(6):907–915.

23. Gisolfi CV, Summers RW, Lambert GP, et al. Effect of beverage osmolality on intestinal fluid absorption during exercise. *J Appl Physiol.* 1998;85(5):1941–1948.

24. Houmard JA, Egan PC, Johns RA, et al. Gastric emptying during 1 h of cycling and running at 75% VO$_{2 \text{ max}}$. *Med Sci Sports Exerc.* 1991;23(3):320–325.

25. Leiper JB, Prentice AS, Wrightson C, et al. Gastric emptying of a carbohydrate-electrolyte drink during a soccer match. *Med Sci Sports Exerc.* 2001;33(11):1932–1938.

26. Rehrer NJ, Beckers E, Brouns F, et al. Exercise and training effects on gastric emptying of carbohydrate beverages. *Med Sci Sports Exerc.* 1989;21(5):540–549.

27. Brouns F, Saris WHM, Rehrer NJ. Abdominal complaints and gastrointestinal function during long-lasting exercise. *Int J Sports Med.* 1987;8:175–189.

28. Rehrer NJ. Fluid and electrolyte balance in ultra-endurance sport. *Sports Med.* 2001;31(10):701–715.

29. Lambert GP, Lang JA, Bull AJ, et al. Fluid tolerance while running: effect of repeated trials. *Int J Sports Med.* 2008;29:878–882.

30. Neufer PD, Young AJ, Sawka MN. Gastric emptying during exercise: effects of heat stress and hypohydration. *Eur J Appl Physiol.* 1989;58:433–439.

31. Rehrer NJ, Beckers EJ, Brouns F, et al. Effects of dehydration on gastric emptying and gastrointestinal distress while running. *Med Sci Sports Exerc.* 1990;22(6):790–795.

32. Cooper H, Levitan R, Fordtran JS, et al. A method for studying absorption of water and solute from the human small intestine. *Gastroenterology.* 1966;50:1–7.

33. Thomson ABR, Keelan M, Thiesen A, et al. Small bowel review: normal physiology part 1. *Dig Dis Sci.* 2001;46:2567–2587.

34. Kellett GL. The facilitated component of intestinal glucose absorption. *J Physiol.* 2001;531.3:585–595.

35. Stevens BR. Vertebrate intestine apical membrane mechanisms of organic nutrient transport. *Am J Physiol.* 1992(263):R458–R463.

36. Ugolev A, Zaripov B, Iezuitova N, et al. A revision of current data and views on membrane hydrolysis and transport in the mammalian small intestine based on comparison of techniques of chronic and acute experiments: experimental re-investigation and critical review. *Comp Biochem Physiol A Comp Physiol.* 1986;85A:593–612.

37. Madara JL, Pappenheimer JR. Structural basis for physiological regulation of paracellular pathways in intestinal epithelia. *J Memb Biol.* 1987;100:149–164.

38. Fordtran JS, Saltin B. Gastric emptying and intestinal absorption during prolonged severe exercise. *J Appl Physiol.* 1967;23(3):331–335.

39. Lang JA, Gisolfi CV, Lambert GP. Effect of exercise intensity on active and passive glucose absorption. *Int J Sport Nutr Exerc Metab.* 2006;16:485–493.

40. Lambert GP, Mason B, Broussard L, et al. Intestinal absorption and permeability during exercise with aspirin: effects of glutamine in replacement beverages. *FASEB J.* 1998;12(4):A370.

41. Hegarty JE, Fairclough PD, Clark ML, et al. Jejunal water and electrolyte secretion induced by L-arginine in man. *Gut.* 1981;22:108–113.

42. Fordtran JS. Stimulation of active and passive sodium absorption by sugars in the human jejunum. *J Clin Invest.* 1975;55:728–737.

43. Gisolfi CV, Summers RD, Schedl HP, et al. Effect of sodium concentration in a carbohydrate-electrolyte solution on intestinal absorption. *Med Sci Sports Exerc.* 1995;27(10):1414–1420.

44. Gisolfi CV, Spranger KJ, Summers RW, et al. Effects of cycle exercise on intestinal absorption in humans. *J Appl Physiol.* 1991;71(6):2518–2527.

45. Loo DDF, Zeuthen T, Chandy G, et al. Cotransport of water by the Na+/glucose cotransporter. *Proc Natl Acad Sci.* November 1996;93:13367–13370.

46. Krofchick D, Huntley SA, Silverman M. Transition states of the high-affinity rabbit Na+/glucose cotransporter SGLT1 as determined from measurement and analysis of voltage dependent charge movements. *Am J Physiol Cell Physiol.* 2004;287:C46–C54.

47. Lambert GP, Lanspa S, Welch R, et al. Combined effects of glucose and fructose on fluid absorption from hypertonic carbohydrate-electrolyte beverages. *J Exerc Physiol.* 2008;11(2):46–55.

48. Shi X, Summers RW, Schedl HP, et al. Effects of carbohydrate type and concentration and solution osmolality on water absorption. *Med Sci Sports Exerc.* 1995;27(12):1607–1615.

49. Leiper JB, Maughan RJ. Comparison of absorption rates from two hypotonic and two isotonic rehydration solutions in the intact human jejunum. *Clin Sci.* 1988;75(suppl 19):22P.

50. Leiper JB, Maughan RJ. The effect of luminal tonicity on water absorption from a segment of the intact human jejunum. *J Physiol.* 1986;378:95P.

51. Gisolfi CV, Summers RW, Schedl HP, et al. Human intestinal water absorption: direct vs. indirect measurements. *Am J Physiol.* 1990;258:G216–G222.

52. Leiper JB, Maughan RJ. Absorption of water and electrolytes from hypotonic, isotonic, and hypertonic solutions. *J Physiol.* 1986;373:90P.

53. Shi X, Summers RW, Schedl HP, et al. Effects of solution osmolality on absorption of select fluid replacement solutions in human duodenojejunum. *J Appl Physiol.* 1994;77(3):1178–1184.

54. Rolston DD, Mathan VI. Jejunal and ileal glucose-stimulated water and sodium absorption in tropical enteropathy: implications for oral rehydration therapy. *Digestion.* 1990;46:55–60.

55. Beaumont DM, Cobdent L, Sheldon WL, et al. Passive and active carbohydrate absorption by the aging gut. *Age Ageing.* 1987;16:294–300.

56. Keeling WF, Martin BJ. Gastrointestinal transit during mild exercise. *J Appl Physiol.* 1987;63(3):978–981.

57. Keeling WF, Harris A, Martin BJ. Orocecal transit during mild exercise in women. *J Appl Physiol.* 1990;68(4):1350–1353.

58. van Nieuwenhoven MA, Brouns F, Brummer RJ. The effect of physical exercise on parameters of gastrointestinal function. *Neurogastroenterol Motil.* 1999;11(6):431–439.

59. Soffer EE, Summers RW, Gisolfi C. Effect of exercise on intestinal motility and transit in trained athletes. *Am J Physiol: Gastrointest Liver Physiol.* 1991;260(23):G698–G702.

60. Feldman M, Nixon JV. Effect of exercise on postprandial gastric secretion and emptying in humans. *J Appl Physiol: Respirat Environ Exercise Physiol.* 1982;53(4):851–854.

61. Cheskin LJ, Crowell MD, Kamal B, et al. The effects of acute exercise on colonic motility. *J Gastrointest Motil.* 1992;4:173–177.

62. Rao SSC, Beaty J, Chamberlain M, et al. Effects of acute graded exercise on human colonic motility. *Am J Physiol.* 1999;276:G1221–G1226.

63. Harris A, Lindeman AK, Martin BJ. Rapid orocecal transit in chronically active persons with high energy intake. *J Appl Physiol.* 1991;70(4):1550–1553.

64. De Schryver AM, Keulemans YC, Peters HP, et al. Effects of regular physical activity on defecation pattern in middle aged-patients complaining of chronic constipation. *Scand J Gastroenterol.* 2005;40(4):422–429.

65. Markiewicz K, Cholewa M, Górski L, et al. Effect of physical exercise on gastric basal secretion in healthy men. *Acta Hepatogastroenterol (Stuttg).* 1977;24(5):377–380.

66. Minato K. Effect of endurance training on pancreatic enzyme activity in rats. *Eur J Appl Physiol.* 1997;76:491–494.

67. Zsinka AJ, Frenkl R. Exocrine function of the pancreas in regularly swimming rats. *Acta Physiol Hung.* 1983;62(2):123–129.

68. Baumgart D, Dignass A. Intestinal barrier function. *Curr Op Clin Nutr Metab Care.* 2002;5:685–694.

69. Nagler-Anderson C. Man the barrier! Strategic defences in the intestinal mucosa. *Nature Rev.* 2001;1:59–67.

70. Lambert GP. Stress-induced gastrointestinal barrier dysfunction and its inflammatory effects. *J Anim Sci.* 2009;87:E101–E108.

71. Lambert GP, Murray R, Eddy D, et al. Intestinal permeability following the 1998 Ironman triathlon. *Med Sci Sports Exerc.* 1999;31(5):S318.

72. Pals KL, Chang RT, Ryan AJ, et al. Effect of running intensity on intestinal permeability. *J Appl Physiol.* 1997;82(2):571–576.

73. Lambert GP, Boylan MW, Laventure JP, et al. Effect of aspirin and ibuprofen on GI permeability during exercise. *Int J Sports Med.* 2007;28(9):722–726.

74. Halvorsen FA, Ritland S. Gastrointestinal problems related to endurance event training. *Sports Med.* 1992;14(3):157–163.

75. Keefe EB, Lowe DK, Goss JR, et al. Gastrointestinal symptoms of marathon runners. *West J Med.* 1984;141:481–484.

76. Moses FM, Brewer TG, Peura DA. Running-associated proximal hemorrhagic colitis. *Ann Int Med.* 1988;108(3):385–386.

77. Oektedalen O, Lunde OC, Opstad PK, et al. Changes in the gastrointestinal mucosa after long distance running. *Scand J Gastroenterol.* 1992;27:270–274.

78. Lambert GP. Intestinal barrier dysfunction, endotoxemia, and gastrointestinal symptoms: the "canary in the coal mine" during exercise-heat stress? In: Marino F, ed. *Thermoregulation and Human Performance: Physiological and Biological Aspects.* New York: Karger; 2008:61–73.

79. Lambert GP, Broussard LJ, Mason BL, et al. Gastrointestinal permeability during exercise: effects of aspirin and energy-containing beverages. *J Appl Physiol.* 2001;90:2075–2080.

80. Lambert GP, Lang JA, Bull AJ, et al. Fluid restriction increases GI permeability during running. *Int J Sports Med.* 2008;29(3):194–198.

CHAPTER 13

The Metabolic Systems: Control of ATP Synthesis in Skeletal Muscle

Ronald A. Meyer and Robert W. Wiseman

Abbreviations

ADP	Adenosine diphosphate	MRI	Magnetic resonance imaging
AMP	Adenosine monophosphate	NAD	Nicotinamide adenine dinucleotide
ATP	Adenosine triphosphate	NADH	Reduced nicotinamide adenine dinucleotide
ATPase	Adenosine triphosphatase		
CoA	Coenzyme A	NMR	Nuclear magnetic resonance
CK	Creatine kinase	PCr	Phosphocreatine
DNP	Dinitrophenol	PDH	Pyruvate dehydrogenase
ΔG_{ATP}	Free energy of ATP hydrolysis (Δ = change)	P_i	Inorganic phosphate
		SERCA	Sarcoplasmic-endoplasmic reticulum calcium ATPase
GP	Glycogen phosphorylase		
IMP	Inosine monophosphate	SR	Sarcoplasmic reticulum
K_{CK}	CK equilibrium constant in a certain direction		

Introduction

The transition from rest to tetanic contraction imposes a unique burden on the metabolism of skeletal muscle compared to most other tissues. During this transition, which can occur within 30 ms in a fast muscle, the adenosine triphosphate (ATP) utilization rate can increase from approximately 0.01 μmol ATP $\cdot$ g^{-1} $\cdot$ s^{-1} at rest to nearly 10 μmol ATP $\cdot$ g^{-1} $\cdot$ s^{-1}, a 1000-fold increase! The ATP content of mammalian fast skeletal muscles is 7 to 8 μmol $\cdot$ g^{-1}. Thus, the entire ATP content of a fast muscle fiber could, in principle, be depleted after a 1-second contraction. In reality, however, net depletion of muscle ATP is observed only during the most intense heavy exercise regimens and even then rarely exceeds 30% to 40% of the available muscle ATP content. This chapter explains how this tight coupling of ATP synthesis to ATP utilization in skeletal muscle emerges from the integrated response of the metabolic system to changes in work intensity. It is only by considering the response of the system as a whole that one can understand phenomena such as the oxygen deficit at the onset of exercise and the dependence of lactate production on exercise intensity.

Many excellent textbooks and monographs, for example, Hochachka (1), provide introductions to exercise biochemistry. Therefore, we assume you are already familiar with basic aspects of metabolism, such as the pathways of glycolysis, the citric acid cycle, and the principles of enzyme kinetics. This chapter focuses on intracellular control mechanisms and the regulation of ATP free energy. The importance of adequate oxygen and carbon substrate delivery to muscle cells during exercise is considered in other chapters of this book.

The Rate of ATP Use during Contraction

The ATP hydrolysis rate during a muscle contraction and ultimately during repetitive exercise depends on two factors: (a) fiber type, or more specifically, the myosin and SERCA (sarcoplasmic-endoplasmic reticulum calcium adenosine triphosphatase [ATPase]) isoform types; and (b) the peak force and mechanical nature of the contraction. Myosin ATPase accounts for 70% of contractile ATP use, and SERCA activity accounts for most of the remaining 30%. Thus, variations in the kinetic properties of these two enzymes are the major source of the variation in the intrinsic ATP cost of muscle contraction, both within a species and across species. Of course, differences in myosin and SERCA isoform expression, along with differences in metabolic profile, are also the key features distinguishing the mammalian fiber types (see Chapter 4). Mammalian fibers with the fastest myosin kinetics (fast twitch white fibers with type IIB/IIX myosin heavy chain) and fastest SERCA (type 1) develop force quickly, shorten at the highest velocity, and relax most rapidly after a contraction. At the other extreme, slow twitch red fibers (type I myosin heavy chain, type 2A SERCA) develop force, shorten, and relax relatively slowly.

The profound effect of fiber type on contractile ATP cost (ATP use divided by force times time integral) or economy (the reciprocal of ATP cost) is not subjectively apparent to an exercising human, first because intact human muscles are generally composed of a mix of fiber types and second because the fastest fibers are organized in large motor units recruited only during the heaviest efforts. However, the limbs of rodents and some other quadrupeds have muscles with relatively uniform fiber type. For example, the soleus muscle of mice, rats, and cats consists of predominantly slow-twitch fibers, whereas the anterior tibialis or biceps brachii muscles consist of predominantly fast fiber types. Studies of these animal muscles demonstrate that slow fibers can maintain isometric force with more than three times the economy of fast fibers (2). For example, the ATP cost of a fused isometric tetanus is 2.4 μmol $\cdot$ (g muscle)$^{-1}$ $\cdot$ (kg force)$^{-1}$ $\cdot$ s^{-1} in intact cat soleus muscle (95% slow twitch) versus 8.0 in cat biceps brachii muscle (>70% fast twitch white, 20% fast twitch red). Analogous measurements have not been performed in intact human muscles; for example, no one has made a study of subjects with genetically diverse fiber compositions. However, based on studies of ATP turnover during activation of glycerinated, skinned single fibers isolated from human subjects (i.e., fibers from which the sarcolemma and all internal cell membranes are removed by glycerin treatment), the difference in contractile economy between fiber types in humans is similar to the difference in economy between fiber types in other mammalian species (3). This difference in contractile economy between fiber types has important implications for understanding the energetic cost of locomotion (4) and also for understanding individual differences in performance. For example, the association between elite performance in endurance sports and a high percentage of slow fibers may be largely due to the greater economy of slow fibers rather than to differences in mitochondrial content between human fiber types. In fact, in human muscles, the mitochondrial contents of fast red and slow fibers are not substantially different. Endurance training can dramatically increase mitochondrial content

in all the fibers recruited by a training regimen (see Chapter 18), but there is little evidence that exercise training alone can significantly change an individual's fiber type distribution. Of course, the downside to the high economy of slow fibers is their slower shortening velocity, hence lower peak mechanical power output (power equals force times velocity). Thus, individuals endowed with the slow fiber type predominance appropriate for low-power activities, such as long distance running, are necessarily at a disadvantage for events requiring a high power output, such as sprinting.

KEY POINT

Contractile cost is a larger determinant of endurance than mitochondrial density between red and white muscle fibers.

The second major determinant of contractile ATP cost is the force and mechanical nature (*e.g.*, isometric vs. isotonic) of the contraction. For isometric contractions lasting several seconds, contractile ATP use increases linearly with the force times time integral, and for series of twitch contractions, steady-state ATPase rate is proportional to peak twitch force times twitch rate (5). To a good approximation these relationships hold during fatigue; that is, as peak force decreases during a series of fatiguing contractions, the ATP rate decreases. Finally, contractile ATP cost varies with the type of contraction. For example, ATPase rate of isolated muscles or skinned fibers is up to twice as high during shortening contractions than during isometric contractions, which is consistent with models of the kinetics of myosin crossbridge cycling at various velocities (3). Conversely, the ATPase rate in isolated muscles decreases during lengthening (eccentric) compared to isometric contractions, although this effect is not apparent in a study of ATP cost in human muscles during voluntary contractions (6).

In intact rat fast twitch skeletal muscle the *peak cellular* ATPase rate during a fused tetanus has been estimated to exceed 10 μmol $\cdot$ g^{-1} $\cdot$ s^{-1} (5). This estimate is based on gated phosphorus nuclear magnetic resonance (NMR) studies that were validated by comparison to steady-state measurements of muscle oxygen consumption at lower contraction intensities. Unfortunately, analogous measurements during maximal activation in intact human muscles are not easy to obtain. The estimated ATP cost of maximum voluntary contractions in human muscle ranges from 0.5 to 2 μmol $\cdot$ g^{-1} $\cdot$ s^{-1}. Unfortunately, these measurements are the average from an unknown mixed fiber population, and there is no assurance that all motor units are recruited or that all units are maximally active during a maximum voluntary contraction. Electrical stimulation of motor nerves at rates sufficient to achieve a fused tetanus would be quite painful, and the force generated from synchronous discharge of all motor units in a human muscle could be damaging. Therefore, the peak cellular ATPase rate in fast human muscle fibers can at present be estimated only by comparison with animal studies. For example, extrapolating from comparison of the ATP cost of a twitch in human mixed versus rat fast muscle (0.15 vs. 0.26 μmol $\cdot$ g^{-1} for human and rat, respectively [5,7]), the maximal ATP turnover in tetanized human fast fibers must be at least 5 μmol $\cdot$ g^{-1} $\cdot$ s^{-1}. Of course, this maximal rate, which would correspond to an oxygen consumption of more than 1000 mL oxygen (kg muscle)$^{-1}$ $\cdot$ min^{-1}, cannot be continuously sustained for long (discussed later). During realistic repetitive exercises, the average rate of muscle ATP turnover is somewhat less. For example, the rate of oxygen consumption during heavy cycling exercise in well-trained subjects is around 3600 mL oxygen per minute. Assuming 10 kg of active leg muscle and assuming six muscle ATPs produced per oxygen consumed, this corresponds to an average muscle ATP turnover of around 1.6 μmol (g muscle)$^{-1}$ $\cdot$ s^{-1}.

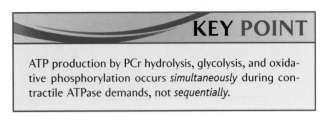

> ## KEY POINT
>
> The ATP demands during activity in muscle depend on the mechanical nature and intensity of the contraction.

Summary
The energetic cost of muscle contraction during exercise depends on the intrinsic contractile economy of the fiber types recruited in the active muscles, and also on the peak fiber force, shortening velocity, and repetition rate of contractions. The most energetically economical exercises involve isometric contractions of muscles at low to moderate force during which primarily slow fibers are recruited.

The Capacity of ATP Synthesis Pathways in Muscle

The pathways for ATP production in vertebrate skeletal muscle are the same as in most other tissues: (a) direct phosphorylation of adenosine diphosphate (ADP) to ATP by phosphocreatine (PCr), (b) glycolytic ATP production, and (c) mitochondrial ATP production. Exercise physiology books traditionally present these pathways in a hierarchy from the most rapidly activated but shortest lasting source of ATP (PCr utilization) to the most slowly activated but longest lasting source (mitochondrial ATP production). Although this hierarchy correctly characterizes the relative total capacities of the three pathways for ATP generation, it obscures the key feature of the integrated metabolic response at the onset of exercise. In fact, *fluxes through all three pathways occur simultaneously*, and the **control** of each depends on the **regulated** response of

the whole system to a change in ATPase rate. Nonetheless, it is useful to summarize this traditional hierarchy.

> ## KEY POINT
>
> ATP production by PCr hydrolysis, glycolysis, and oxidative phosphorylation occurs *simultaneously* during contractile ATPase demands, not *sequentially*.

High-energy Phosphate (ATP and PCr) Stores

Direct phosphorylation of ADP to ATP occurs via the reactions catalyzed by creatine kinase (CK):

$$\text{PCr} + \text{ADP} \leftrightarrow \text{ATP} + \text{creatine}$$

and adenylate kinase:

$$\text{ADP} + \text{ADP} \leftrightarrow \text{ATP} + \text{AMP}$$

(For simplicity, we largely omit the important dependence of these and the subsequent reactions on pH and cation concentration, and hence on the ionic distribution of the substrates. For an example, consult Harkema and Meyer [8].) In skeletal muscle, the total cytoplasmic activities of these enzymes are quite large, and so these reactions are typically assumed to be near equilibrium during contraction. In fact, calculations suggest that the CK reaction is significantly displaced from equilibrium during tetanic contractions (5). However, equilibrium is reestablished within less than a second after a tetanus, so the equilibrium assumption is reasonable when averaged over a repetitive exercise regimen.

The well-known consequence of these near-equilibrium reactions is that even in the absence of other ATP-regenerating pathways, ADP accumulation is limited, first by PCr depletion and, ultimately, by adenosine monophosphate (AMP) accumulation. Furthermore, in skeletal muscle, AMP accumulation is limited by its deamination to inosine monophosphate (IMP), catalyzed by AMP deaminase:

$$\text{AMP} \rightarrow \text{IMP} + \text{NH}_3$$

Thus, in the absence of any other source of ATP regeneration, hydrolysis of ATP results in discharge of the energy stored as PCr and ATP and, ultimately, in partial depletion of the adenine nucleotide pool to IMP. This occurs with minimal drop in energy *potential,* because the increase in ADP is minimized, and the free energy of ATP hydrolysis (ΔG_{ATP}), which decreases with increased ADP, is largely preserved (Fig. 13.1). The ΔG_{ATP} is the energy available from the reaction to do work, and at 37°C, pH 7 is:

$$\Delta G'_{ATP} = \Delta G'_{ATP} + RT \ln([\text{ADP}][\text{Pi}]/[\text{ATP}])$$
$$= -32 \text{ kJ/mol} + 2.58 \ln([\text{ADP}][\text{Pi}]/[\text{ATP}])$$

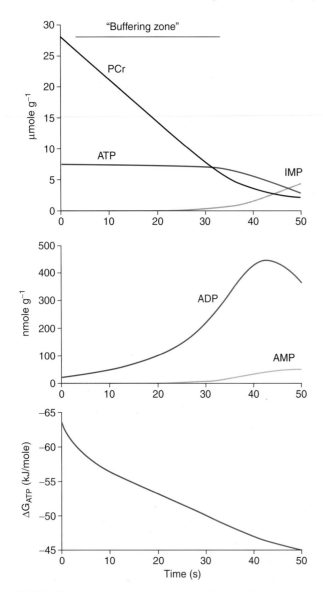

The total capacity of this high energy phosphate system in a fast muscle, assuming complete depletion of PCr (about $25-30\ \mu mol \cdot g^{-1}$) and ATP ($7.5\ \mu mol \cdot g^{-1} \times 2$, assuming depletion to AMP and IMP) is around $40\ \mu mol \cdot g^{-1}$, or in principle enough to sustain a maximal contraction at $10\ \mu mol \cdot g^{-1} \cdot s^{-1}$ for about 4 seconds.

Glycolytic ATP Synthesis

The net reaction of anaerobic glycolysis from glycogen-stored glucose to lactate is

$$(glucose)_n + 3\ ADP + 3\ P_i \rightarrow (glucose)_{n-1} + 3\ ATP + 2\ lactic\ acid$$

Assuming only stored glycogen as substrate ($50-100\ \mu mol$ glucose units $\cdot g^{-1}$), the total capacity for ATP generation by this pathway alone is thus around 150 to 300 μmol ATP g^{-1}, or enough to sustain maximal contraction for up to 30 seconds. Despite the low yield of ATP, this pathway is not thermodynamically inefficient because, as emphasized by Brooks (9), most of the available free energy remains in lactate, which can be further oxidized in the muscle or in other tissues.

Surprisingly, some authors have suggested that lactic acid production via glycolysis is not the cause of muscle acidosis, because hydrogen ion release actually occurs earlier in the pathway and ATP hydrolysis also produces hydrogen ions. However, with respect to its effect on pH balance in the muscle, all that matters is the net reaction. Because glycolytic ATP production is balanced by ATP utilization so that the net change in ATP is minor (and, as illustrated in Fig. 13.1, any significant ATP depletion is largely balanced by IMP and ammonia production, not ADP accumulation), the net glycolytic reaction in an active muscle is just glucose → 2 lactic acid.

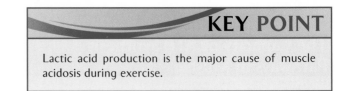

Lactic acid production is the major cause of muscle acidosis during exercise.

FIGURE 13.1 Computed time course of phosphocreatine (PCr) and adenine nucleotide depletion in a fast twitch skeletal muscle hydrolyzing adenosine triphosphate (ATP) at a steady-state rate of $1\ \mu mol \cdot g^{-1} \cdot s^{-1}$, assuming there is no source for ATP resynthesis except high-energy phosphate stores. Metabolite contents were computed using a kinetic model for CK and adenylate kinase fluxes (25). Adenosine monophosphate (AMP) deaminase flux assumed a simple Michaelis-Menten type of dependence on substrate AMP concentration with Km = 0.7 mM and V_{max} = 5 mM $\cdot s^{-1}$. The maximum contents of PCr, ATP, and IMP (*top panel*, in $\mu mol \cdot g^{-1}$) are much greater than the maximum contents of ADP and AMP (*middle panel*, in nmol $\cdot g^{-1}$). The buffering zone is the operating region before substantial net ATP depletion, when both PCr and free energy of ATP hydrolysis (ΔG_{ATP}) (*bottom panel*) decrease nearly linearly with time or with net high energy phosphate depletion. This is in the range of muscle metabolite levels observed during steady-state submaximal exercise.

The functional consequences of intracellular lactic acidosis are complex and not necessarily deleterious. For example, although acidosis does slow muscle relaxation rate after contractions, the idea that muscle fatigue is caused by direct effects of lactic acidosis on myofibrillar actin-myosin interaction and force generation has been largely abandoned (10). Certainly acidosis inhibits many enzymes and ion channels and may decrease the maximum rate of mitochondrial ATP production in intact muscle. On the other hand, acidosis actually appears to increase the mitochondrial energy potential for ATP synthesis (8). One might naively assume that acidosis lowers the cytosolic ΔG_{ATP}, because net ATP hydrolysis yields a fractional hydrogen ion above pH 6.5:

$$ATP \rightarrow ADP + Pi + \alpha H^+$$

where α is the molar fraction of hydrogen ions released per mole of ATP hydrolyzed.

However, if ATP hydrolysis is thermodynamically coupled to PCr hydrolysis via the CK reaction, acidosis has the opposite net effect on ATP free energy. Assuming equilibrium of the CK reaction, the ΔG_{ATP} must equal that of PCr hydrolysis, and the free energy of PCr hydrolysis increases (*i.e.*, is more negative) as pH falls (8). Stated another way, the pH dependence of the CK reaction over the physiologic range is as follows:

$$PCr + ADP + \beta H^+ \leftrightarrow ATP + creatine$$

where β is the molar fraction of hydrogen ion consumed per mole of PCr hydrolyzed, ranging from about 0.9 to 0.6 from pH 7 to pH 6. This tends to lower ADP as a muscle becomes acidic. For example, assuming equilibrium of the CK reaction, constant muscle [PCr]/[Cr] = 1, and [P_i] = 15 mM (reasonable values during moderately heavy exercise) (where P_i is inorganic phosphate), a decrease in pH from 7.1 to 6.5 increases the free energy of PCr and ATP hydrolysis from −55.8 to −57.7 kJ · $mole^{-1}$ (8).

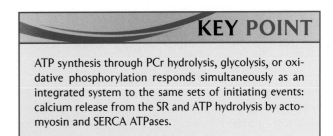

KEY POINT

In the presence of the CK system, lactic acidosis actually blunts the decline in ATP free energy that would otherwise occur with depletion of PCr.

Summary

The temporal buffering of ATP free energy by hydrolysis of PCr and the incomplete oxidation of glucose to 2 lactate ions are not independent. For didactic purposes, it is relatively easy to instruct students on this topic by first outlining ATP buffering through the CK system and then ATP buffering via glycolysis, but this has lead to naïve understanding of the integrated metabolic network. In a coupled system where CK and glycolysis are operational, this occurs simultaneously not sequentially and, further, these mechanism for ATP production are chemically linked through proton ion production and the stoichiometries of their respective chemical reactions.

Oxidative Phosphorylation

Finally, the net reaction for complete oxidation of glycogen-derived pyruvate (including the reduced nicotinamide adenine dinucleotide [NADH] yield from glycolysis) is as follows:

$$2\ C_3H_5O_3 + 6O_2 + 2\ NADH + 33\ ADP + 33\ P_i \rightarrow$$
$$6\ CO_2 + 6\ H_2O + 2\ NAD + 33\ ATP$$

The corresponding net reaction for complete oxidation of the 16-carbon saturated fatty acid palmitate is:

$$C_{16}H_{32}O_2 + 23\ O_2 + 129\ ADP + 129\ P_i \rightarrow 16\ CO_2 +$$
$$16\ H_2O + 129\ ATP$$

Clearly mitochondrial oxidative phosphorylation, particularly using fatty acid substrates, is the only source of ATP production with the capacity to support prolonged exercise, and in this respect the traditional presentation is correct.

The tempting inference from this traditional hierarchy is that these pathways are controlled independently and that their relative importance at the onset of exercise is related to the speed at which they can be activated and how long each can last. This inference is *not* correct. For example, although it is correct that net PCr hydrolysis accounts for most of the ATP used during the first seconds at the onset of contractions, this fact does not demonstrate that there is any intrinsic delay or inertia for activation of either glycolysis or mitochondrial ATP production.

KEY POINT

ATP synthesis through PCr hydrolysis, glycolysis, or oxidative phosphorylation responds simultaneously as an integrated system to the same sets of initiating events: calcium release from the SR and ATP hydrolysis by actomyosin and SERCA ATPases.

Control Versus Regulation in Muscle Metabolism

It is important to distinguish between metabolic *control* and metabolic *regulation*. *Control* is the effect of a signal on the flux through an enzyme or pathway, where changes in the signal result in a change in the rate of the enzyme or pathway, but where the signal concentration is an independent variable. In contrast, *regulation* is the maintenance of some parameter in a relatively constant state, despite changes in external signals or in fluxes through the pathways in which the parameter is involved. By these definitions, the central external *controlling* element in muscle metabolism is the input from the motor neuron, reflected intracellularly by release of calcium from the sarcoplasmic reticulum (SR), and by activation of myosin and SERCA ATPases. The central *regulated* parameter is not the ATP hydrolysis rate or pathway fluxes per se but rather the cytoplasmic ΔG_{ATP}. This regulation arises from the entire network behavior of both the ATP synthesizing pathways and the dominant ATPases in the cell, that is, myosin and SERCA. Its effectiveness is illustrated by the fact that the maximum drop in ATP free energy observed in human muscle even during the heaviest exercise is only 14 kJ · mole^{-1} (to −50 kJ · mole^{-1} from near −64 kJ · mole^{-1} at rest) (11).

The physiologic importance of *regulating* cytoplasmic ATP free energy can be appreciated by considering the energy required to maintain ion gradients across the sarcolemma and SR. For example, ignoring electrical effects and assuming a stoichiometry of two calcium ions pumped per ATP hydrolyzed by the SERCA pump, the maximum cytoplasmic to SR luminal calcium gradient that can be developed depends on ΔG_{ATP}:

$$[Ca^{++}]_{SR}/[Ca^{++}]_{CYTO} = exp[(-\Delta G_{ATP}/(2 \times RT))]$$

where RT is the gas constant times absolute temperature (2.58 kJ · mole^{-1} at 37°C). Thus, a 14 kJ · mole^{-1} drop in ATP free energy would reduce this maximum gradient by more than 93%. If ΔG_{ATP} were to fall to less than −48 kJ · mole^{-1}, there would not be sufficient energy to sequester calcium against the normal 10,000-fold gradient after a contraction (12), and the muscle might fail to relax, with obviously disastrous effects on locomotion. Similarly, the maximum sodium gradient that can be maintained across the cell membrane by Na-K ATPase, assuming three sodium ions pumped per ATP hydrolyzed, depends on ΔG_{ATP}:

$$[Na^{+}]_{out}/[Na^{+}]_{in} = exp((-\Delta G_{ATP}/3 - F \times Em)/RT)$$

where Em is the membrane potential (−80 mV) and F is Faraday's constant and ignoring the small additional energy needed to cotransport potassium, which is near electrochemical equilibrium across the membrane. Thus, failure of the sarcolemmal Na-K ATPase to maintain the normal 20-fold sodium gradient across the sarcolemma would also occur near −48 kJ · mole^{-1}, with equally disastrous consequences for the muscle. In the absence of tight control of ATP supply by ATP demand, regulation of ATP free energy potential would be lost, and cellular ion gradients crucial to control of muscle activation and relaxation would fail.

The concept that muscle ATPase rate controls the rate of ATP production is easy to apply to the direct production of ATP from PCr and ADP. In this case, it is obvious that no other control mechanism is required, because the CK and adenylate kinase near-equilibrium reactions simply respond by mass action to the change in adenine nucleotide concentrations when ATP is hydrolyzed.

It may seem impossible to apply the same concept to control of more complex pathways such as glycolysis or fatty acid and amino acid catabolism because of the entrenched view that control of these pathways must reside at specific rate-limiting or irreversible reaction steps. For example, in the case of control of glycolysis, the conventional textbook presentation is that control resides at the "irreversible" reactions catalyzed by glycogen

phosphorylase (GP), phosphofructokinase, and pyruvate kinase. However, no enzymatic reaction is irreversible on the molecular level, although the thermodynamic drive for the reaction might point very heavily in one direction in vivo. Lambeth and Kushmerick (13) exploited this basic consideration in a simulation of glycogenolysis and glycolysis in skeletal muscle. The simulation assumed that all of the reactions between glycogen and lactate production were reversible, that glycogen concentration was constant, and that lactate removal equaled lactate production, so that pH effects were not considered. The simulation was run to steady state at three ATPase activities corresponding to rest, moderate exercise, and heavy exercise (up to 1 mM ATP · second^{-1}, equivalent to 224 mL O^2 · kg muscle^{-1} · min^{-1}), and the steady-state sensitivities of glycolytic flux to each enzyme's activity were computed. Sensitivity is the ratio of percentage change in a pathway's steady-state flux to percentage change in an enzyme's activity, and in the formalism of metabolic control analysis, it is also known as the flux control coefficient (14) (discussed later). The main conclusion from these computations was that flux control over glycolysis resided almost entirely (>95%) in the ATPase over the entire range considered. At the highest ATPase rate, the small proportion of flux control contributed by glycolytic enzymes was widely distributed over the whole pathway, whereas at rest it was confined to GP and phosphofructokinase. Increasing the percentage of GP in the active (a) form from 1% to 40% (similar to the activation observed at the onset of exercise in human muscle) had no effect on the overall flux but did shift the minor flux control exerted by glycolytic enzymes to include greater contributions from enolase and pyruvate kinase. The latter result explains some previously puzzling experimental results; for example, the observations that the inactivation of GP after a few minutes of exercise does not decrease glycolytic flux and that activation of GP by administration of epinephrine does not necessarily increase glycolytic flux. Despite the greater complexity of the pathways for fatty acid and amino acid catabolism, this basic consideration must apply to those pathways as well.

KEY POINT

If a pathway is tightly coupled to ATP synthesis, the flux through this pathway cannot increase unless the ATPase rate increases or the contribution from some other ATP-producing pathway decreases.

The concept that calcium-activated ATPases are central to the control of muscle mitochondrial ATP production was examined by Jeneson and associates (15) using metabolic control analysis. Metabolic control analysis is a quantitative method for analyzing the distribution of flux control within a steady-state network of reactions using a mathematical approach distinct from the conventional focus on isolated "control" points (14). In this method, the relative contribution to control of each enzyme or functional element of a pathway's flux is characterized by its sensitivity or flux control coefficient, as defined earlier. The effects of a shared substrate on each element's activity are characterized by elasticity coefficients. Elasticity is analogous to a reaction's order with respect to a substrate. For example, the elasticity of a simple Michalis-Menten type of enzymatic reaction to a saturating substrate is zero because the reaction's rate does not increase with further increases in the substrate. Finally, the concentration control coefficient of an enzyme on a pathway's shared substrate is just the relative change in that substrate's concentration with a change in the enzyme's activity. These coefficients are related by several algebraic constraints; for example, that the sum of control coefficients for a pathway flux must equal one and the sum of concentration control coefficients for a substrate must equal zero. In practice, the mathematics of metabolic control analysis becomes formidable for networks with more than a few elements, and calculation of elasticity coefficients in vivo from enzyme kinetic data in vitro is not always straightforward. Nonetheless, Jeneson and associates (15) solved this algebraic problem for a three-element network of myosin ATPase, SERCA, and mitochondrial ATP production, assuming ATP and ADP as the only common substrates that link these elements, and using flux estimates derived from studies of human muscle during twitch stimulation. As might be expected, all three elements exerted some concentration control over the ATP: ADP ratio. However, over the range from mild to moderate stimulation intensities, *flux control* over the mitochondria (the only ATP-generating element in the model) resided almost entirely within the myosin and SERCA ATPases. Only when the calculations were extrapolated to very high stimulation rates did control over mitochondrial ATP generation shift to the mitochondrial element itself. The conceptual result is that the entire system adapts to increased flux with minimal perturbation in ATP free energy.

Summary

The ATP synthesis rate in muscle is tightly coupled to the ATP hydrolysis rate during contractions because the flux from each of the three ATP sources (high energy phosphate stores, glycolysis, and oxidative phosphorylation) is controlled by the ATP hydrolysis rate itself over most of the physiologic range. The effect of this tight control is regulation of the intracellular free energy available from ATP hydrolysis.

The Control of Muscle Respiration

The argument that mitochondrial ATP production and respiration rate are controlled by muscle ATPases is not likely to satisfy many readers because it does not specify any distinct biochemical signaling mechanism acting at the mitochondria. Mitochondrial ATP production occurs in a complicated membrane-bound organelle and involves the coordinated activity of dozens of nonvectorial and vectorial reaction steps. (Vectorial reactions are those that occur with a spatial orientation, such as ion transport.) Therefore, the idea that specific signals are required to control mitochondria is appealing, and enormous effort has been spent to determine what controls muscle respiration. Consideration of the candidates requires a summary of the mechanism and energetics of mitochondrial ATP production.

Mitochondria

Mitochondria are small organelles (0.5–1 μm across) composed of two lipid bilayers (Fig. 13.2). The outer membrane is smooth and permeable to the free diffusion of substrates such as carbon fuels, ADP, ATP, P_i, creatine, PCr, and ions (including hydrogen ions) and dissolved gases. The inner membrane is relatively impermeable and highly invaginated, essential properties for mitochondrial function. The invaginations, termed *cristae*, vary with the oxidative capacity of the mitochondrion because of the high density of respiratory complexes and specific transporters embedded within this membrane. Thus, energetically important metabolites such as ATP, ADP, and P_i freely diffuse through the outer membrane but require carriers for their transport across the inner membrane, as do the monocarboxylic and dicarboxylic acid carbon substrates. The inner membrane encompasses the mitochondrial matrix, a lumen that contains all the enzymes, and substrates and cofactors necessary for the function of the citric acid cycle. Mitochondria produce ATP by converting the energy in chemical bonds from the oxidation of carbohydrates and fats into NADH, which is used by the electron transport system to create a hydrogen ion electrochemical gradient. This gradient is generated across the inner membrane by pumping hydrogen ions out of the matrix and into the inner membrane space using the respiratory complexes. The flow of hydrogen ions back down this energy gradient into the matrix rapidly alters the conformation of F0/F1-ATP synthase, thus transferring the energy from the gradient into the terminal phosphate bond of ATP. Finally, the exchange of cytoplasmic ADP for matrix ATP via the adenine nucleotide transporter is in effect driven by the energy of the hydrogen ion gradient.

The conceptual flux and energetic relationships through mitochondria are depicted in Figure 13.3 by a sequence of pipes and reservoirs. Each element of the overall mechanism has an associated flux (illustrated by the size of the black arrows in the pipes) and a maximum flux capacity (illustrated by the diameters of the pipes). The energetic state of the system is characterized by several free energy potentials, depicted by the relative heights of the shaded areas in each potential reservoir. For example, the redox potential is the free energy available in oxidation of NADH to nicotinamide adenine dinucleotide (NAD); that is:

$$\Delta G_{REDOX} = \Delta G^{\circ}_{REDOX} + RT \ln([NAD]/[NADH])$$

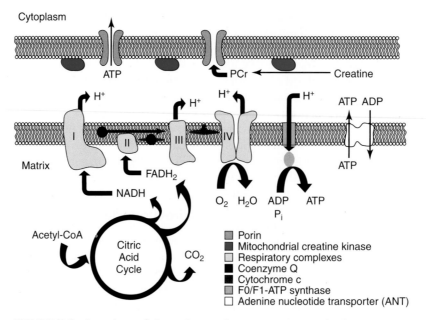

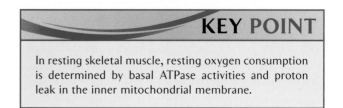

FIGURE 13.2 Locations of the major respiratory components in the mitochondrial membranes and matrix. ATP, adenosine triphosphate; PCr, phosphocreatine; ADP, adenosine diphosphate; $FADH_2$ reduced flavin adenine dinucleotide; P_i inorganic phosphate; NADH, reduced nicotinamide adenine dinucleotide; CoA, coenzyme A.

The standard free energy, $\Delta G°_{REDOX}$, is about $-218\,kJ \cdot mole^{-1}$, so even at an NAD/NADH ratio of 1, there is more than enough potential energy to synthesize three ATPs at a cytoplasmic ATP free energy of -60 to $-65\,kJ \cdot mole^{-1}$. The hydrogen ion electrochemical potential depends on the hydrogen ion gradient across the inner membrane and membrane potential according to the following:

$$\Delta G_{H+} = 2.303 \times RT\,(pH_{matrix} - pH_{cyto}) + F \times Em$$

The ATP free energy inside and outside the mitochondria can be computed as in Eq. 13.1. (In this conceptual diagram, we have ignored the fact that the ATP/ADP ratio and therefore the ΔG_{ATP} are lower in the matrix of mitochondria than in the cytoplasm. The additional potential in the cytoplasm is gained by the exchange of ATP^{4-} for ADP^{3-} in the adenine nucleotide transporter, energetically driven by the hydrogen electrochemical potential gradient.) These various potentials are coupled but can change relative to each other depending on the magnitude of the connecting fluxes relative to their maximum flux capacities. In the steady state, the flux into and out of each element is equal, and the steady-state flux through the system could in principle be limited at any element.

Figure 13.3A depicts the situation in skeletal muscle at resting or basal state, or in isolated mitochondria near the classic state 4; that is, with unlimited carbon fuel and oxygen but relatively little drain from the terminal cytoplasmic free energy reservoir by cytoplasmic ATP hydrolysis. In state 4, all of the potentials are charged, and the only drain on the system is the uncoupled leak of hydrogen ions back into the

mitochondrial matrix. (By leak we mean any dissipation of the hydrogen ion gradient that is not coupled to ATP synthesis and export.) The situation in a skeletal muscle at rest approximates the situation in state 4 except that the basal resting ATP synthesis rate is normally much greater than the leak, and the ratio of ATP synthesized to oxygen consumed approaches the optimal coupling ratio of 6.

Now consider the effect on this system if the cytoplasmic ATP hydrolysis rate is increased (Fig. 13.3B), for example, to 50% of the muscle cell's maximum possible oxidative capacity. The cytoplasmic ΔG_{ATP} will fall, ADP and P_i concentrations will increase, the transport of these substrates into the matrix will increase, and the rate of ATP synthase will increase. This will in turn lower the hydrogen ion potential and flux through the electron transport chain will increase, and so on back through the entire sequence. The potential energy at every step will decrease to an extent determined by the kinetic properties and maximum capacity of the flux elements into and out of those potentials. Ultimately, a new steady state with equally higher flux into and out of each element will be established. Of course, each element will behave in a fashion consistent

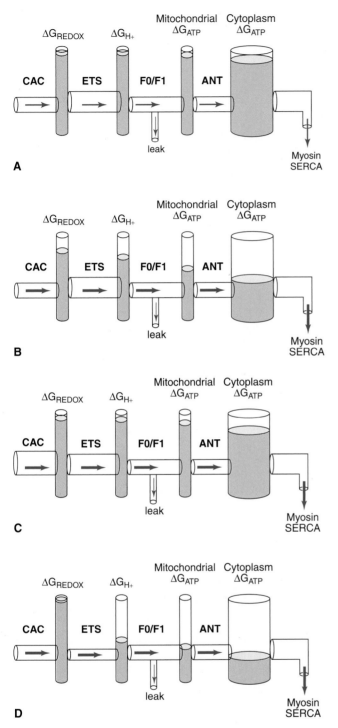

A

B

C

D

FIGURE 13.3 The steady-state relationship between intramitochondrial and extramitochondrial energy potentials and the pathway conductances connecting them under various conditions. **A.** State 4, or resting skeletal muscle. **B.** Skeletal muscle during submaximal exercise. **C.** Effect of mitochondrial dehydrogenase activation during submaximal exercise. **D.** Effect of hypoxia during submaximal exercise. ANT, adenine nucleotide transporter; CAC, citric acid cycle; ETS, electron transport system; Fo/F₁, an ATP synthase; SERCA, sarcoplasmic-endoplasmic reticulum calcium ATPase.

with its kinetic properties. For example, the steady-state transport of nucleotides by adenine nucleotide transporter will be consistent with its binding affinities for ADP and ATP, and the synthesis of ATP by F1/F0-ATP synthase will be consistent with its affinities for ADP and P_i. Thus, under some specific set of experimental conditions (*e.g.*, isolated mitochondria saturated with all other substrates), a plot of ADP concentration versus steady-state respiration rate might be best fit by a simple Michaelis-Menten type of first order (hyperbolic) relationship, with the apparent Michaelis constant near that of the adenine nucleotide transporter binding constant for ADP. Under some other set of conditions, the relationship between ADP and respiration rate might be best fit by a higher order (sigmoidal) function, reflecting kinetic elasticity to ADP at more than one site; for example, at both adenine nucleotide transporter and ATP synthase (16), or cooperative binding at the adenine nucleotide transporter itself. If phosphate is initially low, there might be a satisfying relationship between phosphate concentration and steady-state respiration rate.

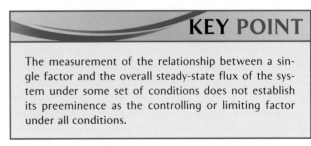

TEST **YOURSELF**

Dinitrophenol (DNP) is a mitochondrial uncoupling agent that was sold years ago as a dietary aid. As a weight loss pill, it worked magnificently because the subjects who took the compound did actually lose weight. However, an unwanted side effect was often hyperthermia, and even death of a subject.

1. Which element shown in Figure 13.3 is directly influenced by DNP?
2. What effect would DNP have on the ATP:O_2 ratio; that is, the ratio of ATP's synthesized per O_2 consumed?
3. Assuming a constant cytoplasmic ATPase rate, how would DNP alter the potentials depicted in Figure 13.3?

KEY POINT

The measurement of the relationship between a single factor and the overall steady-state flux of the system under some set of conditions does not establish its preeminence as the controlling or limiting factor under all conditions.

Now consider the effect of calcium activation on this system (Fig. 13.3C). In addition to the activation of cytoplasmic ATPases, calcium has effects at four possible sites within the mitochondria: pyruvate dehydrogenase (PDH), α-ketoglutarate dehydrogenase, isocitrate dehydrogenase, and ATP synthase (17). Of these, the evidence is most complete for PDH, so for simplicity we consider only the effect of calcium at that site. PDH (actually a 3-megadalton complex of enzymes) catalyzes the following net reaction:

$$\text{Pyruvate} + \text{NAD} + \text{CoA} + \text{acetyl-CoA} + \\ \text{NADH} + \text{CO}_2$$

Thus, this reaction both contributes to the redox potential and provides input of acetyl-coenzyme A (CoA) to the citric acid cycle. Calcium-stimulated dephosphorylation of the complex effectively increases the maximum flux capacity, an effect illustrated in Figure 13.3C by increased diameter of the flux connection into the redox potential. *Ignoring* the effect of increased calcium on cytoplasmic ATPases results in a new steady state with higher redox potential and higher hydrogen ion and ATP free energy potentials (assuming constant leak) and with no change in the steady-state rate of ATP production. *Including* the parallel effect of calcium on cytoplasmic ATPases, results in a new steady state with higher flux throughout the system. In that case, the changes in potential accompanying the increased flux would depend on the balance between calcium's effects at the various sites. For example, in a tightly coupled system with densely packed mitochondria operating at high flux rates (*e.g.,* cardiac muscle) flux control might reside predominantly in the calcium-sensitive dehydrogenases. In that case, changes in respiratory flux can occur with little or no change in cytoplasmic ATP free energy (18).

Finally, consider the effect of low oxygen concentration on this system (Fig. 13.3D). The result is restriction of flow in the electron transport chain. The system might still be able to support the same steady-state flux, but the upstream redox potential would increase, and the downstream hydrogen ion and ATP potentials would fall. Therefore, changes in oxygen concentration can alter the steady-state relationship between cytoplasmic phosphate metabolites and respiratory rate (19).

Thus, we arrive by a different route to the view presented in the previous section: over the submaximal range, the steady-state rate of skeletal muscle respiration is largely controlled by the rate of cytoplasmic ATP hydrolysis, signaled to the mitochondria primarily by the increase in ADP and to some extent by P_i. Under the conditions prevalent in mammalian fast muscle over the submaximal range of exercise intensities, these signaling mechanisms translate into the experimentally observed quasi-linear relationship between respiratory rate and cytoplasmic ΔG_{ATP} (Fig. 13.4). Other factors, such as oxygen or carbon substrate availability, activation of PDH, and altered mitochondrial content after exercise training or deconditioning, can effectively alter the maximum flux capacity or change the overall thermodynamic drive for mitochondrial ATP synthesis and thereby modulate the steady-state relationship between cytoplasmic nucleotides and respiratory flux. Nonetheless, in skeletal muscle the control resides primarily in the ATPases.

The Limit to Muscle Respiratory Response Time

The response time for the increase in oxygen consumption to a new steady state in human skeletal muscle at the onset

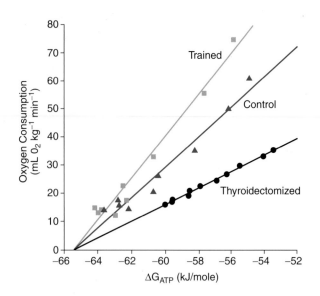

FIGURE 13.4 Relationships between cytoplasmic free energy of ATP hydrolysis (ΔG_{ATP}) and estimated oxygen consumption during recovery after submaximal stimulation in gastrocnemius muscles from trained (highest muscle mitochondrial content), control, and chemically thyroidectomized (lowest mitochondrial content) rats. Assuming resting oxygen consumption of 12.5 mL oxygen per kilogram per minute in all groups. (Redrawn with permission from Paganini AT, Foley JM, Meyer RA. Linear dependence of muscle phosphocreatine kinetics on oxidative capacity. *Am J Physiol.* 1997;272[41]:C501–C510.)

of submaximal exercise is 30 seconds or more (20). In contrast, at 37°C the response time of isolated mitochondria to a step increase in external ADP or P_i concentration is less than 3 seconds (17), an order of magnitude faster. What accounts for this difference?

TEST YOURSELF

Myxothiazol is an antibiotic that has also been administered to animals in higher doses to study mitochondrial metabolism (28). What is the mechanism of action of myxothiazol? Assuming a constant cytoplasmic ATPase rate, how would myxothiazol administration alter the potentials depicted in Figure 13.3?

The main part of the answer is implicit in Figure 13.3. Any transition from one respiratory rate to another (*e.g.,* from rest, as in Figure 13.3A, to submaximal exercise, as in Fig. 13.3B) is accompanied by a change in the height of one or more of the potential reservoirs. The speed with which these changes can occur depends on the volume, or *capacitance,* of the reservoirs and on the maximum flow capacity, or *conductance,* of the connecting pipes. Thus, each metabolic potential has an associated capacitance that influences how fast that potential, and therefore the net flux through the whole pathway, can change. If all of the potentials change, the response time of the whole system will be dominated by the potential with the largest capacitance.

The concept of metabolic capacitance can be quantitatively applied to each of the potentials depicted in Figure 13.3. In the presence of the CK reaction, the capacitance of the cytoplasmic ΔG_{ATP} potential over most of the submaximal range (the buffering zone of Fig. 13.1) just depends on the total creatine content (PCr + creatine). Total creatine is about 35 to 45 μmol $\cdot$ g^{-1} in mammalian fast muscle and somewhat less in slow twitch muscle. This greatly exceeds the total capacitance associated with all of the other intramitochondrial potentials depicted in Figure 13.3, because all of these capacitances are restricted to the relatively small volume of the mitochondrial matrix (at most 8% of skeletal muscle cell volume). For example, the capacitance of the mitochondrial matrix adenine nucleotide pool is not augmented by a CK system. Therefore, its maximum capacitance is just equal to the total intramitochondrial adenine nucleotide content, or at most 1.6 μmol $\cdot$ g^{-1} of muscle, assuming 20 mM total nucleotide concentration in the matrix compartment. Similarly, the capacitance associated with the mitochondrial redox potential just depends on total mitochondrial NAD and NADH content. Even assuming the entire NAD and NADH content in skeletal muscle is in the matrix, this is less than 1 μmol $\cdot$ g^{-1} of muscle. The capacitance associated with the hydrogen ion electrochemical potential just depends on the pH buffering capacity of the matrix (again limited by the small matrix volume) plus a very minor contribution from the electrical capacitance of the inner membrane. Finally, the capacitance associated with the PDH reaction itself is trivial, because the total content of CoA in skeletal muscle is less than 0.02 μmol $\cdot$ g^{-1}.

Because the metabolic capacitance of the cytoplasmic CK system so greatly exceeds all other potential capacitances associated with mitochondrial ATP production, the time-dependent behavior of the system in Figure 13.3, and therefore of muscle respiration, can be shown by collapsing all the intramitochondrial potentials and conductances into single elements. To a good approximation, the time dependence can be modeled by a three-element circuit composed of a single lumped mitochondrial potential (represented by a battery), a single mitochondrial conductance, and a single parallel capacitance representing the cytoplasmic CK system (Fig. 13.5A). The main feature of this circuit is that after a step increase in load (*i.e.*, increased cytoplasmic ATP hydrolysis rate), the flux through the conductance (mitochondrial ATP production) and the flux from the capacitance (PCr hydrolysis) both approach a new steady state along exponential time courses, with time constant just equal to capacitance divided by conductance (21). Therefore, this model explains the observation that the kinetics of PCr and oxygen consumption at the onset of and after submaximal exercise are mirror images (Fig. 13.5B).

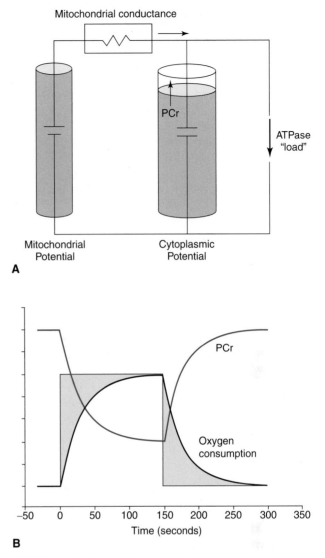

FIGURE 13.5   A. Collapsed three-element potential, conductance, and capacitance model of respiratory kinetics with an overlaid electrical circuit analogue. **B.** Relationships between muscle phosphocreatine (PCr) (*blue line*), muscle oxygen consumption rate (*black line*), and the associated muscle oxygen deficit (*initial shaded area*) and recovery oxygen debt (*second shaded area*) at the onset of and after exercise requiring a steady-state increase in muscle adenosine triphosphatase (ATPase) rate.

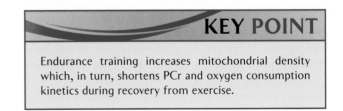

KEY POINT

Endurance training increases mitochondrial density which, in turn, shortens PCr and oxygen consumption kinetics during recovery from exercise.

In this model, the increase in muscle mitochondrial content that occurs in response to aerobic exercise training corresponds to increased conductance of the mitochondrial element; that is, adding more mitochondria corresponds to adding more conductance elements in parallel. Because the time constant is inversely dependent on total mitochondrial conductance, the model explains the fact that aerobic training shortens the time constants for both PCr and oxygen consumption kinetics during submaximal exercise, in addition to increasing the maximum respiratory rate and increasing the slope of the relationship between cytoplasmic ΔG_{ATP} and respiratory rate (Fig. 13.4). Interestingly, increased mitochondrial content appears to have no effect on the lumped mitochondrial potential in rat fast muscle. As shown in Figure 13.4, extrapolations of the relationships between estimated respiratory rate and ΔG_{ATP} to zero respiratory rate yield the same potential independent of mitochondrial content. This no-load potential is an estimate of the lumped intramitochondrial potential for ATP synthesis in this muscle type (-65 kJ $\cdot$ mole^{-1}).

The Oxygen Deficit and Metabolic Inertia

Inasmuch as the circuit model of Figure 13.5A explains the coincidence of PCr and oxygen consumption kinetics at the onset of submaximal exercise, it also explains the oxygen deficit at the onset of submaximal exercise and the oxygen debt after it (the shaded areas in Fig. 13.5B). According to this view, the oxygen deficit results from the time dependence of the whole system and does not represent "the period when the energy demand of contraction *cannot* [emphasis added] be met solely by mitochondrial ATP generation" (22). This explanation for the oxygen deficit suggests that some intrinsic delay or inertia must be overcome before mitochondrial ATP production can be activated and that PCr hydrolysis just makes up the deficit caused by the slow mitochondrial response. The inertial delay in mitochondrial activation has variously been attributed to delayed oxygen delivery, to a need to prime the citric acid cycle with substrates (anaplerosis), and most recently to a delay in activation of the PDH complex and production of acetyl-CoA (22).

In fact, the observation that PCr and oxygen consumption kinetics are both faster in muscles with higher mitochondrial content provides prima facie evidence that this alternative explanation for the oxygen deficit must be largely incorrect. If there was a long *intrinsic* delay in mitochondrial activation, then, all other things being equal, having more mitochondria would have no effect on the delay, although it still would increase maximum steady-state oxygen consumption. Clear evidence against this explanation comes from the effect of depleting total creatine content on muscle PCr kinetics. If PCr and oxygen consumption kinetics were both determined by an intrinsic delay in mitochondrial activation, partial depletion of total creatine content would have no effect on the time constant for PCr depletion, provided that sufficient PCr remained to make up the deficit. In contrast, if the kinetics are determined by mitochondrial conductance and CK capacitance together, as argued earlier, then decreasing total creatine content, and hence the capacitance of the system, should hasten the kinetics of both PCr and oxygen consumption. This experiment was performed over a decade ago (23). The result was that the time constant for PCr changes decreased nearly linearly with depletion of total

creatine. Similarly, inhibition of CK shortens the time constant for changes in oxygen consumption with increased workload in isolated hearts (24). A dramatic decrease in respiratory response time likely occurs in skeletal muscle of mice with genetic knockout of cytoplasmic CK (25).

Of course, the simplified model of Figure 13.5 omits important modulating effects considered in the previous section, such as the effects of hypoxia or PDH activation. For example, if acetyl-CoA production via PDH was the conductance element limiting maximum oxygen consumption in muscle, then pharmacologic activation of PDH with a drug such as dichloroacetate would effectively hasten the kinetics of oxygen consumption at the onset of submaximal exercise. However, recent evidence indicates that dichloroacetate does not alter the kinetics of either PCr or oxygen consumption in human muscle (26). Instead, the reported effects of PDH activation (decreased net PCr hydrolysis and lactate accumulation during exercise in some [22] but not all [27] studies) are most likely related to an effect on mitochondrial redox potential. Higher redox potential would drive the same steady-state respiration with less decrease in cytoplasmic ΔG_{ATP} and therefore relatively less drive on the PCr and glycogenolysis pathways.

Summary

The response time of mitochondrial ATP production at the onset of submaximal exercise is determined by the muscle's mitochondrial content or maximum respiratory capacity *and* by the capacitance of the cytoplasmic CK system. Evidence that other "inertial" factors significantly limit respiratory kinetics in well-oxygenated skeletal muscle is scanty. In any case, use of the term *inertia* to describe metabolic kinetics should be discouraged. Inertia refers to the property of a mass to continue in constant motion unless some energy is applied or dissipated to alter that motion. The electrical analogue of inertia is inductance; that is, energy must be applied or dissipated to *change* the current in a coil of wire. It is difficult to imagine how a metabolic flux could have inertia or inductance, because metabolic flux always dissipates some energy and must cease when there is no driving free energy potential. To put it another way, the inertia of your body's mass might carry you across the finish line, but a slow start cannot be blamed on the inertia of your metabolites.

TEST YOURSELF

Creatine supplementation for 5 days increases total muscle creatine content by up to 20% in human subjects. Assuming creatine supplementation does not induce any other adaptation in muscle, based on the model of Figure 13.5A, what effect would you predict creatine supplementation to have on:

1. The time constant for PCr recovery after submaximal exercise?
2. The initial rate of PCr recovery after submaximal exercise?

The Limits to Maximum Sustainable ATP Turnover Rate in Muscle

As described earlier, the maximum *instantaneous* rate of ATP utilization during contraction depends on the muscle's myosin and SERCA isoform types and on the extent of their activation by calcium. Of course, in the absence of any balancing ATP production, this rate cannot be sustained for long. Because of fatigue processes, force generation and therefore the ATP hydrolysis rate will decrease, attenuating the drop in cytoplasmic ΔG_{ATP}. Fatigue, therefore, plays a crucial role in the regulation of ΔG_{ATP} in healthy skeletal muscle. If fatigue processes did not limit ATP hydrolysis, a muscle cell could work itself to death. The precise mechanism or mechanisms of muscle cell fatigue are not fully understood. However, most recent evidence suggests that decreased force during heavy repetitive exercise regimens (*e.g.*, weightlifting) is largely due to decreased SR calcium release (see Chapter 5).

It follows that the maximum *sustainable* rate of ATP utilization in muscle cells depends on the maximum flux capacity of the pathways for ATP production, along with the duration over which the rate must be sustained. For contraction regimens of relatively short duration, the sustainable rate can be highest, because all three pathways for ATP production can contribute significantly to the total. In that case, the balance between the three pathways is determined by their maximum flux capacities relative to each other (which varies with fiber type and training status) *and* by the interplay between their differing elasticities to calcium and/or net ATP hydrolysis. Thus, PCr hydrolysis contributes the most to muscle ATP synthesis during the first seconds of exercise *at any intensity* because the response of the CK reaction to the initial change in ATP:ADP ratio is the greatest, not because the response times of glycolysis and oxidative respiration are intrinsically slow. The contribution of glycolysis to ATP production is greatest during short duration heavy exercises, both because the maximum oxidative capacity of recruited fibers is limited *and* because the type IIB and IIX fibers recruited at high intensities have the greatest complement of glycolytic enzymes. On the other hand, for prolonged exercise, which must rely on the high *total* ATP-producing capacity of mitochondria, the maximum sustainable rate depends directly on mitochondrial content, or more specifically on the activity of inner mitochondrial membrane complexes (28).

Of course, maximum sustainable ATPase rate might be reduced further if oxygen or carbon substrate supply is limited, for example, by poor blood flow or by limited diffusion of these substances to the muscle cells. Although these possibilities are beyond the scope of this chapter, there is a related question about intracellular energy. Does the intracellular diffusion of ATP and ADP between sites of ATP use (*e.g.*, myofibrils and SERCA) and ATP production (*e.g.*, mitochondria) limit the maximum sustainable ATPase rate?

Intracellular Diffusion as a Limit to Maximum Sustainable ATPase Rate

Assuming no specific diffusion barrier for adenine nucleotides compared to other similar-sized molecules, this question can be answered by considering the nature of molecular diffusion. Diffusion is just the statistical result of random molecular motions. From this it can be shown that on average, the time (t) it takes an individual molecule to randomly move some distance (d) increases with the *square* of the distance:

$$t = d^2 / 2D \text{ (for one-dimensional diffusion)}$$

Therefore, the effectiveness of diffusion as a transport mechanism depends critically on the diffusion distance. The diffusion coefficient, D, depends on the effective radius of the diffusing molecule, and on the medium in which it is diffusing. For example, the diffusion coefficient of P_i in solution at 37°C (about 1×10^{-6} cm$^2 \cdot$ s^{-1}) is higher than that of ATP (about 0.5×10^{-6} cm$^2 \cdot$ s^{-1}). Both molecules diffuse more slowly in muscle cells than in water, presumably because of the tortuosity of the diffusion path around myofilaments and other intracellular structures. The familiar Fick law of steady-state diffusion also follows directly from the statistical average of random molecular motions. In one dimension, Fick's law is as follows:

$$J = D \times dC / dx$$

where J is the diffusive flux across some plane and dC/dx is the concentration gradient perpendicular to that plane. Thus, the concentration gradient required to maintain some steady-state flux depends on the diffusion coefficient. For example, for any steady-state flux, the phosphate gradient from myofibrils to mitochondria is less than the ADP gradient (and also less than the ATP gradient in the opposite direction).

It seems plausible that ADP would be the metabolite limiting intracellular flux between myofibrils or SERCA and mitochondria, because the concentration of ADP is much lower than the concentration of ATP and P_i. If a substantial gradient for ADP was required, ADP would have to be substantially higher at the myofibrils and SERCA than at the mitochondria, which might inhibit calcium uptake and slow shortening velocity. However, despite the intuitive plausibility of this notion, the truth depends critically on the actual diffusion distance between the organelles. Calculations show that for distances less than several micrometers (e.g., the axial distance across several myofibrils), the required ADP gradient could not be energetically significant. On the other hand, over longer distances (e.g., in a 50-μm-diameter muscle fiber with mitochondria clustered in the periphery) the gradient could become significant to energy (5). However, in both of these cases, the CK reaction actually decreases the required ADP diffusion gradients to insignificance. Because specific CK isozymes are localized in mitochondria and in myofibrils (in addition to the soluble CK in between), the CK system provides an additional path for metabolite diffusion: the creatine shuttle (29,30).

The Creatine Shuttle

The fact that most of the diffusive flux of high energy phosphate between sites in muscle cells is actually carried by creatine and PCr rather than by ADP and ATP is now widely accepted. However, the *reason* the creatine shuttle works so effectively is sometimes misunderstood. Certainly, the concentration of free creatine in muscle (up to 20 μmol $\cdot$ g^{-1} at the upper end of the submaximal buffering range illustrated in Fig. 13.1) is much higher than the concentration of ADP (less than 0.2 μmol $\cdot$ g^{-1} over the submaximal range). Therefore, development of the same absolute diffusion gradient requires a much smaller percent difference in creatine. Furthermore, the diffusion coefficient of creatine is about twice as large as that of the larger molecular weight nucleotides, so the creatine gradient required to support the same diffusive flux would be less. The product of diffusion coefficient times concentration is sometimes called diffusivity, and clearly the diffusivity of creatine is much higher than that of ADP in skeletal muscle. However, this difference in diffusivity does not fully convey the key underlying factor that determines the effectiveness of the creatine shuttle. In fact, most of its effectiveness arises from the high apparent equilibrium constant of the CK reaction. It has been shown (30) that, assuming near equilibrium of the CK reaction, the ratio of steady-state diffusive fluxes carried by creatine versus ADP (and PCr vs. ATP) across any surface between sites of ATP hydrolysis and ATP synthesis varies according to

$$J_{Cr} / J_{ADP} = (D_{Cr} / D_{ADP}) \times (\text{total creatine} / \text{total nucleotide}) \times K_{CK} \times [(R + 1) / (R + K_{CK})]^2$$

where D is the diffusion coefficients, K_{CK} is the CK equilibrium constant in the direction shown above, and R is the ATP/ADP ratio. The ratio of diffusion coefficients is approximately 2, and the ratio of total creatine to total adenine is about 4. In contrast, K_{CK} is approximately 100. Therefore, this is by far the dominant term as long as the ATP/ADP ratio is high. Stated another way, the creatine shuttle is extremely effective because small spatial *differences* in ADP concentration translate into much larger *differences* in creatine

concentration via the CK equilibrium. The CK system does not simply add another diffusing pair of metabolites; it greatly amplifies the effective diffusion gradient.

The importance of considering K_{CK} rather than just diffusivity in the effectiveness of the creatine shuttle can be illustrated by considering the expected result of increasing muscle total creatine content, for example, by creatine supplementation. Creatine supplementation can increase muscle total creatine content in some individuals by up to 30%. If one considered only the effect of this increase on creatine diffusivity, one might imagine that this could in principle increase the shuttle's effectiveness by 30% and (assuming diffusion limits aerobic capacity) increase aerobic power by 30%. However, because K_{CK} is so dominant, a 30% increase in total creatine would not significantly add to the shuttle's already overwhelming effectiveness. Therefore, even if creatine supplementation did increase aerobic capacity, this effect could not be attributed to enhancement of the creatine shuttle. In fact, there is no convincing evidence that creatine supplementation increases muscle aerobic capacity. On the contrary, chronic creatine depletion or genetic ablation of cytoplasmic CK results in increased skeletal muscle mitochondrial content and aerobic capacity, presumably because of an adaptive response to the increased pulsatility of nucleotide levels that must occur in the absence of CK buffering (25).

> ### KEY POINT
>
> The effectiveness of CK shuttle derives from an amplification of the ADP signal to a creatine signal through the high K_{eq} of CK.

All of this assumes that there is no specific barrier to nucleotide diffusion to the inner mitochondrial membrane. Although no such barrier is evident in isolated mitochondria, it has been suggested that the outer membrane is much less permeable to nucleotides in vivo than in vitro. This view is largely based on studies of respiration in permeabilized muscle fibers or bundles of fibers, whose sarcolemma is made permeable to small molecules but not to larger molecules, such as proteins, after treatment with a mild detergent (34). The experimental observation is that addition of creatine to the bath surrounding the fiber bundles enhances the respiration rate at submaximal ADP concentrations, increasing the apparent affinity of the mitochondria for ADP. Conversely, addition of PCr suppresses respiration and decreases the apparent affinity for ADP in this experimental situation. Thus, it is proposed that PCr and creatine traverse the outer mitochondrial membrane more freely than the nucleotides and are the metabolites that actually control muscle respiration (31). Unfortunately, there is now good evidence (32) that the diffusion barrier in permeabilized fiber experiments lies not at the outer membrane but is instead simply due to the

A MILESTONE OF DISCOVERY

The First Phosphorus NMR Spectra of Skeletal Muscle

Researchers now routinely use NMR spectroscopy to measure the time course of many metabolic events in exercising human skeletal muscle. The first phosphorus NMR spectra of intact skeletal muscle (reproduced below) were published by David Hoult and his colleagues at the University of Oxford in 1974. At that time there were no NMR magnets large enough to accommodate a human subject or even a whole rat. This paper reported the time course of metabolic changes in ischemic hind limb muscles freshly excised from anesthetized rats and placed in a magnet designed for spectroscopy of organic chemicals in small test tubes. Nonetheless, many future applications of phosphorus NMR to exercise physiology were clearly foreshadowed in this paper. For example, the faster depletion of PCr (peak III in the figure) than ATP (peaks IV, V, and VI are the γ-, α-, and β-phosphates of ATP, respectively) was evident over time, and the extent of muscle acidification (from pH 7.1 in the freshly excised muscle down to pH 6.2

after 160 minutes of ischemia at 20°C) was determined from the changing position of the inorganic phosphate peak (peak II). Furthermore, the authors correctly deduced that the breadth of the phosphate peak compared to the PCr peak was due to pH heterogeneity within the muscle and hinted that this pH heterogeneity might be used to characterize the fiber compartments of the muscle.

As exciting as these first results were to researchers interested in muscle metabolism, it is not likely that by themselves they would have led to the widespread availability of human-sized NMR magnets. Fortunately, the paper describing the principle of magnetic resonance imaging (MRI) had been published just a year earlier (35), and within 10 years human MRI magnets were available at most major medical centers. Hoult and his colleagues at Oxford went on to make many important contributions to MRI, as well as to muscle spectroscopy.

Hoult DI, Busby SJW, Gadian DG, et al. Observation of tissue metabolites using 31P nuclear magnetic resonance. Nature. 1974;352:285–287.

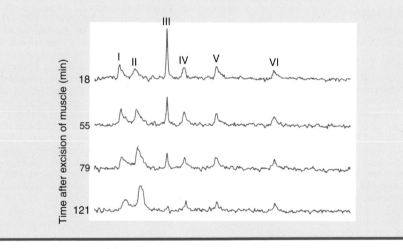

CHAPTER SUMMARY

relatively long path from the bath to the core of the fibers in these experiments (50 μm or more). This is exactly the situation in which ADP diffusion alone is likely to become rate limiting.

The main message of this chapter is that cytoplasmic ATPases control muscle ATP production at work rates below the maximal sustainable rate. As exercise intensity approaches the maximum sustainable rate, control increasingly depends on the limited maximum capacity of the ATP-generating pathways themselves. Of course, many important questions remain to be answered. For example, although it is unlikely that the intracellular

diffusion of small molecules such as ADP limits metabolic rate, it is quite possible that the spatial arrangement of large metabolic enzymes and enzyme complexes is important for flux control. For example, more than 20 years ago, it was suggested that glycogen particles and associated glycogenolytic enzymes may be in close proximity to SR ATPases, which may explain the observed coupling between glycogenolysis and contraction (33). With the tools of modern molecular biology, it should now be possible to test this idea in vivo by genetically mutating the interacting domains of these enzyme complexes. Similarly, the possibility that energy-related signals, such as AMP, are important for control of muscle gene expression and the adaptations to exercise training has just begun to be explored (34). These are exciting times for those interested in muscle metabolism.

REFERENCES

1. Hochachka PW. *Muscles as Molecular and Metabolic Machines*. Boca Raton, FL: CRC Press; 1994.
2. Harkema SJ, Adams GR, Meyer RA. Acidosis has no effect on the ATP cost of contraction in cat fast- and slow-twitch skeletal muscles. *Am J Physiol*. 1997;272(41):C485–C490.
3. He ZH, Bottinelli R, Pellegrino MA, et al. ATP consumption and efficiency of human single muscle fibers with different myosin isoform composition. *Biophys J*. 2000;79:945–961.
4. Taylor CR. Relating mechanics and energetics during exercise. *Adv Vet Sci Comp Med*. 1994;38A:181–215.
5. Meyer RA, Foley JM. Cellular processes integrating the metabolic response to exercise. In: Rowell LB, Shepherd JT, eds. *Handbook of Physiology, Section 12: Exercise: Regulation and Integration of Multiple Systems*. New York: Oxford University; 1996:841–869.
6. Ryschon TW, Fowler MD, Wysong RE, et al. Efficiency of human skeletal muscle in vivo: comparison of isometric, concentric, and eccentric muscle action. *J Appl Physiol*. 1997;83:867–874.
7. Blei ML, Conley KE, Kushmerick MJ. Separate measures of ATP utilization and recovery in human skeletal muscle. *J Physiol (Lond)*. 1993;465:203–222.
8. Harkema SJ, Meyer RA. Effect of acidosis on control of respiration in skeletal muscle. *Am J Physiol*. 1997;272(41):C491–C500.
9. Brooks GA. The lactate shuttle during exercise and recovery. *Med Sci Sports Exerc*. 1986;18:360–368.
10. Brooks GA. Lactate doesn't necessarily cause fatigue: why are we surprised? *J Physiol (Lond)*. 2001;536:1.
11. Jeneson JA, Bruggeman FJ. Robust homeostatic control of quadriceps pH during natural locomotor activity in man. *FASEB J*. 2004;18:1010–1012.
12. Chen W, London R, Murphy E, et al. Regulation of the Ca^{++} gradient across the sarcoplasmic reticulum in perfused rabbit heart: a 19F nuclear magnetic resonance study. *Circ Res*. 1998;83:898–907.
13. Lambeth MJ, Kushmerick MJ. A computational model for glycogenolysis in skeletal muscle. *Ann Biomed Eng*. 2002;30:808–827.
14. Cornish-Bowden A. *Fundamentals of Enzyme Kinetics*. London: Portland; 1995.
15. Jeneson JAL, Westerhoff HV, Kushmerick MJ. A metabolic control analysis of kinetic controls in ATP free energy metabolism in contracting skeletal muscle. *Am J Physiol*. 2000;279:C813–C832.
16. Jeneson JAL, Wiseman RW, Westerhoff HV, et al. The signal transduction function for oxidative phosphorylation is at least second order in ADP. *J Biol Chem*. 1996;271:27995–27998.
17. Territo PR, French SA, Dunleavy MC, et al. Calcium activation of heart mitochondrial oxidative phosphorylation: rapid kinetics of mVO2, NADH, and light scattering. *J Biol Chem*. 2001;276:2586–2599.
18. Balaban RS, Kantor HL, Katz LA, et al. Relation between work and phosphate metabolite in the in vivo paced mammalian heart. *Science*. 1986;232:1121–1123.
19. Hogan MC, Richardson RS, Haseler LJ. Human muscle performance and PCr hydrolysis with varied inspired oxygen fractions: a 31P-MRS study. *J Appl Physiol*. 1999;86:1367–1373.
20. Rossiter HB, Ward SA, Doyle VL, et al. Inferences from pulmonary O2 uptake with respect to intramuscular phosphocreatine kinetics during moderate exercise in humans. *J Physiol (Lond)*. 1999;518:921–932.
21. Meyer RA. A linear model of muscle respiration explains monoexponential phosphocreatine changes. *Am J Physiol*. 1988;254(23):C548–C553.
22. Greenhaff PL, Campbell-O'Sullivan SP, Constantin-Teodosiu D, et al. An acetyl group deficit limits mitochondrial ATP production at the onset of exercise. *Biochem Soc Trans*. 2002;30:275–280.
23. Meyer RA. Linear dependence of muscle phosphocreatine kinetics on total creatine content. *Am J Physiol*. 1989;257(26):C1149–C1157.
24. Harrison GJ, van Wijhe MH, de Groot B, et al. CK inhibition accelerates transcytosolic energy signaling during rapid workload steps in isolated rabbit hearts. *Am J Physiol*. 199;276(45):H134–H140.
25. Roman BB, Meyer RA, Wiseman RW. Phosphocreatine kinetics at the onset of contractions in skeletal muscle of MM creatine kinase knockout mice. *Am J Physiol Cell Physiol*. 2002;283:C1776–C1783.
26. Rossiter HB, Ward SA, Howe FA, et al. Effects of dichloroacetate on VO2 and intramuscular 31P metabolite kinetics during high-intensity exercise in humans. *J Appl Physiol*. 2003;95:1105–1115.
27. Savasi I, Evans MK, Heigenhauser GJF, et al. Skeletal muscle metabolism is unaffected by DCA infusion and hyperoxia after the onset of intense aerobic exercise. *Am J Physiol Endocrinol Metab*. 2002;283:E108–E115.
28. McAllister RM, Terjung RL. Acute inhibition of respiratory capacity of muscle reduces peak oxygen consumption. *Am J Physiol*. 1990;259(28):C889–C896.
29. Bessman SP, Geiger PJ. Transport of energy in muscle: the phosphorylcreatine shuttle. *Science*. 1981;211:448–452.
30. Meyer RA, Sweeney HL, Kushmerick MJ. A simple analysis of the "phosphocreatine shuttle." *Am J Physiol*. 1984;246(15):C365–C377.
31. Walsh B, Tonkonogi M, Soderlund K, et al. The role of phosphorylcreatine and creatine in the regulation of mitochondrial respiration in skeletal muscle. *J Physiol (Lond)*. 2001;537:971–978.
32. Kongas O, Yuen TL, Wagner MJ, et al. High km of oxidative phosphorylation for ADP in skinned muscle fibers: where does it stem from? *Am J Physiol*. 2002;283:C743–C751.
33. Entman ML, Keslensky SS, Chu A, et al. The sarcoplasmic reticulum-glycogenolytic complex in mammalian fast twitch skeletal muscle: proposed in vitro counterpart of the contraction-activated glycogenolytic pool. *J Biol Chem*. 1980;255:6245–6252.
34. Zong H, Ren JM, Young LH, et al. AMP kinase is required for mitochondrial biogenesis in skeletal muscle in response to chronic energy deprivation. *Proc Natl Acad Sci USA*. 2002;99:15983–15987.
35. Lauterbur PC. Image formation by induced local interactions: examples using nuclear magnetic resonance. *Nature*. 1973;242:190–191.

CHAPTER 14

The Metabolic Systems: Carbohydrate Metabolism

Mark Hargreaves

Abbreviations

ADP	Adenosine diphosphate	GLUT4	Glucose transporter isoform 4
AICAR	Aminoimidazole-4-carboxamide-1-β-D-riboside	MAPK	Mitogen-activated protein kinase
		MCT	Monocarboxylate transporter
AMP	Adenosine monophosphate	NADH	Reduced nicotinamide adenine dinucleotide
AMPK	AMP-activated protein kinase		
ATP	Adenosine triphosphate	PDH	Pyruvate dehydrogenase
CHO	Carbohydrate	PDK	Pyruvate dehydrogenase kinase
CoA	Coenzyme A	P_i	Inorganic phosphate
FFA	Free fatty acid	PKC	Protein kinase C

Introduction

Carbohydrate (CHO) is the preferred substrate for contracting skeletal muscle during strenuous exercise, and the importance of available CHO for endurance exercise performance has been recognized since the early 1900s. In the ensuing years, considerable experimental effort has further characterized the effects of exercise on CHO metabolism and the systemic and cellular factors that regulate CHO mobilization and utilization. In animal tissues, CHO is stored as glycogen, a branched polymer of glucose with a mixture of α-1,4 and α-1,6 linkages between glucose units. The liver has the highest concentration of glycogen, but by virtue of its mass, skeletal muscle contains the largest store of glycogen (Table 14.1). The size of both the liver and muscle glycogen reserves is influenced by interactions between levels of exercise and dietary CHO intake. Because the endogenous CHO stores are relatively low and are utilized to a large extent during athletic competition and training, adequate dietary CHO intake is essential to ensure optimal CHO availability before, during, and after exercise. A focus on CHO intake, together with energy and fluid balance, is a cornerstone of performance and sports nutritional programs.

During exercise, liver and muscle glycogen stores are mobilized, and muscle glycogen use and glucose uptake increase with increasing intensity of exercise. At exercise intensities greater than 50% to 60% $\dot{V}o_{2max}$, muscle glycogen is the major substrate for oxidative metabolism (1,2) (Fig. 14.1). As exercise duration is extended, liver and muscle glycogen levels decrease and uptake of glucose increases progressively until, in the absence of CHO supplementation, falling blood glucose levels limit glucose uptake. Reduced intramuscular glycogen availability and hypoglycemia are associated with the development of fatigue during prolonged strenuous exercise, and nutritional strategies to enhance endurance performance focus on increasing CHO availability before (3) and during (4) such exercise.

The relative contributions of muscle glycogen and blood glucose to substrate oxidation are determined by various factors, notably exercise intensity and duration, and training status. CHO ingestion increases the contribution of glucose to substrate oxidation, but this appears to be a result of lower fat oxidation, secondary to reduced lipolysis and mitochondrial fatty acid oxidation, because there is no significant effect of CHO ingestion on muscle glycogen utilization as assessed by either direct muscle

| | Weight or volume | Concentration | |
Tissue	(kilograms or liters)	(mmol · kg⁻¹ or · *L⁻¹)	CHO store (g)

TABLE 14.1   Sites and Amount of Carbohydrate Stored in a Rested, Moderately Active 70-kg Man with 40% of Body Mass as Skeletal Muscle

Tissue	Weight or volume (kilograms or liters)	Concentration (mmol · kg⁻¹ or · *L⁻¹)	CHO store (g)
Liver	1.8	250 (0–500)	80 (0–160)
ECF	10.0	5*	9
Muscle	28.0	100 (0–200)	500 (300–700)

Numbers in parentheses represent possible range depending on exercise, training, and dietary carbohydrate (CHO) intake.
ECF, extracellular fluid.

sampling (4) or the use of indirect calorimetry and glucose tracers (5,6). During 120 minutes of exercise at ~70% peak pulmonary oxygen uptake ($\dot{V}O_{2peak}$) in the fasted state, total CHO oxidation was 361 g, of which 60 g were from blood glucose (17% CHO oxidation, 12% of total energy) derived from liver glucose output (~60 g). When CHO was ingested, total CHO oxidation was not significantly different (375 g), but glucose oxidation increased to 96 g or 26% of total CHO oxidation and 19% of total energy, with a significant reduction in liver glucose output to 29 g. There was no significant difference in estimated muscle glycogen oxidation (6).

This chapter briefly describes the effects of exercise on CHO mobilization and utilization, the important regulatory mechanisms, and aspects of CHO metabolism during the postexercise recovery period. In most instances, reference will be made to studies undertaken in human subjects, and the focus is on dynamic exercise. Although relatively less studied, muscle glycogen is also utilized during resistance exercise, especially at high loads when increased intramuscular pressure can occlude blood supply, thereby reducing oxygen delivery and increasing muscle glycogenolysis.

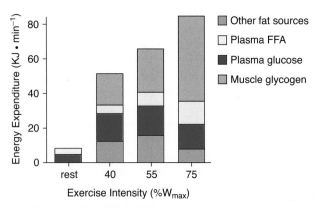

FIGURE 14.1 Contributions from muscle glycogen and plasma glucose to total energy expenditure during 20 minutes of dynamic exercise bouts of increasing intensity, expressed as %W$_{max}$. FFA, free fatty acid (Reprinted with permission from Van Loon LJC, Greenhaff PL, Constantin-Teodosiu D, et al. The effects of increasing exercise intensity on muscle fuel utilization in humans. *J Physiol [Lond]*. 2001;536:301.)

Muscle Glycogen Utilization during Exercise

The utilization of muscle glycogen is most rapid at the onset of exercise and increases exponentially with increasing exercise intensity (Fig. 14.1). During very intense exercise, the rate of muscle glycogenolysis can be as high as 40 mmol · kg⁻¹ · min⁻¹ of wet mass, whereas during prolonged submaximal exercise it can be as low as 1 to 2 mmol · kg⁻¹ · min⁻¹ (7,8). Thus, the regulation of glycogenolysis is exquisitely sensitive to the metabolic rate of skeletal muscle during exercise. With exercise, rapid activation of glycogen phosphorylase, the enzyme that catalyzes the rate-limiting step in muscle glycogenolysis, results from covalent modification, allosteric regulation, and changes in intramuscular concentrations of substrates. As exercise duration increases, the rate of muscle glycogenolysis declines as glycogen availability and phosphorylase activity decrease, intramuscular [H⁺] increases (during intense exercise), and the availability of other substrates for oxidative metabolism, such as glucose and free fatty acids (FFAs), increases. During prolonged exercise at power outputs eliciting 60% to 75% $\dot{V}O_{2max}$, muscle glycogenolysis occurs predominantly in type I muscle fibers, with increasing glycogen degradation in type II fibers as the type I fibers are depleted of glycogen. Fatigue during such exercise is often associated with muscle glycogen depletion (see Chapter 6 on Fatigue) (7,8). With increasing exercise intensity there is a greater rate of glycogenolysis in type I fibers, together with recruitment of type II fibers, such that at exercise intensities approaching and exceeding $\dot{V}O_{2max}$, glycogenolysis occurs in all muscle fiber types but at a higher rate in type II fibers.

In addition to intensity and duration of exercise, major factors influencing the rate of muscle glycogenolysis during dynamic exercise are preceding diet and training status. Increased dietary CHO intake is associated with greater muscle glycogen utilization, whereas increased fat intake results in a lower muscle glycogen use during subsequent exercise. These effects are mostly related to changes in intramuscular glycogen availability, although alterations in plasma hormone (see Chapter 19) and substrate concentrations may also contribute. However, 5 days on a high fat diet resulted in reduced muscle glycogen use during dynamic exercise, compared with 5 days on a high CHO diet, despite muscle glycogen levels before exercise being similar following consumption of a high CHO diet for 24 hours before exercise in both trials (9). This suggests that metabolic adaptations to a high fat diet, independent of muscle glycogen availability, result in an attenuation of muscle glycogenolysis during exercise following such a diet. Muscle glycogenolysis during dynamic exercise is reduced ~40% following a period of endurance training, despite an increase in resting muscle glycogen levels. The well described increase in muscle oxidative capacity is generally believed to be responsible for this alteration in muscle glycogen metabolism (10).

Morphologic studies have characterized a heterogeneous intramuscular distribution of glycogen and its association with the sarcolemma, sarcoplasmic reticulum, mitochondria, and myofibrils. Glycogen granules, or glycosomes, are also physically associated with a number of proteins, including glycogen phosphorylase, phosphorylase kinase, glycogen synthase, glycogenin, protein phosphatases, and adenosine monophosphate (AMP)-activated protein kinase (AMPK), that are involved in the metabolism of glycogen itself and other substrates, such as glucose (11). Furthermore, glycogen is associated with key organelles, notably the sarcoplasmic reticulum, and its availability has been linked with calcium homeostasis and fatigue (12). Thus, glycogen is not only a substrate for oxidative metabolism during dynamic exercise, but has a key role in metabolic regulation and muscle function.

Regulation of Muscle Glycogenolysis

The activity of glycogen phosphorylase is regulated by the interplay between intramuscular factors related to muscle contractile activity and metabolism and by systemic hormonal and substrate availability. This dual control (13) ensures that muscle glycogenolysis is closely matched to the energetic demands of dynamic exercise. In the resting state, glycogen phosphorylase exists primarily in the inactive b form. With the onset of dynamic exercise, phosphorylase kinase phosphorylates the b form to the active a form in response to elevated calcium levels and binding of epinephrine to β-adrenergic receptors on the sarcolemma. The activity of both forms of the enzyme can be increased allosterically by AMP and adenosine diphosphate (ADP) and by increases in inorganic phosphate (P_i). Because the rate of muscle glycogenolysis is not always closely associated with the percent phosphorylase a (14), these latter posttransformational factors enhance the glycogenolytic rate during exercise of increasing intensity and following reversal of phosphorylase transformation during prolonged exercise.

Local Factors

The increase in sarcoplasmic calcium during excitation-contraction coupling results in conversion of phosphorylase b as a result of calcium binding to the calmodulin subunit

of phosphorylase kinase and to troponin C. The increase in percent phosphorylase a is rapidly reversed (13) despite ongoing contractile activity, and this may be partly related to the decline in muscle glycogen, conformational changes in glycogen phosphorylase and/or phosphorylase kinase, and/or decreased muscle pH, which inhibits enzyme activity. The maintenance of glycogenolytic activity during ongoing dynamic exercise, especially at high intensities, is due to increased intramuscular concentrations of P_i, a substrate for phosphorylase, and AMP and ADP, which allosterically activate both phosphorylase a and b.

Substrate Availability

The availability of P_i and glycogen, the substrates for glycogen phosphorylase, has been shown to affect glycogen phosphorylase activity and glycogenolysis during dynamic exercise. Increases in intramuscular P_i during muscle contractions stimulate glycogen phosphorylase activity and contribute to enhanced glycogenolysis during exercise. Glycogen can bind to glycogen phosphorylase, thereby increasing its activity, and this may explain the linear relationship between muscle glycogen levels before exercise and its utilization during submaximal exercise. Despite the greater glycogenolysis, increased muscle glycogen availability prior to dynamic exercise enhances performance in endurance events lasting more than 90 minutes (3). The influence of muscle glycogen is less apparent during very intense exercise, and results in the literature are conflicting. Increased blood glucose availability may reduce glycogenolysis because increases in glucose-6-phosphate have the potential to inhibit glycogen phosphorylase activity; however, this does not occur during prolonged, strenuous cycling exercise (4,15), and there are conflicting data on the effect of CHO ingestion on muscle glycogen use during treadmill running. The ergogenic effects of CHO ingestion appear to be due to elevated blood glucose levels, which contribute to maintenance of skeletal muscle CHO oxidation (4) and cerebral glucose supply and energy turnover. Reduced blood glucose levels may increase reliance on muscle glycogen use, although this has not been tested directly. Hyperinsulinemia before exercise results in a fall in blood glucose with the onset of dynamic exercise, and this has sometimes been associated with increased muscle glycogen use (15); however, because hyperinsulinemia also inhibits lipolysis, this effect could equally be due to reduced plasma FFA levels, which also increases reliance on muscle glycogen during exercise. In contrast, elevated plasma FFA levels are associated with reduced muscle glycogenolysis, an effect that appears to be due to lower glycogen phosphorylase activity secondary to attenuated increases in ADP, AMP, and P_i during dynamic exercise.

Hormonal Regulation

In addition to local intramuscular factors, glycogen phosphorylase is also subject to regulation by epinephrine, which binds to sarcolemmal β-adrenergic receptors and results in cyclic AMP-mediated activation of glycogen phosphorylase kinase. Increased epinephrine is associated with greater glycogen phosphorylase activity and glycogenolysis during muscle contraction in the perfused rat hind limb (13) and with greater glycogenolysis during moderate exercise in humans (16). During heavy dynamic exercise, epinephrine infusion does not further increase muscle glycogenolysis, probably because of sufficient activation of glycogenolysis by endogenous epinephrine secretion and increases in intramuscular concentrations of ADP, AMP, and P_i.

Summary

The rate of muscle glycogenolysis increases exponentially with exercise intensity and decreases with increasing exercise duration. Glycogenolysis is regulated by local factors (Ca^{2+}, Pi, ADP, AMP, IMP, glycogen) and epinephrine. Blood glucose availability has relatively little influence on muscle glycogenolysis, whereas reduced FFA availability enhances glycogen use during exercise.

TEST YOURSELF

What are the major local and endocrine factors that control the rate of muscle glycogenolysis during exercise? How does the rate of muscle glycogenolysis change with increasing exercise intensity?

Muscle Glucose Uptake during Dynamic Exercise

During exercise skeletal muscle glucose uptake can increase several fold, depending on exercise intensity and duration (17,18) (Fig. 14.1). This is a consequence of enhanced glucose delivery to contracting skeletal muscle as a result of increased muscle blood flow and capillary recruitment and increased glucose extraction as measured by a greater arteriovenous glucose difference. Glucose extraction is increased by enhanced sarcolemmal glucose transport and activation of the glycolytic and oxidative pathways responsible for glucose metabolism. Sarcolemmal glucose transport is increased following translocation of the glucose transporter isoform 4 (GLUT4) from intracellular sites to the plasma membrane with exercise (17) (Fig. 14.2). The importance of GLUT4 is demonstrated by the almost complete abolition of contraction-stimulated glucose uptake in transgenic mice with selective deletion of GLUT4 from skeletal muscle (20). In addition to translocation to the sarcolemma, it is possible that exercise also increases the intrinsic activity of GLUT4, but this is more contentious. Once inside the cell, glucose is rapidly phosphorylated by hexokinase and further metabolized

in the glycolytic and oxidative pathways. There is little, if any, intracellular accumulation of glucose during exercise except at power outputs close to or at $\dot{V}O_{2max}$, when glucose utilization may be less than glucose transport (17). One possible explanation for reduced glucose utilization is an increase in concentration of muscle glucose-6-phosphate, an inhibitor of hexokinase, as a result of enhanced muscle glycogenolysis (15). With increasing exercise duration, there is a progressive increase in muscle glucose uptake associated with increased sarcolemmal GLUT4 (19) (Fig. 14.2) and reduced muscle glycogen levels (15). During prolonged heavy exercise in the absence of CHO supplementation, blood glucose levels decline and become limiting for muscle glucose uptake, which is then reduced. If CHO is ingested, blood glucose levels and CHO oxidation are maintained (4–6), exercise duration is increased (4), and glucose uptake increases continuously to the point of volitional fatigue (6).

Increased dietary CHO and fat intakes are generally associated with enhanced and reduced muscle glucose uptake, respectively, secondary to changes in plasma glucose and insulin levels. When muscle glycogen levels are equalized after such dietary intakes, the effect of preceding diet on glucose uptake is negligible (9). Dynamic endurance exercise training results in a lower

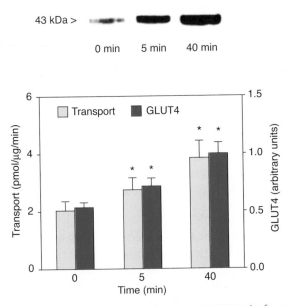

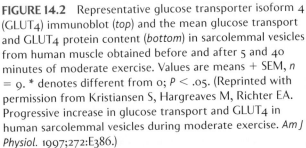

FIGURE 14.2   Representative glucose transporter isoform 4 (GLUT4) immunoblot (*top*) and the mean glucose transport and GLUT4 protein content (*bottom*) in sarcolemmal vesicles from human muscle obtained before and after 5 and 40 minutes of moderate exercise. Values are means + SEM, n = 9. * denotes different from 0; $P < .05$. (Reprinted with permission from Kristiansen S, Hargreaves M, Richter EA. Progressive increase in glucose transport and GLUT4 in human sarcolemmal vesicles during moderate exercise. *Am J Physiol.* 1997;272:E386.)

muscle glucose uptake during exercise at the same absolute power output (21), an effect that is less apparent during exercise at the same relative exercise intensity. In fact, with exercise intensity approaching $\dot{V}O_{2max}$, there may even be an increased muscle glucose uptake after training. This enhanced glucose uptake capacity is partly due to increased skeletal muscle GLUT4 protein expression after training, an adaptation that also contributes to greater insulin-stimulated skeletal muscle glucose uptake in trained subjects.

Regulation of Skeletal Muscle Glucose Uptake

Increased skeletal muscle blood flow and capillary recruitment enhance glucose supply to contracting skeletal muscle, but local factors within muscle have the major role. In particular, sarcolemmal glucose transport and glucose phosphorylation are key regulated processes (22). Exercise results in the rapid GLUT4 translocation to the muscle surface membranes and is a fundamental event increasing muscle glucose uptake. Glucose transport is regulated by signals related to excitation-contraction coupling, most notably the increase in sarcoplasmic calcium, and by feedback signals that reflect the metabolic state of the muscle cell, including AMP, phosphocreatine, and glycogen levels (23). Calcium has long been recognized as a stimulator of muscle glucose transport (24), although the downstream events that ultimately increase glucose transport have not been fully described. It is possible that calcium interacts directly with proteins involved in the trafficking of GLUT4 vesicles to the sarcolemma. Alternatively, or in addition, calcium may act via calcium-sensitive signaling pathways such as the conventional isoforms of protein kinase C (PKC α, β, γ) and the calcium/calmodulin-dependent protein kinase (23). Muscle contractions increase PKC translocation to the membrane fraction (where it is active) as well as intracellular levels of diacylglycerol (DAG), an activator of both the conventional and novel (δ, ϵ, θ, η) isoforms of PKC. Furthermore, the PKC inhibitor calphostin C partially inhibits contraction-stimulated glucose transport, suggesting a role for the diacylglycerol-sensitive conventional and novel isoforms (23). In addition, it has recently been demonstrated that treadmill running increases atypical (ζ, ι/λ) PKC activity in mouse skeletal muscle.

KEY POINT

Several lines of evidence implicate PKC activation in the contraction-induced stimulation of muscle glucose transport, although additional studies are required to better define the importance of the various PKC isoforms.

There has been interest in the possible role of AMPK in the regulation of muscle glucose uptake during dynamic exercise. This enzyme is activated by increases in ADP and AMP within skeletal muscle during moderate to heavy dynamic exercise, hypoxia, and starvation. Pharmacologic activation of the enzyme by aminoimidazole-4-carboxamide-1-β-D-riboside (AICAR) increases sarcolemmal GLUT4 and muscle glucose uptake via an insulin-independent mechanism. Furthermore, exercise increases AMPK activity, in particular the α_2-isoform, although during very intense exercise the α_1-isoform is also activated. These observations have led to the suggestion that AMPK is responsible for the exercise-induced increase in muscle glucose uptake. However, mice expressing a dominant negative (inactive) form of AMPK in skeletal muscle retained 60% to 70% of their contraction-stimulated glucose transport despite abolition of hypoxia- and AICAR-stimulated glucose transport. Furthermore, contraction-stimulated glucose transport was not affected in muscle from either α_2-AMPK or α_1-AMPK knockout mice, suggesting that neither isoform is essential for glucose transport during muscle contractions (23). Thus, whereas activation of AMPK increases muscle glucose uptake, the importance of this protein in regulating muscle glucose uptake during dynamic exercise remains to be fully clarified. Knockout of the kinase upstream from AMPK, LKB1, reduces contraction-stimulated glucose transport in skeletal muscle suggesting that other LKB1 substrates, including AMPK-related kinases, may be involved in this process (25).

Other stimuli that potentially regulate muscle glucose transport during exercise include the mitogen-activated protein kinases (MAPK), reactive oxygen species and nitric oxide. Muscle contraction increases the activities of MAPK pathways, including the extracellular regulated kinases and the stress-activated protein kinases JNK and p38. Inhibition of a kinase upstream from extracellular regulated kinases does not affect glucose transport during muscle contraction, casting some doubt on the importance of these kinases. More research is required to elucidate the importance of the MAPK pathways in the activation of glucose transport during dynamic exercise. Contracting skeletal muscle produces nitric oxide and some studies have shown that inhibition of nitric oxide synthase attenuates the contraction-induced increase in glucose transport in vitro and the exercise-induced increase in muscle glucose uptake in humans (26). Reactive oxygen species, the production of which is increased during strenuous exercise, may also stimulate muscle glucose transport during exercise (26), but more studies are warranted. Finally, the identification of two related Rab-GTPase-activating proteins, AS160 (also known as TBC1D4–TBC1 domain family, member 4) and TBC1D1, as potential targets of protein kinases in both the insulin (Akt/protein kinase B) and exercise (26) signaling pathways has stimulated interest in their roles in linking the proximal and distal components of the respective signaling pathways and in mediating the well described interactions between them (27).

Hormonal Regulation of Muscle Glucose Uptake during Dynamic Exercise

The increase in muscle glucose uptake during exercise occurs via a mechanism that involves some or all of the signaling pathways identified earlier but does not require activation of the insulin signaling pathway. Despite early suggestions that a "permissive" level of insulin was required for muscle glucose transport to increase with contractions, it is now clear that insulin is not required for the contraction-induced increase in muscle glucose transport. Indeed, the effects of insulin and muscle contractions on GLUT4 translocation and glucose transport in skeletal muscle are additive (24). The preservation of the exercise-sensitive pathway in insulin-resistant states, such as type 2 diabetes and obesity, provides a rationale for the promotion of regular physical activity in the management of patients with these metabolic disorders. Furthermore, the additive nature of the exercise and insulin stimuli on muscle glucose uptake accounts for the observations of increased muscle glucose uptake and premature hypoglycemia when exercise is commenced with an elevated plasma insulin (e.g., after a high CHO meal or insulin injection in a type 1 diabetic) and increased glucose uptake and oxidation when CHO is ingested during prolonged heavy dynamic exercise (4).

Increased epinephrine inhibits muscle glucose uptake during exercise (16), an effect that appears to be due to its stimulatory effect on muscle glycogenolysis and the consequent increase in muscle glucose-6-phosphate, an inhibitor of hexokinase and glucose phosphorylation. However, the inhibitory effect of epinephrine during exercise is still present when muscle glycogen levels are low before exercise, which results in a blunted increase in glucose-6-phosphate. This implies a potential direct effect on sarcolemmal glucose transport, and there are data suggesting that epinephrine, via cyclic AMP, may inhibit GLUT4 intrinsic activity. β-Adrenergic blockade results in enhanced glucose disposal during dynamic exercise, consistent with removal of the inhibitory effect of epinephrine.

Substrate Availability

Because muscle glucose uptake occurs by facilitated diffusion, increases and decreases in blood glucose availability have the expected effects on muscle glucose uptake. During prolonged low intensity exercise in the absence of CHO supplementation, the decline in blood glucose results in reduced muscle glucose uptake (18,28). When blood glucose levels are maintained or increased by CHO ingestion during exercise, muscle glucose uptake and oxidation are increased. There are data demonstrating that hyperglycemia can enhance sarcolemmal GLUT4 translocation, but factors unrelated to glucose also contribute to the increased muscle glucose uptake under these conditions, most notably the higher plasma insulin. There is an inverse relationship between muscle glycogen availability and glucose uptake during exercise (15,29). This is due to effects on both intramuscular glucose metabolism, mediated via glucose-6-phosphate, and membrane glucose transport because sarcolemmal GLUT4 translocation in response to muscle contraction is greater with low muscle glycogen. Low muscle glycogen before exercise also results in greater activation of AMPK during exercise, which may also partly contribute to the enhanced muscle glucose uptake (29). Plasma FFA availability may also influence muscle glucose uptake during exercise, although the weight of evidence in human exercise studies supports a conclusion that plasma FFA has a relatively minor influence on muscle glucose uptake during dynamic exercise. The classical glucose–fatty acid cycle hypothesis proposed by Randle and colleagues predicts an inhibitory effect of elevated plasma FFA on muscle glucose uptake (see Chapter 16). Although this has been observed in one human study, there are several in the literature demonstrating reduced muscle glycogen use but no effect of increased FFA on glucose uptake. Similarly, although inhibition of adipose tissue lipolysis by nicotinic acid has been shown to increase glucose disposal slightly, the major effect was to increase muscle glycogenolysis, which accounted for almost all of the observed increase in CHO oxidation during exercise under conditions of reduced FFA availability.

Summary

Muscle glucose uptake is influenced by exercise intensity and duration. It occurs by facilitated diffusion and the sites of regulation include glucose delivery (blood flow and glucose), sarcolemmal glucose transport, and glucose disposal (phosphorylation and subsequent metabolism). GLUT4 translocation to the muscle surface is a fundamental event increasing muscle glucose uptake during exercise. Regulatory mechanisms include, but may not be limited to Ca^{2+}, PKC, calcium/calmodulin-dependent protein kinase, AMPK, MAPK, nitric oxide, and reactive oxygen species. Insulin and contraction effects on muscle glucose uptake are independent and additive.

KEY POINT

There is an inverse relationship between muscle glycogenolysis and glucose uptake; hyperglycemia enhances muscle glucose uptake and increased FFA reduces glucose uptake.

TEST YOURSELF

Is sarcolemmal glucose transport, mediated by GLUT4, rate-limiting for skeletal muscle glucose uptake during exercise?

What happens to blood glucose levels when a patient with type 1 diabetes commences exercise soon after injecting insulin?

Liver Glucose Output during Dynamic Exercise

The maintenance of blood glucose during exercise in the face of large increases in muscle glucose uptake is achieved by a concomitant increase in liver glucose output. The increase in liver glucose output is also dependent on exercise intensity and duration (Fig. 14.3) in a manner very similar to muscle glucose uptake; however, at higher exercise intensities, liver glucose output may exceed muscle glucose uptake, resulting in hyperglycemia. The early increase in liver glucose output is due to stimulation of liver glycogenolysis, and analysis of liver biopsy samples obtained

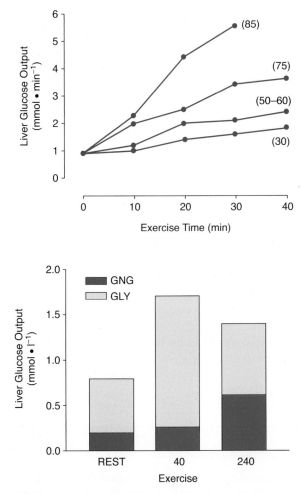

FIGURE 14.3 Liver glucose output during cycling exercise at varying exercise intensities (*top*) and during prolonged exercise at about 30% $\dot{V}O_{2max}$ (*bottom*), with estimated contributions from either glycogenolysis (GLY) or gluconeogenesis (GNG). Parenthetical numbers in top panel refer to exercise intensity, expressed as %$\dot{V}O_{2max}$. (Top panel redrawn from Hultman E, Harris RC. Carbohydrate metabolism. In: Poortmans JR, ed. *Principles of Exercise Biochemistry*. Basel: Karger; 1988:78–119. Data for bottom panel from Ahlborg G, Felig P, Hagenfeldt L, et al. Substrate turnover during prolonged exercise in man. *J Clin Invest*. 1974;53:1080–1090.)

before and after 1 hour of heavy exercise demonstrated a decline in liver glycogen from the normal postabsorptive value of 270 to 125 mmol · kg^{-1} (8). As exercise duration increases, the liver glycogen level decreases, and its contribution to liver glucose output is reduced (Fig. 14.3). There is enhanced uptake of gluconeogenic precursors, such as lactate, pyruvate, glycerol, and alanine (18,28), and activation of liver gluconeogenic enzyme activity. The result is that the contribution of gluconeogenesis to total liver glucose output increases from about 25% in the resting state to 45% to 50% after 4 hours of low-intensity exercise (16,26) (Fig. 14.3). Tracer-derived estimates of the contribution of gluconeogenesis to liver glucose output during 120 minutes of exercise at 60% $\dot{V}O_{2peak}$ are ~23% (30). The increase in gluconeogenesis cannot completely compensate for decreased liver glycogen availability and liver glucose output is reduced, resulting in a falling blood glucose level and muscle glucose uptake. Nevertheless, the importance of gluconeogenesis, at least in exercising rodents, is demonstrated by the observation that inhibition of liver gluconeogenesis reduces endurance capacity by about 30%. Given that endogenous liver glucose output cannot sustain glucose availability during prolonged strenuous exercise, endurance athletes ingest CHO to enhance performance, and under these circumstances gut-derived glucose augments, and may completely replace, endogenous liver glucose output. Following endurance training, liver glucose output during dynamic exercise at the same absolute power output is reduced in parallel with the decrease in muscle glucose uptake and oxidation (21). Liver glucose output was reduced ~42%, with the contribution from gluconeogenesis falling from 23% to 14% of total glucose output (30). These training-induced changes in liver glucose output were associated with higher insulin, but lower glucagon and catecholamine, levels and reduced gluconeogenic precursor (lactate, glycerol) availability (30).

Regulation of Liver Glucose Output

The regulation of liver glucose output involves complex, interactive, and redundant mechanisms and it is unlikely that a single factor is responsible for the stimulation of liver glucose output during dynamic exercise. Rather, neural and hormonal factors function together to ensure that it increases in an attempt to maintain glucose supply to active skeletal muscle and to the central nervous system. The close association between liver glucose output and muscle glucose uptake during moderate exercise raised the possibility of intricate feedback from contracting skeletal muscle, mediated by small decreases in blood glucose, afferent nerve activity, or even a circulating factor released from active muscle. In contrast, during heavy dynamic exercise, the increase in liver glucose output often precedes and is greater than the increase in muscle glucose uptake, which suggests a so-called feed-forward regulation. The neuroendocrine pathways responsible for enhanced liver glucose output are activated in parallel with motor cortical activation of skeletal muscle (central command) in a manner similar to that described for the cardiovascular and respiratory responses to exercise (31). Evidence in support of this is the exaggerated liver glucose output during dynamic exercise under conditions of relative muscle weakness and enhanced central command (31). This does not diminish the importance of feedback control; rather, both mechanisms work together to ensure that liver glucose output is appropriate for the prevailing exercise intensity and duration and glucose availability. Indeed, when both central command and afferent nerve feedback are abolished by electrically induced cycling in the presence of complete epidural blockade, plasma glucose levels are lower than during voluntary dynamic exercise at the same oxygen uptake.

KEY POINT

There is an interaction between feed-forward and feedback regulation; for example, increased blood glucose blunts the rise in liver glucose output to a lesser extent during high-intensity exercise than during exercise of low to moderate intensity.

Pancreatic Hormones

Insulin and glucagon are important regulators of liver glucose output in the resting state and remain so during exercise (22). The decline in plasma insulin levels allows liver glucose output to increase, whereas elevated plasma glucagon levels late in prolonged exercise stimulate gluconeogenesis. It is difficult to directly assess the role of glucagon in human subjects given that the portal vein samples cannot be obtained; however, because portal vein glucagon levels are presumably higher here than those measured in peripheral blood due to pancreatic glucagon release and reduced hepatic blood flow, and there is increased hepatic sensitivity to glucagon during exercise (22), this hormone appears to play a key role in liver glucose output during exercise. Thus, insulin and glucagon are important regulators of liver glucose output during dynamic exercise (22), but other factors appear to be involved in stimulating the liver to increase glucose output (32).

Sympathoadrenal Activity

In many exercise situations (e.g., intense exercise with hypoxia, exercise in the heat, with addition of arm exercise to leg exercise), the increase in liver glucose output is often closely correlated with enhanced sympathoadrenal activity, as reflected by increases in plasma epinephrine and norepinephrine. However, in many studies in which sympathoadrenal activity has been inhibited (adrenergic blockade, adrenalectomy, liver nerve resection), there has been no significant attenuation of the exercise-induced increase

in liver glucose output. Exogenous infusion of epinephrine can stimulate liver glucose output, either directly or by increasing plasma lactate, a gluconeogenetic precursor, secondary to enhanced muscle glycogenolysis. However, increased sympathoadrenal activity does not appear to be absolutely required for the increase in liver glucose output during dynamic exercise (33). Again, these results suggest complex redundancy in the regulation of liver glucose output and the interactions between sympathoadrenal activity, pancreatic hormones, and other as yet unidentified mediators of liver glucose output during dynamic exercise.

Carbohydrate Availability

Liver glucose output during dynamic exercise is higher after a CHO-rich diet than after a CHO-poor diet, consistent with marked differences in liver glycogen availability prior to exercise (8). Similarly, after a prolonged fast (60 hours) liver glucose output during exercise was about 65% lower than after an overnight fast, with gluconeogenesis contributing 78% and 13% to total liver glucose output, respectively (8). During intense exercise exogenous glucose infusion at a rate that equaled the average liver glucose output in a previous control trial abolished the normal exercise-induced increase in liver glucose output (34). Similar results have been obtained with CHO ingestion during dynamic exercise. Thus, blood glucose availability provides powerful feedback regulation of liver glucose output during exercise.

Summary

Liver glucose is determined by exercise intensity and duration and is usually closely coupled to muscle glucose uptake. At higher exercise intensities, feed-forward stimulation of liver glycogenolysis can produce hyperglycemia. Decreased insulin and increased glucagon, along with elevated catecholamines, enhance liver glucose output during exercise. Liver glucose output is exquisitely sensitive to feedback inhibition by increased blood glucose.

KEY POINT

Redundancy exists between various control mechanisms for glucose uptake and glycogenolysis, which emphasizes the importance of glucoregulation during exercise.

TEST YOURSELF

Which is the most important hormone involved in the regulation of liver glucose output during exercise?
What happens to liver glucose output when CHO is ingested during prolonged, strenuous exercise?

Regulation of Carbohydrate Oxidation during Dynamic Exercise

The degradation of glycosyl units, derived from either muscle glycogen or blood glucose, in glycolysis yields pyruvate, which can be either oxidized or converted to a number of other metabolites, such as lactate and alanine. For pyruvate to be oxidized, it must be first converted to acetyl-coenzyme A (CoA) in a reaction catalyzed by pyruvate dehydrogenase (PDH), a multienzyme complex within the mitochondrial matrix. Thus, PDH regulates the entry of CHO into the tricarboxylic acid cycle and its subsequent oxidation. The PDH complex comprises three enzymes and a kinase (PDH kinase or PDK) and a phosphatase (PDH phosphatase) that catalyze phosphorylation (inhibition) and dephosphorylation (activation) of the PDH enzyme, respectively. Increased ratios of adenosine triphosphate (ATP) to ADP, acetyl-CoA to CoASH, and reduced nicotinamide adenine dinucleotide (NADH) to NAD$^+$ activate PDH kinase and increased pyruvate inhibits it, whereas increased sarcoplasmic calcium activates PDH phosphatase (35). During exercise, the major activators of PDH are increased calcium and ADP, both of which also stimulate glycolysis and the production of pyruvate, another activator of PDH (35). These changes account for the close agreement between greater PDH activation and CHO oxidation with increasing exercise intensity (14) (Fig. 14.4). Increasing glycolytic flux and the rate of pyruvate production during exercise, either by increasing muscle glycogen prior to exercise or by infusing epinephrine (16), results in greater PDH activation and CHO oxidation. Conversely, increased FFA availability and a high-fat diet, together with glycogen-depleting exercise, reduced PDH activation during exercise (35). During exercise lasting several hours reduced pyruvate production, secondary to diminished glycolytic flux as muscle glycogen and glucose uptake are reduced, together with increased PDK activity,

are the most likely explanations for the observed decreases in PDH activation and CHO oxidation under these conditions. Collectively, these results indicate that PDH activation is the key step by which exercise intensity and duration modulate CHO oxidation.

PDH activation is also important at the onset of exercise. During the transition from rest to exercise there is a lag in oxygen uptake, and the energy demands of exercise are met by phosphocreatine degradation and glycolytic ATP production. The lag in oxidative energy production has traditionally been attributed to the slow increase in oxygen delivery to contracting skeletal muscle. Recent findings suggest that a delay in PDH activation may also partly contribute because pharmacologic activation of PDH by dichloroacetate resulted in reduced phosphocreatine degradation and lactate production (35).

> ### KEY POINT
>
> PDH is an extremely complex enzyme system that is important for CHO and fat oxidation, as well as the interplay between these substrates during exercise.

> ### TEST YOURSELF
>
> Why does CHO oxidation decrease during prolonged exercise?
> Dichloroacetate is a compound that increases PDH activity. How might it affect substrate level phosphorylation during the transition from rest to exercise?

Summary

PDH activation is a key step in the regulation of CHO oxidation by exercise intensity and duration. PDH is regulated by many substrates and cofactors, but calcium and pyruvate are the major activators of PDH during exercise.

Lactate Metabolism during Dynamic Exercise

Perhaps one of the most studied responses to exercise is blood lactate during incremental exercise. The exponential increase in blood lactate closely follows the increased glycolytic flux and reliance on muscle glycogenolysis during exercise of increasing intensity. There has been ongoing debate in the exercise physiology literature on the underlying cause of lactate production during exercise at intensities well below maximal oxygen uptake and on the possible links between muscle hypoxia, blood lactate, and ventilatory control, as articulated in the anaerobic

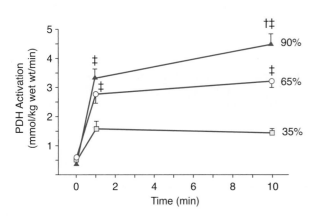

FIGURE 14.4 Pyruvate dehydrogenase (PDH) activation at rest and during 10 minutes of exercise at varying power outputs, expressed as %$\dot{V}O_{2max}$. (Reprinted with permission from Howlett RA, Parolin ML, Dyck DJ, et al. Regulation of skeletal muscle glycogen phosphorylase and PDH at varying exercise power outputs. *Am J Physiol.* 1998;275:R420.)

threshold hypothesis. Irrespective of underlying mechanisms, measurement of blood lactate during dynamic exercise has become widespread in the physiologic evaluation of endurance athletes and, indeed, lactate variables (*e.g.*, lactate threshold, onset of blood lactate accumulation, and maximal lactate steady state) are often better predictors of endurance exercise performance than maximal oxygen uptake. This reflects the close associations between lactate threshold, muscle oxidative capacity, and the rate of CHO utilization during dynamic exercise (36). Furthermore, the right shift in the blood lactate–power output curve is the classical marker of metabolic adaptation to endurance training. During prolonged dynamic exercise above the lactate threshold, there is a continuous rise in blood lactate, indicating a sustained rate of lactate production due to a greater reliance on CHO and/or reduced lactate removal. In contrast, below the lactate threshold, a steady-state blood lactate level is achieved as a result of a balance between the rates of lactate production and release into the bloodstream and lactate removal, and the level may even approach resting levels during prolonged exercise.

Although for many years lactate was considered simply a metabolic byproduct of glycolysis, there are now convincing data that lactate is an important metabolic intermediate during and after exercise, being a substrate for oxidative metabolism in contracting skeletal and cardiac muscle and a gluconeogenic precursor. The concept of a lactate shuttle has been developed (37), and there is evidence in support of exchange of lactate between active and inactive muscles during exercise. Contracting skeletal muscle is a major site of lactate oxidation during exercise, which contributes as much as 30% of the total CHO oxidation (38), although there remains some debate on the biochemical mechanisms underlying mitochondrial lactate oxidation (39,40). Thus, lactate can be simultaneously released and taken up by contracting skeletal muscle during exercise, with uptake closely linked with delivery. There is also evidence that noncontracting muscle releases lactate, particularly during the latter stages of prolonged dynamic exercise, thereby providing a mechanism for supplying additional carbon for oxidation and/or gluconeogenesis. It has been suggested that increases in epinephrine stimulate glycogenolysis in and lactate release from inactive muscle.

The transport of lactate across the sarcolemma is mediated by proton-linked monocarboxylate transporters (MCTs), and as many as eight isoforms have been identified (41). In human skeletal muscle, the most abundant isoform is MCT1, followed by MCT4. MCT1 expression correlates closely with muscle oxidative capacity and appears to be responsible for lactate uptake, whereas MCT4 is more abundant in type II fibers and may be important for lactate efflux from muscles with a greater reliance on glycolysis (41). Endurance training increases MCT1 expression in skeletal muscle and, together with the increase in muscle oxidative capacity, it contributes to enhanced lactate uptake and oxidation.

As mentioned earlier, there has been debate on the regulation of lactate production during exercise and the role of oxygen availability (42). In many situations in which oxygen delivery to contracting skeletal muscle is reduced (hypoxia, anemia, carbon monoxide exposure) during exercise, blood and muscle lactate levels are increased. It has been suggested that this is a necessary consequence of increases in ADP, P_i, and NADH that not only act to stimulate mitochondrial respiration but also activate glycolysis and conversion of pyruvate to lactate in the lactate dehydrogenase reaction (42). Because this reaction is stimulated by pyruvate via a mass action effect, lactate is produced whenever there is a mismatch between the rate of pyruvate production in the glycogenolytic–glycolytic pathway and the ability of PDH and mitochondrial shuttle systems to remove pyruvate and NADH, respectively, from the cytosol for oxidation (43). During the transition from rest to exercise or from a lower power output to a higher one, insufficient oxygen delivery and/or inadequate PDH activation result in a greater reliance on phosphocreatine and glycolytic ATP and lactate production. Similarly, manipulations of lactate production at a given level of oxygen consumption during exercise (*e.g.*, epinephrine infusion, increased muscle glycogen availability, heat stress) result in higher muscle and blood lactate accumulation (16).

Summary

Lactate is produced whenever there is a mismatch between the rate of pyruvate production in the glycogenolytic–glycolytic pathway and the ability of PDH and mitochondrial shuttle systems to remove pyruvate and NADH, respectively, from the cytosol for oxidation.

KEY POINT

Lactate is an important metabolic intermediate during and after exercise, being a substrate for oxidative metabolism as well as a gluconeogenic precursor.

TEST YOURSELF

Is lactate a metabolic end point or a metabolic intermediate?
Is muscle hypoxia an obligatory requirement for lactate production during exercise?

CHO Metabolism after Exercise

The postexercise period is characterized by the need to replenish muscle glycogen stores. Although exercise-induced glycogen depletion activates glycogen synthase (44), significant resynthesis of muscle glycogen is dependent on ingestion of CHO, which increases blood glucose and insulin levels. In particular, insulin stimulates GLUT4 translocation to the sarcolemma and further activates glycogen synthase. Studies in transgenic mice overexpressing either GLUT4 or glycogen synthase in skeletal muscle have demonstrated that both are critical for muscle glycogen synthesis, although the enhanced muscle glycogen storage observed in trained athletes appears to be more related to increased skeletal muscle GLUT4 expression (24). An increase in both GLUT4 gene and protein expression has been observed immediately after exercise, and this appears to be linked to the restoration of muscle glycogen (24). Glycogen synthase activity is increased after exercise, the increase in activity being greater with more extensive glycogen depletion (44). Interestingly, exercise commenced with very low muscle glycogen levels that resulted in no further glycogen degradation did not increase glycogen synthase activity over the already elevated basal level (44). The mechanisms responsible for this association between muscle glycogen and glycogen synthase activity remain to be fully elucidated, but they may be related to the intracellular location of glycogen synthase within muscle and/or the activity of protein phosphatase 1 (PP1), an enzyme that dephosphorylates glycogen synthase, thereby increasing its activity (44). There is evidence that this enzyme may be bound to glycogen, and particular interest has focused on the G_M targeting subunit. The exercise-induced increase in glycogen synthase activity is critically dependent on G_M-PP1 activity, and it has been suggested that the activity of this complex is inhibited by high muscle glycogen levels.

The postexercise period is also characterized by enhanced insulin sensitivity that may persist for up to 2 days. This enhanced insulin action partly arises from enhanced sarcolemmal GLUT4 and activation of glycogen synthase, and it allows for restoration of muscle glycogen to levels above the normal resting levels, a phenomenon known as glycogen supercompensation that was first reported in humans in 1966 (see *A Milestone of Discovery* at the end of this chapter). Enhanced insulin sensitivity is closely linked to glucose availability after exercise because glucose deprivation prolongs the time course of elevated insulin action, whereas CHO feeding speeds the reversal of enhanced insulin action, an observation made in both rodents (24) and humans (45). These changes in insulin action are linked with muscle glycogen availability because there is an association between muscle glycogen use during exercise and the increment in muscle glucose uptake during physiologic hyperinsulinemia 3 hours after exercise (46) (Fig. 14.5). Low muscle glycogen enhances glycogen synthase activity (44) and insulin-stimulated muscle glucose transport (46). The cellular mechanisms responsible for this latter observation are not completely understood, but GLUT4 translocation to the sarcolemma in response to insulin stimulation is enhanced by prior muscle glycogen depletion (24,46).

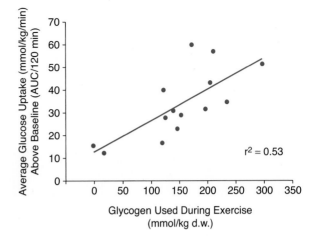

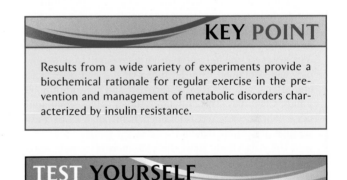

FIGURE 14.5 Relationship between glucose uptake during hyperinsulinemia 3 hours after exercise and the amount of glycogen used during exercise. (Reprinted with permission from Richter EA, Derave W, Wojtaszewski JFP. Glucose, exercise and insulin: emerging concepts. *J Physiol [Lond].* 2001;535:317.)

However, enhanced insulin action persists after restoration of muscle glycogen stores (24), implying that other factors must contribute to the effects of exercise on insulin action.

KEY POINT

Results from a wide variety of experiments provide a biochemical rationale for regular exercise in the prevention and management of metabolic disorders characterized by insulin resistance.

TEST YOURSELF

Is enhanced insulin action after exercise due to increased insulin signaling in skeletal muscle?
What are the interactions between blood glucose and insulin levels and muscle glycogen during the postexercise recovery period?

CHAPTER SUMMARY

Previous exercise increases muscle insulin sensitivity. Increased postexercise insulin action is due to both glycogen-dependent and independent mechanisms. Postexercise glycogen resynthesis is dependent on activation of glycogen synthase by muscle contraction and elevated insulin, secondary to CHO ingestion. Increased GLUT4 expression in the postexercise period contributes to glycogen storage.

Muscle glycogen and blood glucose derived from liver glycogenolysis and gluconeogenesis are the major oxidative substrates for contracting skeletal muscle during heavy exercise, and fatigue often coincides with depletion of these CHO stores. The rates of muscle glycogen utilization, muscle glucose uptake, and liver glucose output are determined primarily by exercise intensity and duration, but they can be modified by the preceding diet and training status. Key regulatory mechanisms include local control by intramuscular levels of calcium and metabolic intermediates; alterations in

glycogen, glucose, and FFA availability; and neural and hormonal control. Redundancy exists between various control mechanisms, emphasizing the importance of glucoregulation during exercise. Lactate is an important metabolic intermediate during and after exercise, being a substrate for oxidative metabolism and a gluconeogenic precursor. During the postexercise period, restoration of muscle glycogen stores,

A MILESTONE OF DISCOVERY

The Swedish scientists Jonas Bergström and Eric Hultman (Fig. 14.6) pioneered the use of the percutaneous needle biopsy in studies of muscle metabolism during exercise in human volunteers. In the late 1960s, they published a number of papers in which they examined aspects of phosphocreatine and glycogen metabolism in human skeletal muscle during exercise and the effects of various nutritional interventions. They collaborated with Lars Hermansen and Bengt Saltin on further exercise studies that verified and extended the classic studies of Christensen and Hansen and established the theoretical basis of dietary regimens for increasing muscle glycogen availability and enhancing endurance exercise performance.

For their 1966 *Nature* article, Bergström and Hultman conducted an elegant experiment on themselves in which they were placed on either side of a cycle ergometer and performed single-leg exercise to deplete the muscle glycogen stores of one leg as the other leg rested. Muscle samples were obtained from both legs at the end of exercise and after 1, 2, and 3 days of recovery and consumption of a high CHO diet. The muscle glycogen values (millimoles per kilogram wet mass) obtained from analysis of these samples are summarized in Table 14.2.

The data clearly show the utilization of muscle glycogen during exercise, rapid resynthesis of glycogen to preexercise levels within 24 hours in the previously exercised leg,

and glycogen supercompensation when a high CHO intake was continued for another 2 days. These results provided the theoretical basis for future studies on muscle glycogen loading and exercise performance and initial insights into the possible influence of muscle glycogen on substrate metabolism and insulin action after exercise. The authors concluded:

Exercise with glycogen depletion enhances the resynthesis of glycogen. The factor operates locally in the exercised muscle and the effect persists for at least 3 days. The nature of the mechanisms involved is unknown. It could be that a stimulation of one or more of the factors directly involved in glycogen synthesis takes place or that an effect is provided on the cell membrane, stimulating glucose uptake. It is possible that some of the beneficial effects of exercise in normal and diabetic subjects are mediated by this factor, thus promoting the storage of carbohydrate as glycogen instead of fat.

In the years since this study, many investigators have further characterized glycogen metabolism after exercise and elucidated the important role for muscle glycogen in the activation of glycogen synthase, insulin- and contraction-stimulated GLUT4 translocation and glucose uptake, skeletal muscle GLUT4 expression, and enhanced insulin sensitivity (24).

Bergström J, Hultman E. Muscle glycogen synthesis after exercise: an enhancing factor localized to the muscle cells in man. Nature. 1966;1210:309–310.

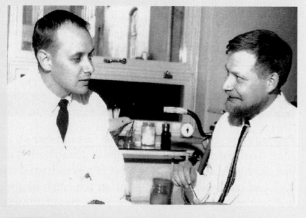

FIGURE 14.6 The late Jonas Bergström (*left*) and Eric Hultman in their laboratory at St. Erik's Hospital, Stockholm, in 1967. (Reproduced with permission from Professor Eric Hultman.)

| TABLE 14.2 | Muscle Glycogen Levels Before and After Select Days on a High Carbohydrate Intake Following Single-Leg Exercise |

Subject	Leg	Time (day)			
		0	1	2	3
JB	Rested	72.3	94.5	83.4	111.2
	Exercised	5.6	116.8	177.9	216.8
EH	Rested	77.8	94.5	94.5	100.1
	Exercised	5.6	116.8	189.0	205.7

Units are mmol · kg^{-1} wet mass.

which takes precedence, is dependent on the ingestion of CHO. Enhanced muscle glycogen synthesis and sarcolemmal glucose transport, along with increased GLUT4 expression, contribute to enhanced insulin action in the postexercise period and partly account for the beneficial effects of acute and chronic exercise in insulin-resistant states.

REFERENCES

1. Romijn JA, Coyle EF, Sidossis LS, et al. Regulation of endogenous fat and carbohydrate metabolism in relation to exercise intensity and duration. *Am J Physiol*. 1993;265:E380–E391.
2. Van Loon LJC, Greenhaff PL, Constantin-Teodosiu D, et al. The effects of increasing exercise intensity on muscle fuel utilization in humans. *J Physiol (Lond)*. 2001;536:295–304.
3. Hawley JA, Schabort EJ, Noakes TD, et al. Carbohydrate-loading and exercise performance: an update. *Sports Med*. 1997;24:73–81.
4. Coyle EF, Coggan AR, Hemmert MK, et al. Muscle glycogen during prolonged strenuous exercise when fed carbohydrate. *J Appl Physiol*. 1986;61:165–172.
5. Jeukendrup AE, Raben A, Gijsen A, et al. Glucose kinetics during prolonged exercise in highly trained human subjects: effect of glucose ingestion. *J Physiol (Lond)*. 1999;515:579–589.
6. McConell G, Fabris S, Proietto J, et al. Effect of carbohydrate ingestion on glucose kinetics during exercise. *J Appl Physiol*. 1994;77:1537–1541.
7. Gollnick PD, Piehl K, Saltin B. Selective glycogen depletion pattern in human muscle fibres after exercise of varying intensity and at varying pedalling rates. *J Physiol (Lond)*. 1974;241:45–57.
8. Hultman E, Harris RC. Carbohydrate metabolism. In: Poortmans JR, ed. *Principles of Exercise Biochemistry*. Basel: Karger; 1988: 78–119.
9. Burke LM, Angus DJ, Cox GR, et al. Effect of fat adaptation and carbohydrate restoration on metabolism and performance during prolonged cycling. *J Appl Physiol*. 2000;89:2413–2421.
10. Chesley A, Heigenhauser GJ, Spriet LL. Regulation of muscle glycogen phosphorylase activity following short-term endurance training. *Am J Physiol*. 1996;270:E328–E335.
11. Graham TE. Glycogen: an overview of possible regulatory roles of the proteins associated with the granule. *Appl Physiol Nutr Metab*. 2009;34:488–492.
12. Nielsen J, Schrøder HD, Rix CG, et al. Distinct effects of subcellular glycogen localization on tetanic relaxation time and endurance in mechanically skinned rat skeletal muscle fibres. *J Physiol (Lond)*. 2009;587:3679–3690.
13. Richter EA, Ruderman NB, Gavras H, et al. Muscle glycogenolysis during exercise: dual control by epinephrine and contractions. *Am J Physiol*. 1982;242:E25–E42.
14. Howlett RA, Parolin ML, Dyck DJ, et al. Regulation of skeletal muscle glycogen phosphorylase and PDH at varying exercise power outputs. *Am J Physiol*. 1998;275:R418–R425.
15. Hargreaves M. Interactions between muscle glycogen and blood glucose during exercise. *Exerc Sport Sci Rev*. 1997;25:21–39.
16. Watt MJ, Howlett KF, Febbraio MA, et al. Adrenaline increases skeletal muscle glycogenolysis, PDH activation and carbohydrate oxidation during moderate exercise in humans. *J Physiol (Lond)*. 2001;534:269–278.
17. Katz A, Broberg S, Sahlin K, et al. Leg glucose uptake during maximal dynamic exercise in humans. *Am J Physiol*. 1986;251:E65–E70.
18. Wahren J. Glucose turnover during exercise in man. *Ann NY Acad Sci*. 1977;301:45–55.
19. Kristiansen S, Hargreaves M, Richter EA. Progressive increase in glucose transport and GLUT4 in human sarcolemmal vesicles during moderate exercise. *Am J Physiol*. 1997;272:E385–E389.
20. Zisman A, Peroni AD, Abel ED, et al. Targeted disruption of the glucose transporter 4 selectively in muscle causes insulin resistance and glucose intolerance. *Nat Med*. 2000;6:924–928.
21. Coggan AR, Kohrt WM, Spina RJ, et al. Endurance training decreases plasma glucose turnover and oxidation during moderate-intensity exercise in men. *J Appl Physiol*. 1990;68:990–996.
22. Wasserman DH. Four grams of glucose. *Am J Physiol*. 2009;296:E11–E21.
23. Rose AJ, Richter EA. Skeletal muscle glucose uptake during exercise: how is it regulated? *Physiology*. 2005;20:260–270.
24. Hollozy JO. A forty-year memoir of research on the regulation of glucose transport into muscle. *Am J Physiol*. 2003;284:E453–E467.
25. Koh HJ, Brandauer J, Goodyear LJ. LKB1 and AMPK and the regulation of skeletal muscle metabolism. *Curr Opin Clin Nutr Metab Care*. 2008;11:227–232.
26. Merry TL, McConell GK. Skeletal muscle glucose uptake during exercise: a focus on reactive oxygen species and nitric oxide signaling. *IUBMB Life*. 2009;61:479–484.
27. Cartee GD, Funai K. Exercise and insulin: convergence or divergence at AS160 and TBC1D1? *Exerc Sport Sci Rev*. 2009; 37:188–195.
28. Ahlborg G, Felig P, Hagenfeldt L, et al. Substrate turnover during prolonged exercise in man. *J Clin Invest*. 1974;53:1080–1090.
29. Wojtaszewski JFP, MacDonald C, Nielsen JN, et al. Regulation of 5'AMP-activated protein kinase activity and substrate utilization in exercising human skeletal muscle. *Am J Physiol*. 2003;284:E813–E822.
30. Coggan AR, Swanson SC, Mendenhall LA, et al. Effect of endurance training on hepatic glycogenolysis and gluconeogenesis during prolonged exercise in men. *Am J Physiol*. 1995;268:E375–E383.
31. Kjaer M, Secher NH, Bach FW, et al. Role of motor center activity for hormonal changes and substrate mobilization in humans. *Am J Physiol*. 1987;253:R687–R695.
32. Coker RH, Wasserman DH, Simonsen L, et al. Stimulation of splanchnic glucose production during exercise in humans contains a glucagon-independent component. *Am J Physiol*. 2001;280:E918–E927.
33. Kjaer M, Engfred K, Fernandes A, et al. Regulation of hepatic glucose production in humans: role of sympathoadrenergic activity. *Am J Physiol*. 1993;265:E275–E283.
34. Howlett KF, Angus DJ, Proietto J, et al. Effect of increased blood glucose availability on glucose kinetics during exercise. *J Appl Physiol*. 1998;84:1413–1417.
35. Spriet LL, Heigenhauser GJF. Regulation of pyruvate dehydrogenase (PDH) activity in human skeletal muscle during exercise. *Exerc Sport Sci Rev*. 2002;30:91–95.
36. Coyle EF, Coggan AR, Hopper MK, et al. Determinants of endurance in well-trained cyclists. *J Appl Physiol*. 1988;64:2622–2630.
37. Brooks GA. Intra- and extra-cellular lactate shuttles. *Med Sci Sports Exerc*. 2000;32:790–799.
38. Van Hall G, Jensen-Urstad M, Rosdahl H, et al. Leg and arm lactate and substrate kinetics during exercise. *Am J Physiol*. 2003;284:E193–E205.
39. Hashimoto T, Brooks GA. Mitochondrial lactate oxidation complex and an adaptive role for lactate production. *Med Sci Sports Exerc*. 2008;40:486–494.
40. Yoshida Y, Holloway GP, Ljubicic V, et al. Negligible direct lactate oxidation in subsarcolemmal and intermyofibrillar mitochondria obtained from red and white rat skeletal muscle. *J Physiol (Lond)*. 2007;582:1317–1335.
41. Juel C, Halestrap AP. Lactate transport in skeletal muscle: role and regulation of the monocarboxylate transporter. *J Physiol (Lond)*. 1999;517:633–642.
42. Katz A, Sahlin K. Regulation of lactic acid production during exercise. *J Appl Physiol*. 1988;65:509–518.
43. Spriet LL, Howlett RA, Heigenhauser GJF. An enzymatic approach to lactate production in human skeletal muscle during exercise. *Med Sci Sports Exerc*. 2000;32:756–763.
44. Nielsen JN, Richter EA. Regulation of glycogen synthase in skeletal muscle during exercise. *Acta Physiol Scand*. 2003;178:309–319.
45. Bogardus C, Thuillez P, Ravussin E, et al. Effect of muscle glycogen depletion on in vivo insulin action in man. *J Clin Invest*. 1983;72:1605–1610.
46. Richter EA, Derave W, Wojtaszewski JFP. Glucose, exercise and insulin: emerging concepts. *J Physiol (Lond)*. 2001;535:313–322.

CHAPTER 15

The Metabolic Systems: Lipid Metabolism

Lawrence L. Spriet

Abbreviations

AC	Adenylate cyclase	FAD, FADH$_2$	Flavin adenine dinucleotide
ADP	Adenosine diphosphate	FAT/CD36	Fatty acid translocase
AMP	Adenosine monophosphate	FATP 1-6	Fatty acid transport proteins 1 through 6
AMPK	AMP-activated protein kinase	FFA	Free fatty acid
ATGL	Adipose triacylglycerol lipase	G$_i$	Inhibitory G protein
ATP	Adenosine triphosphate	GPAT	Glycerol-phosphate acyltransferase
Ca^{2+}	Calcium	HSL	Hormone-sensitive lipase
CaMKII	Calcium/calmodulin kinase II	IMTG	Intramuscular triacylglycerol
cAMP	Cyclic AMP	M-CoA	Malonyl-CoA
CGI-58	Comparative gene identification 58	MG	Monoacylglycerol
CHO	Carbohydrate	MRS	Magnetic resonance spectroscopy
CoA	Coenzyme A	NAD$^+$, NADH	Nicotinamide adenine dinucleotide;
CPT I, II	Carnitine palmitoyltransferase I and II		oxidized and reduced forms
DG	Diacylglycerol	NE	Norepinephrine
DGAT	Diacylglycerol acyltransferase	P$_i$	Inorganic phosphate
EPI	Epinephrine	PKA	Protein kinase A
ERK	Extracellular signal regulated kinase	RER	Respiratory exchange ratio
ETC	Electron transport chain	RQ	Respiratory quotient
FABP$_C$	Cytoplasmic fatty acid-binding protein	$\dot{V}O_{2max}$	Maximal oxygen uptake
FABP$_{PM}$	Plasma membrane fatty acid-binding FACS	TCA	Tricarboxylic acid
	Fatty acyl-CoA synthetase	TG	Triacylglycerol
FACS	Fatty acyl-CoA synthetase		

Introduction

It is now accepted that lipid is an important substrate for the aerobic production of energy in human skeletal muscle during light, moderate, and even heavy dynamic exercise. However, it was not until the work of Christensen and Hansen was published in 1939 that the controversy over whether lipid (fat) could be used as a substrate for exercise was finally solved by Assmussen (1). The authors demonstrated, through a series of elegant studies, that both fat and carbohydrate (CHO) could be used as substrate for muscular contractions and that the amount of fat and CHO used depended on several factors. The preceding diet was the main factor during short duration dynamic exercise of low to moderate intensity. As exercise intensity increased, the proportion of fat oxidation decreased and CHO oxidation increased such that fat use was virtually absent at a power output that elicited 100% of maximal oxygen uptake ($\dot{V}O_{2max}$). However, during prolonged moderate intensity dynamic exercise, the relative fat contribution increased due to the increasing availability of plasma free fatty acid (FFA) and decreasing CHO stores. Later studies used more direct experimental approaches to demonstrate the importance of plasma FFA and fat derived from stores inside the muscle as substrates for oxidation during exercise (see *A Milestone of Discovery* at the end of this chapter [2]).

Fat is often the dominant fuel for skeletal muscle at rest and during light to moderate intensity exercise. In absolute terms, the contribution of fat to the total energy production increases from low power outputs to a maximum between ~50% to 65% $\dot{V}o_{2max}$ and then decreases as the exercise intensity increases to ~85% $\dot{V}o_{2max}$ and above (3,4) (see Chapter 14, Fig. 14.1). Consequently, fat is the less important of the two substrates during heavy dynamic exercise as CHO becomes the dominant substrate. Although CHO can provide all the substrate required for exercise at ~100% $\dot{V}o_{2max}$ when no fat is available, fat can only provide substrate at a rate to sustain ~60% to 75% $\dot{V}o_{2max}$ when calculated as if no CHO is available. However, fat is an energy dense fuel with a high yield per unit mass and is stored in large quantities in the body. Therefore, fat can provide a substantial and increasing amount of energy during prolonged dynamic exercise at light to moderate intensities. Aerobic training also increases the maximal rate that fat oxidation can produce energy in skeletal muscle and increases the proportion of energy produced from fat oxidation at any absolute power output (5,6). It is also important to remember that fat metabolism is not activated as quickly as CHO metabolism at the onset of exercise and that it cannot be used to generate "anaerobic" energy during heavy exercise near or above 100% $\dot{V}o_{2max}$ (sprint exercise).

Large quantities of fat are stored as triglyceride or triacylglycerol (TG) in numerous adipose tissue sites in the body. Smaller amounts of fat are also stored directly in muscle cells. Due to the high energy density of fat, the fat stored in muscle can provide almost as much fuel as muscle glycogen (~67%–100%) (see Chapter 14, Fig. 14.1). Therefore, the intramuscular TG (IMTG) store is not trivial, especially during exercise situations, where it is readily available as a fuel source. Fat is also found in numerous forms in the circulation. However, it appears that the FFA bound to albumin is the predominant source of circulatory fat that is readily available for uptake and oxidation by skeletal muscle during dynamic exercise. Circulating TG in the form of chylomicrons and very low density lipoproteins appear to contribute less than 5% to 8% of the fat oxidized during dynamic exercise (2). At rest when the need for FFA uptake is low, circulating TGs can be degraded and provide FFA for storage and oxidation in the muscle.

Until very recently, the regulation of skeletal muscle fat metabolism was not studied as thoroughly as CHO metabolism. Most textbooks in use today still claim that the only sites of control in the regulation of fat metabolism are the release of FFA into the blood from adipose tissue and the transport of FFA across the mitochondrial membranes of the muscle cell. However, it is now clear that the regulation of fat metabolism involves many additional sites of control in adipose tissue and skeletal muscle and that the regulation at every site is complex. The focus of this chapter is to outline the present knowledge regarding the regulation of fat metabolism in skeletal muscle. The chapter focuses on the events that lead to the production of energy from the oxidation of fat in human skeletal muscle during dynamic exercise, although skeletal muscle research from additional mammalian species and muscle cell lines is heavily cited. The chapter begins with an overview of the pathways involved in the control of fat metabolism. Subsequent sections provide more detail regarding the putative sites and mechanisms of regulation and other issues related to fat metabolism.

Overview of Fat Metabolism

A major source of fat for the working muscle during exercise is the delivery of long chain FFA to the muscle from adipose tissue (7). The degradation of FFA from adipose tissue TG and the release and removal of FFA from adipose tissue are regulated processes. The FFAs bind to albumin in the blood and the bulk transport of FFA to the muscle (FFA × blood flow) plays a role in the ability of muscle to take up FFA (Fig. 15.1). A common theme with the transport of FFA in the blood, and inside skeletal muscle cells, is the need to provide a protein chaperone. Unbound FFAs interfere with electrical transmission and enzyme function and also act as a detergent. Therefore, at every step involved in the transport and metabolism of FFA, there are protein chaperones that bind the so-called "free" fatty acids. Although the fat is free from its stored or "esterified" form, the vast majority is always coupled to a binding protein. Only a small fraction of the FFAs are believed to be truly free in order to promote binding to albumin in adipose tissue and unbinding for transport into skeletal muscle.

Recent evidence suggests that the majority of the FFAs that enter muscle cells are transported or assisted across the muscle membrane by transport proteins, most notably the fatty acid translocase (FAT/CD36) protein, the plasma membrane fatty acid-binding (FABP$_{PM}$), and members of the fatty acid transport proteins (FATP) family (8) (see Fig. 15.2). A smaller portion appears to diffuse across the membrane. Once inside the muscle, FFAs are chaperoned by cytoplasmic fatty acid-binding proteins (FABP$_C$). The FFAs destined for storage as IMTG or for oxidation in the mitochondria must first be "activated" via binding with coenzyme A (CoA) through the activity of fatty acyl-CoA synthase (FACS) (7). This may occur at several sites in the cytoplasm, including the plasma membrane, the outer mitochondrial membrane, and near the IMTG droplet. A second major source of fat is via the release of FFA from IMTG. The evidence that IMTG contributes substrate for energy production during exercise is now convincing, but the quantitative importance at varying intensities and durations of exercise remains somewhat equivocal (9). The first events in regulating muscle lipolysis are activation of

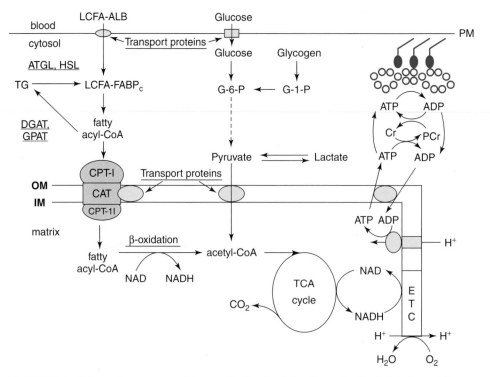

FIGURE 15.1 Schematic overview of fat metabolism in skeletal muscle. *Shaded circles* and *boxes* depict transport proteins. ALB, albumin; ATGL, adipose triglyceride lipase; CAT, carnitine-acylcarnitine translocase; CoA, coenzyme A; CPT I & II, carnitine palmitoyltransferase I & II; Cr, creatine; DGAT, diacylglycerol acyltransferase; ETC, electron transport chain; FABPc, cytoplasmic fatty acid-binding protein; G-6-P, G-1-P, glucose 6- and 1-phosphate; GPAT, glycerol-phosphate acyltransferase; HSL, hormone-sensitive lipase; LCFA, long chain fatty acid; NAD^+, NADH, oxidized and reduced nicotinamide adenine dinucleotide; OM, IM, outer and inner mitochondrial membranes; PCr, phosphocreatine; PM, plasma membrane; TCA, tricarboxylic acid; TG, triacylglycerol. (Adapted with permission from Spriet LL. Regulation of skeletal muscle fat oxidation during exercise in humans. *Med Sci Sports Exerc.* 2002;34:1477–1484.)

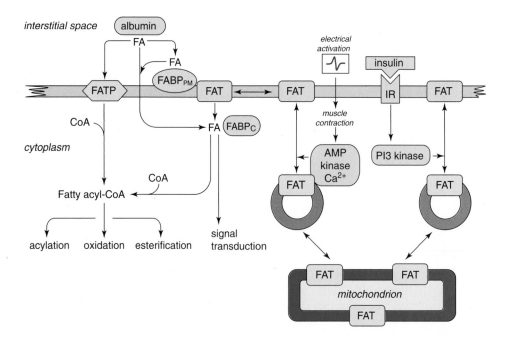

FIGURE 15.2 Schematic diagram of potential mechanisms for long chain fatty acid uptake across the muscle and mitochondrial membranes. FA, fatty acid; $FABP_{PM}$, plasma membrane fatty acid-binding protein; FAT, FAT/CD36 fatty acid translocase; $FABP_C$, cytoplasmic fatty acid-binding protein; FATP, fatty acid transport protein; IR, insulin receptor. (This figure was kindly provided by Dr. Jan Glatz.)

the TG lipases, including the recently discovered adipose TG lipase (ATGL) and hormone-sensitive lipase (HSL). Additional regulatory steps appear to include movement of the ATGL-HSL complex to the lipid droplet, and penetration of a protective perilipin-like protein layer around the lipid droplet.

For oxidation to occur, all of the cytoplasmic $FABP_C$-FFA, whether derived from outside the cell (plasma FFA) or inside the muscle cell (IMTG), must be transported to the outer mitochondrial membrane (Fig. 15.1). It is then activated with CoA, if not already activated, and converted to fatty acylcarnitine by carnitine fatty acyltransferase I (commonly referred to as carnitine palmitoyltransferase I, or CPT I; Fig. 15.3) (10). This compound is moved across the mitochondrial membranes via a translocase, whereas carnitine moves in the opposite direction. Recent evidence also suggests that the transfer of fatty acylcarnitine complex is aided across the membranes in some unidentified manner by the fat transport protein, FATCD36. Inside the mitochondria, carnitine is removed and the CoA is rebound to the long chain fatty acid by the enzyme, carnitine palmitoyltransferase II (CPT II). The fatty acyl-CoA molecules are then metabolized in the β-oxidation pathway with the production of acetyl-CoA and reducing equivalents (reduced nicotinamide adenine dinucleotide [NADH], reduced flavin adenine dinucleotide [$FADH_2$]). The reducing equivalents are directly used in the electron transport chain (ETC), whereas the acetyl-CoA is further metabolized in the tricarboxylic acid (TCA) pathway with the production of additional reducing equivalents. The ETC accepts the reducing equivalents to generate a proton motive force, which provides the chemical energy to synthesize adenosine triphosphate (ATP) from inorganic phosphate (P_i) and adenosine diphosphate (ADP) while consuming oxygen in the process of oxidative phosphorylation.

The potential sites that control skeletal muscle fat metabolism and oxidation during dynamic exercise appear to include:

1. Adipose tissue lipolysis, FFA release from adipose tissue, and FFA delivery to the muscle
2. FFA transport across the muscle membrane
3. Binding and transport of FFA in the cytoplasm
4. IMTG lipolysis
5. FFA transport across the mitochondrial membranes
6. Possibly, regulation associated within the β-oxidation pathway

Lastly, an overarching aspect of the regulation of fat metabolism and oxidation is the skeletal muscle mitochondrial volume (total protein contents of the CPT complex and the β-oxidation enzymes) which determines the overall capacity to oxidize fat.

> ## KEY POINT
>
> The regulation of fat metabolism involves many sites of complex regulatory control in adipose tissue and skeletal muscle. This complexity allows the body to deal with a wide range of physiologic conditions, from postprandial rest to prolonged high intensity exercise.

It is expected that the regulation of fat metabolism during an acute dynamic exercise bout lasting several minutes would involve control by both hormonal signals and signals originating inside the muscle. The blood catecholamine and insulin concentrations are major hormonal regulators. Inside the muscle, three classes of signals are generally associated with the acute activation of energy-producing metabolic pathways: (a) calcium (Ca^{2+}), which is released to initiate muscle contraction, but also serves as an early warning or feed-forward signal for the activation of metabolic processes; (b) feedback from byproducts related to the breakdown of ATP, often referred to as the "energy state" of the muscle—these include the free concentrations of the high energy phosphates ATP, ADP, adenosine monophosphate (AMP), and P_i; and (c) feedback from the involvement of the reduction-oxidation (redox)

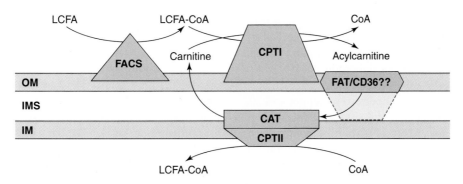

FIGURE 15.3 Schematic diagram of proposed regulation of long chain fatty acid (LCFA) transport into the mitochondria. CAT, carnitine-acylcarnitine translocase; CPT I and II, carnitine palmitoyltransferase I and II; CoA, coenzyme A; FACS, fatty acyl-CoA synthase; FAT/CD36, fatty acid translocase; IMS, intermitochondrial membrane space; OM, IM, outer and inner mitochondrial membranes. (Figure has been adapted from Kiens B, Essen-Gustavsson B, Christensen NJ, et al. Skeletal muscle substrate utilization during submaximal exercise in man: effect of endurance training. *J Physiol.* 1993;469:459–478, with permission from the American Physiological Society.)

couple (NAD$^+$/NADH) at many sites in the mitochondria. These signals and regulators have been well studied and heavily implicated in controlling the cytoplasmic pathways involved in the metabolism of CHO and also in the TCA cycle in the mitochondria, which accepts acetyl-CoA as a substrate from both CHO and fat metabolism. However, until very recently, there had not been many investigations examining the potential for these regulators to also control cytoplasmic and mitochondrial aspects of fat metabolism.

Adipose Tissue Lipolysis

The ability of adipose tissue to respond to dynamic exercise by activating TG hydrolysis and releasing FFA into the blood is important for increasing and maintaining the delivery of FFA to the working muscle. The sequential hydrolysis of TG by specific enzymes results in the liberation of a FFA at each step with the generation of diacylglycerol (DG), monoacylglycerol (MG), and glycerol. For many years, HSL was presumed to be the rate-limiting enzyme controlling this process. Studies over the past two decades demonstrated the important role of phosphorylation by hormone and muscle activated protein kinases in controlling HSL intracellular localization, enzyme activity, and interaction with the regulatory protein perilipin A to coordinate the control of adipose tissue lipolysis (11,12). However, studies reporting that HSL-null mice accumulated DG and were able to retain some β-adrenergic stimulated lipolysis and that HSL exhibited a greater affinity for DG versus TG substrate suggested that another important TG lipase existed (12). In 2004, three laboratories identified and characterized a new enzyme as desnutrin, phospholipase A2-ζ, and ATGL (13–15). The latter name is now commonly used and the findings of this work suggested that ATGL and HSL work hierarchically to regulate complete TG hydrolysis. ATGL is believed to initiate lipolysis by specifically removing the first FFA from TG to produce DG. HSL then hydrolyzes DG to generate an additional FFA and MG, which is converted to FFA and glycerol by MG lipase in the final step of lipolysis. Although ATGL and HSL appear to be nonequilibrium enzymes and regulated by external factors, MG lipase appears to be a near-equilibrium enzyme and regulated by only substrates and products.

At present, it seems unequivocal that ATGL mediates basal and β-adrenergic TG lipolysis in adipocytes as ATGL deletion induces obesity and ATGL over-expression produces a lean phenotype (16,17). In addition, inhibition of ATGL in human adipose tissue lysates reduced total TG lipase activity by 80%, indicating an important role for ATGL in human adipocyte lipolysis (12). Little is known about the kinases that phosphorylate ATGL, but it does not appear to be directly regulated by protein kinase A (PKA) phosphorylation (15).

The role of HSL in the regulation of adipose tissue lipolysis has been relegated to a secondary but still important step that catalyzes the breakdown of DG to MG and FFA

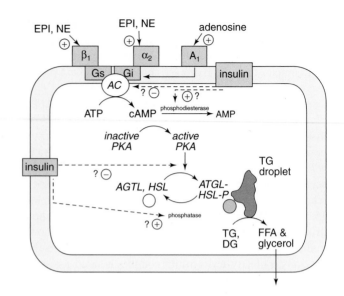

FIGURE 15.4 Schematic diagram outlining the major regulation of adipose tissue lipolysis during exercise. ATGL, adipose triglyceride lipase; cAMP, cyclic AMP; DG, diacylglycerol; EPI, epinephrine; FFA, free fatty acid; Gs and Gi, stimulatory and inhibitory G proteins; HSL, hormone-sensitive lipase; NE, norepinephrine; PKA, protein kinase A; TG, triacylglycerol. (Adapted with permission from Spriet LL. Regulation of skeletal muscle fat oxidation during exercise in humans. *Med Sci Sports Exerc.* 2002;34:1477–1484.)

(Fig. 15.4). It exists in an active, phosphorylated form and a less active, dephosphorylated form. The exact amount of active and less active HSL at any point in time is controlled by the relative activities of PKA, which phosphorylates the enzyme and a phosphatase, which dephosphorylates the enzyme.

TEST YOURSELF

Speculate on why the control of TG lipolysis would be designed to have two regulated enzymes in series to initiate the degradation of lipid.

The phosphorylation and regulation of ATGL and HSL are not the only control steps in the degradation of TG. The activated enzymes may move to the vicinity of the lipid droplets (11) and interact in some way with regulatory proteins like perilipin A that work to encase or protect the lipid droplet (18) from degradation. Phosphorylation of perilipin A may remove this inhibition and allow ATGL and HSL access to the lipid. A major advance in understanding the regulation of lipolysis was the discovery that ATGL required the protein, comparative gene identification 58 (CGI-58), for full activation. The interaction of CGI-58 with ATGL increased adipose tissue TG lipolysis several fold (12,19). CGI-58 resides on the surface of lipid droplets and also interacts with perilipin A under basal conditions. After β-adrenergic stimulation, perilipin A is phosphorylated and CGI-58 rapidly disperses into the cytoplasm and appears to associate with ATGL to increase its activity.

Physiologic Regulation of Resting Lipolysis

Adipose tissue lipolysis is maintained at a low rate while the body is at rest through the inhibitory influences by several hormones (7,20). The plasma catecholamines, norepinephrine (NE) and epinephrine (EPI), exert an inhibitory effect on lipolysis at low concentrations through a cascade of events ending in the maintenance of ATGL and HSL in less active forms (Fig. 15.4). Low NE and EPI levels activate the α-2 adrenergic receptor, which stimulates the inhibitory G protein (G_i), decreases the activity of adenylate cyclase (AC), and decreases the production of cyclic AMP (cAMP). A low cAMP level, in turn, decreases PKA and HSL activities and may indirectly decrease ATGL activity, ultimately reducing the degradation of TG. Adenosine also contributes to the resting inhibition of lipolysis by binding to adenosine receptors and activating the G_i protein. This process can be antagonized by caffeine when present in the blood, as caffeine competes for the adenosine binding sites, prevents the activation of G_i, and often leads to increased lipolysis and plasma FFA levels at rest. On the other hand, nicotinic acid (NA; vitamin B_3) reduces lipolysis by binding to HM74 receptors that are coupled to G_i proteins, decreasing cAMP levels and preventing activation of HSL, leading to decreased systemic FFA release. These compounds have been used to examine the effects of increased and reduced plasma FFA availability on skeletal muscle metabolism. It is not currently known how these physiologic signals control ATGL at rest.

The presence of insulin in the blood can also inhibit lipolysis and may be the most important regulator at rest (Fig. 15.4). Insulin exerts a strong antilipolytic effect following a meal containing significant amounts of CHO as the body attempts to reduce the use of fat while oxidizing and storing the ingested CHO. Insulin binds to receptors on the adipose tissue and is believed to inhibit lipolysis at several sites:

1. Direct inhibition of AC activity
2. Activation of phosphodiesterase activity and the removal of cAMP
3. Direct inhibition of PKA, reducing the activation of HSL
4. Activation of phosphatase, which deactivates HSL

The potential links between insulin and ATGL regulation have not been elucidated.

TEST YOURSELF

How do hormones keep the rate of fat breakdown (lipolysis) in adipose tissue low at rest?

Physiologic Regulation of Lipolysis during Exercise

Dynamic exercise is associated with an increase in sympathetic nervous system activity resulting in an accumulation of EPI and NE in the blood. EPI originates mainly from the adrenal medulla, whereas NE escapes from activated sympathetic nerve terminals. The increased catecholamine concentrations during exercise exert powerful effects to increase lipolysis and override the combined inhibitory influences that dominate at rest (Fig. 15.4). The increases in plasma NE and EPI during exercise bind to β-adrenergic receptors and activate the stimulatory G protein. This antagonizes and overrides the effects of the G_i protein and insulin to increase AC activity, cAMP production, PKA activity, and ultimately phosphorylation of HSL, perilipin, and possibly ATGL. The subsequent release of FFA can lead to the re-esterification to TG or, preferably during exercise, release from the adipose tissue into the blood. The escape of the FFA into the blood is dependent on membrane fat transport proteins and the availability of albumin in the blood. This process does not appear to be limiting in most dynamic exercise situations, but may be limiting during heavy exercise, as discussed later.

FFA Release from Adipose Tissue and Delivery to Muscle

The delivery of FFA to contracting muscle is a function of the plasma [FFA] and muscle blood flow. Because muscle blood flow increases as a function of exercise intensity, even the maintenance of a constant [FFA] means that muscle FFA delivery increases several fold during exercise. During prolonged low to moderate intensity exercise, the blood [FFA] increases within 10 to 30 minutes and also contributes to the increased FFA delivery, as FFA release from adipose tissue slightly exceeds its removal from the plasma. Increased FFA delivery to the muscle correlates with increased muscle FFA uptake and oxidation during dynamic exercise, although the relationship is not linear during all exercise situations. The movement of FFA across the muscle membrane appears to be a saturable process in both rodent and human skeletal muscle and is discussed in a following section.

TEST YOURSELF

Why do catecholamines inhibit adipose tissue lipolysis at rest and yet stimulate lipolysis during exercise?

Adipose Tissue Lipolysis and FFA Release during Light, Moderate, and Intense Exercise

To study the importance of adipose tissue lipolysis and FFA release, simultaneous measurements or estimations of plasma [FFA], adipose tissue lipolysis, and muscle oxidation of plasma FFA have been made during dynamic exercise at increasing power outputs in well-trained cyclists (4,21). Lipolysis increased as a function of the power output at 25% and 65% $\dot{V}O_{2max}$ and the plasma [FFA] remained high during exercise at these two intensities (pre-exercise FFA were already high at ~0.8 to 1.0 mM, due to an overnight fast). Therefore, FFA delivery to the contracting muscles increased from rest to exercise at 25% $\dot{V}O_{2max}$ and again from 25% to 65% $\dot{V}O_{2max}$ and correlated with the maintenance of high plasma FFA uptake and oxidation rates at these two intensities.

These same relationships did not hold during intense exercise (21). During 30 minutes of exercise at 85% $\dot{V}O_{2max}$, adipose tissue lipolysis was maintained at the same rate as 65% $\dot{V}O_{2max}$, but the oxidation rate of plasma FFA decreased at 85% $\dot{V}O_{2max}$. The prediction from these results would be an increase in plasma FFA, but the [FFA] actually decreased by ~50%. The explanation for these results was that a decrease in adipose tissue blood flow prevented much of the liberated FFA from reaching the blood, in spite of a maintained lipolytic rate at 85% $\dot{V}O_{2max}$. The reduced blood flow decreased the availability of albumin, which is necessary to bind FFA and permit transport in the blood. Therefore, the uptake of FFA by the muscles continued at a higher rate than the release from adipose tissue and accounted for the lower plasma [FFA].

It is likely that the large fall in [FFA] during dynamic exercise from 65% to 85% $\dot{V}O_{2max}$ also outweighed the increase in muscle blood flow, resulting in a decrease in FFA delivery to the contracting muscles at 85% $\dot{V}O_{2max}$, although this was not measured. This correlated with a significant decrease in plasma FFA uptake and oxidation at 85% $\dot{V}O_{2max}$. However, it is important to remember that these results do not exclude other factors, including FFA muscle and mitochondrial membrane transport or metabolism related changes, from also contributing to the reduced fat oxidation at the higher power output.

To assess the importance of FFA delivery to the contracting muscles during exercise, the plasma [FFA] at 85% $\dot{V}O_{2max}$ was artificially maintained at the higher level found at 65% $\dot{V}O_{2max}$ by infusing a TG emulsion and heparin solution (22). The plasma FFA uptake and oxidation rates were increased at 85% $\dot{V}O_{2max}$ when FFA delivery was maintained, but did not reach the same rates as at 65% $\dot{V}O_{2max}$. These findings implied that other factors, related to membrane transport or metabolism inside the muscle, also play an important role in determining the rate of plasma FFA uptake and oxidation at higher exercise intensities.

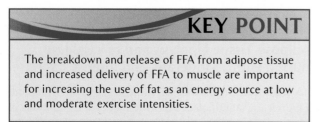

KEY POINT

The breakdown and release of FFA from adipose tissue and increased delivery of FFA to muscle are important for increasing the use of fat as an energy source at low and moderate exercise intensities.

FFA Transport Across the Muscle Membrane

Until recently, it was believed that FFA simply diffused through the bilipid layer of the muscle membrane into the muscle cell. The plasma [FFA] and/or the rate of FFA delivery to the muscles were believed to be the only controlling factors. Over the last 15 years, strong evidence has emerged that a major portion of the FFAs that enter muscle do so via protein-mediated mechanisms (8,23). This may involve actual transport of FFA across the muscle membrane by carrier proteins and/or facilitation of their movement across the membrane by initial binding to transport proteins. The presence of proteins that transport or assist the movement of FFA into muscle cells implies that this is a major site of regulation for fat metabolism (Fig. 15.2).

Three types of transport proteins have been identified: (a) a ~40 kDa peripheral, $FABP_{PM}$) located on the outer leaflet of the plasma membrane; (b) a family of ~63 kDa FATPs (mainly FATP 1, 4) that have at least six transmembrane domains; and (c) a glycosylated ~88 kDa fatty acid translocase (FAT/CD36) that has two transmembrane domains.

Research has attempted to measure the gene expression (messenger RNA), protein abundance, and functional significance of these proteins in response to a variety of physiologic stimuli that alter the uptake of FFA in skeletal muscle. Much of the pioneering research has been done in red and white rodent skeletal muscle where the investigators have tried to determine if there is a strong relationship between the expression and protein content of the putative transporters and actual FFA uptake (8,24). The giant sarcolemmal vesicle technique has been very useful to measure pure FFA transport in a controlled environment. The skeletal muscle vesicles are entirely right side out and contain ample $FABP_C$ to sequester incoming FFA during the uptake measurements. Direct measurements of FFA uptake have shown that all the FFAs that moved into the vesicle are bound to $FABP_C$. None of the incoming FFAs are metabolized in this preparation, such that FFA uptake can be measured without the confounding influence of ongoing metabolism. Measurements of the abundance of muscle membrane transporter protein can also be made on the vesicles to correlate with actual transport rates. It has been reported that mRNA abundance and protein content of the FFA transporters in the plasma membrane and FFA transport capacity were several fold higher in red oxidative rodent muscle (high capacity for fat metabolism) versus white glycolytic muscle (24). The transport of FFA also appeared to be a saturable process in sarcolemmal vesicles prepared from both red and white rat muscles. This correlated with earlier work in rat hind limb and human skeletal muscle exposed to high FFA availability (6,25).

There is an increase in FFA uptake and oxidation during dynamic exercise as both FFA and CHO metabolism increase to meet the demand for ATP. There is also a well-documented increase in the capacity to oxidize plasma FFA following aerobic training (5,6). Chronic electrical stimulation has been shown to increase the expression of FAT/CD36 mRNA and protein, vesicle fatty acid transport, and fatty acid oxidation in rodent red and white muscle. Exercise training in humans also increased total muscle $FABP_{PM}$ and FAT/CD36 protein contents (3,26,39) and the plasma membrane content of $FABP_{PM}$, but not the content of FAT/CD36. Several studies have also shown that protein modifying agents and inhibitors of the putative transport proteins markedly decreased the rate of FFA transport across membranes (23,27,28).

An exciting finding was the report that the FAT/CD36 protein was acutely translocated from an intracellular pool to the muscle membrane (28) during a single bout of muscle contractions, in a manner similar to that reported for the GLUT4 transporter. The increased FAT/CD36 content in the membrane correlated with increased fatty acid transport into vesicles prepared from the contracted muscle. More recently, it has also been shown that muscle contractions acutely increased the plasma membrane content of $FABP_{PM}$, FATP1, and FATP4 proteins in mouse skeletal muscle (29). Another recent study reported that the membrane content of FAT/CD36, $FABP_{PM}$, and FATP4, but not FATP1, correlated highly with the capacities for oxidative metabolism, FFA oxidation, and TG esterification in six different rat skeletal muscles (30). The authors then independently over-expressed each of the four transport proteins within a normal physiologic range, without affecting the total or plasma membrane content of the other three transport proteins. All transport proteins increased FFA transport, but FAT/CD36 and FATP4 were two times more effective than $FABP_{PM}$ and FATP1. Over expression of the transporters failed to increase TG esterification. Finally, all transporters increased the rates of FFA oxidation, but FAT/CD36 and $FABP_{PM}$ were three times more effective than FATP1 and FATP4. Collectively, these data strongly suggest that the ability to acutely and chronically translocate fat transport proteins to the muscle membrane is part of a complex and highly regulated system for promoting fat uptake during exercise.

Previous work reported that insulin can also translocate FAT/CD36 to the muscle membrane and that membrane FAT/CD36 content is greater in obese versus lean rats without an increase in total protein content (8). A very recent study reported that both insulin and muscle contraction increased plasma membrane FAT/CD36, $FABP_{PM}$, FATP1, and FATP4, but not FATP6 in mouse skeletal muscle (30). Only FAT/CD36 and FATP1 were stimulated in an additive manner by insulin and by muscle contraction. Palmitate transport was also stimulated independently and additively by insulin and muscle contraction. These data underscore the importance of measuring fatty acid transport protein abundance directly in the muscle plasma membrane and not simply in the whole muscle homogenate.

KEY POINT

The movement of fat into skeletal muscle is a highly regulated process that involves several transport proteins during exercise and responds to the acute and chronic increases in the need for fat as a fuel source.

At this point, the student may realize that the design and control systems in place to regulate the movement of fat into skeletal muscle are remarkably similar to the design and regulation of moving carbohydrate into muscle (Chapter 14). Transport proteins on the membrane facilitate the movement of fat and CHO into muscle and their abundance correlates with the need for the specific fuel and the ability of the muscle to oxidize the fuel. Situations that require more energy production in muscle, such as acute exercise, lead to rapid translocation (minutes) of more transport protein to the membrane and increased fuel transport into the muscle. In addition, a repeated stress such as daily exercise leads to chronic adaptations that increase the amount of transport protein on the membrane and the ability to transport fat and CHO into the muscle.

TEST YOURSELF

What is the evidence that transport proteins are important in moving both fat and CHO (Chapter 14) into skeletal muscle during exercise?

There has been little work to date identifying the factors that activate the translocation of fat transporter proteins to the membrane during exercise (31). It is expected that Ca^{2+} and the factors related to the energy status of the cell (e.g., free ADP, P_i, and AMP-activated protein kinase [AMPK] activity) would be involved because they are important in activating the pathways that metabolize CHO in the cytoplasm. However, the time course of the changes involved in upregulating FFA uptake and oxidation appears to be slower than the activation of glucose uptake, glycogen breakdown, and CHO metabolism during exercise. There has been a significant amount of research examining the importance of AMPK in activating both CHO and fat metabolism. AMPK appears to function as an energy sensor, being sensitive to decreases in muscle phosphocreatine content and increases in free AMP (32). Activation of AMPK with AMP analogues has been repeatedly demonstrated to correlate with activated CHO metabolism and increased fat oxidation in resting skeletal muscle, suggesting that AMPK may be the key energy sensor in skeletal muscle at rest. However, its role during exercise in the presence of powerful additional signals for stimulating metabolism, is less clear. Increases in Ca^{2+} and reductions in the energy state of the cell during the onset of exercise activate CHO metabolism rapidly at many sites of regulation that are independent of AMPK. These same signals appear to play a smaller role in activating fat metabolism (turns on slower than CHO metabolism) and it may be that AMPK plays a more powerful role in activating fat metabolism during the onset of exercise.

Binding and Transport of FFA in the Cytoplasm

Once inside the muscle cell, FFAs are bound to a cytoplasmic fatty acid-binding protein $FABP_C$, which functions as an intracellular chaperone in a manner similar to albumin in the plasma (33). The $FABP_C$ binds with high affinity to saturated and unsaturated FFA and appears responsible for transferring FFA to cytoplasmic (for storage as IMTG) and mitochondrial (for oxidation) sites for further processing. The content of $FABP_C$ is proportional to the oxidative capacity of the muscle fibers in rodent skeletal muscle, but similar in most human skeletal muscles. This is likely due to the reasonably high aerobic capacity of the two dominant fiber types in human skeletal muscles, the type I and IIa, and the low abundance of type IIb fibers. $FABP_C$ content is also sensitive to physiologic stimuli and increases following aerobic training and high fat diets (33).

The role that $FABP_C$ plays in the regulation of fat transport appears to be necessary, but permissive (33). Experiments with knock-out animals have shown that skeletal muscle $FABP_C$ can be decreased by ~67% without altering fat transport as measured in giant sarcolemmal vesicles. However, if $FABP_C$ is completely removed, fat transport is severely reduced. This argues that $FABP_C$ is in great excess in the cytoplasm and plays a permissive role in fat transport. Estimates suggest that only 2% of the total $FABP_C$ protein is bound to FFA at any point in time.

The $FABP_C$-FFA complex is "activated" by the addition of a CoA group through the action of the enzyme FACS most likely at several sites in the cell (Fig. 15.2). The resultant fatty acyl-CoA then appears to attach to an additional binding protein, the aptly named acyl-CoA-binding protein. This new complex is then the suitable substrate for either esterification into IMTG in the cytoplasm or transport into the mitochondria for oxidation.

Synthesis of Muscle Triacylglycerol

FFA that has been transported into the cell or was previously released from IMTG in the cell can be oxidized, used for other cell functions or esterified back to IMTG (re-esterified). The substrates to complete re-esterification include glycerol 3-phosphate and, ultimately, three moieties of fatty acyl-CoA. There are four reactions in the synthesis pathway with glycerol 3-phosphate acting as a backbone in the first step to accept one fatty acyl-CoA to produce acylglycerol-3-phosphate (7). Additional fatty acyl-CoA moieties are added at steps 2 and 4. The enzymes that add fatty acyl-CoA to the structure are acyltransferases and the process is referred to as acylation. The phosphatidic acid produced at step 2 is the substrate for the final acylation step, but also can be a substrate for phospholipid production in the cell. The enzymes involved in this pathway were originally thought to have no external regulators and simply controlled by substrate and product concentrations. However, recent evidence suggests that the enzymes at steps 1 and 4, glycerol-phosphate acyltransferase (GPAT) and diacylglycerol acyltransferase (DGAT), can be phosphorylated and are externally regulated (7). Insulin appears to play a role in activating these enzymes.

TEST YOURSELF

Design a study that would examine whether insulin activates GPAT and DGAT and leads to increased TG synthesis in skeletal muscle.

There has been interest in determining how much of the fat coming into the cell traffics directly to IMTG synthesis or oxidation at rest and during exercise and also how much cycling may occur between IMTG breakdown and re-esterification in skeletal muscle both at rest and during dynamic exercise. A recent study found that incoming FFAs were largely trafficked to IMTG before they entered the long-chain fatty acylcarnitine pools at rest (34), but little is known about these events during exercise. The existence of "TG-fatty acid cycling" has also been demonstrated in a variety of muscle preparations at rest. However, it appears that FFA re-esterification is minimized during exercise when there is net utilization of IMTG as an energy substrate, because a recent study using a dual tracer approach reported that FFA re-esterification was only ~7% of IMTG breakdown during moderate intensity exercise (35).

The Use of IMTG as a Substrate during Dynamic Exercise

There has been controversy regarding whether IMTG contributes a significant amount of energy during exercise situations where FFA oxidation provides a major portion of the energy. However, recent studies using several techniques for measuring IMTG have led to the general consensus that IMTG is an important substrate during prolonged moderate-intensity dynamic exercise (~50%–65% $\dot{V}O_{2max}$) in both men and women, and up to ~85% $\dot{V}O_{2max}$ in well-trained athletes (9,36).

Estimating IMTG Use during Dynamic Exercise

Four approaches have been used to study the use of IMTG in muscle (9). Two direct approaches use muscle sampled with a biopsy needle, followed either by extraction of the lipid from the sample and biochemically measuring TG, or histochemically staining of the sampled muscle for lipid (36). A third approach has been to estimate the whole body fat oxidation rate (from VO_2 and respiratory exchange ratio) and also measure the rate of disappearance of plasma FFA with a tracer. Assuming that skeletal muscle metabolism is dominating whole body metabolism during moderate exercise, an indirect estimation of IMTG use is the difference between whole body fat oxidation and that provided from the plasma. The fourth approach is indirect and noninvasive and uses [1]H-magnetic resonance spectroscopy (MRS) on the surface of muscle to distinguish between intramuscular and extramuscular TG (9).

Generally, the results using all four techniques have reported significant decreases in IMTG during exercise where fat oxidation is a primary source of energy (9,36). Some muscle biopsy studies have not been able to measure net decreases in IMTG during exercise because of two factors: (a) a significant variability between muscle biopsy samples in human skeletal muscle, although this is less in aerobically trained subjects; and (b) the high energy density of fat means that the IMTG used during 90 to 120 minutes of cycling at 50% to 65% $\dot{V}O_{2max}$ will not be large (~2–4 mmol kg dm [dry muscle weight] or only 10%–15% of the total TG store). However, a recent study employed three techniques for the estimation of IMTG use simultaneously (all but MRS) and reported that 3 hours of cycling at ~60% $\dot{V}O_{2max}$ in men produced consistent and significant decreases in IMTG with all techniques (36). It also seems apparent from these recent studies that adipose tissue contamination of the biochemical estimates of IMTG is either not present or minimal because the measured values are in the same range or lower than the estimated IMTG values reported using the ^{1}H-MRS technique. Therefore, in summary, there is general consensus that IMTG is a significant source of substrate during moderate intensity exercise in active and trained men and women. This may extend to heavy exercise (~85% $\dot{V}O_{2max}$) in aerobically trained individuals.

TEST YOURSELF

Why does aerobic exercise have to last a long time (2–3 hours) before we can measure significant decreases in muscle stores of TG?

Is Lipid Ingestion after Exercise Important?

There has been a new concern regarding postexercise lipid ingestion raised by a series of experiments examining the replenishment of IMTG following exercise. If IMTG is used during dynamic exercise sessions, then it will need to be replenished during the recovery period. A contemporary research question is whether beginning an exercise session with an IMTG store that is less than normal will actually limit the ability to perform exercise of moderate intensity? However, it seems logical that an inability to replenish the IMTG store over repeated dynamic exercise sessions could lead to such a situation, as has been documented for muscle glycogen. The few studies that have examined the replenishment of IMTG following prolonged dynamic exercise reported that high levels of fat intake (35%–57% of total energy intake) replenished IMTG stores more quickly than low levels of fat (10%–24%). The amount of ingested fat needed to produce complete IMTG repletion has been estimated to be ~2 g · kg body mass · day (37). However, the high fat intake may compromise the ability to restore muscle glycogen and impair dynamic exercise performance if the total energy intake is not high. Additional studies examining fat intake following exercise in the range of 20% to 30% of the total energy intake are needed to clarify this issue. When 2 days are available for recovery, a diet of 25% to 30% fat, 15% protein, and 55% to 60% CHO of the total energy intake may be optimal. However, if prolonged exercise occurs nearly every day, it has been recommended that the diet in the initial 6 to 8 hours postexercise should be high in CHO and low in fat to replace muscle and liver glycogen first. Following this time period, higher amounts of fat can then be added in the form of regular meals (37).

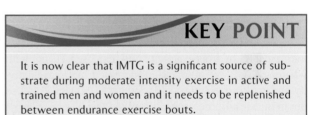

KEY POINT

It is now clear that IMTG is a significant source of substrate during moderate intensity exercise in active and trained men and women and it needs to be replenished between endurance exercise bouts.

Regulation of Muscle Lipolysis

A significant amount of fat is stored in human skeletal muscle, usually in the range of 20 to 40 mmol · kg dry muscle or enough energy to account for ~67% to 100% of the energy stored as glycogen in a well-fed person. Exercise training has generally reported that IMTG is elevated (9). In skeletal muscle as in adipose tissue, there are three reactions leading to the degradation of IMTG to 3 FFA and glycerol. The newly identified ATGL also exists in skeletal muscle (15,38) and is believed to initiate lipolysis by removing the first FFA from TG to produce DG. HSL then hydrolyzes DG to generate an additional FFA and MG, which is converted to FFA and glycerol by MG lipase in the final step of muscle lipolysis (Fig. 15.5).

The research examining the existence and regulatory role of ATGL in skeletal muscle and responses to acute and chronic exercise exposure is just beginning to appear.

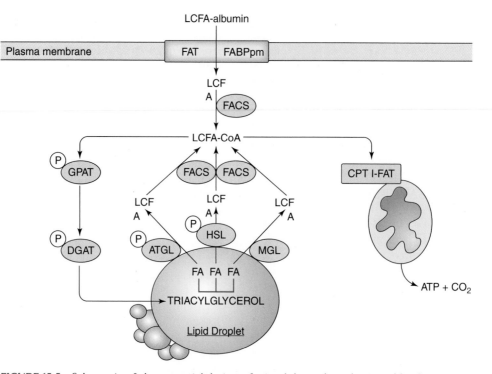

FIGURE 15.5 Schematic of the potential design of triacylglycerol synthesis and lipolysis in skeletal muscle. ATGL, adipose triglyceride lipase; CoA, coenzyme A; CPT I, carnitine palmitoyltransferase I; DGAT, diacylglycerol acyltransferase; FA, fatty acid; FABP$_{PM}$, plasma membrane fatty acid-binding protein; FACS, fatty acyl-CoA synthase; FAT, FATCD36 fatty acid translocase; GPAT, glycerol-phosphate acyltransferase; HSL, hormone-sensitive lipase; LCFA, long chain fatty acid; MGL, monoacylglycerol lipase.

However, ATGL does appear to be essential for muscle lipolysis; reducing the expression of ATGL in myotubes increased TG hydrolase activity and increased TG content, whereas ATGL over-expression increased hydrolase activity and reduced TG mass (19). When ATGL was knocked out in mouse adipose tissue, it resulted in a blunted plasma [FFA] and muscle ATGL content increased fourfold above control animals to compensate for the reduction in FFA delivery to the muscle (39). In addition, a recent study identified ATGL in human skeletal muscle and reported a twofold increase in ATGL content following 8 weeks of exercise training (38). However, the content of CGI-58, the activating protein of ATGL, was not changed following training. This preliminary work suggests that ATGL plays a similar role in skeletal muscle as in adipose tissue and is responsible for the degradation of TG to DG and FFA.

A skeletal muscle version of HSL has also been identified. It is activated by kinases that add a phosphate (PKA and extracellular signal regulated kinase [ERK]) and deactivated by phosphatases that remove a phosphate at the "activating" sites (11,40,41). There are also kinases that phosphorylate the enzyme at "inhibitory" sites (AMPK and calcium/calmodulin kinase II, CaMKII) and make phosphorylation at the "activating" PKA and ERK sites more difficult.

In human skeletal muscle at rest, there is a high constitutive level of HSL activity. The combination of low EPI and Ca^{2+} concentrations and resting levels of insulin appear to determine the levels of HSL activity measured at rest. During the initial minute of low and moderate intensity dynamic exercise, HSL is activated by a combination of EPI and contractions at moderate and intense exercise (40,41). The contraction-induced activation appears related to increased protein kinase C (PKC) and ERK activity by Ca^{2+} and/or other unknown activators and the activation by EPI through the cAMP cascade and increased PKA activity. With prolonged moderate intensity exercise beyond 1 to 2 hours and sustained heavy exercise, HSL activity decreased in spite of continuing increases in EPI, possibly due to increasing accumulations in free AMP, activation of AMPK, and phosphorylation of "inhibitory" sites on HSL (42). Taken together, the human muscle data suggest that intramuscular factors dominate the control of HSL activity with hormonal factors playing a smaller role.

The existing work in human skeletal muscle also supports the idea of numerous levels of regulation involved in the degradation of IMTG, with control points downstream from ATGL and HSL activation also being important. However, factors distal to these steps are also important in determining the actual rate of IMTG degradation. For example, HSL can be allosterically inhibited during prolonged exercise due to the accumulation of long-chain fatty acyl-CoA. It has been proposed that the actual movement to or association of ATGL and HSL with the lipid droplet in the cytosol must also occur for lipolysis to proceed. The existence of CGI-58, the activating protein of ATGL, is also known to be involved. Lastly, the phosphorylation of proteins that encapsulate the lipid droplet (*i.e.*, perilipin, adipose differentiation-related protein) may also be necessary to permit the physical "docking" of ATGL and HSL with the lipid droplet for muscle lipolysis to occur. In summary, our current understanding of the regulation of IMTG lipolysis is rudimentary at best, but also provides a fruitful area for future research.

FFA Transport across the Mitochondrial Membranes

It has long been known that the carnitine palmitoyltransferase (CPT) complex, consisting of CPT I, acylcarnitine translocase, and CPT II, plays an important regulatory role in the transport of long chain fatty acids into the mitochondria (10) for subsequent β-oxidation in skeletal muscle (Fig. 15.3). CPT I appears to span the outer mitochondrial membrane and catalyze the transfer of a variety of long chain fatty acyl groups from CoA to carnitine. The generated acylcarnitine then permeates the inner membrane, via the acylcarnitine/carnitine translocase in some unknown manner. The fatty acyl-CoA is then reformed in the matrix of the mitochondria by CPT II. This enzyme is located on the inner mitochondrial membrane and catalyzes the transfer of the acyl group from carnitine to CoA and the re-formed acyl-CoA enters the β-oxidation pathway.

Regulation of Mitochondrial FFA Transport by Malonyl-CoA?

CPT I has been considered the rate-limiting step in the oxidation of long chain fatty acids as it is regulated by external factors. It is reversibly inhibited by malonyl-CoA (M-CoA), the first committed intermediate in fatty acid synthesis (10,27). Thus, there has been considerable interest in the potential role of M-CoA in regulating mitochondrial FFA uptake and oxidation in skeletal muscle. Research in rodent skeletal muscle suggests that muscle M-CoA levels are highest at rest to inhibit CPT I activity and maintain low rates of mitochondrial fatty acid transport. During exercise, when increased mitochondrial FFA transport and oxidation are needed, M-CoA levels decrease and release the inhibition of CPT I (43).

Another line of research has proposed that fat metabolism is regulated by the level of glycolytic activity occurring in the muscle (44). Increases in glycolytic flux rates, as the aerobic exercise intensity increases, correlate with decreasing rates of FFA oxidation. It was proposed that signals related to the increased glycolytic flux down-regulate FFA metabolism inside the muscle cell and that increases in [M-CoA] could be the regulator that inhibits mitochondrial FFA uptake and oxidation during heavy dynamic exercise.

However, research has demonstrated that M-CoA levels do not change during low to moderate intensity exercise of varying durations in human skeletal muscle despite large increases in fatty acid oxidation rates (45). In addition, increasing the exercise intensity from 65% to 90% $\dot{V}_{O_{2max}}$ was not associated with an increase in muscle [M-CoA] despite large decreases in FFA oxidation. Therefore, the conclusion at the present time is that M-CoA is not involved in the upregulation of mitochondrial FFA transport from rest to low and moderate intensity exercise and also not responsible for down-regulating mitochondrial FFA transport when transitioning to intense exercise. This suggests some other potential "exercise" regulators may be involved in activating CPT I activity and fat oxidation at the onset of exercise.

Other Mechanisms that may Regulate Mitochondrial FFA Transport

These findings in human muscle suggest that the regulation of CPT I activity is more complex than simply control by [M-CoA]. Interestingly, several general regulators of metabolism, including Ca^{2+} and free ADP and AMP, were without effect on CPT I activity when studied in isolated, intact subsarcolemmal and intermyofibrillar mitochondria from rat and human skeletal muscle (4). Additional metabolites that accumulate (acetyl-CoA, acetylcarnitine) or decrease (CoA) during dynamic exercise were also without effect. However, CPT I activity was inhibited by small, physiologically relevant decreases in pH (7.0 to 6.8) (27). This sensitivity to pH may explain the decrease in mitochondrial FFA transport and metabolism that occurs when moving from moderate to heavy dynamic exercise. Collectively, this work suggested that other factors, including substrate-enzyme interactions, structural changes in the binding of M-CoA to CPT I, and/or the presence of additional, presently unknown regulators may be important for increased mitochondrial FFA transport during exercise.

One interesting and recent development has been the report that a CPT I isoform that is insensitive to M-CoA exists in rodent skeletal muscle (46). A recent study investigated the effects of exercise (120 minutes of cycling at ~60% $\dot{V}_{O_{2max}}$) on CPT I-M-CoA kinetics and found that although whole body fat oxidation rates progressively increased during exercise, M-CoA inhibition of CPT I was progressively attenuated (47). Compared to rest, 120 minutes of cycling reduced the inhibition of varying [M-CoA] by 16% to 34%. These data suggest that control system(s) independent of M-CoA account for the upregulation of mitochondrial FFA transport and oxidation during exercise.

It has also been proposed that the level of free carnitine may regulate mitochondrial FFA uptake during heavy dynamic exercise as it is a substrate for the CPT I reaction (4). The carnitine content decreases as a function of increasing dynamic exercise intensity and increased glycolytic flux. The decreasing free carnitine level may limit the ability to transport FFA into the mitochondria and ultimately limit

FFA oxidation during dynamic exercise when glycolytic flux is high (Fig. 15.3). However, no experimental model has been able to test whether this is a causal relationship. It is also not currently known how much free carnitine is needed in the cytoplasm to maintain the CPT I-mediated FFA transport into the mitochondria. However, the highest rates of FFA oxidation occur when the carnitine levels are already substantially lower than resting levels and carnitine is not consumed in the transport process, but recycled back into the cytoplasm. These factors make it unlikely that free carnitine availability limits FFA oxidation.

TEST YOURSELF

If you were able to alter the muscle (carnitine), what experiment would you do to test that hypothesis that the availability of free carnitine limits fat oxidation during exercise at 80% VO_{2max}?

The Role of Fat Transport Proteins in Mitochondrial FFA Transport

An exciting development over the past 5 years has been the demonstration of the presence of FAT/CD36 associated with the mitochondrial membranes of rodent and human skeletal muscle (47–49). Most of the work has been done with FAT/CD36, although $FABP_{PM}$ has been measured in mitochondria and work is continuing to determine if the FATP proteins are present. However, it is currently believed that $FABP_{PM}$ does not contribute to mitochondrial FA oxidation as a transport protein because $FABP_{PM}$ is identical in structure to malate-aspartate aminotransferase, a key enzyme in the shuttling of reducing equivalents across the mitochondrial membranes. This interpretation is supported by the observation that acute over-expression of $FABP_{PM}$ in rodent muscle increased mitochondrial $FABP_{PM}$ content and malate-aspartate aminotransferase activity proportionately without altering mitochondrial FA oxidation rates (50). The suggestion was the same in a second study where muscle malate-aspartate aminotransferase activity and $FABP_{PM}$ both increased in proportion to increases in mitochondrial content following an exercise training regimen (26).

FAT/CD36 represents a potential alternative level of regulation for mitochondrial FFA transport as gain of function (over-expression of FAT/CD36 in myotubes) and loss of function (FAT/CD36 null animals) experiments resulted in increased and decreased palmitate oxidation rates in isolated mitochondria, respectively (Fig. 15.3) (23,51). In addition, translocation of FAT/CD36 to mitochondrial membranes during acute muscle contraction coincides with increased FA oxidation rates (Fig. 15.2) (47,49,51).

It is important to note that both mitochondrial FAT/CD36 content and mitochondrial CPTI activity have been positively correlated with mitochondrial FA oxidation rates, and these two proteins immunoprecipitate together in both human and rodent skeletal muscle, suggesting a close physical relationship (23). Therefore, FAT/CD36 appears to be an important regulatory protein for movement of fat into the mitochondria, working in conjunction with CPTI in an unknown manner. In the bigger picture, FAT/CD36 may also represent a unique protein capable of coordinating plasma membrane fatty acid transport with mitochondrial membrane transport and ultimate oxidation to produce energy.

KEY POINT

The movement of LCFAs across the mitochondrial membranes is highly regulated in skeletal muscle and appears to involve several transport proteins.

TEST YOURSELF

Do you think that the presence and location of fat transport proteins may also be influenced by diet? What experiment would you do to see if eating a high-fat diet increased the content of FAT/CD36 in various locations in skeletal muscle?

β-oxidation

The fatty acylcarnitine moved into the matrix of the mitochondria is reconverted to fatty acyl-CoA via CPT II and the released carnitine is free to move back out of the mitochondria. The fatty acyl-CoA then passes through the β-oxidation pathway where a series of four reactions remove two carbons to form one molecule of acetyl-CoA with the production of reducing equivalents (one NADH and one $FADH_2$) along the way (7). The NADH and $FADH_2$ are immediate substrates for the ETC where they ultimately produce ~3 ATP/NADH and ~2 ATP/$FADH_2$. The remaining fatty acyl-CoA is now two carbon atoms shorter and repeatedly passes through the pathway until totally degraded. Therefore, an 18 carbon fatty acyl-CoA (i.e., stearic acid) provides 9 acetyl-CoA, 8 NADH, and 8 $FADH_2$ in the β-oxidation pathway. Because each acetyl-CoA also goes on to provide additional reducing equivalents (3 NADH, 1 $FADH_2$) and 1 GTP in the TCA cycle, the energy density of each fatty acyl-CoA molecule becomes very clear.

At the present time, there is little evidence that the enzymes in the β-oxidation pathway are regulated by the same signals (Ca^{2+}, free ADP and AMP, redox state, etc.) that regulate many other metabolic pathways. This suggests that the rate of β-oxidation is regulated by the availability of pathway substrates (fatty acyl-CoA, H_2O, NAD^+, FAD, and free CoA) and products (NADH, $FADH_2$, and acetyl-CoA) (7). It is likely that the provision of fatty acyl-CoA, NAD^+, and FAD are the dominant activators and that the products are not powerful inhibitors because NADH, $FADH_2$, and acetyl-CoA are quickly used in the ETC and TCA cycle, respectively. In addition, acetyl-CoA, which is a product of the pathway, actually increases during exercise and the flux in the β-oxidation pathway increases several fold. The reality of substrate control is that β-oxidation will proceed when fatty acyl-CoA is delivered to the mitochondrial matrix. It also moves the site of β-oxidation regulation and, ultimately, the last step in the regulation of fat oxidation upstream to the movement of fatty acyl-CoA across the mitochondrial membranes. There has been a recent suggestion that the enzymes in the β-oxidation pathway may be regulated by factors other than their substrates and products, but there currently is no direct evidence to support this (52).

The most effective way to change the control or increase the capacity of the β-oxidation pathway is to increase the mitochondrial content, as occurs with dynamic exercise training. It is common to measure the maximal activity of the third enzyme in the β-oxidation pathway, β-hydroxyacyl-CoA dehydrogenase, to assess the adaptation to dynamic exercise training programs. Other representative enzymes or proteins are measured to assess the changes in other mitochondrial pathways.

KEY POINT

The mitochondrial content of muscle and the movement of fat into the mitochondria play large roles in determining the rate of fat oxidation that will occur during exercise.

CHAPTER SUMMARY

Lipid is an important substrate for the aerobic production of energy in human skeletal muscle during low and moderate dynamic exercise in most individuals and even heavy exercise in well-trained individuals. FFA that is released from adipose tissue and delivered to contracting muscles is a major source of substrate for the muscle during dynamic exercise. Fat is also stored inside the muscle as TG and can be degraded to FFA during exercise to provide substrate for oxidation. Although CHO can provide all the substrate required for dynamic exercise at $\sim$100% $\dot{V}_{O_{2max}}$ when no fat is available, fat can only provide substrate at a rate to sustain $\sim$60% to 75% $\dot{V}_{O_{2max}}$ when the calculation assumes no CHO is available. However, fat is an energy dense fuel with a high yield per unit mass and is stored in large quantities in the body. Therefore, fat can provide a substantial and increasing amount of energy during prolonged exercise at low to moderate intensities. Aerobic training also increases the maximal rate that fat oxidation can produce energy in skeletal muscle by increasing the availability of fuel and upregulating several of the control steps in fat metabolism, including increasing mitochondrial volume. Training also increases the proportion of energy produced from fat oxidation at any absolute power output. It is also important to remember that fat metabolism is not activated as quickly as CHO metabolism at the onset of exercise and that it cannot be used to generate "anaerobic" energy during heavy exercise near and above 100% $\dot{V}_{O_{2max}}$ (sprint exercise).

For many years, the regulation of fat metabolism in human skeletal muscle during exercise was not well studied or understood. Traditionally, it was believed that the regulation of fat metabolism was mainly at the level of FFA provision to the muscle (adipose tissue lipolysis) and transport of long chain fatty acids into the mitochondria (CPT I activity). It is now known that the regulation of fat metabolism is far more complex and involves additional sites of control, including the transport of FFA into the muscle cell, the binding and transport of FFA in the cytoplasm, the regulation of muscle lipolysis activity within the cell, and the transport of fat into the mitochondria. The past 10 years have seen an exponential rise in research interest examining the regulation of fat metabolism in skeletal muscle. This work has led to several exciting findings, including the discovery of proteins that assist in transporting fat across the plasma and mitochondrial membranes, the ability of these proteins to translocate to these membranes when the need for fat transport increases acutely or chronically, and the discovery of the role of ATGL in regulating adipose tissue and muscle lipolysis.

A MILESTONE OF DISCOVERY

Havel and coworkers published a series of papers in the 1960s designed to examine the importance of plasma FFAs as a substrate source for skeletal muscle at rest and during dynamic exercise. Their findings also had large implications for the importance of fat stored inside the muscle as a substrate for exercise. It was already quite clear at the time of this publication that plasma FFA accounted for a significant portion of the oxidative metabolism both at rest and during low- to moderate-intensity dynamic exercise. This study took a more direct approach to assessing substrate use during leg exercise in four active men. The subjects reported to the laboratory following a 13- to 15-hour overnight fast and catheters were placed in the brachial artery of one arm and the brachial vein of the other arm. A catheter was also placed in the femoral vein to sample the blood draining the contracting muscles of the leg. A constant infusion of ^{14}C-palmitate allowed for the estimation of FFA uptake, oxidation, and release from the leg region during dynamic exercise. Expired air was sampled to measure the content of $^{14}CO_2$ and for the estimation of pulmonary O_2 uptake. Arterial and femoral venous blood samples were analyzed for O_2 and CO_2 content using the classic Van Slyke method. Subjects then exercised for 90 to 120 minutes at low dynamic exercise intensities. The increase in O_2 uptake measured at the mouth from rest to exercise was assumed to originate entirely from the region drained by the femoral vein. Leg blood flow was then estimated using the Fick equation: leg blood flow = increase in pulmonary O_2 uptake/arterial-femoral venous O_2 difference.

The fraction of FFA extracted by the leg decreased during exercise, but the influx of FFA into the leg increased. A net uptake of FFA by the leg was constantly observed during dynamic exercise. The output of ^{14}C in the blood CO_2 almost equaled the FFA input from the plasma following 1 hour of exercise. The pulmonary respiratory exchange ratio was 0.81 ± 0.03 and the leg respiratory quotient averaged 0.80 ± 0.11 during the exercise, suggesting that fat provided ~60% to 65% of the total oxidized substrate. The authors suggested that the large standard deviation for leg respiratory quotient was a function of the dependence on four measurements and underscored the problems that researchers still face today when making these same measurements. Plasma FFA accounted for ~50% and plasma TG less than 8% of the FFA oxidized during dynamic exercise. This provided strong evidence that other fat sources accounted for the remainder of the oxidized FFA. It led the authors to suggest that, "either local stores of triglyceride in fat cells which deliver fatty acids directly to muscle without traversing the general circulation, or lipids within muscle cells (*i.e.*, IMTG) are utilized for oxidative metabolism of working skeletal muscle." Subsequent research in the intervening years has supported the latter contention that IMTG is degraded and oxidized during low and moderate intensity dynamic exercise. This study presented the strongest data at the time to demonstrate that FFA, derived from both outside and inside the muscle cell, could be oxidized during dynamic exercise, as had been previously shown for carbohydrate. It was also interesting to note that the subjects were overnight fasted in this study and began exercise with high resting FFA concentrations of ~0.6 mM, which would bias metabolism toward using more fat and less carbohydrate. Therefore, the results must be examined in this light and, as a result, controversy continues as to whether subjects for metabolic research should be studied in a fed or fasted state.

Havel RJ, Pernow B, Jones NL. Uptake and release of free fatty acids and other metabolites in the legs of exercising men. J Appl Physiol. 1967;23(2):90–99.

REFERENCES

1. Asmussen E. Muscle metabolism during exercise in man. A historical survey. In: *Muscle Metabolism During Exercise.* New York: Plenum Press; 1971:1–11.
2. Havel RJ, Pernow B, Jones NL. Uptake and release of free fatty acids and other metabolites in the legs of exercising men. *J Appl Physiol.* 1967;23:90–99.
3. Perry CGR, Heigenhauser GJF, Bonen A, et al. High-intensity aerobic interval training increases fat and carbohydrate metabolic capacities in human skeletal muscle. *Appl Physiol Nutr Metab.* 2008;33:1112–1123.
4. VanLoon LJ, Greenhaff PL, Constantin-Teodosiu D, et al. The effects of increasing exercise intensity on muscle fuel utilization in humans. *J Physiol.* 2001;536:295–304.
5. Kiens B, Essen-Gustavsson B, Christensen NJ, et al. Skeletal muscle substrate utilization during submaximal exercise in man: effect of endurance training. *J Physiol.* 1993;469:459–478.
6. Turcotte L, Richter EA, Kiens B. Increased plasma FFA uptake and oxidation during prolonged exercise in trained vs. untrained humans. *Am J Physiol.* 1992;262:E791–E799.
7. VanderVusse GJ, Reneman RS. Lipid metabolism in muscle. In: Rowell LB, Shepherd JT, eds. *Handbook of Physiology, Section 12, Exercise: Regulation and Integration of Multiple Systems.* New York: Oxford University Press; 1996:952–994.
8. Bonen A, Chabowski A, Luiken JJ, et al. Is membrane transport of FFA mediated by lipid, protein, or both? Mechanisms and regulation of protein-mediated cellular fatty acid uptake: molecular, biochemical, and physiological evidence. *Physiologist.* 2007;22:15–29.
9. Watt MJ, Heigenhauser GJF, Spriet LL. Intramuscular triacylglycerol utilization in human skeletal muscle during exercise: is there a controversy? *J Appl Physiol.* 2002;93:1185–1195.
10. McGarry JD, Brown NF. The mitochondrial carnitine palmitoyltransferase system: from concept to molecular analysis. *Eur J Biochem.* 1997;224:1–14.
11. Holm C, Osterlund T, Laurell H, et al. Molecular mechanisms regulating hormone-sensitive lipase and lipolysis. *Ann Rev Nutr.* 2000;20:365–393.
12. Watt M, Spriet LL. Triacylglycerol lipases and metabolic control: implications for health and disease. *Am J Physiol.* 2010; 299:E162–E168.
13. Jenkins CM, Mancuso DJ, Yan W, et al. Identification, cloning, expression, and purification of three novel human calcium-independent phospholipase A2 family members possessing triacylglycerol lipase and acylglycerol transacylase activities. *J Biol Chem.* 2004;279:48968–48975.
14. Villena JA, Roy S, Sarkadi-Nagy E, et al. Desnutrin, an adipocyte gene encoding a novel patatin domain-containing protein, is induced by fasting and glucocorticoids: ectopic expression of desnutrin increases triglyceride hydrolysis. *J Biol Chem.* 2004,279:47066–47075.
15. Zimmermann R, Strauss JG, Haemmerle G, et al. Fat mobilization in adipose tissue is promoted by adipose triglyceride lipase. *Science.* 2004;306:1383–1386.
16. Ahmadian M, Duncan RE, Varady KA, et al. Adipose overexpression of desnutrin promotes fatty acid use and attenuates diet-induced obesity. *Diabetes.* 2009;58:855–866.
17. Haemmerle G, Lass A, Zimmermann R, et al. Defective lipolysis and altered energy metabolism in mice lacking adipose triglyceride lipase. *Science.* 2006;312:734–737.
18. Mottagui-Tabar S, Ryden M, Lofgren P, et al. Evidence for an important role of perilipin in the regulation of human adipocyte lipolysis. *Diabetologia.* 2003;46:789–797.
19. Watt MJ, van Denderen BJ, Castelli LA, et al. Adipose triglyceride lipase regulation of skeletal muscle lipid metabolism and insulin responsiveness. *Mol Endocrinol.* 2008;22:1200–1212.

20. Carey, G. Mechanisms regulating adipocyte lipolysis. In: *Skeletal Muscle Metabolism in Exercise and Diabetes*. Plenum Press: New York: Plenum Press; 1998:157–170.

21. Romijn JA, Coyle EF, Sidossis LS, et al. Regulation of endogenous fat and carbohydrate metabolism in relation to exercise intensity and duration. *Am J Physiol*. 1993;265:E380–E391.

22. Romijn JA, Coyle EF, Sidossis LS, et al. Relationship between fatty acid delivery and fatty acid oxidation during strenuous exercise. *J Appl Physiol*. 1995;79:1939–1945.

23. Holloway GP, Luiken JJ, Glatz JF, et al. Contribution of FAT/CD36 to the regulation of skeletal muscle fatty acid oxidation: an overview. *Acta Physiol*. 2008;194:293–309.

24. Bonen, A, Luiken JJ, Liu S, et al. Palmitate transport and fatty acid transporters in red and white muscles. *Am J Physiol*. 1998;275:E471–E478.

25. Turcotte L, Kiens B, Richter EA. Saturation kinetics of palmitate uptake in perfused skeletal muscle. *FEBS Lett*. 1991;279:327–329.

26. Talanian, JL, Holloway GP, Snook LA, et al. Exercise training increases sarcolemmal and mitochondrial fatty acid transport proteins in human skeletal muscle. *Am J Physiol*. 2010;299: E180–E188.

27. Bezaire V, Heigenhauser GJF, Spriet LL. Regulation of CPT I activity in intermyofibrillar and subsarcolemmal mitochondria from human and rat skeletal muscle. *Am J Physiol*. 2004;286:E85–E91.

28. Bonen A, Luiken JJ, Arumugam T, et al. Acute regulation of fatty acid uptake involves the cellular redistribution of fatty acid translocase. *J Biol Chem*. 2000;275:14501–14508.

29. Jain SS, Chabowski A, Snook LA, et al. Additive effects of insulin and muscle contraction on fatty acid transport and fatty acid transporters, FAT/CD36, FABPpm, FATP1, 4, and 6. *FEBS Lett*. 2009;583:2294–2300.

30. Nickerson JG, Alkhateeb H, Benton CR, et al. Greater transport efficiencies of the membrane fatty acid transporters FAT/CD36 and FATP4 than FABPpm and FATP1, and differential effects on fatty acid esterification and oxidation in rat skeletal muscle. *J Biol Chem*. 2009;284:16522–16530.

31. Nickerson JG, Momken I, Benton CR, et al. Protein-mediated fatty acid uptake: regulation by contraction, AMP-activated protein kinase, and endocrine signals. *Appl Physiol Nutr Metab*. 2007;32:865–873.

32. Winder WW. Energy-sensing and signaling by AMP-activated protein kinase in skeletal muscle. *J Appl Physiol*. 2001;91:1017–1028.

33. Glatz JFC, Schapp FG, Binas B, et al. Cytoplasmic fatty acid-binding protein facilitates fatty acid utilization by skeletal muscle. *Acta Physiol Scand*. 2003;178:367–372.

34. Kanaley JA, Shadid S, Sheehan MT, et al. Relationship between plasma free fatty acid, intramyocellular triglycerides and long-chain acylcarnitines in resting humans. *J Physiol*. 2009;587:5939–5950.

35. Guo Z, Burguera B, Jensen MD, et al. Kinetics of intramuscular triglyceride fatty acids in exercising humans. *J Appl Physiol*. 2000;89:2057–2064.

36. Stellingwerff, T, Boon H, Jonkers RS, et al. Significant intramyocellular lipid use during prolonged cycling in endurance-trained males as assessed by three different methodologies. *Am J Physiol*. 2007;292:E1715–E1723.

37. Decombaz, J. Nutrition and recovery of muscle energy stores after exercise. *Sportmedizin und Sporttraumatologie*. 2003;51:31–38.

38. Alsted TJ, Nybo L, Schweiger M, et al. Adipose triglyceride lipase in human skeletal muscle is upregulated by exercise training. *Am J Physiol Endocrinol Metab*. 2009;296:E445–E453.

39. Huijsman E, van de Par C, Economou C, et al. Adipose triacylglycerol lipase deletion alters whole body energy metabolism and impairs exercise performance in mice. *Am J Physiol*. 2009;297:E505–E513.

40. Talanian, JL, Tunstall RJ, Watt MJ, et al. Beta-adrenergic regulation of human skeletal muscle hormone sensitive lipase activity during exercise onset. *Am J Physiol*. 2006;291:R1094–R1099.

41. Watt MJ, Heigenhauser GJF, Spriet LL. Effects of dynamic exercise intensity on the activation of hormone-sensitive lipase in human skeletal muscle. *J Physiol*. 2003;547:301–308.

42. Watt, MJ, Heigenhauser GJF, O'Neill M, et al. Hormone-sensitive lipase activity and fatty acyl-CoA content in human skeletal muscle during prolonged exercise. *J Appl Physiol*. 2003;95:314–321.

43. Winder WW, Arogyasami J, Barton RJ, et al. Muscle malonyl-CoA decreases during exercise. *J Appl Physiol*. 1989;67:2230–2233.

44. Coyle EF, Jeukendrup AE, Wagenmakers AJM, et al. Fatty acid oxidation is directly regulated by carbohydrate metabolism during exercise. *Am J Physiol*. 1997;273:E268–E275.

45. Odland LM, Howlett RA, Heigenhauser GJF, et al. Skeletal muscle malonyl-CoA content at the onset of exercise at varying power outputs in humans. *Am J Physiol*. 1998;274:E1080–E1085.

46. Kim JY, Koves TR, Yu GS, et al. Evidence of a malonyl-CoA-insensitive carnitine palmitoyltransferase I activity in red skeletal muscle. *Am J Physiol*. 2002;282:E1014–E1022.

47. Holloway GP, Bezaire V, Heigenhauser GJ, et al. Mitochondrial long chain fatty acid oxidation, fatty acid translocase/CD36 content and carnitine palmitoyltransferase I activity in human skeletal muscle during aerobic exercise. *J Physiol*. 2006;571:201–210.

48. Bezaire V, Bruce CR, Heigenhauser GJ, et al. Identification of fatty acid translocase on human skeletal muscle mitochondrial membranes: essential role in fatty acid oxidation. *Am J Physiol*. 2006;290:E509–E515.

49. Campbell S, Tandon N, Woldegiorgis G, et al. A novel function for fatty acid translocase (FAT)/CD36: involvement in long chain fatty acid transfer into the mitochondria. *J Biol Chem*. 2004;279:36235–36241.

50. Holloway GP, Lally J, Nickerson JG, et al. Fatty acid binding protein facilitates sarcolemmal fatty acid transport but not mitochondrial oxidation in rat and human skeletal muscle. *J Physiol*. 2007;582:393–405.

51. Holloway GP, Jain SS, Bezaire V, et al. FAT/CD36-null mice reveal that mitochondrial FAT/CD36 is required to upregulate mitochondrial fatty acid oxidation in contracting muscle. *Am J Physiol*. 2009;297:R960–R967.

52. Sahlin K. Control of lipid oxidation at the mitochondrial level. *Appl Physiol Nutr Metab*. 2009;34:382–388.

CHAPTER 16

The Metabolic Systems: Interaction of Lipid and Carbohydrate Metabolism

Graham P. Holloway and Lawrence L. Spriet

Abbreviations

ACC	Acetyl-CoA carboxylase	HK	Hexokinase
ADP	Adenosine diphosphate	HSL	Hormone-sensitive lipase
AMP	Adenosine monophosphate	P_i	Inorganic phosphate
AMPK	AMP kinase	IMTG	Intramuscular triacylglycerol
ATGL	Adipose triacylglycerol lipase	M-CoA	Malonyl-CoA
ATP	Adenosine triphosphate	NADH	Nicotinamide adenine dinucleotide
Ca^{2+}	Calcium	PFK	Phosphofructokinase
CHO	Carbohydrate	PHOS	Phosphorylase
CPTI	Carnitine palmitoyltransferase I	PDH	Pyruvate dehydrogenase
CoA	Coenzyme A	PDHa	Pyruvate dehydrogenase in active form
FAT/CD36	Fatty acid translocase	PDK	Pyruvate dehydrogenase kinase
FATP 1	Fatty acid transport protein 1	RG	Red gastrocnemius
FFA	Free fatty acid	RER	Respiratory exchange ratio
G-6-P	Glucose-6-phosphate	SOL	Soleus
G-FA	Glucose-fatty acid	TG	Triacylglycerol
GLUT	Glucose transporter		

Introduction

The previous chapters outlined the regulation of lipid and carbohydrate (CHO) metabolism and established that both are important substrates for oxidative phosphorylation. The oxidation of any one fuel at rest or during dynamic exercise rarely occurs in isolation and skeletal muscle, like other systems in the body, is an integrative organ and many aspects of metabolism are simultaneously active at any point in time. It has long been known that both CHO and lipid are oxidized at rest to provide the energy required for basal metabolic processes in skeletal muscle and that there is a reciprocal relationship between the utilization of CHO and lipid. At rest, these shifts in fuel use typically occur despite largely unchanged metabolic demand and are heavily influenced by the availability of each substrate. For example, increasing the availability of

CHO in the blood increases the uptake and oxidation of CHO while concomitantly decreasing the availability and oxidation of fat in skeletal muscle, with little change in metabolic rate.

The situation during the onset of exercise is quite different than rest because the metabolic rate increases several fold over the resting rate. Therefore, the need for energy also increases several fold and the metabolic pathways that oxidize both fat and CHO must be activated simultaneously. Once dynamic exercise of a given intensity and metabolic demand has been established (steady state), there is some room for reciprocal shifts in the proportion of CHO and fat that are oxidized. The reciprocal nature and interaction between CHO and fatty acid oxidation is largely dependent on the intracellular metabolic environment and substrate availability, both of which are influenced by exercise intensity and the overall rate at which energy is required.

This chapter attempts to answer the question of how skeletal muscle is able to regulate the proportion of fuel that is derived from CHO and fat. The focus is on information obtained in human skeletal muscle, but findings from other mammalian skeletal muscle models are cited where human information is lacking. Although descriptive studies documenting changes in the proportion of fat and CHO utilization are numerous, the mechanisms regulating these shifts in fuel use have not been thoroughly elucidated. We first discuss the classical studies that attempted to independently alter fuel availability and, subsequently, consider alterations in the intracellular environment. Importantly, these mechanisms are not mutually exclusive and it is impossible to independently alter fuel availability without changing the intracellular metabolites that regulate cytosolic enzymes. Nevertheless, these approaches have yielded invaluable insight into the interaction of CHO and lipid metabolism at rest and during exercise.

Classic Carbohydrate-Fatty Acid Interaction Studies

Fuel Selection in Cardiac and Diaphragm Muscles

The pioneering work by Randle, Garland, and Newsholme in the early 1960s introduced the concept of a reciprocal relationship between fat and CHO oxidation in muscle (1,2). They termed this relationship the glucose-fatty acid (G-FA) cycle and used it to explain the interaction between CHO and lipid metabolism in disease states (see the Milestone in Discovery at the end of this chapter). Their early experiments examined the regulation of fuel interaction in muscle using perfused, contracting heart muscle and incubated, resting diaphragm muscle from rodents. These seminal experiments characterized the effects of altering fuel availability and the reciprocal nature of CHO and lipid metabolism, while also providing evidence that the intracellular environment participates in this fuel selection interaction. These experiments showed that by increasing the availability of lipids, muscles increased fat oxidation and reduced CHO oxidation.

> ### KEY POINT
>
> Increasing the availability of fat shifts fuel preference to favor fatty acid oxidation while simultaneously decreasing CHO oxidation.

This shift in fuel preference occurs concurrently with increased contents of muscle acetyl-coenzyme A (CoA), citrate, and glucose-6-phosphate (G-6-P) (Fig. 16.1). Previous in vitro or "test tube" work had established

that acetyl-CoA inhibited the activity of the mitochondrial enzyme pyruvate dehydrogenase (PDH), by activating PDH kinase (PDK), the enzyme that phosphorylates PDH to its less active form. Therefore a rise in acetyl-CoA decreases PDH activity and pyruvate oxidation, shifting fuel reliance to fatty acids. Additional in vitro work identified citrate as a potent inhibitor of the cytoplasmic enzyme phosphofructokinase (PFK), predicting an in vivo or "intact muscle" effect. However, the notion that citrate is a primary regulator of the G-FA cycle assumes that the free fatty acid (FFA)-induced increase in mitochondrial citrate can "escape" to the cytoplasm to inhibit PFK. Lastly, G-6-P had also been shown to inhibit hexokinase (HK) in vitro. By combining the findings from their isolated muscle experiments with the in vitro enzyme studies, Randle et al. (1,2) established a mechanistic basis for their G-FA cycle, which explained the reciprocal relationship between fat and CHO oxidation.

Summary of glucose-fatty acid cycle

The G-FA cycle suggests that an increased FFA availability results in an accumulation of muscle acetyl-CoA and citrate leading to a down-regulation (or inhibition) of the activities of two key glycolytic enzymes, PDH and PFK. The inhibition of these two rate-limiting enzymes will reduce flux through the glycolytic pathway, causing an accumulation of G-6-P (essentially the starting point of glycolysis). The accumulation of G-6-P will inhibit HK activity (HK phosphorylates glucose to G-6-P and G-6-P and has been shown to inhibit HK activity in the test tube, as discussed previously), and thus glucose phosphorylation and further production of G-6-P. The resulting accumulation of "free" glucose will dissipate the concentration gradient of glucose across the plasma membrane, and therefore glucose uptake by skeletal muscle will be reduced (Fig. 16.1). Although excess fatty acids increase the reliance on fatty acid oxidation, mechanistic insight into potential activation of processes involved in regulating fatty acid oxidation is virtually nonexistent, and instead our understanding relies exclusively on "clamping down" CHO oxidation and, by default, increasing our reliance on fatty acids. Although some of the mechanisms proposed in these seminal studies have been challenged, the fundamental tenet that fatty acid and CHO oxidation display a reciprocal relationship during steady-state conditions (rest or exercise) has been accepted as a general truth.

> ### TEST YOURSELF
>
> What were the key mechanisms proposed by Randle and colleagues that regulate the reciprocal relationship between CHO and fat oxidation in contracting heart and resting diaphragm muscles?

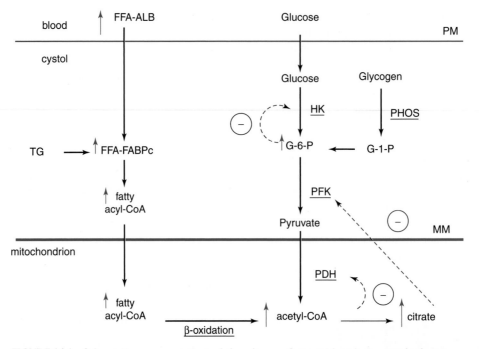

FIGURE 16.1   Schematic representation of the glucose-fatty acid cycle in muscle. Increasing availability of plasma free fatty acid (FFA) increases fat metabolism and ultimately fat oxidation. It also elevates mitochondrial contents of acetyl-CoA and citrate, which feedback to inhibit (−) pyruvate dehydrogenase (PDH) and phosphofructokinase (PFK) activities. Decreased glycolytic activity then leads to increased glucose-6-phosphate content and inhibition (−) of hexokinase (HK) activity, decreased glucose phosphorylation, and ultimately decreased glucose uptake. ALB, albumin; FABP, fatty acid-binding protein; G-1-P, glucose-1-phosphate; MM, mitochondrial membranes; PHOS, glycogen phosphorylase; PM, plasma membrane.

Fuel Selection in Resting and Contracting Skeletal Muscles

As mentioned, most of the early support for the G-FA cycle was obtained from contracting heart or resting diaphragm muscle from rodents while bathed in, or perfused with, a medium that contained either no FFA or conversely very high FFA concentrations. The chronic low metabolic demands placed on these tissues (heart and diaphragm) are very different from the large variations seen in skeletal muscle. In addition, the continuous rhythmical contractions, or duty cycle, of the heart and diaphragm muscles dictate that the majority of the oxidizable substrate used to produce energy by these muscles must be delivered from outside the cell (CHO from the liver and FFA from adipose tissue). In contrast, most human skeletal muscles contain two primary sources for CHO and lipid supply: the circulation (glucose and FFA) and fuel stored within the muscle (glycogen and intramuscular triacylglycerol [IMTG]). Therefore, the mechanisms elucidated by Randle and colleagues in heart and diaphragm muscles may not be directly transferable to peripheral skeletal muscles, especially considering that during moderate and high-intensity aerobic exercise the majority of oxidizable fuel originates from fuel stores inside the cells, not the circulation.

KEY POINT

The original G-FA cycle proposed mechanisms to account for fuel interactions in diaphragm and cardiac muscles, which may be different in peripheral skeletal muscles given the greater reliance on fuels from inside the cell that exists during prolonged exercise.

Holloszy and colleagues (3,4) advanced our understanding of fuel selection (CHO and fatty acid interactions) by examining the existence and regulation of the G-FA cycle in skeletal muscle of exercising rats. Animals were fed corn oil followed by infusions of heparin (which releases lipoprotein lipase from the endothelium to dramatically increase FFA) to increase preexercise FFA fivefold (3). This increase in circulating FFAs resulted in longer run times to exhaustion, decreased the contribution of both sources of CHO—most notably less glycogen utilization in skeletal muscle (soleus [SOL], red vastus lateralis, and red gastrocnemius [RG]) and the liver—and less glucose uptake by active muscles. Similar to Randle's observation in cardiac and diaphragm muscles, citrate content was elevated during exercise in the skeletal muscles exposed to high FFA concentrations, providing a potential mechanism to decrease CHO utilization. Rennie and Holloszy (5) also perfused rat hind limbs with either 1.8 mM oleate or control conditions with no fat. These highly controlled experiments once again showed that high FFA minimized CHO oxidation, as evidenced by decreased (a) hind limb glucose uptake, (b) glycogen utilization (33%–50%), (c) lactate release, and (d) lactate accumulation (~50%) during 10 minutes of electrical stimulation in the SOL and RG muscles. The reduction in muscle CHO use coincided with elevations in G-6-P and citrate contents in SOL and RG muscles. These results suggested that the G-FA cycle did operate in contracting red skeletal muscle and that the "citrate" arm of the cycle functioned as originally proposed for contracting heart and resting diaphragm muscles, whereas the role of PDH in regulating CHO and fatty acid interaction during exercise was not studied. However, a number of other studies utilizing similar methodologies (perfusion and electrical stimulation at various intensities) across a wide range of hind limb oxygen uptakes and glycogenolytic rates have not been able to demonstrate the existence of the G-FA cycle in contracting rodent skeletal muscle (6,7), creating some controversy.

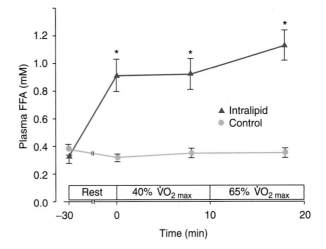

FIGURE 16.2   Plasma FFA during 10 minutes of cycling at 40% and 10 minutes at 65% $\dot{V}O_{2max}$ with intralipid (and heparin) infusion or control. Values are mean ± SE. *Significant main effect between trials. (Reproduced with permission from Holloway GP, Jain SS, Bezaire VS, et al. FAT/CD36 null mice reveal that mitochondrial FAT/CD36 is required to up-regulate mitochondrial fatty acid oxidation in contracting muscle. *Am J Physiol Regul Integr Comp Physiol.* 2009;297:R960–R967.)

Increased Lipid Availability during Dynamic Exercise in Humans

Research in human skeletal muscle has consistently supported the notion of a reciprocal relationship between CHO and fatty acid oxidation, however, not always via the original mechanisms proposed by Randle and colleagues, defined as the G-FA cycle. Most of what we know regarding the ability of fat to down-regulate CHO metabolism has been derived from studies that used experimental manipulations to increase or decrease the plasma FFA availability, without affecting many other processes. Although many models have been used with varying success—including high fat meals and diets, short- and long-term aerobic training, caffeine and nicotinic acid ingestion, fasting, and prolonged dynamic exercise—the acute infusion of a lipid solution coupled with periodic heparin administration has been most commonly and effectively used. This technique has the advantage of acutely (~30 minutes) increasing the plasma [FFA] without significant alterations in other substrates, metabolites, and hormones (8,9) (Fig. 16.2). In contrast, dietary attempts at acutely increasing the availability of endogenous FFA to the working muscles in humans immediately prior to or during exercise in an attempt to spare CHO have been largely unsuccessful. This is a response to fat not being digested quickly, and therefore prolonged alterations in the normal diet are required to alter the IMTG stores and spare CHO. As a result, these practices are not in use by athletes.

TEST YOURSELF

What approaches have scientists taken to study the G-FA cycle in skeletal muscle?

If a reciprocal relationship between CHO and fat oxidation does exist in skeletal muscle, it would be expected that any fat-induced down-regulation (inhibition) of CHO oxidation would target the key sites (transport, enzymatic reactions) regulating CHO metabolism and oxidation. In the muscle, these would include sarcolemmal glucose transporter (GLUT1, 4), glucose phosphorylation (HK), glycogenolysis (glycogen phosphorylase, PHOS), glycolysis (PFK), and conversion to acetyl-CoA (PDH). These enzymes (at least PHOS, PFK, and PDH) have been shown to be regulated through similar allosteric activators located in the cytosol, enabling the entire glycolytic pathway to be coordinated and regulated by a small number of metabolic regulators (Fig. 16.3). These metabolic regulators include, but are not limited to, calcium (Ca^{2+}), adenosine diphosphate (ADP), adenosine monophosphate (AMP), and inorganic phosphate (P_i) and can activate the rate-limiting enzymes directly (allosterically) or indirectly through secondary phosphorylation events.

Effects of Increased Plasma FFA on Carbohydrate Metabolism in Human Skeletal Muscle

The experiments examining the interaction between fat and CHO in human skeletal muscle demonstrated that it

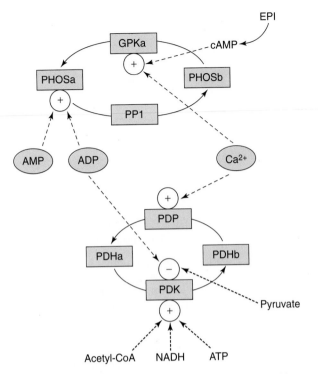

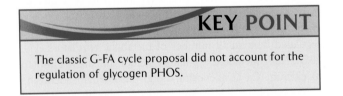

FIGURE 16.3 Schematic overview of the regulation of key enzymes in carbohydrate metabolism, glycogen phosphorylase (PHOS), and pyruvate dehydrogenase (PDH) a and b, active and less active form of enzymes. AMP, adenosine monophosphate; cAMP, cyclic AMP; EPI, epinephrine; GPK, glycogen phosphorylase kinase; PDK and PDP, pyruvate dehydrogenase kinase and phosphatase; PPi, glycogen pyrophosphatase.

is possible to alter the proportions of fat and CHO oxidation during exercise, but the mechanisms controlling these shifts are largely different from those originally proposed in the G-FA cycle. This is mainly the result of the original work by Randle et al. (1,2) not involving the regulation of muscle glycogen degradation. Contracting heart and resting diaphragm muscles are less dependent on muscle glycogen as a substrate than skeletal muscle.

KEY POINT

The classic G-FA cycle proposal did not account for the regulation of glycogen PHOS.

During exercise at ~80% $\dot{V}O_{2max}$ in moderately active individuals the majority of energy is derived from CHO use, and during the first 20 to 30 minutes particularly from muscle glycogen. The mechanisms proposed in the classic G-FA cycle can obviously not account for fuel shifts at this intensity of exercise because the original work only considered extracellular fuel sources. However, exercising at this high level of intensity in the presence of artificially raised

FFA levels has been shown to decrease net glycogen use by ~50% in the initial 15 minutes of exercise and increase fat oxidation by ~15% during 30 minutes of exercise (9,10), suggesting mechanisms beyond those originally proposed by Randle and colleagues (2). Insight into the allosteric regulation of the rate-limiting enzymes in CHO oxidation has revealed important roles for increased levels of free ADP, free AMP, and Ca^{2+} in this context. Importantly, the muscle contents of free ADP and free AMP, activators of glycogen PHOS, were significantly reduced (did not increase as much) in the high FFA and exercise conditions discussed previously and appeared to explain the decreased glycogen use. There were no effects on muscle citrate, acetyl-CoA, and G-6-P contents or the proportion of PDH in the active form (PDHa) (8,10), and whole body glucose disappearance (glucose uptake) was also unaffected by elevated FFA at this intensity (9). Therefore, at this intense aerobic power output, the fat-induced down-regulation of CHO oxidation was regulated at the level of glycogen PHOS. Because the diaphragm and cardiac muscles rely almost exclusively on exogenous substrates, the original G-FA cycle proposed by Randle and colleagues did not consider PHOS activity, and instead focused on enzymes distal to G-6-P, namely PFK and PDH.

TEST YOURSELF

Why would the controlling mechanisms in human skeletal muscle be different from the results with rodent diaphragm and heart muscle?

When these same experiments were repeated at lower exercise power outputs (~40% and 65% $\dot{V}O_{2max}$), as well as during dynamic knee extension, high fat provision again down-regulated (or inhibited) CHO oxidation, suggesting this fuel interaction is not dependent on intensity of exercise. Although the mechanism(s) of action responsible for the shift in fuel utilization again involved PHOS activity at lower power outputs, the small increase in citrate and the lower PDHa levels suggest the mechanisms also involve PFK and PDH activities (11). Although the rise in citrate supports one of Randle's original hypotheses, test tube studies examining the inhibitory effects of citrate on PFK activity suggest that the small increase in citrate in the high fat trials would have minimal effect in contracting human skeletal muscle and likely is not a mechanism to shift fuel preference (12). A recent study taking the opposite approach, decreasing the availability of plasma FFA while exercising at ~60% $\dot{V}O_{2max}$ by ingesting nicotinic acid, reported an increased respiratory exchange ratio (RER), glycogen use, and PDHa (13). However, there was no effect on metabolic byproducts typically associated with the G-FA cycle, namely muscle citrate, acetyl-CoA, or pyruvate contents.

Summary

These experiments clearly demonstrated that altering substrate availability changed the intracellular environment in human skeletal muscle, creating a reciprocal relationship between CHO and lipid oxidation. However, although these shifts in fuel selection involve changes in the activation of PHOS, PFK, and PDH, the exact signals that cause these are not clearly defined. Potential mediators of these enzymes and a theory are discussed later.

Potential Intracellular Signals that Regulate Fuel Preference during Dynamic Exercise

Interestingly, the previously discussed studies characterizing fuel interactions by increasing the availability of exogenous FFA also reported that the increase in free ADP, AMP, and P_i levels of the muscle that normally occurs during dynamic exercise was attenuated. This was assessed by measuring muscle phosphocreatine, creatine, adenosine triphosphate (ATP), and lactate (to predict [hydrogen ion]) and calculating muscle free ADP, AMP, and P_i contents. Because P_i is a substrate for PHOS, and free ADP and AMP are direct allosteric regulators (activators) of the active form of PHOS, the noted reductions in these regulators could account for the decreased glycogenolysis with high fat provision (8,14) (Figs. 16.3 and 16.4). Less free ADP accumulation would also make it more difficult for PDH to convert to the active form during exercise at 40% and 65% $\dot{V}O_{2max}$, as a high ATP/ADP ratio activates PDK activity and decreases (or inhibits) PDHa (Figs. 16.3 and 16.4). A similar situation arises during steady-state exercise following aerobic training, where an increase in mitochondrial content has been shown to attenuate rises in free ADP, decreasing the activation of CHO oxidation and increasing the reliance on fatty acid oxidation. However, in the acute studies where substrate delivery was experimentally altered (*e.g.*, intralipid + heparin infusion) mitochondrial content was not altered, and, therefore, a key question that remains to be answered is why does the provision of exogenous fat provide an attenuated rise in free ADP, AMP, and P_i and a decreased reliance on CHO during exercise?

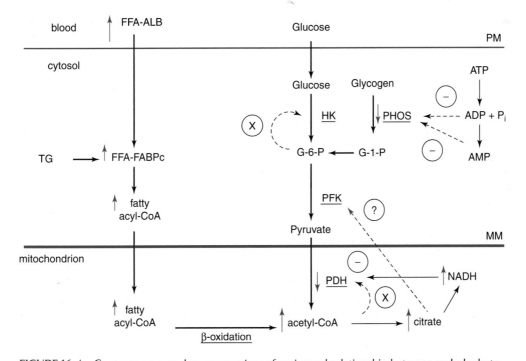

FIGURE 16.4 Contemporary and summary view of reciprocal relationship between carbohydrate and fat oxidation during exercise at power outputs of 40%, 65%, and ~80% $\dot{V}O_{2max}$. Increasing the availability of plasma free fatty acids (FFA) has no effect on acetyl-coenzyme A (CoA) and glucose-6-phosphate (G-6-P) contents (X) at any power outputs and increased citrate content only at 40% and 65% $\dot{V}O_{2max}$. Reduced FFA availability did reduce pyruvate dehydrogenase (PDH) activity at 40% and 65% $\dot{V}O_{2max}$ and the flux through glycogen phosphorylase (PHOS) at all power outputs. The effect on PHOS flux was dominant at ~80% $\dot{V}O_{2max}$ and less important at 40% and 65% $\dot{V}O_{2max}$ (see text). The accumulation of free adenosine diphosphate (ADP), adenosine monophosphate (AMP), and inorganic phosphate (P_i) was reduced during exercise (−) in the presence of increased FFA availability. One theory suggests that mitochondrial nicotinamide adenine dinucleotide (NADH) is more abundant with high fat provision during the onset of exercise, increasing the aerobic production of adenosine triphosphate (ATP) and reducing the mismatch between ATP demand and supply and accounting for the reduced accumulation of ADP, AMP, and P_i. ALB, albumin; FABP, fatty acid-binding protein; G-1-P, glucose-1-phosphate; HK, hexokinase; PFK, phosphofructokinase.

The major inputs for aerobic ATP production in the mitochondria are ADP and P_i, oxygen, and reduced nicotinamide adenine dinucleotide (NADH-reducing equivalents). An increase in NADH at a given energy demand (power output) may allow for the blunted accumulation of free ADP and P_i during exercise while maintaining a constant drive for mitochondrial respiration. The blunted rise in free ADP and Pi, in addition to high NADH levels, would be expected to decrease activation of both PHOS and PDH. As a result, it has been proposed that enhanced fat availability increases the provision of NADH from fat, resulting in a higher NADH concentration in the mitochondria (11,14), and hence, a decreased CHO oxidation in a classical reciprocal relationship. Unfortunately, it is difficult to test this theory because mitochondrial NADH is not easy to measure in intact human skeletal muscle, and much controversy surrounds the various techniques that have been employed. Nevertheless, when NADH was estimated using the whole muscle homogenate technique, it was elevated at rest and at 1 minute of exercise at 40% $\dot{V}o_{2max}$ when extra fat was provided (11). However, after 10 minutes at 40% $\dot{V}o_{2max}$ and again after 10 minutes at 65% $\dot{V}o_{2max}$, NADH was no longer higher than the control condition. Therefore, although the mitochondrial NADH theory for explaining the reciprocal control of fuel use when fat availability is increased or decreased during exercise is attractive, a more thorough testing of this theory awaits improved techniques for measuring mitochondrial NADH content.

TEST YOURSELF

Why would a fatty acid-induced increase in mitochondrial NADH content decrease the reliance on CHO?

Increased FFA Availability during Prolonged Dynamic Exercise

When dynamic exercise of moderate intensity is prolonged beyond 1 to 2 hours the availability of plasma FFA increases to high levels while the availability of muscle glycogen decreases (15). Not surprisingly, fat oxidation rises and CHO oxidation falls. This scenario provides another opportunity to study the reciprocal control of fat and CHO oxidation during exercise. During prolonged dynamic exercise PDHa decreased along with CHO oxidation, but surprisingly, no changes in the energy status of the cell or decreases in pyruvate content accompanied the decrease in PDHa and glycogenolysis (15). It is possible that a reduction in the availability of substrate was responsible for the decreased PHOS and PDHa activities because the glycogen content was low and the production of pyruvate was decreased even though it did not translate into a decreased content in the muscle. However, an alternate possibility to explain the decreased PDHa involves the rapid upregulation of PDK activity (the enzyme regulating phosphorylation and inhibition of PDH).

High Fat Availability Upregulates PDK Activity and Decreases PDH Activity

Situations that chronically decrease CHO availability and increase the reliance of skeletal muscle on fat produce increases in the mRNA and protein contents of the PDK 4 isoform and the activity of PDK (16). This ultimately leads to a decreased fraction of PDH in the active form at rest and decreased whole body CHO oxidation. Although these changes occurred over hours and days, the question arose as to whether more rapid fat-induced upregulation of PDK activity could occur during prolonged dynamic exercise and explain the down-regulation of PDH that occurred during 4 hours of moderate exercise? Recent research examined this question and demonstrated that PDK activity was increased after 4 hours of moderate exercise, but without increases in PDK 2 and 4 protein contents (17). This suggested that incorporation of existing PDK protein loosely associated with the PDH complex increases the intrinsic PDK activity. This increased PDK activity appeared to contribute to the down-regulation of PDH during prolonged dynamic exercise, but it is presently not clear what regulates these changes. It may be that activation of signals secondary to the increasing FFA concentrations and/or diminishing CHO (glycogen store and insulin concentration) supply may be involved.

Increased Intramuscular Fat Availability

Skeletal muscle is "exposed" to two sources of fat: circulating FFA and IMTG. The muscle does not differentiate between the fatty acids that are either taken up into the muscle from the circulatory system or hydrolyzed from IMTG sources. Therefore, it is possible that altering the content of IMTG (a common aerobic training adaptation), similar to increasing FFA, may decrease CHO oxidation. The most common method to alter the IMTG availability is via chronic dietary manipulations. IMTG can be increased by 50% to 80% following the consumption of high fat diets where fat supplies 50% to 70% of the total energy intake, and IMTGs can be decreased when dietary fat intake is reduced from 22% to 2% of caloric intake (18,19). Using these dietary interventions, it has been shown that long-term high fat diets reduce muscle glycogen utilization and total CHO oxidation rates during moderate-intensity exercise, without altering glucose uptake (20). Conversely, when IMTGs are reduced after a low fat diet (2% of total energy intake), whole body CHO oxidation and muscle glycogen utilization are also increased without altering whole body glucose uptake (18). These data suggest that IMTG has no effect on muscle glucose uptake during exercise, but does influence muscle glycogen utilization. However, low-fat diets also contain a higher proportion of calories from CHO sources, and therefore although IMTG concentrations are reduced, reciprocally glycogen concentrations are increased, which is likely to have also contributed to the increased CHO oxidation and reduced fat utilization in the foregoing study. Clearly, to elucidate the possible interaction between the IMTG store and CHO fuel metabolism, studies must employ interventions that induce acute changes in IMTG content independent of alterations in the availability of other substrates (*e.g.*, muscle glycogen, plasma FFA). Burke et al. (21) moved their work in this direction, and demonstrated that the effects of a high fat diet on reducing glycogen use during dynamic exercise persisted, even after muscle glycogen stores were returned to normal levels. In this model, participants consumed either a high CHO diet (9.6 g · kg-1 · day-1 CHO and 0.7 g · kg-1 · day-1 fat) or an isoenergetic high fat diet (2.4 g · kg-1 · day-1 CHO and 4.0 g · kg-1 · day-1 fat) for 5 days while undergoing aerobic training. On the sixth day all participants consumed a high CHO diet that normalized muscle glycogen levels prior to the exercise trial that commenced on day 7. Regardless of the "normalized" glycogen level, a portion of the "CHO-sparing" effect of the high fat diet was still present during the exercise trial. The subjects in this study, and others by the same authors, were well trained and continued to exercise at a very high level during the 5-day high fat/low CHO diet intervention. Typical high fat dietary interventions are not associated with continued and uncompromised training, and, therefore, the ability to maintain and/or increase fatty acid oxidation (aerobic training) while consuming a high fat diet may be extremely important for inducing these metabolic shifts. At the present time, the mechanisms responsible for these persistent effects of the high fat diet are not known, but it is reasonable to speculate that a redistribution of fatty acid transport proteins to the plasma membrane and mitochondria may contribute.

TEST YOURSELF

What is a typical confounding variable in studies utilizing a high fat diet to study the reciprocal relationship of CHO and fatty acid oxidation in skeletal muscle?

Increased Muscle Glycogen Availability

In contrast to the numerous studies that have demonstrated a regulatory role of skeletal muscle glycogen content on muscle glycogenolysis, glucose uptake, and CHO oxidation, there is relatively little information regarding the influence of muscle glycogen on FFA uptake, IMTG metabolism, and FFA oxidation. One study reported similar rates of FFA uptake between exercising legs, 12 hours after glycogen-depleting exercise in one leg (22). Glycerol release from the low glycogen leg was ~60% greater than the control leg, suggesting a possible increase in IMTG hydrolysis with low muscle glycogen, although this difference was not statistically significant. When muscle glycogen was increased after 7 weeks of training and consumption of a CHO rich diet (65% CHO, 20% fat), leg FFA and very low-density lipoprotein uptake were both lower during cycling exercise than in subjects who performed

similar training, but consumed a fat rich diet (62% fat, 21% CHO [15]). Another study observed increased leg FFA uptake when muscle glycogen was low, but FFA clearance was similar, suggesting that dietary/hormonal effects on adipose tissue lipolysis and plasma (FFA) were the main factors modulating muscle FFA uptake (23). However, these authors also observed greater AMP kinase (AMPK) activity and acetyl-CoA carboxylase (ACC) phosphorylation with low glycogen content, which may have contributed to enhanced intramuscular fat oxidation, as well as potential mobilization of FFA from the IMTG store. Thus, although it is possible that muscle glycogen plays a role in determining substrate oxidation through interaction with modulators and key enzymes of fat metabolism, these possibilities have not been thoroughly examined.

Increased Carbohydrate Availability and Dynamic Exercise

Several studies have demonstrated that increasing the availability of exogenous CHO before and during dynamic exercise, and the availability of endogenous CHO (glycolytic flux) during exercise, increases CHO and reciprocally decreases fat oxidation (24,25). However, it is disappointing that few of these studies have examined the mechanisms underlying these shifts in fuel selection. Potential mechanisms explaining the effect of glucose ingestion on fat oxidation during dynamic exercise are given in Figure 16.5.

Increased Exogenous Glucose Availability

Preexercise CHO ingestion reduces fat oxidation during a subsequent bout of low to moderate dynamic exercise, and there is accumulating evidence to support a direct inhibitory role of increased exogenous glucose availability on fat utilization during exercise. The reduction in fat metabolism following glucose ingestion appears to be due to the combined effects of decreased FFA availability, secondary to decreased adipose lipolysis, and to direct effects on fatty acid oxidation in the muscle.

Research has examined the effects of CHO ingestion on adipose tissue lipolysis during low to moderate intensity exercise (24). During exercise in the fasted state, adipose tissue lipolysis exceeded skeletal muscle fat oxidation, whereas CHO ingestion resulted in elevated plasma insulin, reduced adipose tissue lipolysis, and decreased fat oxidation (Table 16.1). Preexercise CHO ingestion also increased glycolytic flux and CHO oxidation and reduced both plasma-derived FFA and IMTG oxidation (24). The magnitude of the decreased fat oxidation equaled the reduction in lipolysis, suggesting a limitation of FFA availability for fat oxidation. However, these investigators also used palmitate and octanoate tracers and concluded that CHO ingestion also exerted an inhibitory effect

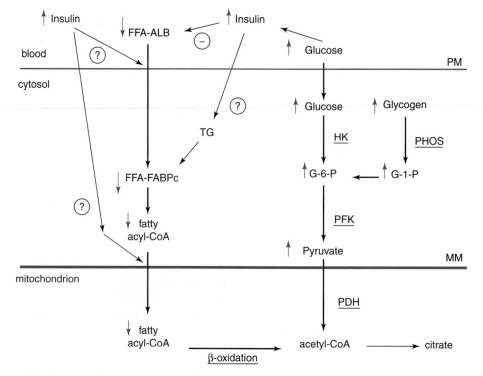

FIGURE 16.5 Schematic representation of potential effects of carbohydrate ingestion prior to dynamic exercise in decreasing plasma free fatty acid (FFA) concentration and down-regulating fat metabolism in skeletal muscle. Ingested glucose increases the release of insulin, which inhibits adipose tissue lipolysis and reduces the plasma [FFA]. Increased insulin may also inhibit FFA transport across the plasma (PM) and mitochondrial (MM) membranes and decrease triacylglycerol (TG) breakdown in the muscle. Carbohydrate oxidation, possibly from plasma glucose and/or muscle glycogen, is increased. ALB, albumin; FABP, fatty acid-binding protein; G-6-P and G-1-P, glucose 6- and 1-phosphate; HK, hexokinase; PDH, pyruvate dehydrogenase; PFK, phosphofructokinase.

on fat oxidation in the muscle (24). Glucose ingestion reduced long chain FFA (palmitate) uptake and oxidation (dependent on membrane transport), but not oxidation of the medium chain fatty acid octanoate (independent of membrane transport). These data suggest that there is an inhibitory effect of CHO oxidation on the transport of FFA across the muscle membrane and/or the mitochondrial membranes, and ultimately, the oxidation of fat.

TABLE 16.1 Effect of Glucose Ingestion (Glc) Compared to Fasting (Fast) on Various Aspects of Fat Metabolism During Exercise

		μmol/kg/min				
Trial	Time (min)	Total fat oxidation	R_a FFA	R_d FFA	Plasma FFA oxidation	FA oxidation from intramuscular TG
Fast-palmitate	20–30	30.9 ± 2.1	12.2 ± 1.0	12.0 ± 1.0	10.5 ± 0.8	20.4 ± 2.1
	30–40	32.1 ± 1.6	12.8 ± 1.0	12.7 ± 1.0	10.9 ± 0.8	21.2 ± 1.9
Glc-palmitate*	20–30	19.7 ± 1.5	8.3 ± 0.8	8.2 ± 0.8	5.7 ± 0.4	14.0 ± 1.8
	30–40	21.1 ± 1.6	8.2 ± 0.6	8.1 ± 0.5	5.7 ± 0.4	15.4 ± 1.8

*Glc-palmitate trial is significantly lower than Fast-palmitate trial at that time; $P < 0.05$.

Values are mean + SE for 6 subjects. [1-^{13}C]palmitate was intravenously infused during both trials. R_a and R_d rates of appearance and disappearance of plasma free fatty acids (FFA), respectively. Plasma FFA oxidation is calculated as the product of R_d FFA and percent of infused palmitate tracer oxidized. Fatty acid oxidation from intramuscular triglyceride (TG) is calculated as the difference between total fat oxidation and plasma FFA oxidation.

With permission from Chesley A, Heigenhauser GJ, Spriet LL. Regulation of muscle glycogen phosphorylase activity following short-term endurance training. *Am J Physiol.* 1996;270:E328–335 (6).

Increased insulin concentration

The reduction in fat metabolism following glucose ingestion appears to be due to decreased adipose tissue lipolysis and the resulting decreased FFA availability, as well as to direct effects on fatty acid oxidation in the muscle. Both effects may be the result of the increased plasma insulin levels. The elevated plasma insulin levels exert a powerful inhibitory effect on hormone-sensitive lipase (HSL) in adipose tissue, reducing the breakdown of triacylglycerol (TG) and decreasing the circulating plasma FFA concentrations. These changes translate into reduced delivery of FFA to the muscles during exercise and a decrease in FFA uptake and oxidation.

Insulin has been shown to increase the content of fat transport proteins in the muscle membrane to facilitate transport. Although at first the increase in transport seems to support increased fat oxidation, insulin may also stimulate esterification of FFA and decrease IMTG lipolysis in skeletal muscle, and, therefore, direct incoming FFA toward storage and away from oxidation, as occurs in adipose tissue. Although there has generally been little done on the regulation of IMTG hydrolysis in human skeletal muscle, HSL activity is reduced when CHO is ingested during exercise (26), suggesting insulin may regulate HSL activity, and therefore IMTG hydrolysis, in human skeletal muscle. Although an elevated insulin concentration may exert these effects following glucose ingestion, it would not explain the decrease in fat oxidation that occurs when the power output increases from 40% to 80% $\dot{V}_{O_{2max}}$, for example.

TEST YOURSELF

It is possible that increased plasma insulin has direct inhibitory effects on other regulatory sites of fat metabolism and oxidation in skeletal muscle. Which sites would be logical candidates?

Increased Muscle Glycogen Use during Dynamic Exercise

The studies discussed previously in this chapter related largely to small reciprocal changes in CHO and fatty acid oxidation during steady conditions (either resting or during exercise). However, as previously noted, exercise intensity can also influence substrate availability and intracellular metabolites that regulate the key enzymes, PHOS and PDH.

Fat oxidation increases from rest to low and moderate-intensity exercise (maximum at ~64% $\dot{V}_{O_{2max}}$), but decreases substantially at power outputs above ~75% $\dot{V}_{O_{2max}}$ (27,28). Increasing the exercise power output above ~50% $\dot{V}_{O_{2max}}$ also increases the use of the endogenous CHO store, muscle glycogen. Blood glucose levels, muscle glycogenolysis, glycolytic flux, PDH activation, and CHO oxidation are all increased during exercise at higher, compared with moderate, exercise power outputs (29,30). Lower plasma FFA availability, secondary to reduced adipose tissue blood flow and FFA release, may contribute to the decreased fat oxidation at these higher intensities of exercise. However, when plasma FFA availability during heavy dynamic exercise was increased by intravenous lipid and heparin infusion, normalizing FFA levels to those observed during moderate-intensity exercise, FFA oxidation was increased, but not fully restored (9). These data suggest mechanisms within muscle also limit fatty acid oxidation at these higher exercise intensities.

Potential Mechanisms for Down-regulated Fat Oxidation at Higher Intensities of Exercise

Like CHO oxidation, fatty acid oxidation involves several sites of regulation and, therefore, it would be expected that the CHO mediated down-regulation of fatty acid oxidation within skeletal muscle would target one or more of these sites: (a) TG degradation (HSL and adipose triacylglycerol lipase [ATGL] regulated) and release of FFA from adipose tissue; (b) transport of FFA to the active skeletal muscle; (c) the transport of FFA into the cell (largely a protein-mediated phenomenon); (d) the release of FFA from IMTG (HSL and ATGL regulated); and (e) the transport of FFA into the mitochondria (carnitine palmitoyltransferase 1 [CPT1] and likely additional transport proteins).

Carbohydrate-Induced decrease in long chain FFA transport into muscle

As mentioned previously, blood flow to the adipose tissue during high-intensity exercise may partially compromise fatty acid oxidation by reducing the delivery of FFA to the active muscle. Long chain FFA (but not medium chain FFA) transport into skeletal muscle is a highly regulated process involving several fatty acid transport proteins (see *Fat Metabolism* for more details). Some of these transport proteins have been shown to translocate to the plasma membrane during muscle contraction, acutely increasing the ability of skeletal muscle to transport FFA into the cell. The movement of these transporters to the plasma membrane, and the subsequent rate of FFA transport, has been shown to increase linearly with various electrical stimulation protocols designed to optimize fatty acid metabolism. However, to date, the response of these transporters has not been examined during higher intensities of exercise, and it remains to be determined if FFA transport into muscle is compromised by both declining FFA concentrations, as well as the amount of fatty acid transport proteins on the plasma membrane. Although this response has not been directly studied, one study has examined fatty acid metabolism of varying chain lengths during moderate (~40% $\dot{V}_{O_{2max}}$) and heavy (~80% $\dot{V}_{O_{2max}}$) intensity exercise (25), and shown that increasing the exercise intensity reduces long chain FFA uptake and oxidation, but not the oxidation or uptake of medium chain fatty acids (25). This suggested an inhibitory effect of increased glycolytic flux on the oxidation of long chain FFA, likely involving plasma membrane transport and/or transport into mitochondria, both of which appear to be highly regulated for long chain but not medium chain FFAs.

Decreased IMTG hydrolysis with higher intensities of exercise

The exact regulation of IMTG hydrolysis involves HSL, ATGL, and perilipins (for a complete reference list see Watt [31]). AMPK has been suggested to phosphorylate and inactivate HSL at higher power outputs, decreasing IMTG hydrolysis. Although ATGL has been implicated in regulating IMTG hydrolysis in human skeletal muscle, no data regarding the acute regulation of this enzyme is currently available, and, therefore, its role in decreasing fat oxidation at higher power outputs is purely speculative. Proteins known as perilipins coat lipid droplets and separate IMTGs from the lipolytic enzymes HSL and ATGL, yielding low rates of lipolysis. Phosphorylation of perilipin is involved in recruiting both HSL and ATGL to the lipid droplet, enhancing rates of IMTG hydrolysis. It is, therefore, possible that phosphatase-induced dephosphorylation of perilipin could decrease IMTG hydrolysis at higher exercise intensities; however, this remains to be tested. Regardless of the speculative nature of ATGL and perilipin, the whole body and HSL data indicate that the decreased fat oxidation during heavy dynamic exercise is partially due to a reduction in FFA availability. Reductions in mitochondrial fatty acid oxidation would exacerbate the decreased FFA delivery, and could also contribute to the decreased fat oxidation that occurs above ~75% $\dot{V}O_{2max}$.

TEST YOURSELF

Why is skeletal muscle FFA delivery reduced at higher intensities of exercise? (Information relevant to this question is also found in Chapter 15.)

Fat transport into mitochondria

The transport of long chain fatty acids into mitochondria appears to be a key step in regulating the overall rate that skeletal muscle can oxidize fatty acids. Historically, the regulation of fatty acid oxidation at the level of mitochondria has been solely attributed to the relationship between CPTI and malonyl-CoA (M-CoA) concentrations. It is well known that an abundant CHO supply and high insulin levels cause an elevation of M-CoA content in lipogenic tissues (e.g., liver) via stimulation of ACC activity (32). In the liver, M-CoA has a clearly defined role in inhibiting CPTI activity

and the transport of lipid into mitochondria when CHO is abundant. However, M-CoA has also been detected in human skeletal muscle (33) and a muscle isoform of ACC, which appears to be regulated differently from hepatic ACC, has been discovered in skeletal muscle. Because skeletal muscle is not capable of de novo fat synthesis, it is not clear what role M-CoA plays in regulating the entry of FFA into the mitochondria at rest and during exercise in this biologic tissue. The unique challenge that skeletal muscle faces during exercise is the need to greatly increase the production of energy from both fat and CHO oxidation, not simply switch between fuels. This is quite different from the reciprocal changes in CHO and fat oxidation that occur in resting skeletal muscle and other tissues that do not experience large increases in metabolic demand.

The M-CoA theory, extended to the findings in rodent skeletal muscle, suggests that resting M-CoA levels are high enough to limit FFA transport into the mitochondria. It is clear that M-CoA levels decrease during muscle contractions in rodent skeletal muscle, when energy production from fat oxidation is increased (34). This suggests that the decrease in M-CoA during exercise may be important in relieving the inhibition of CPTI that normally exists in resting skeletal muscle.

Summary

In both liver and skeletal muscle the transport of LCFAs into mitochondria is carnitine dependent, and largely regulated by the activity of CPTI. During exercise in rodent skeletal muscle the increased demand for energy is affiliated with a reduction in M-CoA content, which removes the inhibition of CPTI, increasing the transport of LCFAs into mitochondria and the rate of fatty acid oxidation.

Fat transport into mitochondria in human skeletal muscle

Measurements of M-CoA content in human skeletal muscle during dynamic exercise have consistently demonstrated that M-CoA content is largely unaffected by exercise at varying power outputs (35%–100% $\dot{V}O_{2max}$) and rates of fat oxidation (5,35). In addition, the well-established role for AMPK in regulating the reductions in M-CoA in rodent muscle is now being challenged, because mice expressing a dominant AMPK isoform that is inactive (essentially an AMPK knock-out or null model) retain the ability to phosphorylate ACC and reduce M-CoA content during exercise (36). Taken together, these results do not support a regulatory role for M-CoA content in fat oxidation during exercise in human skeletal muscle, and suggest that the regulation of CPTI activity during the onset of dynamic exercise is more complex, and likely additional regulation of CPTI (e.g., M-CoA sensitivity) and/or other transport proteins exist on mitochondrial membranes.

KEY POINT

Reductions in skeletal muscle M-CoA may account for increases in fatty acid oxidation in contracting rodent muscle, but not in human skeletal muscle.

Experiments with isolated mitochondria have shown that mitochondrial fatty acid oxidation can be increased without alterations in CPTI activity (37). This observation suggested there are likely additional proteins that contribute to the regulation of mitochondrial fatty acid oxidation. Fatty acid translocase (FAT)/CD36, a plasma membrane fatty acid transport protein, has been found on skeletal muscle mitochondrial membranes (38,39). Support that FAT/CD36 regulates mitochondrial fatty acid oxidation comes from a number of observations, including (a) mitochondrial fatty acid oxidation rates are lower in FAT/CD36 animals with no FAT/CD36 (40); (b) exercise increases mitochondrial fatty acid oxidation and FAT/CD36 protein content (41); (c) FAT/CD36 co-immunoprecipitates with CPTI (26,39); and (d) over-expression of FAT/CD36 increased fatty acid oxidation in L6E9 myotubes (42). More recently, another putative plasma membrane fatty acid transport protein, aptly named fatty acid transport protein 1 (FATP1), was also identified on mitochondrial membranes in L6E9 myotubes, and over-expression of FATP1 increased mitochondrial fatty acid oxidation. Although evidence is mounting to suggest a regulatory role for FAT/CD36 and FATP1 in mitochondrial fatty acid oxidation, this research is novel and there remains controversy as to the exact role of these proteins. In addition, the effect of exercise intensity on regulating mitochondrial FAT/CD36 and FATP1 has not been examined. This research does not negate the importance of CPTI in mitochondrial fatty acid oxidation, but rather indicates a complexity in mitochondrial fatty acid transport not previously examined.

TEST YOURSELF

What data are available to suggest that the regulation of fatty acid oxidation at the level of the mitochondrion is different in the skeletal muscle of rodents and humans?

As previously mentioned, intralipid infusions of various chain length fatty acids have shown that increasing the exercise intensity from 40% to 80% $\dot{V}O_{2max}$ reduced long chain FFA uptake and oxidation, but not the medium chain fatty acid octanoate oxidation (25). We have discussed these data with respect to plasma membrane transport; however, the data also suggest that increasing the intensity of exercise inhibits the transport of long chain (but not medium chain) fatty acids across the mitochondrial membranes. Although these authors did not examine potential mechanisms, it has been suggested the small reductions in pH associated with dynamic exercise at moderate to heavy power outputs may account for this inhibition at the mitochondria (30). Studies in mitochondria isolated from resting human skeletal muscle showed that small decreases in pH from 7 to 6.8 caused large reductions in CPTI activity (43), and this may contribute to decreased fatty acid oxidation during dynamic exercise at higher power outputs. More research is required to clarify the regulation of CPTI activity during exercise in order to determine the mechanisms, whereby increasing glycolytic activity could down-regulate fat oxidation at this step. Surprisingly, increasing concentrations of Ca, and free ADP, AMP, and P_i, which occur with increasing exercise intensities and increased CHO use, did not inhibit CPTI activity in mitochondria isolated from human skeletal muscle.

Summary

It appears that fat oxidation is compromised at higher intensities of exercise as a result of (a) decreased blood flow to adipose tissue, (b) decreased release of FFA into the plasma and decreased delivery of FFA to skeletal muscle, (c) decreased hydrolysis of IMTGs, (d) decreased delivery of FFA to skeletal muscle mitochondria, and (e) reductions in muscle pH, decreasing FFA transport into mitochondria. The roles of plasma membrane transport, ATGL, perilipin, and mitochondrial fatty acid transport proteins in regulating this decrease in fatty acid oxidation at higher intensities of exercise, although plausible, remain speculative.

The effects of pharmacologic agents on CHO and fatty acid fuel selection

The ingestion of pharmacologic agents has also been used to either promote or decrease the use of fat during exercise, while simultaneously probing for the mechanisms regulating shifts in fuel utilization. Caffeine has been used to increase adipose tissue fat mobilization and skeletal muscle oxidation, but the response to this procedure has been variable between subjects, limiting what can be concluded on a group basis. When effective, caffeine appears to antagonize the normal inhibitory effects of adenosine on adipose tissue lipolysis at rest, resulting in measurable increases in plasma FFA concentrations before exercise begins. The increased FFA delivery to and oxidation by the working muscles during exercise appears to spare the use of muscle glycogen in some individuals (14). However, the caffeine-induced increase in plasma FFA seen at rest is not able to increase adipose tissue lipolysis above the exercise effect, and no further glycogen sparing occurs beyond the first 15 to 20 minutes of exercise. Conversely, nicotinic acid has been administered to decrease the availability of plasma FFA, because binding with receptors on adipose tissue leads to powerful and rapid inhibition of lipolysis (13). Again the response to this drug is variable. Some subjects respond with large decreases in fat oxidation and increases in CHO oxidation during dynamic exercise, whereas others appear to replace the "missing" plasma fat with IMTG-derived fat, resulting in no shift in the proportional use of fat and CHO.

The effects of training on CHO and fatty acid fuel selection

Although genetics is a requirement for elite athletic ability, Holloszy's research in the late 1960s and early 1970s demonstrated the remarkable plasticity of skeletal muscle, and the power of training with respect to altering muscle characteristics (for review, see Holloszy and Coyle [44]). One of the seminal findings from Holloszy's landmark studies was that repeated bouts of exercise over days and months induced mitochondrial proliferation. This chapter does not discuss how these biogenic events are initiated (see Chapter 18), however the expansion of mitochondrial content has profound effects on CHO and fatty acid oxidation, and represents another example of a shift in fuel use where the increased fat oxidation in effect "spares" the use of CHO. After aerobic training the maximal capacity for fat

A MILESTONE OF DISCOVERY

The English scientists Randle, Garland, Newsholme, and Hales published several papers in the 1960s that examined the regulation of glucose uptake and carbohydrate (CHO) metabolism in muscle and the abnormalities that accompanied changes in insulin sensitivity and diabetes mellitus (1,2). In their research, they noticed that abnormalities of CHO metabolism were often accompanied by increases in the concentrations of plasma free fatty acid (FFA) and ketone bodies. Interestingly, many of these abnormalities were the same ones that we are still studying and attempting to explain today—diabetes, starvation, CHO deprivation, and obesity! They wished to determine if these high levels of circulating FFA and ketone bodies could produce the same abnormalities as reported in these diseases: decreased glucose uptake, glycolysis, and pyruvate oxidation in muscle. A series of in vitro and in vivo studies led to the formation of the idea of the glucose-fatty acid (G-FA) cycle. Dr. Randle outlined his recollection of the essential components of the G-FA cycle in the CIBA Medal Lecture on "Fuel selection in animals" in London, England, in December of 1985 (47): "(1) the relationship between glucose and fatty acid metabolism is reciprocal and not dependent; (2) in vivo, the oxidation of fatty acids and ketone bodies released into the circulation in diabetes or starvation may inhibit the catabolism of glucose in muscle; (3) in vitro, the oxidation of fatty acids released from muscle triglyceride may play a similar role; (4) the effects of fatty acid and ketone body oxidation are mediated by inhibition of the pyruvate dehydrogenase (PDH) complex, phosphofructokinase-1 (PFK) and hexokinase (HK); (5) the essential mechanism is an increase in the mitochondrial ratio of [acetyl-CoA]/[CoA], which inhibits the PDH complex and by indirect means leads to inhibition of PFK by citrate and of HK by glucose-6-phosphate (G-6-P); (6) the effect of low concentrations of insulin to accelerate glucose transporter is inhibited by oxidation of fatty acids or ketone bodies."

These authors formed their theory by combining the results from in vivo studies using perfused, contracting heart muscle and incubated, resting diaphragm muscle from rodents, with in vitro or test tube muscle homogenate experiments, that examined the ability of certain modulators to affect the activity of the key glycolytic enzymes. When the FFA availability to the muscles was increased, fat oxidation increased and CHO oxidation decreased, and muscle acetyl-CoA, citrate, and G-6-P contents increased. The in vitro work had already established that acetyl-CoA inhibited the activity of PDH by activating PDH kinase, which phosphorylates PDH to its less active form, that citrate was a potent inhibitor of PFK, and finally that G-6-P inhibited HK.

These early experiments were performed with heart and diaphragm muscles that have regular contraction cycles and derive the majority of the required oxidizable substrate from outside the cell. It is important to note that this situation is different from the working conditions of most peripheral skeletal muscles, and especially human skeletal muscle. These muscles are often quiet for long periods of time. When muscles do contract, the high energy demands of moderate and heavy aerobic exercise dictates that the majority of oxidizable substrate must come from fuel stores inside the cells, representing a very different paradigm from this seminal work in cardiac and diaphragm muscles. However, these landmark experiments provided a testable theory for future experimenters to study and attempt to explain the relationship between CHO and fat use in contracting skeletal muscle at various exercise intensities and durations, and under varying nutritional states.

The fundamental tenet of the pioneering work by Randle and colleagues, namely the reciprocal relationship between CHO and fat oxidation, has been shown to exist in skeletal muscle. However, our understanding of the interaction between CHO and fat oxidation in skeletal muscle has expanded to include the role of free ADP, free AMP, and P_i on the regulation of both glycogen PHOS and PDH. Although these mechanisms were not accounted for by Randle and colleagues, and therefore are not technically part of the G-FA cycle, they provide further mechanistic insight into fuel interactions in resting and contracting skeletal muscle.

Randle PJ, Garland PB, Hales CN, et al. The glucose fatty-acid cycle. Its role in insulin sensitivity and the metabolic disturbances of diabetes mellitus. Lancet. 1963;1:785–789.

oxidation, as well as the proportion of energy derived from fat oxidation at any given absolute exercise intensity where steady state is achieved, are increased. Holloszy theorized that the increase in mitochondrial volume would result in a smaller increase in free ADP, decreasing the activation of PHOS and PDH, and increasing the reliance on fat. This notion has been supported in exercising humans (45,46).

TEST YOURSELF

Why would a decrease in free ADP following training result in a greater reliance on fatty acid oxidation during a subsequent steady-state bout of exercise?

CHAPTER SUMMARY

CHO and fat are the primary metabolic substrates oxidized during dynamic exercise. The notion that increasing the availability of CHO can increase the oxidation of CHO, and increasing the exogenous FFA availability can increase fat oxidation, are well supported. There are data to suggest that increasing fat availability at rest decreases CHO oxidation. However, during dynamic exercise, the classic G-FA cycle does not explain this interaction. Instead, increasing fat availability down-regulates muscle glycogenolysis and PDH activity, possibly by increasing mitochondrial NADH availability and ultimately buffering the exercise-induced increases in free ADP, AMP, and P_i accumulation. During prolonged dynamic exercise, increased plasma [FFA] may upregulate PDK activity and thereby attenuate the activation of PDH. There is also evidence demonstrating that altering exogenous CHO availability can decrease fat oxidation, via an increase in plasma insulin and decreased FFA availability, and also by decreasing the rate of fat transport into the muscle and/or the mitochondria. Increasing the dynamic exercise intensity stimulates a greater reliance on CHO as a fuel and appears to down-regulate fat metabolism through mechanisms based both within and external to the muscle. Future studies examining membrane fat transport, muscle TG lipolysis (HSL and ATGL activity), and mitochondrial fat transport (CPTI activity and fatty acid transport proteins) in human skeletal muscle and the effects of altered endogenous fuel availability (IMTG and muscle glycogen contents) on the interaction between CHO and fat metabolism during dynamic exercise are clearly needed.

REFERENCES

1. Randle PJ, Garland PB, Hales CN, et al. The glucose fatty-acid cycle. Its role in insulin sensitivity and the metabolic disturbances of diabetes mellitus. *Lancet.* 1963;1:785–789.
2. Randle PJ, Newsholme EA, Garland PB. Regulation of glucose uptake by muscle. Effects of fatty acids, ketone bodies and

3. pyruvate, and of alloxan-diabetes and starvation, on the uptake and metabolic fate of glucose in rat heart and diaphragm muscles. *Biochem J.* 1964;93:652–665.
3. Hickson RC, Rennie MJ, Conlee RK, et al. Effects of increased plasma fatty acids on glycogen utilization and endurance. *J Appl Physiol.* 1977;43:829–833.
4. Rennie MJ, Holloszy JO. Inhibition of glucose uptake and glycogenolysis by availability of oleate in well-oxygenated perfused skeletal muscle. *Biochem J.* 1977;168:161–170.
5. Odland LM, Howlett RA, Heigenhauser GJ, et al. Skeletal muscle malonyl-CoA content at the onset of exercise at varying power outputs in humans. *Am J Physiol.* 1998;274:E1080–E1085.
6. Dyck DJ, Peters SJ, Wendling PS, et al. Effect of high FFA on glycogenolysis in oxidative rat hindlimb muscles during twitch stimulation. *Am J Physiol.* 1996;270:R766–R776.
7. Richter EA, Ruderman NB, Gavras H, et al. Muscle glycogenolysis during exercise: dual control by epinephrine and contractions. *Am J Physiol.* 1982;242:E25–E32.
8. Dyck DJ, Peters SJ, Wendling PS, et al. Regulation of muscle glycogen phosphorylase activity during intense aerobic cycling with elevated FFA. *Am J Physiol.* 1996;270:E116–E125.
9. Romijn JA, Coyle EF, Sidossis LS, et al. Relationship between fatty acid delivery and fatty acid oxidation during strenuous exercise. *J Appl Physiol.* 1995;79:1939–1945.
10. Dyck DJ, Putman CT, Heigenhauser GJ, et al. Regulation of fat-carbohydrate interaction in skeletal muscle during intense aerobic cycling. *Am J Physiol.* 1993;265:E852–E859.
11. Odland LM, Heigenhauser GJ, Spriet LL. Effects of high fat provision on muscle PDH activation and malonyl-CoA content in moderate exercise. *J Appl Physiol.* 2000;89:2352–2358.
12. Peters SJ, Spriet LL. Skeletal muscle phosphofructokinase activity examined under physiological conditions in vitro. *J Appl Physiol.* 1995;78:1853–1858.
13. Stellingwerff T, Watt MJ, Heigenhauser GJ, et al. Effects of reduced free fatty acid availability on skeletal muscle PDH activation during aerobic exercise. Pyruvate dehydrogenase. *Am J Physiol Endocrinol Metab.* 2003;284:E589–E596.
14. Chesley A, Heigenhauser GJ, Spriet LL. Regulation of muscle glycogen phosphorylase activity following short-term endurance training. *Am J Physiol.* 1996;270:E328–E335.
15. Watt MJ, Heigenhauser GJ, Spriet LL. Intramuscular triacylglycerol utilization in human skeletal muscle during exercise: is there a controversy? *J Appl Physiol.* 2002;93:1185–1195.
16. Wu P, Peters JM, Harris RA. Adaptive increase in pyruvate dehydrogenase kinase 4 during starvation is mediated by peroxisome proliferator-activated receptor alpha. *Biochem Biophys Res Commun.* 2001;287:391–396.
17. Watt MJ, Heigenhauser GJ, LeBlanc PJ, et al. Rapid upregulation of pyruvate dehydrogenase kinase activity in human skeletal muscle during prolonged exercise. *J Appl Physiol.* 2004;97:1261–1267.
18. Coyle EF, Jeukendrup AE, Oseto MC, et al. Low-fat diet alters intramuscular substrates and reduces lipolysis and fat oxidation during exercise. *Am J Physiol Endocrinol Metab.* 2001;280:E391–E398.
19. Hawley JA. Effect of increased fat availability on metabolism and exercise capacity. *Med Sci Sports Exerc.* 2002;34:1485–1491.
20. Helge JW, Watt PW, Richter EA, et al. Fat utilization during exercise: adaptation to a fat-rich diet increases utilization of plasma fatty acids and very low density lipoprotein-triacylglycerol in humans. *J Physiol.* 2001;537:1009–1020.
21. Burke LM, Angus DJ, Cox GR, et al. Effect of fat adaptation and carbohydrate restoration on metabolism and performance during prolonged cycling. *J Appl Physiol.* 2000;89:2413–2421.
22. Blomstrand E, Saltin B. Effect of muscle glycogen on glucose, lactate and amino acid metabolism during exercise and recovery in human subjects. *J Physiol.* 1999;514(pt 1):293–302.
23. Wojtaszewski JF, MacDonald C, Nielsen JN, et al. Regulation of 5'AMP-activated protein kinase activity and substrate utilization in exercising human skeletal muscle. *Am J Physiol Endocrinol Metab.* 2003;284:E813–E822.
24. Coyle EF, Jeukendrup AE, Wagenmakers AJ, et al. Fatty acid oxidation is directly regulated by carbohydrate metabolism during exercise. *Am J Physiol.* 1997;273:E268–E275.
25. Sidossis LS, Stuart CA, Shulman GI, et al. Glucose plus insulin regulate fat oxidation by controlling the rate of fatty acid entry into the mitochondria. *J Clin Invest.* 1996;98:2244–2250.

26. Schenk S, Horowitz JF. Coimmunoprecipitation of FAT/CD36 and CPT I in skeletal muscle increases proportionally with fat oxidation after endurance exercise training. *Am J Physiol Endocrinol Metab.* 2006;291:E254–E260.

27. Romijn JA, Coyle EF, Sidossis LS, et al. Regulation of endogenous fat and carbohydrate metabolism in relation to exercise intensity and duration. *Am J Physiol.* 1993;265:E380–E391.

28. van Loon LJ, Greenhaff PL, Constantin-Teodosiu D, et al. The effects of increasing exercise intensity on muscle fuel utilization in humans. *J Physiol.* 2001;536:295–304.

29. Gollnick PD, Piehl K, Saltin B. Selective glycogen depletion pattern in human muscle fibres after exercise of varying intensity and at varying pedalling rates. *J Physiol.* 1974;241:45–57.

30. Howlett RA, Parolin ML, Dyck DJ, et al. Regulation of skeletal muscle glycogen phosphorylase and PDH at varying exercise power outputs. *Am J Physiol.* 1998;275:R418–R425.

31. Watt MJ. Triglyceride lipases alter fuel metabolism and mitochondrial gene expression. *Appl Physiol Nutr Metab.* 2009;34:340–347.

32. McGarry JD, Brown NF. The mitochondrial carnitine palmitoyltransferase system. From concept to molecular analysis. *Eur J Biochem.* 1997;244:1–14.

33. Odland LM, Heigenhauser GJ, Lopaschuk GD, et al. Human skeletal muscle malonyl-CoA at rest and during prolonged submaximal exercise. *Am J Physiol.* 1996;270:E541–E544.

34. Winder WW, Arogyasami J, Barton RJ, et al. Muscle malonyl-CoA decreases during exercise. *J Appl Physiol.* 1989;67:2230–2233.

35. Roepstorff C, Halberg N, Hillig T, et al. Malonyl-CoA and carnitine in regulation of fat oxidation in human skeletal muscle during exercise. *Am J Physiol Endocrinol Metab.* 2005;288:E133–E142.

36. Dzamko N, Schertzer JD, Ryall JG, et al. AMPK-independent pathways regulate skeletal muscle fatty acid oxidation. *J Physiol.* 2008;586:5819–5831.

37. Koves TR, Noland RC, Bates AL, et al. Subsarcolemmal and intermyofibrillar mitochondria play distinct roles in regulating skeletal muscle fatty acid metabolism. *Am J Physiol Cell Physiol.* 2005;288:C1074–C1082.

38. Bezaire V, Bruce CR, Heigenhauser GJ, et al. Identification of fatty acid translocase on human skeletal muscle mitochondrial membranes: essential role in fatty acid oxidation. *Am J Physiol Endocrinol Metab.* 2006;290:E509–E515.

39. Campbell SE, Tandon NN, Woldegiorgis G, et al. A novel function for fatty acid translocase (FAT)/CD36: involvement in long chain fatty acid transfer into the mitochondria. *J Biol Chem.* 2004;279:36235–36241.

40. Holloway GP, Jain SS, Bezaire VS, et al. FAT/CD36 null mice reveal that mitochondrial FAT/CD36 is required to up-regulate mitochondrial fatty acid oxidation in contracting muscle. *Am J Physiol Regul Integr Comp Physiol.* 2009;297:R960–R967.

41. Holloway GP, Bezaire V, Heigenhauser GJ, et al. Mitochondrial long chain fatty acid oxidation, fatty acid translocase/CD36 content and carnitine palmitoyltransferase I activity in human skeletal muscle during aerobic exercise. *J Physiol.* 2006;571:201–210.

42. Sebastian D, Guitart M, Garcia-Martinez C, et al. Novel role of FATP1 in mitochondrial fatty acid oxidation in skeletal muscle cells. *J Lipid Res.* 2009;50:1789–1799.

43. Starritt EC, Howlett RA, Heigenhauser GJ, et al. Sensitivity of CPT I to malonyl-CoA in trained and untrained human skeletal muscle. *Am J Physiol Endocrinol Metab.* 2000;278:E462–E468.

44. Holloszy JO, Coyle EF. Adaptations of skeletal muscle to endurance exercise and their metabolic consequences. *J Appl Physiol.* 1984;56:831–838.

45. Cadefau J, Green HJ, Cusso R, et al. Coupling of muscle phosphorylation potential to glycolysis during work after short-term training. *J Appl Physiol.* 1994;76:2586–2593.

46. Phillips SM, Green HJ, Tarnopolsky MA, et al. Progressive effect of endurance training on metabolic adaptations in working skeletal muscle. *Am J Physiol.* 1996;270:E265–E272.

47. Randle PJ. Fuel selection in animals. *Biochem Soc Trans.* 1986;14:799–806.

The Metabolic Systems: Protein and Amino Acid Metabolism in Muscle

Anton J. M. Wagenmakers

Abbreviations

Akt	Protein kinase B (also PKB)		for measurements made with the amino acid incorporation method
AICAR	5-aminoimidazole-4-carboxamide 1-β-D-ribonucleoside	mRNA	Messenger ribonucleic acid
AMP	Adenosine monophosphate	mTOR	Mammalian target of rapamycin, a kinase
AMPK	AMP-activated protein kinase		
ATP	Adenosine triphosphate	MURF1	Muscle specific ubiquitin ligase, upregulated in muscle wasting
BCAA	Branched-chain amino acid		
Ca²⁺	Calcium ion	PKB	Protein kinase B, also called Akt
CrP	Creatine phosphate	PI3-kinase	Phosphatidylinositol-3-kinase
eEF	Eukaryotic elongation factor	p70^{S6K}	Ribosomal protein S6 kinase
eIF	Eukaryotic initiation factor	rRNA	Ribosomal nucleic acid
4E-BP1 (or 4EBP1)	eIF4E binding protein-1	Ser	Serine
EDL	Extensor digitorum longus	S6	Ribosomal protein S6
FoxO	Forkhead box subgroup O transcription factor	TA	Tibialis anterior
		Thr	Threonine
FSR	Fractional protein synthesis rate, usually expressed in % per day	5'-TOP mRNA	mRNA with a tract of oligopyrimidines at the 5' end
IGF-1	Insulin-like growth factor 1	tRNA	Transfer ribonucleic acid
MAFbx	Muscle specific ubiquitin ligase, also called atrogin-1, upregulated in muscle wasting	W_{max}	Maximal aerobic workload during dynamic exercise
MPS	Mixed muscle protein synthesis rate, in this chapter the abbreviation is only used		

Introduction

The ability of humans to walk, run, and perform physical work is critically dependent on the presence and maintenance of an appropriate muscle mass. However, skeletal muscle exhibits a very high plasticity. In a young adult lean 70-kg male, skeletal muscle mass is 28 to 35 kg, and his body contains 12 kg of protein, of which ≥7 kg is present in the skeletal muscles (1–3). Therefore, skeletal muscle is regarded to be the main protein reserve that can at least partially be used to supply amino acids to other tissues during periods of starvation and long-term illness. Most of the muscle protein is accounted for by the myofibrils, the contractile elements that enable the muscle to contract, and thus generate force, movement, and work. High intensity resistance training is known to lead to muscle hypertrophy and to increases in the number of myofibrils per muscle fiber and strength, whereas physical inactivity has the opposite effect. Sarcopenia is the involuntary but physiologic loss of muscle mass that progressively develops during aging. Sarcopenia occurs in every individual, including those that are healthy and successfully maintain physical activity (4,5). Sarcopenia is a cause of muscle weakness and reduces mobility and fatal, accidental falls in the elderly population have an immense impact on national health care budgets. In many acquired chronic diseases (*e.g.*, cardiovascular disease, type 2 diabetes, chronic obstructive pulmonary disease, rheumatoid arthritis, kidney disease, cancer) patients develop a clinical condition called cachexia, which is derived from the Greek *kakos hexis*, literally meaning "bad condition." In cachexia the loss of muscle mass, strength, and function is much larger and faster than in sarcopenia, severely disabling and massively reducing the quality of life of those affected (6,7).

TEST YOURSELF

Explain the difference between sarcopenia and cachexia (using information provided in later sections of this chapter).

Skeletal muscle not only exhibits a high plasticity in protein mass, but also in the identity of the constituent proteins. In the 1960s, it was shown that endurance training both in rats (8) and humans (9) substantially increases the content of enzymes with a role in oxidative metabolism (mitochondrial enzymes and those with a role in substrate transport and mobilization). High concentrations of these oxidative enzymes give world class endurance runners the capacity to run a marathon in just over 2 hours. Inactivity and chronic disease on the other hand reduce the content of the oxidative enzymes, limit maximal aerobic workload to 50 to 60 watt, and prevent participation in normal daily living activities such as walking to local shops (10). Very important also is that a high muscle oxidative capacity is intrinsically related to insulin sensitivity and (cardio)vascular health via mechanisms that we at least partially understand (11).

The aim of this chapter is to give an integrative overview of the pathways and mechanisms that regulate muscle protein synthesis and degradation and determine the balance between the two. As exercise and nutrition are the most important natural tools available to every human being to maintain muscle mass and oxidative capacity during our lifespan, the focus is on the interaction between nutrition and exercise of various intensities and duration. This chapter is an entry into the large body of sometimes complex and confusing literature in this area and provides the knowledge that is required to make contributions to the design of novel strategies to prevent or limit muscle protein and quality loss in health and disease over the course of the human lifespan.

The Importance of Protein Turnover

Amino acids occur in nature in the form of proteins (amino acid polymers connected by peptide linkages) and free amino acids. There are 20 different amino acids that can be charged to an aminoacyl-transfer ribonucleic acid (tRNA) and be used for protein synthesis. The body of a 70-kg man contains 12 kg of protein and 200 to 230 g of free amino acids (1–3). About 120 g of the free amino acids are present intracellularly in skeletal muscle. There is a continuous exchange of amino acids between the free amino acid pool and the protein pool as proteins are constantly being synthesized and simultaneously being degraded (this cyclic exchange process is called protein turnover). Protein turnover at whole body level amounts to 280 g per day in humans (3) and consumes about 20% of the resting energy expenditure. Protein turnover is an essential prerequisite for survival as otherwise proteins damaged by toxic compounds, free radicals, peroxidation, ultraviolet light exposure, or extreme contraction forces would not be replaced with new functionally intact proteins.

KEY POINT

Protein turnover is essential because damaged proteins have a reduced activity and need to be replaced with new functional proteins.

Mechanisms to Alter Muscle Protein Content and Protein Composition

A net gain in the total protein content of a muscle fiber can be achieved by an increase in protein synthesis or a decrease in protein degradation and by any combination of changes in which the protein balance is positive (protein synthesis > protein degradation). A net gain of the total protein content by definition also leads to hypertrophy of muscle cells and gain of muscle mass. A negative protein net balance (protein synthesis < protein degradation) will lead to a net loss of the protein content and muscle fiber atrophy.

A change in the protein composition of a muscle cell in response to a physiologic stimulus such as exercise or nutrition on a theoretical base can be achieved by the following mechanisms:

1. A change of the gene expression profile leading to the appearance of a different set of messenger ribonucleic acids (mRNAs) or a change in the relative concentration of mRNAs in the expressed profile
2. A change in the breakdown rate of specific mRNAs leading to a change in the relative concentration of mRNAs in the expressed profile
3. A selection of specific mRNAs for translation initiation and protein synthesis
4. A selection of specific proteins for preferential degradation by the proteolytic systems that operate in muscle

This implies that part of the control of the proteins that are ultimately present in muscle is at the DNA transcription level, part at the level of the stability and turnover of the expressed mRNAs, and part at the level of protein synthesis and of protein degradation. The first two levels are addressed in Chapter 5. In this chapter, the latter two levels are described.

Methods to Measure In Vivo Rates of Protein Synthesis and Degradation in Humans

The methodology that is used in humans to measure protein synthesis and degradation rates at whole body level and in individual tissues and proteins has been described in earlier reviews (3,12). In brief, the most accurate, reliable, and direct method to measure the synthesis rate of mixed muscle protein synthesis (MPS) or of individual proteins is the amino acid incorporation technique. In most human studies, a continuous infusion of 3 to 6 hours is given of an amino acid with a stable isotope label (^{13}C-, ^{15}N- or ^2H-). The increase in enrichment in time is divided by the enrichment of the amino acid precursor pool and the incorporation time to give the fractional protein synthesis rate (FSR) in percentage per day or per hour. In rats and mice most laboratories use radioactively labeled amino acid tracers to measure FSRs. The method has successfully been used to measure the synthesis rate of mixed muscle protein and to investigate the control of protein synthesis by fasting/refeeding and hormones (3,12,13). However, very few laboratories worldwide are technically able to apply it to muscle protein subfractions (14) and individual proteins. This is the primary reason why our insight in the time course of the increases in the synthesis rate of myofibrillar proteins, mitochondrial proteins, and important transporter proteins such as glucose transporter 4 after various modes of exercise is still limited today.

The net balance approach across a forearm or a leg has been developed to simultaneously measure MPS and degradation rates. A tracer amino acid is given by a primed continuous intravenous infusion until the plasma concentration and enrichment are constant (in tracer steady-state) and then a set of replicates are obtained both from arterial blood and venous blood draining the forearm or the leg. In most cases, an amino acid is used that is not transaminated or oxidized in muscle such that the amino acid can only disappear from the muscle compartment via incorporation into muscle protein and release to the blood, and appear in the muscle compartment via uptake from the blood and protein degradation. A set of formula

is then used to calculate the net balance of the tracee (the amino acid that is being traced) and of the tracer. This gives two equations with protein synthesis and degradation as unknowns and these can, therefore, be calculated. It should be kept in mind though that tissues other than muscle (skin, bone, and adipose tissue) are present in arms and legs and significantly contribute to the indicated net balances. A limitation of the method is that the calculation of protein synthesis depends on the measurement of minimally four variables each with a confidence limit. The estimate of protein synthesis, therefore, tends to be less accurate and have a greater variance than with the incorporation method. The tissue net balance method also can only look at the total protein pool (muscle and other tissues) in the sampled compartment and not at synthesis and degradation rates of individual muscle proteins or subfractions. The methodologic and technical limitations of the tissue net balance and of later modifications of it (*e.g.*, the three pool model of Biolo et al. [15]) have been previously discussed in great detail (3).

Despite the indicated limitations in the methodologies involved, both methods have made significant contributions to our present insight in the control of MPS and degradation in humans in vivo (3,12,13).

Human Skeletal Muscle Proteins Have a Low Turnover Rate

Mixed muscle protein in overnight fasted humans has a turnover rate of 1.15% per day (Table 17.1). This is much lower than in tissues like liver and gut and 400 times lower than the value of very low density lipoprotein apo-B100, which is the protein with the highest reported turnover rate in humans. Subfractionation of muscle protein has shown that the myofibrillar proteins have the lowest turnover rates at close to 1% per day, whereas mitochondrial proteins and the cytosolic enzymes generally have slightly

TABLE 17.1	Fractional Protein Synthesis Rates (FSR) in Humans[a]	
	FSR (% per day)	Q_{wb} (%)[a]
Mixed muscle protein	1.15	29
Mitochondrial protein	2.50	—
Mixed liver protein	12.1	11
Plasma albumin	5–6	2.4
VLDL apo-B100	425	0.12

[a]Measured as the incorporation of a tracer labeled amino acid in the indicated protein fraction during a continuous intravenous infusion and calculated contributions of individual tissues to whole body protein turnover (Q_{wb}).

[b]Q_{wb} is assumed to be 280 g of protein per day.

VLDL, very low density lipoprotein.

The data in this table have originally been published by Wagenmakers (3). For details of the assumptions, calculations, and the literature sources, see Wagenmakers (3).

higher turnover rates (Table 17.1). It has particularly been speculated that important, key enzymes have higher protein turnover rates because relatively small changes in either protein synthesis or degradation in that case can lead to a rapid adjustment of the concentration of that enzyme in response to a physiologic stimulus and can, thus, contribute to metabolic regulation. A mean turnover rate of 1.15% per day for mixed muscle protein implies that in a 70-kg man with 7 kg of muscle protein, 70 g of muscle protein is being synthesized and degraded every day. This also implies that muscle, despite its enormous protein mass, contributes only about 30% to whole body protein turnover (estimated at 280 g per day; see Table 17.1).

TEST YOURSELF

Are these statements true?
1. All proteins in skeletal muscle have the same protein turnover rate.
2. There are proteins in the human body of which the entire protein pool is replaced with newly synthesized molecules within 6 hours.
Name an example of the latter.

Effects of Nutrition and Exercise on Muscle Protein Synthesis, Protein Degradation, and Net Balance

Diurnal Cycling of Protein Synthesis and Degradation

In a person in energy and protein balance, the muscle and whole body protein mass will be constant. In muscle, as in other tissues, there is, however, a diurnal cycle in the size of the protein pool with some protein being deposited in the feeding period (first shown by Rennie et al. [16]) and the same amount being lost during overnight fasting. The high plasma insulin concentration that is present in the postprandial state, especially after ingestion of a mixed protein-containing meal, in combination with increases in the intracellular concentration or arterial availability of the essential amino acids, stimulates protein synthesis and reduces protein degradation in tissues like muscle and liver (3,12,13,17–19). When we, on the basis of published data (3), assume that in the feeding period MPS is increased by about 10% to 20% and protein degradation reduced by 20%, then a quick calculation learns that between 7 g and 14 g of protein is deposited in the combined skeletal muscles in the feeding period. This is only 0.1% to 0.2% of the total amount of muscle protein. At whole body level estimates indicate that 35 g of protein is deposited in the feeding period on a normal protein intake (0.7 g · kg · day^{-1}) and 90 g on a high protein intake (2.5 g · kg · day^{-1}). Diurnal cycling in other words increases with protein intake. It is generally assumed that gut and liver are the main sites where these proteins are temporarily deposited, in part, as digestive enzymes and enzymes involved in amino acid oxidation and urea synthesis, following ingestion of protein-containing meals. Part of these enzymes concern digestive enzymes and liver enzymes involved in amino acid oxidation and urea synthesis, which become redundant in the postabsorptive state (3). It is assumed that breakdown of these splanchnic proteins in the overnight fasting period will make the meal derived amino acids more evenly available in the 24-hour period to other tissues like heart, kidney, brain, and muscle, such that these tissues will show only minimal changes in the size of the protein pool during the night.

TEST YOURSELF

A human individual is ingesting 200 g of protein per day, which is much more than the protein requirement. Part of the ingested protein is oxidized and part is incorporated into tissue proteins. Which tissue will take the majority of the incorporated protein?

Acute Effects of Resistance Exercise

The methodology in use to measure protein synthesis in humans only allows for the accurate detection of changes that are prolonged (>1 h) and do not involve rapid changes in pool size, amino acid enrichment, and protein turnover rates (3,13). This is the reason that today only a limited number of studies have attempted to estimate MPS rates during acute bouts of resistance exercise. Dreyer et al. (20) observed a 30% decrease during an acute bout of resistance exercise lasting 1 hour and performed in the overnight fasted state. Beelen et al. (21) extended the resistance exercise to a 2-hour period by using an intermittent protocol to obtain a more accurate value of MPS. During carbohydrate ingestion they observed an MPS that corresponded to a normal resting value, whereas the combined ingestion of carbohydrate and a protein hydrolysate increased the MPS by 30% during the resistance exercise bout in comparison to only carbohydrate.

Summary

Collectively, these data suggest that there are only small or no decreases in MPS during resistance exercise in humans in the fasted state, whereas amino acid or protein ingestion before the exercise bout increases MPS above basal rates.

Acute Effect of Endurance Exercise

Nineteenth century nitrogen balance studies failed to show increased protein oxidation.

In the 1840s, the German physiologist Von Liebig hypothesized that muscle protein was the main fuel used to achieve muscular contraction, which, of course, would imply that protein oxidation and net protein breakdown (degradation–synthesis) would substantially increase during exercise. As early as the 1870s this hypothesis was invalidated when nitrogen balance studies failed to show an increase in nitrogen losses during and following prolonged periods of heavy exercise (3). Also, in recent literature, most of the carefully controlled nitrogen balance studies in trained athletes show that only minimal increases in nitrogen loss occurs during prolonged dynamic exercise lasting 1 to 4 hours at intensities between 30% and 75% $\dot{V}O_{2max}$. Minor increases in nitrogen excretion (reflecting 5–10 g of protein oxidation) have only been observed when the glycogen stores had deliberately been emptied before the start of exercise.

Stable isotope tracer studies show a small decrease or no change in muscle protein synthesis rates during cycling and running

With the introduction of stable isotope amino acids, new techniques became available to investigate protein metabolism during exercise in man. Wolfe and colleagues (22) used L-[1-^{13}C]leucine as a tracer to follow whole body protein metabolism. Leucine flux and whole body protein degradation were similar at rest and during 1 hour of exercise at 30% $\dot{V}O_{2max}$, but leucine oxidation increased nearly threefold. Because flux equals synthesis plus oxidation in the mathematical whole body tracer model used (3), it was concluded that protein synthesis decreased during exercise. There was a discrepancy though with a second method used in this study. Whole body urea production estimated

from the dilution of isotopically labeled urea, which should increase when protein oxidation is increased, was exactly similar both at rest and during exercise. The increase in leucine oxidation seems to be specific for leucine only (3), and does not seem to point at a general increase in protein or amino acid oxidation during endurance exercise as originally assumed (22). Direct measurement of MPS by the same group (18) did not show a difference between a 4-hour rest period and 4 hours of treadmill running at 40% $\dot{V}O_{2max}$. The few direct MPS measurements that have been made during running and cycling in humans either show no change or a limited decrease (13).

KEY POINT

During endurance exercise, there is very little change or a slight decrease in whole muscle rates of protein synthesis in normal subjects.

Lessons from knee extensor kicking exercise and exercise in patients with McArdle's disease

There are two conditions in which the balance between MPS and protein breakdown is clearly negative during prolonged endurance exercise. Van Hall et al. (23) have investigated the exchange of amino acids during 90 minutes of one-leg knee extensor kicking exercise in trained human subjects and observed a 10-fold increase in the release of amino acids that are not transaminated or oxidized in muscle (phenylalanine, tyrosine, threonine, lysine, methionine, and glycine). This large change in amino acid net balance seems to indicate that protein synthesis must fall far below protein degradation. During one-leg knee extensor kicking exercise the workload and oxygen consumption per kg muscle is twofold to threefold higher than during normal cycling, implying that absolute intensity is much higher and the energy status is more likely to be disturbed as adenosine triphosphate (ATP) consumption may exceed ATP production. Another condition with an even larger imbalance between MPS and protein degradation is normal bicycling exercise in patients with McArdle's disease (1). These patients do not have access to muscle glycogen during exercise because they lack an active form of glycogen phosphorylase in muscle. In patients with McArdle's disease, there is convincing evidence that there is a massive energy disturbance in skeletal muscle that leads to excessive decreases in the ATP and creatine phosphate (CrP) concentration, and large increases both in adenosine monophosphate (AMP) concentration and AMP-activated protein kinase (AMPK) activity. Substantial parallel decreases in the muscle ATP and CrP content and in the MPS rate have also been observed by Bylund-Fellenius et al. (24) in rat hind leg muscles subjected to electrical stimulation. As explained in a later section, activation of AMPK is likely to inhibit mammalian target of rapamycin (mTOR) phosphorylation and have a negative impact on the MPS rate via this mechanism (24–27). Also, there are a number of steps in the protein synthesis process that are ATP dependent and that may slow down in muscles with a massive energy deficit.

Summary

Resistance exercise and endurance exercise in human beings lead to minimal energy disturbances in skeletal muscle and maintenance of the net protein balance, whereas in conditions in which fuel oxidation does not match the ATP turnover requirements (examples mentioned previously) the energy disturbance is large and protein synthesis falls far below the protein breakdown rate.

TEST YOURSELF

What are the mechanisms that lead to a decrease in protein synthesis during exercise in McArdle's disease and why is the decrease in protein synthesis only minimal during resistance and endurance exercise in healthy individuals?

Effects of Exercise and Nutrition on Protein Synthesis and Degradation in the Period after Resistance Exercise

Using the amino acid incorporation technique, two groups (28,29) have measured MPS rates after a single bout of resistance exercise in untrained subjects. Both observed substantial increases in MPS for periods of more than 24 hours. In one of the studies (28), the FSRs were measured during ingestion of a mixed protein-containing meal (in repeated boluses to assure maintenance of a tracer steady state) and in the other (29) in the fasted state. The highest increase in both studies was seen in the first 2 to 6 hours after exercise with the maximal values of fractional protein synthesis being about twofold to threefold higher than in the basal period before exercise. Phillips et al. (29) also reported increases in fractional protein degradation rates for more than 24 hours.

Several attempts have also been made to investigate whether amino acid ingestion or infusion or carbohydrate ingestion can further increase muscle protein anabolism in the postresistance exercise situation in placebo-controlled studies. Only the results of studies, that have used the amino acid incorporation technique to measure mixed MPS (as FSR) are summarized. Roy and colleagues (30) investigated the effect of glucose ingestion ($1 \text{ g} \cdot \text{kg}$) immediately and 1 hour after resistance exercise in comparison to a placebo control and observed a 36% increase over basal control values in MPS measured over the first 10 hours following exercise when glucose had been ingested. Biolo and colleagues (6) infused a balanced amino acid mixture ($0.15 \text{ g} \cdot \text{kg} \cdot \text{h}^{-1}$) in the 1- to 4-hour period following either rest or resistance exercise. In the basal postabsorptive state, MPS was 1.58% per day. This value increased to 2.40% per day and to 3.45% per day during the amino acid infusion in the rest trial and after resistance exercise respectively. Tipton and colleagues (31) have measured MPS over a 24-hour period in a study with a complex design involving two trials. In the first trial the subjects were resting throughout the day, in the second trial they performed a bout of resistance exercise at noon (6 hours after the start of the study) while ingesting 15 g of an essential amino acid supplement both immediately before and after the exercise bout. In both trials, they also ingested a mixed protein-containing meal 2 to 3 hours before the time of the exercise bout and a second mixed protein-containing meal in repeated boluses (to assure a tracer steady state) in a 2-hour period about 5 to 7 hours after exercise. MPS rates were found to be higher in the exercise trial in three periods:

1. In the period involving the first meal, the exercise bout and the intake of the essential amino acid supplements (1.40% vs. 1.14% per day);
2. During the 2-hour period of ingestion of the second meal (4.51% vs. 1.82% per day); and
3. During the night following ingestion of the second meal (1.70% vs. 1.32% per day).

The majority of these studies seem to suggest that the ingestion of a mixed protein-containing meal is required to increase FSRs to maximal values and these go as high as 200% to 400% of the normal postabsorptive control value of 1.15% per day. This conclusion also is confirmed by a number of recent leg balance studies of the Wolfe group (32). However, some of the conclusions of these studies may be a bit unsecure because they investigated the effect of the oral ingestion of boluses of drinks containing amino acids or amino acid/carbohydrate mixtures. The use of bolus feedings implies that there are no proper steady-state conditions and, in that case, failure to correct for changes in the concentration or enrichment of amino acids in the blood and muscle pool will bias the results. For this reason, some of the messages and conclusions—for example, on the optimal timing and composition of the amino acid/protein/carbohydrate drinks to be taken after exercise for an optimal anabolic effect—are waiting for confirmation by studies using a more pertinent methodology.

KEY POINT

After resistance exercise there is a simultaneous increase in both protein synthesis and degradation that lasts for >24 hours after exercise.

Many studies in humans have been performed in the fasted state and it is now generally agreed that one bout of resistance exercise in that case results in 40% to150% increases in MPS rates with significant increases still being present until 48 hours after the exercise (13,17–19). A study by Wilkinson et al. (14) has shown that the stimulation of MPS by resistance exercise occurs in both the myofibrillar and mitochondrial fraction in untrained subjects, but only in the myofibrillar fraction when the untrained subjects have participated in a 10-week resistance exercise training program. The physiologic meaning of this observation is not clear. Despite a marked increase in MPS in the fasted state, muscle net protein balance remains negative due to a simultaneous increase in muscle protein degradation (17,29) and, therefore, it is not entirely clear to the author of this chapter what the physiologic meaning of the increased MPS rate after resistance exercise in the fasted state is and whether the size of this increase is a measure of the anabolic effect that is observed when resistance exercise is combined with a mixed meal or protein ingestion in the postexercise period. As explained previously, when amino acid availability is increased in the period after resistance exercise either via intravenous infusion or oral ingestion, there are larger increases in MPS than in muscles that have been resting. As muscle protein breakdown rates are suppressed when the resistance exercise is combined with exogenous amino acids this then leads to a period of net protein deposition after each resistance exercise bout of a training session. It is assumed that the largest benefit of this extra anabolic effect of exogenous amino acid ingestion is present in the first 6 to 8 hours after the exercise bout, although hard evidence to support this claim is currently lacking.

TEST YOURSELF

What would be the difference in results (in terms of changes in MPS) if you measured MPS after resistance exercise in the fasted versus fed state (in your answer consider food intake before, during, and after exercise)?

Effects of Exercise and Nutrition on Protein Synthesis and Degradation Rates after Endurance Exercise

All measurements of MPS (measured as FSR) made during recovery from endurance exercise have been made in the overnight fasted state. Carraro et al. (33) observed a significant 30% increase in mixed MPS rates during 4 hours of recovery from 4 hours of treadmill running at 40% $\dot{V}O_{2max}$. A few other studies (18) either do not show increases or used amino acid incorporation periods of <1 hour, which

are unlikely to generate solid data. Wilkinson et al. (14) measured the FSR in the muscle mitochondrial and myofibrillar protein fraction and observed a 200% increase in the mitochondrial fraction and no increase in the myofibrillar fraction during the 1- to 4-hour recovery period after 45 minutes of single leg cycling at 75% $\dot{V}O_{2max}$. The latter observation is extremely important because, in response to endurance exercise training, there is not an increase in total muscle protein mass, but a selective increase in the mitochondrial density and protein content. The observation made by Wilkinson et al. (14) suggests that increases in protein synthesis following an acute bout of endurance exercise are entirely restricted to the mitochondrial protein fraction. As this was the case both in the untrained state and after 10 weeks of endurance training, the study suggests that such increases occur after each session in a 10-week training period and that the sum of the increases in mitochondrial content at the end of the training result in the well-known increases in $\dot{V}O_{2max}$ and the performance benefits of endurance exercise (8,9). The increase in mixed MPS observed by Carraro et al. (33) during recovery from 4 hours of treadmill running most likely is fully accountable by the large increase in the synthesis rate of mitochondrial protein. Information on the effects of meal or protein ingestion on the increase in FSR of the mitochondrial protein regretfully is not available to the best of the author's knowledge.

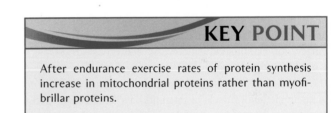

KEY POINT

After endurance exercise rates of protein synthesis increase in mitochondrial proteins rather than myofibrillar proteins.

Age- and Disease-related Changes in the Regulation of Muscle Protein Metabolism by Exercise and Nutrients

A reduced physical activity with increasing age plays an important role in the mechanisms that lead to sarcopenia and loss of oxidative capacity (mitochondrial density) in elderly individuals. Elderly individuals tend to avoid weight-bearing exercise, implying that they miss regular exposure to the anabolic stimulus of resistance exercise in comparison to young adults. They also tend to avoid walking and cycling, implying that they miss a regular increase in the expression of mitochondrial enzymes that is required to maintain mitochondrial biogenesis and density (34). A less than optimal protein content of the diet has also been suggested to contribute to the age-related loss of muscle mass (19,35).

Early studies reported decreased basal mixed MPS rates in the elderly compared to young subjects. There, however, seems to be consensus now (13,19,36) that basal mixed MPS are normal. However, many recent publications have shown that the anabolic response to meal ingestion is blunted leading to reduced increases in MPS and reduced suppression of muscle protein degradation (13,19). The resultant continuous small reduction in muscle protein accretion in the period following meal ingestion is currently suggested to be the major cause of sarcopenia. Although there are suggestions that single bouts of exercise (37) and resistance training (38) have beneficial effects in elderly individuals, Kumar et al. (39) have suggested that the response of elderly individuals to resistance exercise is blunted in the fasted state and leads to smaller increases in MPS in the postexercise period in the elderly compared to the young.

Disuse and bed rest make substantial contributions to the muscle atrophy that occurs in patients with chronic disease and cachexia mentioned in the introduction. In many of these diseases, the imbalance between protein synthesis and protein degradation is much larger than in elderly individuals and leads to a much more rapid loss of muscle mass and strength. The molecular mechanisms are discussed in the following sections.

Biochemical Pathways, Signals, and Signaling Cascades that Control MPS

The biochemical pathways by which mRNAs are translated into proteins and their control by signaling events and cascades have primarily been identified in a large variety of established eukaryotic cell lines (26,40–42). Kimball and colleagues (47) were the first to investigate the regulation of these pathways by hormones and amino acids in skeletal muscle of rats and have contributed most to the early insights into the role of nutrition in the control of MPS. The groups of Esser (43–45) and Jefferson and Farrell (25,46,47) and several others performed early study in rats investigating the acute effects of exercise and the anabolic effect of resistance exercise in the postexercise period and generated pioneering information on the anabolic signaling pathways. An exponential growth has occurred in the last 5 to 6 years in the number of human studies making parallel measurements of MPS rates and activation of the anabolic signaling routes and these have complemented our current insight in the molecular mechanisms regulating protein synthesis. For exhaustive review of the latter the interested reader is referred to a series of recent reviews by the leading laboratories in the field published in the *Journal of Applied Physiology* (48).

The Three Phases of Protein Synthesis (Translation of mRNA)

Translation of mRNA into proteins can be divided into three phases: initiation, elongation, and termination. Initiation and elongation are the main regulatory sites. Together they control the translation rate in response to most physiologic stimuli. The process of translation initiation (Fig. 17.1) occurs via a series of discrete steps and is mediated by a dozen proteins referred to as eukaryotic initiation factors (eIFs). The end result of the process is the assembly of a translationally competent ribosome at the AUG start site near the 5′ end of the mRNA. Translation initiation can be functionally divided into three stages:

1. The binding of initiator methionyl-tRNA° to the 40S ribosomal subunit to form the 43S preinitiation complex;
2. The binding of the mRNA capped with eIF4E, eIF4A, and eIF4G to the 43S preinitiation complex to form the 48S preinitiation complex; and
3. The binding of the 60S ribosomal subunit to the 48S preinitiation complex to form the active 80S initiation complex (Fig. 17.1).

In each of these steps some of the involved eIFS can be phosphorylated by regulatory kinases leading either to an increased or decreased formation rate of translationally competent ribosomes.

In the elongation phase of mRNA translation the polypeptide is assembled. This phase consumes a substantial amount of metabolic energy with at least four high energy bonds being consumed for each amino acid added to the nascent peptide chain (26,40,41). Translation elongation is mediated by a set of nonribosomal proteins called eukaryotic elongation factors or eEFs. Several of the eEFs can also be phosphorylated—among them are eEF1A and eEF1B, which are activated by phosphorylation and are involved in the recruitment of amino acyl-tRNAs to the ribosome, and eEF2, which mediates ribosomal translocation along the mRNA and is inhibited by phosphorylation (26).

Role of Nutrients and Hormones in the Translational Control of MPS

Hormones and amino acids are among the major signals that modulate the involved kinases and phosphatases that control protein synthesis. Insulin and insulin-like growth factor 1 (IGF-1) were first shown to stimulate protein synthesis via their action on key signaling molecules downstream of phosphatidylinositol-3-kinase (PI-3 kinase) and protein kinase B (PKB or Akt) in the insulin-signaling cascade. An important finding was that the rapamycin-sensitive mTOR signaling pathway played an important role further downstream in the control of translation by insulin and IGF-1 (40,47). Insulin and IGF-1 via mTOR activation among others stimulate the phosphorylation state of the eIF4E binding protein 1 (4E-BP1) and of ribosomal protein S6 kinase (p70^{S6K}). 4E-BP1 binds to eIF4E, thereby reducing its availability for the capping of the mRNA (Fig. 17.1) and formation of the 48S preinitiation complex. Phosphorylation of 4E-BP1 prevents its binding to eIF4E and thereby enhances formation of the mRNA complex capped with eIF4E, eIF4A, and eIF4G and thus accelerates

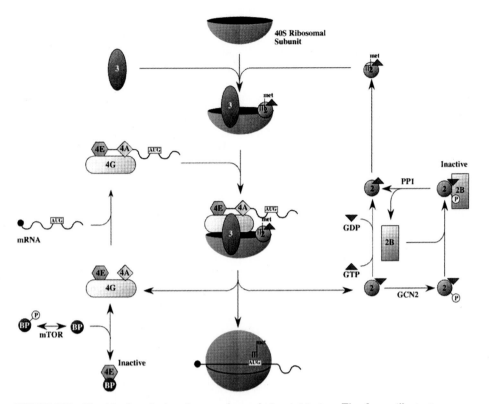

FIGURE 17.1   The biochemical pathways of translation initiation. The figure illustrates the three stages of translation initiation that have been explained in the text (binding of methionyl-tRNA$_i$ [met] to the 40S ribosomal subunit, followed by binding of the messenger ribonucleic acid [mRNA], and finally binding of the 60S ribosomal subunit). The translation initiation factors that participate in the individual stages are depicted as different geometric shapes and are labeled with a number or number and letter on the basis of the identity of the factor. For example, eukaryotic initiation factor (eIF) eIF4E is depicted as a hexagon with the label 4E in the center of the shape. In addition, the regulation of eIF2B activity by phosphorylation of the α-subunit of eIF2 and the sequestration of eIF4E by eIF4E binding protein-1 (4E-BP1) are illustrated. eIF2B is the protein that recharges the eIF2-guanosine diphosphate (GDP) complex with guanosine triphosphate (GTP), such that the eIF2B-guanosine triphosphate (GTP) complex can bind to a new molecule of met-tRNA$_i$ and start a new initiation cycle. Phosphorylation of 4E-BP1 by the mTOR (mammalian target of rapamycin) signaling pathway (see text for details) prevents its binding to eIF4E and thus enhances the capping of the mRNA with the relevant eIF4s. AUG (the nucleoside triplet adenosine, uridine, guanosine) is encoding for the start site of translation of the mRNA. GCN2, general control nonderepressing eIF2a protein kinase 2. (This figure was originally published by Kimball and colleagues [47]. We thank Dr. Kimball and the American Physiological Society for permission to use it.)

the formation of translationally competent ribosomes and polyribosomes. p70^{S6k} is a kinase that acts upon protein S6 of the small ribosomal subunit. Phosphorylation of S6 has been shown to switch on a mechanism that allows the preferential initiation and translation of a set of mRNA termed the 5′-TOP (tract of oligopyrimidine) (40,41) that, among others, includes those encoding for each of the ribosomal proteins and for eEF1A and eEF2 (25,40,41). Via this mechanism, refeeding of fasted rats (34) rapidly increases the concentration of ribosomal subunits (both proteins and rRNA) and eEFs and thus regenerates the capacity of the protein synthetic machinery that is reduced during prolonged fasting. Insulin stimulated and IGF-1 stimulated

phosphorylation of p70^{S6k} also results in suppression of the activity of the kinase that phosphorylates eEF2 (26) and, via this mechanism, is able to increase elongation rates independent of increases in the capacity of the protein synthetic machinery.

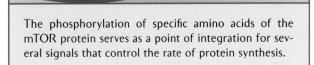

KEY POINT

The phosphorylation of specific amino acids of the mTOR protein serves as a point of integration for several signals that control the rate of protein synthesis.

The following important observation was that amino acids, and particularly leucine, also are able to activate mTOR via an insulin independent mechanism. Amino acids can thus directly cause phosphorylation of 4E-BP1 and p70^{S6K} but in muscle this seems to require the presence of a minimal amount of insulin (47). It has also been shown that activation of PKB/Akt and insulin are not able to phosphorylate and activate mTOR in muscle cells that are deprived of amino acids (40). Therefore, phosphorylation of mTOR seems to represent an important point of integration of the signals arising from insulin, IGF-1, and amino acids (Fig. 17.2). It seems at this point that the fine-tuning occurs of the control of the rate of initiation (which determines the proportion of ribosomes attached to mRNAs), the rate of elongation (efficiency of translation), and of the rate of synthesis of ribosomal proteins and eEFs (upgrading the capacity of the protein synthetic machinery).

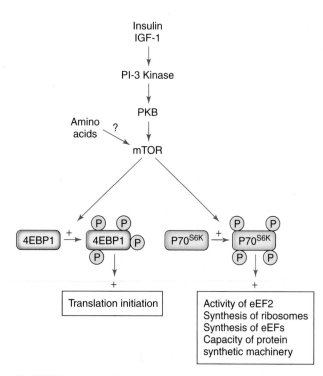

FIGURE 17.2 Signal transduction pathways leading to hyperphosphorylation of eIF-4E binding protein-1 (eIF-4E) binding protein-1 (4E-BP1) and p70^{S6k}. Hyperphosphorylation of 4E-BP1 leads to increased formation rates of translationally competent polyribosomes (see Fig. 17.1). Hyperphosphorylation of ribosomal protein S6 kinase (p70^{S6k}) activates this kinase and leads to phosphorylation of the ribosomal protein S6. As a consequence, S6 will select the messenger ribonucleic acids (mRNAs) encoding for the ribosomal proteins and for eukaryotic elongation factors (eEFs) for preferential translation, thus, increasing the synthesis of ribosomes, the capacity for recruitment of aminoacyl-tRNAs to the mRNA and for translocation of ribosomes along the mRNA. This increase in the overall capacity of the protein synthetic machinery is estimated to take at least 1 or 2 hours as these proteins first have to be synthesized. Hyperphosphorylation of p70^{S6k} also results in suppression of the activity of the kinase that phosphorylates and inactivates eEF2 and via this mechanism is able to increase elongation rates instantaneously independent of time-dependent increases in the capacity of the protein synthetic machinery.

Role of Exercise in the Translational Control of Protein Synthesis in Skeletal Muscle

Acute effects of resistance exercise on the main anabolic signals during exercise

Bylund-Fellenius et al. (24) subjected rat hind leg muscles to electrical stimulation via the sciatic nerve for 10 minutes. The procedure led to maximal isometric contractions and resulted in substantial decreases both in the muscle ATP and CrP content and in the MPS rate compared to the resting situation. Clear evidence has been obtained in many cultured cell types that an acute energy deficit down-regulates the activity of kinases that play a crucial role in both translation initiation (40–42) and elongation (26,40,41). AICAR (5-aminoimidazole-4-carboxamide 1-β-D-ribonucleoside) is an organic compound that is taken up by most cell types and converted to an analogue of AMP, thereby activating AMPK. Addition of AICAR to hepatocytes (26) gave rise to a rapid and robust increase in the phosphorylation state of eEF2 and acutely down-regulated the translation elongation rate. Bolster and colleagues (25) injected rats with AICAR and this doubled the activity of AMPK in skeletal muscle by 51% and reduced the MPS rate to less than half. Substantial parallel reductions were also seen in the phosphorylation status (main activation sites) of PKB/Akt, mTOR, p70^{S6k}, and 4E-BP1.

Three human studies have investigated the acute effect of resistance exercise on the anabolic signals in human muscle sampled immediately after exercise. Dreyer et al. (20) observed a 75% increase in AMPK enzyme activity, no change in PKB/Akt and mTOR phosphorylation, a 30% reduction in 4E-BP1 phosphorylation, a nonsignificant 20% increase in eEF2 phosphorylation (note phosphorylation leads to inactivation of this enzyme), and a nonsignificant doubling of p70^{S6K} phosphorylation at threonine (Thr) 389. (It should be noted that p70^{S6K} has several phosphorylation sites and that not all human studies have measured the same site. Thr 389 is the main mTOR activation site of the enzyme and is measured in most studies. Phosphorylation at Thr 421 and serine [Ser] 424 is required for altering the conformation of p70^{S6K} and making Thr 389 available for phosphorylation by mTOR, thereby fully activating the enzyme [49].) Dreyer et al. (20) suggested that the reduction in 4EBP1 phosphorylation explained the observed 30% decrease in MPS during the 1-hour resistance exercise period. Koopman et al. (50) observed a 300% increase in AMPK phosphorylation, a 75% decrease in 4E-BP1 phosphorylation, a twofold increase in Thr 421/Ser 424 phosphorylation of p70^{S6K} (that is the conformational change required to make the enzyme accessible to mTOR), and a threefold nonsignificant increase in S6 phosphorylation. Deldicque et al. (49) observed a 60% to 90% down-regulation of PKB/Akt and 4EBP1 phosphorylation, a decrease in Thr 389 phosphorylation of p70^{S6K}, and a 20-fold increase in Thr 421/Ser 424 phosphorylation of p70[S6K].

Despite the large variation in the reported anabolic signaling events, collectively, the rat and human studies seem to lead to a number of firm conclusions. The first is that activation of AMPK during resistance exercise reduces 4E-BP1 phosphorylation and that this, via its inhibiting effect on translation initiation, might lead to a small reduction in mixed MPS as observed by Dreyer et al. (20) in a 1-hour protocol. However, Beelen et al. (21) in an intermittent and, therefore, less intense 2-hour exercise protocol did not observe a decrease in mixed MPS, so this decrease in MPS is not always present. The electrical stimulation protocol used in rats by Bylund-Fellenius et al. (24) leads to much larger decreases in muscle ATP and CrP than routinely observed in human resistance exercise protocols. Such a large energy deficit may well lead to a shut down of the energy demanding protein synthetic machinery in skeletal muscle via a dual mechanism involving both reduced 4E-BP1 phosphorylation (reducing translation initiation) and increased eEF2 phosphorylation (reducing translation elongation). This latter dual molecular mechanism may also be responsible for the large imbalance between MPS and protein degradation observed during one leg knee extensor kicking exercise in healthy individuals (23) and during dynamic cycling exercise in patients with McArdle's disease (1)—conditions that are both known to lead to large energy deficits and increased AMPK activation (1–3).

Finally, two of the human studies (49,50) observe that resistance exercise leads to Thr 421/Ser 424 phosphorylation of p70[S6K]. This phosphorylation event is known to alter the conformation of the enzyme and make Thr 389 available for phosphorylation and activation by mTOR. This implies that at the end of the resistance exercise bout p70[S6K] is ready for mTOR activation as soon as mTOR itself is activated by food intake or amino acid ingestion (see next section).

Summary

During resistance exercise of a high intensity, leading to AMPK activation, there is a decrease in MPS. The mechanism behind this decrease in MPS is that the AMPK activation leads to a shut down of the energy demanding protein synthetic machinery in skeletal muscle via a dual mechanism involving both reduced 4E-BP1 phosphorylation (reducing translation initiation) and increased eEF2 phosphorylation (reducing translation elongation). During resistance exercise p70[S6K] is phosphorylated on the Thr 421/Ser 424 residues. This phosphorylation event is known to alter the three-dimensional structure of the enzyme and make Thr 389 available for phosphorylation and activation by mTOR. This implies that, as soon as mTOR is activated by protein or food intake in the period after the exercise (see next section), there will be an extra increase in protein synthesis which explains, at least in part (see end of next section), the anabolic effect of resistance exercise.

Effects of resistance exercise and nutrient intake on anabolic signals in the postexercise period

The early observation in humans that MPS rates (FSR) are increased for periods as long as 48 hours after a single acute bout of resistance exercise (28,29) has led to an intense search for the underlying molecular mechanism. The first muscle studies measuring candidate signaling intermediates that might be in control of the increased anabolic response used rat models of resistance exercise. Baar and Esser (43) used an intermittent high frequency electrical stimulation protocol to create high intensity lengthening contractions of the extensor digitorum longus (EDL) and tibialis anterior (TA) muscles. This protocol, in a 6-week training program, led to 14% increase in wet mass of the EDL and TA, 7% in the plantaris, and no change in the soleus. The protocol was also used to study the effect of a single bout of exercise covering the 0- to 36- hour period after exercise with the rats having free access to food before and after but not during the stimulation protocol. Six hours after a single exercise bout, there was a massive increase in the fraction of the muscle RNA that was present in the polyribosome fraction (in comparison to rested muscle in the other leg) indicating that more translationally competent (poly)ribosomes had been formed and were actually synthesizing proteins. This observation was restricted to the muscles that showed hypertrophy in the training study. Baar and Esser (43) also measured the enzyme activity of p70[S6K] in the muscles. It was increased substantially at the end of the exercise bout and rose to maximal values (similar to those seen following insulin stimulation) 3 and 6 hours after exercise and remained increased far above resting control levels at 36 hours, that is for a period as long as the anabolic effect of resistance exercise is known to last in untrained humans. Again this observation was restricted to the muscles that showed hypertrophy in the training protocol and the degree of p70[S6K] phosphorylation after 6 hours was proportional to the size of the hypertrophy. To investigate whether this increase in p70[S6K] was of functional significance, Chen et al. (44) using the same exercise model isolated the polyribosome fraction and showed that the mRNA encoding for elongation factor EF1A (one of the 5′-TOP mRNAs known to be selected for translation by phosphorylated ribosomal protein S6) was preferentially translated 6 hours after exercise (Fig. 17.3).

Kimball, Jefferson, Farrell, and colleagues (25,46,47) have used another model of resistance exercise in which rats repeatedly lift a weight carried in a backpack while standing on their hind legs. The time course of mixed MPS rates, enzyme activities of PI3-kinase activity, and p70[S6k] all failed to show changes 1 and 3 hours after exercise. PI3-kinase activity (sevenfold) and p70[S6k] activity (threefold) were significantly increased 6 hours after exercise and remained elevated until 24 hours, whereas protein synthesis rates were only increased by about 25% 12 and 24 hours after exercise. Hernandez et al. (30) therefore concluded that there was an exercise effect on protein synthesis in this model, but that there was a delay of at least 12 hours

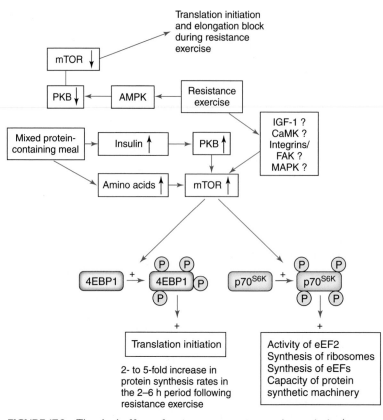

FIGURE 17.3 The dual effect of resistance exercise on the anabolic (protein kinase B (PKB/Akt)-mammalian target of rapamycin (mTOR) signaling pathway and muscle protein synthesis (MPS). During resistance exercise the PKB/Akt-mTOR signaling pathway is inhibited by AMP-activated protein kinase (AMPK) leading to a fall in MPS, but 10–20 minutes after resistance exercise this inhibition is relieved and is changing into an activation (see text for details). The largest increases in protein synthesis after resistance exercise are seen in the 2- to 7-hour period when a mixed protein-containing meal is ingested. IGF-1, insulin-like growth factor 1; CaMK, calcium/calmodulin-dependent protein kinase; FAK, focal adhesion kinase; MAPK, mitogen-activated protein kinase; 4EBP1, eIF-4E binding protein-1; p70^{S6K}, ribosomal protein S6 kinase; eEF2, eukaryotic elongation factor 2.

before it became effective. However, as protein synthesis rates were routinely made in this study after 5 hours of fasting, the data may also imply that food intake is required as an additional stimulus to switch the anabolic exercise signals on and increase MPS rates. Because of the nutritional design chosen the animals that were studied 1 and 3 hours after exercise did not receive food before and after exercise, whereas the 6-hour animals had free access to food before exercise and for 1 hour after exercise. The animals, studied 12 and 24 hours after exercise, had free access to food both before exercise and for 7 hours and 19 hours after exercise.

In another recent study of the same group (51), using the same exercise model, the rats were fasted for 5 to 8 hours before exercise and in the hour after exercise. A brief transient increase was seen in the hour after exercise in the phosphorylation state of PKB/Akt, mTOR, 4E-BP1, p70^{S6k}, and ribosomal protein S6. The increase was not present at the end of exercise, was maximal in the 10- to 20-minute period, and had returned for most signaling intermediates to control levels after 60 minutes. The difference in time course and degree of activation (phosphorylation) of p70^{S6K} between this study and those of Baar and Esser (43) in which the animals had free access to food before and immediately after exercise is striking.

TEST YOURSELF

Based on the information presented, predict the change in the state of phosphorylation of 4EBP1 and eEF2 2 to 4 hours after a single bout of resistance exercise in the fed state.

KEY POINT

Access to food after resistance exercise is critical to prolonged increases in rates of protein synthesis in the recovery period.

Collectively, the rat studies seem to suggest that food should be ingested before and after the resistance exercise to bring PI3-kinase and p70[S6K] in the activated (phosphorylated) form in the period after resistance exercise and to keep them in the activated form for 24 to 36 hours after the resistance exercise.

The information on signaling events in the human studies is somewhat confusing because the majority of the studies have been done in the fasted state and show increases in MPS in contrast to the observations made by Hernandez et al. (46). However, as explained before, also in the human studies, maximal increases in mixed MPS only occur after the intake of amino acids or complete meals and, in that case, the effects remain for periods up to 24 hours (28,31). Although Phillips et al. (29) made the MPS measurements at 24 and 48 hours in the fasted state, meals had been taken in the intervening periods and increases in MPS were still present after 48 hours. Deldicque et al. (49) took a muscle biopsy in the fasted state 24 hours after one bout of resistance exercise, while their subjects had eaten a complete set of meals on the first day after the exercise bout. There was still a 10-fold increase in Thr 421/Ser 424 phosphorylation of p70[S6K] implying that the enzyme remained in the conformation that could be activated by mTOR whenever food or amino acids were taken in the postexercise period. Glover et al. (52) combined resistance exercise in one leg with ingestion of a small mixed meal and observed that the meal increased the phosphorylation of PKB/Akt in both legs (rest and exercised) and the exercise increased phosphorylation of PKB/Akt, Thr 389 of p70[S6K], and ribosomal protein S6 with the largest increases seen in the exercised leg during feeding. No increases in mTOR neither by feeding or exercise were observed in this study (52). Larger increases in mTOR phosphorylation in combination with increased phosphorylation of p70[S6K] and ribosomal protein S6 have also been observed in human studies when branched-chain amino acid (BCAA) ingestion was combined with resistance exercise (53). These observations are in striking contrast to human studies performed in the fasted state in which MPS and small increases in Thr 389 phosphorylation of p70[S6K] often return to resting levels within 3 to 4 hours after the resistance exercise bout (13).

Summary

The combined rat and human data both on increases in postexercise MPS and activation of the anabolic signaling intermediates seem to suggest that resistance exercise preactivates p70[S6K] via Thr 421/Ser 473 phosphorylation and that a full mixed meal or essential amino acids should then be taken (either before, during, or immediately after the resistance exercise bout) to activate PI3-kinase and mTOR and lead to full activation of p70[S6K] via Thr 389 phosphorylation. At this moment, it is highly unlikely that this is the full molecular mechanism as information on the time course of activation—for example, of 4E-BP1 and eEF2 after resistance exercise in the fed state—is lacking and it is clear that initiation, elongation, and ribosome synthesis should all increase in parallel to achieve maximal MPS rates. We also should not forget that after a single bout of resistance and endurance exercise, there is the well-known increase in insulin-stimulated glucose uptake that also lasts for about 48 hours in humans and has been suggested to be at least, in part, the consequence of increased activation of the insulin signaling cascade (14).

Acute effects of endurance exercise on anabolic signals in muscle

No clear picture emerges from the few studies that have measured the anabolic signaling intermediates during dynamic endurance exercise. The relevance of the repeated observation of Rose and Richter (27) that the phosphorylation of eEF2 increases during endurance exercise is not clear as it has not been related to MPS rates measured simultaneously. Furthermore, several other laboratories have failed to observe decreases in MPS during endurance exercise.

Effects of endurance exercise on anabolic signals in the postexercise period

The most important adaptation in the first hours after endurance exercise is the upregulation of transcription factors that control the expression of genes encoding for mitochondrial proteins. This will be followed in the 2- to 24-hour period after endurance exercise by increases in mRNAs that encode for the mitochondrial enzymes (34). Due to a rapid increase in the relative contribution of these mRNAs to the total mRNA pool, there will be an increased synthesis rate of the mitochondrial enzymes whenever a protein-containing meal is consumed in the period that these mRNA are present in a high concentration. Today it is not known whether there are molecular mechanisms to preferentially select the mRNAs encoding for the mitochondrial proteins for translation. The observation of Rose and Richter (27) that the phosphorylation of eEF2 is reduced immediately after endurance exercise is very important, because it otherwise might prevent translation of the mRNA encoding for the mitochondrial enzymes.

Effects of functional overload and disuse

Bodine et al. (70) provided clear evidence that the PKB/Akt-mTOR pathway also plays a major role in the muscle hypertrophy that is caused by chronic functional overloading and that repression of the pathway leads to muscle atrophy. They created a functional overload of the plantaris muscle in rats by synergist ablation. After

14 days this resulted in a substantial muscle hypertrophy. The amount of PKB/Akt, and the phosphorylation status of PKB/Akt, 4E-BP1, and p70^{S6k} were markedly increased after 14 days. The effects were achieved via the mTOR signaling pathway as rapamycin could reverse the increase in phosphorylation status of 4E-BP1 and p70^{S6k} and severely blunt the hypertrophy. Unloading of the plantaris via hind limb suspension (a model of disuse) after 14 days caused a decreased phosphorylation of PKB/Akt and p70^{S6k} and an increase in 4E-BP1–eIF4E complex assembly thus inhibiting capping of the mRNA with the relevant eIF4s. The role of the PKB/Akt-mTOR signaling route in the development of muscle hypertrophy was also demonstrated by overexpression of PKB/Akt by plasmid DNA injection. Such treatment caused muscle hypertrophy in adult mice and blunted the atrophy seen during hind limb suspension.

The anabolic signals in aging and chronic disease and the effects of exercise upon it

Several studies (13,18,36) have provided convincing evidence that blunting occurs of the signals of insulin, IGF-1, and amino acids in the muscle of elderly compared to young human muscles. It has also been observed that, in order to achieve an anabolic effect of resistance exercise, the timing of the food ingestion after exercise should start earlier after exercise in elderly individuals than in young adults (54). Old muscles have also been suggested to have a reduced capacity to produce the muscle-specific isomers of IGF-1 in response to high-intensity contractions, a local anabolic hormone that may play an important role in the anabolic effect of resistance exercise, and decrease in the capacity of the muscle for regeneration after damage or periods of disuse. There is only one published but convincing study that observed that one single bout of aerobic exercise was able to restore the impaired response to insulin of the phosphorylation of anabolic signaling intermediates (PKB, mTOR, 4EBP1, and p70^{S6k}) and the MPR in parallel in elderly individuals (37). Although this result is extremely promising, the conclusion is that we need more research to investigate the potential of various modes and intensities of exercise and of training intervention programs to restore the anabolic responsiveness of the muscle of elderly individuals.

Summary

The PKB/Akt-mTOR pathway plays a major role in muscle hypertrophy resulting from functional overload, whereas hind limb suspension as model of inactivity (disuse) suppresses this pathway. In elderly individuals, the anabolic signals of insulin and amino acids on the PKB/Akt-mTOR signaling pathway and protein synthesis are blunted, but there is limited early evidence that only one bout of endurance type exercise may restore these anabolic signals.

Biochemical Pathways, Signals, and Signaling Cascades that Control Muscle Protein Degradation

Proteins in skeletal muscle undergo a continuous cycle of synthesis and degradation (protein turnover), which regulates both the overall protein mass and the levels of specific proteins. Increased rates of protein degradation, among others, contribute to the muscle wasting seen with fasting and in many pathologic states. Despite potentially being equal in importance in the control exerted on protein quantity and quality, we are just beginning to unravel the pathways, signal routes, and mechanisms that regulate protein degradation (6,55–62).

Like other mammalian tissues, skeletal muscle contains multiple proteolytic systems. The lysosomal, calcium ion (Ca^{2+})-activated, and ubiquitin-proteasome–dependent pathways have the highest enzyme activities and are quantitatively the most important in the daily response to nutrients, hormones, and exercise and also seem to control the selection of proteins for degradation.

The Lysosomal/Autophagy Pathway

The historically best-known proteolytic system is the lysosomal pathway. Lysosomes are vacuolar organelles surrounded by a membrane. They are particularly abundant in liver and are able to create an internal milieu with a low pH. They contain a variety of enzymes that have a maximum activity at low pH and that play a role in the clearance not only of proteins but also of other macromolecules (glycogen, RNA, DNA). Lysosomes collaborate with autophagosomes in the removal of long-lived proteins, macromolecular aggregates, and damaged intracellular organelles. Autophagosomes themselves also are membrane-surrounded structures and, because they have a limited degrading capacity, they rely on fusion with lysosomes for protein degradation to occur. As skeletal muscle only contains a relatively low number of lysosomes, it has been assumed for a long time that the major lysosomal proteinases (cathepsins B, H, L, and D) did not play a role of significance in skeletal muscle proteolysis (55,56,63). However, thorough microarray analyses by Lecker et al. (58) have identified a set of atrophy-specific genes ("atrogenes") that were upregulated in four mouse and rat models characterized by rapid muscle atrophy (starvation, cancer, type 2 diabetes, and kidney failure). The identified atrogenes were commonly expressed in all these conditions and, among others, encompassed cathepsin L, all the proteins important for autophagy, and the ubiquitin ligases MAFbx/atrogin-1 and MURF, which are critical for the rate of ubiquitin-proteasome proteolysis. Coordinated expression of these atrogenes seems to suggest that the two systems collaborate in the breakdown of damaged proteins in conditions characterized by disuse and disease and rapid muscle atrophy. It has subsequently been discovered that skeletal muscle constitutively contains unusually small autophagosomes that had not been recognized before (62). Two recent papers (59,61) have now provided hard evidence that forkhead box subgroup O (FoxO) transcription factors are essential for muscle atrophy. Activation of FoxO3 using molecular techniques (gain of function and loss of function approaches) caused dramatic atrophy of cultured myotubes and muscles via transcription of the full set of atrogenes. Today, it is not known whether autophagy plays a role of significance in the degradation of myofibrillar, mitochondrial, or other protein fractions in healthy physically active individuals, but this without doubt will be a priority area for future research.

calpain degradation and that the processing of protein kinase C is controlled by calpains, implying that the programmed activation of calpains has a role in modulating the activity of the insulin signaling cascade (1). Calpains also play key roles in the disassembly of sarcomeric proteins (actin, myosin, nebulin, titin, troponin, and tropomyosin) and in Z-band disintegration (55,56,63,64). Our knowledge of the physiologic role of the calpains and their control by nutrients and hormones regretfully still is in its infancy and the effect of exercise and training are not known at all. Proteins that have undergone limited proteolysis by calpains most likely subsequently undergo complete hydrolysis in muscle by the ubiquitin-proteasome and the lysosomal/autophagy systems (55,56,63,64).

Summary

Until recently, it was assumed that the lysosomal/autophagy pathway was not important in skeletal muscle because the number of lysosomes is much smaller than in other tissues like liver. However, gene expression microarray analysis has now shown that the expression of most lysosomal and atrophy genes are upregulated in all rapid muscle wasting conditions investigated so far. In addition to that unusually small autophagosomes have recently been discovered in skeletal muscle. On the basis of these recent observations, this pathway is now considered to be very important in conditions characterized by rapid muscle wasting and cachexia, but of minor importance in situations in which the muscle mass is maintained.

Summary

The Ca^{2+}-activated proteinases do not contribute significantly to the bulk of muscle protein breakdown in normal conditions and chronic muscle wasting conditions with exception of the muscular dystrophies. However, this pathway has been suggested to play an important role in the selection (via breakage of only limited number of peptide bonds) of proteins for complete digestion by the ubiquitin-proteasome and the lysosomal/autophagy systems.

Calcium Activated Proteinases

The two major Ca^{2+}-activated proteinases are μ-calpain and m-calpain (55,63,64). The activity of both of these ubiquitous cysteine proteinases is regulated by Ca^{2+} and by an endogenous inhibitor called calpastatin. In skeletal muscle a third calpain, p94, is also expressed abundantly (55,63). The Ca^{2+}-dependent proteolysis does not contribute significantly to the bulk of protein breakdown in muscle in normal conditions. The activity of the calpains is not upregulated in chronic muscle wasting conditions, with one clear exception of the muscular dystrophies. Calpain activity is upregulated in sepsis and some cancers (64). The Ca^{2+}-dependent proteinases have been suggested to have an important role in the selection of proteins for proteolysis. Many short-lived proteins contain negatively charged PEST (Pro, Glu, Ser, Thr) sequences that may bind Ca^{2+} and thus create a microenvironment of higher Ca^{2+} concentration that is favorable to calpain-mediated proteolysis. Suggestions have been made that the insulin receptor substrate (IRS-1) has such a PEST sequence that is susceptible to

Caspase System

Caspases are cysteine proteases, but they do not require Ca^{2+} for activation like the calpains. It is currently assumed that the caspases also do not contribute significantly to the bulk of protein breakdown in muscle in normal conditions (63). The caspases are activated by events that initiate apoptosis (programmed cell death of myonuclei). This is the case in the chronic diseases mentioned in the introduction characterized by inflammation, cachexia, and rapid muscle atrophy (type 2 diabetes, chronic obstructive pulmonary disease, rheumatoid arthritis, kidney disease, cancer) and it, therefore, is in these conditions that they are expected to contribute to the rapid muscle mass loss. Once a significant number of myonuclei have lost their transcription capacity, this will also have a negative impact on the total protein synthesis capacity of the skeletal muscle fibers.

The Ubiquitin-Proteasome System

The ubiquitin-proteasome pathway is primarily responsible for bulk protein breakdown in muscle and also for the breakdown of the myofibrillar proteins, actin and myosin. The pathway is activated in most conditions characterized by rapid muscle mass loss and in most diseases characterized by cachexia and muscle atrophy. These, among others, include fasting, protein deficiency, glucocorticoid treatment, and the acute response to cancer, kidney failure, trauma, and sepsis (55–58). In more chronic wasting conditions such as aging, Cushing's syndrome (chronic high levels of glucocorticoids), progressive stages of renal failure, and the muscular dystrophies the pathway is not further upregulated. This suggests that the ubiquitin-proteasome pathway is especially involved in acute and rapid changes in bulk protein content of the muscle (potentially, in parallel with the recently discovered lysosomal/autophagy system on which we have less information).

The proteolytic machinery of the ubiquitin-proteasome pathway consists of several hundreds of proteins. These include the ubiquitination/deubiquitination enzymes (200–300), the proteasome subunits (about 50), and endogenous proteasome activators and inhibitors. The pathway performs housekeeping functions in basal protein turnover and in the elimination of miscoded, misfolded, damaged, or mislocalized abnormal proteins. Schematically there are two main steps in the pathway:

1. Covalent attachment of a polyubiquitin chain to the protein substrate, under the control of ubiquitination and deubiquitination enzymes, to thus tag proteins that should be broken down
2. Specific recognition of proteins tagged with a polyubiquitin chain and degradation of the tagged proteins by the 26S proteasome (Fig. 17.4)

Ubiquitination of proteins both has proteolytic and nonproteolytic functions. The most important examples of the latter functions are membrane trafficking, protein kinase activation, DNA repair, and chromatin dynamics (65). A common mechanism underlying these functions is that the ubiquitin tag of proteins serves as a signal to

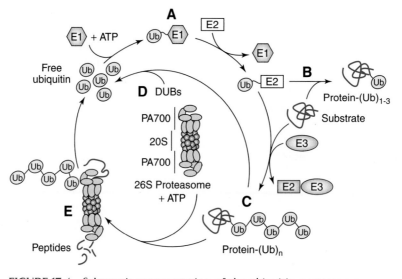

FIGURE 17.4   Schematic representation of the ubiquitin-proteasome pathway. **A.** Ubiquitin (Ub) is a 76 amino acid marker polypeptide. It is first activated by a single enzyme called the ubiquitin-activating enzyme (E1) and then transferred on to one of the ubiquitin-conjugating enzymes (E2s). **B.** An E2 covalently attaches 1, 2, or 3 ubiquitin moieties to a selected protein (Protein-$(Ub)_{1-3}$). The first ubiquitin molecule is attached via an isopeptide bond between the activated C-terminal glycine residue of ubiquitin and the ϵ-amino group of a lysine residue in the substrate. Protein molecules carrying an ubiquitin chain of 1, 2, or 3 molecules are not targeted for protein breakdown. **C.** With (and in some cases also without) the help of one of the ubiquitin protein ligases (E3s) the E2 can form a polyubiquitinated protein (Protein-$(Ub)_n$) carrying 4 or more ubiquitin moieties. E3s also have an important function in recognizing and selecting proteins that should be broken down. **D.** Protein-$(Ub)_n$ can either be deubiquinated by the deubiquitinating enzymes (DUBs) to be saved from proteolysis, or (**E**) is recognized by the proteasome multienzyme complex, unfolded, and injected into the 26S proteasome proteolytic subunit unit, and degraded into peptides. Note that the pathway consumes ATP both in steps A and E. In humans about 10% of resting energy expenditure is used to drive the ubiquitin-proteasome pathway at whole body level. (This figure was originally published by Attaix and colleagues (6). We thank Dr. Attaix and CABI Publishing, Wallingford, Oxon, UK, for permission to use it.)

recruit proteins harboring ubiquitin-binding domains, thereby bringing together ubiquitinated proteins and ubiquitinated receptors to execute specific biologic functions. A polyubiquitin chain of ≥4 is a signal for proteolysis. Polyubiquitination is a complex multiple step process that is explained in Figure 17.4. Molecular details of the involved ubiquitination enzymes (E1 and the superfamilies of E2 and E3), the deubiquitinating (DUB) superfamily, the proteasome subunits, and of the complex structural and functional organization of the proteasome multienzyme complex (containing specific and multiple subunits and sites for recognition, unfolding, a cylindrical proteolytic core, and regulation by specific activator and inactivator proteins) are given by Attaix and colleagues (6,55,56).

Summary

The ubiquitin-proteasome pathway is primarily responsible for bulk protein breakdown in muscle. The pathway is activated in most conditions characterized by rapid muscle mass loss and in most diseases characterized by cachexia and muscle atrophy. Because this pathway has been assumed to be far more important than the other named pathways, we know by far the most about its molecular actions and regulation mechanisms.

TEST YOURSELF

If you were planning a study that sought to determine the effects of exercise on protein degradation of the muscle proteins most involved in hypertrophy, which proteolytic pathways would you choose to measure?

Regulation of the Proteolytic Pathways by Hormones and Nutrients

Insulin and amino acids have a well-known antiproteolytic effect in incubated rat muscle preparations (6,55–57) and in vivo. The suppression of protein degradation by insulin in fact is regarded to be quantitatively more important for the anabolic effect of feeding than the relatively small stimulation of protein synthesis by insulin (3,36). However, until recently the proteolytic pathways that are affected have not been identified. Refeeding after prolonged starvation of rats with carbohydrates/amino acids was noted to down-regulate the expression of several enzymes of the ubiquitin-proteasome system (56). This probably is an important mechanism to limit the activity of the ubiquitin-proteasome system in well-fed human individuals, but because it took more than 12 hours to adjust the protein concentration of the involved enzymes, it did not explain the immediate antiproteolytic response in incubated rat muscles to insulin.

KEY POINT

Proteolysis in skeletal muscle is controlled by several pathways that were once believed to be separate but now are known to work cooperatively to maintain correct levels of protein degradation.

Considerable progress has recently been made in this area with the discovery that autophagy and lysosomal protein breakdown are more important in muscle than previously assumed. This has subsequently led to the identification of two insulin-induced control mechanisms of lysosomal autophagy (Fig. 17.5). It should be kept in mind that these mechanisms have been identified in cultured myotubes, incubated rat muscles, and in animal muscles in vivo and still need confirmation in human beings, but the evidence that they may explain the rapid muscle wasting that is observed in fasting, disuse, denervation, and many chronic human diseases characterized by severe cachexia is quite convincing (59,61,62; Fig. 17.5). The first mechanism operates at the transcriptional level and is mediated by the transcription factor FoxO3. Under normal (anabolic) conditions in well-fed healthy individuals PKB/Akt is known to phosphorylate and inactivate the FoxOs. However, in the indicated conditions with rapid muscle wasting PKB/Akt will be inactivated and lead to dephosphorylation and translocation of FoxO3 to the nucleus. Here it has been shown to induce the coordinated transcription of the ubiquitin ligases MAFbx/atrogin-1 and MuRF1, of the lysosomal proteolytic enzyme cathepsin L, and of all the proteins that are required for lysosomal autophagy.

Because transcription is a relatively slow process, this mechanism is unlikely to play a role in the acute effects of insulin in the diurnal feeding cycle or in isolated muscles incubated with insulin in vitro. The second mechanism is direct (nontranscriptional) inhibition of autophagy by activated mTOR as recently observed (59). This insulin action is expected to be a fast process similar to the effect of insulin on MPS. This mechanism will be fast enough to explain the increase in muscle protein degradation during overnight fasting. As amino acid ingestion and infusion has been shown to be able to activate mTOR in human beings independent of insulin, this mechanism is also likely to explain the well-described reduction of muscle protein degradation by exposure of incubated rat muscles to high amino acid concentrations (3).

Summary

The ubiquitin-proteasome pathway and the recently discovered lysosomal/autophagy pathway are jointly responsible for bulk protein breakdown in skeletal muscle, probably in a perfectly coordinated way. Both of these pathways are suppressed by insulin via mechanisms summarized in Figure 17.5. The simultaneous suppression of these pathways by insulin probably makes an important contribution to the rapid anabolic effect of insulin in the transition of the fasted to the fed state.

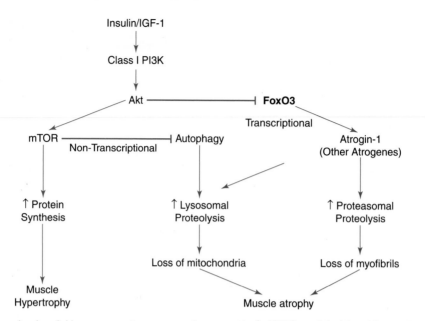

FIGURE 17.5 The central role of Akt, mammalian target of rapamycin (mTOR), and forkhead box subgroup O3 (FoxO3) in the coordinated regulation of muscle protein breakdown by lysosomal and proteasomal pathways during hypertrophy and atrophy. Two recent independent studies using different experimental approaches (59,61) have generated convincing evidence that these mechanisms operate in cultured myotubes, in isolated muscle fibers, and in animal muscle in vivo. To test the relevance of the proposed mechanism, the authors also have verified that denervation and starvation activates FoxO3 in the atrophying muscles of mice and induces expression of the autophagy genes and other atrogenes. It has more recently been proposed (62) that these mechanisms are crucial in the control and coordinated regulation of muscle proteolysis by insulin and hormones and may explain the rapid muscle atrophy that is observed in many of the acquired chronic diseases characterized by disuse and rapid muscle atrophy. The figure illustrates that regulation of these pathways occurs via two major mechanisms. The first operates at the transcriptional level and is mediated by transcription factor FoxO3. Under normal (anabolic) conditions Akt/PKB phosphorylates and inactivates FoxO3. However, in insulin-resistant states and the mentioned conditions with rapid muscle wasting inactivation of Akt/PKB leads to dephosphorylation and translocation of FoxO3 to the nucleus, where it induces the coordinated transcription of the ubiquitin ligases MAFbx/atrogin-1 and MuRF1 and of the proteins that are required for lysosomal autophagy. As transcription is a relatively slow process, this mechanism is unlikely to play a role in the acute effects of insulin in the diurnal feeding cycle or when insulin is added to the medium of an isolated muscle incubated in vitro. The second mechanism is direct (nontranscriptional) inhibition of autophagy by activated mTOR. This insulin action is expected to be a fast process similar to the effect of insulin on MPS. This mechanism will be fast enough to explain the increase in muscle protein degradation during overnight fasting. As amino acid ingestion and infusion has been shown to be able to activate mTOR in human beings independent of insulin, this mechanism is also likely to explain the well-described reduction of muscle protein degradation by exposure to high amino acid concentrations. The reader should also note that as resistance exercise has been shown to potentiate the activation of mTOR by amino acids in the period after exercise, it is also possible that suppression of autophagy beside the observed increases in MPS contribute to the anabolic effect of resistance exercise. It is possible that mTOR can lead to activation of one or more of the enzymes of the ubiquitin-proteasome system or on the other proteolytic systems in muscle, but no other mechanisms have been identified to date. The suggestion that mitochondria are the target of autophagy in skeletal muscle is based on indirect evidence (59), but could well explain the rapid loss of oxidative capacity that is commonly observed in patients with severe muscle atrophy and inflammation.

Regulation of the Proteolytic Pathways by Exercise, Chronic Overloading, Disuse, Aging, and Disease

Effects of acute resistance and endurance exercise

Research in animal models has shown that eccentric damaging exercise stimulates muscle proteolysis. Several studies in humans accordingly have shown that eccentric exercise in humans resulted in increased levels of free ubiquitin and ubiquitin conjugates and in increased proteasome activities when the exercise is performed repeatedly. Endurance exercise in rats for 5 days in a row, on the other hand, resulted in downregulation of the rate of proteolysis and a parallel reduction in proteasome activity (66). Also, in humans, some studies indicate that the expression of the components of the ubiquitin-proteasome system is down-regulated by regular endurance exercise. It is not known whether this leads to a reduced global protein degradation rate or only of specific proteins that play a role in the adaptation to endurance exercise. There is very little information on the effects of exercise on the other pathways.

Role of the ubiquitin-proteasome system in the remodeling of skeletal muscle

Changes in functional load and in pattern of contractile activity are known to lead to a muscle remodeling that involves the increased expression of some proteins and the disappearance of others (*e.g.*, the well-known shifts in myosin heavy chain isomer expression). Protein breakdown and the proteasome also appear to play an important role in this remodeling process (67). Ordway et al. (68) observed a marked and coordinated increase in mRNA and protein levels of the proteasome subunits and in proteasome activity in rabbit tibialis anterior muscle that had been subjected to chronic electrical stimulation for up to 28 days. Taillandier et al. (69) investigated the adaptation that occurs when hind limb suspended rats are reloaded. After 18 hours of reloading of the hind limbs, the components of the ubiquitin-proteasome system were actively expressed and translated as shown by analysis of the polyribosome fraction. Protein synthesis and protein degradation measured in muscles from these animals incubated in vitro were both increased. Following 7 days of reloading there still was an increased amount of ubiquitin conjugates in the myofibrillar fraction. The upregulation of the proteasome pathway in these cases is presumably required to tag and target specific proteins (*e.g.*, damaged proteins or the MHC-isomers that were present before the reloading) for rapid elimination and/or replacement.

Summary

Upregulation of the ubiquitin-proteasome system plays an important role in the molecular adaptation mechanisms in response to a change in muscle load or chronic electrical stimulation. The role in this case is to target the proteins that have become redundant—for example, clearing fast myosin heavy chain isomers during the transition to a slow muscle or the other way around.

Effects of immobilization, denervation, disuse, aging, and disease

Immobilization, denervation, and hind limb suspension in rodents are highly catabolic treatments and are attended by a massive parallel upregulation of most components of the ubiquitin-proteasome system. The mRNAs encoding for the ubiquitin-proteasome system are preferentially translated in these conditions. MAFbx/atrogin-1 and MURF, the muscle-specific ubiquitin protein ligases (E3s), are also overexpressed in immobilization, denervation, and hind limb suspension (8).

It is quite clear that regular exercise is needed to maintain muscle mass and muscle oxidative capacity (mitochondrial protein content) in all stages of the human life and also in pathologic conditions, which by definition are attended by extended periods of bed rest and inactivity (1–4,7–11,54). Some of the changes that occur in these conditions simply are the consequence of the disuse that occurs but some also are clearly related to the aging process or to disease-specific changes (4).

Apart from the fact that the anabolic effect of insulin and amino acids is blunted in the elderly, the consensus is that the proteolytic pathways to include the ubiquitin-proteasome system are not upregulated. Both basal rates of protein synthesis and protein degradation remain similar with aging, but the blunting of the insulin and amino acid signals on both leads to a reduced muscle protein accretion in the period after meal ingestion and explains the slow progressive loss of muscle mass, which we call sarcopenia (3,4,36).

KEY POINT

In the basal state, the activity of proteolytic pathways is not different in the elderly. However, in the postprandial state there is blunting of inhibition of proteolysis by insulin and amino acids which over time can lead to muscle loss as we age.

In many chronic diseases, the loss of muscle mass and function are much more prominent than can be expected on the basis of bed rest and disuse alone. In several disease processes, acute and chronic inflammation has been shown to lead to a decrease of the membrane potential of muscle and nerve (7), thus leading to a functional denervation of the muscle or at least to changes in the 24-hour profile of the signals that travel between the central nervous system and the muscle and back (reflex loops not only have roles in muscle coordination, but also in the regulation of muscle gene expression and metabolism). Inflammation may play a major role in the massive parallel upregulation of the lysosomal autophagy and ubiquitin-proteasome pathways (Fig. 17.4). In patients with trauma and sepsis (severe chronic inflammation) a very low protein content of myosin, low myosin/actin protein ratios, acute down-regulations of the mitochondrial content, and a massive upregulation of the ubiquitin-proteasome system have been observed (7). In patients with cancer, chronic obstructive pulmonary disease, chronic heart failure, and chronic kidney failure, we simply do not know what the molecular and electrophysiologic changes are and how they explain the extreme weakness and fatigability of the peripheral muscles of these patients (7). It is quite likely though that there are both abnormalities in gene expression and mRNA translation and that these abnormalities lead to chronic changes both in protein content and composition that impair muscle contractile function, insulin sensitivity, and metabolism. Another factor not discussed in this chapter that needs to be considered in all conditions with inflammation is that there may be impairments in the endothelial function of the microvasculature in skeletal muscle that may reduce the supply of insulin, glucose, and amino acids. Impairments in endothelial function of the muscle microvasculature and transendothelial transport, potentially, can have a large impact both on signal generation and on amino acid supply (11,71) and, therefore, may contribute to the blunting of the anabolic signals that is observed in aging, obesity, and insulin resistance (11,16,19,71).

Summary

A massive upregulation of the ubiquitin-proteasome system is seen after immobilization, denervation, hind limb suspension, trauma, and sepsis and severe inflammation, which are all attended by rapid muscle wasting. In healthy aging (sarcopenia) and conditions attended by a slow progressive loss of muscle mass the upregulation of the ubiquitin-proteasome system is limited to nonexistent.

TEST YOURSELF

1. Which discoveries have led to the conclusion that the lysosomal/autophagy pathway contributes to muscle protein breakdown in conditions with high rates of muscle wasting?
2. With the knowledge currently available, can you decide if decreases in muscle protein synthesis or increases in protein degradation contribute more to the muscle atrophy that occurs in rats during hind limb suspension? Define the most important missing information.
3. With the knowledge currently available, can you decide if the ubiquitin proteasome or the lysosomal/autophagy pathway contributes more to bulk protein breakdown in conditions with rapid muscle wasting and patients with cachexia? Define the most important missing information.
4. Discuss the most important mechanisms that lead to sarcopenia taking both changes in the regulation of muscle protein synthesis and degradation in the fed and fasted state into account.

Muscle Amino Acid Metabolism

In the 1840s, the German physiologist Von Liebig hypothesized that muscle protein was the main fuel used to achieve muscular contraction. After this view had been invalidated by experimental data (for review see 1–3), many exercise physiologists took the opposite stand and disregarded the amino acid pool in muscle as playing any role of significance in exercise and energy metabolism. Therefore, the final part of this chapter gives a brief overview of the role that muscle is playing in the handling and metabolism of amino acids in the overnight fasted state, following ingestion of protein-containing meals, and during exercise.

Amino acids in muscle not only are the precursor for protein synthesis and the product of protein degradation, but muscle is also actively involved in the metabolism of some amino acids. A detailed review is given elsewhere (1,2), therefore only a brief summary follows. A schematic representation of the major pathways of muscle amino acid metabolism is given in Figure 17.6.

Only six amino acids are substantially metabolized in resting and exercising skeletal muscles. These are the BCAAs (leucine, isoleucine, and valine), asparagine, aspartate, and glutamate. These amino acids together provide the amino groups and the ammonia for the synthesis of glutamine and alanine, which are released in excessive amounts both in the postabsorptive state and during ingestion of protein-containing meals. Only leucine and part of the isoleucine molecule are converted to acetyl-coenzyme A in muscle and can, therefore, be oxidized and contributed to the synthesis of ATP. The other carbon skeletons are used solely for de novo synthesis of tricarboxylic acid cycle intermediates and glutamine. Stable isotope tracer studies have shown that the carbon atoms of the released alanine originate primarily from glycolysis of blood glucose and from muscle glycogen breakdown followed by glycolysis. In resting conditions, these processes contribute each about half of the required amount of pyruvate, whereas glycogen breakdown is the main source during exercise at intensities $>50\%$ W_{max}. After consumption of a protein-containing meal, most amino acids are taken up and metabolized in the splanchnic area (gut and liver). However, the BCAAs and glutamate escape from the splanchnic area and are primarily taken up by muscle to be converted to glutamine. About half of the glutamine released from muscle originates from glutamate taken up from the blood, both after overnight fasting, prolonged starvation, and after consumption of a mixed protein-containing meal, whereas the remainder of the glutamine is generated by de novo synthesis from the six amino acids that are metabolized in muscle. Glutamine produced by muscle is an important fuel for mucosa cells and immune system cells and provides the nitrogen for the synthesis of DNA and RNA in all rapidly dividing cells. Glutamine in several cells is also able to activate the mTOR pathway and, therefore, plays a role in the signal routes and regulation mechanisms that have been discussed in this chapter. Conditions in which the muscle is not able to keep up the glutamine production are often characterized by a weakened immune function and wasting of muscle mass.

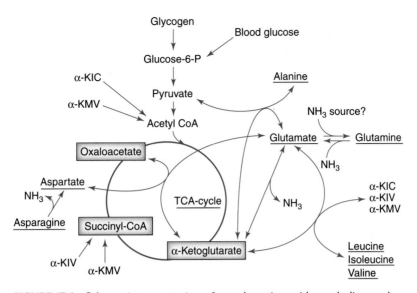

FIGURE 17.6   Schematic presentation of muscle amino acid metabolism and of the interactions of amino acids with the tricarboxylic acid (TCA)-cycle. The transamination products of leucine, isoleucine, and valine are α-ketoisocaproic acid (α-KIC), α-ketomethylvaleric acid (α-KMV), and α-ketoisovaleric acid (α-KIV). G-6-P, glucose-6-phosphate. (Reproduced with permission of Van Hall G, Saltin B, Wagenmakers AJ. Muscle protein degradation and amino acid metabolism during prolonged knee-extensor exercise in humans. *Clin Sci (Lond)*. 1999;97:557–567. © The Biochemical Society.)

The alanine aminotransferase reaction functions to establish and maintain high concentrations of tricarboxylic acid (TCA)-cycle intermediates in muscle during the first few minutes of exercise, and during subsequent work rate increments. Pyruvate primarily originating from glycogen breakdown and glycolysis and glutamate present in the muscle pool and taken up from the blood are used in that case to generate the carbon skeletons of TCA-cycle intermediates (pyruvate + glutamate ↔ alanine + α-ketoglutarate). The increase in concentration of TCA-cycle intermediates probably is needed to increase the flux of the TCA-cycle and meet the increased energy demand of exercise. There, however, are many other reactions that control the flux into and through the TCA-cycle and the relative importance of the TCA-cycle anaplerosis (synthesis of TCA-cycle intermediates leading to increases in their concentration) via conversion of amino acids is under a continued debate. In glycogen-depleted muscles (23) and in muscles of patients with McArdle's disease (muscle glycogen phosphorylase deficiency [1,2]) deamination of the six mentioned amino acids and glutamine synthesis present alternative anaplerotic mechanisms, but only contributes to exercise metabolism at intensities up to 40% to 50% of W_{max}. Together these observations indicate that the metabolism of amino acids in muscle fulfills a number of important roles in the regulation of energy metabolism both at rest and during exercise and in the support of mucosa and immune system cells with a continuous supply of glutamine.

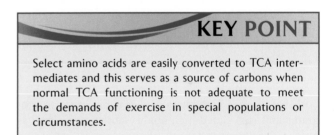

KEY POINT

Select amino acids are easily converted to TCA intermediates and this serves as a source of carbons when normal TCA functioning is not adequate to meet the demands of exercise in special populations or circumstances.

CHAPTER SUMMARY

Resistance training leads to muscle hypertrophy and an increase in the number of myofibrils per muscle fiber. Elderly subjects and patients with chronic diseases on the other hand show a slow progressive muscle atrophy, which makes them immobile and weak, leading to social isolation and a dramatic reduction in their quality of life. Endurance training leads to an increase in the number of mitochondria per muscle volume, whereas immobility and disuse have the opposite effect. Therefore the trained athlete has an enhanced endurance performance, but many elderly humans cannot walk for more than 500 m without a need for a break. This chapter identified the most important pathways and signaling routes that lead to the anabolism of strength training and to the atrophy of disuse. This knowledge opens the way for the development of new therapeutic approaches

A MILESTONE OF DISCOVERY

Dr. David Halliday in 1975 was the first to combine a continuous intravenous infusion of L-[a-^{15}N]lysine in five human subjects with serial biopsies of the vastus lateralis muscle using the percutaneous Bergstrøm needle. Serial samples of plasma were also used for purification of albumin. The infusion solution contained the tracer amino acid and also a mixture of essential and nonessential amino acids. The subjects ingested carbohydrate drinks every 2 hours during the infusions that lasted for 21 to 30 hours and, therefore, they were in an artificial state of continuous feeding. This design enabled Halliday and McKeran to make the first simultaneous estimates of skeletal muscle protein synthesis, plasma albumin synthesis, and total body protein turnover. This early study was one of the most thorough and complete amino acid incorporation studies that have been performed today, despite of the fact that the required analytical techniques were very complex and labor intensive and required great analytical skills both in the chemical and in the mass spectrometry laboratory. We should also keep in mind that the sensitivity of the used isotope ratio mass spectrometer (IRMS) was much lower than it is today and that GC-combustion-IRMS systems, which combine the separation of amino acids online with the generation and analysis of nitrogen, did not yet exist. A separation was made between the myofibrillar protein fraction, which represents the bulk of the muscle protein, and the sarcoplasmic proteins, the soluble enzymes present in the cytosol of muscle fibers. The main result of the study was that, in continuously fed humans, the fractional synthetic rate was 1.46% per day in the myofibrillar protein fraction, 3.80% in the sarcoplasmic protein fraction, 13.2% in plasma albumin, and total body protein turnover was 250 g per day. This paper set the scene for more detailed investigations of the regulation of muscle protein synthesis by feeding, fasting, hormones, and by (prior) exercise. Cheng and coworkers in 1985 (72) also were the first to report a simultaneous estimate of muscle protein synthesis and protein degradation in humans by combining the use of a continuously infused L-[1-^{13}C, ^{15}N]-leucine tracer with deep venous and arterialized blood sampling of the forearm. Similar tracer methodologies today still are the only available technique to make estimates of muscle protein degradation in humans and laboratory animals and as such are essential to further our understanding of the role of muscle protein degradation in the protein adaptation to exercise and training. Professor David Halliday and his collaborators not only made important contributions to the development of stable isotope tracer methodologies, but also have made a major contribution to the current insight in the regulation of muscle amino acid and protein metabolism in humans.

Halliday D, McKeran RO. Measurement of muscle protein synthetic rate from serial muscle biopsies and total body protein turnover in man by continuous intravenous infusion of L-[α-^{15}N] lysine. Clin Sci Mol Med. 1975;49:581–590.

both based on a combination of feasible exercise programs and well-timed high quality nutrition, as well as on the development of new pharmaceutical strategies. Although we know less about the enzymes that control muscle proteolysis, it is quite clear that they also make important contributions to changes in muscle mass and the adaptation of the protein profile to a change in physical activity. Our knowledge about the role that protein synthesis and degradation play in the control of the molecular adaptation to endurance training and the loss of the mitochondrial oxidative enzymes in disuse, aging, and disease still is in its infancy. There is hard evidence though that chronic exercise and training (preferentially, a mixture of resistance and endurance exercise) can prevent most of muscle function loss seen with aging and chronic disabling diseases, greatly improve health, well-being, and quality of life, and reduce the frequency of the most common chronic age-related diseases (cardiovascular disease, obesity, and type 2 diabetes). So the final message is that all human beings of all ages should exercise as frequently as possible to thus keep the protein composition of their muscles and blood vessels optimal while simultaneously being rewarded with immense performance and health benefits.

REFERENCES

1. Wagenmakers AJM. Muscle amino acid metabolism at rest and during exercise: role in human physiology and metabolism. *Exerc Sport Sci Rev.* 1998;26:287–314.
2. Wagenmakers AJM. Protein and amino acid metabolism in human muscle. *Adv Exp Med Biol.* 1998;441:307–319.
3. Wagenmakers AJM. Tracers to investigate protein and amino acid metabolism in human subjects. *Proc Nutr Soc.* 1999; 58:987–1000.
4. Combaret L, Dardevet D, Béchet D, et al. Skeletal muscle proteolysis in ageing. *Curr Opin Clin Nutr Metab Care.* 2009;12:37–41.
5. Doherty TJ. Invited review: aging and sarcopenia. *J Appl Physiol.* 2003;95:1717–1727.
6. Attaix D, Combaret L, Béchet D, et al. Role of the ubiquitin-proteasome pathway in muscle atrophy in cachexia. *Curr Opin Support Palliat Care.* 2008;2:262–266.
7. Wagenmakers AJM. The primary target of nutritional support: body composition or muscle function? *Nestlé Nutr Workshop Ser Clin Perform Programme.* 2002;7:219–234.
8. Holloszy JO. Biochemical adaptations in muscle. *J Biol Chem.* 1967;242:2278–2282.
9. Salti B, Henriksson J, Nygaard E, et al. Fiber types and metabolic potentials of skeletal muscles in sedentary man and endurance runners. *Ann N Y Acad Sci.* 1977;301:3–29.
10. Wagenmakers AJM, Coakley JH, Edwards RHT. The metabolic consequences of reduced habitual activities in patients with muscle pain and disease. *Ergonomics.* 1988;31:1519–1527.
11. Wagenmakers AJM, van Riel NAW, Frenneaux MP, et al. Integration of the metabolic and cardiovascular effects of exercise. *Essays Biochem.* 2006;42:193–210.

12. Liu Z, Barrett EJ. Human protein metabolism: its measurement and regulation. *Am J Physiol.* 2002;283:E1105–E1112.

13. Kumar V, Selby A, Rankin D, et al. Age-related differences in the dose-response relationship of muscle protein synthesis to resistance exercise in young and old men. *J Physiol (London).* 2009;587:211–217.

14. Wilkinson SB, Phillips SM, Atherton PJ, et al. Differential effects of resistance and endurance exercise in the fed state on signaling molecule phosphorylation and protein synthesis in human muscle. *J Physiol.* 2008;586:3701–3717.

15. Biolo G, Tipton KD, Klein S, et al. An abundant supply of amino acids enhances the metabolic effect of exercise on muscle protein. *Am J Physiol.* 1997;273:E122–E129.

16. Rennie MJ, Edwards RHT, Halliday D, et al. Muscle protein synthesis measured by stable isotope techniques in man: the effects of feeding and fasting. *Clin Sci (Lond).* 1982;63:519–523.

17. Burd NA, Tang JE, Moore DR, et al. Exercise training and protein metabolism: influences of contraction, protein intake, and sex-based differences. *J Appl Physiol.* 2009;106:1692–1701.

18. Drummond MJ, Dryer HC, Fry CS, et al. Nutritional and contractile regulation of human skeletal muscle protein synthesis and mTORC1 signaling. *J Appl Physiol.* 2009;106:1374–1384.

19. Koopman R, van Loon LJC. Aging, exercise, and muscle protein metabolism. *J Appl Physiol.* 2009;106:2040–2048.

20. Dreyer HC, Fujita S, Cadenas JG, et al. Resistance exercise increases AMPK activity and reduces 4E-BP1 phosphorylation and protein synthesis in human skeletal muscle. *J Physiol.* 2006;576:613–624.

21. Beelen M, Koopman R, Gijsen AP, et al. Protein coingestion stimulates protein synthesis during resistance-type exercise. *Am J Physiol Endocrinol Metab.* 2008;295:E70–E77.

22. Wolfe RR, Goodenough RD, Wolfe MH, et al. Isotopic analysis of leucine and urea metabolism in exercising humans. *J Appl Physiol.* 1982;52:458–466.

23. Van Hall G, Saltin B, Wagenmakers AJM. Muscle protein degradation and amino acid metabolism during prolonged knee-extensor exercise in humans. *Clin Sci.* 1999;97:557–567.

24. Bylund-Fellenius A-C, Ojamaa KM, Flaim KE, et al. Protein synthesis versus energy state in contracting muscles of perfused rat hindlimb. *Am J Physiol.* 1984;246:E297–E305.

25. Bolster DR, Crozier SJ, Kimball SR, et al. AMP-activated protein kinase suppresses protein synthesis in rat skeletal muscle through down-regulated mammalian target of rapamycin (mTOR) signaling. *J Biol Chem.* 2002;277:23977–23980.

26. Browne GJ, Proud CG. Minireview: regulation of peptide-chain elongation in mammalian cells. *Eur J Biochem.* 2002;269:5360–5368.

27. Rose AJ, Richter EA. Regulatory mechanisms of skeletal muscle protein turnover during exercise. *J Appl Physiol.* 2009;106:1702–1711.

28. Chesley A, MacDougall JD, Tarnopolsky MA, et al. Changes in human muscle protein synthesis after resistance exercise. *J Appl Physiol.* 1992;73:1383–1388.

29. Phillips SM, Tipton KD, Aarsland A, et al. Mixed muscle protein synthesis and breakdown after resistance exercise in humans. *Am J Physiol.* 1997;273:E99–E107.

30. Roy BD, Tarnopolski MA, MacDougall JD, et al. Effect of glucose supplement timing on protein metabolism after resistance training. *J Appl Physiol.* 1997;82:1882–1888.

31. Tipton KD, Borsheim E, Wolf SE, et al. Acute response of net muscle protein balance reflects 24-h balance after exercise and amino acid ingestion. *Am J Physiol.* 2003;284:E76–E89.

32. Miller SL, Tipton KD, Chinkes DL, et al. Independent and combined effects of amino acids and glucose after resistance exercise. *Med Sci Sports Exerc.* 2003;35:449–455.

33. Carraro F, Stuart CA, Hartl WH, et al. Effect of exercise and recovery on muscle protein synthesis in human subjects. *Am J Physiol Endocrinol Metab.* 1990;259:E470–E476.

34. Hood DA. Mechanisms of exercise-induced mitochondrial biogenesis in skeletal muscle. *Appl Physiol Nutr Metab.* 2009;34:465–472.

35. Campbell WW, Johnson CA, McCabe GP, et al. Dietary protein requirements of younger and older adults. *Am J Clin Nutr.* 2008;88:1322–1329.

36. Rennie MJ, Selby A, Atherton P, et al. Facts, noise and wishful thinking: muscle protein turnover in aging and human disuse atrophy. *Scand J Med Sci Sports.* 2010;20:5–9.

37. Fujita S, Rasmussen BB, Cadenas JG, et al. Aerobic exercise overcomes the age-related insulin resistance of muscle protein metabolism by improving endothelial function in Akt/mammalian target of rapamycin signaling. *Diabetes.* 2007;56:1615–1622.

38. Yarasheski KE, Zachwieja JJ, Bier DM. Acute effects of resistance exercise on muscle protein synthesis rate in young and elderly men and women. *Am J Physiol.* 1993;265:E210–E214.

39. Kumar V, Selby A, Rankin D, et al. Age-related differences in the dose-response relationship of muscle protein synthesis to resistance exercise in young and old men. *J Physiol (London).* 2009;587:211–217.

40. Proud CG. Minireview: regulation of mammalian translation factors by nutrients. *Eur J Biochem.* 2002;269:5338–5349.

41. Proud CG. mTORC1 signaling and mRNA translation. *Biochem Soc Trans.* 2009;37:227–231.

42. Sonenberg N, Hershey JWB, Mathews MB. *Translational Control of Gene Expression.* Cold Spring Harbor, NY: Cold Spring Harbor Laboratory Press; 2000.

43. Baar K, Esser K. Phosphorylation of p70S6k correlates with increased skeletal muscle mass following resistance exercise. *Am J Physiol.* 1999;276:C120–C127.

44. Chen Y-W, Nader GA, Baar KR, et al. Response of rat muscle to acute resistance exercise defined by transcriptional and translational profiling. *J Physiol (London).* 2002;545:27–41.

45. Nader GA, Esser KA. Intracellular signaling specificity in skeletal muscle in response to different modes of exercise. *J Appl Physiol.* 2001;90:1936–1942.

46. Hernandez JM, Fedele MJ, Farrell PA. Time course evaluation of protein synthesis and glucose uptake after acute resistance exercise in rats. *J Appl Physiol.* 2002;88:1142–1149.

47. Kimball SR, Farrell PA, Jefferson LS. Invited review: role of insulin in translational control of protein synthesis in skeletal muscle by amino acids and exercise. *J Appl Physiol.* 2002;93:1168–1180.

48. Rasmussen BB, Richter EA. The balancing act between the cellular processes of protein synthesis and breakdown: exercise as a model to understand the molecular mechanisms regulating muscle mass. *J Appl Physiol.* 2009;106:1365–1366.

49. Deldicque L, Atherton P, Patel R, et al. Decrease in Akt/PKB signaling in human skeletal muscle by resistance exercise. *Eur J Appl Physiol.* 2008;104:57–65.

50. Koopman R, Zorenc AHG, Gransier RJJ, et al. Increase in S6K1 phosphorylation in human skeletal muscle following resistance exercise occurs mainly in type II muscle fibres. *Am J Physiol Endocrinol Metab.* 2006;290:E1245–E1252.

51. Bolster DR, Kubica N, Crozier SJ, et al. Immediate response of mTOR-mediated signaling following acute resistance exercise in rat skeletal muscle. *J Physiol (London).* 2003;553:213–220.

52. Glover EI, Oates BR, Tang JE, et al. Resistance exercise decreases eIF2Bε phosphorylation and potentiates the feeding-induced stimulation of p70S6K1 and rpS6 in young men. *Am J Physiol Regul Integr Comp Physiol.* 2008;295:R604–R610.

53. Blomstrand E, Eliasson J, Karlsson HKR, et al. Branched-chain amino acids activate key enzymes in protein synthesis after physical exercise. *J Nutr.* 2006;136:269S–273S.

54. Esmarck B, Andersen JL, Olsen S, et al. Timing of postexercise protein intake is important for muscle hypertrophy with resistance training in elderly humans. *J Physiol (London).* 2001;535:301–311.

55. Attaix D, Taillandier D. The critical role of the ubiquitin-proteasome pathway in muscle wasting in comparison to lysosomal and Ca²⁺-dependent systems. *Adv Mol Cell Biol.* 1998;27:235–266.

56. Attaix D, Combaret L, Kee AJ, et al. Mechanisms of ubiquitination and proteasome-dependent proteolysis in skeletal muscle. In: Zempleni J, Daniel H, eds. *Molecular Nutrition.* Wallingford, Oxon: CABI Publishing; 2003:219–235.

57. Hasselgren PO, Wray C, Mammen J. Molecular regulation of muscle cachexia: it may be more than the proteasome. *Biochem Biophys Res Comm.* 2002;290:1–10.

58. Lecker SH, Jagoe RT, Gilbert A, et al. Multiple types of skeletal muscle atrophy involve a common program of changes in gene expression. *FASEB J.* 2004;18:39–51.

59. Mammucari C, Milan G, Romanello V, et al. FoxO3 controls authophagy in skeletal muscle in vivo. *Cell Metab.* 2007;6:458–471.

60. Sandri M, Sandri C, Gilbert A, et al. Foxo transcription factors induce the atrophy-related ubiquitin ligase atrogin-1 and cause skeletal muscle atrophy. *Cell.* 2004;3:399–412.

61. Zhao J, Brault JJ, Schild A, et al. FoxO3 coordinately activates protein degradation by the autophagic/lysosomal and proteasomal pathways in atrophying muscle cells. *Cell Metab.* 2007;6:472–483.

62. Zhao J, Brault JJ, Schild A, et al. Coordinate activation of authophagy and the proteasome pathway by FoxO transcription factor. *Authophagy.* 2008;413:378–380.

63. Goll DE, Thompson VF, Li H, et al. The calpain system. *Physiol Rev.* 2003;83:731–801.

64. Smith IJ, Lecker SH, Hasselgren PO. Calpain activity and muscle wasting in sepsis. *Am J Physiol Endocrinol Metab.* 2008;295:E762–E771.

65. Chen ZJ, Sun LJ. Nonproteolytic functions of ubiquitin in cell signaling. *Mol Cell.* 2009;33:275–286.

66. Kee AJ, Taylor AJ, Carlsson AR, et al. IGF-1 has no effect on postexercise suppression of the ubiquitin-proteasome system in rat skeletal muscle. *J Appl Physiol.* 2002;92:2277–2284.

67. Murton AJ, Constantin D, Greenhaff PL. The involvement of the ubiquitin proteasome system in human skeletal muscle remodelling and atrophy. *Biochim Biophys Acta.* 2008;1782:730–743.

68. Ordway GA, Neufer PD, Chin ER, et al. Chronic contractile activity upregulates the proteasome system in rabbit muscle. *J Appl Physiol.* 2000;88:1134–1141.

69. Taillandier D, Aurousseau E, Combaret L, et al. Regulation of proteolysis during reloading of the unweighted soleus muscle. *Int J Biochem Cell Biol.* 2003;35:665–675.

70. Bodine SC, Latres E, Baumhueter S, et al. Identification of ubiquitin ligases required for skeletal muscle atrophy. *Science.* 2001;294:1704–1708.

71. Rattigan S, Bradley EA, Roberts SM, et al. Muscle metabolism and control of capillary blood flow: insulin and exercise. *Essays Biochem.* 2006;42:133–144.

72. Cheng KN, Dworzak F, Ford GC, et al. Direct determination of leucine metabolism and protein breakdown in humans using L-[1–13C, 15N]-leucine and the forearm model. *Eur J Clin Invest.* 1985;15(6):349–354.

CHAPTER 18

Mitochondrial Biogenesis Induced by Endurance Training

David A. Hood, Michael F. N. O'Leary,
Giulia Uguccioni, and Isabella Irrcher

Abbreviations

ADP	Adenosine diphosphate	mRNA	Messenger ribonucleic acid
ADP_f	Free ADP	MSF	Mitochondrial import–stimulating factor
AICAR	5-aminoimidazole-4-carboxamide-1-β-D-ribofuranoside	mtDNA	Mitochondrial DNA
		mtHSP	Mitochondrial HSP
ALAs	δ-aminolevulinic acid synthase	MHC	Myosin heavy chain
AMP	Adenosine monophosphate	NRF -1/-2	Nuclear respiratory factor -1/-2
AMPK	AMP-activated protein kinase	NUGEMPs	Nuclear-encoded mitochondrial proteins
ATP	Adenosine triphosphate	PGC-1α	Peroxisome proliferator-activated recep-
ATPase	Adenosine triphosphatase		tor-γ coactivator-1α
CaMK	Calcium/calmodulin-dependent protein kinase	PGC-1β	Peroxisome proliferator-activated recep-tor-γ coactivator-1β
cAMP	Cyclic-AMP	POL-γ	DNA polymerase γ
CBP	CREB-binding protein	PPAR-α	Peroxisome proliferation-activated
COX	Cytochrome oxidase		receptor-α
CPK	Creatine phosphokinase	PPAR-γ	Peroxisome proliferation-activated
CPN	Chaperonin		receptor-γ
ETC	Electron transport chain	PRC	PGC-1β- and PGC-1α-related coactivator
FTR	Fast-twitch red	ROS	Reactive oxygen species
FTW	Fast-twitch white	SR	Sarcoplasmic reticulum
HSP	Heat shock protein	STR	Slow-twitch red
IMF	Intermyofibrillar	SS	Subsarcolemmal
MAP	Mitogen-activated protein	Tfam	Transcription factor A, mitochondrial
MAPK	Mitogen-activated protein kinase	TOM complex	Translocase of the outer membrane
Mfn1/2	Mitofusin 1/2	TIM complex	Translocase of the inner membrane

Introduction

Our understanding of the relevance of structure, function, and biogenesis of mitochondria has increased tremendously over the last 15 years. Indeed, it is very exciting to be involved in a research program that is devoted to mitochondria. The organelle, long known for its vital role in cellular energy production, is now an established participant in cell signaling events leading to apoptosis. In addition, it is now recognized that mitochondrial dysfunction, brought about by either nuclear or mitochondrial DNA (mtDNA) mutations, can lead to a broad variety of pathophysiologic conditions affecting the nervous system, the heart, and/or skeletal muscle. Thus, cell biologists and clinicians alike have become keenly interested in how mitochondrial function and dysfunction contribute to cell signaling and maladaptation. In skeletal muscle, the term *plasticity* was coined (1) to describe the remarkable capability of this tissue to alter its gene expression profile and phenotype in response to changes in functional demand. The first convincing demonstration that mitochondrial content in muscle had the potential to increase in response to a change in functional demand (endurance training) was provided by John Holloszy (2) (see *A Milestone of Discovery* at the end of this chapter). Contractile-activity–induced adaptations in muscle are highly specific and depend on the type of exercise (*i.e.*, dynamic or resistance), as well as its frequency, intensity, and duration. It is now well established that repeated bouts of endurance exercise interspersed with recovery periods result in altered expression of a wide variety of gene products, leading to an altered muscle phenotype and improved fatigue resistance (3–5). This improved endurance is highly correlated with the increase in muscle mitochondrial density and enzyme activity. In addition, it has been established for many years that conditions of muscle disuse (*e.g.*, microgravity, denervation, immobilization, sedentary lifestyle, and aging) lead to diminished mitochondrial content and compromised energy production. These findings are very important for exercise physiologists interested in the cellular basis of endurance performance and are of practical importance for athletes in training programs. More importantly, this adaptation in mitochondrial content permits us to be optimistic about the role of training in ameliorating the functional capacity of previously sedentary individuals, in altering processes that lead to cell death and myonuclear decay, and in reversing the pathophysiology of mitochondrial disease in skeletal muscle. Thus, the expansion of the mitochondrial network within muscle cells as induced by chronic exercise is now recognized to have implications for a broader range of health issues than the enhancement of athletic performance. In addition, the process itself can serve as a valuable cellular model of organelle assembly within eukaryotic cells. Our understanding of the mechanisms of mitochondrial adaptation, broadly termed *mitochondrial biogenesis*, has progressed rapidly in recent years. This is because of the following:

1. The combined use of human, animal, and cell culture models to study mitochondrial adaptations
2. Improvements in microscopy techniques, which permit better resolution of organelle structure
3. The development of physiologic and molecular techniques that permit measures of mitochondrial function and gene expression in single cells or in isolated organelles (3)

This chapter describes the established cellular mechanisms involved in mitochondrial biogenesis and their physiologic relevance.

Physiology of Muscle Mitochondrial Biogenesis

Skeletal muscle falls into three classes of fibers based on metabolic and contractile properties:

1. Slow-twitch red (STR) fibers containing largely the myosin heavy chain (MHC) type I isoforms
2. Fast-twitch red (FTR) fibers containing mainly MHC type IIA isoforms
3. Fast-twitch white (FTW) fibers, possessing mainly MHC type IIB or IIX isoforms, depending on the species

Each of these muscle fiber types has a varying steady-state mitochondrial content that contributes to the intensity of their red appearance and their endurance capacity. In humans, the STR fibers have the largest volume fraction of mitochondria, followed by FTR and FTW fibers, respectively (4). Although considerable overlap exists, there is an approximate threefold to fourfold difference in the capacity for oxidative metabolism between red and white muscle. Repeated bouts of dynamic exercise in the form of endurance training can induce increases in the mitochondrial content (*i.e.*, mitochondrial biogenesis) of all three muscle fibers types (6), provided that the training program has been tailored toward the recruitment of both fast- and slow-motor units. Mitochondrial adaptations will not occur in muscle fibers that are not recruited during the exercise bout, consistent with the idea that mitochondrial biogenesis produced by exercise is initiated by stimuli within the contracting muscle, independent of humoral influences.

Traditional endurance training protocols in humans and other mammals have been shown to produce an increase in mitochondrial content usually ranging from 30% to 100% within about 4 to 6 weeks. This results in improved endurance performance that is largely independent of the much smaller 10% to 20% training-induced changes in maximal volume of oxygen consumed ($\dot{V}o_{2max}$) (7). The extent of the increase in mitochondrial content in muscle cells depends on the initial mitochondrial content. A muscle fiber with a low oxidative white phenotype (FTW, type IIB or IIX fiber) will increase its mitochondrial content by a greater amount than an FTR (type IIA) muscle fiber. The conversion of phenotype from a white muscle to one with a visibly red appearance is brought about by enhanced synthesis of the red pigment heme and its incorporation into myoglobin and mitochondrial cytochromes. Recent work has also indicated that mitochondrial biogenesis can occur in response to high intensity, interval training exercise bouts (8). Thus, high intensity, low duration exercise appears to represent a viable alternative for the induction of mitochondrial biogenesis in muscle.

Mitochondrial biogenesis can also be replicated using models of simulated exercise, such as chronic contractile activity produced by electrical stimulation of the motor nerve. This model has the advantage of producing relatively large changes in mitochondrial biogenesis that can occur in a shorter time (1–4 weeks) (9). Thus, both chronic endurance exercise training and chronic stimulation are the most commonly used models for the study the cellular processes involved in mitochondrial biogenesis. In addition, cell culture models of muscle contraction can provide additional insight. Chronically stimulated cardiac or skeletal muscle myocytes (10) have more recently been used to advantage in describing some of the gene expression responses which precede mitochondrial biogenesis. In this chapter, the term *chronic contractile activity* describes the role and effects of exercise in all of these experimental models, with an appreciation for the limitations and advantages of each technique.

Summary

Exercise increases the mitochondrial content of muscle in a fiber type-specific manner, dependent on motor unit recruitment. A number of experimental models have been developed to study the molecular mechanisms that regulate this important cellular process.

KEY POINT

Mitochondria adapt differently in muscle fiber types depending on their recruitment.

TEST YOURSELF

What are the reasons why understanding mitochondrial biogenesis is important? What fiber types have the highest mitochondrial content and which fibers adapt most to exercise training?

Mitochondrial Subfractions in Skeletal Muscle

Electron microscopic views of both cardiac cells and skeletal muscle fibers has revealed that the mitochondrial reticulum is distributed primarily in two distinct geographic locations: concentrated under the sarcolemma, termed subsarcolemmal (SS) mitochondria, and interspersed throughout the myofibrils, called intermyofibrillar (IMF) mitochondria (Fig. 18.1A and B).

Although fiber types and species differ, the relative proportion of IMF mitochondria is usually at least 75%

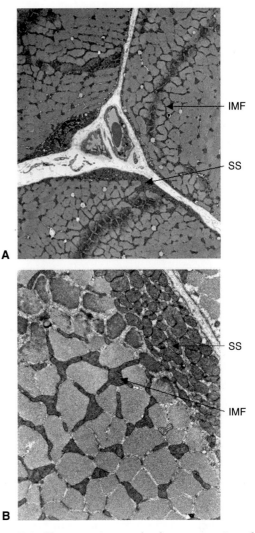

FIGURE 18.1 Electron micrograph of a cross-section of human skeletal muscle. Mitochondria are divided into two separate subfractions in skeletal muscle. **A.** Lower magnification of three muscle fibers adjoining a capillary. **B.** Higher magnification of a single muscle fiber. Note the different cellular locations and shapes of subsarcolemmal (SS) and intermyofibrillar (IMF) mitochondria. SS mitochondria are concentrated below the sarcolemma; IMF mitochondria are distributed between myofibrils. (Modified with permission from Hoppeler H. *Kraft- und Ausdauertraining: funktionelle und strukturelle Grundlagen. In Der Muskel.* Uelzen: Medizinisch Literarische Verlagsgesellschaft (Medical Literary Publishing); 1989:9–17.

of the total mitochondrial volume. We speculate that the IMF mitochondria are particularly useful in delivering adenosine triphosphate (ATP) for the myofibrillar adenosine triphosphatase (ATPase), thereby powering actin and myosin interactions, whereas the ATP produced by SS mitochondria may be more easily delivered to the sarcolemma or to peripheral myonuclei, structures that are in close proximity. This ATP would be used to provide energy for membrane pumps (*e.g.*, Na-K ATPase) or for energy-requiring events within the nucleus (*e.g.,* transcription or messenger ribonucleic acid (mRNA) splicing). It is notable that these mitochondrial subfractions differ in their adaptability to a stimulus (*e.g.,* training), suggesting that their location within the cell makes them differentially sensitive to a common cellular signal. Variations in chronic muscle use and disuse have revealed that SS mitochondria consistently adapt to a greater degree, or sooner, than IMF mitochondria. Under pathologic conditions of mtDNA disease, SS mitochondria proliferate preferentially, leading to histochemically defined "ragged red" fibers. When subcellular fractionation techniques are used to isolate SS and IMF mitochondria, these subfractions exhibit subtle differences in functional, biochemical, and compositional properties (11). This is not surprising, given that many examples of continuous membrane networks differing in their protein composition exist within cells (*e.g.,* the sarcolemma at the neuromuscular junction, or the sarcoplasmic reticulum (SR) at the junction with the T-tubule). In isolated mitochondria, oxygen consumption is usually measured in the absence of adenosine diphosphate (ADP) (resting respiration, termed *state 4*) and in the presence of nonlimiting amounts of ADP (activated respiration, termed *state 3*). State 3 and 4 respiration rates are typically higher in IMF than in SS mitochondria. The resulting ATP concentration inside the organelle is about twofold greater in IMF mitochondria (11). The reasons for this difference in respiration rate may be related to their divergent enzyme and lipid compositions. In turn, these biochemical and physiologic differences may be due to the local proximity of SS mitochondria to peripheral myonuclei and to a differential capacity of each mitochondrial subfraction for protein synthesis and import (discussed later in the chapter).

The Mitochondrial Reticulum within the Cell is a Balance of Organelle Fission and Fusion Processes

Research has indicated that mitochondria in muscle exist in an interconnected network, or reticulum (see Fig. 18.1B) (12). The extensiveness of this reticulum appears to depend on the overall oxidative capacity of the tissue and may differ between SS and IMF regions within the muscle cell (13). When considering the underlying mechanisms that induce mitochondrial biogenesis, it is now well accepted that mitochondria are dynamic organelles that undergo constant cycles of reticulum fission and fusion. The biologic function of these processes is thought to permit the exchange of mitochondrial proteins, lipids, and mtDNA within a preexisting mitochondrial network. In addition, it also appears that this process functions as a quality control mechanism, which allows the removal of damaged portions of the mitochondrial reticulum without requiring the loss of an entire network (14). The fission proteins, fission protein 1

and dynamin-related protein 1, and the fusion proteins, mitofusin 1/2 (Mfn1/2) and optic atrophy factor 1, control these important remodeling processes. The correct functioning of these proteins is critical for normal mitochondrial dynamics because their dysregulation leads to pathology and mitochondrial dysfunction (15). An interesting scenario is whether fission and fusion dynamics are differentially regulated within the SS and IMF mitochondrial subfractions and whether this could account for some of the reported differences in their adaptability to muscle use and disuse and apoptotic susceptibility. In the context of exercise, it is currently unknown whether exercise modulates mitochondrial fission/fusion dynamics. At least some aspects of mitochondrial fusion are altered with exercise because Mfn2 mRNA levels were reported to increase in humans in the recovery phase following a single bout of exercise (16). Mfn2 promoter activation and mRNA expression depends, at least in part, on the actions of peroxisome proliferator-activated receptor-γ coactivator (PGC)-1α, a coactivator that is increased with exercise. It will be interesting to see whether some of the mitochondrial changes associated with aging and physical inactivity are attributed not only to alterations in mitochondrial content, but also to the dysregulation of mitochondrial dynamics.

Summary

Mitochondria exist largely as a membrane network within muscle cells. The extent of this network depends on the species investigated, the oxidative capacity of the fiber, and on the dynamic processes of organelle fission and fusion. When mitochondria are isolated from muscle for study, subtle differences exist in their functional and biochemical properties depending on whether they are located near the sarcolemma or between the myofibrils. Mitochondria in these subcellular locations also differ in their adaptability to exercise and disease.

KEY POINT

Mitochondria are dynamic organelles within muscle, exhibiting varying shapes, sizes, and locations.

Mitochondrial Composition Can Change in Response to Contractile Activity

Mitochondrial content can be measured directly, using morphometric estimates of organelle volume in relation to total cellular volume. More commonly, and with much less effort, mitochondrial content is estimated by the change in maximal activity of a typical marker enzyme such as citrate synthase or by the change in content of a protein like cytochrome c. This is valid under most conditions because changes in mitochondrial volumes estimated morphometrically parallel the changes in enzyme V_{max} values. The measurement of single proteins or enzyme activities has been useful for determining rates of mitochondrial turnover, assuming that the behavior of the protein resembles that of the organelle as a whole. The caveat in this approach is the recognition that mitochondrial protein composition can be altered in response to chronic exercise, particularly during the imposition of additional confounding situations, such as iron deficiency or mitochondrial disease.

Mitochondrial proteins turnover with a half-life of about 1 week following the onset of a new level of muscle contractile activity (*e.g.*, greater intensity, duration, or frequency per week) (17). Mitochondrial phospholipid content changes occur with an even shorter half-life (about 4 days), suggesting that the assembly and/or degradation of the organelle could be initiated by changes in phospholipid composition. In the absence of normal rates of cytochrome synthesis and incorporation into the inner membrane during iron deficiency, imposed contractile activity appears to lead to continued membrane lipid synthesis, producing an increased mitochondrial volume with markedly reduced and abnormal protein content. These data point to the independent synthesis of proteins and phospholipids during mitochondrial biogenesis. However, very little is known regarding the synthesis of mitochondrial phospholipids during exercise.

TEST YOURSELF

Describe the morphology and characteristics of mitochondria in skeletal muscle. In response to exercise, how can mitochondrial composition and morphology change?

Mitochondrial Content Can Influence Metabolism during Exercise

The increased endurance performance that results from mitochondrial biogenesis is a consequence of changes in muscle metabolism during exercise. At the onset of exercise, the calcium-induced activation of myosin ATPase results in an elevated concentration of free ADP (ADP$_f$; Fig. 18.2). This molecule serves to activate:

1. The creatine phosphokinase (CPK) reaction toward the formation of ATP and creatine
2. Glycolysis
3. State 3 mitochondrial respiration

Because endurance training increases the mitochondrial content of skeletal muscle without large effects on CPK or glycolytic enzymes, the result is that a greater fraction of the energy required at a given exercise intensity will be derived from mitochondrial metabolism and a lower concentration of ADP$_f$ will be required to attain the same level of oxygen consumption. This lower ADP$_f$ concentration at a given $\dot{V}_{O_2}$ will reduce the rates of glycolysis and lactic acid formation, lower rates of adenosine monophosphate (AMP) formation, and permit the sparing of phosphocreatine (3). Reduced synthesis of AMP should lead to lower allosteric activation of phosphorylase and preserve glycogen. In addition, the activation of AMP kinase should be attenuated, reducing signal transduction that mediates downstream events, such as the translocation of glucose transporter 4 to the plasma membrane. These adaptations, along with increased activities of mitochondrial β-oxidation enzymes, predispose the individual toward greater lipid and less carbohydrate oxidation during exercise, resulting in an enhanced endurance performance.

Summary

The greater the mitochondrial content, the more the reliance on lipid, rather than carbohydrate metabolism, during exercise, and the lower the lactic acid production and phosphocreatine utilization.

KEY POINT

Having more mitochondria results in a greater endurance capacity.

Overview of the Cellular Events in Mitochondrial Biogenesis

The morphologic manifestation of mitochondrial biogenesis produced by multiple exercise bouts performed over several weeks can be visualized by electron microscopy as an expansion of the mitochondrial reticulum in both SS and IMF regions of each muscle fiber. However, the requirement for weeks of training to achieve this new steady-state mitochondrial content is not a reflection of the early molecular events that ultimately lead to those measurable morphologic changes. The final phenotypic adaptation (*i.e.*, elevated muscle mitochondrial content) is the cumulative result of a complex series of events that begins with the very first bout of exercise in a training program. As discussed later, the time between the onset of the first exercise bout and the ultimate mitochondrial adaptation is characterized by intermittent contraction-induced signaling events (18). These signals are known to activate protein kinases, acetates, and phosphatases that modify the activity of proteins, resulting in an increase in the mRNA expression of nuclear-encoded mitochondrial proteins (NUGEMPs) (Fig. 18.3).

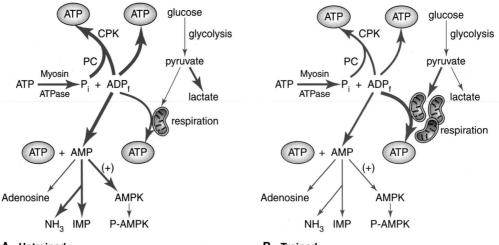

FIGURE 18.2   A. Acute exercise in untrained individuals triggers accelerated metabolism via the formation of free adenosine diphosphate (ADP_f) by the myosin adenosine triphosphatase (ATPase) reaction. ADP_f simultaneously activates the creatine phosphokinase (CPK) reaction, glycolytic flux, and mitochondrial respiration to maintain adenosine triphosphate (ATP) levels constant. Two molecules of ADP_f can be converted to ATP and adenosine monophosphate (AMP) in the myokinase (MK) reaction. In fast-twitch muscle fibers, AMP is metabolized to inosine monophosphate (IMP) and ammonia (NH_3) by AMP deaminase. In slow-twitch muscle fibers, AMP is largely converted to adenosine. The increase in AMP and the drop in phosphocreatine (PC) activate AMP kinase (AMPK) activity. **B.** Acute exercise elicits the same response in an endurance-trained individual. However, the trained muscle has a greater mitochondrial content as a result of organelle biogenesis, with very little change in the V_{max} of key reactions in other pathways. Thus, more ATP can be provided via mitochondrial respiration. This reduces the consumption of PC, attenuates the rate of glycolysis and lactic acid production, reduces the formation of AMP and NH_3, and decreases the activation of AMPK. This, along with the concomitant training-induced increase in mitochondrial fatty acid oxidation enzymes, promotes carbohydrate sparing and enhances endurance performance. Line thicknesses illustrate approximate shifts from one pathway to another with training. P_i, inorganic phosphate.

Following mRNA translation, the resulting nuclear-encoded proteins are chaperoned to the mitochondria and imported into the different compartments, such as the matrix space or the inner or outer membrane. A subgroup of these proteins is transcription factors that act directly on mtDNA to increase the mRNA expression of mitochondrial gene products and mtDNA copy number. mtDNA is critical because it encodes vital proteins involved in the mitochondrial respiratory chain. Because mtDNA contains no introns, point mutations within the genome have severe consequences. Thus, to produce an organelle that is functional in providing cellular ATP, contractile activity-induced mitochondrial biogenesis requires (a) the integration of a multitude of contraction-induced cellular signals and (b) the cooperative and timely expression of the nuclear and mitochondrial genomes.

TEST YOURSELF

Why does a higher mitochondrial content lead to a greater endurance performance, or a reduced fatigability? Describe the fundamental gene expression pathways that must be invoked to produce an increase in mitochondrial content.

Cellular Mechanisms of Mitochondrial Biogenesis

Contractile Activity Initiates Cell Signaling Events

The molecular signals linking acute exercise responses to subsequent long-term increases in mitochondrial content are beginning to be defined. The intensity and duration of the contractile effort determines the magnitude of the signal or signals. This signaling can affect the following:

1. The activation or inhibition of transcription factors
2. The activation or inhibition of mRNA stability factors that mediate changes in mRNA degradation
3. Alterations in translational efficiency
4. The posttranslational modification of proteins
5. Changes in the kinetics of the transport of newly made proteins from the cytosol into the mitochondria (protein import)
6. Alterations in the rate of folding or assembly of proteins into multisubunit complexes

Signaling to these cellular events likely occurs via a variety of enzymatic processes, but the most commonly studied ones are those mediated by the activation of protein kinases and phosphatases, which covalently modify proteins by phosphorylation and dephosphorylation, respectively. Exercise is now known to be a potent activator of these enzymes (18,19). Among those discussed later in the chapter that appear to be involved in mitochondrial biogenesis include calcium/calmodulin-dependent protein kinase (CaMK), p38 mitogen-activated protein (MAP) kinase (MAPK), and AMP-activated protein kinase (AMPK) (Fig. 18.3). There are three fundamental cellular processes that occur during each acute exercise bout that lead to the activation of these kinases. These include (a) ATP turnover,

leading to the formation of AMP and the activation of AMP kinase; (b) an increase in cytosolic calcium, released from the SR; and (c) the production of reactive oxygen species (ROS), derived from a number of sources within muscle, including mitochondria themselves.

ATP turnover

Exercise increases the rate of ATP turnover within muscle cells. This alters the ratio of ATP to ADP_f and stimulates muscle metabolic rate. ADP_f can be converted to AMP via the myokinase reaction. This change in energy status

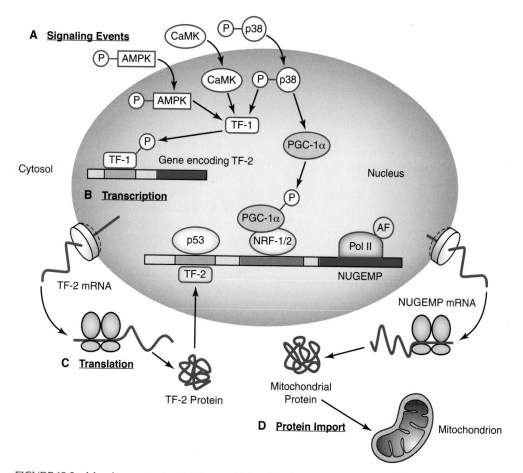

FIGURE 18.3 Muscle contraction initiates cell signals, which activate protein kinases, such as p38, AMP-activated protein kinase (AMPK), and calmodulin-dependent protein kinase (CaMK). Once activated, these kinases can translocate to the nucleus to phosphorylate transcription factors. In a hypothetical example, transcription factor-1 (TF-1) is activated by phosphorylation, which enhances its DNA-binding activity. TF-1 subsequently affects the rate of transcription of other transcription factors (e.g., TF-2). Once TF-2 messenger ribonucleic acid (mRNA) is produced, it is exported and translated into TF-2 protein in the cytosol. It can then be targeted to the nucleus to modify the rate of transcription of genes, which encode mitochondrial proteins. In a more specific case, exercise is known to affect the expression of the transcription factor nuclear respiratory factor-1 (NRF-1), as well as the coactivator peroxisome proliferator–activated receptor (PPAR) γ-coactivator-1α (PGC-1α). The transcription factor p53 is also an important regulator of organelle biogenesis. These proteins alter the transcription rates of nuclear-encoded mitochondrial proteins (NUGEMPs) by directly interacting with the basal transcription machinery. This multisubunit enzyme complex consists of the RNA polymerase II (Pol II) and a number of associated factors (AF). The mRNA representing the nuclear-encoded mitochondrial protein is translated into protein in the cytosol and targeted to the mitochondria via molecular chaperones, followed by import into the organelle (see Fig. 18.5).

of the muscle cell can also be achieved without exercise through the uncoupling of the mitochondrial respiratory chain, by mtDNA depletion, with iron deficiency, by genetic disruption of the creatine phosphokinase system, or with prolonged use of the agent β-guanidinopropionic acid. The rise in muscle AMP levels and the decreases in phosphocreatine and ATP concentrations associated with these conditions lead to the activation of AMPK. AMPK can also be activated pharmacologically using the adenosine analogue 5-aminoimidazole-4-carboxamide-1-β-D-ribofuranoside (AICAR). This drug is frequently used to mimic the metabolic effects of exercise in muscle. The chronic activation of AMPK activation is known to increase mitochondrial protein levels, including cytochrome c and δ-aminolevulinic acid synthase (ALAs). Cytochrome c is an important component of the electron transport chain (ETC), whereas ALAs is the rate-limiting enzyme in the synthesis of heme, the cytochrome prosthetic group. These downstream effects are probably mediated by an increase in the expression of the coactivator PGC-1α, as well as the activation of the transcription factor nuclear respiratory factor-1 (NRF-1) (discussed later) and its subsequent binding to a DNA sequence in the promoter regions of these genes.

Calcium

Ca^{2+} is released from the SR as a result of motoneuron-induced depolarization. Ca^{2+} then mediates actin and myosin interaction and muscle contraction. It also acts as a second messenger to couple the initial electrical events to subsequent alterations in gene expression. Disturbances in mitochondrial ATP production, evident from studies of mtDNA depletion or in mitochondrial myopathy patients, also result in elevated intracellular Ca^{2+} levels. These Ca^{2+} changes modify the activities of a multitude of calcium-dependent protein kinases and phosphatases, including CaMK, protein kinase C, and calcineurin, among others. Initial experiments with muscle cells in culture illustrated that chronic elevations in cytosolic Ca^{2+} resulted in increases in mitochondrial enzyme activities, as well as increases in the mRNA and protein expression of the ETC component cytochrome c, the important transcriptional coactivator PGC-1α (20,21), and mitochondrial biogenesis. In addition, transgenic mice selectively expressing a constitutively active form of CaMK IV in muscle showed an increase in mtDNA copy number and expression of a wide variety of genes involved in mitochondrial biogenesis. These included gene products directly involved in oxidative phosphorylation, fatty acid metabolism, and PGC-1α (22). These data imply that Ca^{2+} released from the SR during each action potential could serve as an important second messenger leading to mitochondrial biogenesis. However, the amplitude, duration, and temporal pattern of the Ca^{2+} signals necessary to provoke such changes must be established under more physiologic conditions.

Mitochondrially Derived Reactive Oxygen Species

Mitochondria consume oxygen to make ATP, which provides the cell with energy for survival. When the demand for ATP increases, such as during exercise, there is an elevation in mitochondrial oxygen consumption and an increase in the rate of ATP production. In fact, during exercise, skeletal muscle oxygen consumption can increase 30-fold and this results in an increase in ROS production (23). Mitochondrially derived ROS are formed when electrons traveling through the ETC are donated to oxygen from either complex I or III. If ROS are not properly regulated they can have deleterious effects on cellular function because they (a) promote the degradation of proteins and other macromolecules, (b) lead to the accumulation of somatic mutations and oxidative damage to mtDNA, and (c) activate apoptosis. To counteract these effects, muscle cells are equipped with both cytosolic and mitochondrial antioxidant proteins that function to prevent ROS accumulation. Therefore, ROS concentrations in muscle are determined by the balance between ROS production and their removal by antioxidant proteins and other ROS scavengers.

Muscle cells appear to convert approximately 0.2% to 0.8% of the total oxygen consumed into ROS. At this level of production, it is likely that ROS act as contributors to the signaling, which then leads to muscle phenotype adaptations to exercise. For example, ROS have been shown to activate both nuclear factor-kappa B and activator protein-1, which are transcription factors involved in the expression of PGC-1α, NRF-1, manganese superoxide dismutase, copper-zinc superoxide dismutase, and catalase (23). Indeed, the treatment of muscle cells with exogenous ROS activates the PGC-1α promoter, leading to a greater mRNA expression via both AMP kinase-dependent and -independent pathways (24). It has also been shown that exposure of cells to increases in ROS leads to an expansion of the mitochondrial reticulum and an increase in NRF-1 expression (25). These are important steps involved in mitochondrial biogenesis and the results clearly show that ROS, at non–death-provoking levels within the cell, can provide a physiologic advantage in signaling phenotype adaptations. Indeed, the inability to generate ROS does not permit cellular adaptations to be fully manifest.

Summary

The findings to date suggest that contractile activity simultaneously brings about the activation of AMPK, increases ROS production, and modifies intracellular Ca^{2+} levels. It is likely that all three of these signaling pathways are instrumental in producing mitochondrial biogenesis, in part, via the transcriptional coactivator PGC-1α.

Contractile Activity Affects the Transcription of Nuclear Genes Encoding Mitochondrial Proteins

Mitochondria are the only organelles to contain their own DNA, termed mtDNA. This genome encodes 13 of the approximate 1500 proteins required for proper mitochondrial function. Therefore, the process of mitochondrial biogenesis relies heavily on the additional expression of NUGEMPs to expand the organelle network. The regulation of nuclear gene expression is a dynamic process involving alterations in transcription (the synthesis of mRNA from DNA) or posttranscriptional mRNA modifications. Central to the basis of gene transcription is the activity and expression of proteins known as transcription factors (Fig. 18.3). Transcription factors are involved in the regulation of gene transcription via the ability of these proteins to interact with and bind to specific DNA consensus sequences in the promoter region of downstream target genes. Most nuclear genes, including those involved in mitochondrial biogenesis, are transcribed by the RNA polymerase II multisubunit enzyme complex. The recruitment of this enzyme complex to the promoter sequence, along with the interaction of transcription factors that modify RNA polymerase transcriptional activity, forms the basic platform from which a change in gene expression can occur.

Numerous transcription factors have been implicated in mediating the physiologic and metabolic adaptations associated with contractile activity. Those involved in the regulation of mitochondrial biogenesis include the NRF-1 and -2, peroxisome proliferation-activated receptor-α and receptor-γ (PPAR-α and PPAR-γ), estrogen-related receptor-α, p53, specificity protein 1, and the products of the immediate early genes c-jun and c-fos (26). This variety of transcription factors is important to satisfy the transcriptional process of the diverse number of genes required for the expansion of the mitochondrial network. Contractile activity has been shown to induce increases in the mRNA and/or protein levels of several transcription factors, consistent with their roles in mediating phenotypic changes as a result of chronic exercise. For example, both contractile activity in vitro and exercise in vivo have been shown to induce NRF-1 mRNA expression. In addition, the exercise-induced increase in NRF-1 expression precedes the increase of cytochrome c mRNA, an important component of the ETC in mitochondria.

The promoter regions of several nuclear genes encoding mitochondrial proteins have considerable sequence variability, meaning that the different NUGEMPs do not use the same transcription factors to regulate their expression. This variability suggests that the coordinated regulation of both the nuclear and mitochondrial genomes with contractile activity most likely involves a handful of regulatory proteins. Beyond the array of transcription factors involved in the regulation of NUGEMPs for mitochondrial biogenesis, transcriptional coactivators have emerged as potent regulatory proteins of gene expression. Coactivators lack the ability to bind DNA, but instead dock onto transcription factors and alter transcription via chromatin remodeling and interactions with transcription machinery. In fact, the PGC-1 family of coactivators is a very well studied example. These proteins have emerged as critical regulators of multiple cellular processes, including adaptive thermogenesis, glucose metabolism, muscle fiber type specialization, and oxidative phosphorylation across a wide range of tissues (27). PGC-1α was the first discovered member of the family of PGC-1 coactivators involved in the regulation of mitochondrial oxidative metabolism. PGC-1β- and PGC-1α-related coactivator (PRC) also comprise this family and both share a relatively similar involvement in the regulation of mitochondrial content and function. Specifically in muscle, strong evidence suggests that among the three PGC-1 members, PGC-1α most likely is the dominant regulator of mitochondrial function, respiration, and biogenesis. This effect is mediated, in part, by the powerful ability of PGC-1α to coactivate multiple transcription factors involved specifically in the regulation of NUGEMPs (27). In particular, coactivation of NRF-1, NRF-2, and estrogen-related receptor-α by PGC-1α results in the transactivation of genes involved in the ETC and transcription factors of mtDNA, such as transcription factor A, mitochondrial (Tfam) (26). Artificial overexpression of PGC-1 in skeletal muscle cells augments nuclear (e.g., cytochrome c, cytochrome oxidase [COX] subunit IV) and mitochondrially encoded (e.g., COX subunit II) ETC mRNA levels and amplifies mtDNA copy number. Thus, PGC-1α acts to orchestrate the expression of a variety of genes encoded by the nucleus, as well as mtDNA, leading to mitochondrial biogenesis. PGC-1β and PRC resemble PGC-1α in that they are able to bind to and coactivate NRF-1, thereby leading to increased gene expression of mitochondrial proteins (26). Increased protein of PGC-1β and PRC results in elevated levels of mtDNA transcription factors, as well as mRNA expression of nuclear and mitochondrial proteins of the ETC. The ability of PGC-1α, as well as -β and PRC, to integrate the transcriptional activity of these and several other nuclear transcription factors is what provides the coactivators with the capacity to coordinate the large number of genes required for mitochondrial biogenesis.

PGC-1α: An Important Regulator of Mitochondrial Function and Content in Muscle

PGC-1α mRNA expression and protein levels are induced in a variety of tissues in response to developmental, nutritional, hormonal, and environmental stimuli (Fig. 18.4) (28). The tissues in which PGC-1α mRNA is most highly expressed are those that rely mainly on oxidative metabolism for ATP production. These mitochondria-enriched tissues include skeletal muscle, heart, and brain. In skeletal muscle, the effects of exercise on PGC-1α mRNA and protein levels have been observed following a single bout or with chronic exercise (28,29). At least in the case of

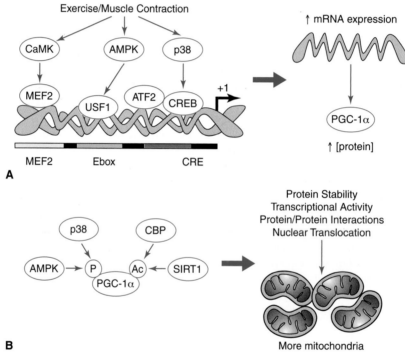

FIGURE 18.4 Peroxisome proliferator-activated receptor-γ coactivator-1α (PGC-1α) transcriptional **(A)** and posttranslational **(B)** regulation. **A.** Important protein kinases, transcription factors, and DNA sequence elements that affect the activity of the PGC-1α promoter. The intracellular signals produced by exercise or muscle contraction induce the activation of kinases such as calcium/calmodulin-dependent protein kinase (CaMK), adenosine monophosphate (AMP)-kinase (AMPK), and p38 mitogen-activated protein kinase (p38). These kinases target myocyte enhancer factor (MEF), upstream stimulatory factor 1 (USF1), activating transcription factor 2 (ATF2), and cAMP responsive element binding protein (CREB), respectively, and enhance transcription factor binding to specific DNA sequence elements within the PGC-1α promoter such as the MEF2, EBox, and the cyclic AMP response element (CRE). The number +1 represents the transcription start site. **B.** Posttranslational modifications that affect the biologic activity of PGC-1α via phosphorylation (P) or acetylation/deacetylation (Ac). AMPK and p38 MAPK directly phosphorylate PGC-1α to increase protein stability, transcriptional activity, and nuclear translocation. Acetylation of PGC-1α by CBP/p300 (CBP) and, conversely, deacetylation by the nicotinamide adenine dinucleotide-dependent deacetylase silent information regulator-1 (SIRT1) result in decreased and increased biologic activity of PGC-1α, respectively. Enhanced PGC-1α biologic activity and/or expression are important for the induction of mitochondrial biogenesis.

chronic exercise, the upregulation of PGC-1α mRNA and protein levels coincided with increases in mitochondrial biogenesis. The beneficial effects of increasing PGC-1α at the protein level in skeletal muscle also include increased cellular respiration and a tendency toward producing a fast-to-slow fiber type transformation. In the absence of PGC-1α, mitochondrial content and respiratory function decline, endurance performance deteriorates, and mitochondria are more susceptible to releasing pro-apoptotic proteins (29–31). However, mitochondrial biogenesis during exercise is not severely compromised because PGC-1α knockout animals can still increase mitochondrial biogenesis via endurance training (32). This suggests that other regulatory proteins exist that serve to compensate for the lack of PGC-1α during an exercise stimulus. Nonetheless, a complete understanding of how PGC-1α expression is regulated, and how its activity is controlled, can go a long way to improving our comprehension of the overall process of mitochondrial biogenesis and function during health, disease, and exercise.

The changes in PGC-1α mRNA expression in response to exercise and other stimuli can be largely accounted for by the activation of signaling pathways that target transcription factors and their regulatory elements within the PGC-1α promoter. Thus far, the best characterized pathways are those occurring through a proximal cyclic AMP (cAMP)-responsive element via the actions of cAMP-responsive element binding protein and activating transcription factor 2, both cAMP-responsive element binding factors, as well as a more distal adenine/thymine (A/T)-rich element that binds the myocyte enhancer factors (33). Additional transcription factors and regulatory elements within the PGC-1α promoter that have been shown to effect changes in PGC-1α mRNA levels include the forkhead transcription factor, and an Ebox, binding the upstream stimulatory factor 1 transcription factor (34). Although the use of pharmacologic agents to activate intracellular signals normally induced by contractile activity (see Fig. 18.6) have been very successful in defining the mechanisms leading to the activation of the PGC-1 promoter, the direct effect of contractile activity, the accompanying activation of these intracellular signals, and the ensuing effect on PGC-1α promoter activity and gene expression remain to be fully resolved.

Posttranslational modifications of the PGC-1α protein also account for many of the mechanisms that underlie PGC-1α-mediated actions on mitochondrial biogenesis. A growing list of protein kinases are involved in regulating the biologic activity of PGC-1α either through enhanced protein stability, transcriptional activity, and changes in subcellular localization (35). In skeletal muscle, the activation of both p38 MAPK and AMPK pathways resulted in the direct phosphorylation of PGC-1α on multiple serine/threonine sites, an effect that was required for the PGC-1α dependent recruitment, interaction, and coactivation of proteins to induce gene expression. In the case of PGC-1α-mediated phosphorylation by p38 MAPK, distinct dual actions of this kinase result in enhanced protein stabilization via direct phosphorylation and increased transcriptional activity, a result of the disruption between PGC-1α and a repressor. Other less characterized posttranslational modifications to PGC-1α, such as acetylation, may represent an important mechanism by which its transcriptional activity can be modulated. For example, associations with histone acetyl-transferases such as CBP/p300 or with the nicotinamide adenine dinucleotide-dependent deacetylase silent information regulator 1 could serve to decrease and increase transcriptional activity, respectively.

Summary

Although much work remains to be done to elucidate the effects of exercise on the regulation of PGC-1α expression in skeletal muscle, it is clear that enhanced stability, transcriptional activity, and nuclear translocation of the PGC-1 protein via posttranslational modifications are also important for the chronic effects of exercise on mitochondrial content within skeletal muscle.

TEST YOURSELF

How do members of the PGC-1 family act to promote mitochondrial biogenesis in muscle?

KEY POINT

PGC-1α has emerged as the most important single regulator of mitochondrial content thus far discovered.

Contractile Activity Influences mRNA Stability

mRNA levels are a function of the rate of production (*i.e.*, gene transcription) and the rate of degradation (*i.e.*, mRNA stability). Thus, in addition to the transcription of genes that produces mRNA transcripts leading to protein expression, the stabilization of mRNA molecules can also lead to phenotype adaptations. The ability of an mRNA molecule to resist degradation can provide a longer lasting substrate for the process of protein synthesis, resulting in greater protein levels within the cell. Thus, mRNA stability has emerged as an important regulatory component of gene expression. However, this process generates much less scientific attention than the events of gene transcription, partly because the methods for its assessment are less familiar. The stability of mRNA is usually mediated by protein factors that interact at the 3' untranslated region of the transcript to either stabilize or destabilize the mRNA. These are expressed in a tissue-specific fashion, leading to wide variations in the stability of mRNA across tissues. In general, nuclear transcripts encoding mito-chondrial proteins appear to be least stable in liver and most stable in skeletal muscle. For example, the mRNA encoding ALAs, the heme metabolism enzyme, has a very short half-life ($t_{1/2}$) of 22 minutes in liver but has a $t_{1/2}$ of approximately 14 hours in skeletal muscle. Thus, mRNA stabilization may have the greatest consequence for mito-chondrial biogenesis in liver because modest increases in stability can have a marked effect on mRNA levels in this tissue.

Contractile Activity–Induced Increases in Cytochrome *c* Expression are Mediated by Changes in Transcription and mRNA Stability

Cytochrome *c* has long been used as an indicator of mus-cle mitochondrial adaptations. Its expression is decreased by muscle disuse and increased by variations in exercise intensity and duration. Studies in vivo have examined cytochrome *c* expression in skeletal muscle and have revealed roles for contractile activity–induced changes in both gene transcription and mRNA stability. A cyto-chrome *c* promoter–reporter DNA construct was injected into tibialis anterior muscles of animals undergoing uni-lateral chronic electrical stimulation (3 hours to days) for 1 to 7 days (36). This technique, along with an mRNA decay assay in vitro, revealed time-dependent changes in both transcriptional activity and mRNA stability. The results indicated that the increase in cytochrome *c* mRNA observed as a result of chronic contractile activity was initially due to an induced increase in mRNA stability (2–4 days) and that this was followed by transcriptional activation leading to an increase in cytochrome *c* mRNA and protein. Whether this sequence of events holds for other proteins of the mitochondrial inner membrane remains to be determined, but the data suggest that the processes of transcription and mRNA stability should be considered when contractile-induced changes in gene expression are observed.

Summary

mRNA expression is regulated by transcription (synthe-sis) and mRNA turnover or stability (degradation) pro-cesses. Mechanisms of mRNA stability in muscle have been relatively ignored thus far and are fruitful areas for future investigation.

TEST YOURSELF

What is mRNA stability? How can this mechanism alter the phenotype of muscle?

Contractile Activity Affects Mitochondrial Protein Import

Description of the Protein Import Machinery

Of the approximate 1500 proteins within mitochondria, only 13 are encoded by mtDNA. Therefore, an elaborate sys-tem is required to transport nuclear-derived proteins from the cytosol into mitochondria (Fig. 18.5) (37), and this pro-cess is absolutely vital for organelle synthesis. The targeting pathway of these proteins depends on their ultimate location in the organelle (*i.e.*, matrix, outer or inner membrane, inter-membrane space). Many proteins are fabricated as precur-sor proteins with a signal sequence, often at the N-terminus. The most established and widely studied pathway is the one that directs proteins to the matrix space. In this case, the positively charged N-terminal signal sequence of the pre-cursor interacts with a cytosolic molecular chaperone that unfolds it and directs it to the outer membrane import recep-tor complex, termed the translocase of the outer membrane (Tom complex; Fig. 18.5). Cytosolic chaperones include heat shock proteins 70 and 90 kDa (HSP70, HSP90) and mitochondrial import–stimulating factor (MSF). Precursors are directed via these chaperones to either the Tom20 and Tom22 receptors, or to the Tom70–Tom37 heterodimer. They are then transferred to Tom40 and the small Tom proteins 5, 6, and 7, which form an aqueous channel through which the precursor protein passes to be sorted to the outer mem-brane, the inner membrane, or to the translocase of the inner membrane (Tim complex). The key Tim complex proteins include Tim17, Tim23, and Tim44. Tim17 and Tim23 span the inner membrane and have domains associated with both the matrix and intermembrane space. In a manner analogous to the Tom complex, Tim17 and Tim23 bind the precursor protein and form a pore through which the precursor can travel. Upon emerging on the inner face of the inner mem-brane, the precursor is pulled into the matrix by the ratchet-like action of mitochondrial HSP70 (mtHSP70). Once in the matrix, the N-terminal signal sequence of the precursor is cleaved by a mitochondrial processing peptidase to form the mature protein. It is then folded into its active conformation by HSP 60 kDa (HSP60) and chaperonin 10 kDa (cpn10). Apart from the import machinery itself, the translocation process into the matrix requires the presence of an intact membrane potential ($\Delta\Psi$, negative inside) across the inner membrane to help pull the positively charged presequence into the matrix. In addition, ATP is required for cytosolic unfolding in the cytosol and for the action of mtHSP70 in the matrix.

Most of the pioneering work that has led to discovery of the mechanisms of protein import described here was resolved in lower eukaryotes such as the yeast *Saccharomy-ces cerevisiae* and the fungus *Neurospora crassa*. More recent work, described next, has revealed that the mechanisms of import are similar in mammalian tissues, such as skeletal muscle and heart.

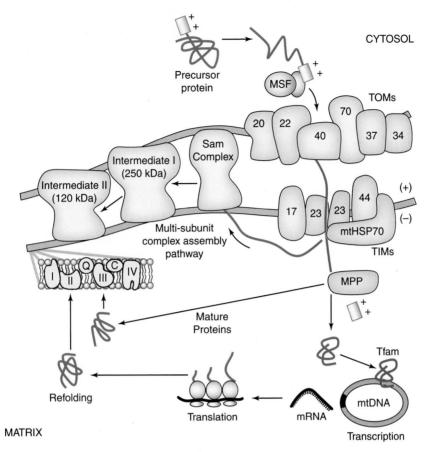

FIGURE 18.5   Nuclear-encoded proteins destined for the mitochondria are synthesized as precursor proteins in the cytosol containing a positively charged N-terminal presequence to which molecular chaperones bind. Chaperones such as mitochondrial import–stimulating factor (MSF) guide the precursor protein to the outer membrane translocase complex (Tom complex). The precursor protein is unfolded and directed through the outer membrane aqueous pore mainly consisting of Tom40. The precursor then interacts with the inner membrane phospholipid cardiolipin (*not shown*) and the translocase of the inner membrane (Tim complex). The matrix chaperone mitochondrial heat shock protein 70 (mtHSP70) pulls in the precursor and the signal sequence is cleaved by the mitochondrial processing peptidase (MPP), thereby forming the mature protein in the matrix. It is refolded by chaperonins heat shock protein 60 (HSP60) and chaperonin 10 (*not shown*). The number within each import machinery component refers to its size in kilodaltons. One important regulatory protein is mitochondrial transcription factor A (Tfam), which controls mitochondrial DNA (mtDNA) replication and transcription. ATP is required for multiple steps during the import process, including cytosolic unfolding and mtHSP70-directed movements. Imported proteins can combine with mtDNA-encoded gene products to form multisubunit complexes like cytochrome *c* oxidase (COX), or they can be inserted into the inner membrane and follow a pathway of multisubunit complex assembly within the membrane. This involves interaction with a sorting and assembly machinery (SAM) complex, followed by reorganization of the protein into different intermediates that are specific for each multisubunit holoenzyme. Chronic contractile activity accelerates the import process, in part, via the induction of important components of the import machinery, including MSF, Tom20, mtHSP70, and the refolding proteins. An adaptive increase in the rate of transcription and translation within a muscle cell could also increase the rate of import by providing more precursor substrate for the translocation process. mtDNA transcription is initiated by mitochondrial transcription factor A (Tfam) binding to a DNA sequence in the regulatory D-loop region. mRNA transcripts are translated within the organelle (protein synthesis) to form a total of 13 proteins. These are incorporated directly into the respiratory chain as single proteins, or they combine with nuclear-encoded imported proteins to form multisubunit complexes.

Import Studies in Skeletal Muscle Mitochondria

The first studies performed with isolated muscle mitochondria indicated that the kinetics of precursor protein import into the matrix of skeletal muscle SS and IMF mitochondrial subfractions differed by about twofold. IMF mitochondria import precursor proteins more rapidly than SS mitochondria and there is a close relationship between the rate of mitochondrial respiration and ATP production and the rate of protein import (11). This may contribute, in part, to the subtle differences in the biochemical characteristics of these mitochondrial subfractions.

Adaptations in the protein import machinery have relevance for mitochondrial biogenesis in skeletal muscle. In response to chronic contractile activity, a number of protein import machinery components are induced, up to approximately twofold. These include the cytosolic chaperones MSF and HSP70; the intramitochondrial proteins mtHSP70, HSP60, and cpn10; and the import receptors Tom20 and Tom34. Coincident with these changes are parallel contractile activity–induced increases in the rate of import into the matrix (38). Tom20 seems to be particularly important in this respect because experiments in muscle cells in which this outer membrane protein was artificially overexpressed and underexpressed led to parallel concomitant changes in the rates of protein import into the matrix. A very similar adaptation in the protein import pathway has been observed in cardiac mitochondria as result of thyroid hormone treatment. This indicates that the adaptive response is not unique to a contractile stimulus. Rather, it is common to other stimuli that increase mitochondrial biogenesis. The physiologic value of this adaptation is that the capacity for protein import is increased, producing mitochondria that are more sensitive to small changes in precursor protein concentration. Thus, at any given upstream production rate of cytosolic precursor proteins via transcription and translation, a higher rate of protein import would occur—a situation that would be advantageous for mitochondrial biogenesis. This would be of particular benefit during conditions of impaired mitochondrial protein import (a situation that could arise during chronic muscle disuse or disease) or during reductions in muscle cell ATP levels (such as those produced by severe contractile activity) or in cells with mtDNA mutations in which ATP production is reduced.

Summary

The protein import pathway is a complex protein targeting and transfer system, which is vital for organelle biogenesis, given the limited coding capacity of mtDNA. This capacity of this pathway increases in response to chronic exercise.

KEY POINT

The import of mitochondrial proteins from the cytosol into the organelle is critical for the assembly of multisubunit complexes within mitochondrial network.

TEST YOURSELF

Why is protein import vital for mitochondrial biogenesis? Describe the intricacies of this pathway, beginning with the translation of a nuclear-encoded precursor protein destined for the matrix.

The Expression and Copy Number of mtDNA

One of the most interesting aspects of mitochondrial biogenesis is that it requires the cooperation of the nuclear and mitochondrial genomes (Figs. 18.5 and 18.6). Mitochondria are unique in the fact that they house multiple copies of a small circular DNA molecule (mtDNA) comprising 16,569 nucleotides. Although mtDNA is minuscule in comparison to the 3 billion nucleotides found in the nuclear genome, it nonetheless contributes 13 mRNA, 22 tRNA, and 2 rRNA molecules that are essential for mitochondrial biogenesis and function. The 13 mRNA molecules all encode protein components of the respiratory chain, responsible for electron transport and ATP synthesis. The import of nuclear-encoded mtDNA maintenance proteins is necessary to transcribe and replicate this genome. These proteins include Tfam, mtRNA polymerase, DNA polymerase γ (POL-γ), mitochondrial single-stranded binding protein, RNA processing enzymes, and mitochondrial transcription factor B. Tfam has been studied most extensively because of its importance in both mtDNA transcription and replication. The level of Tfam correlates well with mtDNA abundance, and its loss, either in patients with mitochondrial myopathies or produced by experimental disruption of the Tfam gene, which results in partial or total depletion of mtDNA. Homozygous Tfam knockout animals die prior to birth and they are characterized by abnormal mitochondria and low rates of oxidative phosphorylation (39). Animals possessing heart- and muscle-specific disruptions of Tfam exhibit reduced levels of mtDNA and mtRNA and they display characteristics found in the mitochondrial disease Kearns-Sayre syndrome, such as dilated cardiomyopathy, abnormal mitochondrial morphology, and atrioventricular conduction block. These data provide evidence for the importance of Tfam in normal cardiac function, perhaps because the heart possesses the highest amount of mitochondria of all tissues.

The pioneering work of Williams and associates (40) showed that chronic contractile activity induces increases in mtDNA copy number, mtRNA transcripts, and the proportion of triplex DNA structure in the D-loop region. These data suggest that the replication of mtDNA into multiple copies regulates the level of mitochondrial gene expression in skeletal muscle cells. The increase in mtDNA copy number observed as a result of chronic contractile activity is accompanied by the augmented expression of mitochondrial single-stranded binding protein, but not POL-γ. These data suggest that POL-γ is sufficiently abundant and not limiting for the transcription of mtDNA. In addition, contractile activity induces an early and rapid increase in Tfam mRNA and protein expression in muscle. This is followed by an accelerated rate of Tfam import into mitochondria, accompanied by an increase in Tfam-mtDNA binding. This leads to an

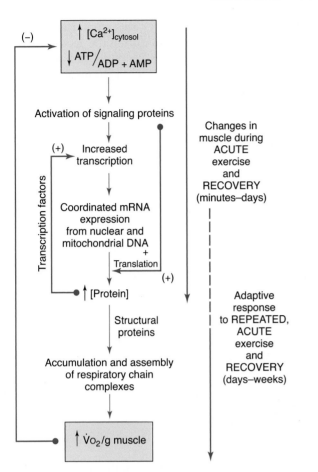

FIGURE 18.6 Summary of time-dependent changes in muscle cell signaling, gene expression, and assembly of multisubunit proteins (*e.g.*, COX), resulting in functional (increased $\dot{V}O_2$ per gram of muscle) and phenotypic (white to red) adaptations in muscle. Acute exercise increases intracellular calcium, ROS production, and the turnover of adenosine triphosphate (ATP). The magnitude of these signals depends on the intensity and duration of the exercise stimulus. Within minutes, these changes can activate signaling proteins (*e.g.*, CaMK, AMPK), which covalently modify proteins involved in transcription, translation, or messenger ribonucleic acid (mRNA) stability (*not shown*). The altered rates of transcription of nuclear and mitochondrial DNA result in the coordinated expression of mRNAs derived from both genomes. Over time, the mRNAs accumulate and are translated to protein, which becomes detectable after several days to weeks. The resulting proteins can contribute further to the adaptive changes in the pathway of gene expression (*e.g.*, if they are synthesized as nuclear-encoded transcription factors), or they can be assembled into components of metabolic pathways within the organelle, such as Krebs cycle enzymes, cytochromes, or multisubunit complexes of the respiratory chain. The resulting increased capacity for oxygen consumption (after several weeks of training) leads to the metabolic and performance alterations described in Fig. 18.2 and attenuates the exercise stress signal as mitochondrial biogenesis proceeds. ADP, adenosine diphosphate; AMP, adenosine monophosphate.

enhanced transcription of mtRNA and increased activity of enzymes possessing mtDNA-encoded subunits (*e.g.*, COX) (41). When combined with the actions of PGC-1α and NRF-1 on the nuclear genome, these changes are largely responsible for the observed coordination between nuclear and mitochondrial mRNA responses to chronic contractile activity. This serves to maintain the correct stoichiometry between nuclear-encoded and mitochondrially encoded subunits during the assembly of respiratory chain complexes.

Deletions or mutations of mtDNA leading to defective or absent gene products result in impaired respiration and mitochondrial disease of which a large number have now been documented (42). These are largely tissue-specific diseases and they predominate in organs with high energy demands, such as brain, heart, and muscle. In skeletal muscle, the result of an mtDNA abnormality is termed mitochondrial myopathy and it is characterized by exercise intolerance, fatigue, and exaggerated lactic acid production. An important yet unresolved question is whether exercise training can improve this situation in mitochondrial myopathy patients. Recent studies have begun to shed some light on the adaptive potential of exercise training. Most mtDNA-induced mitochondrial myopathy patients have a mixture of wild-type and mutant mtDNA, a situation known as mtDNA heteroplasmy. The extent of the pathophysiology is dependent on the ratio of mutant to normal, wild-type mtDNA copies per cell. It has been shown that aerobic training can induce increased levels of respiratory enzymes and proteins in mitochondrial myopathy patients (43,44). This increase led to an improvement in oxidative capacity and work performance. However, the endurance training protocol also produced an increase in the relative fraction of mutated mtDNA as well as an increase in signs of oxidative stress in most of the patients. Thus, although an improvement in work capacity is certainly beneficial, further examination of the effect of training is necessary in this population of patients with heteroplasmic mtDNA. Interestingly, a recent study appears to indicate the value of resistance training on oxidative capacity in this population of subjects (45). It is evident that more research using different training regimens and in a greater number and variety of mitochondrial myopathy patients is necessary to establish the utility of this approach for improving the quality of life for patients with mitochondrial disease.

Summary

mtDNA encodes 13 proteins that are vital for ETC function and ATP production. mtDNA copy number can increase as a result of chronic exercise, thereby helping to coordinate the synthesis of mitochondrial protein complexes that require both nuclear- and mtDNA-encoded subunits.

TEST YOURSELF

What does mtDNA encode? Why is this important and why do mutations have serious consequences?

Intramitochondrial Protein Synthesis and Contractile Activity

Because an impairment of mitochondrial protein synthesis can lead to disease, it is not surprising to learn that the process is vital for normal organelle adaptation to exercise. mRNA transcripts derived from mtDNA are employed along with the rRNAs and tRNAs in mitochondrial translation. Unfortunately, this process is not widely studied in muscle; however, recent advances in methodology may permit more extensive evaluations (46). Measurements using isolated muscle mitochondrial subfractions have revealed that IMF mitochondria synthesize protein at a greater rate than SS mitochondria, consistent with their greater oxidative capacity. In response to acute (5-minute), intense contractile activity, protein synthesis within SS mitochondria decreases, possibly as a result of the contraction-induced reduction of ATP within the organelle. Rates of protein synthesis are restored to normal during the recovery period (47). These data indicate that intramitochondrial protein turnover is influenced by acute contractile activity. To evaluate whether chronic contractile activity altered the rates of protein synthesis or degradation, skeletal muscle was chronically stimulated for 14 days to produce a significant increase in COX activity. Surprisingly, no adaptive increases in protein synthesis or degradation were observed (47). Thus, either the changes in protein turnover that occur as a result of exercise happen relatively early in the adaptation process, or they remain unaffected and, ultimately, do not limit the mitochondrial biogenesis response to contractile activity. More research in this area of mitochondrial biogenesis is warranted.

Exercise-Induced Changes in Gene Expression Are Most Evident during Recovery

It has long been suspected that adaptive responses to exercise manifest during the recovery phase following the exercise period. A wealth of evidence shows that the most pronounced changes occur during this time. This may be because when exercise stops, the energy required for contractile activity purposes is redirected to processes such as gene expression and protein synthesis (i.e., anabolism). The augmented gene expression during recovery is evident with respect to key events involved in mitochondrial biogenesis, such as the induction of PGC-1α (48) and the

transcription factor NRF-1. Other events related to muscle adaptation that increase during the recovery period include total muscle protein synthesis and degradation, increased activity of a variety of kinases involved in translation and cell signaling, and increases in mRNAs encoding important proteins involved in transcription (e.g., c-jun, c-fos) and glucose metabolism (e.g., glucose transporter 4, glycogenin), among others. These changes are usually preceded by increased rates of gene transcription (5), but this is not always the case.

Summary

Most of the data support the idea that the mitochondrial adaptations to contractile activity are a result of an accumulation of adaptive responses that originate from an acute exercise bout, but that are not manifest until the recovery period, when the muscle is at rest. The accumulation of gene products, usually during the recovery phase, resulting from repeated bouts of contractile activity, leads to the formation of more mitochondria via the mechanisms described in this chapter.

Skeletal Muscle Disuse

Thus far in this chapter, we have discussed the mechanisms of exercise-induced mitochondrial adaptations in muscle. In contrast to this, it is also important to recognize the mitochondrial changes that take place during chronic muscle disuse. The most well known and documented alteration that occurs in response to muscle disuse is the loss of skeletal muscle mass (49). The etiology of this is likely multifactorial and includes increases in protein degradation, autophagy, and myonuclear apoptosis, along with reductions in protein synthesis. From a mitochondrial perspective, muscle disuse leads to a decrease in mitochondrial content per gram of muscle, thereby contributing to the reduction in muscle endurance performance. Paradoxically, mitochondrially mediated apoptotic signalling is increased. During denervation-induced muscle disuse, mitochondrial respiration is reduced and ROS production is increased. ROS stimulate the release of at least two pro-apoptotic proteins: cytochrome c and apoptosis-inducing factor (AIF). Apoptosis-inducing factor release and translocation to the nucleus will cause DNA fragmentation. Cytochrome c release will lead to the activation of caspase enzymes, which also eventually result in DNA fragmentation. This can potentially lead to a reduction in myonuclear number and contribute to skeletal muscle atrophy. Interestingly, chronic contractile activity has been shown to have some protective effects against disuse-induced apoptosis because mitochondrial content is increased and pro-apoptotic protein release appears to be attenuated.

The reduction in mitochondrial content during muscle disuse may be partly due to ROS-induced autophagy. In response to increases in oxidative stress, like those observed during muscle disuse, autophagic proteins were shown to translocate to mitochondria and target them for autophagic degradation (50), a process that has been termed mitophagy. The impact of autophagy/mitophagy on skeletal muscle atrophy is not known, but it is reasonable to conclude that chronic muscle disuse activates several cellular signaling pathways that function to collectively reduce the cellular content of mitochondria, along with skeletal muscle mass. More research is required in this exciting area of muscle plasticity.

KEY POINT

Mitochondrial content is reduced during periods of muscle disuse. This affects muscle endurance and metabolism.

TEST YOURSELF

When mitochondrial content is reduced during chronic muscle disuse, can this contribute to muscle atrophy? Describe how.

What is mitochondrially mediated apoptosis? What is a likely trigger for this event?

CHAPTER SUMMARY

Chronic exercise training produces a well-established adaptation in skeletal muscle termed mitochondrial biogenesis. The physiologic benefit of this is enhanced endurance performance. This is advantageous for athletic endeavors and it improves the quality of life and functional independence of previously sedentary individuals. This chapter reviews the benefits of this adaptation with respect to

A MILESTONE OF DISCOVERY

Does endurance exercise training improve respiratory enzyme activity and result in enhanced oxygen uptake of skeletal muscle? Until 1967, properly designed studies using an appropriate duration per day, frequency per week, and intensity per exercise bout to test this hypothesis had not been completed. Limited evidence from comparative studies of birds and mammals indicated a relationship between the activity of a muscle and the content of respiratory enzymes. In addition, it was known that mitochondrial content in skeletal muscle could be increased by administration of thyroid hormone. In light of this, Holloszy hypothesized that the improvement in endurance performance observed with training could be due to an adaptive process of mitochondrial synthesis. At the time, only two studies had addressed the adaptability of mitochondrial enzyme activity and oxidative capacity to an exercise stimulus. Examination of the exercise intensities used in those investigations suggested that although a daily exercise program lasting 5 to 8 weeks should have been sufficient to provoke an adaptive response, the intensity and duration (daily 30-minute bout of swimming) were insufficient to provoke an adaptive response. Therefore, Holloszy used a treadmill training program that progressively increased in intensity and duration over 12 weeks. Muscles were then removed from the animals and homogenates and isolated mitochondrial fractions were prepared for oxygen consumption and enzyme activity measurements. One of the key findings of this study is shown in the table here. Oxygen uptake, expressed as microliters of oxygen per hour per gram, in mitochondria isolated from 1 g fresh muscle was twice as high in the trained (exercising) group as in comparable samples from sedentary muscles.

Group	Oxygen Uptake ($\mu L \cdot g^{-1}$)	Respiratory Control Index	P:O Ratio
Sedentary	506 ± 53	14.7 ± 2.6	2.7 ± 0.2
Exercising	1022 ± 118	16.1 ± 2.2	2.6 ± 0.1

Increases in oxygen uptake also coincided with 60% increases in the yield of total mitochondrial protein and a remarkable sixfold improvement in run time to exhaustion compared to the sedentary group. Holloszy was the first to predict that this improved performance could be a result of lower concentrations of ADP in the cytoplasm due to the greater rate of oxidative phosphorylation, which reduced lactate formation during exercise. This prediction was subsequently confirmed experimentally and this idea is now central to our understanding of the adaptations associated with endurance training. The novelty of the training program and the insight and interpretation provided by Holloszy in this study led to a remarkable advance in our knowledge of muscle adaptations to exercise. This work set the stage for literally hundreds of subsequent investigations on muscle plasticity, phenotype differences among muscle fiber types, and alterations in gene expression as a result of exercise. It also provided a new experimental model for the study of mitochondrial biogenesis. Finally, it shed light on the potential contributions of muscle adaptations to changes in whole body $\dot{V}o_{2max}$ and, ultimately, on the role of these adaptations in the overall health of the individual.

Holloszy JO. Biochemical adaptations in muscle: effects of exercise on mitochondrial oxygen uptake and respiratory enzyme activity in skeletal muscle. J Biol Chem. 1967;242:2278–2282.

metabolism and focuses on the underlying molecular basis for mitochondrial biogenesis in skeletal muscle subjected to models of exercise training. This includes a discussion of the following:

1. The initial signals arising in contracting muscle
2. The transcription factors involved in mitochondrial and nuclear DNA transcription
3. The posttranslational import mechanisms required for organelle synthesis

A summary of our understanding of the molecular and cellular mechanisms that govern the increases in mitochondrial volume with repeated bouts of exercise is shown in Figure 18.6. Further insights into the mechanisms involved may lead us to alternative therapeutic interventions that will benefit those with mitochondrial diseases and those unable to perform regular physical activity.

ACKNOWLEDGMENTS

We are grateful to Dr. Hans Hoppeler (University of Berne, Switzerland) for the provision of the electron micrographs of muscle mitochondria. Research in our laboratory is supported by the Natural Science and Engineering Research Council of Canada (NSERC), the Canada Research Chairs program, and the Canadian Institutes for Health Research (CIHR). Giulia Uguccioni is the recipient of a Heart and Stroke Foundation of Canada Fellowship and Isabella Irrcher is the recipient of a CIHR Post-Doctoral Fellowship. David A. Hood is the holder of a Canada Research Chair in Cell Physiology.

REFERENCES

1. Pette D, ed. *Plasticity of Muscle*. Berlin: Walter de Gruyter; 1980.
2. Holloszy JO. Biochemical adaptations in muscle. *J Biol Chem*. 1967;242:2278–2282.
3. Hood DA. Invited review: contractile activity-induced mitochondrial biogenesis in skeletal muscle. *J Appl Physiol*. 2001;90:1137–1157.
4. Hoppeler H. Exercise-induced ultrastructural changes in skeletal muscle. *Int J Sports Med*. 1986;7:187–204.
5. Pilegaard H, Ordway GA, Saltin B, et al. Transcriptional regulation of gene expression in human skeletal muscle during recovery from exercise. *Am J Physiol*. 2000;279:E806–E814.
6. Baldwin KM, Klinkerfuss GH, Terjung RL, et al. Respiratory capacity of white, red, and intermediate muscle: adaptive response to exercise. *Am J Physiol*. 1972;222:373–378.
7. Henriksson J, Reitman JS. Time course of changes in human skeletal muscle succinate dehydrogenase and cytochrome oxidase activities and maximal oxygen uptake with physical activity and inactivity. *Acta Physiol Scand*. 1977;99:91–97.
8. Gibala MJ, McGee SL. Metabolic adaptations to short-term high-intensity interval training: a little pain for a lot of gain? *Exerc Sport Sci Rev*. 2008;36:58–63.
9. Ljubicic V, Adhihetty PJ, Hood DA. Application of animal models: chronic electrical stimulation-induced contractile activity. *Can J Appl Physiol*. 2005;30:625–643.
10. Connor MK, Irrcher I, Hood DA. Contractile activity-induced transcriptional activation of cytochrome *c* involves Sp1 and is proportional to mitochondrial ATP synthesis in C2C12 muscle cells. *J Biol Chem*. 2001;276:15898–15904.
11. Takahashi M, Hood DA. Protein import into subsarcolemmal and intermyofibrillar skeletal muscle mitochondria. *J Biol Chem*. 1996;271:27285–27291.
12. Kirkwood SP, Packer L, Brooks GA. Effects of endurance training on a mitochondrial reticulum in limb skeletal muscle. *Arch Biochem Biophys*. 1987;255:80–88.
13. Ogata T, Yamasaki Y. Ultra-high-resolution scanning electron microscopy of mitochondria and sarcoplasmic reticulum arrangement in human red, white, and intermediate muscle fibers. *Anat Rec*. 1997;248:214–223.
14. Twig G, Hyde B, Shirihai OS. Mitochondrial fusion, fission and autophagy as a quality control axis: the bioenergetic view. *Biochim Biophys Acta*. 2008;1777:1092–1097.
15. Herzig S, Martinou JC. Mitochondrial dynamics: to be in good shape to survive. *Curr Mol Med*. 2008;8:131–137.
16. Cartoni R, Leger B, Hock MB, et al. Mitofusins 1/2 and ERRalpha expression are increased in human skeletal muscle after physical exercise. *J Physiol*. 2005;567:349–358.
17. Terjung RL. The turnover of cytochrome *c* in different skeletal-muscle fibre types of the rat. *Biochem J*. 1979;178:569–574.
18. Ljubicic V, Hood DA. Specific attenuation of protein kinase activation in muscle with a high mitochondrial content. *Am J Physiol Endocrinol Metab*. 2009;297:E749–E758.
19. Röckl KS, Witczak CA, Goodyear LJ. Signaling mechanisms in skeletal muscle: acute responses and chronic adaptations to exercise. *IUBMB Life*. 2008;60:145–153.
20. Wright DC, Geiger PC, Han DH, et al. Calcium induces increases in peroxisome proliferator-activated receptor gamma coactivator-1alpha and mitochondrial biogenesis by a pathway leading to p38 mitogen-activated protein kinase activation. *J Biol Chem*. 2007;282:18793–18799.
21. Freyssenet D, Di Carlo M, Hood DA. Calcium-dependent regulation of cytochrome c gene expression in skeletal muscle cells. Identification of a protein kinase c-dependent pathway. *J Biol Chem*. 1999;274:9305–9311.
22. Wu H, Kanatous SB, Thurmond FA, et al. Regulation of mitochondrial biogenesis in skeletal muscle by CaMK. *Science*. 2002;296:349–352.
23. Powers SK, Jackson MJ. Exercise-induced oxidative stress: cellular mechanisms and impact on muscle force production. *Physiol Rev*. 2008;88:1243–1276.
24. Irrcher I, Ljubicic V, Hood DA. Interactions between reactive oxygen species and AMP kinase activity in the regulation of PGC-1α expression in skeletal muscle cells. *Am J Physiol Cell Physiol*. 2009;296:C116–C123.
25. Hood DA, Irrcher I, Ljubicic V, et al. Coordination of metabolic plasticity in skeletal muscle. *J Exp Biol*. 2006;209:2265–2275.
26. Scarpulla RC. Transcriptional paradigms in mammalian mitochondrial biogenesis and function. *Physiol Rev*. 2008;88:611–638.
27. Handschin C, Spiegelman BM. Peroxisome proliferator-activated receptor gamma coactivator 1 coactivators, energy homeostasis, and metabolism. *Endocr Rev*. 2006;27:728–735.
28. Ljubicic V, Joseph AM, Saleem A, et al. Transcriptional and post-transcriptional regulation of mitochondrial biogenesis in skeletal muscle: effects of exercise and aging. *Biochim Biophys Acta*. 2009;1800:223–234.
29. Arany Z. PGC-1 coactivators and skeletal muscle adaptations in health and disease. *Curr Opin Genet Dev*. 2008;18:426–434.
30. Adhihetty PJ, Uguccioni G, Leick L, et al. The role of PGC-1alpha on mitochondrial function and apoptotic susceptibility in muscle. *Am J Physiol Cell Physiol*. 2009;297:C217–C225.
31. Handschin C, Chin S, Li P, et al. Skeletal muscle fiber-type switching, exercise intolerance, and myopathy in PGC-1alpha muscle-specific knock-out animals. *J Biol Chem*. 2007;282:30014–30021.
32. Leick L, Wojtaszewski JF, Johansen ST, et al. PGC-1alpha is not mandatory for exercise- and training-induced adaptive gene responses in mouse skeletal muscle. *Am J Physiol Endocrinol Metab*. 2008;294:E463–E474.
33. Yan Z, Li P, Akimoto T. Transcriptional control of the Pgc-1alpha gene in skeletal muscle in vivo. *Exerc Sport Sci Rev*. 2007;35:97–101.
34. Irrcher I, Ljubicic V, Kirwan AF, et al. AMP-activated protein kinase-regulated activation of the PGC-1alpha promoter in skeletal muscle cells. *PLoS ONE*. 2008;3:e3614.
35. Wright DC, Han DH, Garcia-Roves PM, et al. Exercise-induced mitochondrial biogenesis begins before the increase in muscle PGC-1alpha expression. *J Biol Chem*. 2007;282:194–199.

36. Freyssenet D, Connor MK, Takahashi M, et al. Cytochrome c transcriptional activation and mRNA stability during contractile activity in skeletal muscle. *Am J Physiol.* 1999;277:E26–E32.

37. Mokranjac D, Neupert W. Thirty years of protein translocation into mitochondria: unexpectedly complex and still puzzling. *Biochim Biophys Acta.* 2009;1793:33–41.

38. Takahashi M, Chesley A, Freyssenet D, et al. Contractile activity-induced adaptations in the mitochondrial protein import system. *Am J Physiol.* 1998;274:C1380–C1387.

39. Larsson NG, Wang J, Wilhelmsson H, et al. Mitochondrial transcription factor A is necessary for mtDNA maintenance and embryogenesis in mice. *Nature Gen.* 1998;18:231–236.

40. Williams RS. Genetic mechanisms that determine oxidative capacity of striated muscles: control of gene transcription. *Circulation.* 1990;82:319–331.

41. Gordon JW, Rungi AA, Inagaki H, et al. Effects of contractile activity on mitochondrial transcription factor A expression in skeletal muscle. *J Appl Physiol.* 2001;90:389–396.

42. Wallace DC. A mitochondrial paradigm of metabolic and degenerative diseases, aging, and cancer: a dawn for evolutionary medicine. *Annu Rev Genet.* 2005;39:359–407.

43. Taivassalo T, Shoubridge EA, Chen J, et al. Aerobic conditioning in patients with mitochondrial myopathies: physiological, biochemical, and genetic effects. *Ann Neurol.* 2001;50:133–141.

44. Adhihetty PJ, Taivassalo T, Haller RG, et al. The effect of training on the expression of mitochondrial biogenesis- and apoptosis-related proteins in skeletal muscle of patients with mtDNA defects. *Am J Physiol Endocrinol Metab.* 2007;293:E672–E680.

45. Murphy JL, Blakely EL, Schaefer AM, et al. Resistance training in patients with single, large-scale deletions of mitochondrial DNA. *Brain.* 2008;131:2832–2840.

46. Jaleel A, Short KR, Asmann YW, et al. In vivo measurement of synthesis rate of individual skeletal muscle mitochondrial proteins. *Am J Physiol Endocrinol Metab.* 2008;295:E1255–E1268.

47. Connor MK, Bezborodova O, Escobar CP, et al. Effect of contractile activity on protein turnover in skeletal muscle mitochondrial subfractions. *J Appl Physiol.* 2000;88:1601–1606.

48. Pilegaard H, Saltin B, Neufer PD. Exercise induces transient transcriptional activation of the PGC-1alpha gene in human skeletal muscle. *J Physiol.* 2003;546:851–858.

49. Adhihetty PJ, O'Leary MF, Hood DA. Mitochondria in skeletal muscle: adaptable rheostats of apoptotic susceptibility. *Exerc Sport Sci Rev.* 2008;36:116–121.

50. Dagda RK, Zhu J, Kulich SM, et al. Mitochondrially localized ERK2 regulates mitophagy and autophagic cell stress: implications for Parkinson's disease. *Autophagy.* 2008;4:770–782.

CHAPTER 19

The Endocrine System: Integrated Influences on Metabolism, Growth, and Reproduction

Abbreviations

ADP	Adenosine-5′-diphosphate	GH	Growth hormone
AICAR	5-Aminoimidazole-4-carboxamide-1 β-riboside, an activator of AMPK	GLUT4	Glucose transporter protein found in muscle
AMP	Adenosine-5′-monophosphate	GnRH	Gonadotropin-releasing hormone
AMPK	AMP-activated protein kinase, the cell's energy sensor	HAAF	Hypoglycemia-associated autonomic failure
aPKC	Atypical protein kinase C, a downstream component of the insulin signaling pathway	HEC	Hyperinsulinemic euglycemic clamp
		HOMA	Homeostatic Model Assessment
		HSL	Hormone-sensitive lipase
AR	Androgen receptor	IGF-I	Insulin-like growth factor-1
AS160	A 160 kD downstream component of the insulin signaling pathway parallel to aPKC	IMFSIGT	Insulin-modified, frequently sampled intravenous glucose tolerance test
		ISGD	Insulin-stimulated glucose disposal
ATP	Adenosine-5′-triphosphate	IVGTT	Intravenous glucose tolerance test
BAT	Brown adipose tissue	LH	Luteinizing hormone
BMI	Body mass index	LPL	Lipoprotein lipase
CaMK	Ca/calmodulin-dependent protein kinase, a component of the Ca^{++} signaling pathway	MAPK	Mitogen-activated protein kinase, a component in the insulin signaling pathway
CaMKK	CaMK kinase, a component of the Ca^{++} signaling pathway	MGF	Mechano growth factor
		MHC	Myosin heavy chain
CoA	Coenzyme A, a vitamin involved in the metabolism of fatty acids and glucose	MLC	Myosin light chain
		mRNA	Messenger ribonucleic acid
CoQ	Coenzyme Q, a vitamin that transports protons across the inner mitochondrial membrane	mtDNA	Mitochondrial DNA
		NEFA	Nonesterified fatty acid
		NISGD	Non–insulin-stimulated glucose disposal
CRH	Corticotropin-releasing hormone	NTX	N-terminal telopeptide of type I collagen
FA	Fatty acid	OGTT	Oral glucose tolerance test
FFA	Free fatty acid	QUICKI	Quantitative Insulin Sensitivity Check Index
FFM	Free fatty mass		
FSH	Follicle-stimulating hormone	PI3K	Phosphatidylinositol 3-kinase, an upstream component of the insulin signaling pathway
FSIGT	Frequently sampled intravenous glucose tolerance test		
GD	Glucose disposal	PICP	Type I procollagen carboxy-terminal propeptide
GDR	Glucose disposal rate		

PINP	Type I procollagen amino-terminal propeptide	SERCA	Sarcoplasmic/endoplasmic reticulum Ca^{++}-ATPase pump
PKC	Protein kinase C, a component of the Ca^{++} signaling pathway	T_3	Triiodothyronine, the active form of thyroid hormone
PVN	Paraventricular nucleus of the hypothalamus	TG	Triglyceride (triacylglycerol)
Ras	A family of protooncogenes of the regulatory proteins in signal transduction	UCP	Uncoupling protein (UCP-1, UCP-2, and UCP-3)
rhGH	Recombinant human GH	WAT	White adipose tissue
RMR	Resting metabolic rate	VLDL	Very low density lipoproteins

Introduction

Working muscle requires a supply of metabolic fuels from which it can extract the energy to do the work of overcoming or adapting to mechanical loads and repairing the damage caused by those loads. Physical activities differ greatly in the intensity, duration, and frequency of the loads they impose, and they stimulate specific adaptations to themselves. Exercise training remodels the body, and athletes maximize their performance, in part, by managing this remodeling process to acquire a sport-specific (and, in some team sports, position-specific) optimal body size, body composition, and mix of energy stores. Thus, consciously, intentionally, and intelligently or not, all athletes are bodybuilders.

Over the past few decades, much has been learned about the endocrine mechanisms that mediate the influences of diet and exercise on the availability of metabolic fuels for remodeling skeletal muscle and other tissues, and for athletic performance and health. Hormones stimulate or suppress intracellular signaling pathways by attaching to specific receptors on the surface or in the cytoplasm, mitochondrion, or nucleus of the target cell. During exercise, hormones regulate the mobilization of metabolic fuels from energy stores in various tissues throughout the body and the uptake and utilization of those fuels by working muscle. After exercise, hormones regulate the replenishment of those stores, as well as the repair and remodeling of skeletal muscle and other tissues, to better cope with repetitions of mechanical loads.

Despite the responsiveness of endocrine mechanisms, when the metabolic demands of exercise exceed the availability of metabolic fuels, the eventual result is fatigue, and when the demands of exercise training persistently exceed the supply of energy in the diet, the eventual result is illness. Dietary energy is used in six fundamental physiologic functions: basal metabolism, thermoregulation, growth and repair, immunity, locomotion, and reproduction. Energy that is consumed for one of these functions is not available for the others. In athletes, the amount of energy that is habitually consumed by working muscle for locomotion can reduce the availability of metabolic fuels (and especially the availability of glucose, which is the principal metabolic fuel of the brain) to the point that other functions are impaired.

Two terms recur often in this chapter: energy availability and carbohydrate availability. In the field of bioenergetics, energy availability can be generically defined as the amount of dietary energy that remains for other physiologic functions after subtracting the energy consumed by any particular function of interest, such as thermoregulation or immune function. In exercise physiology, it is appropriate to define, quantify, and control energy availability as dietary energy intake minus exercise energy expenditure. Defined in this way, energy availability can be thought of as the amount of dietary energy that remains after exercise training for all other physiologic functions. Analogously, it is useful to define carbohydrate availability as dietary carbohydrate intake minus carbohydrate oxidation during exercise. Because most energy is expended in fat-free mass (FFM), both quantities are best normalized to FFM, in units of kilocalories per kilogram of FFM per day (kcal/kgFFM/day). In adults, energy balance and resting metabolic rate (RMR) occur at energy availabilities of ~45 and ~30 kcal/kgFFM/day, respectively. Therefore, for typical Western diets containing ~55% carbohydrate, these energy availabilities correspond to carbohydrate availabilities of ~22 and ~15 kcal/kgFFM/day.

Undernutrition is especially common in endurance, esthetic, and weight-class sports. To prevent adverse effects on the competitive performance, physical health, growth, and development of wrestlers, the American College of Sports Medicine (ACSM) published a position stand in 1996 recommending measures to educate coaches and wrestlers about sound nutrition and weight control behavior, to curtail weight cutting, and to establish rules limiting weight loss (1). The National Collegiate Athletic Association (2) adopted such rules in 1997 after three wrestlers collapsed and died in the presence of coaches, because the wrestlers were cutting weight to qualify for competition. In 1997, ACSM published another position stand warning athletes, coaches, and parents about the female athlete triad, a syndrome in which severe undernutrition can lead to amenorrhea and osteoporosis (3). This position stand was revised in 2007 to update information about the endocrine mechanisms of these disorders and to provide current guidance for their prevention and treatment (4).

As described in detail below, the endocrine response to exercise and the physiologic consequences of that response depend on nutritional status. This is true acutely in response to a single exercise bout, and chronically in response to exercise training. Historically, this interaction of diet and exercise has been largely ignored in exercise physiology research. As a result, much less is known about the specific effects of exercise, independent of energy availability, than has been widely assumed (5). This chapter focuses attention on the resulting lack of consensus within the field of exercise endocrinology as a subdiscipline of exercise physiology. The literature for exercise endocrinology includes inconsistent experimental results and conflicting interpretations, and in some areas, descriptive studies have yet to lay a foundation for mechanistic experiments. Therefore, this chapter raises as well as answers questions.

KEY POINT

Because the confounding effects of energy availability on physiologic systems have been largely ignored in exercise physiology research, the specific effects of exercise and exercise training, independent of energy availability, remain obscure.

In addition to integrating the influences of diet and exercise on regulating the remodeling of the musculoskeletal system and the fueling of athletic performance, the endocrine system also integrates the influences of other factors, such as cold exposure and hypoxia, on energy availability, immune function, fluid and electrolyte balance, erythropoiesis, and reproductive function. Students should seek more detailed information about those topics in other chapters of this book. A thorough understanding of the current state of knowledge about the regulation of metabolism requires familiarity with the important roles of the sympathetic nervous system. Because this chapter only occasionally touches upon this subject, students should consult other sources for more complete information (6–9). Finally, this chapter assumes a familiarity with the basic endocrinology of hormone classification, chemistry, synthesis, secretion, transport, feedback, receptor interactions, and intracellular signaling. Students should consult other textbooks for information on those topics.

KEY POINT

Along with the sympathetic nervous system, the endocrine system mediates the influences of environment and behavior (including diet and exercise behavior) on all physiologic processes, including glucose homeostasis, muscle plasticity, mitochondrial biogenesis and coupling, bone turnover, and reproductive function.

Regulation of the Storage and Mobilization of Metabolic Fuels

Glucose Homeostasis

Compared with other mammalian brains, the human brain has an extremely high, nearly constant rate of energy consumption, accounting for ~20% of basal metabolism in adults and ~50% in children, even though it comprises only ~2% of body weight. The brain depends almost exclusively on glucose as a metabolic fuel for energy, and because it has virtually no glucose storage capacity, it depends on a constant supply of glucose from the bloodstream. At a normal plasma glucose concentration of ~5 mM, brain glucose uptake is about twice the rate of brain glucose utilization (~100 g day), so that as much glucose is recycled to the bloodstream as is oxidized and otherwise utilized. Because brain glucose uptake is proportional to plasma glucose concentration, however, a declining plasma glucose concentration eventually becomes limiting on brain metabolism. This occurs at a concentration of ~3.6 mM.

Plasma glucose concentration falls during prolonged exercise, with the magnitude of the drop being directly related to the absolute intensity of the work performed and the duration of the exercise bout. Furthermore, the fall in blood glucose is more extreme during successive bouts of exercise, even when the duration and workload are identical (10). For example, in one study (11), five times as much glucose had to be infused to maintain plasma glucose concentrations during the second of two 90-minute exercise bouts at 50% of $\dot{V}O_{2max}$ on the same day, even though glycogen stores were replenished after the first bout.

Between meals, the brain relies on the mobilization of glucose by the liver for its supply of glucose, because skeletal muscle lacks the enzyme to return glucose from muscle glycogen stores to the bloodstream. Liver glycogen stores (~50 g/kg tissue ≈ 90 g) can supply the brain energy requirement for less than 1 day, however, and they are also used to meet the metabolic demands of working muscle. Thus, working muscle competes directly with the brain for glucose, and it competes very aggressively. During a 2-hour marathon race, working skeletal muscle consumes as much glucose as the brain consumes in a week.

Despite this metabolic peril, human beings have survived because the brain has evolved multifaceted, redundant (i.e., highly reliable) endocrine mechanisms for preventing hypoglycemia. Rapidly responsive mechanisms activated by acute glucose deficiency between meals and during exercise mobilize glucose from glycogen and protein stores, while more slowly responding mechanisms activated by chronic glucose deficiency conserve available glucose for the brain by suppressing the utilization of glucose by skeletal muscle and other peripheral tissues.

Glucose counterregulation

The defenses against the isolated influence of hypoglycemia are triggered at so-called glycemic thresholds (*i.e.*, arterialized venous plasma glucose concentrations) (12), with insulin secretion being suppressed as a first line of defense at ~4.5 mM. Glucagon, epinephrine, and growth hormone (GH) secretion are stimulated at ~3.7 mM, and cortisol secretion is stimulated at ~3.6 mM as a second line of defense when brain glucose uptake becomes limiting on brain metabolism. If the plasma glucose concentration falls further, neural glucose deprivation can cause perceptible neurogenic symptoms (*e.g.*, sweating, hunger, tingling, tremor, heart pounding, and anxiety) and neuroglycopenic symptoms (*e.g.*, warmth, weakness, confusion, drowsiness, faintness, dizziness, difficulty speaking, and blurred vision) to stimulate eating as a third line of defense at ~3.0 mM before cognitive dysfunction occurs at ~2.6 mM.

Plasma glucose concentration is the primary determinant of insulin secretion by pancreatic islet β cells, with increases in plasma glucose increasing secretion and decreases decreasing secretion. This responsiveness of β cells to plasma glucose concentration is suppressed by α_2-adrenergic sympathetic stimulation by epinephrine from the adrenal medulla and by norepinephrine from sympathetic nerve terminals. Thus, the rise in catecholamines that occurs during exercise suppresses insulin secretion even when the plasma glucose concentration is maintained at 5.3 mmol/L by an exogenous glucose infusion (Fig. 19.1) (13).

Plasma glucose concentration is also the primary determinant of glucagon secretion by pancreatic islet α cells, with increases in plasma glucose reducing secretion and decreases increasing secretion. Whether glucagon secretion in humans is stimulated directly by catecholamines is a matter of dispute. Because glucagon secretion is inhibited by the paracrine intra-islet tonic influence of insulin, however, the rise in catecholamines that occurs during exercise appears to act indirectly via insulin to raise glucagon concentrations even when euglycemia is maintained by exogenous glucose infusion (Fig. 19.1) (13).

Plasma glucose concentration also regulates the secretion of epinephrine by the adrenal medulla, GH by the pituitary, and cortisol by the adrenal cortex, in all cases mediated by glucose sensors in the central nervous system (7). Increases in plasma glucose decrease secretion, and decreases increase secretion. Exercise also activates these hormones even when euglycemia is maintained by exogenous glucose infusion (Fig. 19.1) (13).

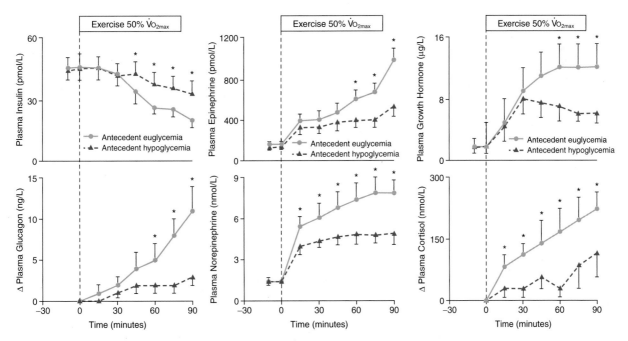

FIGURE 19.1 Acute insulin, glucagon, epinephrine, norepinephrine, growth hormone, and cortisol responses to 90 minutes of exercise at 50% V̇O₂max under clamped euglycemic conditions after clamped euglycemia (5.3 mM) and after two 90-minute bouts of clamped hypoglycemia (3.0 mM) on the previous day. Exercise responses occurred despite clamped euglycemia. Antecedent hypoglycemia blunted all of the responses. (Reprinted with permission from Davis SN, Galassetti P, Wasserman DH, et al. Effects of antecedent hypoglycemia on subsequent counterregulatory responses to exercise. *Diabetes.* 2000;49:76–77.)

Even though increases in GH and cortisol are part of the counterregulatory response to exercise and contribute to the prevention of hypoglycemia, their contribution is of secondary importance (12,14). The rapid mobilization of metabolic fuels that prevents acute hypoglycemia is accomplished by increases in sympathetic activity and glucagon secretion, whereas GH and cortisol responses do not begin to affect glucose production or plasma glucose levels until four hours later, long after the increased metabolic demands of most exercise bouts have ceased. Nor is either GH or cortisol necessary for recovery from hypoglycemia, given that plasma glucose concentrations have been shown to rise equally rapidly after several hours of insulin-induced hypoglycemia in patients with hypopituitarism (but normal pancreatic function) and in normal control subjects. Thus, when insulin and glucagon responses are operative, GH and cortisol are not involved in the correction of brief hypoglycemia or in the prevention of hypoglycemia during an exercise bout, and they contribute in only a minor way to the defense against slowly developing hypoglycemia during an overnight fast or in chronic undernutrition.

Although there is consensus about the primacy of insulin and the relative unimportance of GH and cortisol in the prevention of severe hypoglycemia and the recovery of euglycemia, the importance of catecholamines for glucoregulation during exercise in humans continues to be a matter of dispute. Results from experiments that prevent the action of sympatho-adrenal mechanisms by severing nerves or pharmacologically blocking receptors have been interpreted as implying that these mechanisms make little contribution to glucose production during exercise until after at least 90 minutes of moderate intensity exercise (Fig. 19.2) (15). Recently, however, other experiments investigating the effects of prolonged hypoglycemia and prolonged exercise on subsequent glucose counterregulation have left sympatho-adrenal mechanisms intact. These experiments seem to imply that sympatho-adrenal mechanisms operate in a subtle manner almost from the onset of exercise (6).

Hypoglycemia-associated autonomic failure

The glycemic thresholds mentioned above are dynamic in that they shift higher after sustained hyperglycemia and lower after episodes of hypoglycemia or prolonged exercise (16). As Figure 19.1 illustrates, two 90-minute episodes of insulin-induced hypoglycemia on 1 day lower glycemic thresholds in response to prolonged exercise the next day, thereby blunting glucose counterregulatory hormone responses, hepatic glucose production, and lipolysis by 50%, and impairing the body's ability to maintain normal plasma glucose levels (13). This effect is reciprocal in that two 90-minute bouts of 50% $\dot{V}_{O_{2max}}$ exercise on one day have the same effects on insulin-induced hypoglycemia the following day (17).

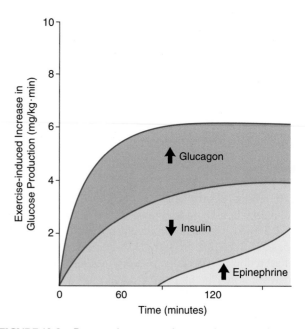

FIGURE 19.2   Rise in glucose production during moderate exercise and the contributions to it by decreased insulin and increased glucagon and epinephrine. Epinephrine becomes increasingly important as exercise is prolonged. (Reprinted with permission from Wasserman DH, Cherrington AD. Regulation of extra muscular fuel sources during exercise. In: LB Rowell, JT Shephard, eds. *Handbook of Physiology, Section 12: Exercise: Regulation and Integration of Multiple Systems.* Oxford: Oxford University; 1996.)

These experiments have a practical relevance for endurance athletes who may do two-a-day workouts during an intensive training regimen. Because the threshold for neurogenic and neuroglycopenic symptoms is reduced along with those for the counterregulatory hormones, the affected individual is unaware of the hypoglycemia on the second day. Consequently, a vicious cycle may ensue in which the absence of symptoms leads to episodes of more severe hypoglycemia, which further lower glycemic thresholds, and so on. The hazard in progressively lowering glycemic thresholds is that eventually, further hypoglycemia will elicit symptoms too late for behavioral or medical intervention. This hazard is especially serious for people with type 1 diabetes, who lack both the first (insulin) and second (glucagon) lines of defense against hypoglycemia.

The mechanism of this effect, which is termed hypoglycemia-associated autonomic failure (HAAF), involves a decline in adrenomedullary and sympathetic activation as reflected in lower plasma catecholamine concentrations and reduced skeletal muscle sympathetic nerve activity (18). As shown in Figure 19.1, cortisol responses are blunted as early as 15 minutes after the onset of exercise.

Although it is associated with hypoglycemia, HAAF is not caused directly by hypoglycemia, for it occurs even when plasma glucose concentrations are maintained by exogenous infusion of glucose during antecedent prolonged exercise (19). The factor that directly suppresses sympathetic activity is the stimulation of corticosteroid receptors in the brain. This is evidenced by the facts that HAAF does not occur in patients with Addison's disease, who lack the ability to secrete cortisol (16), and it can be induced in rats by infusing a low dose of cortisol into the paraventricular nucleus (PVN) of the brain under euglycemic systemic conditions, and prevented by infusing a corticosteroid antagonist during antecedent episodes of hypoglycemia (16). This effect lasts as long as cortisol remains bound to PVN corticosteroid receptors, which may be several days (16).

This corticosteroid-mediated suppression of sympathetic activity appears to explain why HAAF occurs in men but not in eumenorrheic women (17), and in postmenopausal women but not in those who are receiving estrogen replacement (20). By binding to corticosteroid receptors in the brain, estrogen accentuates cortisol responses to stress (21) and stimulates corticotropin-releasing hormone (CRH) gene expression in the PVN (22). Thus, the effect of HAAF is to reduce the normally greater counterregulatory hormonal responses and the resulting greater hepatic glucose production and skeletal muscle glucose oxidation of men and postmenopausal women to those of eumenorrheic women (17). The suppression of adrenomedullary and sympathetic activity in HAAF blunts the mobilization of lactate, glycerol, and free fatty acids (FFAs) in men compared with eumenorrheic women, thereby impairing gluconeogenesis and the conversion of skeletal muscle fuel selection from glucose to FFAs. As a result, men require a much greater exogenous supply of glucose than do eumenorrheic women to maintain normal plasma glucose levels during the late stages of prolonged exercise (17).

Exercise training effects

Besides raising a new caution about intensive endurance training programs, the discovery of HAAF raises some new questions about the mechanisms of endurance exercise training effects. It has been known for almost 30 years that exercise-induced decreases in insulin and increases in counterregulatory hormones are all blunted by exercise training; however, the reason for this is not well understood. Basal and glucose-stimulated insulin levels are also reduced in trained individuals as a result of decreased insulin secretion. Because sensitivity to insulin is increased while sensitivity to the counterregulatory hormones is not, the reduced counterregulatory responsiveness is probably due to the reduction in insulin concentration (23). Training effects on insulin are essentially complete in less than 2 weeks after the onset of training, and lost in less than 2 weeks after training stops. Because removal of the adrenal medulla blocks the effect of training on insulin in rats (24), questions arise about whether endurance exercise training effects and HAAF are related. From a practical perspective, it would also be of interest to learn whether training effects suppress

the awareness of hypoglycemia and thereby create a hazard for some endurance athletes who are unaware of lower and lower plasma glucose concentrations. It would also be of interest to learn whether athletic performance could be improved if such effects could be prevented or reduced.

Cortisol responses to exercise

If it were desirable to minimize HAAF, one way to do so might be to consume carbohydrates during exercise. Exogenous glucose administration reduces the responses to exercise of all glucoregulatory hormones (i.e., insulin plus the counterregulatory hormones), including cortisol (25,26). In one study (26), infusion of glucose to establish and maintain a hyperglycemic 12 mM plasma glucose concentration entirely abolished the cortisol response to 120 minutes of 70% $\dot{V}_{O_{2max}}$ exercise, but the same effect was achieved during 50% $\dot{V}_{O_{2max}}$ exercise to exhaustion by infusing only enough glucose to maintain the preexercise glucose concentration (25). Glucose infusions were used in these experiments to achieve precise control of plasma glucose concentrations, and to avoid limitations and variations in the absorption of orally administered glucose, but the same effect was also achieved during a 21-km hill walk by increasing the consumption of biscuits, chocolate bars, flapjacks, and cheese sandwiches (27).

TEST YOURSELF

Design a controlled experiment to test the hypothesis that counterregulatory hormone responses to exercise are entirely attributable to the energy cost of the exercise.

Anyone who takes a quantitative interest in cortisol responses to exercise will want to measure those responses accurately. In the first successful effort to explain previous inconsistent assessments of cortisol responses to exercise, Davies and Few (28) found that cortisol responses were roughly proportional (r = 0.62) to the relative rather than the absolute exercise workload (28). After 60 minutes of exercise, cortisol levels were higher or lower than preexercise levels in proportion to the extent to which relative workloads were greater or less than 60% of $\dot{V}_{O_{2max}}$, respectively (Fig. 19.3A).

As might have been expected from a finding that explained only $R^2 = 38\%$ of the observed variance, however, this insight did not bring an end to inconsistencies in measurements of cortisol responses to exercise. Brandenberger and Follenius (29) soon demonstrated what appeared to be very large cortisol responses to 90 minutes of exercise at 55% of $\dot{V}_{O_{2max}}$ by obtaining measurements every 10 minutes for 10 hours (Fig. 19.3B). Nevertheless,

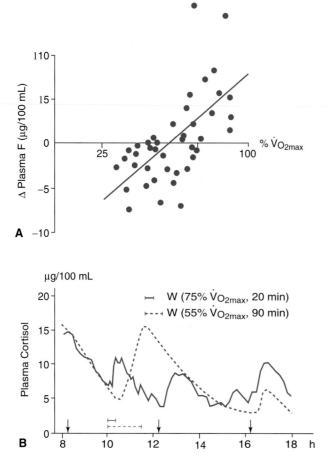

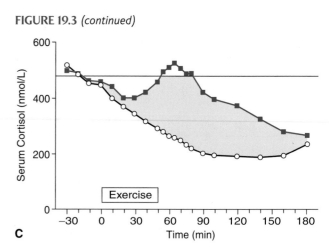

FIGURE 19.3 (continued)

FIGURE 19.3   A. Serum cortisol responses to 60 minutes of aerobic exercise, calculated by subtracting pre-exercise concentrations from postexercise concentrations. Responses appear to be more or less than zero in proportion to the degree to which exercise intensity is more or less than 60% $\dot{V}O_{2max}$. (Reprinted with permission from Davies CT, Few JD. Effects of exercise on adrenocortical function. *J Appl Physiol.* 1973;35:889.) **B.** Serum cortisol concentrations measured at 10-minute intervals for 10 hours on separate days when a subject performed 75% $\dot{V}O_{2max}$ exercise for 20 minutes and 55% $\dot{V}O_{2max}$ exercise for 90 minutes beginning at 10 hours. The response to 55% $\dot{V}O_{2max}$ exercise appears to be much greater than zero and the response to 75% $\dot{V}O_{2max}$ exercise. (Reprinted with permission from Brandenberger G, Follenius M. Influence of timing and intensity of muscular exercise on temporal patterns of plasma cortisol levels. *J Clin Endocrinol Metab.* 1975;40:848.) **C.** Serum cortisol concentrations before, during, and after 50 minutes of 70% $\dot{V}O_{2max}$ exercise at 8 AM (*solid squares*) and at the same times of another day at rest (*open circles*). The baseline before exercise is drawn as a horizontal line through the mean of samples drawn before exercise. The shaded portion of the cortisol response to exercise was not detected by calculating the response relative to concentrations before exercise. (Reprinted with permission from Thuma JR, Gilders R, Verdun M, et al. Circadian rhythm of cortisol confounds cortisol responses to exercise: implications for future research. *J Appl Physiol.* 1995;78:1660.)

for the next 20 years, many exercise physiologists continued to assess cortisol responses to exercise as Davies and Few had done, by comparing a single measurement after exercise with a single measurement before exercise. Then the magnitude of the errors incurred by this method were shown to be as much as 93% when compared with responses calculated relative to the diurnal rhythm of cortisol on another day at rest (Fig. 19.3C) (30). Even the sign of the response can be wrong (appearing to indicate a reduction in cortisol secretion rather than an increase) if the postexercise measurement is taken in the morning as the diurnal rhythm is declining rapidly (when Davies and Few performed their experiment) and the postexercise elevation in cortisol above the resting diurnal rhythm at the same time of a day at rest does not exceed the preexercise level.

TEST **YOURSELF**

Applying the pre-/postcalculation of Davies and Few (28) to the data in Figure 19.3C, what cortisol responses to the same exercise intensity are calculated from postexercise blood samples drawn at times of 50, 60, and 90 minutes?

Thus, cortisol and other glucoregulatory hormone responses to exercise have yet to be comprehensively quantified. Acquiring this basic descriptive information will require a series of experiments spanning a wide range of exercise durations and intensities, at different times of day, in different nutritional states, with and without antecedent exercise or hypoglycemia, and in trained and untrained men and women, with responses calculated by reference to the diurnal rhythm on another resting day for a sufficiently long period to capture the entire response. With such research as a foundation, we may be able to better help athletes mobilize and extend their endogenous supplies of metabolic fuels to maximize performance in endurance events.

Glucose Production

The effectiveness of insulin and glucagon in maintaining glucose homeostasis by regulating hepatic glucose production is partially accounted for by the fact that the pancreatic vein into which they are secreted drains into the portal vein, which carries them directly to the liver before they enter the general circulation via the hepatic vein (31). Although changes in each of these hormones are correlated with changes in hepatic glucose production, the ratio between glucagon and insulin has a stronger correlation with hepatic glucose production than does either hormone alone (14). Thus, the fall in insulin between meals and during prolonged exercise sensitizes the liver to the effects of glucagon. Indeed, in the absence of glucagon, the fall in insulin does not stimulate hepatic glucose production (32). Conversely, the rapid postprandial rise in insulin quickly lowers the glucagon-to-insulin ratio to inhibit glucose production (see also Chapter 14).

The rate of hepatic glycogenolysis is determined by the activity of the enzyme phosphorylase a, which is stimulated by two mechanisms: one involving glucagon and one involving α-adrenergic stimulation (6). By comparison, the regulation of hepatic gluconeogenesis is more complicated because it depends on the mobilization of gluconeogenic precursors, their extraction by the liver, and the efficiency of their conversion to glucose within the liver. Exercise stimulates all of these processes. The accelerated proteolysis, lipolysis, and glycolysis that occur during exercise increase amino acid, glycerol, lactate, and pyruvate precursors, and the rise in glucagon increases the fractional extraction of these precursors and the efficiency of their conversion into glucose. The endocrine mediation of proteolysis and lipolysis is discussed in later sections of this chapter.

During prolonged exercise, gluconeogenesis provides a supply of glucose beyond the capacity of liver glycogen stores. Sequentially, glycogenolysis precedes gluconeogenesis. During the first hour of exercise or hypoglycemia, glycogenolysis predominates, accounting for ~85% of glucose production. Later, as glycogen stores are depleted and gluconeogenic precursors become available, gluconeogenesis predominates and accounts for ~85% of glucose production after ~6 hours (33). Gluconeogenesis also occurs in every individual every day in intervals between meals and during sleep to maintain glucose availability to the brain.

Skeletal muscle glucose uptake

The rate-limiting step for glucose uptake by skeletal muscle is the rate of glucose transport across the cell membrane (see also Chapter 14). Glucose passes through the skeletal muscle cell membrane by facilitated diffusion, that is, down a concentration gradient through a channel in a specialized protein known as glucose transporter 4 (GLUT4). GLUT4 transporters are continuously and simultaneously cycled in the membranes of vesicles between the muscle cell's external plasma membrane, where they facilitate glucose transport, and the internal membranes of certain endosomal compartments, where they are stored (Fig. 19.4A). The amount of GLUT4 that is present in the cell membrane at any given time, and thus the rate of glucose uptake, reflects the dynamic equilibrium between the separately regulated rates of GLUT4 exocytosis and endocytosis, both of which consume energy (34). At rest, only 5% to 10% of a skeletal muscle cell's GLUT4 content is on the cell surface.

KEY POINT

The rate of skeletal muscle glucose uptake reflects the equilibrium between the exocytosis and endocytosis of GLUT4 transporters.

REGULATION OF GLUT4 CYCLING   A rise in plasma insulin concentration brings 20% of GLUT4 transporters to the cell surface within a few minutes by increasing the rate of exocytosis. Insulin mediates its action through a membrane receptor and a complicated series of protein kinases to exert its effects (35). The insulin receptor in the cell membrane is a hormone-activated protein tyrosine kinase that catalyzes the transfer of phosphate groups from adenosine-5′-triphosphate (ATP) to tyrosine residues of proteins. As indicated in Figure 19.4B, phosphatidylinositol-3-kinase (PI3K) is the critical step in the pathway. Rapid exocytosis of GLUT4 to the cell membrane is regulated by two protein kinases farther downstream in the insulin signaling pathway: a 160-KD protein known as AS160, and atypical protein kinase C (aPKC). Insulin also acts more slowly through a separate pathway involving mitogen-activated protein kinase (MAPK) to stimulate transcription and a delayed increase in GLUT4 translocation.

Several other physiologic and pharmacologic factors also rapidly increase the population of GLUT4 transporters in the skeletal muscle plasma membrane (Fig. 19.4B). Knowledge in this field is rapidly advancing. Only a few years ago, these other factors were thought to operate through alternative pathways that are entirely independent of insulin, but current knowledge suggests that these pathways converge at the protein kinases AS160 and aPKC, which are downstream in the insulin-signaling pathway (35).

Muscle contraction increases GLUT4 translocation to the plasma membrane in two ways. First, the energy required for muscle contraction is derived from the conversion of

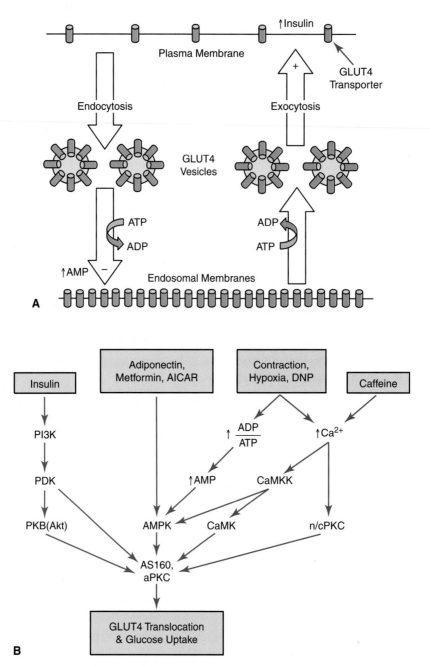

FIGURE 19.4 **A.** Glucose transporter 4 (GLUT4) cycling in skeletal muscle. The GLUT4 cycles constantly in vesicles between the plasma membrane, where it facilitates glucose uptake, and intracellular endosomal membranes, where it is stored. The amount of GLUT4 that is active on the plasma membrane reflects the absolute and relative rates of exocytosis, which is accelerated by insulin, and endocytosis, which is decelerated by adenosine-5′-monophosphate (AMP). **B.** Energy is consumed in both exocytosis and endocytosis. Regulation of GLUT4 translocation. Insulin-mediated, energy-dependent, and Ca^{2+} signaling pathways regulating GLUT4 translocation converge on two protein kinases (AS160 and atypical protein kinase C [aPKC]). ATP, adenosine triphosphate; ADP, adenosine diphosphate; AICAR, 5-aminoimidazole-4-carboxamide-1 β-riboside; DNP, 2,4-Dinitrophenol; PDK, Pyruvate dehydrogenase kinase; PKB(Akt), protein kinase B; AMPK, AMP-activated protein kinase; CaMK, calcium/calmodulin-dependent protein kinase.

high-energy ATP to lower energy adenosine-5′-diphosphate (ADP) and adenosine-5′-monophosphate (AMP). Elevated AMP levels activate a protein kinase (AMPK) that acts as the cell's energy sensor. AMPK influences GLUT4 translocation via the same two downstream protein kinases, AS160 and aPKC, through which insulin acts. In contrast to insulin, which accelerates GLUT4 exocytosis to accelerate glucose uptake for storage when plasma glucose is abundant, activation of AMPK during energy deficiency decelerates GLUT4 endocytosis, thereby reducing cellular energy expenditure while simultaneously increasing glucose uptake for oxidation.

Second, the depolarization of the muscle cell and T-tubule membranes associated with muscle contraction releases Ca^{2+} from the sarcoplasmic reticulum into the cytoplasm, thereby activating a sequence of calcium-mediated second messengers. These messengers also act, at least in part, through AS160 and aPKC. Activation of novel and conventional isoforms of PKC (n/cPKC) by membrane depolarization has been shown to increase AS160 phosphorylation. Calcium also activates two protein kinases, known as Ca/calmodulin-dependent protein kinase (CaMK) and protein kinase C (PKC), but the same kinase (CaMKK) that activates CaMK also activates AMPK and hence AS160 and aPKC. Experiments on AMPK-deficient animals have demonstrated that CaMKK can also stimulate glucose uptake independently of AMPK. The implied parallel pathway mediating the AMPK-independent influence of CaMK on GLUT4 translocation has yet to be identified, but it appears to be independent of AS160 at least. The mechanisms by which AS160 and aPKC influence GLUT4 cycling are not yet well understood.

Other factors that impair mitochondrial production of ATP, such as hypoxia and uncoupling of oxidative phosphorylation from the electron transport chain by depolarization of the inner mitochondrial membrane, also raise AMP levels and release Ca^{2+} into the cytoplasm, this time from the mitochondrial phosphate (36). Uncoupling can be induced pharmacologically with 2,4-dinitrophenol. AMPK can be selectively activated independently of Ca^{2+} by drugs such as metformin and 5-aminoimidazole-4-carboxamide-1 β-riboside (AICAR). Metformin activates AMPK by raising AMP levels, whereas AICAR is converted to ZMP, an analog of AMP. Adiponectin, a protein hormone that acts in opposition to leptin, is secreted by adipose tissue in inverse proportion to body fatness. It binds to receptors in the plasma membrane, like insulin, and acts through a series of second messengers to activate AMPK. Conversely, Ca^{2+} pathways can be selectively activated by caffeine. The effects of caffeine and AICAR are additive, and the combined effect is similar to that caused by contraction.

INSULIN SENSITIVITY   There is continuing controversy about the influence of exercise on insulin sensitivity. This controversy persists, in part, because of confusion arising from differences in the definitions of and techniques for measuring insulin sensitivity, from inadequate

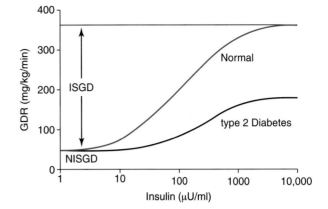

FIGURE 19.5   Nonlinear dependence of the GDR on insulin concentration in normal healthy subjects and patients with type 2 diabetes. Results from persons with insulin resistance lie between these curves. ISGD, insulin stimulated-glucose disposal; NISGD, non–stimulated-glucose disposal.

experimental designs and controls, and from misunderstandings about energy deficiency.

Glucose disposal.   Figure 19.5 illustrates how the glucose disposal (GD) rate (GDR) from the systemic circulation depends on insulin concentrations in normal subjects and in patients with type 2 diabetes under euglycemic conditions. GD is comprised of two components: insulin-stimulated GD (ISGD) and non–insulin-stimulated GD (NISGD). In fasting euglycemia (glucose 4–5 mmol/L), ISGD occurs primarily in skeletal muscle, and NISGD occurs primarily in brain, liver, and kidneys.

GD occurs passively as glucose diffuses down a concentration gradient into tissues and ultimately through cell membranes via GLUT transporters. As described in the previous section, insulin and other factors influence GD by altering the rates of GLUT transporter exocytosis or endocytosis, thereby altering the numbers of GLUT transporters on cell membranes and in intracellular storage vesicles. Thus, graphs of GDR, such as those in Figure 19.5, actually illustrate the variable census of GLUT transporters on cell membranes.

Figure 19.6 illustrates the only four ways in which any factor and its physiologic mechanism could possibly influence the census of GLUT transporters. First, they could alter the slope of the GDR curve, as shown in Figure 19.6A, reflecting an altered increment of GLUT transporters on cell membranes per unit increase in insulin. Second, they could shift the insulin offset of the GDR curve into lower and higher ranges of insulin concentration, as shown in Figure 19.6B. Third, they could alter the height of the GDR curve (i.e., ISGD) by changing the maximum number of GLUT transporters available for insulin to bring to the cell membrane, as illustrated in Figure 19.6C. This might result from a more or less extreme equilibrium between exocytosis and endocytosis, or an alteration of the total population of GLUT transporters. Fourth, they could alter the GDR offset of the GDR curve (i.e., NISGD), as illustrated in Figure 19.6D, by altering

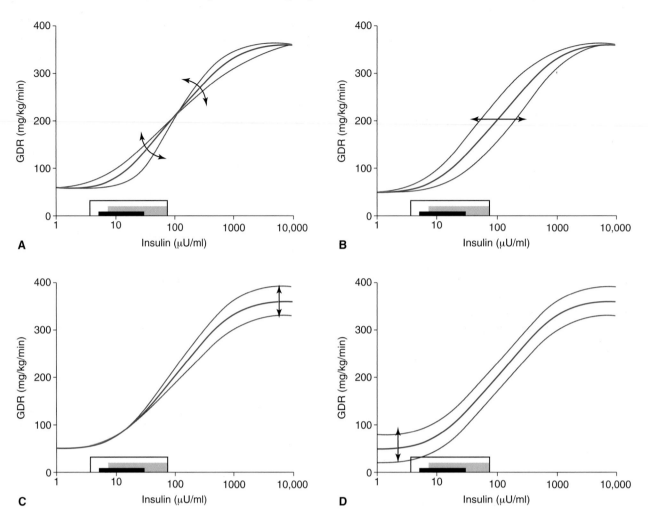

FIGURE 19.6   The four fundamental effects that any factor and its physiologic mechanism could have on glucose disposal. **A.** The slope of the glucose disposal rate (GDR) curve could change. **B.** The location of the GDR curve on the insulin axis could change. **C.** The height of the GDR curve could change. **D.** The location of the GDR curve on the GDR axis could change. Any actual effect of any factor and its physiologic mechanism on GD results from various combinations of these four fundamental effects. Physiologic ranges of insulin: *Black box:* normal subjects; *hatched box:* obese subjects; *white box:* type 2 diabetes patients.

the number of GLUT transporters on the surfaces of cells independently of insulin, as occurs in skeletal muscle during exercise. It is important to note that this last effect on GDR is qualitatively different from the other three, in that it alters GDR without altering the influence of insulin on GDR.

The controversy about the influence of exercise on GDR, therefore, can be reduced to three questions: First, does GDR increase during exercise training? Second, if it does, does it do so in an insulin-mediated manner, as illustrated in Figure 19.6A–C, or does it do so independently of insulin, as illustrated in Figure 19.6D? Third, however GDR increases, does the increase disappear if dietary energy intake is increased in compensation for the energy cost of exercise? If the latter is true, then the apparent effect of exercise is actually an artifact of energy deficiency.

Definitions.   In pursuing answers to these questions, our understanding is impaired by loose usage of the terms "insulin sensitivity" and "index of insulin sensitivity" to refer to several different quantities, some of which are illustrated in Figure 19.7. Some investigators use these terms to refer to the maximum rate of GD (in units of mg/min or mg/min/kg of body weight, FFM, or skeletal muscle mass), indicated in Figure 19.7 as S1. Others use them to refer to the concentration of insulin at which the rate of GD is half maximal (in units of μU/mL), indicated in Figure 19.7 as S2. Still others use these terms to refer to the incremental increase in GD per unit increase in insulin concentration, indicated in Figure 19.7 as S3. Some define S3 as the fractional disappearance of glucose from the bloodstream, that is, the rate of disappearance of glucose divided by the total amount of glucose in the glucose distribution space per unit increase in insulin concentration (in units of [1/min]/[μU/mL]). Others define S3 as the fractional clearance of glucose from the bloodstream, that is, the rate of disappearance divided by the concentration of glucose per unit body surface area per unit increase in insulin concentration (in units of [dL/min/m^2]/[μU/mL]). These two defi-

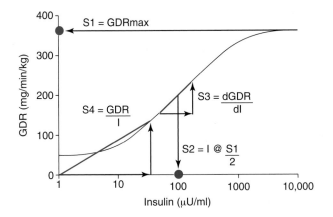

FIGURE 19.7   Some definitions of the term *insulin sensitivity* in relation to the GDR. S_1 = maximum GDR. S_2 = insulin concentration at half of the maximum GDR. S_3 = incremental increase in GD per unit increase in insulin concentration. S_4 = GDR at a particular insulin concentration.

nitions of S3 are distinguished as S3a and S3b, respectively, in the text below. Understanding is further confounded by the fact that high values and increases in S3 are accompanied by low values and decreases in S2 (37,38). Some authors use the terms in reference to the ratio of the rate of glucose uptake at a particular insulin concentration to that insulin concentration (in units of [mg/min]/[μU/mL]), indicated in Figure 19.7 as S4.

Additional confusion is generated when these terms are also used to refer to quantities that do not appear in Figure 19.7, including the inverse of insulin concentration (S5); the ratio of fasting glucose to insulin concentrations (S6); two other calculations (QUICKI and HOMA) based on fasting glucose and insulin concentrations, as discussed below (S7 and S8); and the time required to clear a standard oral dose of glucose from the bloodstream (S9). There are more.

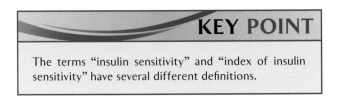

KEY POINT

The terms "insulin sensitivity" and "index of insulin sensitivity" have several different definitions.

Measurement techniques.   The only technique that can measure the entire GDR curve in Figure 19.7 is the euglycemic clamp test. In this test, endogenous insulin secretion is suppressed as exogenous insulin is infused at a series of increasing rates. At each insulin infusion rate, glucose is also infused at whatever rate is necessary to maintain blood glucose at a normal fasting level while blood samples are collected for the measurement of insulin concentrations. The glucose infusion rates and insulin concentrations define the GDR curve. The entire test takes a few hours to complete.

Even though the euglycemic clamp test is the only one that measures the entire GDR curve, the test that is regarded as the gold standard for assessing insulin sensitivity is the hyperinsulinemic euglycemic clamp (HEC) test (39), which collects data under conditions equivalent to those shown on the extreme right side of Figure 19.5. Insulin is infused at a high rate and glucose is infused as necessary to maintain euglycemia while blood samples are collected for a period of 2 hours. The resulting hyperinsulinemia suppresses hepatic glucose production and endogenous insulin secretion, and the euglycemia suppresses hepatic glucose uptake. Thus, the test is specific for GD in peripheral tissue (*i.e.*, skeletal muscle). The rate of glucose infusion that maintains euglycemia is S1.

The HEC test is rigorous, requires sophisticated equipment and highly trained personnel, and is costly and labor-intensive. Therefore, other tests have been developed to diagnose insulin resistance and type 2 diabetes in clinical practice. In the oral glucose tolerance test (OGTT), a bolus of glucose is swallowed and a series of blood samples are drawn to determine how quickly the glucose is cleared from the blood (S9). However, the results are unavoidably confounded by hepatic glucose production and uptake. Other clinical tests are based on measurements of insulin and glucose in a single fasting blood sample, and do not measure GDR. Because they have been shown to correlate to various degrees with S1, however, they are referred to as "indices of insulin sensitivity," meaning indices of S1. The quantities calculated in these tests include 1/insulin, the glucose-to-insulin ratio (G/I), the Homeostatic Model Assessment (HOMA = G*I/405), and the Quantitative Insulin Sensitivity Check Index (QUICKI = 1/[log(G) + log(I)]). QUICKI and log(HOMA) are the most robust and accurate indices and have greater clinical utility (40). QUICKI increases and log(HOMA) decreases as S1 increases.

To overcome the inadequacies of the OGTT while still avoiding the experimental demands of the HEC test for research, researchers developed several different methods, known as the intravenous glucose tolerance test (IVGTT); the frequently sampled IVGTT (FSIGT); and the insulin-modified, frequently sampled IVGTT (IMFSIGT) (41–43). In all of these tests, a bolus dose of glucose is injected to induce a spike in glucose and insulin concentrations, and then glucose and insulin concentrations are measured in a series of blood samples drawn over a period of 3 hours as insulin concentrations return to normal. In the IMFSIGT, insulin is also injected 20 minutes after the glucose bolus. Measurements of declining glucose and insulin concentrations in these samples are then fitted to a so-called "minimal" mathematical model of the distribution of insulin and glucose in body compartments to determine S3a. In one study, the IMFSIGT used to estimate S3a, and the euglycemic clamp test was used to measure S3b in a group of 10 subjects (44). After the two quantities were converted to the same units, S3a and S3b were found to be highly correlated, with the slope and intercept not significantly different from 1 and 0, respectively. The investigators claimed, therefore, that the two methods measure exactly the same thing. They acknowledged the possibility of bias in the IMFSIGT measurements but claimed it was small and attributed it to insulin suppression of hepatic glucose production, which the IMFSIGT cannot distinguish from ISGD.

Correlation, slope, and intercept are not sufficient for comparing two methods that measure the same thing, however, and the Bland-Altman analysis is now accepted as the gold standard for this purpose (45). The Bland-Altman analysis plots differences between pairs of measurements made by the two methods against the average of the pairs. These differences should be randomly, uniformly, and narrowly distributed across the range of averages, and the average difference should not be significantly different from zero. For the data comparing S3a and S3b, the differences are not uniformly, randomly, or narrowly distributed. The coefficient of variation is 28% of the grand average, and thus the confidence interval of differences is 128% of the grand average. Moreover, the mean is significantly biased high by 23% of the grand average. Therefore, in comparison with S3b, S3a is imprecise and highly biased.

TEST YOURSELF

The various techniques used to assess insulin sensitivity measure different features of the GD curve. In Figure 19.6, which types of change is each technique unable to detect or to distinguish from other changes?

Effects of Exercise Training.   The idea that exercise might improve insulin sensitivity arose from cross-sectional comparisons of trained and untrained men that indicated that S9 was faster (47), S3b tended to be higher, and S2 tended to be lower in trained men than in untrained men (37). This idea seemed to be confirmed by long-term studies of exercise training that revealed declining insulin levels in obese men (48) and cardiac patients (49), and shorter S9 in patients with type 2 diabetes (50,51).

These long-term training studies were not fully persuasive, however, because they were confounded by the shortcomings of the OGTT and by weight loss. Indeed, later randomized controlled trials in overweight men (52) and women (53) revealed that increases in S1 after 12 weeks of exercise training did not occur in subjects whose diet was supplemented to prevent weight loss. Other long-term studies showed that S3a (54,55) and S9 (54,55) improved during weight loss but returned to baseline when the reduced weight was maintained. When liposuction was found not to improve S1 (56), suspicion about the factor that might have improved GD in the long-term exercise training studies turned from weight loss to the energy deficiency that causes weight loss.

In two recent long-term clinical trials, investigators sought to determine whether energy deficiency can account for the apparent effects of exercise training on insulin sensitivity. In one trial, three interventions were administered to overweight men and women for 6 months (57,58): 25% caloric restriction (CR), 12.5% CR with exercise expending 12.5% of pre trial daily energy expenditure (CREX), or a low-calorie diet (LCD) of 890 kcal/day until the subjects had lost 15% of body weight, followed by a diet that maintained the lower weight. In comparison with an untreated control group, similar significant reductions in body weight and body fat occurred in all three treatment groups. S3a increased in all three groups ($P = 0.08$) in CR, insulin secretion decreased in all three groups, and there were no significant differences in these responses among the treatment groups (57). Thus, this trial yielded very little evidence of an energy-independent effect of exercise training. However, every intervention in this study involved some degree of CR.

The other trial avoided this shortcoming by administering contrasting energy balance and energy deficiency treatments, and contrasting exercise training and sedentary treatments in a 2×2 experimental design (59). Overweight and obese but otherwise healthy adults were randomized to CR, exercise training with weight loss matched to CR (EWL), exercise training without weight loss (EX), and energy-balanced sedentary treatments (controls) for

TEST YOURSELF

S3b	S3a
0.003	0.016
0.009	0.015
0.012	0.025
0.034	0.038
0.043	0.054
0.045	0.035
0.050	0.068
0.051	0.070
0.055	0.047
0.063	0.090

Verify the above data about S3a by performing a Bland-Altman analysis of the numbers (45).

Recently, Black et al. (46) employed a stable isotope technique for quantitative investigations of S4, insulin secretion, and S1. In this method, glucose labeled with a stable isotope is infused continuously for 2.5 hours as frequent blood samples are drawn. Measurements of rising and then steady-state glucose and insulin concentrations are fitted to a model of GD that is more sophisticated than Bergman's minimal model. This method yields direct measurements of the steady-state rates of appearance and disappearance of glucose, enabling calculation of both whole body GD (S4) and hepatic glucose production.

6 months. A stable-isotope methodology revealed that ISGD was unchanged in the controls and significantly increased in all three treatment groups. The similar increases in CR and EWL (~33%) were significantly larger than that in EX (~14%). The interaction in these results suggests that the influence of exercise training on ISGD may depend on energy status: under energy-deficient conditions, exercise training may have no effect on ISGD beyond the impact of its energy cost, but it may have a small energy-independent effect on energy balance.

An unexpected observation in the early long-term training studies was that improvements in insulin sensitivity disappeared only a few days after the study ended, suggesting that these improvements may have been due to the acute effects of the last exercise bout. This insight led investigators to conduct short-term exercise training studies to avoid significant reductions in body weight and to collect data within 24 hours after training stopped. The results of these studies were mixed, but so were the experimental designs and protocols used.

Some of these short-term studies compared the effects of exercise training with those of CR, which has been shown to increase S3a (57), ISGD (59), and S1 (60) in long-term studies. One such short-term study found that S1 increased more after exercise training than after CR (61), even though the 50% CR was much more extreme than the 20% increase in energy expenditure during exercise training.

Other short-term studies have directly addressed the question of whether apparent effects of exercise on insulin sensitivity disappear when dietary energy intake is increased in compensation for the energy cost of exercise. One indicated that S3a increased in subjects who exercised for an hour a day to expend 450 calories each day for 7 days, even though they were immediately refed those 450 calories in the laboratory (62). Another administered very similar (500 kcal) treatments for 6 days and found that S4 increased 40% in the subjects who exercised without dietary supplementation and was unchanged in those with dietary supplementation (46). A third study compared the effects of slight overfeeding (OF) and extreme underfeeding (UF) on subjects who exercised for 3 hours a day for 7 days (63). These investigators did not measure effects on insulin sensitivity, but indices of S1 can be calculated from the fasting glucose and insulin data they reported. QUICKI values increased more and log(HOMA) values decreased more during UF than OF, indicating a greater increase in S1 during UF, but a small increase in S1 also appears to have occurred during OF.

Another short-term experiment (64) provided evidence that S1 increases in a dose-dependent manner as energy deficiency becomes more extreme. In that study, healthy young women exercised to expend the same amount of energy (15 kcal/kgFFM) each day at a balanced energy availability of 45 kcal/kgFFM/day and at three deficient energy availabilities of 30, 20, and 10 kcal/kgFFM/day (64). When calculated from reported fasting glucose and insulin data measured after 5 days of treatment, the QUICKI values progressively increased and log(HOMA) values progressively decreased as energy availability declined.

TEST YOURSELF

Verify the QUICKI and log(HOMA) results described above using the data in the tables below.

| | Glucose (mg/dL) | | Insulin (µU/mL) | |
Day	OF	UF	OF	UF
0	84	85	7.6	7.9
1	83	74	7.8	6.0
2	85	75	7.5	6.0
3	88	73	6.0	5.4
4	84	74	5.9	4.8
5	84	74	6.0	5.4
6	84	75	6.5	5.0
7	85	77	7.0	5.5

Data from Nemet et al. (63).

EA (kcal/kg FFM/day)	Glucose (mg/dL)	Insulin (µU/mL)
10	68	1.8
20	72	3.3
30	77	4.2
45	83	4.8

Data from Loucks and Thuma (64).

The well-established enhancement of S1 and other measures of insulin sensitivity by CR in sedentary subjects and by low energy availability in exercising subjects over periods of 7 days to 6 months stands in sharp contrast to the equally well-established suppression of S1 by fasting for 48 to 72 hours (65–69). In fasting, of course, energy availability and carbohydrate availability are both 0 kcal/kgFFM/day. Metabolism is in rapid transition during the first few days of starvation as hepatic glycogen stores are depleted and peripheral tissues shift from glucose to fat and ketone metabolism to conserve scarce glucose for the brain (70). Perhaps the immediate suppressive effect of fasting on S1 is transitory and is followed by an enhancement of S1 after this transient is completed, in time to match the effects seen in short-term studies of CR and energy-deficient exercise a few days later. Or perhaps the difference between energy availabilities of 10 and 0 kcal/kgFFM/day is sufficient to markedly affect S1. In the subjects mentioned above, who were exercising at energy availability of 10 kcal/kgFFM/day, energy intake was 25 kcal/kgFFM/day and carbohydrate intake was ~13 kcal/kgFFM/day (64). It is possible that the availability of that exogenous carbohydrate has large effects on S1.

Summary

Numerous short-term prospective experiments and long-term clinical trials have demonstrated increases in various measures of insulin sensitivity during exercise training. Evidence as to whether these increases are an artifact of energy deficiency is mixed, and perhaps the preponderance of evidence, like beauty, is still in the eye of the beholder. The lack of comprehensive data on GD from euglycemic clamp studies, and especially the lack of data on NISGD, limits our ability to draw conclusions about whether these increased measures of insulin sensitivity correspond to changes in the cycling of GLUT4 transporters that are actually mediated by insulin, as in Figure 19.6A–C, or not, as in Figure 19.6D.

Fat Metabolism

Fatty acid cycling by adipose tissue

Adipose tissue plays an important role in whole body energy metabolism because it is the only tissue that is able to release nonesterified FAs (NEFAs) into the circulation (see Chapters 15 and 16). During prolonged exercise, plasma NEFAs are the major energy source for working muscle. In almost all physiologic circumstances, all of the FAs released by adipose tissue were previously taken up from circulating chylomicrons carrying dietary fat and very low density lipoproteins (VLDLs) carrying triglycerides (TGs) secreted by the liver. The energy equivalent of this cycling of FAs between adipose tissue and the circulation amounts to ~1200 kcal/day in normal human subjects. This includes substantial re-esterification of released NEFAs, the regulation of which enables the rapid amplification of adipose tissue NEFA output in response to metabolic demand. This regulation is achieved by the integrated effects of blood flow through the tissue, autonomic nervous system activity, and the levels of hormones and substrates circulating in the blood (71,72).

Unless it is unavailable, the energy source for adipose tissue is glucose. Glucose availability is also rate-limiting for TG synthesis because adipocytes lack the enzyme glycerokinase and cannot re-esterify the glycerol released by lipolysis. Therefore, the glycerol-3-phosphate used for esterifying TGs is obtained by glycolysis. This is not an important GD pathway, however; it accounts for only ~4% of an oral glucose load, whereas skeletal muscle accounts for ~35%. Considering the small amount of energy in the form of glucose required to control such a large amount of energy in the form of NEFAs, adipose tissue is the most efficient energy storage tissue in the body. Glucose uptake by adipocytes is accomplished by insulin-dependent GLUT4 transporters and insulin-independent GLUT1 transporters. However, insulin has no physiologically important effect on adipose tissue glucose uptake, because the insulin concentration for half-maximal stimulation of glucose uptake in adipose tissue is only ~13 pM (73). (For comparison with normal values, see Fig. 19.10A.)

Thus, the major function of adipose tissue is the storage and release of chemical energy in the form of NEFAs. The direction of this energy flow is determined by the coordinated regulation of the enzymes hormone-sensitive lipase (HSL) and lipoprotein lipase (LPL). Insulin inhibits and the counterregulatory hormones stimulate HSL, which catalyzes the hydrolysis of stored TG to release NEFAs and glycerol. Because half-maximal suppression of HSL by insulin occurs at a concentration of only ~120 pM, the release of NEFAs is substantially suppressed within 30 minutes and is essentially zero within 60 to 90 minutes after a mixed meal (Fig. 19.10A).

By contrast, a rise in insulin stimulates LPL and a rise in catecholamines (6) inhibits LPL, which hydrolyzes VLDL-TG in the adipose tissue capillary bloodstream and releases NEFAs into the plasma, where they are available for uptake by adipocytes. Synthesized in and secreted by adipocytes, LPL migrates to the adipose tissue capillary lumen, where it attaches to endothelial cells by proteoglycan chains such that it comes into contact with circulating chylomicrons and VLDL-TG. Because insulin also stimulates the esterification of FAs in adipose tissue (74), the precipitous postprandial rise in insulin after a mixed meal raises the plasma concentration and lowers the intracellular adipocyte NEFA concentration, creating a concentration gradient down, which the NEFAs flow from the bloodstream into adipocytes for esterification. The gradual fall in insulin after a meal and during prolonged exercise slowly releases the inhibition of HSL and suppresses esterification and LPL activity, thereby gradually reversing the concentration gradient and the direction of NEFA flow.

Coordination of NEFA release with the sudden increase in metabolic demand at the onset of exercise is mediated by β-adrenergic effects of sympathetic activation (75). Norepinephrine released from sympathetic nerves is the important stimulus because the effect is retained after adrenomedullation (76). As exercise continues, adrenergic stimulation of lipolysis and inhibition of VLDL hydrolysis is reinforced by the gradual decline in insulin and rise in GH and cortisol (77). These stimuli also reduce the re-esterification of NEFA to approximately zero within 60 minutes during exercise at 50% to 60% of $\dot{V}O_{2max}$ further increasing the concentration gradient driving NEFA output. By contrast, muscular contractions and catecholamines stimulate muscle LPL to promote lipid uptake during exercise and postabsorptive conditions.

Adipose tissue blood flow responds rapidly to nutrient ingestion, facilitating TG disposal (78), and β-adrenergic stimulation has vasodilator effects in adipose tissue. Nevertheless, during exercise, adipose tissue blood flow is insufficient to absorb all of the NEFAs released, and the rate of appearance of NEFA in the bloodstream declines as exercise intensity increases despite the associated increase in β-adrenergic drive (79). As a result, at the end of exercise, an accumulated backlog of NEFAs in adipose tissue is suddenly released into the circulation (77).

Ketogenesis

Hepatic ketogenesis is a reflection of the energy state of the liver. As a marker of hepatic fat oxidation, which is a key source of energy for gluconeogenesis, ketogenesis occurs in acute and chronic circumstances that require high rates of gluconeogenesis. The rate of ketogenesis is determined by the mobilization of NEFAs by adipose tissue, by the uptake of NEFAs by the liver, and by the efficiency with which

NEFAs are converted to ketone bodies in the liver. Therefore, by regulating the mobilization of NEFAs, the exercise responses of insulin and the glucose counterregulatory hormones also contribute to the regulation of ketogenesis.

Insulin also inhibits the fractional extraction of NEFA from the bloodstream by the liver. Therefore, the fall in insulin during exercise further contributes to ketogenesis by increasing hepatic NEFA uptake (80). Meanwhile, the rise in glucagon increases the activity of the key enzyme in ketone production: carnitine acyltransferase (i.e., palmitoylacyltransferase), which transfers FAs in the cytoplasm from coenzyme A (CoA) to carnitine for transportation into the mitochondrial matrix. The ratio of ketone body output to NEFA uptake is an index of the NEFA-to-ketone conversion efficiency. During 60 minutes of moderate intensity exercise, this ratio increases from 20% to 40% in normal healthy subjects, and from 60% to 100% in poorly controlled insulin-dependent diabetics (81).

Initially, ketones in the liver are taken up from the blood and metabolized by the heart, kidney, and skeletal muscle so that circulating levels in the blood remain low. If glucose deficiency continues for only a few days, however, glucose and ketone utilization by these tissues declines and plasma ketone concentrations rise to levels exceeding those of plasma glucose, making substantial amounts of ketones available as an alternative metabolic fuel for the brain. Hepatic ketone production capacity is uniquely high in human beings, and this is what maintains brain metabolism in humans during chronic dietary carbohydrate deficiency. When plasma ketone levels begin to rise, some ketones pass through the kidneys into the urine, where they can be detected to monitor carbohydrate availability without the need for invasive blood sampling.

Summary

In this section on the regulation of the storage and mobilization of metabolic fuels, we have drawn attention to how much of what has been widely accepted about blood glucose regulation and the effects of exercise on skeletal muscle fuel selection has been confounded by concurrent and preceding energy deficiency. The decrease in insulin and increase in counterregulatory hormones during exercise and at rest after exercise training may be, to some yet-to-be-determined degree, artifacts of acute and chronic energy deficiency. The specific effects of exercise, independent of energy deficiency, remain obscure. We now turn our attention to the similarly strong influence of nutrition on the endocrine-mediated adaptation of skeletal muscle to mechanical loading.

KEY POINT

Certain metabolic hormones carry information from peripheral tissues to the central nervous system about the availability of metabolic fuels, whereas others carry instructions from the central nervous system to peripheral tissues that regulate the storage, mobilization and utilization of those fuels.

Regulation of Muscle Plasticity

Protein Turnover

Of the three macronutrients, protein is unique in that there is no pool of stored protein that is not serving important physiologic purposes. As might be expected, therefore, protein is the least oxidized of the three metabolic fuels for meeting daily energy requirements. Nevertheless, even though the energy required to synthesize protein is twice as great as that required to synthesize glycogen or TGs, the daily turnover of protein (~37 mmol/kg/day) greatly exceeds the turnover of carbohydrates (~15 mmol/kg/day) and TGs (~24 mmol/kg/day) (82). This protein turnover is equivalent to the protein content of 1 to 1.5 kg of muscle and accounts for ~20% of resting energy expenditure, which is as much as the Na^+/K^+ pump. Individual proteins turn over at widely different rates, with half-lives as short as 15 minutes for some regulatory proteins, about 2 weeks for actin and myosin, and as long as 3 months for hemoglobin.

In muscle protein turnover (see Chapter 17), many factors associated with genetics, age, exercise, nutrition, and hormonal regulation influence the intracellular signaling pathways that control gene transcription; messenger ribonucleic acid (mRNA) translation; posttranslational modification and degradation of myofibrillar, mitochondrial, cytosolic, membrane, and extracellular proteins; and the proliferation and differentiation of muscle satellite cells. Muscle growth and atrophy result from small differences in the high rates of protein synthesis and breakdown that constitute the daily turnover of muscle protein. Both protein synthesis and breakdown occur all the time, and they are different, separately regulated processes, not simply the reverse of each other. Both processes are selective with respect to the muscles, fiber types (as well as particular fibers), and proteins that are involved at any given time. It is important to recognize that protein breakdown is a necessary part of fiber type transformation and muscle remodeling in general. Indeed, since proteolysis is performed by proteins, an increase in protein breakdown depends on the increased synthesis of proteolytic proteins.

KEY POINT

Protein synthesis and protein breakdown are different, separately regulated processes that operate at increasing and decreasing rates throughout the day.

The rates of protein synthesis and breakdown in muscle depend in part on the intracellular availability of amino acids, including those derived from the breakdown of intracellular proteins and those transported in both directions across the cell membrane. In addition to supplying amino acids from old proteins as raw materials for the synthesis of new proteins, proteolysis also supplies amino acids for gluconeogenesis and other important physiologic functions. Thus, by imposing huge demands for glucose, prolonged exercise constitutes a leak draining the pool of amino acids available for protein synthesis. Of course, the intracellular availability of amino acids is directly affected by the protein content of the diet. As described above, it is also indirectly affected by exercise and the carbohydrate content of the diet through their influence on glucoregulatory hormones that also affect amino acid transport and protein synthesis and breakdown.

Proteolysis

Over the last 20 years, there has been an explosion of research into the mechanisms of protein breakdown, motivated by the clinical consequences of muscle atrophy in various catabolic conditions, such as cancer, metabolic acidosis, AIDS, sepsis, starvation, diabetes, trauma, surgery, paralysis, and space flight, and by the discovery that most proteolysis occurs in a highly selective, tightly regulated, and therefore controllable process. Different proteolytic mechanisms are involved in skeletal muscle, including the ubiquitin-proteosome system, lysosomes, calpains, and caspases. Each of these mechanisms targets different proteins and is regulated differently (see Chapter 17).

Hormone Effects on Protein Turnover

Goldberg's rats

During the late 1960s and early 1970s, Alfred Goldberg conducted a series of experiments to investigate the mechanism of work-induced hypertrophy of skeletal muscle in rats (83). In these experiments, Goldberg severed the insertion of the gastrocnemius muscle from the Achilles tendon in one hindlimb to eliminate its usual synergistic assistance to the soleus and plantaris muscles in extending the ankle. After only 5 days, the overloaded soleus and plantaris muscles had grown by a surprising ~40% and ~20%, respectively, compared with the corresponding muscles in the sham-operated contralateral limb. What was especially remarkable, however, was that the same growth occurred in hypophysectomized, diabetic, and starving rats. Goldberg concluded that work-induced hypertrophy of skeletal muscle is mediated by mechanisms intrinsic to particular working muscles, unlike developmental growth, which is known to depend on circulating pituitary axis hormones (i.e., GH, insulin-like growth factor-I [IGF-I], testosterone, and thyroxine), insulin, and nutrients. These findings inspired a stream of experiments that continue to this day to elucidate the mechanism by which the autocrine expression of IGF-I mediates the hypertrophy of working muscle.

Wolfe's men

During the 1990s and early 2000s, Robert Wolfe's laboratory conducted another series of experiments investigating the mechanism of work-induced hypertrophy of skeletal muscle in men (84). Whereas Goldberg measured cumulative effects on muscle mass over a period of time, Wolfe used a combination of stable isotope infusion, arterial and venous blood sampling, and muscle biopsy to calculate the rates of protein synthesis and breakdown, and inward and outward amino acid transmembrane transport in the quadriceps muscle at one moment in time. Wolfe and Goldberg drew different conclusions from their studies.

Figure 19.8 summarizes Wolfe's findings on the effects of dietary intake and resistance exercise on protein synthesis and breakdown in men (84). After a 12-hour fast, protein breakdown exceeds protein synthesis (#1). Under such catabolic conditions, resistance exercise increases the rates of both protein synthesis and breakdown 3 hours later, such that breakdown still exceeds synthesis (#2). By contrast, consuming amino acids at rest establishes anabolic conditions by selectively increasing protein synthesis (#3). When amino acids are consumed within 3 hours after a resistance exercise bout, the effects of the two treatments on protein synthesis are additive: synthesis exceeds breakdown and both processes are accelerated (#4). Consuming glucose as well as amino acids at rest accelerates both synthesis and breakdown (#5), and exercise then selectively accelerates protein synthesis to magnify the anabolic effect (#6). Thus, Wolfe's findings indicate that circulating supplies of nutrients, and the hormonal responses to those nutrients, determine whether working muscle will grow or atrophy, with the result that exercise magnifies the anabolic response only when sufficient glucose and (presumably) insulin are available.

TEST YOURSELF

Using the mean values of protein synthesis and breakdown shown in Figure 19.8, calculate the net protein synthesis (synthesis minus breakdown) for each of the six experimental conditions. Then calculate the percentage increase in postexercise net protein synthesis achieved by adding glucose to amino acids in the postexercise meal.

Of course, there are substantial differences between Goldberg's and Wolfe's experiments that may eventually be shown to account for their apparently inconsistent findings. There are profound species differences between rats and humans. Plasma glucose and insulin levels and metabolic rates are substantially higher in rats. Rats are cold at room temperature because the thermoneutral temperature zone for rats is about 8°C higher than that for humans. In addition, their diurnal rhythms are reversed. Energy deficiency lowers GH levels in rats and raises them in humans. Rats eat many small meals per day, and when fasted, can lose up to a third of their body weight within 3 days. In humans, the brain accounts for 20% of resting energy expenditure in adults and 50% in children. In rats,

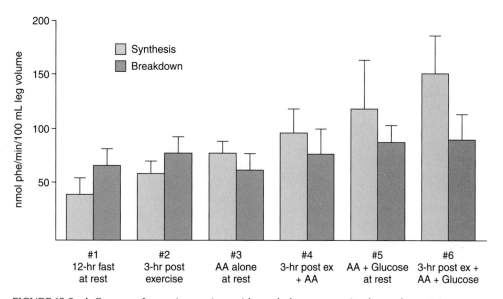

FIGURE 19.8 Influence of exercise, amino acids, and glucose on mixed muscle protein turnover in young volunteers. Under postabsorptive conditions, protein breakdown exceeds synthesis at rest (*#1*), and exercise accelerates both processes (*#2*). A meal of amino acids increases protein synthesis and suppresses protein breakdown at rest, so that synthesis exceeds breakdown (*#3*), and exercise accelerates both processes (*#4*). Adding glucose to the meal further increases synthesis and breakdown at rest (*#5*), and again exercise accelerates both processes to increase net protein synthesis (*6#*). Thus, nutritional status determines whether exercise is anabolic or catabolic. (Reprinted with permission from Rasmussen BB, Phillips SM. Contractile and nutritional regulation of human muscle growth. *Exerc Sport Sci Rev.* 2003;31:131.)

it accounts for only 2%. Because working muscle competes directly against the brain for glucose as a metabolic fuel, the effects of exercise on brains with such different energy requirements may also differ.

Wolfe and Goldberg also used different resistance exercise treatments. Goldberg's treatment was applied constantly for 5 days, whereas Wolfe's was applied only once. Their outcome variables were also different. Wolfe calculated rates of protein synthesis and breakdown at a particular point in time 3 hours after an exercise bout, whereas Goldberg measured the integrated effects of synthesis and breakdown on muscle size and mass over several days. Although the results do not present the complete story about work-induced muscle hypertrophy in humans, Wolfe's men show that the story is not as simple as Goldberg's rats appeared to indicate.

Insulin

Insulin has a major influence on protein turnover, and it is important to recognize that the regulation of protein turnover by insulin and amino acids differs between splanchnic and skeletal muscle beds (85). This can lead to substantial discrepancies between estimates of whole body and skeletal muscle protein turnover. Insulin acts mostly on skeletal muscle, whereas amino acids act on both skeletal muscle and the splanchnic bed.

The most consistently observed effect of insulin on protein metabolism is the suppression proteolysis (86).

This effect is independent of blood glucose levels (87). It is clear, however, that insulin deficiency alone does not cause the breakdown of myofibrillar proteins, because fluxes across the leg and the forearm of the protein breakdown product 3-methyl-hystidine do not change when insulin is administered (88).

All four proteolytic pathways in skeletal muscle (see Chapter 17) are insulin dependent. Insulin deficiency activates the ubiquitination of proteins (89) and stabilizes the lysosomal membrane, thereby reducing free cathepsin activity and limiting protein breakdown (90). Insulin also inhibits caspase (91) and calpain activity (92) by reducing PI3K activity. Only modest increases in plasma insulin are necessary to diminish skeletal muscle protein breakdown. As illustrated in Figure 19.9A, the suppressive effect of insulin on proteolysis in forearm muscles of fasting humans is complete at ~150 pM (~25 uU/mL) (86). (See also Fig. 19.10A for comparison with normal values.)

Observations of the effects of insulin on protein synthesis are less consistent. Insulin increases the rate of amino acid uptake by skeletal muscle (93). Insulin signaling also regulates protein synthesis at both transcription and translation initiation steps. Insulin increases mRNA for selected proteins, including myosin heavy chain (MHC) α in rat skeletal muscle. Peptide chain initiation in muscle is reduced in insulin deficiency and restored by insulin treatment. As a result, decreasing insulin availability by inducing experimental diabetes or starvation reduces the rate of peptide chain initiation by 40% to 50% (82). On

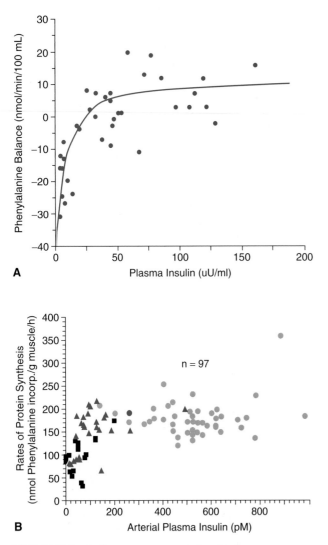

A. Phenylalanine Balance (nmol/min/100 mL) vs Plasma Insulin (uU/ml)

B. Rates of Protein Synthesis (nmol Phenylalanine incorp./g muscle/h) vs Arterial Plasma Insulin (pM), n = 97

FIGURE 19.9 A. Dose-response relationship between plasma insulin and net forearm skeletal muscle amino acid (phenylalanine) balance during postabsorptive rest. Proteolysis occurs below about 150 pM (about 25 uU/mL). Above about 150 pM, insulin has no effect on protein breakdown (1 uU/mL = 6 pM). (Reprinted with permission from Louard RJ, Fryburg DA, Gelfand RA, et al. Insulin sensitivity of protein and glucose metabolism in human forearm skeletal muscle. *J Clin Invest.* 1992;90:2353.) **B.** Dose-response relationship between arterial plasma insulin and rates of protein synthesis after acute resistance exercise in 97 rats. Below about 80 pM, insulin deficiency limits exercise-stimulated protein synthesis. (Reprinted with permission from Fedele MJ, Hernandez JM, Lang CH, et al. Severe diabetes prohibits elevations in muscle protein synthesis after acute resistance exercise in rats. *J Appl Physiol.* 2000;88:105.)

the other hand, hyperinsulinemia can also suppress protein synthesis. Without concurrent amino acid infusion or consumption, insulin administration can lower amino acid concentrations in the blood, reducing the supply of substrate for skeletal muscle protein synthesis and thus lowering the protein synthesis rate.

Peter Farrell's laboratory investigated the effects of insulin on protein synthesis by employing an experimental model similar to those of both Goldberg and Wolfe. Farrell's experimental animal was a rat, and his resistance exercise treatment was also applied periodically over several days. The rats were required to use both hind legs to lift a progressively more heavily weighted vest in order to reach an overhead bar. One exercise treatment required the rats to perform this squat leg press 50 times a day. After several days, Farrell measured protein synthesis rates in the gastrocnemius muscle and insulin levels. As shown in Figure 19.9B, the stimulation of skeletal muscle protein synthesis under physiologic conditions in Farrell's rats is saturated at a fasting insulin concentration of only ~80 pM, corresponding to levels seen in severely diabetic rats after 5 hours of fasting (94). Below this level, insulin deficiency limited the stimulation of protein synthesis by resistance exercise. Thus, Farrell's data indicate that insulin does affect protein synthesis in working skeletal muscle of the rat, but only below what is a very low concentration for a rat. Above 80 pM, protein synthesis increases with amino acid availability and with stimulation by resistance exercise. Were insulin levels higher in Goldberg's diabetic and starving rats? Maybe, but we'll never know, because he did not measure them. We do not yet know whether insulin's stimulation of protein synthesis in working muscle in humans is also saturated at ~80 pM or at some other concentration.

These thresholds, above which insulin's stimulation of protein synthesis in the working muscle of rats (~80 pM) and its inhibition of protein breakdown in the resting muscle of humans (~150 pM) are saturated, are much lower than the concentration at which the insulin's stimulation of skeletal muscle glucose uptake in humans is saturated (>600 pM). Thus, insulin's effects on protein turnover occur in the lower part of its physiologic range. To put these thresholds into a human physiologic perspective, Figure 19.10A shows them in relation to the variations in insulin levels observed in normal, healthy, sedentary individuals consuming three meals a day at 8 AM, 2 PM, and 8 PM. Their insulin levels are almost always below 150 pM, and they fall below 80 pM within 4 hours after the most recent meal. These data illustrate the challenges posed by the need for athletes to manage their diets in such a way as to maintain insulin levels to avoid unnecessary protein breakdown and perhaps also to avoid limiting protein synthesis. The decline in insulin that occurs during prolonged exercise further increases this challenge. These data also emphasize the importance of the carbohydrate content of the diet for optimizing protein turnover.

Cortisol

Cortisol is often credited with being the principal catabolic hormone because of its central role in proteolysis. Because proteolysis increases the availability of amino acids for

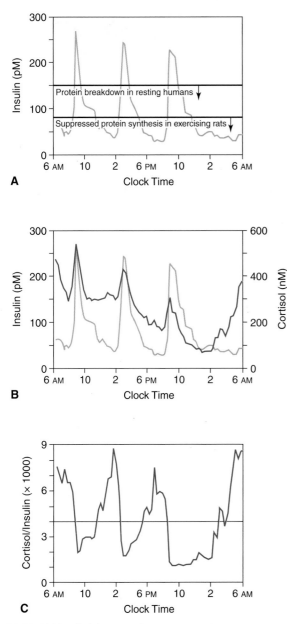

FIGURE 19.10   A. Mean insulin concentrations over a period of 24 hours in eight men and women who consumed three standardized meals at 8:00 AM, 2:00 PM, and 8:00 PM. Horizontal lines indicate the insulin concentrations at which insulin's suppression of protein breakdown in resting humans and stimulation of protein synthesis in exercising rats are saturated. **B.** Mean insulin concentrations (as in **A**) and cortisol concentrations over 24 hours in the same men and women. **C.** Cortisol-to-insulin ratios over 24 hours in the same men and women. Proteolysis is accelerated when the cortisol-to-insulin ratio is above the horizontal line at 4 (×1000). (Adapted with permission from Van Cauter E, Shapiro ET, Tillil H, et al. Circadian modulation of glucose and insulin responses to meals: relationship to cortisol rhythm. *Am J Physiol.* 1992;262:E470.)

gluconeogenesis, the proteolytic and glucoregulatory roles of cortisol are often regarded as two sides of the same coin. Although this is true, the coin is a strange one, because it has different values on its two sides. On one side, the daily turnover of protein is much greater than the turnover of carbohydrates and fats, whereas on the other side, protein is the least oxidized of the three metabolic fuels. That is, cortisol's importance for protein turnover exceeds its importance for glucoregulation.

Elevated physiologic levels of cortisol are necessary but not sufficient to accelerate muscle protein breakdown by the ubiquitin-proteosome system. Cortisol and other glucocorticoids increase the capacity of this system by stimulating the expression of ubiquitin, ubiquitin carrier, and proteosome genes, resulting in increases in ubiquitin, ubiquitin carrier, and proteosome subunit mRNAs and proteins. However, a second factor must be present to activate ubiquitination. In exercise, muscle damage, the release of Ca^{2+} into the cytosol from the sacroplastic reticulum, and elevated reactive oxygen species in the form of incompletely oxidized metabolic fuels are factors inherent in exercise that activate lysosomal, calpain, and caspase proteases to make myofibrillar proteins available for ubiquitination. In type 2 diabetes, fasting, and certain other catabolic conditions, the second factor is low insulin levels (87). In type 2 diabetes, uremia, sepsis, and metabolic acidosis, the second factor is impaired responsiveness to insulin. Thus, over and above the inherent mechanisms by which exercise stimulates proteolysis, undernutrition and the energy cost of exercise drive proteolysis by raising the cortisol-to-insulin ratio.

Table 19.1 shows results obtained by infusing hydrocortisone into six healthy young men for 64 hours (95). Measurements were made under resting conditions immediately before the infusion began 16 hours after their last meal, as well as 12 to 16 hours and 60 to 64 hours after the infusion started. By mobilizing amino acids and promoting gluconeogenesis, the elevation of cortisol concentrations into the upper part of the physiologic range increased plasma glucose levels, which raised insulin levels in response. Nevertheless, because the rise in insulin was not as great as the rise in cortisol, the cortisol-to-insulin ratio rose from 4.1 (×1000) to >7 (×1000), increasing the rates of appearance of amino acids beyond the initial postabsorptive rates.

With that experiment in mind, consider Figure 19.10B, which shows daily variations in cortisol in relation to insulin concentrations in individuals consuming three meals a day. The resulting daily variations in the cortisol-to-insulin ratio are shown in Figure 19.10C. The cortisol-to-insulin ratio exceeds 4 (×1000) for about 6 hours during sleep. This is largely unavoidable and may be beneficial by increasing the availability of amino acids. Eating only three meals per day, however, doubles the number of hours each day during which an elevated cortisol-to-insulin ratio accelerates proteolysis.

TABLE 19.1	Postabsorptive Hormone and Glucose Concentrations and Amino Acid Appearance Rates[a]		
	Before	12–16 h	60–64 h
Hormones			
Cortisol (nM)	280 ± 30	890 ± 120	990 ± 40
Insulin (pM)	68 ± 7	100 ± 4	129 ± 9
Cortisol/insulin (×1000)	4.1	8.9	7.7
Glucose (mM)	4.6 ± 0.1	5.9 ± 0.2	5.6 ± 0.1
Amino acid appearance rates			
Leucine (%)	100	117	113
Phenylalanine (%)	100	114	118
Glutamine (%)	100	139	139
Alanine (%)	100	138	229

[a]Before and during 64 hours of hydrocortisone infusion in six healthy young men. Modified with permission from Darmaun D, Matthews DE, Bier DM. Physiological hypercortisolemia increases proteolysis, glutamine, and alanine production. *Am J Physiol.* 1988;255:E366–E373.

Figure 19.11 shows the effect of an intravenous infusion of glucose on the cortisol-to-insulin ratios that occur during a prolonged exercise bout under postabsorptive conditions at 70% peak $\dot{V}O_2$ (26). Two hours of exercise without the glucose infusion raised the postabsorptive cortisol-to-insulin ratio from ~10 (×1000) to >30 (×1000). By contrast, glucose infusion suppressed the ratio to <4 (×1000). These data demonstrate how strongly proteolysis is stimulated during prolonged exercise in the postabsorptive state.

Growth hormone

Postnatal somatic growth and especially peri- and postpubertal growth depend on the normal pulsatile secretion of GH from the pituitary. GH administration substantially reverses the impaired growth that occurs in hypophysectomized animals, and chronic administration of recombinant human GH (rhGH) restores growth in GH-deficient children and adolescents, and increases lean body mass in GH-deficient adult and elderly patients. In such individuals, GH, unlike insulin, stimulates protein synthesis without affecting proteolysis (96). In growing pigs, GH administration increases circulating insulin and IGF-I concentrations over and above the effect of feeding, and thus its unclear whether GH exerts direct or indirect actions via these other hormones (97). In skeletal muscle, GH exerts its effect by increasing the efficiency of translation initiation (i.e., the amount of protein synthesized per ribosome) rather than by increasing the number of ribosomes. This effect occurs over and above the effect of feeding on translation initiation, but it occurs only in the postprandial and not in the postabsorptive state (97).

In normal, healthy adults, however, GH appears to play only a minor role in promoting muscle hypertrophy and strength (98). Resistance exercise, like aerobic exercise, elicits an acute increase in GH concentrations that declines within an hour or so after exercise stops. The magnitude of this response is in proportion to the associated metabolic demand, but over the next 12 hours GH concentrations are slightly suppressed (99). There is no evidence that these GH responses to resistance exercise have any effect on skeletal muscle growth. Acute local and systemic infusions of rhGH at pharmacologic doses for 6 hours lead to increased protein synthesis in adults. However, when chronically administered for several weeks in combination with resistance exercise training, supraphysiologic doses of rhGH result in increased total body water, lean body mass, and whole body protein synthesis in general without specifically increasing skeletal muscle protein synthesis or skeletal muscle mass, cross-sectional area, fiber size, strength, or power in untrained young men, experienced young weight lifters, or older men (98).

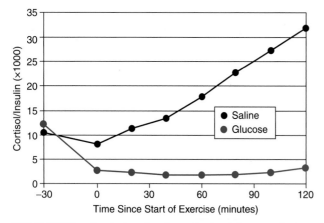

FIGURE 19.11 Cortisol-to-insulin ratios in eight men during 2 hours of exercise in the postabsorptive state at 70% $\dot{V}O_{2max}$ with glucose and saline infusions. The glucose infusion maintained plasma glucose at 12 mM and suppressed the cortisol-to-insulin ratio to <4 (×1000). (Adapted with permission from data in MacLaren DP, Reilly T, Campbell IT, et al. Hormonal and metabolic responses to maintained hyperglycemia during prolonged exercise. *J Appl Physiol.* 1999;87:127–128.)

Insulin-like growth factor-1

The anabolic influence of GH on somatic growth is probably mediated by IGF-I, as indicated by the fact that IGF-I knockout mice remain small despite markedly increased circulating GH levels resulting from the loss of IGF-I negative feedback (100). Seventy-five percent of circulating IGF-I is secreted by the liver in response to GH stimulation via exon-1 of the hepatic IGF-I gene. Although GH also stimulates IGF-I expression in type I fibers of skeletal muscle via exon-2, exercise-induced muscle hypertrophy does not depend on either circulating GH or circulating IGF-I. In one study, increased mechanical loading led to substantial compensatory hypertrophy in the overloaded skeletal muscles of hypophysectomized rats in which both circulating GH and circulating IGF-I were drastically reduced (101). This occurred because type II skeletal muscle fibers have the intrinsic capacity to express IGF-I mRNA and IGF-I peptide via exon-1 of the IGF-I gene in response to mechanical loading, even in the absence of GH stimulation (102). Type II fibers express both a generalized form of IGF-I and a unique isoform of IGF-I known as mechano growth factor (MGF). MGF is only expressed in response to stretch and loading (103) and is hardly detectable in muscle unless the muscle is exercised or damaged.

IGF-I stimulates protein synthesis and reduces protein breakdown in muscle fibers (104). GH-stimulated IGF-I expression maintains and expands slow-twitch type I fibers, whereas exercise-stimulated IGF-I expression maintains and expands fast-twitch type II fibers. Increased mechanical loading, stretch, and eccentric contraction all increase IGF-I and IGF-I mRNA expression in muscle cells (105), and pretreatment with IGF-I antiserum blocks the increase in muscle protein synthesis due to exercise (106). Even without mechanical stimulation, experimental manipulation of IGF-I levels in muscle, either by overexpression or direct infusion, induces hypertrophy both in vitro and in vivo, and interference with intracellular IGF-I signaling prevents this response. Thus, it appears to be the paracrine/autocrine secretion and local action of IGF-I within working muscle cells, and not the hepatic secretion and remote action of circulating IGF-I, that stimulates individual skeletal muscle fibers to adapt to the specific functional demands imposed by diverse physical activities.

Like insulin, IGF-I also reduces glucocorticoid-induced muscle proteolysis by inhibiting cathepsin, calpain, and proteosomal enzyme activities (107). Beyond protein synthesis, sustained muscle hypertrophy requires additional nuclei to be contributed to muscle fibers to maintain a relatively fixed ratio between the volume of muscle fibers and the volume of the nuclei that maintain them. This requirement is met by the proliferation and differentiation of muscle satellite cells and their fusion with enlarging muscle fibers. IGF-I is found in satellite cells (108) and facilitates all of these processes. The proportional and temporal expressions of IGF-I and its MGF isoform are very sensitive to the loading state of the muscle. After muscle damage occurs, MGF is produced for about 24 hours, whereas IGF-I production continues for a longer period. MGF and IGF-I also differ greatly in their capacity to activate satellite cells. In one study, a 25% increase in muscle mass induced by local IGF-I administration over a period of 4 months was achieved by MGF administration in just 2 weeks (109).

Androgens

It has been shown that a bout of high-volume resistance exercise can lower total and free testosterone concentrations by about 10% over a period of 12 hours (110), but regular high-volume resistance exercise training for several weeks does not affect basal testosterone concentrations (111). Hypertrophic responses to resistance exercise in women, whose testosterone concentrations are only ~10% of those in men, appear to confirm Goldberg's findings in hypophysectomized rats (101) that the basal testosterone concentrations normally found in males are not necessary for hypertrophic responses to resistance training. Nevertheless, elevated basal testosterone concentrations do magnify these responses. Under anabolic dietary conditions, resistance training and supraphysiologic exogenous doses of testosterone induce substantial similar and additive gains in FFM, muscle size, and strength (Fig. 19.12) (112).

Testosterone acts by increasing muscle protein synthesis without having any effect on protein breakdown (113). Testosterone has no effect on the transport of amino acids into muscle fibers (113). Acute elevations of testosterone for several hours do not increase protein synthesis, indicating that testosterone acts via the genome by enhancing transcription and not by accelerating translation (114).

Testosterone exerts its effects by binding to the single receptor that binds all androgens in all androgen-sensitive tissues, and different androgen-dependent processes have different testosterone dose-response relationships. The androgen receptor (AR) regulates the transcription of androgen-sensitive target genes, and the concentrations of AR and AR mRNA reflect the degree of androgen responsiveness of a tissue. Testosterone administration has been shown to increase AR concentrations in skeletal muscle (115), and oxandrolone administration to increase AR mRNA concentrations in satellite cells (116).

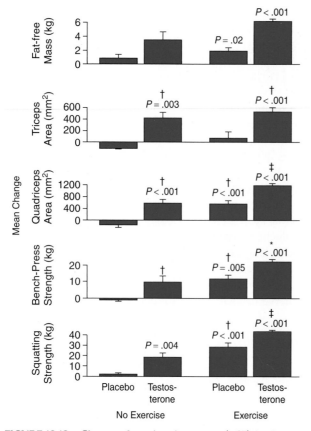

FIGURE 19.12 Changes from baseline mean (+SE) fat-free mass, triceps and quadriceps cross-sectional areas, and muscle strength in bench-press and squatting exercises after 10 weeks in a 2 × 2 design to determine the independent effects of resistance exercise and supraphysiologic testosterone treatments. *P*-values indicate the detection of responses other than zero. Asterisks indicate significant differences (*P* < .05) between the indicated responses and the responses of the no-exercise groups, daggers indicate significant differences between the indicated responses and the response of the no-exercise placebo group, and double daggers indicate significant differences between the indicated responses and the responses of all three other groups. Resistance exercise and supraphysiologic testosterone independently increased muscle size and strength to a similar degree. (Reprinted with permission from Bhasin S, Storer TW, Berman N, et al. The effects of supraphysiologic doses of testosterone on muscle size and strength in normal men. *N Engl J Med.* 1996;335:6.)

Electrical stimulation (117) and resistance exercise (118) also increase skeletal muscle AR mRNA concentrations, explaining, in part at least, why resistance exercise and testosterone have additive effects on muscle growth and strength (112).

Testosterone administration also increases IGF-I mRNA in skeletal muscle (87) and downregulates IGF-I binding proteins (114), thereby further increasing IGF-I bioavailability. Conversely, testosterone suppression reduces muscle strength and IGF-I mRNA concentration, and increases concentrations of IGF-I binding proteins, thereby reducing IGF-I bioavailability (119).

In one study, the dose-response effects of testosterone on several parameters of body and muscle size, strength, and power were measured in subjects who were instructed to continue their usual diet and exercise habits (120). Increases in FFM were related to testosterone concentrations from hypogonadal to supraphysiologic levels, but with rapidly diminishing returns above the physiologic range. Moreover, testosterone accounted for only about half of the variance in the magnitudes of these effects ($100*R^2 = 53\%$; Fig. 19.13). Indeed, the effects on every measured parameter of muscle size, strength, and power were as great in many individuals with physiologic concentrations as they were in individuals with the highest supraphysiologic concentrations.

Some of the variation in these effects of testosterone administration may have been due to individual differences in physiologic factors, such as testosterone metabolism, polymorphisms of the AR, 5-α-reductase, and other muscle growth regulators. However, given what we know about the similar additive effects of exercise and testosterone under anabolic conditions, we can assume that much of the variance was probably due to the intentionally uncontrolled diet and exercise habits of the subjects. Clearly, even supraphysiologic doses of testosterone do not in themselves enhance muscle growth in all individuals who are following their usual diet and exercise habits.

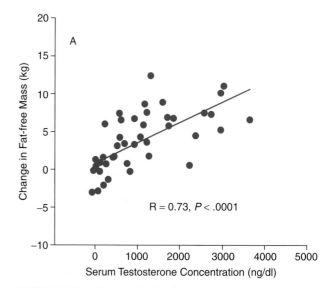

FIGURE 19.13 Changes in fat-free mass in relation to total serum testosterone concentrations in 40 healthy men after 16 weeks of testosterone enanthate administration with uncontrolled diets and physical activity. Testosterone increased fat-free mass in a dose-dependent manner, but supraphysiologic levels did not ensure increases greater than those in the normal physiologic range (300–1000 ng · dL⁻¹). (Adapted with permission from Fig. 2A in Bhasin S, Woodhouse L, Casaburi R, et al. Testosterone dose-response relationships in healthy young men. *Am J Physiol.* 2001;281:E1177.)

Thyroid hormone

Thyroid hormone (triiodothyronine [T_3]) has profound effects on protein turnover and hence the metabolic rate. T_3 exerts its effects on gene expression at transcription, posttranscription, translation, and posttranslation levels (121). T_3 is transported into the nucleus, where it binds to thyroid hormone receptors to affect transcription. These T_3-bound receptors interact as monomers, homodimers, or heterodimers with vitamin D and retinoic acid receptors, or in association with other auxiliary proteins in binding to the thyroid response elements of genes. The complexity of these combinations enables T_3 to exert diverse effects from tissue to tissue. Posttranscriptionally, T_3 appears to influence mRNA stability. T_3 also affects translation efficiency and proteolysis.

Although the responses of Goldberg's hypophysectomized rats indicated that T_3 is not necessary for the hypertrophy of overloaded muscles (101), T_3 does have a profound influence on muscle growth, in that both an excess and a deficiency can cause general muscle wasting. Hepatic production of IGF-I in response to GH stimulation depends on T_3, which is suppressed by carbohydrate deficiency. Low levels of T_3 suppress both proteolysis and synthesis. Moderate levels stimulate protein synthesis and, to a lesser extent, proteolysis, but high levels selectively further stimulate proteolysis. T_3 affects proteolysis because of the ATP dependence of the ubiquitin-proteosome system, and because T_3 stimulates ATP production in mitochondria.

In addition to affecting muscle size, T_3 also alters the distribution of fiber types in muscles, with slow muscles being more sensitive to these effects than fast muscles. Differences in the contractile properties of slow and fast muscles derive in part from differences in their mix of MHC and myosin light chain (MLC) isoforms. Reductions in circulating T_3 increase the expression of the slow type I MHC isoform and decrease expression of the fast type IIB MHC isoform. In type IIA/IIX isoforms, MHC expression shifts bidirectionally depending on the muscle type. In slow muscles and in the red inner regions of fast muscles, reductions in T_3 cause some transformable type IIA/IIX fibers to express the type I MHC isoform, whereas in the white superficial regions of fast muscles, some transformable type IIB fibers revert to the type IIX MHC isoform. Hypothyroidism also upregulates the expression of slow MLC isoforms in both slow and fast muscle, and represses the expression of fast MLC isoforms in type IIA fibers in slow muscle. These effects on the interconversion of fiber types are similar to those of mechanical loading. Hyperthyroidism has the opposite effects, which are similar to those of chronic unloading. When placed in competition with one another, hyperthyroidism completely blocks MHC responses to mechanical loading, and hypothyroidism completely blocks MHC responses to mechanical unloading.

Thyroid hormone also has substantial effects on the sarcoplasmic reticulum, which performs three key functions (Ca^{2+} release, uptake, and storage) in the contraction and relaxation cycle of working muscle. The uptake of Ca^{2+} by the sarcoplasmic/endoplasmic reticulum Ca^{2+}-ATPase pump (SERCA) expends one molecule of ATP for every two Ca^{2+} taken up, an energy cost amounting to ~25% of metabolic energy expenditure during contractile activity. Like the MHC and MLC isoforms, various mixes of both fast SERCA1 and slow SERCA2 mRNA isoforms are expressed in fibers of slow and fast muscle types. In similarity to their effects on MHC and MLC isoforms, hypothyroidism reduces the rate of Ca^{2+} uptake and hyperthyroidism increases it by regulating SERCA mRNA isoform expression in a fiber-type specific manner.

These influences of thyroid hormone on myosin and Ca^{2+}-ATPase pump expression have demonstrable effects on the mechanical properties of skeletal muscle. Hypothyroidism and hyperthyroidism have been shown to respectively reduce and increase the maximum shortening velocity of soleus muscle. Thyroid hormone also influences the relationship between the frequency of stimulation and force a muscle generates. Graphically, the force-frequency relationship of slow muscle fibers lies to the left of that of fast fibers. By completely repressing the expression of fast fibers in the soleus muscle, hypothyroidism shifts its force-frequency relationship further to the left. Conversely, by converting some slow type I fibers to fast type IIA/X fibers, hyperthyroidism shifts the force-frequency relationship of soleus muscle to the right. By comparison, the force-frequency relationship of fast muscles is relatively insensitive to thyroid state. Muscle tension relaxation time is also sensitive to T_3 in a manner reflecting the fiber content of particular muscles. In the predominantly slow fiber soleus muscle, hyperthyroidism reduces relaxation time by ~50% and hypothyroidism increases it by ~100%. These effects are small in predominantly fast fiber muscles and intermediate in mixed fiber muscles. Thus, by reducing shortening velocity and extending relaxation time, the net effect of low thyroid hormone levels is to reduce the capacity of slow muscles to produce mechanical work and power.

Summary

In this section on the regulation of muscle plasticity, we have shown how the same metabolic hormones that regulate blood glucose and skeletal muscle fuel selection can also regulate skeletal muscle amino acid uptake and skeletal muscle protein synthesis and breakdown. The other hormones involved (IGF-I, T_3, and testosterone) are also directly or indirectly dependent on energy and carbohydrates. As a result, variations in energy and carbohydrate intake have large confounding influences on the effectiveness of resistance and endurance exercise training programs for adapting muscle mass and composition to mechanical loads. Much remains to be learned about how we can optimize nutrition to more predictably achieve the desired benefits. We now turn our attention to the mitochondrion and the endocrine regulation of its role in thermogenesis and skeletal muscle fuel selection.

Regulation of Mitochondrial Biogenesis and Coupling

Little is known about endocrine regulation of the effects of endurance training on various processes, including transcriptional and translational processes involved in the biogenesis of mitochondria, coordinated transcription of nuclear and mitochondrial DNA for mitochondrial proteins, upregulation of mitochondrial enzyme systems, increased expression of FA enzyme systems and glucose transporter proteins, and transformation of MHC isoforms (see Chapter 4). Thus, these are fertile areas for future research.

Replication of mitochondrial DNA (mtDNA) depends in part on the transcription factor, Tfam, the expression and function of which are modified by contractile activity (122). Recently, a second transcription factor, p43, was found to bind to both mtDNA and T_3, and to regulate mtDNA independently of Tfam (123). This is of interest because it has been known for many years that mitochondrial biogenesis is also stimulated, independently of contractile activity, by thyroid hormone (124) acting via nuclear and mitochondrial receptors. The response is fiber-type specific, probably resulting from differences in the distribution of thyroid receptors (125).

Sustained, very high (i.e., nonphysiologic) glucocorticoid levels have also been shown to stimulate mitochondrial biogenesis in rat skeletal muscle, suggesting that glucocorticoids may contribute to the elevation in metabolic rate under chronically stressful conditions (126). Exogenous administration of dexamethasone (a potent synthetic glucocorticoid) for 3 days at 1000 nM, but not at 100 nM, elevated mtDNA-encoded transcripts for cytochrome *c* oxidase subunit III selectively in skeletal muscle and doubled the activity of cytochrome *c* oxidase, a marker of total oxidative phosphorylation capacity. These effects on ATP turnover were abolished by the administration of the antiglucocorticoid RU486, implying that they were mediated by glucocorticoid receptors. Dexamethasone had no effect on the coupling state of the respiratory chain, suggesting that the influence of glucocorticoids is to increase mitochondrial mass.

Regulation of the Coupling State of the Respiratory Chain

During the resynthesis of ATP from ADP, the metabolism of metabolic fuels results in the production of NADH and FADH2 in the matrix of the mitochondrion. NADH and FADH2 are then oxidized to NAD+, FAD, and H+ in the respiratory chain located in the inner membrane of the mitochondrion. In the process, protons are transported across the membrane and out of the matrix, establishing a chemical and electrical potential gradient across the membrane (i.e., potential energy). The flow of protons back down this chemical gradient through the F0F1-complex alters the conformation of F0F1 ATP synthase and transfers the associated energy to matrix ADP in the form of a third phosphate bond. Thus, the metabolism and ultimate oxidation of metabolic fuels is coupled to ATP formation (see Chapter 3).

This coupling is not 100% efficient because some protons flow back across the inner mitochondrial membrane without passing through the F0F1-complex, thereby dissipating the associated energy as heat instead of storing it in phosphate bonds. This proton leak regulates the membrane potential and thereby moderates the production of damaging reactive oxygen species, which occurs in proportion to the membrane potential. The leakage of protons through the inner mitochondrial membrane is mediated by so-called uncoupling proteins (UCPs) (127). As described below, T_3 regulates UCPs to protect mitochondrial structure and function during periods of increased FA oxidation.

Uncoupling is increased by lipid infusion, a high-fat diet, cold exposure, and prolonged exercise, all of which increase the availability and oxidation of FAs. Excessive accumulation of FAs in the mitochondrial matrix in the form of acyl-CoA is damaging to mitochondrial structure because acyl-CoA is a surfactant that in high concentrations can damage membranes. Excessive accumulation of acyl-CoA in the mitochondrial matrix also impairs mitochondrial function because the sequestration of CoA in long-chain FA esters inhibits β-oxidation and tricarboxylic acid cycle activity. Under such conditions of high acyl-CoA flux, up-regulation of mitochondrial thioesterase I within the matrix separates FA⁻ anions from CoA, and UCP-mediated uncoupling delivers the supply of protons needed to neutralize FA⁻ anions for their transport out of the matrix through the inner mitochondrial membrane by the same UCP.

The first UCP (UCP-1) was discovered in the mitochondria of brown adipose tissue (BAT) of rats and shown to be responsible for that tissue's thermogenic activity. Cold exposure provokes sympathetic stimulation of lipolysis and increases UCP-1 expression. Overfeeding also up-regulates UCP-1, thereby reducing metabolic efficiency and preventing obesity, whereas fasting decreases UCP-1 expression, increases metabolic efficiency, and conserves energy.

In adult humans, who have little BAT, skeletal muscle is the largest contributor to nonshivering thermogenesis, but UCP-1 is not expressed in skeletal muscle. A second UCP, UCP-2, is expressed in a wide range of tissues, including white adipose tissue (WAT) and skeletal muscle. UCP-2 expression in WAT correlates with RMR, and reduced UCP-2 expression is observed in the WAT and skeletal muscle of obese subjects.

A third UCP, UCP-3, is expressed only in skeletal muscle and BAT, which in humans means specifically in skeletal muscle. Sleeping metabolic rate correlates with UCP-3 expression. UCP-3 expression is increased by consumption of a high-fat diet and is reduced after weight reduction and endurance training, both of which are characterized by reduced metabolic rate and increased metabolic efficiency.

Coenzyme Q (CoQ), an essential cofactor for proton transport in the respiratory chain, is also an obligatory cofactor for proton transport by UCP (128). When activated by CoQ, proton transport by UCP is highly sensitive to the nucleotide ratio ATP/ADP (129). In BAT, where the principal function is thermogenesis, proton transport by UCP-1 is stimulated by a low ATP/ADP ratio. Distributed through diverse tissues, UCP-2 is modulated like UCP-1. In skeletal muscle, however, where abundant heat generation by contraction makes additional heating unnecessary, proton transport by UCP-3 is inhibited by a low ATP/ADP ratio and stimulated at rest by a high ATP/ADP ratio.

Mitochondrial CoQ content is strongly dependent on T_3 (130). During fasting, when T_3 levels are suppressed by low glucose availability, mitochondrial CoQ content is reduced by more than 80%. As a result, energy expenditure declines and cold tolerance is impaired despite high FA availability and high UCP-3 and mitochondrial thioesterase I expression. Exogenous administration of CoQ or T_3 almost instantly increases UCP-3-mediated uncoupling and heat production.

KEY POINT

The suppression of glucose utilization by skeletal muscle is partially mediated by T_3.

Summary

In this section on the regulation of mitochondrial biogenesis and coupling, we have drawn attention to the prominent role of T_3 in mediating the influence of particular metabolic fuels on the efficiency of skeletal muscle ATP production, and, conversely, on the contribution of skeletal muscle to nonshivering thermogenesis during cold exposure. By promoting the transportation of FAs out of the mitochondrion, T_3 shifts muscle substrate utilization away from FAs to increase metabolic efficiency whenever glucose is abundant. We now turn our attention to the recently recognized influence of metabolic hormones on skeletal health.

Regulation of Bone Turnover

Bone Composition

Bone is a composite material comprised of mineral, extracellular protein, water, and cells. The extracellular protein constitutes a porous matrix, into the pores of which the mineral is deposited. The mechanical strength of bone depends on both the mineral and protein phases (131). Bone mineral gives bone its stiffness (*i.e.*, the extent to which bone bends in response to a laterally applied force), but when separated from the protein, the mineral alone is brittle. By binding the brittle mineral together, bone protein gives bone its toughness (*i.e.*, the amount of energy required to break it).

Most research on skeletal health has focused on bone mineral (see Chapter 3), and clinical guidelines are based on this research. This is so because historically, bone, like adipose tissue before it (132), has been thought of as a passive connective tissue that serves predominantly mechanical functions that are not involved in the general energy economy of the body. Moreover, radiologic techniques for assessing bone mineral density have been readily available for many years, and these techniques have been employed to establish epidemiologic associations between bone mineral density and subsequent fractures in elderly men and women. In the elderly, the incidence of fractures doubles with each decline of one standard deviation from mean peak young adult bone mineral density.

At any given bone mineral density, however, fracture incidence varies widely due to the influence of other factors, such as bone protein. Approximately 90% of bone protein is type 1 collagen, which constitutes the extracellular matrix into which bone mineral is deposited. Most of the rest of bone protein is osteocalcin, which constitutes the glue that binds calcium in the bone mineral to type 1 collagen.

Bone Turnover

Bone is constantly being turned over by specialized cells in coordinated processes, first involving resorption by osteoclasts and then formation by osteoblasts. This turnover occurs at the sites of microcracks in the bone mineral. Millions of such asymptomatic microcracks occur every day as a result of routine mechanical loading. Osteoclasts migrate to and resorb the bone surrounding each microcrack. Then osteoblasts refill the resulting void, first by secreting the porous collagen matrix and then by secreting mineral salts into the pores of that matrix.

We can assess the rates of these processes by measuring the concentrations of certain biochemical markers in the blood. For example, in the synthesis of bone type 1 collagen, C- and N-terminal peptides are cleaved off of a procollagen molecule. Likewise, other C- and N-terminal peptides are cleaved off of bone type 1 collagen in the process of breaking it down. All of these terminal peptides make their way into the bloodstream, and their metabolites appear in the urine. Osteocalcin also appears in the blood, and changes in its concentration may be interpreted as an index of bone formation or resorption depending on the context. Other peptides involved in the intermolecular cross-linking of bone type 1 collagen molecules, and other proteins involved in the formation and resorption of bone are also used as markers of bone turnover.

Energy dependence

Recent results obtained with a new tracer technique that enables direct measurement showed that the rate of bone type 1 collagen synthesis (133) is as rapid as that of mixed skeletal muscle protein synthesis (134). This high rate of synthesis was also shown to be nutritionally modulated. Intravenous infusion of mixed macronutrients (glucose, lipids, and amino acids in the ratio of 55%:30%:15% of energy equivalent to 100% of basal metabolic rate) increased the rate of bone collagen synthesis by 66% (133). The stimulatory effect of feeding lasted for 2 hours, as it does in skeletal muscle.

An investigation of the dose-response relationship between energy availability and biochemical markers of bone turnover revealed specific metabolic hormones that may be involved in the mechanisms modulating bone turnover (135). Dietary energy intake and exercise energy expenditure were controlled to administer energy-balanced and three energy-deficient energy availabilities to habitually sedentary young women for 6 days as bone markers, and several metabolic substrates and hormones were measured before and after the treatment period.

As energy availability was reduced from 45 to 10 kcal/kg of FFM per day, the urinary concentration of N-terminal telopeptide (NTX), a marker of bone type I collagen breakdown, increased and the serum concentration of estradiol fell only at the lowest energy availability. These inverse but otherwise similar dose-response effects of energy availability on NTX and estradiol were consistent with the well-documented role of estradiol in restraining the rate of bone resorption. Reductions in estradiol concentrations after natural and surgical menopause lead to increases in the rate of bone resorption and reductions in bone mineral density.

As energy availability was reduced, both insulin and the serum concentration of type I procollagen carboxy-terminal propeptide (PICP), a marker of bone type I collagen synthesis, declined linearly. A similar effect of energy deficiency on type I procollagen amino-terminal propeptide (PINP) has been observed in men. When trained male runners performed intensive exercise while their dietary energy intake was restricted by 50% in an experimental protocol designed to deplete their muscle glycogen stores, PINP concentrations declined by 30% in 3 days (136). The association between dose-response effects of energy availability on PICP and insulin is consistent with the demonstrated specific causal relationship between insulin and bone type I collagen synthesis in streptozotocin-induced diabetic mice (137).

By contrast, reduction of energy availability had a strongly nonlinear dose-response effect on the plasma concentration of osteocalcin, which declined substantially and abruptly between 30 and 20 kcal/kgFFM/day, as did T_3 and IGF-I. Because osteocalcin declined while NTX was unaffected between 30 and 20 kcal/kgFFM/day, the decline in osteocalcin implies a reduction in bone formation rather than bone resorption. During formation, osteocalcin appears in the blood with the onset of bone matrix mineralization, consistent with its role in binding calcium to collagen. In osteoblast cells in culture, T_3 increases osteocalcin expression in a dose-dependent fashion (138)

without inducing collagen expression (139). This influence of T_3 is mediated by IGF-I (140).

Clinical implications

Insulin, T_3, IGF-I, and estradiol concentrations are all suppressed in amenorrheic athletes (141), who practice training regimens with low energy availabilities (142) and display low bone densities that decline as the number of missed menstrual cycles accumulates and are not fully restored by estrogen supplementation or by the recovery of menstrual cycles (4). Biologists expect to find a reproductive advantage in physiologic processes that have been preserved through millions of years of evolution, but ever since the discovery of skeletal demineralization in amenorrheic athletes, the reproductive advantage of low bone mineral density in undernourished women has been obscure. The discovery that bone protein turns over as quickly as skeletal muscle protein, and that this turnover is nutritionally modulated, clarifies that issue. In energy deficiency, the mobilization of protein from bone, as well as skeletal muscle, favors gluconeogenesis and survival for reproduction at a later date. Thus, the loss of bone mineral is secondary to the loss of bone protein and is an acceptable trade-off for survival.

The rapid, nutritionally modulated turnover of bone protein may also explain the increased prevalence of stress fractures in undernourished athletes. Stress fractures develop after a sustained increase in repetitive mechanical loading, which increases the rate of microcrack formation. To prevent accumulating microcracks at heavily loaded sites from linking together to form a symptomatic macrocrack, the rate of bone turnover must increase, but undernutrition reduces the rate of bone formation. Thus, stress fractures appear to be the losing outcome of a mechanically and nutritionally modulated race between microcrack formation and healing.

Summary

In this section on the regulation of bone turnover, we have described how energy deficiency can undermine the otherwise beneficial effect of mechanical loading on bone strength. The loss of bone mineral and the increased incidence of stress fractures in chronically undernourished athletes appear to be metabolic hormone-mediated side-effects of energy deficiency on bone protein. We now turn our attention to the interactive influence of nutrition and exercise on reproductive health.

Reproduction

Regulation of Reproductive Function

Thirty years ago, very high prevalences of menstrual disorders began to be reported in surveys of female athletes, with the highest prevalences occurring in competitive endurance, aesthetic, and weight-class sports. This became a matter of clinical concern when it was discovered that the low estrogen levels in amenorrheic athletes were causing the athletes to lose bone mass during the very years when they should be accumulating it. As a result, some young amenorrheic athletes had the bone density of a 60-year-old woman.

Of course, virtually all causes of menstrual disorders in the general population are also found in athletes. For this reason, all athletes with menstrual disorders should be differentially diagnosed by a qualified physician to ensure that they receive the appropriate medical care. Because many of these medical conditions are rare, no one expected them to explain the high prevalence of menstrual disorders found among athletes; however, some common medical conditions that confer competitive advantages in particular sports may lead affected women to be overrepresented in those sports. For example, hyperandrogenism may lead women with polycystic ovary disease to self-select into sports in which increased muscle mass conveys a competitive advantage, and women with anorexia nervosa may disproportionately self-select into sports in which a low body weight is thought to convey a competitive advantage.

After all such medical conditions, as well as pregnancy and lactation, were excluded, however, early investigators were left with many athletes whose menstrual disorders were unexplained. Somehow athletic training itself appeared to disrupt reproductive function in otherwise apparently healthy young women. Many hypotheses were proposed. Since then, research has shown that these menstrual disorders, diagnosed by the exclusion of other medical conditions, are caused by low energy availability, which is defined as dietary energy intake minus exercise energy expenditure. Exercise has been shown to have no suppressive effect on reproductive function, apart from the impact of its energy cost on energy availability. Athletes appear to be able to prevent or reverse menstrual disorders by dietary supplementation alone, with no moderation of their exercise regimen (4).

Regulation of the Female Reproductive System

The integrative center that governs ovarian function is a cluster of cells in the arcuate nucleus of the hypothalamus in the brain. These cells secrete pulses of a peptide hormone, gonadotropin-releasing hormone (GnRH), into a network of portal blood vessels that transport these pulses directly to the pituitary. There, gonadotrope cells in the anterior pituitary respond to the arrival of these pulses of GnRH by secreting pulses of follicle-stimulating hormone (FSH) and luteinizing hormone (LH) into the systemic bloodstream. Because the half-life of LH is so much shorter than that of FSH, the pulsatile pattern of GnRH secretion is more faithfully reflected in a corresponding pulsatile pattern of LH concentrations in the blood. Ovarian follicular development depends critically on the frequency at which these pulses appear.

In response to the proper stimulation by LH and FSH in the early follicular phase, several clusters of ovarian cells (ovarian follicles) begin to grow. Within the follicles, thecal cells respond to LH by converting increasing amounts of cholesterol to androgens, and granulosa cells respond to FSH by expressing increasing amounts of aromatase, which converts these androgens to estradiol. Gradually, the increasing negative feedback of estradiol carried in the blood to the pituitary constrains FSH secretion so that only the follicle most sensitive to FSH can continue developing. Eventually, the increasing amount of estradiol secreted into the blood by this dominant follicle exerts a positive feedback on LH secretion. In response, the pituitary gland secretes a surge of LH into the blood, resulting in the rupture of the dominant follicle and the release of an egg cell for fertilization. The remaining cells of the dominant follicle respond to the LH surge by undergoing rapid chemical and morphologic changes to become the corpus luteum. LH receptors appear on granulosa cells, which reduce their aromatase activity as they accumulate large quantities of cholesterol and then synthesize and secrete 10 to 100 times more progesterone than estradiol into the blood. The interval during which a dominant follicle develops, from menses until ovulation, is known as the follicular phase of the menstrual cycle, and the interval during which the corpus luteum is active from ovulation until the next menses is known as the luteal phase.

Estrogen and progesterone have profound influences on the uterine endometrium and many other tissues in the body. Estrogen stimulates endometrial proliferation, and progesterone causes it to become highly vascularized. These are necessary, hospitable conditions for the successful implantation of a fertilized egg. If no fertilization occurs within several days after ovulation, the capacity of the corpus luteum to secrete progesterone becomes exhausted, the structural integrity of the endometrium collapses, and menstruation ensues. Under normal circumstances, the secretory capacity of the corpus luteum is sustained long enough for the rapidly dividing cells derived from a fertilized egg to become implanted in the endometrium 6 or 7 days after fertilization. If the secretory capacity of the corpus luteum is exhausted too soon, the endometrium sloughs off before implantation can occur. The likelihood of this occurring increases when the luteal phase is shorter than 10 days. Thus, infertility can result either from the failure of the ovary to release an egg for fertilization or from the failure of a fertilized egg to become properly implanted in the endometrium.

Characterization of the Ovarian Axis in Female Athletes

Secondary amenorrhea is the cessation of menstrual cycles sometime after they begin at menarche. Athletes with secondary amenorrhea produce low levels of estrogen and

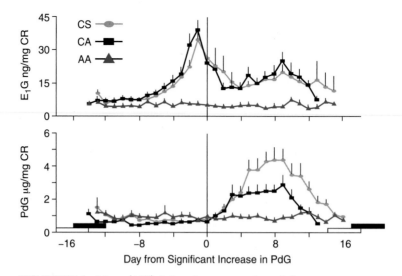

FIGURE 19.14 Mean (+SE) daily urinary excretion of the estrogen metabolite estrone glucuronide (E₁G; *top*) and the progesterone metabolite pregnanediol glucuronide (PdG) in cyclic sedentary (CS) women, cyclic athletes (CA), and amenorrheic athletes (AA). Data are presented over one menstrual cycle for cyclic women and over 30 arbitrary days for amenorrheic women. Days are oriented from a significant increase in urinary PdG excretion, with day 1 being the day of the first significant increase. Solid bar: days of menses in CS; open bar: days of menses in CA. AA display no evidence of follicular development, ovulation, or luteal function. Luteal function is suppressed and abbreviated in CA. (Reprinted with permission from Loucks AB, Mortola JF, Girton L, et al. Alterations in the hypothalamic-pituitary-ovarian and the hypothalamic-pituitary-adrenal axes in athletic women. *J Clin Endocrinol Metab.* 1989;68:408.)

progesterone every day, indicating a complete absence of follicular development, ovulation, and luteal function (Fig. 19.14, AA) (143). By contrast, even the most regularly menstruating eumenorrheic athletes display extended follicular phases and abbreviated luteal phases with blunted progesterone concentrations (Fig. 19.14; cyclic athlete) compared with eumenorrheic sedentary women (Fig. 19.14; cyclic sedentary). This can be observed in eumenorrheic women who run recreationally as little as 12 miles per week.

In eumenorrheic sedentary young women, the 24-hour LH profile in the early follicular phase is characterized by regular, high-frequency pulses of low amplitude (Fig. 19.15; cyclic sedentary) (143). During sleep, the frequency slows and the amplitude increases. Eumenorrheic athletes display a slower, but still regular rhythm of larger pulses (Fig. 19.15; cyclic athlete). Amenorrheic athletes display even fewer pulses at irregular intervals (Fig. 19.15; amenorrheic athlete [AA]).

The prevalence of amenorrhea in endurance, esthetic, and weight-class sports can be as much as 10 times higher than in the general population. The less-severe disorders of ovarian function (follicular and luteal suppression, and anovulation) may display no menstrual symptoms at all, and affected women may be entirely unaware of their condition until they undergo an endocrine workup.

Among eumenorrheic athletes, the incidence of follicular and luteal suppression and anovulation appears to be extremely high. A study involving repeated endocrine workups revealed that 79% of eumenorrheic female runners were luteally suppressed or anovulatory in at least 1 month out of 3 (144).

Hypotheses about the Mechanism of Reproductive Disorders in Athletes

Investigators have performed several different types of experiments to test the many competing hypotheses that have been proposed to explain the menstrual disorders observed in athletes. According to some of these hypotheses, acute endocrine responses to exercise can disrupt the female reproductive system. For example, it has been proposed that androgen responses to exercise may masculinize women, that cortisol responses may indicate that the female reproductive system is being suppressed by stress, and that the vibration of breasts during exercise may elicit a prolactin response similar to that which suppresses the reproductive system in nursing mothers. However, the acute androgen, cortisol, and prolactin responses to exercise turned out to be smaller in amenorrheic athletes than in eumenorrheic athletes.

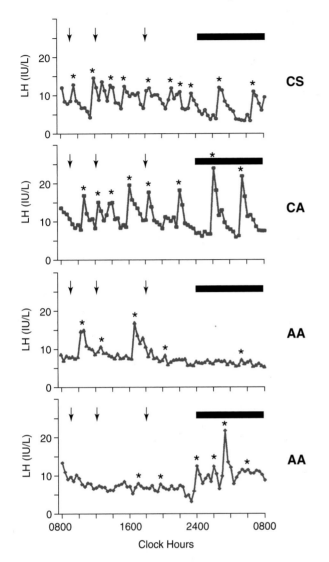

FIGURE 19.15 The 24-hour rhythm of serum luteinizing hormone (LH) levels at 20-minute intervals in a typical cyclic sedentary (CS), a typical cyclic athlete (CA), and two amenorrheic athletes (AA). Asterisks indicate pulses detected by a computer program using objective pulse detection criteria. Arrows indicate mealtimes. Horizontal bars indicate sleep periods. The effects of LH on ovarian function were determined by the frequency of LH pulses, not the average LH concentration. (Reprinted with permission from Loucks AB, Mortola JF, Girton L, et al. Alterations in the hypothalamic-pituitary-ovarian and the hypothalamic-pituitary-adrenal axes in athletic women. *J Clin Endocrinol Metab.* 1989;68:407.)

The body fat hypothesis

The most widely popularized hypothesis to explain menstrual disorders in athletes held that the ovarian axis is disrupted when the amount of energy stored in the body as fat declines below a critical level. This amount of adipose tissue was first postulated to be necessary for the peripheral conversion of circulating androgens to estrogens, even though this conversion also takes place in skeletal muscle, and athletes typically have more muscle

mass than nonathletes. Observations of athletes did not consistently verify the association of menstrual status with body composition (145), however, and did not demonstrate the appropriate temporal relationship between changes in body composition and menstrual function. Eumenorrheic and amenorrheic athletes were also found to span a common range of body compositions that were leaner than most eumenorrheic sedentary women. Among women distance runners, energy balance was found to be a better predictor of estradiol levels than either body mass index (BMI) or percent body fat. Furthermore, when the growth and sexual development of young rats, who have a 4-day estrous cycle, was blocked by dietary restriction, normal LH pulsatility resumed only a few hours after *ad libitum* feeding was permitted, long before any change in body mass or composition was observed, and ovulation occurred within 3 to 4 days (146). In another study, when surgical reduction of the stomachs of severely obese women (body weight ~130 kg, BMI ~47) reduced the amount of food they could eat, rapid weight loss and amenorrhea occurred while the patients were still overweight (body weight ~97 kg, BMI ~35) (147).

Nevertheless, interest in the body composition hypothesis was rejuvenated in the mid-1990s with the discovery of the hormone leptin and the location of leptin receptors in the hypothalamus. Leptin is synthesized and secreted by adipose tissue and was originally thought to communicate information about fat stores. Later, leptin was found to vary profoundly in response to fasting, dietary restriction, refeeding after dietary restriction, and overfeeding before any changes in adiposity occurred. This led to the hypothesis that leptin signals information about dietary (particularly carbohydrate) intake. Indeed, leptin was found to be regulated by the tiny flux of glucose through the hexosamine biosynthesis pathway in muscle and, to a greater extent, adipose tissue. Subsequently, investigators found that the diurnal rhythm of leptin actually depends not on energy intake but on energy availability or, more specifically, carbohydrate availability (148).

The stress hypothesis

According to the stress hypothesis, the stress of exercise activates the adrenal axis, thereby disrupting the GnRH pulse generator. This hypothesis was supported by a considerable amount of animal research demonstrating that GnRH neurons are disturbed by activation of the hypothalamo-pituitary-adrenal axis via pathways involving CRH and endogenous opioid and pro-opiomelanocortin-derived peptides, and by increased cortisol negative feedback. In early experiments, Hans Selye and others induced anestrus and ovarian atrophy in rats by abruptly forcing them to run or swim for prolonged periods, and they interpreted elevated cortisol levels as signs of stress. They concluded that exercise stress had a counterregulatory influence on the female reproductive system (169).

These experiments induced extreme activations of the adrenal axis, however, raising cortisol concentrations by several hundred percent, in contrast to the mild 10%–30% elevations seen in amenorrheic athletes and anorexia nervosa patients. Whether such mild elevations in cortisol influenced the GnRH pulse generator is entirely speculative. Only one experiment successfully employed exercise to induce menstrual disorders in eumenorrheic women (149). The researchers imposed a high volume of aerobic exercise abruptly, in imitation of Selye, causing a large proportion of menstrual disorders in the first month and an even larger proportion in the second. The disorders were more prevalent in a subgroup fed a controlled weight-loss diet than in another subgroup fed for weight maintenance. Even the weight-maintenance subgroup may have been underfed, however, because behavior modification and endocrine-mediated alterations in RMR can counteract the potential influences of dietary energy excess or deficiency on body mass (150).

The first cracks in the stress hypothesis appeared when glucose administration during exercise was found to prevent the cortisol response to exercise in both rats and men. Because all previous animal and human investigations of the influence of the "activity stress paradigm" on reproductive function had confounded the stress of exercise with the stress of forcing animals to exercise (e.g., electroshock or fear of drowning) and/or with energy availability (requiring animals to run farther and farther for smaller and smaller food rewards), there was in fact no unconfounded experimental evidence that the stress of exercise, independently of its energy cost, disrupts reproductive function in voluntarily exercising women. Furthermore, considering that cortisol is a glucoregulatory hormone that is activated by low blood glucose levels, these elevated cortisol levels could also be interpreted as being part of a multifaceted physiologic response to chronic energy deficiency.

The energy availability hypothesis

The energy availability hypothesis recognizes that the expenditure of energy for one physiologic function, such as locomotion, makes that energy unavailable for other purposes, including reproductive development and function. Specifically, this hypothesis holds that failure to provide sufficient metabolic fuels, especially glucose, to meet the energy requirements of the brain causes an alteration in brain function that disrupts the GnRH pulse generator. A considerable amount of data from biologic field trials support the hypothesis that mammalian reproductive function depends on energy availability, particularly in females. In the laboratory, anestrus has been induced in Syrian hamsters by food restriction, the administration of pharmacologic blockers of carbohydrate and fat metabolism,

insulin administration (which shunts metabolic fuels into storage), and cold exposure (which consumes metabolic fuels in thermogenesis) (151). Disruptive effects on the reproductive system were independent of body size and composition. Animal research also suggests that GnRH neuron activity and LH pulsatility are regulated by brain glucose availability via two separate mechanisms involving the area postrema in the caudal brainstem and the vagus nerve (152). Glucose-sensing neurons in the area postrema appear to transmit information to the GnRH pulse generator via neurons containing catecholamines, neuropeptide Y, and CRH. These glucose-sensing neurons are activated by fasting, due in part to reductions in the inhibitory influences of insulin and leptin, as well as glucose.

Cross-sectional comparisons of estimated energy availability in amenorrheic and eumenorrheic athletes support the notion that menstrual function is disrupted by low energy availability (142). Surprisingly, however, amenorrheic and eumenorrheic athletes generally report stable body weights even when their dietary energy intakes are similar to those of sedentary women.

Extensive observational data on the energy and carbohydrate intakes of athletes in many sports (with the notable exception of cross-country skiing) indicate that female athletes consume ~30% less energy and carbohydrates, normalized for body weight, than do male athletes (153). Not surprisingly, therefore, amenorrheic athletes display low levels of plasma glucose, insulin, IGF-I, IGF-I/IGFBP-1 (an index of IGF-I bioavailability), leptin, and T_3, as well as low RMRs. They also display elevated GH and mildly elevated cortisol levels. Compared with eumenorrheic sedentary women, luteally suppressed eumenorrheic athletes also display low levels of insulin, leptin, and T_3, and elevated levels of GH and cortisol, but the magnitudes of these abnormalities are less extreme than in amenorrheic athletes. Thus, metabolic substrates and hormones in amenorrheic and eumenorrheic athletes tell a consistent story of chronic energy and carbohydrate deficiency resulting in the mobilization of fat stores, slowing of the metabolic rate, and a reduction in glucose utilization, with more extreme abnormalities observed in amenorrheic athletes and less extreme abnormalities found in eumenorrheic athletes.

Tests of the exercise stress and energy availability hypotheses

The controversy over whether reproductive disorders in female athletes are caused by the stress of exercise or by low energy availability was resolved by an experiment that determined the independent effects of exercise stress and energy availability on LH pulsatility (154). Energy availability was defined, measured, and controlled operationally as dietary energy intake minus exercise energy expenditure, and exercise stress was defined as everything associated with exercise, except its energy

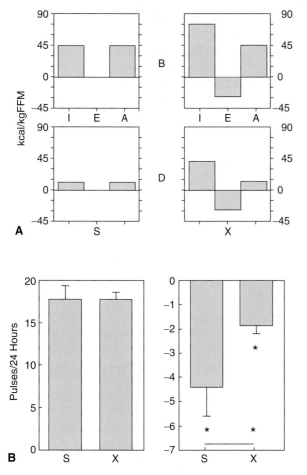

FIGURE 19.16 A. Experimental design for distinguishing the independent effects of exercise stress and energy availability on luteinizing hormone (LH) pulsatility in regularly menstruating, habitually sedentary women. In the sedentary group (S), balanced (B = 45 kcal · kg fat-free mass⁻¹ per day) and deprived (D = 10 kcal · kg fat-free mass⁻¹ per day) energy availabilities (A) were achieved by a dietary intakes (I) of 45 and 10 kcal · kg fat-free mass⁻¹ per day. The exercising group (X) expended 30 kcal · kg fat-free mass⁻¹ per day of energy in supervised exercise on a treadmill in the laboratory. Their balanced (B = 45 kcal · kg fat-free mass⁻¹ per day) and deprived (D = 10 kcal · kg fat-free mass⁻¹ per day) energy availabilities (A) were achieved by dietary intakes (I) of 75 and 40 kcal · kg fat-free mass⁻¹ per day. **B.** LH pulse frequency (*left*) and changes in LH pulse frequency due to low energy availability (*right*) in X and S. Exercise stress had no effect, and low energy availability suppressed LH pulse frequency. (Reprinted with permission from Loucks AB, Verdun M, Heath EM. Low energy availability, not stress of exercise, alters LH pulsatility in exercising women. *J Appl Physiol.* 1998;38:43.)

cost. Figure 19.16A shows the experimental design in which habitually sedentary women of normal body composition were assigned to sedentary (S) or exercising (X) groups and then administered balanced (B = 45 kcal/kgFFM/day) or deprived (D = 10 kcal/kgFFM/day) energy availability treatments in random order under controlled conditions in the laboratory.

Figure 19.16B shows the independent effects of exercise stress, determined by comparing the sedentary and exercising groups, and of energy availability, determined by comparing the balanced and deprived energy availability treatments. Exercise stress had no suppressive effect on LH pulse frequency, and low energy availability suppressed LH pulse frequency regardless of whether the low energy availability was caused by dietary energy restriction alone or by exercise energy expenditure alone. Similar results (not shown) were obtained when half of the reduction in energy availability was caused by dietary energy restriction and the other half was caused by exercise energy expenditure. Low energy availability also suppressed T_3, insulin, IGF-I, and leptin while increasing GH and cortisol (64) in a pattern very reminiscent of that observed in amenorrheic and luteally suppressed eumenorrheic athletes (155).

Since this experiment was first performed, the energy availability hypothesis has also been confirmed by experimental disruptions of ovarian function. Investigators induced amenorrhea in monkeys by training them to run voluntarily on a motorized treadmill for longer and longer periods while their food intake remained constant (156). The monkeys abruptly became amenorrheic within 7 to 24 months after one or two cycles of luteal suppression. When the diet of half of the monkeys was then supplemented without any moderation of their exercise regimen, their menstrual cycles were restored, whereas the other half of the monkeys remained amenorrheic (157). The rapidity of recovery was directly related to the number of calories consumed.

Dose dependence of luteinizing hormone pulsatility on energy availability

The dose-response relationship between energy availability and LH pulsatility in exercising women was also determined by experiment (64). LH pulse frequency was suppressed and pulse amplitude was increased below a threshold of energy availability at ~30 kcal/kgFFM/day, suggesting that athletes may be able to prevent menstrual disorders by maintaining energy availabilities above 30 kcal/kgFFM/day (Fig. 19.16). The top right panel in Fig. 19.17 also shows that the disruption of LH pulsatility was substantially more extreme in women with short luteal phases. If the latter finding is confirmed through further investigations, the screening of women for luteal length may be a convenient way to identify those who need to take extra care to avoid falling below the threshold of energy availability needed to maintain normal LH pulsatility.

The maintenance of normal LH pulsatility in this experiment despite a restriction of energy availability to 30 kcal/kgFFM/day demonstrated that the regulation of the reproductive system in women seems to be robust against reductions in energy availability as large as 33%. Given that the exercise energy expenditure in this experiment was ~840 kcal, these results suggest that women may be able to maintain normal LH pulsatility while running up to 8 miles a day as long as they do not simultaneously reduce their dietary energy intake to <45 kcal/kgFFM/day. If they do reduce their dietary energy intake, as many exercising women do, they will risk falling below the threshold of energy availability needed to maintain normal LH pulsatility.

Figure 19.17 also shows the dose-response effects of energy availability on several metabolic hormones and substrates. Down to 30 kcal/kgFFM/day, the effects of glucoregulatory hormone responses on mobilizing stored metabolic fuels are able to maintain plasma glucose concentrations to within a few percent of energy-balanced levels. Below that threshold, glucose concentrations fall increasingly despite even larger hormone responses and steep increases in fat oxidation and gluconeogenesis, as indicated by the rise in β-hydroxybutyrate. Because hepatic secretion of IGF-I in response to GH stimulation is limited by T_3, the fall in T_3, especially between 20 and 30 kcal/kgFFM/day, makes the liver resistant to GH. Thus, as energy availability declines below 30 kcal/kgFFM/day, we see that progressively more extreme glucoregulatory responses are becoming less and less effective at maintaining plasma glucose levels, and there is progressively more reliance on ketones as the alternative metabolic fuel for brain metabolism.

Age dependence of luteinizing hormone sensitivity to energy availability

The incidence of menstrual disorders declines during the first decade after menarche (158) as fertility rates rise (159). This has long been attributed to the gradual maturation of the HPO axis, but no mechanism for this maturation has been proposed. Furthermore, it has long been recognized that the incidence of amenorrhea is much higher in runners younger than 15 years of gynecologic age than in older runners (160). Recent evidence suggests that the declining incidences of menstrual disorders in the general population and of amenorrhea among runners may both involve a declining sensitivity of LH pulsatility to low energy availability during adolescence as the energy cost of growth decreases (161).

In one study, contrasting energy availabilities of 10 and 45 kcal/kgFFM/day were administered to healthy, habitually sedentary, regularly menstruating, older adolescent women 5 to 8 years of gynecologic age (~20 years of calendar age) and young adult women 14 to 18 years of gynecologic age (~29 years of calendar age) for 5 days (161). Low energy availability suppressed LH pulsatility in the older adolescents but not in the young adults, even though metabolic and endocrine signals of energy deficiency were altered as much or more in the adults as in the adolescents. One possible explanation for this finding is that the sensitivity of the central nervous system to signals of energy deficiency may decline during adolescence. Another possibility is that GH, which responded even more strongly to low energy availability in the adults than in the adolescents in this study, may mobilize more FFAs from adipose tissue in adults than in adolescents. In addition to serving as an energy source for peripheral tissues, long-chain FAs cross the blood–brain barrier in the hypothalamus, where they function as an anorexic signal in opening potassium channels and reducing the firing rate of neurons that stimulate

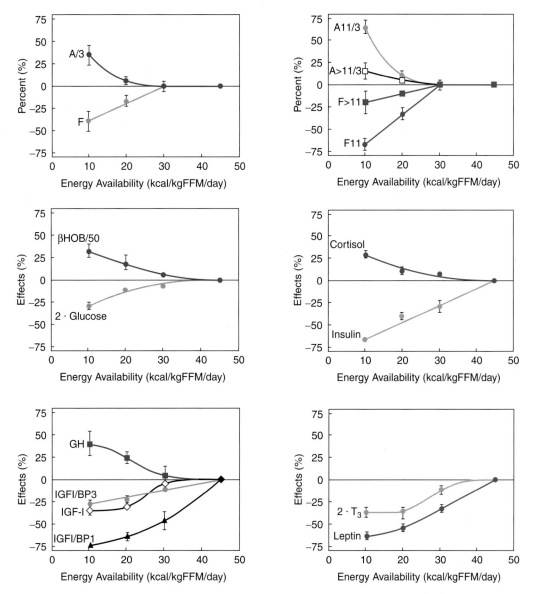

FIGURE 19.17   Incremental effects of energy availability on luteinizing hormone (LH) pulsatility and selected metabolic substrates and hormones in regularly menstruating, habitually sedentary women. All subjects expended 15 kcal · kg fat-free mass⁻¹ per day of energy in supervised exercise on a treadmill in the laboratory. Energy availabilities of 45, 30, 20, and 10 kcal · kg fat-free mass⁻¹ per day were achieved by dietary intakes of 60, 45, 35, and 25 kcal · kg fat-free mass⁻¹ per day. Effects are shown relative to 45 kcal · kg fat-free mass⁻¹ per day. *Top left.* Effects on LH pulse frequency (F) and amplitude (A/3) in all women at each energy availability treatment. Effects on LH pulsatility occurred below about 30 kcal · kg fat-free mass⁻¹ per day. *Top right.* Effects were larger in women with luteal phase lengths of 11 days (F11, A11/3) than in women with luteal phase lengths longer than 11 days (F >11, A >11/3). (Women with luteal lengths less than 11 days were excluded from study.) *Center left.* Incremental effects on the metabolic substrates β-HOB (βHOB/50) and plasma glucose (2 · Glucose). Effects on β-HOB have been divided by 50, and effects on glucose have been doubled for graphical symmetry. Effects on β-HOB and glucose became more extreme as energy availability decreased, despite more extreme responses of the metabolic hormones. *Center right.* Incremental effects on the metabolic hormones cortisol and insulin. Insulin declined linearly with energy availability, whereas effects on cortisol became increasingly extreme as energy availability decreased. *Bottom left.* Incremental effects on the somatotrophic metabolic hormones GH and IGF-I and on the ratios IGF-I/IGFBP-1 (IGFI/BP1) and IGF-I/IGFBP-3 (IGFI/BP3), which are indices of IGF-I bioavailability. GH resistance and elevated IGF-I binding proteins reduced IGF-I bioavailability as energy availability decreased. *Bottom right.* Incremental effects on the metabolic hormones T₃ (2 · T₃) and leptin. Effects on T₃ are doubled for clarity. The decline in T₃ accounts for the GH resistance. (Reprinted with permission from Loucks AB, Thuma JR. Luteinizing hormone pulsatility is disrupted at a threshold of energy availability in regularly menstruating women. *J Clin Endocrinol Metab.* 2003;88:304–306.)

glucose production and feeding (162). Maybe such neurons also suppress LH pulsatility. Yet another possibility is that more energy may be available to adult brains than to adolescent brains under identical energy availability conditions, due to reduced competition for energy from growing peripheral tissues. Calcium balance, which is an index of growth, declines to zero at 14 years of gynecologic age (163), much like the incidence of menstrual disorders.

Reproductive disorders in male athletes

Similar metabolic and analogous reproductive disorders can occur in male athletes, especially those who participate in endurance sports and sports with weight classes, but they are less obvious and less extreme than in women. They are less obvious because men do not present symptoms such as menstrual abnormalities, and they are less extreme in that reproductive development continues in males under conditions in which it is entirely blocked in females.

No 24-hour studies of LH pulsatility in male athletes have been published to date, and shorter, less reliable studies have reported inconsistent results. Nor have any investigators reported observations of semen quality outside the normal range. Reduced total and/or free testosterone levels have been reported by many, but not all, cross-sectional and prospective studies of endurance-trained male athletes, but only one reported levels below the normal range. Statistically significant reductions in reproductive hormones, when noted, were found in the most intensively training athletes. Consequently, the consensus is that reproductive dysfunction is uncommon in male athletes, and the long-term physiologic consequences of a suppressed hypothalamic-pituitary-testicular axis in male athletes probably have little clinical significance.

A prospective study of adolescent male wrestlers revealed reductions in testosterone levels to below the normal range during the wrestling season (164), along with reductions in body weight, fat mass, and strength (165). The wrestlers were consuming only half of their recommended energy intake before the season began, and they did not increase their energy intake during the season. As in female athletes, the failure of these male wrestlers to increase energy intake during the season induced GH resistance with elevated GH and suppressed IGF-I levels. Levels of prealbumin, a classic biomarker of starvation, were also suppressed. As might be expected with reduced anabolic stimulation by testosterone and IGF-I, the wrestlers' fat-free mass and their mid-arm and mid-thigh cross-sectional areas all declined during the wrestling season. As a result, their arm and leg strength and power declined by an average of 13%, contradicting the belief that weight loss conveys a competitive advantage.

Proof that chronic low energy availability, and not exercise stress, disrupts reproductive function in men as it does as in women was provided by a study of young male soldiers participating in an 8-week U.S. Army Ranger training course (166). The course was divided into four 2-week phases conducted in forest, desert, mountain, and swamp environments. The trainees expended 4200 kcal/day as they underwent daily military skill training, 8- to 12-km patrols carrying 32-kg rucksacks, and sleep deprivation (~3.6 hours of sleep/night) while consuming controlled diets that provided ~2000 and ~5000 kcal/day in alternate weeks (Fig. 19.18A). These rigors were so severe that only 30% of the

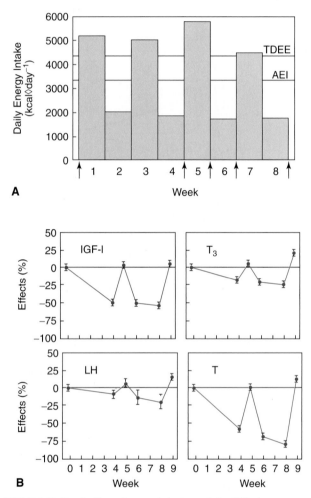

A

B

FIGURE 19.18   A. Experimental design of the U.S. Army Rangers experiment. Ranger candidates trained for 2 weeks each in forest, mountain, desert, and swamp terrain working with a total daily energy expenditure (TDEE) of 4200 kcal · day⁻¹ while consuming an average energy intake (AEI) of 3200 kcal · day⁻¹ in controlled diets that provided about 5000 and 2000 kcal · day⁻¹ in alternate weeks. Blood was sampled at the beginning of the experiment; after the fourth, fifth, sixth, and eighth weeks of training; and after 1 week of ad libitum feeding after training. **B.** Effects of diet, exercise, and other training stresses on IGF-I, T_3, LH, and testosterone (T). One week of ad libitum refeeding after training (week 9) restored normal metabolic and reproductive hormone levels, as did 1 week of controlled refeeding in week 5, despite continued exercise and other training stresses. The restoration of metabolic and reproductive function in week 5 demonstrates that the disruption of reproductive function in men is caused by low energy availability, as it is in women, and not by exercise or other training stresses.

A MILESTONE OF DISCOVERY

As a physician, Hans Selye observed that "any change in surroundings or any unusual strain, such as violent muscular exercise, chronic diseases and even mental stress may disturb the sexual cycle of the female." He also noted that it is "difficult to believe that such entirely different stimuli could all have such similar effects. It seems much more likely that there is some common pathway through which these stimuli influence the gonads." In a 1936 letter, he and a colleague reported for the first time that "diverse nocuous agents" elicited in rats a three-stage general adaptation syndrome of common responses ending in death (167). In 1937, he published a more complete account (168), and in 1939, he described how "the ovaries undergo atrophy and more or less permanent anestrus ensues" (169). Table 19.2 lists Selye's data on ovarian and adrenal weights 40 days into the general adaptation syndrome (169).

From observed effects on the mass, histology, and functions of the ovary and other organs and tissues, Selye concluded that the general adaptation syndrome reflected the influence of (and here he proposed an old word for a new concept in biology) stress. For the next 40 years,

Selye promoted, with increasing success, the utility of the concept of stress in biology. Neither he nor anyone else was ever able to provide a widely accepted empirical definition of stress, however, or to specify its physical units of measure (170). As Selye admitted, "It was only gradually, through habit rather than logic, that the term *stress*, employed in my sense, slipped into common usage, as the concept itself became a popular subject for research" (171).

On his way to positing stress as a useful new concept for explaining physiologic and pathologic responses to the environment, Selye noticed that, in addition to hypertrophy of the adrenal glands, atrophy of the thymus, lymph glands, and spleen, and erosion of the digestive tract, the general adaptation syndrome included cessation of growth and lactation, shrinkage of the liver, loss of muscular tone, a decrease in body temperature, and the disappearance of adipose tissue (167). These changes occurred rapidly during an initial 2-day alarm stage, then slowly, if at all, during a prolonged resistant stage, ending in a rapidly fatal exhaustion stage. Selye also noticed that withholding food shortened the resistant stage when other nocuous agents were

TABLE 19.2	Weights of Ovaries and Adrenal Glands[a]						
Treatment	Animal	Ovaries (grams)	Adrenals (grams)	Treatment	Animal	Ovaries (grams)	Adrenals (grams)
Untreated	1	41	62	Exercise	1	25	100
	2	60	76		2	24	126
	3	41	58		3	24	100
	4	42	72		4	26.2	106
	5	83	70		5	24.2	108
	6	54	71		6	34.2	70
	7	39	50	Average		26.3	101.7
Average		51.4	65.6	Insufficient diet	1	20.1	100
Lima beans	1	15.1	48		2	34	90
	2	10.1	46		3	29.2	60
	3	14	62		4	14.1	90
	4	16	50		5	15.2	64
	5	34.2	47		6	18.2	44
	6	25	43	Average		21.8	74.7
Average		19.1	49.3				
Formaldehyde	1	12.1	144				
	2	22.2	155				
	3	30.2	156				
	4	22.2	74				
	5	23.1	150				
	6	15.6	127				
Average		20.9	134.3				

[a]In rats 40 days into the general adaptation syndrome. Modified with permission from Selye H. The effect of adaptation to various damaging agents on the female sex organs in the rat. *Endocrinology.* 1939;25:615–624.

administered (172). He even hypothesized that "adaptation of the organism is dependent upon a special hitherto unrecognized type of energy," which he called "adaptation energy." Adaptation energy, he argued, is slowly consumed during the resistant stage when the animal "learns to perform adaptive functions more economically and with less dependence on the caloric energy derived from food" (172).

It did not occur to Selye that adaptation energy might be the energy stored in adipose tissue, and this is not surprising, considering that the role of adipose tissue in energy metabolism had not yet been discovered. At the time, it was thought that the only functions of adipose tissue were to provide thermal insulation and mechanical support for certain tissues (132). As a result, it did not occur to Selye that his

nocuous agents all increased energy expenditure or reduced energy intake to the point that his animals were starving. Because others had induced anestrus by forced feeding (169), Selye did not perform any experiments to determine whether increasing dietary intake would prevent the general adaptation syndrome, thereby rendering the empirically vague concept of stress superfluous and distracting from the empirically well-defined bioenergetic regulation of physiologic processes. Sixty years would pass, and tens of thousands of papers would be published about stress, before investigators would begin to do so (170).

Selye H. The effect of adaptation to various damaging agents on the female sex organs in the rat. Endocrinology. 1939;25:615–614.

trainees completed the course. Trainees lost ~12 kg of body weight. As shown in Figure 19.18B, blood samples obtained at the end of selected weeks revealed that T_3, IGF-I, and testosterone levels fell ~20%, ~50%, and ~70%, respectively, during weeks the men consumed diets of 2000 kcal/day and returned to normal initial levels during alternate weeks on diets of 5000 kcal/day, despite continued exposure to all other training stresses.

KEY POINT

Exercise has no suppressive effect on reproductive function beyond the impact of its energy cost on energy availability.

Summary

In this section on reproduction, we have shown how the disruption of reproductive function in many physically active women and some highly physically active men is attributable not to the exercise they do, but rather to the eating they do not do. When exercise energy expenditure increases, dietary energy intake must increase sufficiently to maintain an energy availability in excess of 30 kcal/kgFFM/day in order to preserve normal reproductive function.

CHAPTER SUMMARY

In this chapter, we have focused on the mechanisms by which the endocrine system integrates the influences of diet and exercise on the storage, mobilization, and utilization of metabolic fuels; turnover and growth of skeletal muscle; mitochondrial biogenesis and coupling; turnover of bone protein;

and reproductive function. Similar stories could have been told about how the endocrine system integrates the influences of diet and trauma (or cold exposure or cancer and other processes that consume large amounts of energy) on the availability of metabolic fuels and immune function. All such stories have in common the unique and extreme energy demands of the human brain, which necessitate strict trade-offs among basal metabolism, thermoregulation, locomotion, growth and repair, immunity, and reproduction when dietary energy is scarce. The sympathetic and endocrine mechanisms that implement these trade-offs have made us survivors.

Much of what has passed for the physiology of exercise over the past 50 years has actually been confounded by energy deficiency. Under the fasting conditions employed in many exercise physiology studies, exercise elicits acute glucoregulatory hormone responses to mobilize metabolic fuels and meet the energy requirements of working muscle. By restricting the supply of glucose to the brain, prolonged exercise training and dietary restriction (especially in combination) can also elicit chronic changes in glucoregulatory and other metabolic and reproductive hormones to reduce the metabolic demands of tissues competing with the brain. To optimize their performance and growth, and to preserve their reproductive and skeletal health, athletes need to manage their diet and exercise programs to minimize the frequency and duration of excessively low energy availability. To define the specific physiology of exercise independently of energy deficiency, the next generation of scientific investigators will need to control nutritional status more strictly than previous generations have done.

ACKNOWLEDGMENTS

Research in the author's laboratory was supported in part by Contract No. W81XWH-07-1-0251 from the U.S. Army Medical Research and Material Command (Bone Health and Military Medical Research Program). The content of the information reported in this chapter does not necessarily reflect the position or the policy of the government, and no official endorsement should be inferred.

REFERENCES

1. Oppliger RA, Case HS, Horswill CA, et al. American College of Sports Medicine position stand. Weight loss in wrestlers. *Med Sci Sports Exerc*. 1996;28:ix–xii.
2. Bubb RG. Rule 3. Weight certification, classification and weigh in. In: Halpin T, eds. *2004 NCAA Wrestling Rules and Interpretations*. Indianapolis: National Collegiate Athletic Association; 2003. p. WR-23–WR-35, WI-10–WI-11, and WA-28–WA-33.
3. Otis CL, Drinkwater B, Johnson M, et al. American College of Sports Medicine position stand. The Female Athlete Triad. *Med Sci Sports Exerc*. 1997;29:i–ix.
4. Nattiv A, Loucks AB, Manore MM, et al. American College of Sports Medicine Position Stand: the female athlete triad. *Med Sci Sports Exerc*. 2007;39:1867–1882.
5. Braun B, Brooks GA. Critical importance of controlling energy status to understand the effects of "exercise" on metabolism. *Exerc Sport Sci Rev*. 2008;36:2–4.
6. Nonogaki K. New insights into sympathetic regulation of glucose and fat metabolism. *Diabetologia*. 2000;43:533–549.
7. Routh VH. Glucose-sensing neurons: are they physiologically relevant? *Physiol Behav*. 2002;76:403–413.
8. Kreisman SH, Halter JB, Vranic M, et al. Combined infusion of epinephrine and norepinephrine during moderate exercise reproduces the glucoregulatory response of intense exercise. *Diabetes*. 2003;52:1347–1354.
9. Viguerie N, Clement K, Barbe P, et al. In vivo epinephrine-mediated regulation of gene expression in human skeletal muscle. *J Clin Endocrinol Metab*. 2004;89:2000–2014.
10. Kaciuba-Uscilko H, Kruk B, Szczpaczewska M, et al. Metabolic, body temperature and hormonal responses to repeated periods of prolonged cycle-ergometer exercise in men. *Eur J Appl Physiol Occup Physiol*. 1992;64:26–31.
11. Galassetti P, Mann S, Tate D, et al. Effect of morning exercise on counterregulatory responses to subsequent, afternoon exercise. *J Appl Physiol*. 2001;91:91–99.
12. Cryer PE. The prevention and correction of hypoglycemia. In: Jefferson LS, Cherrington AD, eds. *Handbook of Physiology: Section 7: The Endocrine System Volume II: The Endocrine Pancreas and Regulation of Metabolism*. Oxford: Oxford University Press; 2001: 1057–1092.
13. Davis SN, Galassetti P, Wasserman DH, et al. Effects of antecedent hypoglycemia on subsequent counterregulatory responses to exercise. *Diabetes*. 2000;49:73–81.
14. Wasserman DH, Lickley HL, Vranic M. Interactions between glucagon and other counterregulatory hormones during normoglycemic and hypoglycemic exercise in dogs. *J Clin Invest*. 1984;74:1404–1413.
15. Wasserman DH, Cherrington AD. Regulation of extra muscular fuel sources during exercise. In: Rowell LB, Shephard JT, eds. *Handbook of Physiology: Section 12: Exercise: Regulation and Integration of Multiple Systems*. Oxford: Oxford Press; 1996:1036–1074.
16. Galassetti P. Reciprocity of hypoglycaemia and exercise in blunting respective counterregulatory responses: possible role of cortisol as a mediator. *Diabetes Nutr Metab*. 2002;15:341–347; discussion 347–348, 362.
17. Galassetti P, Neill AR, Tate D, et al. Sexual dimorphism in counterregulatory responses to hypoglycemia after antecedent exercise. *J Clin Endocrinol Metab*. 2001;86:3516–3524.
18. Heller SR, Cryer PE. Hypoinsulinemia is not critical to glucose recovery from hypoglycemia in humans. *Am J Physiol*. 1991;261:E41–E48.
19. Galassetti P, Mann S, Tate D, et al. Effects of antecedent prolonged exercise on subsequent counterregulatory responses to hypoglycemia. *Am J Physiol Endocrinol Metab*. 2001;280:E908–E917.
20. Sandoval DA, Ertl AC, Richardson MA, et al. Estrogen blunts neuroendocrine and metabolic responses to hypoglycemia. *Diabetes*. 2003;52:1749–1755.
21. Young EA. The role of gonadal steroids in hypothalamic-pituitary-adrenal axis regulation. *Crit Rev Neurobiol*. 1995;9:371–381.
22. Roy BN, Reid RL, Van Vugt DA. The effects of estrogen and progesterone on corticotropin-releasing hormone and arginine vasopressin messenger ribonucleic acid levels in the paraventricular nucleus and supraoptic nucleus of the rhesus monkey. *Endocrinology*. 1999;140:2191–2198.
23. Tremblay A, Pinsard D, Coveney S, et al. Counterregulatory response to insulin-induced hypoglycemia in trained and nontrained humans. *Metabolism*. 1990;39:1138–1143.
24. Richter EA, Galbo H, Sonne B, et al. Adrenal medullary control of muscular and hepatic glycogenolysis and of pancreatic hormonal secretion in exercising rats. *Acta Physiol Scand*. 1980;108:235–242.
25. Tabata I, Ogita F, Miyachi M, et al. Effect of low blood glucose on plasm CRF, ACTH, and cortisol during prolonged physical exercise. *J Appl Physiol*. 1991;71:1807–1812.
26. MacLaren DP, Reilly T, Campbell IT, et al. Hormonal and metabolic responses to maintained hyperglycemia during prolonged exercise. *J Appl Physiol*. 1999;87:124–131.
27. Ainslie PN, Campbell IT, Frayn KN, et al. Physiological, metabolic, and performance implications of a prolonged hill walk: influence of energy intake. *J Appl Physiol*. 2003;94:1075–1083.
28. Davies CT, Few JD. Effects of exercise on adrenocortical function. *J Appl Physiol*. 1973;35:887–891.
29. Brandenberger G, Follenius M. Influence of timing and intensity of muscular exercise on temporal patterns of plasma cortisol levels. *J Clin Endocrinol Metab*. 1975;40:845–849.
30. Thuma JR, Gilders R, Verdun M, et al. Circadian rhythm of cortisol confounds cortisol responses to exercise: implications for future research. *J Appl Physiol*. 1995;78:1657–1664.
31. Hirsch IB, Marker JC, Smith LJ, et al. Insulin and glucagon in prevention of hypoglycemia during exercise in humans. *Am J Physiol*. 1991;260:E695–E704.
32. Zinker BA, Mohr T, Kelly P, et al. Exercise-induced fall in insulin: mechanism of action at the liver and effects on muscle glucose metabolism. *Am J Physiol*. 1994;266:E683–E689.
33. Lecavalier L, Bolli G, Gerich J. Glucagon-cortisol interactions on glucose turnover and lactate gluconeogenesis in normal humans. *Am J Physiol*. 1990;258:E569–E575.
34. Antonescu CN, Foti M, Sauvonnet N, et al. Ready, set, internalize: mechanisms and regulation of GLUT4 endocytosis. *Biosci Rep*. 2009;29:1–11.
35. Santos JM, Ribeiro SB, Gaya AR, et al. Skeletal muscle pathways of contraction-enhanced glucose uptake. *Int J Sports Med*. 2008;29:785–794.
36. Klip A, Schertzer JD, Bilan PJ, et al. Regulation of glucose transporter 4 traffic by energy deprivation from mitochondrial compromise. *Acta Physiol (Oxf)*. 2009;196:27–35.
37. Mikines KJ, Sonne B, Farrell PA, et al. Effect of training on the dose-response relationship for insulin action in men. *J Appl Physiol*. 1989;66:695–703.
38. Mikines KJ, Sonne B, Tronier B, et al. Effects of training and detraining on dose-response relationship between glucose and insulin secretion. *Am J Physiol*. 1989;256:E588–E596.
39. DeFronzo RA, Tobin JD, Andres R. Glucose clamp technique: a method for quantifying insulin secretion and resistance. *Am J Physiol*. 1979;237:E214–E223.
40. Quon MJ. Limitations of the fasting glucose to insulin ratio as an index of insulin sensitivity. *J Clin Endocrinol Metab*. 2001;86:4615–4617.
41. Bergman RN, Finegood DT, Ader M. Assessment of insulin sensitivity in vivo. *Endocr Rev*. 1985;6:45–86.
42. Bergman RN, Beard J, Chen M. The minimal modeling method. Assessment of insulin sensitivity and B-cell function in vivo. In: Larner J, Pohl D, eds. *Methods in Clinical Diabetes Research*. New York: Wiley International; 1986:13–20.
43. Welch S, Gebhart SS, Bergman RN, et al. Minimal model analysis of intravenous glucose tolerance test-derived insulin sensitivity in diabetic subjects. *J Clin Endocrinol Metab*. 1990;71:1508–1518.
44. Bergman RN, Prager R, Volund A, et al. Equivalence of the insulin sensitivity index in man derived by the minimal model method and the euglycemic glucose clamp. *J Clin Invest*. 1987;79:790–800.
45. Bland JM, Altman DG. Statistical methods for assessing agreement between two methods of clinical measurement. *Lancet*. 1986;1:307–310.

46. Black SE, Mitchell E, Freedson PS, et al. Improved insulin action following short-term exercise training: role of energy and carbohydrate balance. *J Appl Physiol*. 2005;99:2285–2293.

47. Bjorntorp P, Fahlen M, Grimby G, et al. Carbohydrate and lipid metabolism in middle-aged, physically well-trained men. *Metabolism*. 1972;21:1037–1044.

48. Bjorntorp P, De Jounge K, Sjostrom L, et al. The effect of physical training on insulin production in obesity. *Metabolism*. 1970;19:631–638.

49. Bjorntorp P, Berchtold P, Grimby G, et al. Effects of physical training on glucose tolerance, plasma insulin and lipids and on body composition in men after myocardial infarction. *Acta Med Scand*. 1972;192:439–443.

50. Saltin B, Lindgarde F, Houston M, et al. Physical training and glucose tolerance in middle-aged men with chemical diabetes. *Diabetes*. 1979;28(suppl 1):30–32.

51. Ruderman NB, Ganda OP, Johansen K. The effect of physical training on glucose tolerance and plasma lipids in maturity-onset diabetes. *Diabetes*. 1979;28(suppl 1):89–92.

52. Ross R, Dagnone D, Jones PJ, et al. Reduction in obesity and related comorbid conditions after diet-induced weight loss or exercise-induced weight loss in men. A randomized, controlled trial. *Ann Intern Med*. 2000;133:92–103.

53. Ross R, Janssen I, Dawson J, et al. Exercise-induced reduction in obesity and insulin resistance in women: a randomized controlled trial. *Obes Res*. 2004;12:789–798.

54. Assali AR, Ganor A, Beigel Y, et al. Insulin resistance in obesity: body-weight or energy balance? *J Endocrinol*. 2001;171:293–298.

55. Racette SB, Weiss EP, Obert KA, et al. Modest lifestyle intervention and glucose tolerance in obese African Americans. *Obes Res*. 2001;9:348–355.

56. Klein S, Fontana L, Young VL, et al. Absence of an effect of liposuction on insulin action and risk factors for coronary heart disease. *N Engl J Med*. 2004;350:2549–2557.

57. Larson-Meyer DE, Heilbronn LK, Redman LM, et al. Effect of calorie restriction with or without exercise on insulin sensitivity, beta-cell function, fat cell size, and ectopic lipid in overweight subjects. *Diabetes Care*. 2006;29:1337–1344.

58. Larson-Meyer DE, Redman L, Heilbronn LK, et al. Caloric restriction with or without exercise: the fitness versus fatness debate. *Med Sci Sports Exerc*. 2010;42:152–159.

59. Coker RH, Williams RH, Yeo SE, et al. The impact of exercise training compared to caloric restriction on hepatic and peripheral insulin resistance in obesity. *J Clin Endocrinol Metab*. 2009;94:4258–4266.

60. Capel F, Klimcakova E, Viguerie N, et al. Macrophages and adipocytes in human obesity: adipose tissue gene expression and insulin sensitivity during calorie restriction and weight stabilization. *Diabetes*. 2009;58:1558–1567.

61. Arciero PJ, Vukovich MD, Holloszy JO, et al. Comparison of short-term diet and exercise on insulin action in individuals with abnormal glucose tolerance. *J Appl Physiol*. 1999;86:1930–1935.

62. Houmard JA, Cox JH, MacLean PS, et al. Effect of short-term exercise training on leptin and insulin action. *Metabolism*. 2000;49:858–861.

63. Nemet D, Connolly PH, Pontello-Pescatello AM, et al. Negative energy balance plays a major role in the IGF-I response to exercise training. *J Appl Physiol*. 2004;96:276–282.

64. Loucks AB, Thuma JR. Luteinizing hormone pulsatility is disrupted at a threshold of energy availability in regularly menstruating women. *J Clin Endocrinol Metab*. 2003;88:297–311.

65. Mansell PI, Macdonald IA. The effect of starvation on insulin-induced glucose disposal and thermogenesis in humans. *Metabolism*. 1990;39:502–510.

66. Tsintzas K, Jewell K, Kamran M, et al. Differential regulation of metabolic genes in skeletal muscle during starvation and refeeding in humans. *J Physiol*. 2006;575:291–303.

67. Bergman BC, Cornier MA, Horton TJ, et al. Effects of fasting on insulin action and glucose kinetics in lean and obese men and women. *Am J Physiol Endocrinol Metab*. 2007;293:E1103–E1111.

68. van der Crabben SN, Allick G, Ackermans MT, et al. Prolonged fasting induces peripheral insulin resistance, which is not ameliorated by high-dose salicylate. *J Clin Endocrinol Metab*. 2008;93:638–641.

69. Soeters MR, Sauerwein HP, Dubbelhuis PF, et al. Muscle adaptation to short-term fasting in healthy lean humans. *J Clin Endocrinol Metab*. 2008;93:2900–2903.

70. Cahill GF Jr. Starvation in man. *N Engl J Med*. 1970;282:668–675.

71. Frayn KN, Humphreys SM, Coppack SW. Fuel selection in white adipose tissue. *Proc Nutr Soc*. 1995;54:177–189.

72. Frayn KN. Macronutrient metabolism of adipose tissue at rest and during exercise: a methodological viewpoint. *Proc Nutr Soc*. 1999;58:877–886.

73. Taylor R, Husband DJ, Marshall SM, et al. Adipocyte insulin binding and insulin sensitivity in 'brittle' diabetes. *Diabetologia*. 1984;27:441–446.

74. Leboeuf B. Regulation of fatty acid esterification in adipose tissue incubated *in vitro*. In: Renold AE, Cahill GF, eds. *Handbook of Physiology Section 5: Adipose Tissue*. Washington, DC: American Physiological Society; 1965:385–391.

75. Arner P, Kriegholm E, Engfeldt P, et al. Adrenergic regulation of lipolysis in situ at rest and during exercise. *J Clin Invest*. 1990;85:893–898.

76. Hoelzer DR, Dalsky GP, Schwartz NS, et al. Epinephrine is not critical to prevention of hypoglycemia during exercise in humans. *Am J Physiol*. 1986;251:E104–E110.

77. Hodgetts V, Coppack SW, Frayn KN, et al. Factors controlling fat mobilization from human subcutaneous adipose tissue during exercise. *J Appl Physiol*. 1991;71:445–451.

78. Summers LK, Samra JS, Humphreys SM, et al. Subcutaneous abdominal adipose tissue blood flow: variation within and between subjects and relationship to obesity. *Clin Sci (Lond)*. 1996;91:679–683.

79. Jones NL, Heigenhauser GJ, Kuksis A, et al. Fat metabolism in heavy exercise. *Clin Sci (Lond)*. 1980;59:469–478.

80. Wasserman DH, Spalding JA, Lacy DB, et al. Glucagon is a primary controller of hepatic glycogenolysis and gluconeogenesis during muscular work. *Am J Physiol*. 1989;257:E108–E117.

81. Wahren J, Sato Y, Ostman J, et al. Turnover and splanchnic metabolism of free fatty acids and ketones in insulin-dependent diabetics at rest and in response to exercise. *J Clin Invest*. 1984;73:1367–1376.

82. Liu Z, Barrett EJ. Human protein metabolism: its measurement and regulation. *Am J Physiol Endocrinol Metab*. 2002;283:E1105–E1112.

83. Goldberg AL, Etlinger JD, Goldspink DF, et al. Mechanism of work-induced hypertrophy of skeletal muscle. *Med Sci Sports*. 1975;7:185–198.

84. Rasmussen BB, Phillips SM. Contractile and nutritional regulation of human muscle growth. *Exerc Sport Sci Rev*. 2003;31:127–131.

85. Nygren J, Nair KS. Differential regulation of protein dynamics in splanchnic and skeletal muscle beds by insulin and amino acids in healthy human subjects. *Diabetes*. 2003;52:1377–1385.

86. Louard RJ, Fryburg DA, Gelfand RA, et al. Insulin sensitivity of protein and glucose metabolism in human forearm skeletal muscle. *J Clin Invest*. 1992;90:2348–2354.

87. Mitch WE, Bailey JL, Wang X, et al. Evaluation of signals activating ubiquitin-proteasome proteolysis in a model of muscle wasting. *Am J Physiol*. 1999;276:C1132–C1138.

88. Moller-Loswick AC, Zachrisson H, Hyltander A, et al. Insulin selectively attenuates breakdown of nonmyofibrillar proteins in peripheral tissues of normal men. *Am J Physiol*. 1994;266:E645–E652.

89. Liu Z, Miers WR, Wei L, et al. The ubiquitin-proteosome proteolytic pathway in heart vs skeletal muscle: effects of acute diabetes. *Biochem Biophys Res Commun*. 2000;276:1255–1260.

90. Kettelhut IC, Wing SS, Goldberg AL. Endocrine regulation of protein breakdown in skeletal muscle. *Diabetes Metab Rev*. 1988;4:751–772.

91. Du J, Wang X, Miereles C, et al. Activation of caspase-3 is an initial step triggering accelerated muscle proteolysis in catabolic conditions. *J Clin Invest*. 2004;113:115–123.

92. Pepato MT, Migliorini RH, Goldberg AL, et al. Role of different proteolytic pathways in degradation of muscle protein from streptozotocin-diabetic rats. *Am J Physiol*. 1996;271:E340–E347.

93. Hedge GA, Colby HD, Goodman RI. *Clinical Endocrine Physiology*. Philadelphia: W.B. Saunders; 1987.

94. Fedele MJ, Hernandez JM, Lang CH, et al. Severe diabetes prohibits elevations in muscle protein synthesis after acute resistance exercise in rats. *J Appl Physiol*. 2000;88:102–108.

95. Darmaun D, Matthews DE, Bier DM. Physiological hypercortisolemia increases proteolysis, glutamine, and alanine production. *Am J Physiol*. 1988;255:E366–E373.

96. Russell-Jones DL, Weissberger AJ, Bowes SB, et al. The effects of growth hormone on protein metabolism in adult growth hormone deficient patients. *Clin Endocrinol (Oxf)*. 1993;38:427–431.

97. Bush JA, Kimball SR, O'Connor PM, et al. Translational control of protein synthesis in muscle and liver of growth hormone-treated pigs. *Endocrinology*. 2003;144:1273–1283.

98. Rennie MJ. Claims for the anabolic effects of growth hormone: a case of the emperor's new clothes? *Br J Sports Med*. 2003;37:100–105.

99. Nindl BC, Hymer WC, Deaver DR, et al. Growth hormone pulsatility profile characteristics following acute heavy resistance exercise. *J Appl Physiol*. 2001;91:163–172.

100. Liu JL, Grinberg A, Westphal H, et al. Insulin-like growth factor-I affects perinatal lethality and postnatal development in a gene dosage-dependent manner: manipulation using the Cre/loxP system in transgenic mice. *Mol Endocrinol*. 1998;12:1452–1462.

101. Goldberg AL. Work-induced growth of skeletal muscle in normal and hypophysectomized rats. *Am J Physiol*. 1967;213:1193–1198.

102. Adams GR, Haddad F. The relationships among IGF-1, DNA content, and protein accumulation during skeletal muscle hypertrophy. *J Appl Physiol*. 1996;81:2509–2516.

103. Yang S, Alnaqeeb M, Simpson H, et al. Cloning and characterization of an IGF-1 isoform expressed in skeletal muscle subjected to stretch. *J Muscle Res Cell Motil*. 1996;17:487–495.

104. Fryburg DA. Insulin-like growth factor I exerts growth hormone- and insulin-like actions on human muscle protein metabolism. *Am J Physiol*. 1994;267:E331–E336.

105. Adams GR. Invited review: autocrine/paracrine IGF-I and skeletal muscle adaptation. *J Appl Physiol*. 2002;93:1159–1167.

106. Fedele MJ, Lang CH, Farrell PA. Immunization against IGF-I prevents increases in protein synthesis in diabetic rats after resistance exercise. *Am J Physiol Endocrinol Metab*. 2001;280:E877–E885.

107. Li BG, Hasselgren PO, Fang CH, et al. Insulin-like growth factor-I blocks dexamethasone-induced protein degradation in cultured myotubes by inhibiting multiple proteolytic pathways: 2002 ABA paper. *J Burn Care Rehabil*. 2004;25:112–118.

108. Wilson VJ, Rattray M, Thomas CR, et al. Effects of hypophysectomy and growth hormone administration on the mRNA levels of collagen I, III and insulin-like growth factor-I in rat skeletal muscle. *Growth Horm IGF Res*. 1998;8:431–438.

109. Goldspink G. Methods of treating muscular disorders. US Patent 6,221,842 B1, 2001.

110. Nindl BC, Kraemer WJ, Deaver DR, et al. LH secretion and testosterone concentrations are blunted after resistance exercise in men. *J Appl Physiol*. 2001;91:1251–1258.

111. McCall GE, Byrnes WC, Fleck SJ, et al. Acute and chronic hormonal responses to resistance training designed to promote muscle hypertrophy. *Can J Appl Physiol*. 1999;24:96–107.

112. Bhasin S, Storer TW, Berman N, et al. The effects of supraphysiologic doses of testosterone on muscle size and strength in normal men. *N Engl J Med*. 1996;335:1–7.

113. Ferrando AA, Tipton KD, Doyle D, et al. Testosterone injection stimulates net protein synthesis but not tissue amino acid transport. *Am J Physiol*. 1998;275:E864–E871.

114. Wolfe R, Ferrando A, Sheffield-Moore M, et al. Testosterone and muscle protein metabolism. *Mayo Clin Proc*. 2000;75(suppl):S55–S59; discussion S59–S60.

115. Doumit ME, Cook DR, Merkel RA. Testosterone up-regulates androgen receptors and decreases differentiation of porcine myogenic satellite cells in vitro. *Endocrinology*. 1996;137:1385–1394.

116. Sheffield-Moore M, Urban RJ, Wolf SE, et al. Short-term oxandrolone administration stimulates net muscle protein synthesis in young men. *J Clin Endocrinol Metab*. 1999;84:2705–2711.

117. Inoue K, Yamasaki S, Fushiki T, et al. Rapid increase in the number of androgen receptors following electrical stimulation of the rat muscle. *Eur J Appl Physiol Occup Physiol*. 1993;66:134–140.

118. Bamman MM, Shipp JR, Jiang J, et al. Mechanical load increases muscle IGF-I and androgen receptor mRNA concentrations in humans. *Am J Physiol Endocrinol Metab*. 2001;280:E383–E390.

119. Mauras N, Hayes V, Welch S, et al. Testosterone deficiency in young men: marked alterations in whole body protein kinetics, strength, and adiposity. *J Clin Endocrinol Metab*. 1998;83:1886–1892.

120. Bhasin S, Woodhouse L, Casaburi R, et al. Testosterone dose-response relationships in healthy young men. *Am J Physiol Endocrinol Metab*. 2001;281:E1172–E1181.

121. Caiozzo VJ, Haddad F. Thyroid hormone: modulation of muscle structure, function, and adaptive responses to mechanical loading. *Exerc Sport Sci Rev*. 1996;24:321–361.

122. Gordon JW, Rungi AA, Inagaki H, et al. Effects of contractile activity on mitochondrial transcription factor A expression in skeletal muscle. *J Appl Physiol*. 2001;90:389–396.

123. Wrutniak-Cabello C, Casas F, Cabello G. Thyroid hormone action in mitochondria. *J Mol Endocrinol*. 2001;26:67–77.

124. Winder W, Fitts R, Holloszy JO, et al. Effects of thyroid hormone on different types of skeletal muscle. In: Pette D, ed. *Plasticity of Muscle*. Berlin: Walter de Gruyter; 1980:581–591.

125. Schuler MJ, Pette D. Quantification of thyroid hormone receptor isoforms, 9-cis retinoic acid receptor gamma, and nuclear receptor co-repressor by reverse-transcriptase PCR in maturing and adult skeletal muscles of rat. *Eur J Biochem*. 1998;257:607–614.

126. Weber K, Bruck P, Mikes Z, et al. Glucocorticoid hormone stimulates mitochondrial biogenesis specifically in skeletal muscle. *Endocrinology*. 2002;143:177–184.

127. Schrauwen P, Hesselink M. UCP2 and UCP3 in muscle controlling body metabolism. *J Exp Biol*. 2002;205:2275–2285.

128. Echtay KS, Winkler E, Klingenberg M. Coenzyme Q is an obligatory cofactor for uncoupling protein function. *Nature*. 2000;408:609–613.

129. Echtay KS, Winkler E, Frischmuth K, et al. Uncoupling proteins 2 and 3 are highly active H(+) transporters and highly nucleotide sensitive when activated by coenzyme Q (ubiquinone). *Proc Natl Acad Sci U S A*. 2001;98:1416–1421.

130. Moreno M, Lombardi A, De Lange P, et al. Fasting, lipid metabolism, and triiodothyronine in rat gastrocnemius muscle: interrelated roles of uncoupling protein 3, mitochondrial thioesterase, and coenzyme Q. *Faseb J*. 2003;17:1112–1114.

131. Burr DB. The contribution of the organic matrix to bone's material properties. *Bone*. 2002;31:8–11.

132. Wertheimer H. Introduction—a perspective. In: Renold A, Cahill G Jr., eds. *Handbook of Physiology Section 5: Adipose Tissue*. Washington, DC: American Physiological Society; 1965:5–11.

133. Babraj JA, Smith K, Cuthbertson DJ, et al. Human bone collagen synthesis is a rapid, nutritionally modulated process. *J Bone Miner Res*. 2005;20:930–937.

134. Smith K, Reynolds N, Downie S, et al. Effects of flooding amino acids on incorporation of labeled amino acids into human muscle protein. *Am J Physiol*. 1998;275:E73–E78.

135. Ihle R, Loucks AB. Dose-response relationships between energy availability and bone turnover in young exercising women. *J Bone Miner Res*. 2004;19:1231–1240.

136. Zanker CL, Swaine IL. Responses of bone turnover markers to repeated endurance running in humans under conditions of energy balance or energy restriction. *Eur J Appl Physiol*. 2000;83:434–440.

137. Lu H, Kraut D, Gerstenfeld LC, et al. Diabetes interferes with the bone formation by affecting the expression of transcription factors that regulate osteoblast differentiation. *Endocrinology*. 2003;144:346–352.

138. Rizzoli R, Poser J, Burgi U. Nuclear thyroid hormone receptors in cultured bone cells. *Metabolism*. 1986;35:71–74.

139. Williams GR, Bland R, Sheppard MC. Retinoids modify regulation of endogenous gene expression by vitamin D3 and thyroid hormone in three osteosarcoma cell lines. *Endocrinology*. 1995;136:4304–4314.

140. Huang BK, Golden LA, Tarjan G, et al. Insulin-like growth factor I production is essential for anabolic effects of thyroid hormone in osteoblasts. *J Bone Miner Res*. 2000;15:188–197.

141. Laughlin GA, Yen SSC. Nutritional and endocrine-metabolic aberrations in amenorrheic athletes. *J Clin Endocrinol Metab*. 1996;81:4301–4309.

142. Loucks AB. Low energy availability in the marathon and other endurance sports. *Sports Med*. 2007;37:348–352.

143. Loucks AB, Mortola JF, Girton L, et al. Alterations in the hypothalamic-pituitary-ovarian and the hypothalamic-pituitary-adrenal axes in athletic women. *J Clin Endocrinol Metab*. 1989;68:402–411.

144. De Souza MJ, Miller BE, Loucks AB, et al. High frequency of luteal phase deficiency and anovulation in recreational women runners: blunted elevation in follicle-stimulating hormone observed during luteal-follicular transition. *J Clin Endocrinol Metab*. 1998;83:4220–4232.

145. Redman LM, Loucks AB. Menstrual disorders in athletes. *Sports Med*. 2005;35:747–755.

146. Bronson FH. Food-restricted, prepubertal, female rats: rapid recovery of luteinizing hormone pulsing with excess food, and full recovery of pubertal development with gonadotropin-releasing hormone. *Endocrinology*. 1986;118:2483–2487.

147. Di Carlo C, Palomba S, De Fazio M, et al. Hypogonadotropic hypogonadotropism in obese women after biliopancreatic diversion. *Fertil Steril*. 1999;72:905–909.

148. Hilton LK, Loucks AB. Low energy availability, not exercise stress, suppresses the diurnal rhythm of leptin in healthy young women. *Am J Physiol Endocrinol Metab*. 2000;278:E43–E49.

149. Bullen BA, Skrinar GS, Beitins IZ, et al. Induction of menstrual disorders by strenuous exercise in untrained women. *N Engl J Med*. 1985;312:1349–1353.

150. Leibel RL, Rosenbaum M, Hirsch J. Changes in energy expenditure resulting from altered body weight. *N Engl J Med*. 1995;332:621–628.

151. Wade GN, Schneider JE. Metabolic fuels and reproduction in female mammals. *Neurosci Biobehav Rev*. 1992;16:235–272.

152. Wade GN, Schneider JE, Li HY. Control of fertility by metabolic cues. *Am J Physiol*. 1996;270:E1–E19.

153. Burke LM, Cox GR, Cummings NK, et al. Guidelines for daily carbohydrate intake: do athletes achieve them? *Sports Med*. 2001;31:267–299.

154. Loucks AB, Verdun M, Heath EM. Low energy availability, not stress of exercise, alters LH pulsatility in exercising women. *J Appl Physiol*. 1998;84:37–46.

155. Thong FS, McLean C, Graham TE. Plasma leptin in female athletes: relationship with body fat, reproductive, nutritional, and endocrine factors. *J Appl Physiol*. 2000;88:2037–2044.

156. Williams NI, Caston-Balderrama AL, Helmreich DL, et al. Longitudinal changes in reproductive hormones and menstrual cyclicity in cynomolgus monkeys during strenuous exercise training: abrupt transition to exercise-induced amenorrhea. *Endocrinology*. 2001;142:2381–2389.

157. Williams NI, Helmreich DL, Parfitt DB, et al. Evidence for a causal role of low energy availability in the induction of menstrual cycle disturbances during strenuous exercise training. *J Clin Endocrinol Metab*. 2001;86:5184–5193.

158. Vollman RF. *The Menstrual Cycle*. Philadelphia: W.B. Saunders; 1977.

159. Ellison PT. Advances in human reproductive ecology. *Annu Rev Anthropol*. 1994;23:255–275.

160. Baker ER, Mathur RS, Kirk RF, et al. Female runners and secondary amenorrhea: correlation with age, parity, mileage, and plasma hormonal and sex-hormone-binding globulin concentrations. *Fertil Steril*. 1981;36:183–187.

161. Loucks AB. The response of luteinizing hormone pulsatility to five days of low energy availability disappears by 14 years of gynecological age. *J Clin Endocrinol Metab*. 2006;91:3158–3164.

162. Obici S, Feng Z, Morgan K, et al. Central administration of oleic acid inhibits glucose production and food intake. *Diabetes*. 2002;51:271–275.

163. Weaver CM, Martin BR, Plawecki KL, et al. Differences in calcium metabolism between adolescent and adult females. *Am J Clin Nutr*. 1995;61:577–581.

164. Roemmich JN, Sinning WE. Weight loss and wrestling training: effects on growth-related hormones. *J Appl Physiol*. 1997;82:1760–1764.

165. Roemmich JN, Sinning WE. Weight loss and wrestling training: effects on nutrition, growth, maturation, body composition, and strength. *J Appl Physiol*. 1997;82:1751–1759.

166. Friedl KE, Moore RJ, Hoyt RW, et al. Endocrine markers of semi-starvation in healthy lean men in a multistressor environment. *J Appl Physiol*. 2000;88:1820–1830.

167. Selye H. A syndrome produced by diverse nocuous agents. *Nature*. 1936;138:132.

168. Selye H. Studies of adaptation. *Endocrinology*. 1937;21:169–188.

169. Selye H. The effect of adaptation to various damaging agents on the female sex organs in the rat. *Endocrinology*. 1939;25:615–624.

170. Loucks A. Is stress measured in joules? *Military Psychol*. 2009;21:S101–S107.

171. Selye H. *The Stress of Life*. New York: McGraw-Hill; 1956.

172. Selye H. Adaptation energy. *Nature*. 1938;141:926.

CHAPTER 20

Exercise and the Immune System

Laurie Hoffman-Goetz and Bente Klarlund Pedersen

Abbreviations

A	Adrenaline	IL-6	Interleukin-6
APC	Antigen-presenting cell	LPS	Lipopolysaccharide
BMNC	Blood mononuclear cell	MIP	Macrophage inflammatory protein
C	Cortisol/corticosterone	MHC	Major histocompatibility complex
CAM	Cell adhesion molecule	NE	Norepinephrine
CD	Cluster of differentiation	NFκB	Nuclear factor κ B
CRP	C-reactive protein	NK cell	Natural killer cell
CTL	Cytotoxic T lymphocyte	NKCA	Natural killer cell activity
CVD	Cardiovascular disease	NO	Nitric oxide
E	Epinephrine	PHA	Phytohemagglutinin
GC	Glucocorticoid	ROS	Reactive oxygen species
HEV	High endothelial venule	T_{H1}	Type 1 helper
ICAM-1	Intercellular adhesion molecule-1	T_{H2}	Type 2 helper
IFN-γ	Interferon γ	TNF-α	Tumor necrosis factor-α
IFN-β	Interferon β	TNFR	Tumor necrosis factor receptor
IL-1β	Interleukin-1 β	WBC	White blood cell
IL-2	Interleukin-2		

Introduction

The rationale for studying the impact of physical exercise on the immune system comes from pioneering work on the physiology of stress. The term *stress* refers to the cluster of physiologic responses that arise from the perception of aversive or threatening situations, resulting in fight-or-flight reactions (1). Stress triggers activation of the neocortex, limbic system, and brainstem (with norepinephrine [NE] as the main neurotransmitter), stimulation of the sympathetic nervous system, and consequent secretion into the circulation of epinephrine (E) or adrenaline (A) and NE or noradrenaline from the adrenal medulla. Concurrent stimulation of the paraventricular nucleus of the hypothalamus results in the release of corticotrophin-releasing hormone, release of adrenocorticotrophic hormone from the pituitary, and secretion of glucocorticoids (GCs; cortisol and corticosterone) from the adrenal cortex. The fact that lymphocytes and other immune cells are responsive to stress hormones is not surprising given the constitutive expression of adrenergic receptors and GC receptors. Additional conceptual support for the idea that exercise affects the immune system comes from studies of the general adaptation syndrome (2). Various stimuli, including physical exercise, activate the hypothalamic-pituitary-adrenal axis and influence the number, function, and movement of lymphoid cells. In the early twentieth century, investigators observed leukocytosis in men who had just run a marathon (3), and a lower ability of neutrophils to opsonize and phagocytize bacteria in acutely exercised, infected rabbits (4). Over the last century, hundreds of studies have demonstrated the impact of exercise on the immune system.

Because immunology is usually not part of graduate education in exercise physiology, we begin this chapter with an overview of the immune system. Immunology is a large and complex discipline and is best thought of as a work in progress. This review of the immune system is not intended to be exhaustive, and we have been very selective in describing certain immunologic processes and pathways. We wanted to highlight only those immunologic concepts and relationships that have been studied with respect to exercise. To help guide the reader, we have organized the chapter so that for each section, we first introduce key immune processes and concepts before describing how exercise influences those processes. We hope that by the end of the chapter, you will be able to make connections between exercise physiology and immunology.

Overview of the Immune System

The immune system is the primary physiologic system that mediates resistance and response to harmful exogenous agents (*e.g.*, bacterial products such as endotoxin), endogenous agents (*e.g.*, tumor cells), and pathogens (*e.g.*, viruses). Moreover, research performed during the last decade or so demonstrates that some components of the immune system are also important players in metabolism, and that the immune system is influenced by acute exercise and training adaptation (5,6). The immune system is comprised of central and peripheral organs and tissues, cellular components, and soluble macromolecules. Traditionally, the immune system is divided into two functional divisions or systems: natural host defenses (sometimes referred to as constitutive or innate) and acquired or adaptive host defenses. These systems interact and overlap in a coordinated fashion. The reader is referred to textbooks for more in-depth coverage of immunology (7,8).

Innate Immune Responses

Constitutive host defenses include external and internal components. The external systems include the skin and mucosa, which serve a barrier function, and various antimicrobial substances that are secreted onto the skin and mucus membranes. External factors such as the low pH of the skin provide resistance against penetration of the external surfaces by parasites. The internal systems include a variety of circulating phagocytic cells (principally neutrophils and monocytes) and antimicrobial substances in blood and lymph (acute phase proteins). The innate immune response is typically rapid and highly stereotyped.

Polymorphonuclear phagocytes (primarily neutrophils and eosinophils) arise from pluripotent stem cells in bone marrow and are characterized by the presence of cytoplasmic granules, which contain enzymes such as acid hydrolases, neutral proteases, peroxidases, myeloperoxidase, cationic proteins, lysozyme, and lactoferrin (9). Mononuclear phagocytes (monocytes and macrophages) also develop from stem cells in bone marrow and lose their granules during successive differentiation.

The enzymes found in cytoplasmic granules of neutrophils are involved in oxygen-independent (*e.g.*, hydrolases and lysozyme) or oxygen-dependent (*e.g.*, myeloperoxidase) killing during phagocytosis. Some of these enzymes trigger complement cascades, which in turn facilitate and mediate cytolysis through pore formation at the target plasma membranes. Kinins are also activated by enzymes released from phagocytic granules, and thus indirectly enhance vascular permeability and chemotaxis of phagocytic and other cells.

Oxygen-dependent killing by phagocytic cells is an important pathway for destruction of pathogens. During the respiratory burst, electron transfer from nicotinamide adenine dinucleotide phosphate to oxygen results in the production of superoxide, peroxide, and hydroxyl radicals within the phagosome of neutrophils. This reaction can be detected by chemoluminescence, a method that is often used in exercise immunology studies to measure neutrophil function. The generation of hypohalites via the myeloperoxidase-halide system also contributes to the killing of microorganisms within the phagosome, oxidative decarboxylation of amino acids, generation of toxic aldehydes, and thiol group oxidation, leading to the loss of key microbial enzyme functions (9). When macrophages are activated, such as by exposure to lipopolysaccharide (LPS) or by activation with interferon-γ (IFN-γ) (a cytokine produced by natural killer [NK] cells or T-cells), nitric oxide (NO) synthetase is expressed. This leads to the generation of NO and its metabolites, nitrate and nitrite, which are toxic to microbial organisms. NO and reactive oxygen species (ROS) interact to produce peroxynitrite, which is harmful to microbial cell membranes (9). Later in this chapter, we will turn our attention to a possible regulatory role that ROS may have in metabolism and exercise immunology.

> ### KEY POINT
>
> Innate immunity is stereotyped. It involves physical and physiologic barriers as well as phagocytosis (cellular internalization) and killing of foreign materials by leukocytes. The major types of leukocytes that mediate innate immunity are neutrophils, macrophages, and NK cells.

Acquired Immune Responses

The acquired immune system is characterized by recognition of antigenic determinants or antigenic epitopes (the portion of the antigen molecule that is seen as foreign by the host's immune cells), specificity of antigen recognition (and resultant clonal expansion), and immunologic memory. The cell type that mediates specific or acquired immune responses is the lymphocyte, which is identified by specific surface markers or surface antigens. The most important effector cells involved in specific immune responses are the thymus-derived (T) lymphocyte, the B lymphocyte, and the NK cell (Fig. 20.1).

Immune cells are identified by specific surface markers, referred to as cluster of differentiation (CD) antigens, and different subsets of lymphocytes express different CD antigens at the cell surface. For example, cells expressing the CD8 antigen are T lymphocytes with killer (cytotoxic) properties, CD19 cells are B cells, and CD62L is an adhesion molecule that mediates lymphocyte homing to high endothelial venules (HEVs) and leukocyte rolling on activated endothelium during an inflammatory response. Lymphocytes may be further categorized within a given

CD. For example, all white blood cells (WBCs) can be identified as CD45 positive cells (a marker for the common leukocyte antigen) and can be further separated into $CD45RO^+$ memory cells and $CD45RA^+$ naïve cells. As a point of reference, $CD45RO^+$ lymphocytes allow us to respond rapidly and strongly to a second exposure to an antigen (the basis of vaccination and booster shots), whereas $CD45RA^+$ lymphocytes are our initial first responders to an antigen. In phenotype assays involving the technique of flow cytometry, lymphocytes are frequently identified by the presence of multiple CD antigens. For example, $CD8^+CD56^+$ lymphocytes are a group of unconventional T-NK cells. Lymphocytes can also be characterized by the absence of CD markers; for example, double-positive T lymphocytes are $CD4^+CD8^+$ and indicate an early phase of development of these cells in the thymus gland. Thus, the CD designations provide information about the structure,

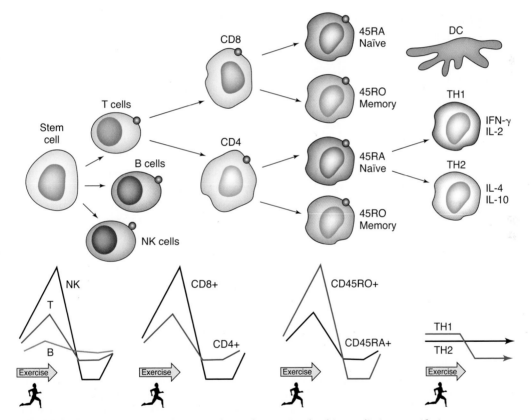

FIGURE 20.1 The major lymphocyte subpopulations involved in mediating specific immune responses. T lymphocytes are effector cells for cell-mediated reactions, and B lymphocytes are effector cells for humoral or antibody-mediated reactions. Natural killer (NK) cells are involved in cytolysis of target cells. After presentation of antigen by dendritic cells (DCs), cluster of differentiation (CD)4 T lymphocytes (45RA naïve) differentiate into type 1 or 2 helper (TH1 or TH2) cells. TH1 cells produce the cytokines interferon-γ (IFN-γ) and interleukin-2 (IL-2), which enhance the cellular immune response. TH2 cells produce the cytokines IL-4 and IL-10, which enhance the synthesis of antibody by B lymphocytes and humoral immunity. During dynamic exercise, there is a decrease in TH1 cells, whereas TH2 cells are relatively unchanged numerically. Naïve (45RA) and memory (45RO) CD4 and CD8 lymphocytes are generated. During dynamic exercise, natural killer (NK) cells in the blood increase more than the T lymphocytes, which increase more than the B lymphocytes. Within the T cell group, CD8 cells increase more than CD4 cells, and memory T cells increase more dramatically than naïve T cells.

TABLE 20.1	CD Antigens Found on Immune Cells Studied in Relation to Exercise	
CD antigen	**Immune cell distribution**	**Major function**
CD2	T-cells and NK cells	Adhesion molecule
CD3	T-cells	T-cell receptor transduction
CD4	T-helper cells	Differentiation marker; T-cell activation
CD8	T-cytotoxic cells	T-cell activation
CD11a	Monocytes, macrophages, lymphocytes	Adhesion
CD11b	Neutrophils, monocytes, NK cells	Adhesion (especially with endothelium)
CD18	Leukocytes	Adhesion
CD19	B-cells and plasma cells	Signal transduction
CD28	T-cells and plasma cells	T-cell proliferation; cytokine production
CD40	B-cells	B-cell growth and differentiation
CD44	Many cells, including leukocytes	Adhesion
CD45	All leukocytes	T- and B-cell activation
CD56	NK cells; some T-cells	Possible role in adhesion
CD62	Peripheral B, T, and NK cells; monocytes/macrophages	Adhesion
CD69	Activated T, B, and NK cells, neutrophils	Early activation marker; role in NK-mediated lysis
CD86	Dendritic cells	Costimulation for T-cells
CD95	Activated T- and B-cells	Apoptosis inducing signal
CD103	Intraepithelial lymphocytes (intestine, bronchi)	Adhesion; accessory molecule for activation

CD, cluster of differentiation; NK cells, natural killer cells.

development, and function of leukocytes. Table 20.1 provides a summary of some of the CD antigens that have been characterized in relation to exercise. However, this list is ever expanding and more than 200 CD antigens have been identified on cells (lymphocytes and other cells). Most immunology textbooks provide detailed and up-to-date descriptions of the known CD antigens.

Another important characteristic of lymphocytes is that they are not fixed within tissues; instead, they constantly recirculate from lymph nodes via efferent lymphatics into lymphatic vessels, lodge in other lymph nodes or specialized regions of secondary lymphoid tissues, or enter the circulation through the major lymphatic ducts. The implications of lymphocyte recirculation are twofold: First, up- or down-expression of cell adhesion molecules (CAMs) on the surface of lymphocytes is essential for the migration of lymphocytes (e.g., for rolling, attachment, and detachment from endothelium). Second, diverse physiologic stimuli, including exercise, affect lymphocyte recirculation by altering the expression of CAMs or by interaction with chemokines (a group of specialized cytokines with chemoattractant properties, affecting cytoskeletal elements of cells). Rehman and colleagues (10) demonstrated the role of adhesion molecules by showing that circulating levels of intercellular adhesion molecule-1 (ICAM-1) in healthy individuals were significantly elevated after exhaustive exercise, and the blood levels of adhesion molecules were affected by catecholamines. (See Chapter 19.)

Another consideration is that any measurement of lymphocytes in one tissue compartment will be an imperfect estimate of lymphocytes in other lymphoid tissues and organs. Although human studies use peripheral blood mononuclear cells (BMNCs) or lymphocytes, circulating WBC responses to exercise may not be representative of WBC responses in tissue compartments (e.g., spleen and lymph nodes) where exposure to antigen occurs. Furthermore, inferences about the number and function of intraepithelial lymphocytes (found in the gastrointestinal, pulmonary, and genitourinary tracts [11]) based on sampling of blood lymphocytes are even more problematic because not all intraepithelial lymphocytes recirculate.

By convention, the specific immune response is described as cell-mediated (involving T-cells) or humoral-mediated (involving B cells and antibody production). In cell-mediated responses, the first step in the induction of a response is the processing of antigen by antigen-presenting cells (APCs), such as macrophages and dendritic cells. After the antigen is internalized into a lysosomal vesicle within the APC, it is fragmented into peptides, some of which are associated with specific cell-membrane proteins known as major histocompatibility complex (MHC) molecules. MHC molecules are derived from proteins found on the surface of cells and are involved in the recognition of antigens by T lymphocytes. There are two main types of MHC molecules: class I and class II. class I molecules are found on all nucleated cells and are recognized by the cytolytic T-cells (CD8). CD8 cells are also called MHC class I restricted T-cells. Class II molecules have a more restricted cell distribution, being expressed constitutively only on APCs. APCs take up the antigen, process or degrade the antigen, and present antigenic determinants to be "seen" at the surface by CD4 T lymphocytes. CD4 cells are also called MHC class II restricted T-cells. In the case of APCs, vesicles return the processed antigen and MHC class II complex (together known as a T-cell epitope) to the cell surface, where it is presented to CD4 lymphocytes (12). Thus, the T-cell epitope provides an induction signal for CD4 lymphocytes, leading to mitosis, activation, and proliferation of memory and effector T-cells. Effector CD4 T cells secrete growth factors that influence the behavior of various cells participating in the immune response. Naïve CD4 lymphocytes are able to differentiate into type 1 helper cells (TH1) or type 2 helper cells (TH2) depending on the types of stimuli and signals received. Naïve CD8 lymphocytes produce a more restricted array of cytokines, and the primary effector function of activated CD8 lymphocytes is the killing of target cells (11).

interacts with the class I molecule and antigen present on the surface of the infected cell. A second, costimulatory signal is normally necessary to activate naïve CD8 lymphocytes into effector CTLs. This signal is transduced by the ligation of B7 (CD80 or CD86) on APCs with CD28 present on CTLs. A third signal is provided by IL-2, a classical TH1 cytokine produced by CD4 lymphocytes. This signal may also be important for the generation of CTLs because IL-2 knockout mice lack CTL-mediated target cell killing (13). Following activation, CTLs kill target cells by a process known as apoptosis, through insertion of a perforin-mediated pore in the target membrane and subsequent release of granzymes (serine proteases), which lead to DNA fragmentation. CTLs express membrane-bound Fas ligand (FasL), which interacts with the Fas receptor found on the surface of target cells (the "Exercise and Lymphocyte Apoptosis" section later in this chapter provides a description of the intrinsic and extrinsic pathways of programmed cell death and their relation to dynamic exercise). CD8 T-cells also produce cytokines, such as IFN-γ, that enhance macrophage involvement as B7-bearing APCs (12).

TEST YOURSELF

Define the following terms: cluster of differentiation, CD4 lymphocyte, and antigen-presenting cell.

TEST YOURSELF

Describe two characteristics that distinguish type 1 and type 2 lymphocytes.

A crucial defining characteristic of CD4 type 1 and type 2 lymphocytes is the type of growth factors or cytokines they produce. Cytokines are low-molecular-weight proteins that influence the direction, intensity, and duration of immune responses. TH1 cytokines, which include IFN-γ and interleukin-2 (IL-2), are associated with cell-mediated responses and down-regulation of TH2 responses. In contrast, TH2 cytokines, such as IL-4 and IL-10, are associated with humoral (antibody) responses and shift immune responses away from cell-mediated immunity. In general, type 1 T-cells mediate protection against intracellular microorganisms such as viruses, whereas type 2 T-cells are important in the defense against extracellular parasites such as helminths. Figure 20.1 illustrates the cytokine profiles for CD4 TH1 and TH2 lymphocytes, and the general effect that dynamic exercise has on these cells. What about CD8 lymphocytes? Once activated, these cells become cytotoxic T lymphocytes (CTLs) that are capable of lysing virally infected cells and tumor targets. Moreover, because CTLs recognize MHC class I molecules found on all nucleated cells, they are capable of eliminating almost any altered cell in the body. Similarly to CD4 T lymphocytes, CD8 T lymphocytes also require multiple signals for activation and proliferation into fully competent effector cells. The first signal is provided by antigenic peptides (e.g., virus antigens) in the infected cell that are bound to MHC class I molecules. The T-cell receptor of CD8 lymphocytes

B-lymphocytes also require two signals to become activated by T-dependent antigens (most proteins are T-dependent antigens). First, the B cell receptor (surface Ig) must interact with antigen, become endocytosed, processed internally, and expressed on the plasma membrane in conjunction with an MHC class II molecule. Once this occurs, CD4 TH2 lymphocytes interact with the T-cell epitope and provide the first signal for antibody synthesis. A second signal is transmitted by the interaction of CD40 (present on B-cells) and CD40L (present on T-cells). Following activation, and with stimulation from growth and differentiation cytokines (TH2 cytokines), the B-cells differentiate into plasma cells and secrete immunoglobulin (Ig) M, IgG, or IgA antibodies. (Plasma cells also synthesize IgE antibody, but this isotype is normally found only in individuals with atopy or allergy.) The primary antibody response (after initial exposure to an antigen) leads to a peak increase in antibody levels within approximately 2 weeks, during which time both effector and memory cells are generated. A subsequent exposure to the antigen (for example, through recall antigen testing) results in a shorter lag time for production of antibody and higher blood antibody concentrations (or titers), reflecting the expansion of existing memory B lymphocytes to active antibody-producing plasma cells. Antibodies mediate a number of effector functions. First, antibodies can bind antigen through precipitation or agglutination reactions and result in neutralization of the antigen. Second, antibodies can promote phagocytosis of an antigen through a process known as opsonization. In opsonization, neutrophils and macrophages bind a portion of the antibody molecule (the Fc domain) at receptors (FcR) found on their surface, whereas the antibody molecule binds the antigen. The entire antibody-antigen complex is then taken up by the phagocytic cell. Third, some antibodies (notably IgM and IgG) activate the complement cascade, resulting in nonspecific lysis of cells that have receptors for the C3b complement component (*e.g.,* red blood cells) (11).

In summary, host defense entails physical and chemical barriers, stereotyped innate responses involving inflammatory cells, and an inducible immune response with the generation of cells such as T-helper (TH1, TH2) and T-cytotoxic cells, and B lymphocytes. These cells provide the major pathway for recognizing and responding to infectious antigens, tumor antigens, and self- or auto-antigens.

> ## KEY POINT
>
> Acquired immunity involves the selective activation of lymphocytes. Lymphocytes can be divided into two types: T-cells, which mediate cellular responses, and B-cells, which mediate antibody responses. Lymphocytes can also be identified by CD markers indicating whether they are memory or naïve cells, or helper or killer cells, and by their cytokine profiles.

Cytokines

Cytokines are an extremely diverse and heterogeneous group of proteins that are secreted by many cells of the immune system. Over the past two decades, research has highlighted the fact that exercise has dramatic effects on the production of cytokines, and that training adaptation and the beneficial effects of exercise are partly mediated by cytokines (14). These proteins mediate, coordinate, and regulate intercellular communication, largely between cells of the immune system. However, cytokines are also involved in other biologic actions, including hematopoiesis, angiogenesis, wound healing, and metabolism. More than 100 cytokines have been identified, and the majority of these have pleiotropic effects on cells or multiple effects on a specific cell type. Among the most important cytokines are the interleukins (such as IL-1, IL-2, IL-6, and IL-10), the interferons (such as IFN-γ and IFN-β), tumor necrosis factor-α (TNF-α), and transforming growth factor-β. As will be described later, interleukins and TNF are especially important during dynamic exercise, and several of the interleukins have proinflammatory effects on target cells. Some cytokines act synergistically, whereas others act antagonistically. Cytokines also have a range of action that is paracrine or autocrine, meaning that the effects are local (this is in distinction to hormones, which have an endocrine range of action on target cells). Cytokine action on target cells is limited by the expression of cytokine receptors (*e.g.,* IL-2 and its receptor IL-2R). When a cytokine binds to its receptor, new gene transcription takes place and specific cellular actions are initiated. Cellular action is quite varied (depending on the target cell) and includes changes in cytoskeleton assembly in neutrophils, the induction of an antiviral state in NK cells, and the production of cytokines that prime T lymphocyte subsets, to name a few. The binding affinity of cytokines with their specific receptors is high and requires minute concentrations (*e.g.,* picomolar and smaller) to lead to physiologic responses. For a complete discussion of cytokines and their action in the immune system, readers are referred to comprehensive immunology textbooks (8).

> ## KEY POINT
>
> Cytokines are intercellular messenger proteins that mediate, coordinate, and regulate complex interactions between components of the immune system. Cytokines are secreted by many cells of the immune system, including lymphocytes, granulocytes, and macrophages, as well as by nonimmune cells.

Dynamic (Acute) Exercise and the Immune Response

The largest body of evidence on exercise and immune responses comes from acute studies in which aerobic exercise protocols were used in humans and animals. Using dynamic exercise protocols, investigators have described patterns of response for the various lymphocyte subpopulations in terms of number and function, NK cell activity (NKCA), B-cell responses, and immunoglobulin production.

Leukocyte and Lymphocyte Subpopulations

In response to acute exercise, blood leukocyte subpopulations react in a highly stereotyped fashion (6,15,16). (The term *stereotyped* is used here to mean a predictable, regular, and circumscribed pattern of reaction.)

Neutrophil concentrations increase during and after exercise, whereas lymphocyte concentrations increase during dynamic exercise and fall below pre-exercise values after long-duration physical work (17). If the exercise has been of moderate intensity and/or short duration, lymphocytes are mobilized to the blood during the exercise and return to pre-exercise levels in the recovery phase of exercise. Several reports describe exercise-induced changes in subsets of BMNCs (6,18–21). The increased lymphocyte concentration observed early after the initiation of an exercise bout is likely due to the recruitment of all lymphocyte subpopulations (T-cells, B-cells, and NK cells) to the vascular compartment. These numerical changes are observed regardless of whether cells are analyzed as a separated buffy coat or as whole blood cultures. NK cells are more sensitive to dynamic exercise than T-cells, which again are more sensitive than B-cells (see Fig. 20.1). During exercise, the CD4/CD8 ratio decreases. This reflects the greater increase in CD8$^+$ lymphocytes than CD4$^+$ lymphocytes. CD4$^+$ and CD8$^+$ cells contain both CD45RO$^+$ memory and CD45RA$^+$ naïve cells, which are identified by the absence of 45RO and the presence of CD62L (22). Data show that the recruitment of T-cells during exercise involves primarily CD45RO$^+$ lymphocytes (23). Thus, the concentrations of CD45RO$^+$ and CD45RO-CD62L increase during exercise, suggesting that memory (but not naïve) lymphocytes are rapidly mobilized to the blood in response to physical exercise (24) (Fig. 20.1). This finding supports the idea that during exercise, lymphocytes are recruited from peripheral compartments, such as the spleen, rather than from the bone marrow. This would explain why splenectomized individuals have an impaired ability to mobilize lymphocytes to the blood during stress.

KEY POINT

Dynamic, heavy exercise leads to rapid increases and decreases in the numbers of circulating neutrophils and lymphocytes, which return to pre-exercise values 24 to 72 hours later. Among the likely mechanisms for these numerical changes are hemodynamic effects and sequestration of immune cells in peripheral tissue pools.

As described in the overview section on the immune system, CD4 TH and the CD8 T-cytotoxic (TC) cells can be divided into type 1 and type 2 cells according to their cytokine profile. CD8 lymphocytes produce a more limited range of cytokines; for example, type 1 CD4 T-cells produce IFN-γ and IL-2, whereas type 2 CD4 T-cells produce IL-4, IL-5, IL-6, and IL-10. type 1 T-cell responses are stimulated by IL-12, and IL-6 has been shown to induce type 2 T-cell responses by stimulating the initial production of IL-4. The process of stimulating T-cells to become either type 1 or type 2 is sometimes called polarization. The term *polarization* refers to the establishment of functionally distinct immune cells, such as cytokines, in response to extracellular signals. Type 1 T-cells mediate protection against intracellular microorganisms such viruses, whereas type 2 T-cells are important in the defense against extracellular parasites such as parasitic worms (helminths). The postexercise decrease in T lymphocyte number is accompanied by a more pronounced decrease in type 1 T-cells (25). The relatively more pronounced decrease in type 1 compared with type 2 T-cells in the recovery period may explain the increased sensitivity to infections after heavy dynamic exercise, as these infections are often caused by viruses.

Telomeres are the extreme ends of chromosomes that consist of TTAGGG repeats. After each round of cell division, telomeric sequence is lost because of the inability of DNA polymerase to fully replicate the 5′ end of the chromosome. Telomere lengths have been used as a marker for replication history and the proliferation potential of cells. In response to exercise, telomere lengths in CD4$^+$ and CD8$^+$ lymphocytes are shorter than those in cells isolated at rest (24). Thus, the initial increase in CD4$^+$ and CD8$^+$ cells after exercise is probably not due to repopulation by newly generated cells, but rather to a redistribution of activated cells.

Natural Killer Cell Activity

NK cells mediate non–MHC-restricted cytotoxicity, with potential resistance to viral infections (26) and cytolysis of some malignant cells (27). A method that is frequently applied to measure NKCA is the ^{51}Cr release assay, for which the percentage of lysed target cells is the end point. IFN and IL-2 enhance the cytolytic activity of NK cells, whereas certain prostaglandins and immune complexes down-regulate the function of NK cells. Dynamic exercise of various types, durations, and intensities induce recruitment to the circulation of cells expressing characteristic NK cell markers (28). NKCA (lysis per fixed number of BMNC) increases in accord with the increased proportions of cells mediating non–MHC-restricted cytotoxicity. After exercise of heavy intensity and long duration (>45 minutes), NKCA is suppressed on a per NK cell basis (29). The maximum reduction in NK cell concentrations, and hence lower NKCA, occurs 2 to 4 hours after dynamic exercise. NKCA is increased when measured immediately after or during both moderate and heavy exercise of a few minutes. The NK cell count and the NKCA are decreased after intense exercise of at least 1 hour of duration. (Of interest, and in marked contrast to acute dynamic exercise, moderate long-term training in animal models is associated with the enhancement of NKCA against tumor targets [30].)

Immunoglobulins

Although IgA accounts for only 10% to 15% of the total immunoglobulin in serum, it is the predominant immunoglobulin class in mucosal secretions, and the level of IgA in mucosal fluids correlates more closely with resistance to upper respiratory tract infections than do serum antibodies (31). In one study, lower concentrations of the salivary IgA were observed in cross-country skiers after a race (32). This finding was confirmed in another study by a 70% decrease in salivary IgA, which persisted for several hours after completion of intense, long-duration ergometer cycling (33). (The importance of this finding for the area of exercise immunology is described in the Milestone of Discovery section at the end of this chapter.) In other investigations, decreased salivary IgA was found after intense swimming (34), running (35), and incremental treadmill running to exhaustion (36). Submaximal exercise had no effect on salivary IgA (36) and the percentage of B-cells among BMNCs did not change in relation to exercise (37).

In Vivo Immune Responses

In a study by Bruunsgaard and colleagues (38), in vivo impairment of cell-mediated immunity and specific antibody production was demonstrated in subjects after intense exercise of long duration (a triathlon race). The cellular immune system was evaluated as a skin test response to seven recall antigens. A recall antigen is an antigen to which an individual has previously been exposed, and the elicited response reflects the activation of memory T or B lymphocytes. The humoral immune system was evaluated as the antibody response to pneumococcal polysaccharide vaccine, which is generally considered to be T-cell-independent, and tetanus and diphtheria toxoids, both which are T-cell-dependent. The skin test response was significantly lower in the subjects who ran a triathlon race compared with triathlete controls and untrained controls who did not participate in the triathlon. No differences in specific antibody titers were found between the groups.

Neutrophils and Phagocytosis

Neutrophils account for 50% to 60% of the total circulating leukocyte pool. These cells are part of the innate immune system, are essential for host defense, and are involved in the pathology of various inflammatory conditions. This inflammatory involvement reflects tissue peroxidation resulting from incomplete phagocytosis (sometimes called the "innocent bystander effect"). One of the more pronounced effects of dynamic exercise on immune parameters is the prolonged neutrocytosis that occurs after acute and prolonged exercise bouts (17). Several reports have shown that exercise triggers a series of changes in the neutrophil population and may affect certain subpopulations differentially. A reduction in the expression of L-selectin (CD62L) immediately after exercise followed by an increase during recovery has been reported (39). This finding supports the observation that in response to the hormonal environment during exercise, neutrophils lose their ability to migrate into tissues (40). Increased expression of the CAMs after exercise may contribute to neutrophil extravasation (i.e., movement out or leakage from the circulation) into damaged tissue, including skeletal muscle. Exercise has both short- and long-term effects on the function of neutrophils. Neutrophils respond to infection by adherence, chemotaxis, phagocytosis, oxidative burst, degranulation, and microbial killing. In general, moderate exercise boosts neutrophil functions, including chemotaxis, phagocytosis, and oxidative burst activity. Maximal exercise, on the other hand, reduces these functions, with the exception of chemotaxis and degranulation, which are not affected (41).

Moderate versus Intense Exercise

During both moderate and intense exercise, lymphocytes are mobilized to the blood compartment. However, dynamic exercise of relatively high intensity lasting more than one hour ($>70\%$ of $\dot{V}_{O_{2max}}$) will induce a decrease in the circulating number of lymphocyte after exercise. Thus, lymphocytes disappear from the circulation in the recovery period, but only if the exercise has been intense. After heavy exercise, lymphocyte and NK cell function is also impaired, as assessed by in vitro assays. Thus, after intense, long-duration exercise, the immune system is temporarily impaired. This period is sometimes called the "open window." During this open window of altered immunity (which may last 3 to 72 hours depending on the parameter measured and the duration and intensity of the exercise), viruses and bacteria may gain a foothold, increasing the risk of subclinical or clinical infection. Results from animal studies support the idea that intense exercise is followed by temporary immune impairment. However, no serious attempt has been made by investigators to demonstrate that athletes who show the most extreme postexercise immunosuppression are those who contract an infection during the ensuing 1 to 2 weeks. The concept of the open window is illustrated in Figure 20.2.

> ### KEY POINT
>
> The decline in the number and function of immune cells with acute, heavy exercise contributes to a clinical phenomenon known as the open window. During this open window of altered immunity (which may last between 3 and 72 hours depending on the parameter measured and the duration and intensity of the exercise), viruses and bacteria may gain a foothold, increasing the risk of subclinical or clinical infection.

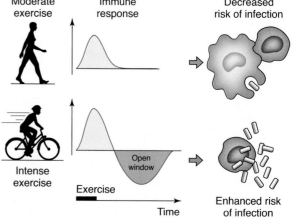

FIGURE 20.2   The open window model, which relates the intensity of exercise to increased or decreased risk of infection (and other clinical conditions). This increased or decreased risk presumably reflects intervening variables of immune system function.

Exercise and Lymphocyte Proliferation

After stimulation with antigen or mitogen, immune cells that are in the quiescent (G_0) phase of the cell cycle undergo activation. A commonly used method for evaluating the activation of lymphocytes is to assess proliferative responses in vitro by measuring the incorporation of [^{3}H] thymidine into DNA after stimulation with an antigen or a mitogen. A mitogen is any substance that nonspecifically stimulates DNA synthesis and mitosis, and typical mitogens for lymphocytes are plant lectins such as phytohemagglutinin (PHA) and bacterial wall products such as LPS. These in vitro studies are performed on either a fixed number of BMNCs or a fixed blood volume, and the results reflect the composition of the lymphocyte subpopulation. Thus, PHA and the mitogen concanavalin A stimulate primarily CD4$^+$ T-cells. Several studies have revealed a decline in the PHA and concanavalin A response during exercise and for a period of up to several hours thereafter (42). This is at least partly due to the increase in NK cells in the circulation and the relative decline of CD4$^+$ cells, as measured by in vitro assays (31,43). Furthermore, the shift in memory/naïve cells and type 1/type 2 cytokine-producing cells will also influence in vitro proliferation. In accordance with this, another study (44) found that 60 minutes of running at 95% of ventilatory threshold decreased mitogen-induced BMNC proliferation but had no effect on NK-depleted BMNCs or BMNCs again adjusted for CD3$^+$ percentage. In contrast, lymphocyte proliferation to B-cell mitogens, pokeweed mitogen, and LPS (which stimulates monocytes) either increases or remains unchanged after exercise (45).

Although studies that measure lymphocyte proliferation, as determined by ^{3}H-thymidine incorporation, suggest that exercise induces changes in the cell cycle, further research is needed to pinpoint specific regulatory components.

Exercise and Lymphocyte Apoptosis

Heavy exercise can have negative effects on the immune system leading to immune suppression and loss of lymphocytes from the circulation. One mechanism that has been proposed for the loss of lymphocytes is cell death. There are two broad pathways of cell death: necrosis and apoptosis. Necrosis is largely a passive process that involves inflammatory phagocytes, which take up and degrade damaged cells, and is irreversible. The end result of necrosis is the slow disintegration of the cell, and this process may be mediated by activation of calpains (46,47). Apoptosis, on the other hand, is an active process that does not involve inflammatory changes. Cell death by apoptosis depends on the activation of a series of intracellular proteases and has been studied in relation to exercise in a variety of cells,

including skeletal muscle and immune cells. However, before we can understand how and why exercise can trigger apoptosis of lymphocytes, we first need to consider some general mechanisms of this process.

Under normal circumstances, apoptosis is tightly regulated and is essential for normal immune system development and regulation (48). Apoptosis may be triggered by radiation, heat, hormonal triggering, various drugs, and intense physical exercise stress. As mentioned above, apoptosis does not lead to an inflammatory response, whereas cell death occurring through necrosis does. During apoptosis, irreversible DNA fragmentation and the formation of membrane-bound apoptotic bodies occur (49). The end result of apoptosis is the cleavage of intracellular proteins that are essential for cell growth and survival.

Apoptosis usually occurs through two pathways: intrinsic and extrinsic. The intrinsic pathway involves the release of cytochrome c from the mitochondria and the initiation of suicide signals through cysteine aspartyl-specific proteases (caspases). Mitochondrial cytochrome c becomes bound to caspase 9 and other molecules to form a complex known as an apoptosome (50). A series of caspases are activated in a cascade-like fashion, leading to proteolysis of downstream targets. Other mitochondrial activators can promote nuclear apoptosis, but in all cases the key mechanism that leads to activation of these proapoptotic proteins is the opening of the mitochondrial permeability transition pore and the resultant loss of mitochondrial transmembrane potential. The opening of the mitochondrial permeability transition pore is regulated by members of the Bcl-2 family of intracellular proteins, which are major components of the apostat (which controls the likelihood that a cell will undergo apoptosis [51]). Lymphocytes undergoing apoptosis are characterized by a number of intracellular changes, including the translocation of nuclear factor κ B (NFκB) (an inducible, nuclear transcriptional activator), the externalization of normally sequestered phosphatidylserine at the cell membrane, and DNA fragmentation (52). How does the activation of the intrinsic pathway of apoptosis relate to exercise? One powerful trigger of this intrinsic pathway is elevated oxidative stress, which occurs with intense aerobic exercise, and both cellular and whole-body respiration contribute to this oxidative stress. We will consider the intrinsic pathway and its relationship to exercise in greater detail later in this section.

Apoptosis also occurs through the extrinsic pathway, which involves activation of cell death receptors (DRs) located at the cell membrane. One of the best-studied DRs is Fas (CD95), which is expressed on the surface of target cells and interacts with its ligand, FasL, found on CTLs. This interaction of Fas-FasL leads to apoptosis of the target cell through initiator caspases (caspase 8 and caspase 10) and caspase 3 activation. DR-mediated apoptosis can also proceed through TNF-α signaling after binding to the TNF receptor (TNFR), which is found on many cells, including lymphocytes. As we describe later in this chapter, intense, muscle-damaging exercise increases the level of many proinflammatory cytokines (such as TNF-α); it is not surprising that apoptosis might also occur when these inflammatory cytokines are elevated.

Control of apoptosis is essential for cell survival and the removal of damaged or injured cells. The intrinsic pathway is partly regulated by shifting or priming the apostat either away from or toward apoptosis. Adjustment to the cell's apostat involves expression of proapoptotic Bcl proteins, such as Bax and Bak, or antiapoptotic Bcl proteins, such as Bcl-2 and Bcl-x$_L$. Other non-Bcl-2 family member proteins (*e.g.*, p53) and inhibitors of apoptosis proteins (*e.g.*, Xiap) likely contribute to the regulation of the intrinsic apoptotic pathway. The extrinsic pathway must also be regulated. One mechanism by which inhibition of the extrinsic pathway occurs is through a protein known as FLIP(L) (53). Both the intrinsic and extrinsic pathways to apoptosis involve the sequential activation of caspases (cysteine proteases) resulting in loss of lymphocyte viability. Figure 20.3 broadly illustrates the two pathways by which apoptosis can occur.

KEY POINT

Apoptosis is a form of controlled cell death that follows specific biochemical pathways and can be triggered by oxidative stress and certain proinflammatory cytokines.

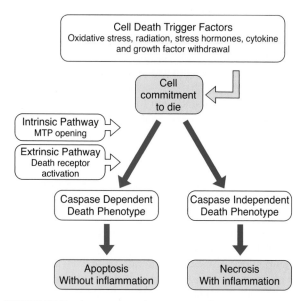

FIGURE 20.3 Apoptosis and necrosis pathways to cell death in response to physiologic and pathophysiologic stimuli. Apoptosis involves activation of the caspase enzyme cascade, triggered through either the intrinsic (mitochondrial) pathway or the extrinsic (death receptor) pathway leading to cell death. Necrosis does not involve caspase enzyme activation. (Modified from Hoffman-Goetz L, Quadrilatero J, Patel H. Cellular life span. In: Mooren FC, Voelker K, eds. *Molecular and Cellular Exercise Physiology.* Champaign, IL: Human Kinetics Press; 2005:19–37.)

Why is apoptosis important to consider with respect to exercise? Maximal exercise influences a number of factors that trigger lymphocyte apoptosis. For example, increased GC secretion, growth factor withdrawal, catecholamine exposure, ROS generation, and increased plasma TNF-α are some of the signals that induce apoptosis in immune cells (48), and these factors (especially GC, catecholamines, and ROS) are notably elevated after strenuous, prolonged, or muscle-damaging exercise. Many studies have demonstrated that heavy exercise can induce lymphocyte apoptosis in humans and animals. In an early study using the terminal deoxyribonucleotidyl transferase-mediated dUTP-digoxigenin nick end labeling assay), Concordet and Ferry (54) observed increased DNA fragmentation of thymic lymphocytes in rats after two treadmill runs to exhaustion (separated by a 24-hour rest). In this classic study, the investigators blocked thymocyte apoptosis by administering a GC receptor antagonist, RU-486 (mifepristone). However, we raise a note of caution regarding interpretation of these findings: DNA fragmentation characterizes many kinds of cell death events, and the detection of DNA fragments may not be entirely specific to apoptosis.

Increased oxygen consumption with exhaustive exercise leads to the generation of ROS and lipid peroxidation of lymphocyte cell membranes. Dynamic exercise ($\dot{V}O_{2max}$ >80%, 60 minutes) increases NFκB activation in human peripheral blood lymphocytes (55), and this transient activation may be explained by oxidative stress and/or GC responses with exercise. Caspase 3 activity is greater in thymocytes after a single intensive bout of dynamic exercise (56), and annexin-V, a marker for phosphatidylserine externalization and early apoptosis, is increased in intraepithelial intestinal T lymphocytes 24 hours after exhaustive exercise (57). In several studies, increased expression of caspase 3 and decreased expression of Bcl-2 proteins, which shift the apostat, occurred in the intestinal lymphocytes of mice that underwent three repeated bouts of exhaustive treadmill exercise (58,59). Moreover, the repeated exercise effect on intestinal lymphocytes did not involve inflammatory changes in the bowel (60), thus ruling out the exercise-associated loss of lymphocytes through necrotic mechanisms.

In other studies, overtraining and acute, muscle-damaging exercise increased the expression of TNF-α (61), triggering lymphocyte apoptosis through the extrinsic pathway. Short-term, high-intensity exercise in men (three consecutive bouts of treadmill running at 85% of $\dot{V}O_{2max}$ for 30 minutes every day) was associated with increased plasma TNF-α and soluble Fas ligand in lymphocytes, and dysfunction of lymphocyte mitochondrial transmembrane potential (which contributes to the initiation of apoptosis); these effects persisted for up to 72 hours after cessation of the exercise (62).

What we can conclude from these studies is that maximal acute exercise induces cell death in circulating and tissue lymphocytes through apoptosis. The loss of lymphocytes by apoptotic cell death after intense exercise may contribute to the greater risk of infections during the open window (see Fig. 20.2) and to the functional changes in lymphocytes that occur with repeated bouts of exercise and/or overtraining.

TEST YOURSELF

Why does acute aerobic exercise increase lymphocyte apoptosis?

Exercise and Lymphocyte Recirculation

Lymphocyte recirculation ensures that the necessary subpopulations are distributed to the appropriate extravascular sites when required. Here we provide a brief overview of lymphocyte recirculation with reference to exercise. For a complete description of the mechanisms of lymphocyte recirculation, the reader is again referred to recent immunology textbooks (7).

Lymphocytes continually move from the circulation and lymph to peripheral lymph nodes and the spleen. Lymphocytes also migrate to tissues that interface with the external environment, such as the skin and the mucosal epithelia of the gastrointestinal, pulmonary, and genitourinary tracts. This continual movement of lymphocytes increases the probability that antigenically committed lymphocytes will contact antigen. Extravasation and recirculation are linked to the expression of numerous CAMs on lymphocytes, granulocytes, and vascular endothelium. In the latter case, CAMs are expressed in postcapillary venules of secondary lymphoid tissues known as HEVs. It has been estimated that >10,000 lymphocytes extravasate per second through HEVs of a single lymph node (11). HEVs express numerous leukocyte-specific CAMs, including selectins, mucin-like adhesion molecules, and adhesion molecules of the immunoglobulin superfamily. Each CAM plays a role in and facilitates WBC recirculation patterns. L-selectin (CD62L), which is found on all leukocytes, is involved in tethering and rolling, whereas the lymphocyte integrin molecule, LFA-1 (CD11a/CD18), is involved in the adhesion and arrest of lymphocytes. ICAM-1 also participates in the movement of inflammatory cells, leukocyte effector functions, adhesion of APCs to T lymphocytes during antigen presentation, and signal transduction by activation of specific tyrosine kinases through phosphorylation with resultant transcription factor activation (63). Thus, in addition to enhancing leukocyte adhesion to vascular and mucosal endothelium, CAMs contribute to the interactions among lymphocytes, APCs, and target cells.

Chemokines, which are small peptides with chemoattractant properties, also influence lymphocyte migration patterns. There are two patterns of chemokine expression: homeostatic and inflammatory. The homeostatic chemokines are constitutively expressed and are involved in regular lymphocyte recirculation. The inflammatory chemokines are expressed only during specific inflammatory stimuli and are involved in recruiting activated lymphocytes and inflammatory cells (64). The interaction of chemokines with specific receptors on lymphocytes initiates abrupt and extensive cytoskeletal changes. An important feature of lymphocyte recirculation is that memory lymphocytes (CD45RO$^+$) home selectively to the tissue in which the antigen was first encountered, whereas naïve CD45RA$^+$ lymphocytes (which have not been exposed to antigen) extravasate nonpreferentially (11).

Various types of exercise affect the expression of CAMs, and the extent of this effect depends on the duration and intensity of the exercise and which CAM is being investigated (65). Generally, there is increased expression on peripheral lymphocytes and neutrophils of CD62L and CD11a molecules, which may contribute to the transient exercise-associated leukocytosis. An increased expression of CD62L and CD11b on blood leukocytes occurs after both interval and eccentric exercise. In contrast, prolonged dynamic exercise does not influence macrophage or neutrophil adherence, but may decrease soluble ICAM-1 levels many hours after completion of the exercise. The impact of dynamic exercise on the expression of the CAM CD103 (found on T lymphocytes in the gastrointestinal intestinal tract) has not been determined, but considering that this compartment may serve as a reservoir for T-cells, this would be important information. Among the potential mechanisms for the changes in the expression of adhesion molecules with dynamic exercise are (a) the action of GC and catecholamines on marginated cell pools (66); (b) the selective apoptosis of leukocytes with a decreased expression of CD62L (67); and (c) the effects of oxidative products, such as endothelium-derived NO, that affect neutrophil adhesion (68).

KEY POINT

Cellular adhesion molecules affect cellular stickiness and allow leukocytes to move between circulation and tissues. The effect of acute exercise on the expression of cellular adhesion molecules on leukocytes depends on the intensity and duration of the exercise.

Dynamic Exercise-Induced Cytokine Production

Cytokines are polypeptides that were originally discovered within the immune system. However, it appears that many cell types produce cytokines, and the biologic roles of cytokines go beyond immune regulation. Recent data suggest that several cytokines have important metabolic functions, and they may exert their effects either locally in an autocrine- or paracrine-like manner or in a hormone-like fashion (5).

As described above, other cytokines—the chemokines—have a chemoattractant effect on blood leukocyte subpopulations and influence cell trafficking. Most of the available information about cytokines has come from sepsis research. In sepsis models, the cytokine cascade consists of increased plasma levels (named in order) of TNF-α, IL-1β, IL-6, IL-1 receptor antagonist (IL-1ra), soluble TNFR (sTNFR), IL-10, and the chemokine IL-8 (chemoattractant for neutrophils), as well as macrophage inflammatory protein 1 (MIP-1) α and β (chemoattractant for lymphocytes). TNF-α and IL-1β are proinflammatory cytokines, whereas sTNFR, IL-1ra, and IL-10 have anti-inflammatory functions. Although IL-6 has been classified as both a proinflammatory and an anti-inflammatory cytokine, recent research suggests that in response to exercise, circulating IL-6 has primarily anti-inflammatory properties (69). IL-6 is the primary inducer of hepatocyte-derived acute-phase proteins, many of which have anti-inflammatory properties. When infused into humans, IL-6 enhances the levels of the anti-inflammatory cytokines IL-1ra and IL-10.

Several cytokines can be detected in plasma during and after heavy or maximal exercise (70,71). Most studies have reported that exercise does not induce an increase in plasma levels of TNF-α and IL-1β. The fact that the classical pro-cytokines TNF-α and IL-1β do not increase, or increase to only a minor degree, is important for distinguishing the cytokine cascade induced by exercise from that induced in response to infections. Typically, the first cytokine that appears in the circulation after exercise is IL-6. The basal plasma IL-6 concentration may increase up to 100-fold, but less dramatic increases are more frequent (see Fig. 20.4) (72,73).

Of note, the exercise-induced increase of plasma IL-6 is not linear over time. Repeated measurements during exercise show an accelerating increase of the IL-6 in plasma in an almost exponential manner. Furthermore, the peak IL-6 level is reached at the end of the exercise or shortly thereafter, followed by a rapid decrease toward pre-exercise levels. Overall, the combination of the mode, intensity, and duration of the exercise determines the magnitude of the exercise-induced increase of plasma IL-6.

The increase in IL-6 is followed by a marked increase in the concentration of IL-1ra and IL-10. Also, the concentrations of the chemokines IL-8, MIP-1α, and MIP-1β may be elevated after a marathon race (74,75). Some components of the early cytokine response to sepsis and exercise are shown in Figures 20.5 and 20.6.

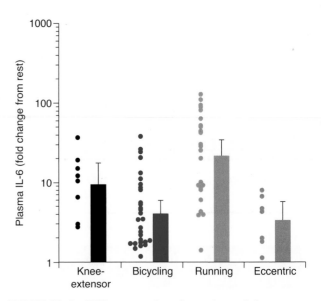

FIGURE 20.4   Different modes of exercise and the corresponding increase in plasma interleukin-6 (IL-6 levels). The graph is based on 73 exercise trials and represents ~800 subjects. Each dot indicates one exercise trial; the corresponding bars represent geometric means with 95% confidence intervals. Although different modes of exercise are associated with different levels of muscle damage, the increase in plasma IL-6 levels after exercise is a consistent finding. (Adapted with permission from Pedersen BK, Fischer CP. Beneficial health effects of exercise—the role of IL-6 as a myokine. *Trends Pharmacol Sci.* 2007;28(4):152–156.)

In studies in which BMNCs were sampled during and after heavy or maximal exercise, or stimulated in vitro to produce cytokines, the in vitro cytokine production was either impaired (76), not changed, or enhanced (77). These findings are likely explained by exercise-induced changes in the composition of the BMNCs.

Initially, it was thought that the exercise-induced elevation of IL-6 was an inflammatory response caused by muscle damage. However, the increase was observed after both concentric contractions (*e.g.*, biking or leg-kicking) without

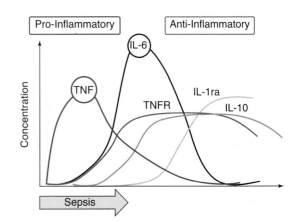

FIGURE 20.5   Schematic presentation of components of the early cytokine responses to sepsis: IL-6, interleukin-6; TNFR, tumor necrosis factor receptor; IL-1ra, interleukin-1 receptor antagonist; IL-10, interleukin-10.

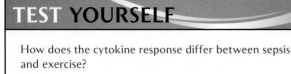

TEST YOURSELF

How does the cytokine response differ between sepsis and exercise?

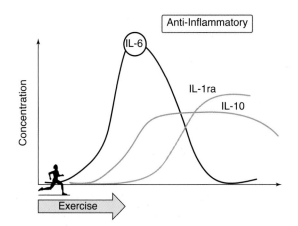

FIGURE 20.6 Schematic presentation of components of the early cytokine responses to endurance exercise: IL-6, interleukin-6; IL-1ra, interleukin-1 receptor antagonist; IL-10, interleukin-10.

muscle damage and eccentric contractions (*e.g.*, strength training or running) in which muscle damage occurs; therefore, the increase in IL-6 could not be due solely to muscle damage. In addition, a comparison of plasma from the femoral artery with plasma from the femoral vein made it clear that the increased levels of plasma IL-6 during exercise originated from skeletal muscle (82). Several pieces of evidence now suggest that muscle fibers per se produce and release

IL-6 and argue for a metabolic role, strictly separated from inflammation, for IL-6. The cytokine responses to exercise and sepsis have many similarities. However, during sepsis, a marked and rapid increase in circulating TNF-α occurs, followed by an increase in IL-6. In contrast, during exercise, the marked increase in IL-6 is not preceded by elevated TNF-α. The IL-6 signaling in macrophages is dependent on activation of the NFκB signaling pathway. In contrast, intramuscular IL-6 expression is regulated by a network of signaling cascades that, along with other pathways, are likely to involve cross talk between the Ca²⁺/nuclear factor of activated T-cells and glycogen/p38 mitogen-activated protein kinase pathways (see Fig. 20.7). The biologic consequence is that the cytokine response in macrophages promotes inflammation, whereas the cytokine response elicited by nondamaging physical exercise has anti-inflammatory and metabolic properties.

KEY POINT

During exercise, the plasma concentration of IL-6 increases in an exponential fashion and declines to the pre-exercise value in the recovery phase of exercise. The increase in plasma IL-6 is followed by the appearance of the cytokine inhibitors IL-1ra and TNFR, and the anti-inflammatory cytokine IL-10. After long-term regular exercise, the circulating resting levels of all cytokines are decreased.

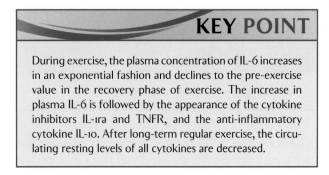
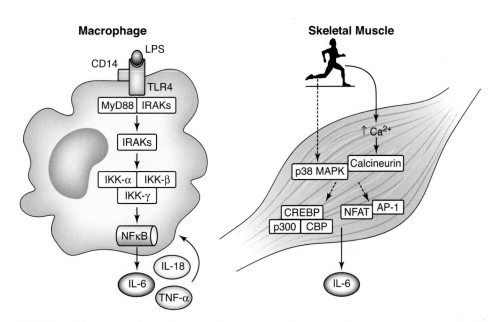

FIGURE 20.7 Proposed cytokine signaling pathways for macrophages and contracting skeletal muscle. Although it is well known that transcription of interleukin-6 (IL-6) and other pro-inflammatory cytokines, such as tumor necrosis factor-α (TNF-α) and IL-β, is principally regulated by the toll-like receptor (TLR) signaling cascade that results in nuclear translocation and activation of nuclear factor κ B (NFκB), evidence from contracting skeletal muscle suggests that contraction leads to increased cytosolic Ca²⁺ and activation of p38 mitogen-activated protein kinase (MAPK) and/or calcineurin, which leads to activation of transcription factors depending on these upstream events. LPS, lipopolysaccharide; CREBP, cAMP responsive element binding protein; NFAT, nuclear factor of activated T-cells; AP-1, activator protein 1. (Adapted with permission from Pedersen BK, Febbraio MA. Muscle as an endocrine organ: focus on muscle-derived interleukin-6. *Physiol Rev.* 2008;88(4):1379–1406.)

Muscle Contraction-Induced Immune Regulation

Skeletal muscle was recently identified as an organ that produces and releases cytokines. Therefore, it has been suggested that cytokines and other peptides that are produced, expressed, and released by muscle fibers and exert paracrine, autocrine, or endocrine effects should be classified as "myokines." Given that skeletal muscle is the largest organ in the human body, the discovery that contracting skeletal muscle secretes proteins establishes a novel paradigm: Skeletal muscle is an endocrine organ that produces and releases myokines in response to contraction, which can influence metabolism in other tissues and organs. The discovery that exercise provokes an increase in a number of cytokines suggests a possible link between skeletal muscle contractile activity and immune changes.

TEST YOURSELF

Why has muscle been described as an endocrine organ?

For most of the last century, researchers have searched for a muscle contraction-induced factor that could mediate certain exercise-induced changes in other organs, such as the liver and adipose tissue. For lack of more precise knowledge, it has been called the "work stimulus" or "work factor" (78). Today, we may prefer to use the term *exercise factor* to cover the effects of muscle contractions (79). It is clear that in addition to the nervous system, there are other signaling pathways from contracting muscles to other organs. Electrical stimulation of paralyzed muscles in patients with spinal cord injuries was shown to induce many of the same physiologic changes observed in intact subjects (80). A recent study showed that exercise induces transcription of metabolic genes in exercising skeletal muscle (81), thus demonstrating that muscle contractions as such may directly influence metabolism. The findings that IL-6 gene transcription takes place locally in contracting skeletal muscle, and that IL-6 is released to the blood in high amounts from an exercising limb (82) raise the possibility that exercise-induced immune changes are directly linked to a factor induced by muscle contractions.

Infusion of recombinant human IL-6 demonstrates that IL-6 enhances cortisol production with the same kinetics and to the same extent as observed during exercise (83). Furthermore, IL-6 induces neutrocytosis and late lymphopenia to the same magnitude and with the same kinetics as during dynamic exercise, suggesting that muscle-derived IL-6 may have a central role in exercise-induced leukocyte recirculation. In addition, many recent findings suggest that muscle-derived IL-6 has important metabolic roles, as illustrated in Figure 20.8. It is now known that skeletal muscle has the capacity to produce and express cytokines that belong to

distinctly different families; to date, the list includes IL-6, IL-8, IL-15, LIF, and brain-derived neurotropic factor. Contractile activity also plays a role in regulating the expression of these cytokines in skeletal muscle (5,84,85).

KEY POINT

Skeletal muscle is a major source of the cytokines IL-6, IL-8, and IL-15. In addition to their contribution to Th1/Th2 immune responses, these cytokines also have a role in metabolism, including insulin sensitivity and glycemic control. Contractile activity is a major regulator of the expression of these cytokines in skeletal muscle.

Endocrine Regulation of Immune Function during Exercise

Exercise induces dramatic changes in the hormonal milieu. Thus, acute, heavy muscular exercise increases the concentrations of a number of stress hormones in the blood, including E, NE, growth hormone, β-endorphins, and cortisol/corticosterone (C), whereas the concentration of insulin slightly decreases (86). In this section, we will describe the evidence for exercise-induced changes in neuroimmune interactions, with an emphasis on catecholamines and cortisol. Our perspective is from the immunologic end. For a more complete introduction to hormonal responses to exercise, the reader is directed to Chapter 19 in this volume.

Catecholamines, Dynamic Exercise, and Lymphocytes

During exercise, E is released from the adrenal medulla, and NE is released from the sympathetic nerve terminals. Arterial plasma concentrations of E and NE increase almost linearly with duration of dynamic exercise and exponentially with intensity, when it is expressed relative to the individual's maximal oxygen uptake (86). The expression of β-adrenoceptors on T-, B-, and NK cells, and macrophages and neutrophils in numerous species provide the molecular basis for these cells to be targets for catecholamine signaling (87). The number of adrenergic receptors in individual lymphocyte subpopulations may determine the degree to which the cells are mobilized in response to catecholamines. In accordance with this hypothesis, it has been shown that different subpopulations of BMNCs have different numbers of β-adrenergic receptors (β-ARs) (88). NK cells contain the highest number of β-ARs, and CD4$^+$ lymphocytes have the lowest number. B-lymphocytes and CD8$^+$ lymphocytes are intermediate between NK cells and CD4$^+$ lymphocytes (89). Acute exercise increases the number of β-ARs expressed on lymphocytes and NK cells (as well as β-AR mRNA levels in these cells). Of interest, NK cells seem to be more responsive to acute exercise than many other subpopulations. CD4$^+$ cells are less sensitive, and CD8$^+$

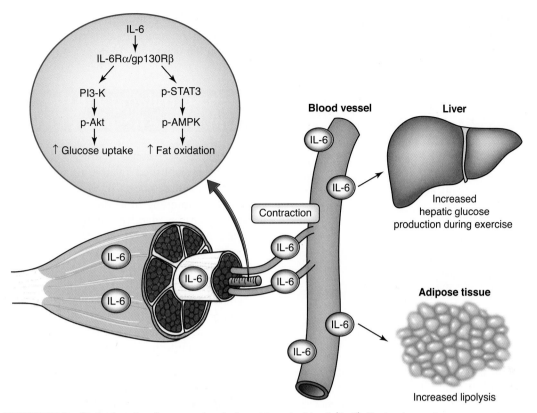

FIGURE 20.8   Biologic role of contraction-induced interleukin-6 (IL-6). Skeletal muscle expresses and releases myokines into the circulation. In response to muscle contractions, both type 1 and type 2 muscle fibers express the myokine IL-6, which subsequently exerts its effects both locally within the muscle (*e.g.*, through activation of adenosine monophosphate (AMP)-kinase) and, when released into the circulation, peripherally in several organs in a hormone-like fashion. In skeletal muscle, IL-6 acts in an autocrine or paracrine manner to signal through a gp130Rβ/IL-6R homodimer, resulting in activation of AMP-kinase and/or phosphatidylinositol 3-kinase (PI3-K) to increase glucose uptake and fat oxidation. IL-6 is also known to increase hepatic glucose production during exercise or lipolysis in adipose tissue. (Adapted with permission from Pedersen BK, Febbraio MA. Muscle as an endocrine organ: focus on muscle-derived interleukin-6. *Physiol Rev.* 2008;88[4]:1379–1406.)

cells and B cells are intermediate (90). Moreover, there is a correlation between the number of β-ARs present in lymphocyte subpopulations and the responsiveness of those subpopulations to exercise. In one study, selective administration of E to obtain plasma concentrations comparable to those obtained during concentric cycling for one hour at 75% of $\dot{V}O_{2max}$, mimicked the exercise-induced effect on BMNC subsets, NKCA, LAK cell activity, and lymphocyte proliferation response (91). However, E infusion caused either a very small or no increase in neutrophil concentrations compared with levels observed after exercise (92). Thus, E seems to contribute to the immediate recruitment of lymphocytes, and particularly NK cells, to the blood during physical exercise. The hormonal responses to exercise are discussed in greater detail in Chapter 19.

Glucocorticoids, Dynamic Exercise, and Lymphocytes

The plasma concentrations of GC increase in relation to exercise of long duration (93). Thus, short-term exercise does

not increase the cortisol concentration in plasma, and only minor changes in the concentrations of plasma GC have been described in relation to acute time-limited exercise stress of less than one hour (93). However, exercise with a significant psychological stress component (*e.g.*, in competition) will lead to elevated cortisol and corticosterone even if the exercise is of short duration. It is well documented that corticosteroids given intravenously to humans cause lymphocytopenia, monocytopenia, eosinopenia, and neutrophilia, which reach their maximum 4 hours after administration (88). The increase in cortisol observed during exercise may be mediated in part by IL-6 (83). A link between exercise-induced lymphocyte changes and an effect of IL-6 on cortisol production has been suggested by studies demonstrating that carbohydrate loading during exercise attenuates both the exercise-induced increase in circulating IL-6 and the dynamic exercise effect on lymphocyte number and function (94).

To summarize, E and, to a lesser extent, NE contribute to the acute effects on circulating lymphocyte subpopulations. GC exerts its effects within a time lag of about 2 hours and contributes to the maintenance of lymphopenia and neutrocytosis after prolonged exercise. GC may contribute to apoptosis in tissue lymphocytes, such as in the thymus and intestinal compartment, observed 24 hours after completion of heavy exercise for 1.5 to 2 hours (57).

TEST YOURSELF

Describe the role of catecholamines and cortisol in the recruitment of lymphocytes and neutrophils to the blood in relation to acute exercise.

Interactions between Immune Function and Metabolism during Exercise

Alterations in metabolism and metabolic factors may contribute to dynamic exercise-associated changes in immune function. It has been hypothesized that reductions in plasma glutamine concentrations due to muscular exercise influence lymphocyte function (95). However, although glutamine in vitro is an important fuel for lymphocytes, a number of glutamine supplementation studies have failed to demonstrate that glutamine can modulate exercise-induced immune changes (96).

Several studies have shown that carbohydrate ingestion attenuates elevations in plasma IL-6 during both running and cycling (94). As a consequence, carbohydrate diminishes the exercise-induced increase in cortisol and fluctuations in lymphocyte and neutrophil numbers. In addition, the increase in IL-6 mRNA and its nuclear transcriptional activity, and protein release from skeletal muscle are augmented when muscle glycogen availability is reduced (97,98). Furthermore, increased expression of IL-6 is associated with increased glucose uptake during exercise (98). This suggests that IL-6 may be involved, at least in part, in mediating glucose uptake during exercise.

TNF-α and IL-6 are tightly linked, and TNF-α stimulates IL-6 production. On the other hand, results from both in vitro (99) and animal (100) studies suggest that IL-6 may inhibit TNF-α production. Recently, it was demonstrated that both physical exercise and rhIL-6 infusion at physiologic concentrations inhibit the production of TNF-α elicited by low-level endotoxemia in humans (101). Although it has been reported that both proinflammatory and anti-inflammatory cytokines are present in the circulation after exercise, it appears that the net result of exercise that involves concentric muscle contractions and is not muscle-damaging is a strong anti-inflammatory effect. The notion that IL-6 plays a central role is supported by the observation that IL-6 infusion enhances plasma levels of IL-1ra and IL-10, and thus markedly contributes to mediation of an anti-inflammatory response. Given that TNF-α induces insulin resistance (102) and non-muscle-damaging

exercise inhibits TNF-α production, it is likely that exercise can also enhance insulin sensitivity via the induction of anti-inflammatory cytokines.

Exercise Training and the Lymphocyte Response

Few studies on exercise training and immune outcomes have been published relative to the body of literature on acute exercise effects in various populations. A comparison of immune function in athletes and nonathletes reveals that the adaptive immune system is largely unaffected by athletic endeavors. The innate immune system appears to respond differentially to the chronic stress of intensive exercise, in that NKCA tends to be enhanced and neutrophil function to be suppressed. However, even when significant changes in the level and functional activity of immune parameters have been observed in athletes, investigators have had little success in linking these to a higher incidence of infection and illness (103).

The Anti-inflammatory Effects of Regular Exercise

The anti-inflammatory effects of regular exercise are likely to be of major clinical importance. Physical inactivity has been associated with low-grade systemic inflammation in cross-sectional studies involving healthy young and elderly individuals (104–111). Moreover, longitudinal studies have shown that regular training induces a reduction in the C-reactive protein (CRP) level (112,113), suggesting that physical activity per se may suppress systemic low-grade inflammation. Several studies have shown that markers of inflammation are reduced after longer term behavioral changes involving both reduced energy intake and increased physical activity (114–118).

In the Finnish Diabetes Prevention Study (119), lifestyle interventions reduced circulating levels of CRP and IL-6. Increases in fiber intake and moderate-to-vigorous leisure time physical activity (but not total leisure time physical activity) predicted decreases in CRP and/or IL-6, and remained associated even after adjustment for baseline body mass index or changes in body mass index during the first year of the study. Changes in carbohydrate or fat intake were either weakly or not linked to reductions in CRP and IL-6 (119). For an in-depth discussion of carbohydrate metabolism and exercise, the reader is referred to Chapter 14.

It appears that exercise may have anti-inflammatory effects that are independent of weight loss; however, the mediators of this effect are unclear. A number of mechanisms have been identified. Exercise increases the release of E, cortisol, growth hormone, prolactin, and other factors that have immunomodulatory effects (120). Furthermore, exercise results in decreased expression of toll-like receptor on monocytes that have been suggested to be involved in mediating whole body inflammation (121). In addition, a recent study showed that long-term freewheel running in mice reduced the expression of the proinflammatory cytokine TNF-α in intestinal lymphocytes (122). In another study, long-term training resulted in the maintenance of mouse intestinal lymphocyte CD4 numbers after an acute exercise bout (which normally induces T-cell apoptosis) (123). The next step is to determine whether this protection from apoptotic loss of intestinal CD4 lymphocytes is due to decreased expression of proinflammatory cytokines or to increased expression of antioxidant defenses.

TEST YOURSELF

Why is regular exercise considered to be anti-inflammatory?

Persistent, low-grade, systemic inflammation is a feature of chronic diseases such as cardiovascular disease, type 2 diabetes, and dementia, and inflammation has been proposed to be a causal factor in the development of insulin resistance and atherosclerosis (124). Regular exercise offers protection against all of these diseases, and recent evidence suggests that the protective effect of exercise may to some extent be ascribed to an anti-inflammatory effect of regular exercise (125). Visceral adiposity contributes to systemic inflammation (126) and is independently associated with the occurrence of cardiovascular disease, type 2 diabetes, and dementia (127,128). A number of studies have suggested that physical activity reduces abdominal and particularly visceral fat in healthy men and women independently of changes in dietary energy intake (129). In a recent study, a group of young, healthy men decreased their daily stepping for 2 to 3 weeks to 1,500 steps from the range recommended for U.S. adults of around 10,000 steps. During this time, the subjects experienced a 7% increase in intra-abdominal fat mass without a change in total fat mass and a decrease in total fat-free mass. Moreover, they developed metabolic changes suggestive of decreased insulin sensitivity and attenuation of postprandial lipid metabolism (130). It is therefore possible that the anti-inflammatory effects of training may be mediated via a long-term effect of exercise leading to a reduction in visceral fat mass and/or by induction of anti-inflammatory cytokines with each bout of exercise.

KEY POINT

Regular moderate exercise has an anti-inflammatory effect that is independent of weight loss and adiposity. This beneficial anti-inflammatory effect may be related to an increased expression of endogenous antioxidants and reduced concentrations of proinflammatory cytokines.

The Role of Reactive Oxygen Species

ROS is a collective name for molecules that contain oxygen, which makes them chemically unstable and reactive. The most reactive ROS are free radicals with one or more unpaired electrons produced as by-products of oxidative metabolism. As their name implies, they are quite reactive and can harm the cell by causing an oxidizing cascade, resulting in DNA damage and protein and lipid oxidation, and ultimately inducing apoptosis or senescence. Indeed, it has been established that ROS play a role in muscle catabolism by inducing the proteasome pathway for protein degradation (131). However, in healthy individuals, ROS are buffered by endogenous antioxidant defense mechanisms such as superoxide dismutase and nitric oxide synthase. ROS levels increase during exercise, and by directly modifying target proteins or changing the intracellular redox state, ROS can initiate cell signaling and induce alterations in gene expression (132). For example, it has been suggested that ROS enhance or are a part of the signaling pathways of growth factors (133). The chronically elevated levels of ROS observed in degenerative disease are likely to be harmful. The finding that regular exercise offers protection against many of these diseases may reflect the fact that physical training is associated with the induction of endogenous antioxidant defense mechanisms (122,134). The long-term effects of regular exercise are completely separate from what occurs during acute exercise. In contrast to the initial view that ROS are potentially damaging, it now seems possible that these substances play important roles in the regulation of cell signaling (135). And despite the previous notion that ROS have a suppressive effect on muscle recovery (which has resulted in an overconsumption of antioxidants among athletes), it is now being argued that increased levels of ROS during exercise may not only be harmless but may even contribute to some of the adaptations that occur after physical exercise (136).

KEY POINT

Regular exercise offers protection against chronic diseases associated with chronically elevated levels of ROS. This may reflect the fact that physical training is associated with the induction of endogenous antioxidant defense mechanisms. Exercise-induced increases in ROS are likely to contribute to some of the adaptations that occur after physical exercise. However, there is no evidence to support a high intake of antioxidants during sports.

Immune Responses to Exercise across the Life Cycle

Less is known about the lymphocyte response to exercise in children as compared with adults. It seems, however, that the mobilization of lymphocytes to the blood compartment in response to exercise follows the same pattern in children as in adults (137). In a study involving children aged 8 to 17 years, swim training was associated with marginally lower baseline NKCA relative to untrained children sampled at rest (138). (This NK response in children is not unlike that observed in adults when NKCA is determined in trained subjects at rest.) It has also been demonstrated that healthy elderly people have a preserved ability to recruit T lymphocytes in response to acute physical stress (24). During the aging process, circulating levels of a number of cytokines increase. Thus, increased plasma levels of TNF-α (139,140), IL-6, IL-1ra (141), and sTNFR (142) have been demonstrated in the elderly. In addition, aging is also associated with increased levels of acute phase proteins such as CRP and serum amyloid A (143), as well as high neutrophil counts (144). Although increases in circulating cytokines and acute phase proteins are only two- to fourfold higher in elderly subjects than in young ones, low-grade inflammation is clearly associated with atherosclerosis, dementia, and diabetes in the elderly (141). Given that exercise, which accentuates concentric muscle contractions, may reduce inflammatory cytokines, it is most likely that some type of exercise would make an important contribution toward controlling chronic low-grade inflammation and associated diseases in elderly people.

CHAPTER SUMMARY

In the years since leukocytosis was first observed in men who had just completed a marathon race, research in the area of exercise immunology has increased exponentially. In this chapter, we have focused on major immunologic changes induced by acute endurance exercise, because such changes are the best documented. Given the scope of exercise immunology, some immunologic issues clearly could not be addressed (*e.g.*, muscle injury and inflammation, exercise in the heat, gender effects, and exercise and chronic diseases). What is apparent, however, is that

A MILESTONE OF DISCOVERY

Are competitive athletes who "overtrain" really at risk for recurrent respiratory infections as a result of reduced mucosal immunity? A widespread belief held by both athletes and the exercising (and nonexercising) public is that repeated, fatiguing exercise will make an individual more susceptible to infection. Is this belief supported by empirical evidence? To what extent do immune changes induced by exercise affect the risk for infection? An early observational report suggested that episodes of respiratory illness in children were related to participation in intense exercise resulting in acute fatigue (145). In later experiments with rats, rabbits, and guinea pigs in investigators sought to determine whether fatiguing exercise increases mortality from bacterial infections (146,147). The results were equivocal and depended on when the exposure took place; thus, fatigue before exposure to bacterial challenge was associated with increased resistance, whereas fatigue after exposure was associated with decreased resistance. Furthermore, these studies' use of revolving drums (which tumbled the animals instead of exercising them, and confounded stress with exercise), lack of measures of fatigue or exercise intensity, and lack of immunologic measures to mediate the increased or decreased resistance made interpretation of these early findings problematic.

Given the role of the mucosal immune system in protecting against upper respiratory tract infections, Mackinnon and colleagues (33) sought to systematically determine whether exhaustive exercise affects the specific immunologic components that provide barrier protection against pathogens at mucosal surfaces. Elite cyclists were exercised for 2 hours at 90% of anaerobic threshold (~75% of each cyclist's maximum exercise capacity), and serum,

salivary, and nasal immunoglobulin titers were measured with the use of modern immunologic techniques, including the enzyme-linked immunosorbent assay. Immediately after the exercise bout and for 1 hour afterward, salivary IgA concentrations (the key antibody in secretions) were significantly lower (9.5 ± 2.8 µg of Ig/mg protein) relative to pre-exercise levels (27.5 ± 6.9 µg of Ig/mg protein) and returned to baseline 24 hours after completion of the bout. In contrast to the salivary IgA and IgM concentrations, the serum and nasal immunoglobulin concentrations were completely unaffected by the exercise bout. The importance of this study is threefold. First, this work (and many subsequent studies by other investigators) provided an immunologic basis for the "open window" model, which relates intensity and duration of exercise to infection risk (see *Exercise Training and the Lymphocyte Response*). Second, this study provided clear, empirical evidence against the assumption that immune responses to exercise that occur in one compartment are mirrored in other tissue compartments, since saliva and serum Ig responses were quite different. Third, by sampling at multiple time points for up to 2 days after the exercise bout, Mackinnon and colleagues rigorously demonstrated that even with exhaustive exercise, immune suppression is transitory and the immune system recovers quickly. The clinical and physiologic meaning of transitory immune changes has been a consideration in the design of exercise-immunology investigations ever since.

Mackinnon LT, Chick TW, van As A, et al. The effect of exercise on secretory and natural immunity. Adv Exp Med Biol. 1987; 216A:869–876.

the field of exercise immunology has moved from descriptions of immune responses to studies on the underlying physiologic, biochemical, and molecular biologic processes involved in these responses, reflecting the maturation of the science. It now appears that the leukocytosis of exercise is likely due to changes in the expression of CAMs, apoptosis, and leukocyte trafficking, which, in turn, reflect the hormonal and cytokine milieu present during exercise. The mechanisms for the leukopenia of long-duration exercise are less clear, although evidence points to apoptosis and changes in trafficking of cells. The role of cytokines, released during exercise, has implications for determining whether cellular or humoral immune responses dominate and whether inflammation or anti-inflammation occurs. Muscle-derived IL-6 may have important metabolic-regulatory effects well beyond the immune system. The strong anti-inflammatory effects of moderate exercise (especially exercise that emphasizes concentric muscle contractions) are likely to be of clinical importance in terms of controlling low-grade inflammation and related disorders such as atherosclerosis and insulin resistance.

ACKNOWLEDGMENTS

This research was supported by the Natural Sciences and Engineering Research Council of Canada (grant 7645 to L.H.G.) and the Danish National Research Foundation (grant 02-512-55 to B.K.P.). The authors thank Inge Holm for her outstanding editorial support with this chapter.

REFERENCES

1. Cannon WB. *The Wisdom of the Body.* New York: Norton; 1939.
2. Seyle H. *The Stress of Life.* New York: McGraw-Hill; 1976.
3. Larrabee RC. Leucocytosis after violent exercise. *J Med Res.* 1902;7:76–82.
4. Abbott AC, Gildersleeve N. The influence of muscular fatigue and of alcohol upon certain of the normal defenses. *Univ Penn Med Bull.* 1910;23:169–181.
5. Pedersen BK, Febbraio MA. Muscle as an endocrine organ: focus on muscle-derived interleukin-6. *Physiol Rev.* 2008;88(4):1379–1406.
6. Pedersen BK, Hoffman-Goetz L. Exercise and the immune system: regulation, integration and adaptation. *Physiol Rev.* 2000;80:1055–1081.
7. Delves PJ, Martin S, Burton D, et al. *Roitt's Essential Immunology.* Oxford: Blackwell Publishing; 2006.
8. Mak TW, Saunders ME. *Primer to the Immune Response.* Burlington: Academic Press/Elsevier; 2008.
9. Baldwin C. Constitutive host resistance. In: Kreier JP, ed. *Infection, Resistance, and Immunity.* 2nd ed. New York: Taylor & Francis; 2002:27–43.
10. Rehman J, Mills PJ, Carter SM, et al. Dynamic exercise leads to an increase in circulating ICAM-1: further evidence for adrenergic modulation of cell adhesion. *Brain Behav Immun.* 1997;11(4):343–351.
11. Goldsby RA, Kindt TJ, Osborne BA, et al. *Immunology.* 5th ed. New York: WH Freeman & Co; 2003.
12. Hickey MA, Taylor DW. The inducible defense system: the induction and development of the inducible defence. In: Kreier JP, ed. *Infection, Resistance, and Immunity.* New York: Taylor & Francis; 2002:113–156.
13. Russell JH, Ley TJ. Lymphocyte-mediated cytotoxicity. *Annu Rev Immunol.* 2002;20:323–370.
14. Brandt C, Pedersen BK. The role of exercise-induced myokines in muscle homeostasis and the defense against chronic diseases. *J Biomed Biotechnol.* 2010;2010:520258.
15. Nieman DC. Current perspective on exercise immunology. *Curr Sports Med Rep.* 2003;2(5):239–242.
16. Gleeson M. Immune function in sport and exercise. *J Appl Physiol.* 2007;103(2):693–699.
17. McCarthy DA, Dale MM. The leucocytosis of exercise. A review and model. *Sports Med.* 1988;6(6):333–363.
18. Nieman DC. Special feature for the Olympics: effects of exercise on the immune system: exercise effects on systemic immunity. *Immunol Cell Biol.* 2000;78(5):496–501.
19. Timmons BW, Cieslak T. Human natural killer cell subsets and acute exercise: a brief review. *Exerc Immunol Rev.* 2008;14:8–23.
20. Kruger K, Mooren FC. T-cell homing and exercise. *Exerc Immunol Rev.* 2007;13:37–54.
21. Lancaster GI, Halson SL, Khan Q, et al. Effects of acute exhaustive exercise and chronic exercise training on type 1 and type 2 T lymphocytes. *Exerc Immunol Rev.* 2004;10:91–106.
22. Bell EB, Spartshott S, Bunce C. CD4+ T-cell memory, CD45R subsets and the persistence of antigen—a unifying concept. *Immunol Today.* 1998;19:60–64.
23. Gabriel H, Schmitt B, Urhausen A, et al. Increased CD45RA+ CD45R0+ cells indicate activated T-cells after endurance exercise. *Med Sci Sports Exerc.* 1993;25(12):1352–1357.
24. Bruunsgaard H, Jensen MS, Schjerling P, et al. Exercise induces recruitment of lymphocytes with an activated phenotype and short telomere lengths in young and elderly humans. *Life Sci.* 1999;65(24):2623–2633.
25. Steensberg A, Toft AD, Bruunsgaard H, et al. Strenuous exercise decreases the percentage of type 1 T-cells in the circulation. *J Appl Physiol.* 2001;91(4):1708–1712.
26. Welsh RM, Vargas-Cortes RM. Natural killer cells in viral infection. In: Lewis CE, McGee JO, eds. *The Natural Killer Cell.* Oxford: Oxford University Press; 1992:108–150.
27. O'Shea J, Ortaldo JR. The biology of natural killer cells: insights into the molecular basis of function. In: Lewis CE, McGee JO, eds. *The Natural Killer Cell.* Oxford: Oxford University Press; 1992:1–40.
28. Mackinnon LT. Exercise and natural killer cells: what is the relationship? *Sports Med.* 1989;7:141–149.
29. Nielsen HB, Secher NH, Kappel M, et al. Lymphocyte, NK, and LAK cell responses to maximal exercise. *Int J Sports Med.* 1996;17(1):60–65.
30. MacNeil B, Hoffman-Goetz L. Chronic exercise enhances in vivo and in vitro cytotoxic mechanisms of natural immunity in mice. *J Appl Physiol.* 1993;74:388–395.
31. Liew FY, Russell SM, Appleyard G, et al. Cross-protection in mice infected with influenza A virus by the respiratory route is correlated with local IgA antibody rather than serum antibody or cytotoxic T cell reactivity. *Eur J Immunol.* 1984;14(4):350–356.
32. Tomasi TB, Trudeau FB, Czerwinski D, et al. Immune parameters in athletes before and after strenuous exercise. *J Clin Immunol.* 1982;2(3):173–178.
33. Mackinnon LT, Chick TW, van As A, et al. The effect of exercise on secretory and natural immunity. *Adv Exp Med Biol.* 1987;216A:869–876.
34. Tharp GD, Barnes MW. Reduction of saliva immunoglobulin levels by swim training. *Eur J Appl Physiol.* 1990;60(1):61–64.
35. Steerenberg PA, van Asperen IA, van Nieuw Amerongen A, et al. Salivary levels of immunoglobulin A in triathletes. *Eur J Oral Sci.* 1997;105(4):305–309.
36. McDowell SL, Hughes RA, Hughes RJ, et al. The effect of exhaustive exercise on salivary immunoglobulin A. *J Sports Med Phys Fit.* 1992;32(4):412–415.
37. Tvede N, Heilmann C, Halkjaer Kristensen J, et al. Mechanisms of B-lymphocyte suppression induced by acute physical exercise. *J Clin Lab Immunol.* 1989;30(4):169–173.
38. Bruunsgaard H, Hartkopp A, Mohr T, et al. In vivo cell mediated immunity and vaccination response following prolonged, intense exercise. *Med Sci Sports Exerc.* 1997;29(9):1176–1181.
39. Kurokawa Y, Shinkai S, Torii J, et al. Exercise-induced changes in the expression of surface adhesion molecules on circulating granulocytes and lymphocytes subpopulations. *Eur J Appl Physiol.* 1995;71(2–3):245–252.

40. Smith JA, Gray AB, Pyne DB, et al. Moderate exercise triggers both priming and activation of neutrophil subpopulations. *Am J Physiol.* 1996;270(4):R838–R845.

41. Brines R, Hoffman-Goetz L, Pedersen BK. Can you exercise to make your immune system fitter? *Immunol Today.* 1996;17(6):252–254.

42. Fry RW, Morton AR, Crawford GP, et al. Cell numbers and in vitro responses of leukocytes and lymphocyte subpopulations following maximal exercise and interval training sessions of different intensities. *Eur J Appl Physiol.* 1992;64(3):218–227.

43. Keast D, Cameron K, Morton AR. Exercise and the immune response. *Sports Med.* 1988;5(4):248–267.

44. Green KJ, Rowbottom DG, Mackinnon LT. Exercise and T-lymphocyte function: a comparison of proliferation in PBMC and NK cell-depleted PBMC culture. *J Appl Physiol.* 2002;92(6):2390–2395.

45. Field CJ, Gougeon R, Marliss EB. Circulating mononuclear cell numbers and function during intense exercise and recovery. *J Appl Physiol.* 1991;71(3):1089–1097.

46. Wang KK. Calpain and caspase: can you tell the difference? *Trends Neurosci.* 2000;23(2):20–26.

47. Hoffman-Goetz L, Quadrilatero J, Patel H. Cellular life span. In: Mooren FC, Voelker K, eds. *Molecular and Cellular Exercise Physiology.* Champaign, IL: Human Kinetics Press; 2005:19–37.

48. Phaneuf S, Leeuwenburgh C. Apoptosis and exercise. *Med Sci Sports Exerc.* 2001;33(3):393–396.

49. Los M, Stroh C, Janicke RU, et al. Caspases: more than just killers? *Trends Immunol.* 2001;22(1):31–34.

50. Ashe PC, Berry MD. Apoptotic signaling cascades. *Prog Neuropsychopharmacol Biol Psychiatry.* 2003;27(2):199–214.

51. Bredesen DE. Key note lecture: toward a mechanistic taxonomy for cell death programs. *Stroke.* 2007;38(suppl 2):652–660.

52. Marchetti P, Castedo M, Susin SA, et al. Mitochondrial permeability transition is a central coordinating event of apoptosis. *J Exp Med.* 1996;184(3):1155–1160.

53. Yu JW, Shi Y. FLIP and the death effector domain family. *Oncogene.* 2008;27(48):6216–6227.

54. Concordet JP, Ferry A. Physiological programmed cell death in thymocytes is induced by physical stress (exercise). *Am J Physiol.* 1993;265(3 pt 1):C626–C629.

55. Vider J, Laaksonen DE, Kilk A, et al. Physical exercise induces activation of NF-kappa B in human peripheral blood lymphocytes. *Antioxid Redox Signal.* 2001;3(6):1131–1137.

56. Patel H, Hoffman-Goetz L. Effects of oestrogen and exercise on caspase-3 activity in primary and secondary lymphoid compartments in ovariectomized mice. *Acta Physiol Scand.* 2002;176(3):177–184.

57. Hoffman-Goetz L, Quadrilatero J. Treadmill exercise in mice increases intestinal lymphocyte loss via apoptosis. *Acta Physiol Scand.* 2003;179(3):289–297.

58. Hoffman-Goetz L, Spagnuolo PA. Effect of repeated exercise stress on caspase 3, Bcl-2, HSP 70 and CuZn-SOD protein expression in mouse intestinal lymphocytes. *J Neuroimmunol.* 2007;187(1–2):94–101.

59. Spagnuolo PA, Hoffman-Goetz L. Lactoferrin effect on lymphocyte cytokines and apoptosis is independent of exercise. *Med Sci Sports Exerc.* 2008;40(6):1013–1021.

60. Spagnuolo PA, Hoffman-Goetz L. Effect of dextran sulfate sodium and acute exercise on mouse intestinal inflammation and lymphocyte cytochrome c levels. *J Sports Med Phys Fitness.* 2009;49(1):112–121.

61. Steinacker JM, Lormes W, Reissnecker S, et al. New aspects of the hormone and cytokine response to training. *Eur J Appl Physiol.* 2003;91:382–391.

62. Tuan TC, Hsu TG, Fong MC, et al. Deleterious effects of short-term, high-intensity exercise on immune function: evidence from leucocyte mitochondrial alterations and apoptosis. *Br J Sports Med.* 2008;42(1):11–15.

63. Hubbard AK, Rothlein R. Intercellular adhesion molecule-1 (ICAM-1) expression and cell signaling cascades. *Free Radic Biol Med.* 2000;28(9):1379–1386.

64. Olson TS, Ley K. Chemokines and chemokine receptors in leukocyte trafficking. Am *J Physiol Regul Integr Comp Physiol.* 2002;283(1):R7–R28.

65. Shephard RJ. Adhesion molecules, catecholamines and leucocyte redistribution during and following exercise. *Sports Med.* 2003;33:261–284.

66. Nakagawa M, Bondy GP, Waisman D, et al. The effect of glucocorticoids on the expression of L-selectin on polymorphonuclear leukocyte. *Blood.* 1999;93(8):2730–2737.

67. Matsuba KT, van Eeden SF, Bicknell SG, et al. Apoptosis in circulating PMN: increased susceptibility in L-selectin-deficient PMN. *Am J Physiol.* 1997;272(6 pt 2):H2852–H2888.

68. Cuzzolin L, Lussignoli S, Crivellente F, et al. Influence of an acute exercise on neutrophil and platelet adhesion, nitric oxide plasma metabolites in inactive and active subjects. *Int J Sports Med.* 2000;21(4):289–293.

69. Xing Z, Gauldie J, Cox G, et al. IL-6 is an antiinflammatory cytokine required for controlling local or systemic acute inflammatory responses. *J Clin Invest.* 1998;101(2):311–320.

70. Ostrowski K, Rohde T, Asp S, et al. Pro- and anti-inflammatory cytokine balance in strenuous exercise in humans. *J Physiol.* 1999;515(pt 1):287–291.

71. Suzuki K, Nakaji S, Yamada M, et al. Systemic inflammatory response to exhaustive exercise. Cytokine kinetics. *Exerc Immunol Rev.* 2002;8:6–48.

72. Fischer CP. Interleukin-6 in acute exercise and training: what is the biological relevance? *Exerc Immunol Rev.* 2006;12:6–33.

73. Pedersen BK, Fischer CP. Beneficial health effects of exercise—the role of IL-6 as a myokine. *Trends Pharmacol Sci.* 2007;28(4):152–156.

74. Niess AM, Sommer M, Schlotz E, et al. Expression of the inducible nitric oxide synthase (iNOS) in human leukocytes: responses to running exercise. *Med Sci Sports Exerc.* 2000;32(7):1220–1225.

75. Ostrowski K, Rohde T, Asp S, et al. Chemokines are elevated in plasma after strenuous exercise in humans. *Eur J Appl Physiol.* 2001;84(3):244–245.

76. Drenth JP, van Uum SH, Van DM, et al. Endurance run increases circulating IL-6 and IL-1ra but downregulates ex vivo TNF-alpha and IL-1 beta production. *J Appl Physiol.* 1995;79(5):1497–1503.

77. Haahr PM, Pedersen BK, Fomsgaard A, et al. Effect of physical exercise on in vitro production of interleukin 1, interleukin 6, tumor necrosis factor-alpha, interleukin 2 and interferon- gamma. *Int J Sports Med.* 1991;12(2):223–227.

78. Winocour PH, Durrington PN, Bhatnagar D, et al. A cross-sectional evaluation of cardiovascular risk factors in coronary heart disease associated with type 1 (insulin-dependent) diabetes mellitus. *Diabetes Res Clin Pract.* 1992;18(3):173–184.

79. Pedersen BK. The diseasome of physical inactivity and the role of myokines in muscle-fat cross talk. *J Physiol.* 2009;587:5559–5568.

80. Mohr T, Andersen JL, Biering-Sorensen F, et al. Long-term adaptation to electrically induced cycle training in severe spinal cord injured individuals. *Spinal Cord.* 1997;35(1):1–16.

81. Pilegaard H, Ordway GA, Saltin B, et al. Transcriptional regulation of gene expression in human skeletal muscle during recovery from exercise. *Am J Physiol Endocrinol Metab.* 2000;279(4):E806–E814.

82. Febbraio MA, Pedersen BK. Muscle-derived interleukin-6: mechanisms for activation and possible biological roles. *FASEB J.* 2002;16(11):1335–1347.

83. Steensberg A, Fischer CP, Keller C, et al. IL-6 enhances plasma IL-1ra, IL-10, and cortisol in humans. *Am J Physiol Endocrinol Metab.* 2003;285(2):E433–E437.

84. Pedersen BK, Pedersen M, Krabbe KS, et al. Role of exercise-induced brain-derived neurotrophic factor production in the regulation of energy homeostasis in mammals. *Exp Physiol.* 2009;94(12):1153–1160.

85. Pedersen BK. Edward F. Adolph distinguished lecture: muscle as an endocrine organ: IL-6 and other myokines. *J Appl Physiol.* 2009;107(4):1006–1014.

86. Kjaer M, Dela F. Endocrine responses to exercise. In: Hoffman-Goetz L, ed. *Exercise and Immune Function.* Boca Raton: CRC Press; 1996:1–20.

87. Madden K, Felten DL. Experimental basis for neural-immune interactions. *Physiol Rev.* 1995;75(1):77–106.

88. Rabin BS, Moyna MN, Kusnecov A, et al. Neuroendocrine effects of immunity. In: Hoffman-Goetz L, ed. *Exercise and Immune Function.* Boca Raton: CRC Press; 1996:21–38.

89. Maisel AS, Harris T, Rearden CA, et al. Beta-adrenergic receptors in lymphocyte subsets after exercise. Alterations in normal individuals and patients with congestive heart failure. *Circulation.* 1990;82(6):2003–2010.

90. Hoffman-Goetz L, Pedersen BK. Exercise and the immune system: a model of the stress response? *Immunol Today.* 1994;15:382–387.

91. Kappel M, Tvede N, Galbo H, et al. Evidence that the effect of physical exercise on NK cell activity is mediated by epinephrine. *J Appl Physiol.* 1991;70(6):2530–2534.

92. Tvede N, Kappel M, Klarlund K, et al. Evidence that the effect of bicycle exercise on blood mononuclear cell proliferative responses and subsets is mediated by epinephrine. *Int J Sports Med.* 1994;15(2):100–104.

93. Galbo H. *Hormonal and Metabolic Adaption to Exercise.* New York: Thieme Verlag; 1983.

94. Nehlsen Cannarella SL, Fagoaga OR, Nieman DC, et al. Carbohydrate and the cytokine response to 2.5 h of running. *J Appl Physiol.* 1997;82(5):1662–1667.

95. Newsholme EA, Parry Billings M. Properties of glutamine release from muscle and its importance for the immune system. *J Parenter Enteral Nutr.* 1990;14(suppl 4):63S–67S.

96. Hiscock N, Pedersen BK. Exercise-induced immunodepression—plasma glutamine is not the link. *J Appl Physiol.* 2002;93(3):813–822.

97. Keller C, Steensberg A, Pilegaard H, et al. Transcriptional activation of the IL-6 gene in human contracting skeletal muscle: influence of muscle glycogen content. *FASEB J.* 2001;15(14):2748–2750.

98. Steensberg A, Febbraio MA, Osada T, et al. Interleukin-6 production in contracting human skeletal muscle is influenced by pre-exercise muscle glycogen content. *J Physiol.* 2001;537(pt 2):633–639.

99. Fiers W. Tumor necrosis factor. Characterization at the molecular, cellular and in vivo level. *FEBS Lett.* 1991;285(2):199–212.

100. Matthys P, Mitera T, Heremans H, et al. Anti-gamma interferon and anti-interleukin-6 antibodies affect staphylococcal enterotoxin B-induced weight loss, hypoglycemia, and cytokine release in D-galactosamine-sensitized and unsensitized mice. *Infect Immunol.* 1995;63(4):1158–64.

101. Starkie R, Ostrowski SR, Jauffred S, et al. Exercise and IL-6 infusion inhibit endotoxin-induced TNF-alpha production in humans. *FASEB J.* 2003;17(8):884–886.

102. Hotamisligil GS, Shargill NS, Spiegelman BM. Adipose expression of tumor necrosis factor-alpha: direct role in obesity-linked insulin resistance. *Science.* 1993;259(5091):87–91.

103. Nieman DC, Pedersen BK. Exercise and immune function. Recent developments. *Sports Med.* 1999;27(2):73–80.

104. Abramson JL, Vaccarino V. Relationship between physical activity and inflammation among apparently healthy middle-aged and older US adults. *Arch Intern Med.* 2002;162(11):1286–1292.

105. Geffken DF, Cushman M, Burke GL, et al. Association between physical activity and markers of inflammation in a healthy elderly population. *Am J Epidemiol.* 2001;153(3):242–250.

106. King DE, Carek P, Mainous AG III, et al. Inflammatory markers and exercise: differences related to exercise type. *Med Sci Sports Exerc.* 2003;35(4):575–581.

107. Smith JK, Dykes R, Douglas JE, et al. Long-term exercise and atherogenic activity of blood mononuclear cells in persons at risk of developing ischemic heart disease. *JAMA.* 1999;281(18):1722–1727.

108. Taaffe DR, Harris TB, Ferrucci L, et al. Cross-sectional and prospective relationships of interleukin-6 and C-reactive protein with physical performance in elderly persons: MacArthur studies of successful aging. *J Gerontol A Biol Sci Med Sci.* 2000;55(12):M709–M715.

109. Wannamethee SG, Lowe GD, Whincup PH, et al. Physical activity and hemostatic and inflammatory variables in elderly men. *Circulation.* 2002;105(15):1785–1790.

110. Bruunsgaard H, Ladelund S, Pedersen AN, et al. Predicting death from tumour necrosis factor-alpha and interleukin-6 in 80-year-old people. *Clin Exp Immunol.* 2003;132(1):24–31.

111. Kelley GA, Sharpe KK. Aerobic exercise and resting blood pressure in older adults: a meta-analytic review of randomized controlled trials. *J Gerontol A Biol Sci Med Sci.* 2001;56(5):M298–M303.

112. Fallon KE, Fallon SK, Boston T. The acute phase response and exercise: court and field sports. *Br J Sports Med.* 2001;35(3):170–173.

113. Mattusch F, Dufaux B, Heine O, et al. Reduction of the plasma concentration of C-reactive protein following nine months of endurance training. *Int J Sports Med.* 2000;21(1):21–24.

114. Tchernof A, Nolan A, Sites CK, et al. Weight loss reduces C-reactive protein levels in obese postmenopausal women. *Circulation.* 2002;105(5):564–569.

115. Marfella R, Esposito K, Siniscalchi M, et al. Effect of weight loss on cardiac synchronization and proinflammatory cytokines in premenopausal obese women. *Diabetes Care.* 2004;27(1):47–52.

116. Dandona P, Weinstock R, Thusu K, et al. Tumor necrosis factor-alpha in sera of obese patients: fall with weight loss. *J Clin Endocrin Metab.* 1998;83(8):2907–2910.

117. Monzillo LU, Hamdy O, Horton ES, et al. Effect of lifestyle modification on adipokine levels in obese subjects with insulin resistance. *Obesity.* 2003;11(9):1048–1054.

118. Seshadri P, Iqbal N, Stern L, et al. A randomized study comparing the effects of a low-carbohydrate diet and a conventional diet on lipoprotein subfractions and C-reactive protein levels in patients with severe obesity. *Am J Med.* 2004;117(6):398–405.

119. Herder C, Peltonen M, Koenig W, et al. Anti-inflammatory effect of lifestyle changes in the Finnish Diabetes Prevention Study. *Diabetologia.* 2009;52(3):433–442.

120. Handschin C, Spiegelman BM. The role of exercise and PGC1[alpha] in inflammation and chronic disease. *Nature.* 2008;454(7203):463–469.

121. Gleeson M, McFarlin B, Flynn M. Exercise and toll-like receptors. *Exerc Immunol Rev.* 2006;12:34–53.

122. Hoffman-Goetz L, Pervaiz N, Guan J. Voluntary exercise training in mice increases the expression of antioxidant enzymes and decreases the expression of TNF-alpha in intestinal lymphocytes. *Brain Behav Immun.* 2009;23:498–506.

123. Davidson SR, Hoffman-Goetz L. Freewheel running selectively prevents mouse CD4$^+$ intestinal lymphocyte death produced after a bout of acute strenuous exercise. *Brain Behav Immun.* 2006;20(2):139–143.

124. Mathur N, Pedersen BK. Exercise as a mean to control low-grade systemic inflammation. *Mediators Inflamm.* 2008;2008:109502.

125. Petersen AM, Pedersen BK. The anti-inflammatory effect of exercise. *J Appl Physiol.* 2005;98(4):1154–1162.

126. Yudkin JS. Inflammation, obesity, and the metabolic syndrome. *Horm Metab Res.* 2007;39(10):707–709.

127. Zhang C, Rexrode KM, van Dam RM, et al. Abdominal obesity and the risk of all-cause, cardiovascular, and cancer mortality: sixteen years of follow-up in US women. *Circulation.* 2008;117(13):1658–1667.

128. Pischon T, Boeing H, Hoffmann K, et al. General and abdominal adiposity and risk of death in Europe. *New Engl J Med.* 2008;359(20):2105–2120.

129. Ross R, Janiszewski PM. Is weight loss the optimal target for obesity-related cardiovascular disease risk reduction? *Can J Cardiol.* 2008;24(suppl D):25D–31D.

130. Olsen RH, Krogh-Madsen R, Thomsen C, et al. Metabolic responses to reduced daily steps in healthy nonexercising men. *JAMA.* 2008;299(11):1261–1263.

131. Arthur PG, Grounds MD, Shavlakadze T. Oxidative stress as a therapeutic target during muscle wasting: considering the complex interactions. *Curr Opin Clin Nutr Metab Care.* 2008;11(4):408–416.

132. Jackson MJ. Reactive oxygen species and redox-regulation of skeletal muscle adaptations to exercise. *Philos Trans R Soc Lond B Biol Sci.* 2005;360(1464):2285–2291.

133. Juarez JC, Manuia M, Burnett ME, et al. Superoxide dismutase 1 (SOD1) is essential for H2O2-mediated oxidation and inactivation of phosphatases in growth factor signaling. *Proc Natl Acad Sci U S A.* 2008;105(20):7147–7152.

134. Gomez-Cabrera MC, Domenech E, Vina J. Moderate exercise is an antioxidant: upregulation of antioxidant genes by training. *Free Radic Biol Med.* 2008;44(2):126–131.

135. Reid MB. Free radicals and muscle fatigue: of ROS, canaries, and the IOC. *Free Radic Biol Med.* 2008;44(2):169–179.

136. Powers SK, Jackson MJ. Exercise-induced oxidative stress: cellular mechanisms and impact on muscle force production. *Physiol Rev.* 2008;88(4):1243–1276.

137. Perez CJ, Nemet D, Mills PJ, et al. Effects of laboratory versus field exercise on leukocyte subsets and cell adhesion molecule expression in children. *Eur J Appl Physiol.* 2001;86(1):34–39.

138. Boas SR, Joswiak ML, Nixon PA, et al. Effects of anaerobic exercise on the immune system in eight to seventeen year old trained and untrained boys. *J Pediatr.* 1996;129(6):846–855.

139. Dobbs RJ, Charlett A, Purkiss AG, et al. Association of circulating TNF-alpha and IL-6 with ageing and parkinsonism. *Acta Neurol Scand.* 1999;100(1):34–41.

140. Paolisso G, Rizzo MR, Mazziotti G, et al. Advancing age and insulin resistance: role of plasma tumor necrosis factor-alpha. *Am J Physiol.* 1998;275(2 Pt 1):E294–E299.

141. Bruunsgaard H, Pedersen M, Pedersen BK. Ageing and proinflammatory cytokines. *Curr Opinion Hematol.* 2001;8(3):131–136.

142. Bruunsgaard H, Andersen-Ranberg K, Jeune B, et al. A high plasma concentration of TNF-alpha is associated with dementia in centenarians. *J Gerontol A Biol Sci Med Sci.* 1999;54(7):M357–M364.

143. Ballou SP, Lozanski FB, Hodder S, et al. Quantitative and qualitative alterations of acute-phase proteins in healthy elderly persons. *Age Ageing.* 1996;25(3):224–230.

144. Bruunsgaard H, Pedersen AN, Schroll M, et al. Impaired production of proinflammatory cytokines in response to lipopolysaccharide (LPS) stimulation in elderly humans. *Clin Exp Immunol.* 1999;118(2):235–241.

145. Cowles WN. Fatigue as a contributory cause of pneumonia. *Boston Med Surg.* 1918;179:555.

146. Nicholls EE, Spaeth RA. The relation between fatigue and the susceptibility of guinea pigs to infections of type I pneumococcus. *Am J Hygiene.* 1922;2:527–535.

147. Oppenheim EH, Spaeth RA. The relation between fatigue and the susceptibility of rats towards a toxin and an infection. *Am J Hygiene.* 1922;2:51–66.

CHAPTER 21

The Body Fluid and Hemopoietic Systems

Gary W. Mack

Abbreviations

Å	Angstrom (0.1 nm)	P_d	Permeability coefficient for a particular molecule (cm/sec)
ANP	Atrial natriuretic peptide		
AVP	Arginine vasopressin	P_{osm}	Plasma osmolality (mOsmol · kg^{-1} H$_2$O)
BIA	Bioelectrical impedance analysis	PRES	hydrostatic pressure
BV	Blood volume	PV	Plasma volume
cap	Capillary	R	Universal gas constant
CFU	Colony-forming unit		(62.363 L · mmHg · K^{-1} · mol^{-1})
ECF	Extracellular fluid	RBC	Red blood cell
EPO	Erythropoietin	RCV	Red cell volume
ESA	Erythropoiesis-stimulating agent	rhEPO	Recombinant human erythropoietin
FFM	Fat-free mass	S	Surface area
GH	Growth hormone	S_aO_2	Hemoglobin saturation of arterial blood
Hb	Hemoglobin (g/dL)	SFO	Subfornical organ
Hct	Hematocrit (volume of packed red cells in percent)	SON	Supraoptic nucleus
		T	Absolute temperature in °K (Kelvin)
ICF	Intracellular fluid	TBV	Total blood volume
ISF	Interstitial fluid	TBW	Total body water
K$^+$	Potassium ion	$\dot{V}O_{2max}$	Maximal rate of oxygen consumption
Na$^+$	Sodium ion		
π	Colloid osmotic pressure or oncotic pressure (mmHg)		

Introduction

Within the human body, optimal cellular function is maintained as long as the internal environment maintains the proper concentration of nutrients (*e.g.*, oxygen and glucose), ions (*e.g.*, sodium (Na$^+$) and potassium (K$^+$)), and other essential constituents (*e.g.*, amino acids). The constancy of the body fluid bathing each cell, or what Claude Bernard called the "milieu intérieur," is determined by an interaction of several sophisticated physiologic control systems that act to attain homeostasis. Regulatory mechanisms involved in fluid homeostasis include the kidney (also see Chapter 22), which ultimately determines the rates of water and electrolyte output, and numerous extrarenal reflexes that modify rates of fluid and salt intake and adjust fluid distribution among various fluid compartments within the body. During exercise, fluid homeostasis is challenged in several ways. Body water is redistributed by fluid shifts between the vascular compartment and the interstitial fluid (ISF) compartment, and movement between the extracellular fluid (ECF) and intracellular fluid (ICF) compartments. During prolonged exercise, the loss of body water due to thermoregulatory sweating provides another impetus for body water redistribution.

The redistribution of body water evokes reflexes that act to restore the constancy of the milieu intérieur. Because the level of circulating blood volume (BV) needs to be protected to ensure adequate circulatory control and stability during exercise, the body also evokes reflexes that act to limit the magnitude of fluid loss from the vascular compartment. Finally, dynamic exercise training and or heat acclimation can alter the absolute size of various fluid compartments and the redistribution of fluids during exercise-induced dehydration. Specifically, exercise-induced hypervolemia (BV expansion) is considered a hallmark adaptation of endurance training. It is clear that the increase in BV provides an individual with a physiologic and thus performance-enhancing advantage during exercise. In this chapter, we will address the general characteristics of the body fluid compartments, the distribution of fluids at rest and during exercise, the impact of exercise on homeostatic control of body fluid balance, and adaptations of the fluid compartments to exercise training. Because the BV is composed primarily of the plasma volume (PV) and red cell volume (RCV), the regulation of RCV and its impact on exercise performance will also be discussed.

Body Fluid Compartments

The majority of total body water (TBW) fluid resides within the cells, or ICF space, and about one third is found in the space surrounding the cells, or ECF space (1). Water moves passively, via osmosis, along with the solutes as they are transported or move across boundary layers. The composition of the ICF is determined by the permeability and transport characteristics of the cell membrane; however, the ICF and EFC spaces have similar total osmolality values ($\approx$286 mOsmol/kg H_2O). The plasma osmolality (P_{osm}) is typically 1 mOsmol/kg H_2O higher than the ISF or ICF osmolality. It is known that the sodium and chloride concentrations in plasma and ISF water are different despite the high permeability of these electrolytes across the capillary interface. The difference in electrolyte concentrations is attributed to the higher protein concentration in the plasma compared with the ISF. The low permeability of protein across the capillary interface is responsible for the difference in electrolyte concentrations between the plasma and ISF, and is known as the Gibbs-Donnan equilibrium. Negatively charged proteins attract positively charged ions (*i.e.*, Na^+ and K^+) while repelling negatively charged ions (*i.e.*, Cl^-). Thus, the passive distribution of theses electrolytes is disturbed in order to maintain electroneutrality in each fluid compartment. The result is that P_{osm} is typically higher than the osmolality of the ISF or ICF compartment. Consequently, alterations in plasma protein concentration will result in changes in the distribution of electrolytes between the plasma and ISF due to the Gibbs-Donnan equilibrium. The ECF is mixed

throughout the body in a two-stage process. First, it is rapidly transported and distributed throughout the body via circulating plasma. Second, it is mixed between the plasma and fluid outside the vascular compartment, or ISF space, by diffusion and bulk transport across the capillary wall. A change in the water content of any of the body's fluid compartments will result in a redistribution of body water and an alteration of the solute concentration in all of the compartments.

We can estimate TBW from a measured dilution space using deuterium with a relative precision of 1.5% or about 0.6 L. Other dilution tracers, such as ethanol, are a viable alternative, but ethanol dilution underestimates TBW by 5% to 10% and the methodology has slightly less precision (2.6%) (2). Bioelectrical impedance analysis (BIA) can also be used to predict TBW; however, such measurements should be made with some caution. Single-frequency (50-kHz series) BIA instruments should be able to predict absolute TBW in a population of normal, healthy individuals as long as the ratio of ECF to ICF compartment size is within a physiologic range. However, these instruments are not accurate if a drug or disease significantly alters the ICF/ECF ratio. Also, single-frequency BIA units cannot detect small changes in TBW. A multifrequency BIA instrument using a 0/∞-kHz parallel Cole-Cole model will better predict small changes in TBW (3).

For the sedentary individual, TBW averages approximately 60% of body weight or about 600 mL/kg body weight (Fig. 21.1). The literature indicates that TBW varies with age, sex, weight, and lean body mass (1). However, when TBW is expressed as a function of fat-free mass (FFM; $\approx$780 $\pm$ 7 mL/kg FFM), it is similar across a wide range of ages (20–90 years), suggesting that differences in

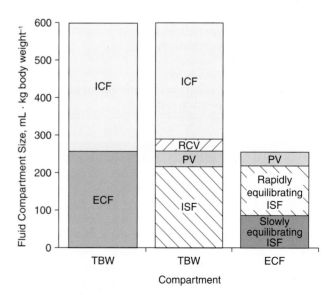

FIGURE 21.1 Schematic representation of the distribution of total body water (TBW) between various fluid compartments. ICF, intracellular fluid; RCV, red cell volume; PV, plasma volume; ISF, interstitial fluid; ECF, extracellular fluid.

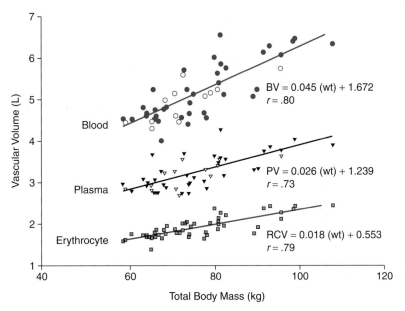

FIGURE 21.2 Plasma volume (PV), red cell volume (RCV), and total blood volume (TBV) as a function of body weight. (From Sawka MN, Young AJ, Pandolf KB, et al. Erythrocyte, plasma, and BV of healthy young men. *Med Sci Sports Exerc.* 1992;24:447–453.)

body composition contribute to most of the reported variability in TBW (4,5). The distribution of TBW between the various fluid compartments is illustrated in Figure 21.1. In combination with the inherent limitations of dilution methodology, heterogeneity within the extracellular compartments prevents precise identification of the other fluid compartment sizes. As such, the values for the distribution of TBW presented in Figure 22.1 should be viewed as only approximate.

The ICF compartment accounts for 55% of the H_2O content of TBW (≈50% for women and 60% for men) and the ECF compartment accounts for the remaining 45% (50% for women and 40% for men). Within the ECF compartment, fluid is distributed between the intravascular and extravascular fluid spaces. In the classical description, the ECF fluid is distributed between the plasma, which contains 7.5% of the TBW, and the ISF compartment, which holds ≈20% of the TBW. However, portions of the ISF space, identified by its inability to rapidly equilibrate with conventional tracer molecules, are

found in dense connective tissue and bone, and account for 7.5% and 7.5% of TBW, respectively (1). In addition, the activity of secretory cells within the body produces a fluid that is not a simple ultrafiltrate of plasma but is still considered a portion of the ISF compartment. This fluid space is identified as the transcellular fluid compartment and accounts for 2.5% of TBW. This distribution of TBW is illustrated in Figure 21.1.

In general, for a 70-kg man, the ECF volume averages 260 mL/kg body weight or 43% of TBW and is determined primarily by the total body sodium content. The ICF volume averages 330 mL/kg body weight or ≈55% of TBW. The PV is ≈17% of the ECF space and averages 45 mL/kg body weight, and RCV averages 31 mL/kg body weight. The result is that BV averages ≈76 mL/kg body weight in sedentary adults. Figure 21.2 illustrates the relationship between vascular compartment size and body weight.

Table 21.1 summarizes the fluid compartment sizes and includes the norms published by the International

TABLE 21.1	Body Fluid Compartment Size in Sedentary Individuals and Trained Athletes						
Category	TBW mL/kg	ICF mL/kg	ECF mL/kg	ISF mL/kg	PV mL/kg	RCV mL/kg	BV mL/kg
NORMS	600	340	260	220	40	31	71
Sedentary	627	366	246	201	45	31	76
Trained athlete	671	424	247	189	58	42	100

Absolute volumes are expressed as milliliter per kilogram of body weight, and relative changes are expressed as a change in volume as a percentage of the appropriate control. The values for TBW, ICF, ECF, and ISF volumes for sedentary and trained athletes represent mean values calculated from limited data available in the literature (52,61,87). The values for PV, RCV, and BV represent the average of reported values in the literature (13,51,57,88,89). The clinical database (NORMS) represents values for the standard human as reported by the International Commission on Radiological Protection in 1975. TBW, total body water; ICF, intracellular fluid space; ECF, extracellular fluid; ISF, interstitial fluid; PV, plasma volume; RCV, red cell volume; BV, blood volume.

Commission on Radiological Protection (6). The compartment sizes for sedentary and exercise-trained individuals reported in Table 21.1 represent average values reported in the literature. A deviation of these numbers from the expected norms will reflect both individual variability and measurement errors associated with the various tracers used to estimate TBW, ECF, PV, and RCV.

It is well established that total exchangeable sodium, total exchangeable potassium, and TBW determine plasma sodium concentration. Edelman et al. (7) first quantified this in a study in which they proposed the following equation to describe the relationship between plasma sodium concentration (mEq · L^{-1} water) and exchangeable sodium, potassium, and TBW:

$$[Na^+]_p = 1.11 \frac{(Na^+_e + K^+_e)}{TBW} - 25.6 \qquad [1]$$

where Na^+_e = total body exchangeable sodium, and K^+_e = total body exchangeable potassium.

Nguyen and Kurtz (8) further explored this relationship and provided a simple approach for using this relationship to examine dysnatremias (a disturbance in sodium balance):

$$[Na^+]_p' = \frac{([Na^+]_p + 23.8)\, TBW_i + 1.03 \times E_{MB}}{TBW_i + V_{MB}} - 23.8 \qquad [2]$$

where $[Na^+]_p$ is the plasma sodium concentration (mEq · L^{-1} plasma) that results from a change in the mass balance of TBW (V_{MB}) and/or a change in the mass balance of exchangeable sodium and potassium (E_{MB}). This simple equation can be used to examine how electrolyte and water balance impact serum sodium levels.

TEST YOURSELF

Using Equation 2 above, predict whether an individual will develop hyponatremia given the following information:

- A 70-kg man with an initial TBW = 25 L.
- Exercise in the heat for 3 hours, and hydration with water to maintain body weight
- Initial plasma sodium concentration = 140 mEq/liter plasma
- Sweat lost = 3 L with a composition of 50 mEq Na$^+$/L and 5 mEq K$^+$/L
- Urine production = 500 mL of urine with a composition of ≈25 mEq Na$^+$/L and 15 mEq K$^+$/L

It is well known that a portion of the exchangeable body sodium is not osmotically active. Such inactive sodium depots have been identified in bone (1) and possibly skin (9). However, it is unclear whether these storage depots are a fixed size or can change in size. These storage sites may take up or release sodium and

thereby influence plasma sodium levels. Heer et al. (10) observed a positive sodium balance in subjects without a change in body weight or expansion of the ECF space. The authors proposed that some of the sodium was inactivated by being taken up by the inactive sodium depots; however, they failed to correct for potassium balance. The modified Edelman equation indicates that a negative potassium balance could easily explain the results obtained by Herr et al. (10). Recent work by Seeliger et al. (11) clearly indicates that when the mass balance of sodium, potassium, and water is taken into consideration during sodium loading experiments, all of the accumulated sodium is in an osmotically active form. At present, the ability to regulate the size of the osmotically inactive sodium pool has not been adequately demonstrated. As such, it is inappropriate to implicate an osmotically inactive sodium pool in the development of a dysnatremia unless the water, sodium, and potassium balance is first taken into account.

Dynamic exercise training, specifically of an endurance nature, causes an increase in most fluid compartments (Table 21.1). Limited data on the measurement of TBW, ICF, and ECF compartment sizes in endurance-trained athletes makes a comparison with sedentary individuals somewhat speculative; however, the data in Table 21.1 provide a reasonable view of the available literature. Because TBW expressed per kilogram of FFM is fairly constant over an individual's life span, it is possible that the differences in TBW (expressed in mL/kg body weight) between trained athletes and untrained individuals will disappear when the data are normalized to FFM (12).

Sufficient data have been published to clearly establish that endurance-trained athletes undergo considerable BV expansion (Table 21.1). A cross-sectional look at the available data indicates that PV, RCV, and BV values are about 30% higher in endurance-trained athletes than in sedentary individuals. In sedentary individuals, PV averages about 45 mL/kg BW or approximately 18% of the ECF compartment size. In endurance-trained athletes, PV averages 58 mL/kg or about 23% of the ECF space. Of importance, data collected from cross-sectional analyses of endurance-trained athletes and sedentary individuals indicate that the increase in BV with endurance training is shared by an increase in PV and RCV. In longitudinal training studies lasting anywhere from 3 to 21 days, the increase in BV is limited to only 10% to 15%. In addition, the increase in PV is usually greater than the increase in RCV (noticeable hemodilution). Figure 21.3 illustrates the time course of the change that occurs in vascular compartments during endurance training. A high BV, even in individuals with no history of exercise training, is associated with a high maximal rate of oxygen consumption ($\dot{V}O_{2max}$) (13). Finally, an individual's state of heat acclimation also contributes to the size and distribution of TBW. Table 21.2 illustrates the ability of heat acclimation to produce a generalized expansion of the ECF compartment, particularly PV and ISF volume, with little impact on ICF compartment size or RCV (14).

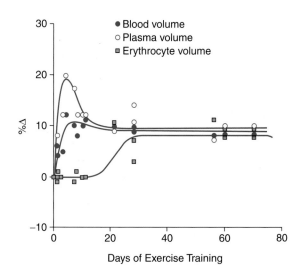

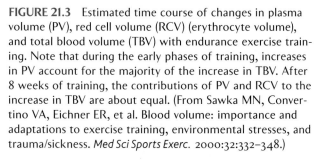

FIGURE 21.3 Estimated time course of changes in plasma volume (PV), red cell volume (RCV) (erythrocyte volume), and total blood volume (TBV) with endurance exercise training. Note that during the early phases of training, increases in PV account for the majority of the increase in TBV. After 8 weeks of training, the contributions of PV and RCV to the increase in TBV are about equal. (From Sawka MN, Convertino VA, Eichner ER, et al. Blood volume: importance and adaptations to exercise training, environmental stresses, and trauma/sickness. *Med Sci Sports Exerc.* 2000:32:332–348.)

Summary

Exercise training results in an increase in TBW and a generalized expansion of both the ECF and ICF compartments. However, when exercise training is combined with heat stress (heat acclimation), we see an additional fluid compartment expansion that is limited to the ECF space. Overall, the increase in ECF compartment size, and particularly the increase in PV, will provide cardiovascular stability in subsequent exercise bouts.

Water Balance and Exercise

Water homeostasis and osmoregulation are critical physiologic functions for the survival of all organisms. Water and salt balance are maintained by behavioral and physiologic reflexes that act to control ingestive behaviors (*e.g.*, water intake and sodium appetite) and water and electrolyte losses. Exercise impacts water and electrolyte homeostasis in several ways. First, exercise causes a fluid shift out of the vascular compartment, initiating reflex responses that act to defend PV and hence BV during exercise. Second, prolonged thermoregulatory sweating during exercise leads to a loss of water and electrolytes, which in turn leads to exercise-induced dehydration and the initiation of osmoregulatory reflexes. Control of urinary excretion of water through osmoregulatory control of arginine vasopressin (AVP) secretion will help limit the magnitude of water loss by the kidney during exercise. Finally, the restoration of water deficits following exercise-induced dehydration is controlled by the sensation of thirst and ingestive behaviors that regulate fluid intake. The maintenance of water and electrolyte homeostasis under any set of conditions (during exercise or recovery from dehydration) reflects the balance between ingestive behaviors that restore lost water (and electrolytes) and water and electrolyte retention by renal mechanisms. In this section, we will examine these three aspects of exercise and fluid balance.

Water Distribution at Rest

The steady-state volumes for each fluid compartment are listed in Table 21.1 and reflect the impact of net water movement under resting conditions. At rest and during exercise, water is continually exchanged between the fluid compartments. The forces guiding these water fluxes are osmotic and hydrostatic. Osmosis is the primary mechanism by which water exchange occurs between the ICF and ISF compartments. The osmotic gradient for water exchange is determined by the concentration gradient of osmotically active substances. The concentration of osmotically active substances or osmolality (expressed as milliosmoles per kilogram of water) is determined by the total solute concentration. Electrolytes contribute predominantly to the transmembrane osmotic gradient. However, as the result of active transport and metabolic processes, the cell contains high concentrations of amino acids, nucleotides, and small organic molecules that are impermeable to the plasma membrane. These molecules are charged and their counterions contribute to the total osmolality of the intracellular compartment (known as the

TABLE 21.2	Changes in Body Fluid Compartment Size with Training and Heat Acclimation						
Category	TBW Δ%	ICF Δ%	ECF Δ%	ISF Δ%	PV Δ%	RCV Δ%	BV Δ%
Training: cross-sectional	7	16	—	−6	29	35	32
Training: longitudinal					11	8	9
Heat acclimation	4	<1	14.4	17.7	15	<1	15

Changes (Δ) in total body water (TBW), intracellular fluid (ICF), extracellular fluid (ECF), interstitial fluid (ISF), plasma volume (PV), red cell volume (RCV), and blood volume (BV). Changes are expressed as a percentage of the initial value. The values for ΔTBW, ΔICF, ΔECF, and ΔISF volumes for sedentary and trained athletes represent mean values calculated from limited data available in the literature (52,61,87). The values for ΔPV, ΔRCV, and ΔBV represent the average of reported values in the literature for longitudinal training programs (13,51,57,88,89).

Heat acclimation data were obtained from Patterson MJ, Stocks JM, Taylor NA. Sustained and generalized extracellular fluid expansion following heat acclimation. J Physiol. 2004;559:327–334.

Donnan effect). van't Hoff's equation defines the relationship between solute concentration and osmotic pressure:

$$\pi = [\text{solute}] \cdot R \cdot T \qquad [3]$$

where π is osmotic pressure in millimeters of mercury (mm Hg), R is the universal gas constant, and T is the absolute temperature.

Intracellular osmolality is controlled by adjusting the rate of transport of solute into (to prevent dehydration) or out of (to prevent overhydration) the cell to regulate cell volume.

Transcapillary exchange of fluid

The distribution of fluid between the intravascular compartment and the ISF space is governed by parameters outlined by Starling in 1896 and experimentally verified by Landis in 1927. Transcapillary fluid movement follows the difference in hydrostatic pressure and osmotic pressure across the capillary, and is described by what is known as the Starling-Landis equation (15):

$$j_V/S = Lp \cdot (PRES_{cap} - PRES_{ISF}) + \sigma_d \, (\pi_{cap} - \pi_{ISF}) \qquad [4]$$

where j_V is the solvent (water) flux across the capillary per unit surface area (S), Lp is the hydraulic conductivity (permeability), S is the capillary surface area, PRES is the hydrostatic pressure in mm Hg, cap is capillary, σ_d is the osmotic reflection coefficient, and π is the colloid osmotic pressure in mm Hg.

Classically, we solve this equation by substituting global values for hydrostatic and colloid osmotic pressures in plasma and tissue ISF. Standard values for the parameters of the Starling-Landis equation under resting conditions are listed in Table 21.3.

At the arteriolar end of the capillary, the net hydrostatic pressure gradient that is trying to force fluid out of the capillary (Δ PRES = 34 mm Hg) exceeds the net colloid osmotic pressure gradient that is pulling fluid into the vascular compartment ($\Delta \pi = -20$ mm Hg). Consequently, fluid filtration out of the vascular compartment occurs. At the venular end of the capillary, the net colloid osmotic pressure gradient that is pulling fluid into the capillary ($\Delta \pi = -20$ mm Hg) exceeds the net hydrostatic pressure gradient that is forcing fluid out of the capillary (Δ PRES = 12 mm Hg). Under these conditions, fluid moves back into the vascular compartment (reabsorption). Normally, the amount of fluid that is filtered only slightly exceeds the volume of fluid that is reabsorbed. The remaining fluid is returned to the vascular compartment via the lymphatic capillaries.

At about the same time that Starling and Landis were describing the biophysical principles that govern transcapillary fluid flow, it was observed that blood composition during exercise showed an increase in red blood cell (RBC) number or hematocrit (Hct). The increase in Hct during exercise was first thought to be the result of an increase in the number of RBCs mobilized from some unknown "vascular storage" site in the abdominal region (i.e., the spleen). However, several scientists were convinced that the increase in Hct during exercise was the result of water movement out of the vascular compartment as described by Starling and Landis. The latter hypothesis soon became the dominant explanation for changes in RBC number during exercise.

Transcapillary exchange of macromolecules

Transcapillary exchange of macromolecules is described by a set of equations derived by Kedem and Katchalsky (16):

$$j_s/S = j_V/S \, (1 - \sigma_d) \cdot [\text{solute}]_{mean} + P_d \cdot ([\text{solute}]_{cap} - [\text{solute}]_{ISF}) \qquad [5]$$

where j_s/S is the solute flux per unit area, and P_d is the diffusional permeability.

This equation describes the important parameters that govern microvascular exchange across a homoporous membrane in a global sense, but it does not directly address the exact structure-function relationship of microvascular transport. Recent advances in the field of microvascular exchange have significantly improved our understanding of this process and should be reviewed by anyone who is interested in the study of fluid balance (17,18). Rippe and Haraldsson (18) proposed a two-pore theory of capillary permeability, which holds that capillary barrier characteristics can be described in terms of pore (channel) size and number. In this model, the pathways for macromolecule transport through microvascular walls of continuous capillaries (i.e., those found in skeletal muscle) are depicted as water-filled pores (or channels) of fixed diameter (small pores with a radius of ≈40 Å and large pores with a radius of 250–200 Å). The spaces between adjacent endothelial cells (interendothelial clefts or slits)

TABLE 21.3	Approximate Starling Forces in Resting Skeletal Muscle							
Capillary	PRES$_{cap}$	PRES$_{ISF}$	ΔPRES	π_{cap}	π_{ISF}	$\Delta\pi$	Net	
Arteriolar	+32	−2	+34	+25	+5	−20	+14	filtration
Venular	+10	−2	+12	+25	+5	−20	−8	reabsorption

Hydrostatic and colloid osmotic pressures are given in mm Hg. PRES$_{cap}$, capillary hydrostatic pressure; PRES$_{ISF}$, ISF hydrostatic pressure gradient; π_{cap}, capillary colloid osmotic pressure; π_{ISF}, ISF colloid osmotic pressure gradient; $_{Net}$, sum of ΔPRES and $\Delta\pi$ (15,18).

are the most likely candidates for these small pores. The large pores are thought to represent either interendothelial clefts that are wider than the typical small pore or large-radius (300–700 Å) transcellular channels. In general, the solute transport across most capillary beds can be described by the presence of small pores that restrict proteins and few non–size-selective large pores. The number and type of pores per unit area can account for differences in permeability between various vascular beds. The two-pore concept is the simplest model to account for most, but not all, of the transport characteristics of capillary macromolecule exchange and fluid flux. More recently, Michel and Curry (17) described a fiber-matrix model of capillary permeability. In this model, the pore size is not determined by the tight junction size (interendothelial clefts) but by the characteristics of a molecular filter (fiber matrix) associated with the endothelial cell glycocalyx. This surface glycocalyx acts as a primary molecular sieve and diffusion barrier for plasma proteins. In the fiber matrix model, the Starling forces that determine fluid exchange are the hydrostatic and oncotic pressure gradients across the glycocalyx or fenestral diaphragm rather than the typical global gradients in hydrostatic and oncotic pressure between plasma and tissue. This view of transcapillary exchange leads to two dramatic changes in our view of the Starling forces. First, local Starling forces are heterogeneous across the length of the capillary. Second, the local protein and tissue pressure just behind the glycocalyx or fenestral diaphragm (endothelial fenestrae spanned by a diaphragm) determine the hydrostatic and oncotic pressure gradients for fluid and solute movement rather than some global tissue pressure or protein concentration. These concepts help to explain large spatial variations in local water flux across the surface glycocalyx. Both models provide a better understanding of the biophysics of capillary exchange.

Fluid Shifts and Dynamic Exercise

In contracting muscles, fluid exchange between the vascular compartment and the interstitial space is controlled by the prevailing Starling forces across microvascular beds and the osmotic gradients between ICF and ECF spaces. It is difficult to measure rapid changes in ECF or ICF spaces in humans; however, rapid fluid shifts into or out of the vascular compartment can be estimated reliably and accurately. One of the first observations associated with the impact of exercise on hematologic variables was an increase in the volume of packed red cells (Hct). The increase in Hct was associated with a shift of protein-free fluid out of the vascular compartment into the tissue ISF space. It is now recognized that this PV shift in response to exercise can be estimated by measuring changes in Hct and hemoglobin (Hb) using the following equation (19):

$$\%\Delta PV = 100 \times \left[\frac{Hb_{CON}}{Hb_t} \times \frac{(1 - Hct_t \times 100)}{(1 - Hct_{CON} \times 100)} \right] - 100$$

[6]

where $\%\Delta PV$ is the percent change in PV, Hb is the hemoglobin concentration in grams per deciliter (g/dL), CON is the control blood sample, and t is the blood sample at time t after the control sample.

This equation describes the change in PV relative to a control condition. It is critical to understand that this calculation is only as accurate as the precision of the control condition. The simple act of changing one's posture from supine to standing is associated with significant hemoconcentration. Thus, the upright posture causes a fluid movement out of the vascular space, with maximal hemoconcentration occurring some 40 to 60 minutes later. This posture-dependent hemoconcentration may or may not mask the impact of exercise on the PV shift. For example, in the upright posture on a cycle ergometer, the PV shift during dynamic exercise of 70% of $\dot{V}O_{2max}$ averages about -17% if the exercise is preceded by a short 10- to 15-minute control period. On the other hand, the PV shift during dynamic exercise will be negligible if the control period lasts 60 minutes or longer. There is no absolute answer as to how long one must maintain a given posture before body fluid equilibrium occurs. If the experiment controls for posture and time spent in the posture before exercise, reasonable comparisons between control and experimental groups can be made. However, a 60-minute postural control period provides an excellent starting point for any experiment designed to measure accurate changes in PV using the Dill-Costill equation (Eq. 6). Contraction of the spleen occurs during exercise in humans; however, release of RBCs by the spleen into the circulation has little impact on circulating erythrocyte volume or peripheral Hct. This means that contraction of the spleen does not influence estimates of PV shifts obtained with the Dill-Costill equation.

Fluid shifts during mild dynamic exercise

Early research clearly showed that PV shifts during exercise interact with posture. Therefore, in this discussion, we will focus primarily on upright cycle ergometer exercise when describing the general phenomenon of fluid shifts during exercise. During upright dynamic cycle ergometer exercise, the PV shift out of the vascular compartment is proportional to the relative exercise intensity (% $\dot{V}O_{2max}$) (20–22). At maximal aerobic power ($\dot{V}O_{2max}$), a fluid volume equal to 20% to 25% of the initial PV will move out of the vascular compartment during the first 5 to 15 minutes of exercise. The plasma composition of electrolytes is unaltered by the fluid shift at exercise intensities lower than 40% $\dot{V}O_{2max}$, indicating that the fluid that leaves the vascular compartment is isotonic with plasma. At the onset of muscle contraction, $PRES_{cap}$ rises rapidly and is sustained at this elevated level for the duration of the exercise (23). The rise in $PRES_{cap}$ during exercise is proportional to the rise in mean arterial blood pressure (MAP). This is an interesting observation because normally $PRES_{cap}$ is autoregulated, such that it changes very little over a wide range of arterial blood pressures. However, during exercise this autoregulation is lost. The coupling of $PRES_{cap}$ to MAP during exercise is most likely related to the large increase in blood flow to active skeletal muscle as a result of metabolic hyperemia and a functional sympatholysis. At the onset of exercise, the rise in $PRES_{cap}$ promotes a rapid efflux of isotonic fluid from the vascular compartment.

Fluid shifts during moderate to heavy dynamic exercise

At higher exercise intensities, hypotonic fluid is shifted out of the vascular compartment, which causes P_{osm} to increase. In addition, increased activity of skeletal muscles results in a local intracellular and interstitial hyperosmolality. During heavy dynamic exercise, the skeletal muscle ICF lactate concentration can increase from 5 to >29 mmol/L, whereas extracellular lactate can increase from 1.3 to >13 mmol/L (24). These increases in lactate concentration create a favorable osmotic gradient for water into the ICF space of the active skeletal muscle cell. During heavy exercise, the increase in skeletal muscle ECF space is about 10 times greater than the increase in ICF space. The lag times in the rate of equilibrium between the ISF and vascular compartment indicate that a rapid increase in interstitial osmolality could also contribute to the movement of water out of the vascular compartment.

During heavy exercise, P_{osm} will increase by 15 mOsmol/kg H_2O. According to van't Hoff's law, this equates to an osmotic gradient of 200 mm Hg. The increase in P_{osm} during exercise acts to limit excessive reductions in PV and thus maintain circulating BV. An interesting observation is that during graded exercise, the rise in plasma sodium concentration is proportional to the rise in plasma lactate (25). The stoichiometry of the increase in lactate and sodium in the plasma during exercise suggests that the negatively charged lactate ion restricts Na^+ efflux from the vascular compartment as its accompanying hydrogen ion is buffered by the carbonic anhydrase reaction. This coupling of Na^+ with the lactate will serve to limit fluid efflux from the plasma compartment and help maintain circulating BV and cardiovascular stability. Figure 21.4 illustrates the general relationship between relative exercise intensity, P_{osm}, and PV during upright cycle ergometer exercise.

Starling equilibrium during prolonged dynamic exercise

As exercise continues, the rate of fluid efflux from the plasma declines and a new Starling equilibrium is established as the result of several adjustments. First, a washout of local ISF solute occurs due to increased blood flow to the active skeletal muscle and a slight rise in local tissue hydrostatic pressure ($PRES_{ISF}$) (26). The rise in ISF hydrostatic pressure is a function of the pressure–volume relationship (or compliance) of the ISF compartment. The rise in capillary filtration and muscle pump activity will also lead to an increase in lymph flow. The increase in lymph flow serves a dual purpose: the increased filtration and lymph flow will flush lymph proteins

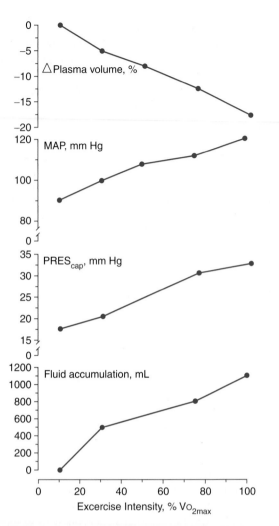

FIGURE 21.4 Impact of relative exercise intensity on plasma volume, plasma osmolality (P_{osm}), and capillary hydrostatic pressure ($PRES_{cap}$), and tissue fluid accumulation during upright cycle ergometer exercise.

into the vascular compartment, causing a small decline in π_{ISF} (27), and the increase in lymph flow will then cause an influx of lymphatic protein into the vascular space and thus increase π_{cap}. In addition, as hypotonic fluid leaves the vascular compartment, there is an accompanying rise in plasma oncotic pressure. This rise in plasma oncotic pressure will oppose the hydrostatic pressure gradient. These adjustments in the Starling forces act to limit fluid efflux from the vascular compartment and maintain circulating BV.

The magnitude of the fluid accumulation in active skeletal muscle immediately after exercise has been measured. During upright cycle ergometer exercise, the total volume of fluid that accumulates in active skeletal muscle averages about 18, 30, and 45 mL/kg active muscle during light, moderate, and heavy exercise, respectively (28). These values represent absolute volume accumulations of about 500, 800, and 1100 mL after light, moderate, and heavy exercise, respectively, for a 70-kg human. During heavy exercise, the net reduction in PV averages about 600 mL or 20% of the initial PV (29). To compensate for the large fluid accumulation that occurs in active skeletal muscle during exercise, the vascular compartment must simultaneously absorb fluid from nonactive tissue to minimize the reduction in PV (30). Again, the driving forces for this fluid absorption are the Starling forces (Eq. 4). Increased sympathetic nerve signals sent to inactive tissues during exercise will result in vasoconstriction. Arteriolar vasoconstriction will cause a reduction in $PRES_{cap}$, causing the $\Delta Press$ gradient to favor absorption of fluid into the vascular compartment. During heavy exercise, the P_{osm} and plasma protein concentration (*i.e.*, π_{cap}) will increase. Thus, both a decrease in hydrostatic pressure gradient and an increase in the osmotic pressure gradient contribute to fluid absorption into the vascular compartment from inactive tissues (*e.g.*, skin, intestines, and noncontracting muscle). Without the absorption of water from inactive tissues, the fall in PV during exercise would likely limit cardiovascular and exercise performance.

Modulation of fluid shifts during dynamic exercise

Although the Starling forces are the primary regulators of fluid exchange during exercise, there are several factors that also modulate fluid shifts. The list of variables that are thought to impact PV regulation during exercise is extensive and includes hormones, exercise mode (*e.g.*, cycling, treadmill walking, and swimming), posture, exercise intensity, muscle mass (arm vs. leg exercise), gender, menstrual cycle phase, hydration status, and fitness level. In this section, we will focus only on the role of a few important factors that act as modulators of fluid shifts during exercise.

Atrial natriuretic peptide (ANP) is known to directly alter capillary permeability to water and albumin, and indirectly alter capillary permeability by increasing the hydrostatic pressure gradient for fluid efflux by changing the ratio of precapillary and postcapillary resistance (arteriolar dilation leads to increase $PRES_{cap}$). During upright exercise (*e.g.*, treadmill walking), the plasma concentration of ANP will increase in proportion to exercise intensity. If the identical treadmill exercise (*i.e.*, with an identical energy cost) is performed in water (up to the xyphoid process), we will see a greater release of ANP and a larger plasma fluid shift out of the vascular space (31). These observations provide evidence that ANP plays a role in modulating the PV shift during dynamic exercise.

The exercise mode has an impact on fluid shifts during exercise. Arm-cranking exercise produces a relatively larger PV shift compared with leg exercise at the same $\dot{V}O_2$ (22). The greater PV shift that occurs during arm exercise is proportional to the larger MAP and thus the greater increase in the critical Starling force, $PRES_{cap}$. At similar absolute exercise intensity (*i.e.*, same $\dot{V}O_2$), swimming and upright cycling produce the same shift in PV out of the vascular compartment (32). Body fluid status prior to exercise will also impact fluid shifts during exercise. During light-intensity treadmill exercise, in-air hemodilution occurs in euhydrated subjects, whereas hemoconcentration occurs in hypohydrated (-5% of body weight) subjects (33).

Summary

The balance of the Starling forces during exercise determines fluid shifts between the intravascular and ISF compartments. During exercise, these Starling forces are influenced not only by exercise intensity but also by gravitational forces (e.g., posture), hydrostatic forces (e.g., water immersion and lower body positive pressure), and/or humoral factors (e.g., ANP). Because of this complex interaction, it is difficult to derive a simple description of fluid shifts during exercise. What is clear is that the maximal degree of PV shift during exercise is limited to about 20%. Therefore, regardless of which factor dominates (exercise or gravity), the fluid shift out of the vascular compartment will be limited and balanced by a rise in $PRES_{ISF}$, P_{osm}, and π_{cap}.

Exercise-Induced Dehydration

As exercise continues, body water is lost due to thermoregulatory sweating and insensible water loss. Body temperatures (core and skin) and ambient conditions determine thermoregulatory sweating during exercise. Maximal whole body sweat loss during dry heat exposure in humans has been reported to be 1.5 to 2.0 kg/hour, but some researchers have reported values as high as 3.0 to 4.0 kg/hour during heavy exercise in the heat (33,34). It should be noted, however, that local sweat rates at different sites on the body surface vary considerably. In humans, water loss from the respiratory system (*i.e.*, insensible water loss) can contribute an additional 0.12 kg/hour of water loss during heavy exercise. Thus, a 70-kg adult could lose on the order of 2.5% of his or her water content ($\approx 60\%$–65% of body mass) per hour of heavy exercise in the heat. The majority of this water loss is due to sweating. However, the loss of body water due to sensible and insensible water loss is offset by the gain of water by the body from metabolism and release of water bound to glycogen. Exercising at an oxygen cost of 42 mL O_2/min/kg body weight will result in the production of about 122 g H_2O/hour. As glycogen is metabolized, the water that is complexed with this molecule (≈ 2.7 g H_2O per 1 g glycogen) is released. Burning 100 g glycogen per hour can liberate 0.3 to 0.4 L of water per hour into the TBW pool. It is important to note that during exercise-induced dehydration,

TEST YOURSELF

A trained runner (age: 21 years; body mass: 65 kg) runs an ultra-distance race at a pace equal to about 71% of his $\dot{V}O_{2max}$. His sweat rate during the race averages 1.2 kg/hour, and the rate of glycogen depletion is about 80 g/hour. He ingests approximately 400 mL of water per hour during the race. What is his body mass at the end of the 3-hour race? Is this runner clinically dehydrated at the end of the race?

an individual can experience a loss of sweat and respiratory water but still maintain TBW by a gain of body water from metabolism (CHO or FAT + $O_2 \rightarrow CO_2 + H_2O$) or the release of water during a reduction in glycogen stores.

Sweat is a hypotonic fluid with an average $[Na^+]$ and $[K^+]$ of 56.4 (range: 30.6–105.7) and 9.6 (range: 6.9–11.5) mEq/liter, respectively (34). Assuming an average sweat concentration of 55 mEq Na^+ per liter, we can estimate that a 70-kg adult will lose $\approx$96 mEq Na^+ per hour or $\approx$3.3% of the total exchangeable Na^+ per hour. Thus, in addition to the loss of water due to sweating, there is a concomitant loss of electrolytes. From previous discussions, it is clear that the ECF and ICF compartments share these exercise-induced water and electrolyte deficits. It is also clear that the ability to mobilize water from the extravascular to the intravascular space during exercise will help maintain circulating BV, an important step in ensuring optimal regulation of both arterial blood pressure and temperature.

Water and electrolyte losses during dynamic exercise

During light dynamic exercise in the heat (with a body weight decrease from 2.0 to 6.0 kg), the water losses are equally distributed between the ECF and ICF spaces (34). Within the ECF compartment, water loss from the plasma averages around 20% of the ECF volume loss. This is expected, because at rest before dehydration occurs, plasma water accounts for about 20% of the ECF volume. Given that extracellular Na^+ content determines the size of the ECF compartment, it is easy to see why the loss of Na^+ from the body would closely predict the decrease in ECF space. During dehydration, the $[Na^+]$ in sweat determines the amount of free water loss from the body via the sweat gland (analogous to free water loss by the kidney) and the subsequent increase in P_{osm} (35). The rise in P_{osm} will contribute to the osmotic gradient between the ICF and ECF compartments in inactive tissue and determine the amount of water mobilized into the vascular compartment by osmosis. The mobilization of fluid from the ICF into the ECF space will act to prevent excessive reductions in PV and circulating BV, and provide cardiovascular stability during dehydration. The mobilization of fluid from the ICF to ECF space cannot prevent the decline in PV, because the reduction in PV during dehydration is generally proportional to the reduction in TBW. However, the magnitude of the reduction in PV during dehydration can be attenuated. The maintenance of circulating BV during exercise-induced dehydration is a function of the body's ability to mobilize fluid from the ICF space, which itself is linked to the sodium concentration in sweat (35). Thus, a more dilute sweat allows a greater conservation of the PV during dehydration, primarily due to the greater movement of water from the ICF compartment. It should be noted that sweat $[Na^+]$ is generally lower in heat-acclimated individuals and trained athletes, indicating an improved ability to maintain circulating BV during exercise-induced dehydration.

Water and electrolyte loss during dynamic exercise is dependent on the environmental conditions. Kozlowski and Saltin (36) showed that thermal dehydration (*e.g.*, from a sauna bath) and mild exercise in the heat produce similar reductions in TBW and ECF, and match the reductions discussed above. However, heavy exercise performed in a cool environment results in a slightly higher loss of total exchangeable potassium and only minimal reductions in ECF (<4% of the reduction in TBW) and PV (36). Most of the reduction in TBW was ascribed to a decrease in ICF volume.

Summary

Water losses during exercise are generally distributed between all fluid compartments and are influenced by the associated electrolyte losses. Exercise intensity and environmental temperature influence the redistribution of TBW after exercise-induced dehydration occurs. It is unclear what role excess potassium losses play in the reduction of ICF during heavy exercise in a cool environment.

Osmoregulatory responses to exercise-induced dehydration

Exercise-induced dehydration results in hyperosmolality and hypovolemia. Physiologic compensation for the reduction in the size and tonicity of the cellular fluid and ECF compartment involves modification of water and sodium losses by the kidney through the action of water- and sodium-retaining hormones and modulation of efferent renal sympathetic nerve activity. Two prominent responses to exercise-induced dehydration are a release of AVP and an increase in plasma rennin activity.

During exercise, plasma levels of AVP increase in a linear fashion after P_{osm} exceeds a certain threshold. At rest, this threshold is $\approx$280 to 285 mOsmol/kg H_2O (37,38), and during exercise it increases in proportion to the exercise intensity (25). The threshold P_{osm} that elicits the increase in AVP is also dependent on the size of the intravascular compartment, such that during dehydration both the increase in P_{osm} and reduction in PV will contribute to the increase in AVP and result in a high AVP level at any given osmotic drive. Several other factors contribute to the release of AVP, including an elevation in body temperature, muscle receptor activation, and elevated plasma levels of angiotensin II. In a study by Convertino et al. (39), during heat stress, elevated body temperature increased plasma AVP from 1.2 to 5.5 pg/mL, while P_{osm} increased only 2.4 mOsmol/kg. The increase in AVP per unit change in P_{osm} observed during passive heat stress was two times greater than predicted from the linear relationship between P_{osm} and AVP during hypertonic saline infusion. Thus, an increase in body temperature provides an additional stimulus for AVP release during exercise (also see Chapter 23).

In humans, after exercise-induced dehydration occurs, urine osmolality is on the order of 1000 to 1400 mOsmol/kg H_2O, which is greater than that seen during infusions of large doses of AVP. Thus, the maximal concentrating ability of the kidney after exercise-induced dehydration is not entirely dependent on the action of elevated AVP. In response to a decrease in PV during dehydration, renin release from the juxtaglomerular cells will be increased in response to a reduction in sodium load to the macula densa (*i.e.*, reduced glomerular filtration rate), reduced arterial blood pressure in afferent arterioles, increased renal sympathetic nerve activity, or increased levels of circulating catecholamines. The activation of the renin-angiotensin-aldosterone axis will enhance renal sodium reabsorption during prolonged exercise in the heat.

Rehydration Following Exercise

After exercise-induced dehydration occurs, water balance is restored by the integration of behavioral and physiologic reflexes that act to control ingestive behaviors (water intake) and urinary excretion (water loss). Control of urinary excretion through osmoregulatory control of AVP secretion will limit water loss by the kidney. However, this control system has no ability to restore lost water. Therefore, the restoration of body fluid balance after dehydration induced by exercise (or any other stress) ultimately depends on reflexes that regulate fluid intake. Unfortunately, the pattern of rehydration in humans displays a distinct delay in the restoration of water balance despite unlimited access to water, a problem referred to as "involuntary dehydration" (40). Such a delay is not seen in all animal species. In fact, a dehydrated dog will drink exactly the required volume of water to restore fluid balance within a 5 minute period (41). However, humans (and other species) are considered to be slow rehydrators. In this section, we will describe the physiologic and behavior control systems that contribute to the restoration of body fluid balance following dehydration, and try to explain the physiologic nature of involuntary dehydration.

Dipsogenic signals

A primary dipsogenic* signal that drives thirst or drinking behavior after dehydration is an increase in P_{osm}. The sensation of thirst and AVP secretion are under similar yet distinct forms of physiologic control (Fig. 21.5). Both are initiated by osmoreceptors located in the circumventricular organs of the anterior third ventricle (42) that respond to changes in P_{osm}, and by sodium sensors in the anterior wall of the third ventricle that respond to changes in cerebrospinal and brain extracellular sodium concentration. Thirst and AVP secretion are controlled such that above a certain osmotic threshold (~280 mOsmol/kg H_2O), there is a linear relationship between the increase in P_{osm} and the increase in $[AVP]_{plasma}$ or thirst (38). In addition, animal studies provide evidence for the existence of peripheral osmoreceptors, possibly in

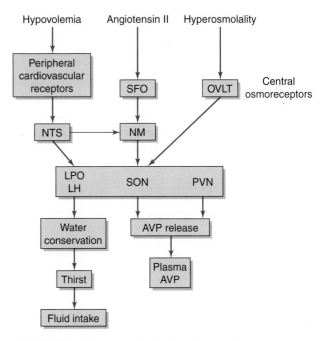

FIGURE 21.5 Schematic depiction of central nervous system integration of inputs (osmotic, volume, and angiotensin II) for control of thirst and arginine vasopressin (AVP) secretion. SFO, subfornical organ; OVLT, organum vasculosum lamina terminalis; NTS, nucleus of the solitary tract; NM, nucleus medians; LPO, lateral preoptic hypothalamus; LH, lateral hypothalamus; SON, supraoptic nucleus; PVN, paraventricular nucleus.

the hepatic portal system. Rapid dilution of hepatic-portal blood could account for some of the rapid adjustments in thirst and AVP secretion observed during the early phase of rehydration (0–60 minutes); however, this hypothesis requires further support, particularly from human studies. The supraventricular and supraoptic nuclei of the hypothalamus also have a high expression of water channels or aquaporin 4, leading to the hypothesis that aquaporin 4 channels may participate in osmoregulation. Further research is also needed to identify and characterize the role of these water channels in osmoregulation.

Thirst and AVP secretion also occur in response to a reduction in ECF volume. The sensory pathway for this reflex is thought to involve an increase in plasma angiotensin II acting on circumventricular organs and neural signals from mechanoreceptors located in the great vessels and atrium of the heart (low-pressure baroreceptors) (42). The sensory information with regard to plasma tonicity and ECF volume influences the supraoptic and paraventricular nuclei within the hypothalamus, and modulates the synthesis and release of AVP. This same sensory information also subserves thirst sensation. Following dehydration, fluid intake is determined in large part by the magnitude of the increase in P_{osm} and decrease in PV. Removing the volume-dependent dipsogenic signal in dehydrated individuals (*e.g.*, by placing the subject in a supine posture or a head-out water immersion position) will markedly

*From the term *dipsas*, a serpent whose bite was fabled to produce a raging thirst.

reduce thirst ratings and attenuate the total volume of fluid ingested. In dehydrated humans, rehydration during head-out water immersion results in only 40% of the fluid intake observed when rehydration occurs in air (43).

The neural pathways involved in the consciousness of thirst have only recently been identified. Results obtained by combining positron emission tomography and magnetic resonance imaging have demonstrated that the sensory input from osmoreceptors feeds into higher brain regions, the anterior cingulate region, and specific sites within the middle temporal gyrus and periaqueductal gray area (44). Activation of these brain regions occurs in proportion to the increase in plasma sodium concentration during hypertonic saline infusion. Specific sites within the anterior cingulate region (Brodmann areas 32, 24, and 31) remain active after a dry mouth is rinsed with water, but disappear rapidly after drinking. The latter brain regions may play an important role in the consciousness of thirst (44).

Preabsorptive signals

Afferent signals originating from the oropharyngeal region influence thirst and AVP secretion. The sensation of a dry mouth provides an important drive for thirst and the initiation of drinking. The sensation of dry mouth (45) is known to rise in proportion to P_{osm} and is closely correlated with an individual's perceived rating of thirst. However, a dry mouth is not a principal physiologic signal that drives fluid intake following dehydration; rather, it is a perceived sensation that can serve to initiate drinking regardless of the body fluid status.

Sensory pathways associated with the oropharyngeal region and the stomach also act to signal termination of thirst, and can modulate osmotic and volume-dependent dipsogenic signals. For example, rinsing a dry mouth with water will transiently reduce thirst ratings despite the persistence of a strong osmotic and/or volume-dependent dipsogenic signal. Rinsing the mouth with water does not appear to significantly influence AVP secretion. The act of swallowing water produces a steep and sudden inhibition of AVP and thirst. This inhibition cannot be attributed to the dilution of plasma or a reduction in osmoreceptor activity, because it occurs before any substantive changes in P_{osm} can be detected. Furthermore, this rapid response cannot be explained by the possible presence of hepatic osmoreceptors, because the rapid reduction in thirst occurs after ingestion of isotonic saline. The rapid inhibition of thirst and AVP secretion appears to be a response to oropharyngeal stimulation as dehydrated subjects swallow water (but not food) by mouth.

The oropharyngeal region is also involved in the restoration of fluid balance by monitoring the rate and/or volume of ingested fluid via a process called oropharyngeal metering. Oropharyngeal metering plays a dominant role in determining total fluid replacement in species that rapidly rehydrate, such as dogs (41). Although humans experience a slower recovery of fluid balance, oropharyngeal metering

does provide important sensory information (45). It has been shown that dehydrated humans who are allowed to drink *ad libitum* but subsequently undergo rapid removal of the ingested fluid from the stomach via a nasogastric tube develop a marked and persistent elevation in P_{osm} and reduction in PV. Despite the presence of marked and persistent dipsogenic signals, *ad libitum* fluid intake is only increased 15%. These data support the hypothesis that in humans, the act of swallowing and oropharyngeal metering provides an integrated signal in proportion to the cumulative volume of ingested fluid that acts to limit the overall rate of fluid ingestion (45). Finally, gastric distention can also provide sensory input to signal termination of fluid intake. However, the importance of gastric distension in the early termination of drinking in humans has not been clearly established.

To summarize, oropharyngeal stimulation contributes to drinking behavior in two general ways. First, it provides a signal for the initiation of drinking via an impact on thirst drive, through the sensation of dryness in the oropharyngeal region. Second, it provides a signal to terminate drinking via two mechanisms: a reflex inhibition of osmotically stimulated thirst and AVP secretion, and oropharyngeal metering.

The hedonic* properties of a fluid can also have a profound impact on the volume that is consumed and the rate at which it is ingested. Specific properties of the ingested fluid, such as flavor and temperature, impact consumption. During exercise in the heat, water intake is markedly reduced if the drinking water temperature is increase to 40°C (46). With persistent dehydration, the impact of temperature becomes smaller as the dipsogenic drive (involving volume and osmotic-dependent factors) overrides the hedonic properties. Following exercise-induced dehydration, maximal rates of rehydration can occur with water at a temperature of 15°C. Flavoring a rehydration fluid will also increase drinking, and this effect is independent of fluid temperature (46). It should be noted that hedonic preferences such as temperature and flavor are culturally influenced. As such, the preferred water temperature or flavor for a given group of individuals can vary considerably.

Involuntary dehydration

Several observations about rehydration in humans provide a background for understanding involuntary dehydration. First, the increase in P_{osm} and reduction in PV as a result of exercise-induced dehydration are proportional to the magnitude of water loss. Second, the overall volume of fluid ingested during rehydration will be proportional to the level of dehydration (40). Third, the rate of fluid intake during the first few minutes of rehydration will be proportional to the peak thirst rating (34). Fourth, the total volume of fluid ingested within a 3-hour rehydration period (without food) will constitute only about 60% to 70% of the fluid

---

*Of or relating to pleasure.

lost during dehydration. These are generalizations that can be applied to many situations; however, it is clear that the magnitude of involuntary dehydration may be manipulated by other factors (*e.g.,* aging and training). To explain this lack of full rehydration in humans, we must look at the time-dependent responses of the principal dipsogenic signals.

In human studies, the rates of fluid intake during the early phase of rehydration (0–60 minutes) appear to be independent of small differences in the volume or osmotic-dependent dipsogenic factors (47). Thus, during this period, the primary dipsogenic signals drive drinking on the basis of their initial intensity just before fluid ingestion. On the other hand, specific preabsorptive factors, such as oropharyngeal metering and gut distension, provide inhibitory signals that will limit drinking during this period. During this early phase of rehydration, one can manipulate the primary dipsogenic drives and cause marked changes in drinking. For example, when the volume-dependent dipsogenic drive is eliminated in dehydrated individuals (*e.g.,* by assumption of a supine posture or immersion in water up to the neck before the onset of drinking), fluid intake is reduced by 40% to 50% (43). In the upright posture, reflexes that want to restore the ECF volume and P_{osm} to normal levels drive the act of drinking.

As drinking continues (for 60–180 minutes), fluid balance and cation balance are linked; that is, if an individual ingests pure water, he or she will replace sufficient fluid to return the ECF space (*i.e.,* P_{osm}) back to its original isotonic level (see Fig. 21.6). However, although this behavior will control P_{osm}, the loss of electrolytes during sweating will result in an absolute reduction in ECF volume. In other words, the degree of rehydration in each fluid compartment

is determined by the ability to restore the ions lost from each compartment during exercise-induced dehydration.

These ideas are reinforced by results in the literature that demonstrate greater fluid restoration following exercise-induced dehydration when individuals ingest sodium-containing fluids (48,49).

Summary

During recovery from moderate whole-body dehydration, the delay in rehydration is caused both by an electrolyte deficit in the intracellular and extracellular spaces and by removal of the volume-dependent dipsogenic drive due to the retention of ingested fluid in the vascular space.

TEST YOURSELF

A new fluid-replacement drink is being marketed for athletes. The company that makes the drink claims it can provide immediate relief for exercise-associated muscle cramps because of its ability to rapidly restore electrolytes lost during exercise. The fluid has a high sodium concentration and a distinct odor that reminds you of pickle juice. Design an experiment that will help you identify the time course of physiologic responses associated with the intake of this high sodium-containing drink. In addition, your experiment should account for any physiologic response associated with oropharyngeal stimulation and/or psychological responses associated with the drink's clearly abhorrent taste.

Exercise-Induced Hypervolemia

PV expansion is a well-described consequence of upright endurance exercise training (50–52). Overall, the literature is an almost universally supportive of the notion that PV expansion is a hallmark of endurance exercise training. It is important to note that a few studies have been unable to document changes in PV with endurance training. There is no clear reason why these studies failed to induce hypervolemia. Short-term exercise training in an environment without full gravitational forces (*e.g.,* supine exercise or exercise in water) does not produce any remarkable hypervolemia. However, although endurance-trained swimmers have larger BVs compared with sedentary controls, they have smaller BVs than endurance-trained runners. It may be that in the absence of gravity, the time course and magnitude of the BV adaptation to training is delayed and/or attenuated. To allow some level of generalization, in this section we will focus on exercise-induced hypervolemia in response to upright cycle ergometer exercise training, and discuss its time course and mechanisms.

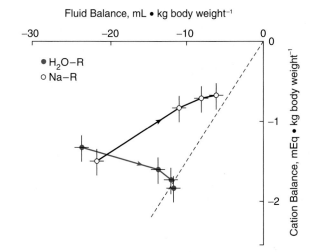

FIGURE 21.6 Relationship between fluid balance and electrolyte (cation) balance during *ad libitum* rehydration with water (H₂O-R) or 0.04% NaCl (Na-R). The dashed line represents a theoretical isotonic line. (Redrawn with permission from Gillen CM, et al. Cardiovascular and renal function during exercise-induced blood volume expansion in men. *J Appl Physiol.* 1994;76:2602–2610.)

Mechanisms of Exercise-Induced Hypervolemia

PV expansion occurs within 24 hours after a high-intensity, intermittent upright exercise bout (51). This hypervolemia is essentially isotonic and occurs in the context of increased intravascular total protein content, approximately 85% of which is in the form of albumin (51). Convertino et al. (50) demonstrated a progressive expansion of plasma albumin content during the first 3 days of an endurance training protocol. Furthermore, Gillen et al. (51,53) showed that albumin content expands 1 hour after exercise to the level it will maintain for the next 48 hours.

Exercise-induced hypervolemia: the role of plasma proteins

There are two possible mechanisms for the immediate increase in PV that occurs 24 hours after heavy exercise: (a) a net decrease in filtrative forces or (b) a net increase in absorptive forces acting across and along the capillary membranes. An elevation of albumin content after exercise would cause an expansion of the intravascular fluid compartment at the expense of the extravascular fluid compartment through the latter mechanism as a result of increased plasma oncotic pressure. Considering that each gram of added albumin will bind approximately 18 mL of H_2O, it is not surprising that the fluid volume associated with a 10% increase in albumin content (15 g) corresponds well to the PV expansion that Gillen et al. (51,53) measured 24 hours after heavy exercise. Therefore, plasma albumin content expansion facilitates PV expansion through albumin's colloid osmotic properties (50,51). The rapid increase in intravascular albumin content cannot be explained by changes in albumin metabolism (synthesis or degradation) or albumin vascular permeability; rather, it must be ascribed primarily to a redistribution of albumin stores from the interstitial to the intravascular compartments. However, the simple act of increasing intravascular albumin content cannot explain the PV expansion at 24 to 48 hours, because direct infusion of 12 g of albumin into the vascular compartment is entirely lost within 24 hours (54).

Several different mechanisms can promote the increase and/or maintenance of this extra protein in the intravascular space and the retention of isotonic fluid. First, a rapid accumulation of albumin in the intravascular space occurs as a result of increased translocation of albumin (protein) from the interstitial compartment to the vascular compartment. Second, the rate of albumin escape from the vascular compartment is reduced (55). Finally, an increase in hepatic albumin synthetic rate can contribute to a long-term increase in plasma albumin content and the maintenance of the expanded PV.

Rapid translocation of fluid and protein into the vascular compartment is critical for the restoration and maintenance of PV immediately after exercise. This phase of fluid balance after exercise is due to the simple reabsorption of isotonic fluid from the interstitium, a process that is primarily regulated by changes in local Starling forces across the capillary wall. Exercise stimulates lymph flow as much as 10-fold, promoting the translocation of protein from the interstitial to the intravascular compartment. The rapid rise in plasma albumin content after exercise must be explained by such a mechanism. Here, it is important to note that under conditions of increased lymphatic outflow pressure (*i.e.*, supine posture), increased lymph flow and albumin return to the vascular compartment are limited. This is because, in the supine posture, an elevated central blood pressure will act to increase lymphatic outflow pressure, thereby limiting lymphatic albumin delivery to the vascular compartment. This may explain, in part, why aerobic training in the supine posture (56) or high-intensity intermittent exercise in the supine posture (57) does not produce a significant PV expansion.

Exercise-induced hypervolemia: Starling forces

In previously active skeletal muscle, the colloid osmotic pressure difference (ISF vs. plasma) is similar before and after exercise, and does not appear to contribute to retention of fluid in the vascular space. However, because of a slight increase in $PRES_{ISF}$, a reduction in the transcapillary hydrostatic pressure gradient in skeletal muscle after exercise favors the movement of fluid into the vascular space. The increase in $PRES_{ISF}$ should also promote increased lymphatic flow and the return of fluid and protein to the vascular space. Over a more prolonged time period, the increase in skeletal muscle lymph flow will lead to oncotic buffering within the interstitial space, producing a small reduction in π_{ISF}. In inactive tissues (*e.g.*, subcutaneous tissue), the transcapillary colloid osmotic pressure difference will increase to favor fluid movement back into the vascular space, primarily due to an increase in π_{plasma}.

The transcapillary clearance of albumin in previously active skeletal muscle declines 24 hours after exercise (55). In addition, the whole body transcapillary escape rate of albumin (measured by the rate of washout from the vascular compartment of labeled albumin) also decreases after exercise (55). Overall, the net accumulation of albumin in the vascular compartment is the result of a translocation of albumin from the interstitial to the vascular compartment and increased retention of the translocated protein.

Changes in albumin metabolism occur too slowly to contribute to the rapid changes in plasma albumin content observed within the first few hours after exercise. At rest, the fractional synthetic rate of albumin is about 5% per day. Twenty-four hours after heavy exercise, a small yet significant increase in fractional synthetic rate to 6% to 7% per day occurs (58,59). This increase in the albumin synthetic rate is insufficient to account for the elevation in albumin content that occurs during the first 6 hours after exercise, but it can fully account for the increase in albumin content observed after a 24-hour recovery period.

Because albumin synthesis is transcriptionally regulated, it is not surprising that albumin gene expression is enhanced in exercise-trained rodents (60). In a recent work by Nagashima et al. (58), the effect of heavy exercise on PV expansion, plasma albumin content, and the albumin fractional synthetic rate were negated when the subjects were in the supine posture during both the exercise and recovery periods. Thus, the rapid expansion of PV was prevented when the subjects were in the supine posture. These observations indicate that the mechanism of exercise-induced hypervolemia is posture-specific and the upright posture provides an important stimulus for an increase in plasma albumin content and PV after heavy exercise.

Exercise-induced hypervolemia: water and salt retention

PV expansion during dynamic exercise training is isotonic (61), indicating that increased sodium and water retention by the kidney contributes to this volume expansion. Plasma aldosterone and plasma renin activity are elevated after moderate to heavy dynamic exercise, and should mediate an increase in renal sodium retention from the distal tubules (50,62). After a single bout of heavy exercise, a reduction in sodium and water excretion by the kidney occurs within 24 hours (62). A heavy dynamic exercise bout increases sodium reabsorption in the proximal and distal tubules. The increased sodium reabsorption in the proximal tubule is most likely mediated by a reduction in renal blood flow. In addition, baroreflex-mediated reductions in fluid-regulating hormones are delayed and attenuated after heavy dynamic exercise. Thus, plasma renin activity, aldosterone, and vasopressin levels remain at control levels despite a 10% to 12% elevation in PV after heavy dynamic exercise. These renal mechanisms complement the role of albumin in the expansion of PV immediately after heavy dynamic exercise. However, the renal adaptation lags behind the increase in plasma albumin content. As such, within the first 24 to 48 hours after heavy dynamic exercise, PV expansion occurs at the expense of the ISF space. With chronic dynamic exercise training, the ECF space expands until it eventually matches the increase in PV. The time course of these adaptations during dynamic exercise training has not been fully identified. However, during heat acclimation in one study, an expansion of the ECF space was noted by the eighth day of acclimatization (14).

In summary, the process of exercise-induced hypervolemia can be described on the basis of acute and long-term adjustments. The acute adjustment, which occurs within the first 24 to 48 hours involves the selective expansion of PV, primarily due to an increase in intravascular albumin content (51,53). On a long-term basis, the size of the intravascular compartment does not appear to be disproportionately larger than the increase in extracellular volume (61). Taken together, these data suggest that the overall adjustments in fluid compartment

sizes require a considerable amount of time, and selective expansion of PV has precedence in this procedure. During the acute phase, the increase in plasma albumin content occurs within 1 to 2 hours of exercise and is subsequently maintained (51,53,57). Another mechanism is the attenuation of volume-regulating reflexes (53,57), characterized by an attenuated cardiopulmonary baroreflex control of peripheral vascular tone 2 hours after exercise (53) and the maintenance of fluid-regulating hormones such as renin and aldosterone (21,57,63). In combination, these mechanisms appear to play a role in exercise-induced hypervolemia by allowing the increased level of fluid volume and albumin content to remain for extended periods. The increase in PV observed 24 hours after exercise is closely related to the increase in plasma albumin content, and the increased albumin synthetic rate contributes to the rise in plasma albumin content.

TEST YOURSELF

Volume-regulating reflexes are attenuated in athletes. Athletes also exhibit the typical 10% to 15% PV expansion 24 hours after a high-intensity exercise protocol or workout. Design an experiment to quantify the importance of an attenuated volume-regulating reflex in determining the magnitude of PV expansion 24 hours after an intense exercise bout. Do athletes show an additional attenuation in volume-regulating reflexes after intense exercise, and does this attenuation contribute to PV expansion?

Regulation of Red Cell Mass and Exercise

The major function of RBCs (i.e., erythrocytes) is to transport the oxygen-carrying molecule Hb from the lungs to the tissues. However, these same RBCs also contribute significantly to the buffering capacity of the blood. RBCs contain a large quantity of the enzyme carbonic anhydrase, which catalyzes the reaction between carbon dioxide and water. Thus, the RBCs promote the transport of large quantities of CO_2, in the form of bicarbonate ion, from the tissues to the lungs. In addition, the Hb molecule itself is an excellent acid–base buffer. The average concentration of RBCs per milliliter of blood is 5.2 million for men and about 4.7 million for women. These numbers equate to an Hct (the proportion of blood volume that is occupied by RBCs) of 45 and 41 for men and women, respectively. The RBCs concentrate Hb to a level of 34 g/dL of ICF volume. Therefore, the average Hb concentration in whole blood averages 16 g/dL blood in men and 14 g/dL in women. Blood also contains white cells (5000–10,000 per mL) and platelets (240,000–400,000 per mL).

Regulation of Erythropoiesis

In adults, circulating RBCs are produced exclusively by the bone marrow from cells called pluripotential hemopoietic stem cells. These pluripotential hemopoietic stems cells reproduce to create differentiated cells (committed stem cells termed *colony-forming units [CFUs]*) that are destined to become different types of circulating blood cells (*e.g.,* erythrocytes, lymphocytes, or monocytes). Multiple proteins, called growth inducers and differentiation inducers, control this process of growth and differentiation. The formation of these inducers is controlled by factors outside the bone marrow.

Role of erythropoietin

The principle factor that stimulates RBC production in bone marrow is a circulating hormone called erythropoietin (EPO; 166 amino acid residues linked to three carbohydrate chains, 34 kDa glycoprotein) (64). In adults, about 90% of the EPO is formed in the kidneys, in either proximal tubular cells or peritubular capillary endothelial cells. Liver hepatocytes account for the remaining 10% of the circulating EPO produced by the body. EPO binds to its receptors on the membranes of the committed erythroid progenitor cells (CFU-erythrocytes) in the bone marrow and increase erythropoiesis by stimulating both the proliferation and maturation of CFU-erythrocytes. EPO levels in resting individuals at sea level average about 15 mU EPO/mL plasma (95% confidence limits, 10–30 mU EPO/mL plasma) (64,65). The principle stimulus for EPO production by the kidney is low oxygen tension in the tissue. The balance of oxygen delivery and oxygen consumption of the renal tissue determines the oxygen tension in the renal tissue. General hypoxemia in the absence of EPO will not stimulate RBC production.

Over the past two decades, several erythropoiesis-stimulating agents (ESAs) have been developed to help manage the anemia associated with chronic kidney disease. The use of such agents to enhance oxygen-carrying capacity is well documented (66,67), and athletes now use ESAs as an ergogenic aid. More importantly, ESA use appears to have replaced conventional "blood doping" as the illicit mechanism of choice to improve oxygen-carrying capacity and aerobic capacity in athletes. ESAs vary in potency primarily because of differences in the half-life of the agents. Recombinant human EPO (rhEPO) is synthesized in culture from a variety of cell types (Chinese hamster ovary, baby hamster kidney, and human fibrosarcoma cells) that carry the cDNA encoding human EPO. rhEPO molecules that possess more N-linked glycosylation chains tend to have a longer half-life and thus more biologic activity (68). The integration of a large methoxy-polyethyleneglycol polymer chain onto the rhEPO molecule (a process called pegylation) also extends the half-life and results in a new rhEPO

called continuous EPO receptor activator (CERA). EPO-mimetic peptides (*e.g.,* Hematide) can also bind to the EPO receptor and produce dose-dependent increases in reticulocytes and Hb concentration. EPO gene expression is stimulated by the hypoxic-inducible transcription factor (HIF). Molecules that act to stabilize HIF have been shown to promote EPO expression; however, clinical trials for such molecules have been plagued by serious side effects.

Hormones that modulate erythropoiesis

Several hormones act to modulate EPO release by modifying the balance between oxygen delivery and oxygen consumption of the renal tissue, or to modulate EPO's effect on the erythroid progenitor cells. Thyroxin increases the rate of EPO production by increasing the rate of oxygen utilization by renal tissue. Angiotensin II impacts EPO production by reducing oxygen delivery to renal tissue via a reduction in renal blood flow, and by increasing renal oxygen consumption by stimulating sodium reabsorption in the proximal tubules. Androgenic steroids do not affect oxygen tension in the renal tissue; rather, they act directly on renal cells to augment production of EPO to a given hypoxic stimulus, and stimulate erythroid precursor cells to stimulate maturation (69). Administration of pharmacologic doses of growth hormone (GH) to both adults and children results in an increase in total BV (TBV) (70). More importantly, GH receptors are known to be located in bone marrow (71). Results from studies that examined the mechanism of action of GH in vitro, based on work with isolated erythroid progenitor cells from humans, indicate that the effects of GH on erythropoiesis are mediated by insulin-like growth factor I (IGF-I). This evidence supports the notion that GH has a role in modulating erythropoiesis.

Dynamic exercise and erythropoiesis: the role of erythropoietin

The oxygen-dependent feedback regulation of EPO production is widely accepted (65). Anemia or hypoxemia signals the renal oxygen sensors and EPO-producing cells to increase EPO production. Increased EPO stimulates bone marrow erythropoiesis and an increase in RBC mass. With the increase in RBC mass and improved oxygen delivery to the tissues, the hypoxic drive for EPO release is reduced. This feedback loop explains the typical response of EPO after acute exposure to altitude (hypobaric hypoxia; see Chapter 24 for more details). In one study, during a sojourn at 4350 m, plasma EPO levels increased to 120 mU EPO/mL by day 3 (65). New RBCs appeared in the circulation within 5 to 7 days, improving oxygen saturation of the blood, and EPO levels began to return toward baseline. A major question is "Is the increased red cell mass associated with exercise training linked to EPO and this same feedback control loop, or is it related to some other nonrenal factor?"

Oxygen desaturation during exercise seems to be a likely candidate for stimulating EPO production during exercise. However, to achieve arterial desaturation at sea level, you must meet two requirements: (a) exercise intensities must be near $\dot{V}_{O_{2max}}$, and (b) you must have highly trained athletes. Acute continuous exposure (5–60 minutes) to normobaric hypoxia (10.5% F_iO_2) does not induce a rise in plasma EPO levels (65). On the other hand, short bursts of supramaximal exercise performed at an altitude of 1000 or 2000 m will result in exercise-induced hypoxemia ($S_aO_2 < 91\%$) and an increase in plasma EPO levels (65). These observations indicate that, aside from simple hypoxemia, there might be an exercise factor that contributes to the EPO response. The problem is that most exercise studies have not observed a measurable change in plasma EPO levels. For example, Schmidt et al. (72) did not see an increase in plasma EPO after 60 minutes of moderate exercise (60% $\dot{V}_{O_{2max}}$) or a maximal exercise test. Klausen et al. (65) failed to alter plasma EPO after 60 minutes of cycle ergometer exercise at 85% to 90% of heart rate max ($S_aO_2 > 95\%$). Any small increase in plasma EPO level (≈ 3 U EPO/L) after exercise would easily fall within the normal diurnal variation observed for plasma EPO. A bioassay used to estimate EPO activity revealed that the rate of iron incorporation into bone marrow cell cultures is increased after exercise (73). In this case, the plasma containing EPO is used to stimulate erythropoietic activity in a cell culture and is thought to indicate EPO activity of the serum. However, the serum after exercise also contains all of the other hormones released during exercise. One interpretation of these findings is that, despite the relatively small increase in EPO after exercise, the serum is able to enhance erythropoietic activity in bone marrow cells.

Dynamic exercise and erythropoiesis: the role of circulating hormones

GH release during exercise may also contribute to EPO-mediated erythropoiesis. The increase in plasma GH during exercise is dependent on the exercise intensity and duration. During graded exercise, the threshold exercise intensities that are necessary to induce an increase in plasma GH or in plasma catecholamine and blood lactate are similar (74). At lower intensities of exercise, the duration of the exercise bout must exceed ≈ 15 minutes before a detectable rise in plasma GH can be seen. Therefore, given an adequate exercise stimulus, a rise in plasma GH after exercise is expected.

Dynamic exercise and red blood cell turnover

The impact of exercise on the erythrocyte life span will influence the time course and magnitude of BV expansion during training. During endurance training, erythrocyte

turnover is increased (76). Endurance training is associated with an increase in reticulocytosis (an increase in the number of immature RBCs) and erythrocyte destruction. Increased erythrocyte turnover dictates that trained athletes will have younger erythrocytes than sedentary individuals. Younger erythrocytes demonstrate a rightward shift in their oxygen-Hb dissociation curve, which explains, in part, the observed rightward shift in their oxygen-Hb dissociation curve of blood from endurance-trained athletes (77,78). The mean erythrocyte life span in male endurance athletes averages <70 days, as compared with 120 days for sedentary individuals.

Several pathways contribute to accelerated erythrocyte loss during exercise training, including gastrointestinal bleeding, dietary iron deficiency, insufficient erythropoiesis, and intravascular hemolysis (79). Of these pathways, intravascular hemolysis is considered the most clinically relevant. Exercise-induced hemolysis has been implicated in the development of sports anemia and suboptimal iron status in endurance-trained athletes. Exercise-induced erythrocyte destruction may be induced by several distinct mechanisms, including mechanical trauma (usually associated with foot strike or compression of erythrocytes within small blood vessels during muscle contraction), elevated body temperature, dehydration, hemoconcentration, and oxidative stress. Exercise-induced oxidative stress may contribute to erythrocyte destruction, and this pathway may be modulated by antioxidant treatment. However, endurance training will enhance the activity of antioxidant enzymes and improve coupling of the electron transport chain. As such, the role of exercise-induced oxidative stress in the destruction of RBCs will be diminished significantly with exercise training. In general, circulatory trauma to RBCs during exercise appears to be the primary contributor to exercise-induced hemolysis. The mechanical trauma of a foot strike during running is considered to be the major contributor to exercise-induced hemolysis (79).

To summarize, an increase in red cell mass with exercise training appears to occur sometime after the first two weeks of training (Fig. 21.5). The timing of the increase in red cell mass with exercise training is similar to that seen during exposure to short-term, intermittent hypobaric hypoxia. In both cases, the hematologic response is a slight rise in EPO levels after exercise, or hypobaric hypoxia repeated for three to four weeks results in an increase in red cell mass. Because the intensity of exercise during most training sessions would be insufficient to evoke clear hypoxemia, the rise in erythropoietic activity of the plasma must result from a combined effect of relative renal hypoxemia and exercise on the hypophyseal-adrenal, hypophyseal-gonadal, GH, IGF-I, and renin-angiotensin axis. It must be the impact of exercise on the erythropoietic activity of the plasma, not simply the increase in EPO levels, that is the critical factor in increasing red cell mass.

Red Cell Expansion and $\dot{V}O_{2max}$

Changes in red cell mass influence aerobic capacity through two important pathways. Changes in the Hb concentration ([Hb]) will affect aerobic capacity by altering the maximal oxygen transport capacity of blood, whereas changes in TBV will affect aerobic capacity by altering the cardiac output (52,80). Reductions in [Hb] in humans via acute and chronic isovolemic anemia cause a reduction in maximal aerobic capacity, but not always a reduction in maximal cardiac output. The removal of 900 mL of blood by phlebotomy results in an 11% reduction in [Hb], which rapidly begins to recover 2 weeks after phlebotomy but requires a total of 5 to 6 weeks for [Hb] to return to control levels (80). The time course of recovery is slightly longer in trained runners (81).

The removed blood can be stored indefinitely by means of a freeze-preservation technique. Autologous infusion of the stored RBCs or blood doping produces an abnormally high [Hb]. Twenty-four hours after infusion of RBCs stored in this manner (a process also referred to as induced erythrocythemia), an 8% increase in [Hb] is observed. More importantly, this elevation in [Hb] is maintained for one week after an autologous infusion of RBCs (80). The [Hb] will gradually return to baseline levels in a somewhat linear manner over the next 12 to 15 weeks. Using this type of autologous blood transfusion technique, Buick et al. (81) were able to demonstrate significant postinfusion increases in [Hb] (9%), maximal aerobic capacity (5%), and run time to exhaustion (34%). Greater improvements can be obtained with larger volumes of blood (i.e., 1350 mL blood); however, this also results in an excessive rise in Hct (80). An alternative approach is to use an rhEPO treatment. A 4-week rhEPO treatment ($150\,IU \cdot kg^{-1}$, once per week, subcutaneous injection) in healthy humans causes a significant increase in both Hb concentration and $\dot{V}O_{2max}$ (66,67).

TEST YOURSELF

Exercise produces a small, transient rise in plasma EPO. Does this rise in plasma EPO account for the increase in RCV with training? Consider the possibility of combining aerobic exercise training with rhEPO therapy. Can you design an experiment to characterize the magnitude of the RCV expansion with training as a function of plasma EPO levels?

Integration of Physiologic Control Systems

Osmotic Control of AVP Secretion with Endurance Training

AVP secretion and thirst are governed by sensory information related to both P_{osm} and BV (42). Osmotic regulation of thirst and AVP secretion is characterized by a threshold level of P_{osm} ($\approx$282 mOsmol/kg), above which thirst or AVP rise in proportion to the increase in P_{osm}. As indicated by animal studies, the stimulus-response curve for P_{osm}-AVP is shifted upward during hypovolemia and downward with hypervolemia. Because endurance training is accompanied by a hypervolemia, one might expect some alteration in the osmotic control plasma AVP (or thirst) in endurance-trained athletes. However, an increase in BV in endurance-trained athletes is also accompanied by an attenuation of low-pressure baroreceptor function (82). Figure 21.7 shows the effect of hypertonic saline infusion (to stimulate thirst and AVP secretion) under three PV conditions (normovolemia, hypovolemia, and hypervolemia) in a group of sedentary and endurance-trained subjects. Isoosmotic hypovolemia was achieved by administering diuretic pills for 3 days prior to

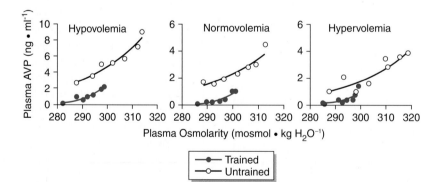

FIGURE 21.7 Unpublished observation of osmotically stimulated arginine vasopressin (AVP) release in sedentary ($n = 5$) and endurance-trained subjects ($n = 4$) under hypovolemic, normovolemic, and hypervolemic conditions. Isoosmotic hypovolemia was induced by diuretic treatment, and isoosmotic hypervolemia was caused by an acute infusion of isotonic saline. Osmotic regulation of AVP secretion is attenuated in the trained group. Hypervolemia did not alter osmotic regulation of AVP secretion for either group. Hypovolemia did not markedly alter osmotic regulation of AVP secretion in the trained group.

testing, and isoosmotic hypervolemia was induced by infusion of isotonic saline equal to 2% of body weight 30 minutes just before hypertonic saline infusion. Osmoregulatory control of thirst was increased during hypovolemia but unchanged during hypervolemia in the sedentary individuals. These observations confirm the role of low-pressure baroreceptors in modulating osmotically stimulated AVP secretion in healthy adults (43). In contrast, osmotically stimulated thirst was not significantly modulated by changes in PV in the endurance-trained individuals. Do these data indicate an alteration in osmotically stimulated AVP secretion in endurance-trained individuals? This question cannot be directly addressed by the present data, because as hypertonic saline is infused into an individual, the rise in P_{osm} is also accompanied by a rise in PV. To answer this question correctly, we must obtain isovolumetric plots of AVP versus P_{osm}.

Osmotic Inhibition of Thermoregulatory Function

Progressive dehydration during exercise produces a decrease in PV, an increase in P_{osm}, and an increase in heat storage. The higher heat storage is a result of a reduced ability to dissipate heat. Figure 21.8 illustrates that hypohydration results in a lower sweat rate at a given body core temperature. This decrement in sweat rate is proportional to the level of hypohydration. The mechanism that is responsible for mediating the reduction in sweat rate during hypohydration is not fully understood. However, it is clear that plasma hypovolemia and plasma hyperosmolality act independently to cause a reduction in evaporative water loss. This is illustrated by the data of Sawka et al. (83), which show a rightward shift of the sweat rate–esophageal temperature relationship in humans following graded hypohydration (also see Chapter 24).

A reduction in the rate of evaporative water loss following thermally induced dehydration has been demonstrated in several animal species. In humans, hypertonic saline infusion during exercise results in a reduced sweat rate at any given body core temperature. These results, in combination with observations in humans and other species of altered thermoregulatory function after dehydration, are consistent with neurophysiologic data demonstrating the modulating influence of osmotic stimuli on thermosensitive neurons in the hypothalamic thermoregulatory center. These data support the hypothesis that modulation of sweating during heat stress may be accomplished by modifying neural information in the thermoregulatory control centers in the hypothalamus, either through the central effects of osmolality or the release of central neural transmitters. A study by Takamata et al. (84) provided an interesting look at this interaction. In their experiments, they induced thermoregulatory sweating in human subjects (by heating the lower legs to 43°C) in an isoosmotic or hyperosmotic state. In the hyperosmotic state, thermoregulatory sweating was attenuated. The subject was then allowed to ingest a single bolus of water (4.3 mL/kg body weight). The ingestion of the water caused a rapid reduction in thirst rating and plasma AVP levels. In addition, there was a marked, albeit transient, increase in local sweat rate. These results demonstrate the vital and dynamic interaction that occurs between osmoregulatory and thermoregulatory systems in humans. Figure 21.9 provides a schematic summary of these interactions.

CHAPTER SUMMARY

The difficulty of maintaining consistency in the volume, composition, and distribution of fluids within the body is a fundamental problem faced by all animal species. With its multiple sensory inputs and integrative capacity, the central nervous system provides the regulatory stability that is necessary to meet this challenge. Exercise simply adds to the already burdensome sensory information that the central nervous system must filter and integrate. In this chapter, we have discussed a variety of specific interactions between homeostatic control systems and their role in body fluid balance during exercise (or in exercise-induced dehydration). In addition, we have reviewed the adaptations of the body fluid system that occur in response to endurance training, and their ability to improve physiologic function. The well-defined expansion of BV is a perfect example. This adaptation within the fluid-regulating system provides greater stability of cardiovascular function during exercise, especially in the heat. Another example is the adaptation in the improved sodium retention by sweat glands after exercise training or heat acclimatization that results in a lower sodium concentration in sweat. This adaptation also enhances the body's ability to maintain circulating BV in the face of a TBW deficit. Thus, exercise-induced adaptations in the fluid regulatory system provide support for the cardiovascular system during subsequent exercise sessions.

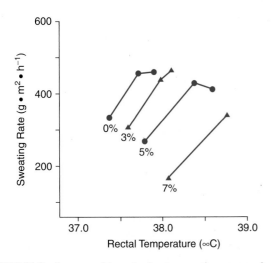

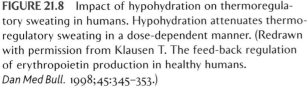

FIGURE 21.8   Impact of hypohydration on thermoregulatory sweating in humans. Hypohydration attenuates thermoregulatory sweating in a dose-dependent manner. (Redrawn with permission from Klausen T. The feed-back regulation of erythropoietin production in healthy humans. *Dan Med Bull.* 1998;45:345–353.)

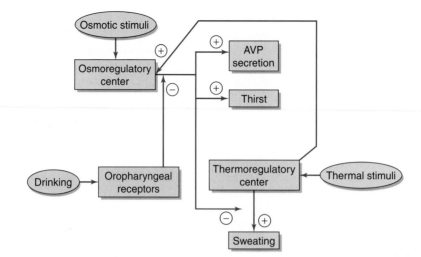

FIGURE 21.9 Schematic model of the interaction between osmoregulatory control of thirst and arginine vasopressin (AVP) secretion and thermoregulatory control of sweating and oropharyngeal stimulation during drinking. Oropharyngeal stimulation during drinking attenuates the osmotic inhibition input into the thermoregulatory center, as well as osmotically stimulated thirst and AVP secretion. Increased body temperature also modulates osmotically stimulated AVP secretion and thirst.

A MILESTONE OF DISCOVERY

After thermal- or exercise-induced dehydration occurs in humans, what causes the long delay in rehydration or involuntary dehydration? Since 1947, the phenomenon of delayed rehydration has puzzled researchers. Earlier studies had indicated that two factors unique to human dehydration contribute to involuntary dehydration: upright posture and Na^+ loss in sweat. Building on a series of animal studies that examined involuntary rehydration in rodents (85), Dr. Hiroshi Nose proposed a unique approach to study involuntary dehydration in humans. Nose et al. (35,47,86) designed an eloquent experiment that quantified the changes that occur in body fluid compartments during dehydration, and monitored the distribution and fate of ingested water during rehydration. They proposed that a high retention of ingested fluids in the vascular space during rehydration would act to rapidly dilute plasma constituents and restore plasma volume (PV), thereby accounting for the rapid removal of osmotic and volume-dependent dipsogenic drives. Nose et al. (35) carefully documented the shift in body fluid compartments following dehydration. Their results demonstrated that the body's ability to maintain circulating BV during dehydration induced by exercise in the heat is a function of the body's ability to mobilize fluid from the intracellular fluid space, which itself is linked to the sodium concentration in sweat. This observation provided insight into the benefit of producing a more dilute sweat during heat adaptation, which is to enhance the individual's ability to maintain circulating BV during exercise in the heat. In this study, even after the subjects were allowed to drink pure water *ad libitum* during a 3-hour observation period, they replaced only 68% of the water that was lost during dehydration. However, a disproportionate amount of the ingested water was retained in the vascular compartment, which restored 78% of the PV deficit following dehydration. This restoration of PV was sufficient to diminish volume-dependent dipsogenic stimulation. The selective retention of water in the vascular compartment also caused a rapid decline in P_{osm}, and hence, rapid removal of the osmotic-dependent dipsogenic drive. The most critical finding of this work was that when the dehydrated subjects drank water *ad libitum* while ingesting sodium chloride capsules (equivalent to a 0.45% NaCl solution), they restored significantly more of their lost body water (47). This experiment demonstrated that the recovery of fluid balance during rehydration is linked to the recovery of cation balance (Fig. 21.6). An important aspect of this experimental design is that fluid recovery was followed for 3 hours, well beyond the time frame of earlier studies. This extended period of observation is important because a difference in fluid balance appears only after approximately 2 hours of rehydration. This work provided a well-defined experimental approach for studying fluid balance in humans and unraveled some of the mysteries behind involuntary dehydration in humans. Overall, the research showed that during recovery from moderate (2.3% body weight loss) whole body dehydration, a delay in rehydration is caused by an electrolyte deficit from the intracellular and extracellular spaces and the rapid removal of a volume-dependent dipsogenic drive due to the selective retention of ingested fluid in the vascular space.

Nose H, Mack GW, Shi X, et al. Role of osmolality and plasma volume during rehydration in humans. J Appl Physiol. 1988;65:325–331.

ACKNOWLEDGMENTS

This research was supported by grants from the Heat, Lung, and Blood Institute of the National Institutes of Health (HL-39818 and HL-20634) and performed at the John B. Pierce Laboratory, Yale University School of Medicine (New Haven, CT), and the Human Performance Research Center, Department of Exercise Sciences, Brigham Young University (Provo, UT).

REFERENCES

1. Edelman IS, Leibman J. Anatomy of body water and electrolytes. *Am J Med.* 1959;27:256–257.
2. Norberg A, Sandhagen B, Bratteby LE, et al. Do ethanol and deuterium oxide distribute into the same water space in healthy volunteers? *Alcohol Clin Exp Res.* 2001;25:1423–1430.
3. Gudivaka R, Schoeller DA, Kushner RF, et al. Single- and multifrequency models for bioelectrical impedance analysis of body water compartments. *J Appl Physiol.* 1999;87:1087–1096.
4. Lesser GT, Markofsky J. Body water compartments with human aging using fat-free mass as the reference standard. *Am J Physiol.* 1979;236:R215–R220.
5. Visser M, Gallagher D, Deurenberg P, et al. Density of fat-free body mass: relationship with race, age, and level of body fatness. *Am J Physiol.* 1997;272:E781–E787.
6. Protection ICoR. *Report of the Task Group on Reference Man.* Elmsford, NY: Pergamon Press; 1975.
7. Edelman IS, Leibman J, O'Meara MP, et al. Interrelations between serum sodium concentration, serum osmolarity and total exchangeable sodium, total exchangeable potassium and total body water. *J Clin Invest.* 1958;37:1236–1256.
8. Nguyen MK, Kurtz I. A new quantitative approach to the treatment of the dysnatremias. *Clin Exp Nephrol.* 2003;7:125–137.
9. Titze J, Lang R, Ilies C, et al. Osmotically inactive skin Na+ storage in rats. *Am J Physiol Renal Physiol.* 2003;285:F1108–F1117.
10. Heer M, Baisch F, Kropp J, et al. High dietary sodium chloride consumption may not induce body fluid retention in humans. *Am J Physiol Renal Physiol.* 2000;278:F585–F595.
11. Seeliger E, Ladwig M, Reinhardt HW. Are large amounts of sodium stored in an osmotically inactive form during sodium retention? Balance studies in freely moving dogs. *Am J Physiol Regul Integr Comp Physiol.* 2006;290:R1429–R1435.
12. Shimamoto H, Komiya S. Comparison of body water turnover in endurance runners and age-matched sedentary men. *J Physiol Anthropol Appl Human Sci.* 2003;22:311–315.
13. Convertino VA. Blood volume: its adaptation to endurance training. *Med Sci Sports Exerc.* 1991;23:1338–1348.
14. Patterson MJ, Stocks JM, Taylor NA. Sustained and generalized extracellular fluid expansion following heat acclimation. *J Physiol.* 2004;559:327–334.
15. Landis EM, Pappenheimer JR. Exchange of substances through the capillary walls. In: Hamilton WF, Dow P, eds. *Handbook of Physiology.* Washington, DC: American Physiological Society; 1963.
16. Kedem O, Katchalsky A. Thermodynamic analysis of the permeability of biological membranes to non-electrolytes. *Biochim Biophys Acta.* 1958;27:229–246.
17. Michel CC, Curry FE. Microvascular permeability. *Physiol Rev.* 1999;79:703–761.
18. Rippe B, Haraldsson B. Transport of macromolecules across microvascular walls: the two-pore theory. *Physiol Rev.* 1994;74:163–219.
19. Dill DB, Costill DL. Calculation of percentage changes in volumes of blood, plasma, and red cells in dehydration. *J Appl Physiol.* 1974;37:247–248.
20. Convertino VA, Keil LC, Bernauer EM, et al. Plasma volume, osmolality, vasopressin, and renin activity during graded exercise in man. *J Appl Physiol.* 1981;50:123–128.
21. Convertino VA, Keil LC, Greenleaf JE. Plasma volume, renin, and vasopressin responses to graded exercise after training. *J Appl Physiol.* 1983;54:508–514.
22. Miles DS, Sawka MN, Glaser RM, et al. Plasma volume shifts during progressive arm and leg exercise. *J Appl Physiol.* 1983;54:491–495.
23. Bjornberg J. Forces involved in transcapillary fluid movement in exercising cat skeletal muscle. *Acta Physiol Scand.* 1990;140:221–236.
24. Saltin B, Sjogaard G, Gaffney FA, et al. Potassium, lactate, and water fluxes in human quadriceps muscle during static contractions. *Circ Res.* 1981;48:118–124.
25. Nose H, Takamata A, Mack GW, et al. Water and electrolyte balance in the vascular space during graded exercise in humans. *J Appl Physiol.* 1991;70:2757–2762.
26. Mohesinin V, Gonzalez RR. Tissue pressure and plasma oncotic pressure during exercise. *J Appl Physiol.* 1984;56:102–108.
27. Aukland K, Reed RK. Interstitial-lymphatic mechanisms in the control of extracellular fluid volume. *Physiol Rev.* 1993;73:1–78.
28. Jacobsson S, Kjellmer I. Accumulation of fluid in exercising skeletal muscle. *Acta Physiol Scand.* 1964;60:286–292.
29. Sawka MN, Francesconi RP, Pimental NA, et al. Hydration and vascular fluid shifts during exercise in the heat. *J Appl Physiol.* 1984;56:91–96.
30. Lundvall J, Mellander S, Westling H, et al. Fluid transfer between blood and tissues during exercise. *Acta Physiol Scand.* 1972;85:258–269.
31. Nagashima K, Nose H, Yoshida T, et al. Relationship between atrial natriuretic peptide and plasma volume during graded exercise with water immersion. *J Appl Physiol.* 1995;78:217–224.
32. McMurray RG. Plasma volume changes during submaximal swimming. *Eur J Appl Physiol Occup Physiol.* 1983;51:347–356.
33. Sawka MN, Pandolf KB. Effects of body water loss on physiological function and exercise performance. In: Gilsolfi CV, Lamb DR, eds. *Fluid Homeostasis during Exercise.* Carmel: Benchmark Press; 1990:1–38.
34. Mack GW, Nadel ER. Body fluid balance during heat stress in humans. In: Blatteis CM, Fregly MJ, eds. *Handbook oif Physiology.* Bethesda, MD: American Physiology Society; 1996:187–114.
35. Nose H, Mack GW, Shi XR, et al. Shift in body fluid compartments after dehydration in humans. *J Appl Physiol.* 1988;65:318–324.
36. Kozlowski S, Saltin B. Effect of sweat loss on body fluids. *J Appl Physiol.* 1964;19:1119–1124.
37. Thompson CJ, Burd JM, Baylis PH. Plasma osmolality of thirst onset is similar to the threshold for vsopression release in man. *Clin Sci.* 1985;69:39P.
38. Baylis PH. Osmoregulation and control of vasopressin secretion in healthy humans. *Am J Physiol.* 1987;253:R671–R678.
39. Convertino VA, Greenleaf JE, Bernauer EM. Role of thermal and exercise factors in the mechanism of hypervolemia. *J Appl Physiol.* 1980;48:657–664.
40. Greenleaf JE, Sargent F. Voluntary dehydration in man. *J Appl Physiol.* 1965;20:719–724.
41. Thrasher TN, Keil LC, Ramsay DJ. Drinking, oropharyngeal signals, and inhibition of vasopressin secretion in dogs. *Am J Physiol.* 1987;253:R509–R515.
42. Johnson AK. Brain mechanisms in the control of body fluid homeostasis. In: Gilsolfi CV, Lamb DR, eds. *Perspectives in Exercise Science and Sports Medicine.* Carmel, ID: Benchmark Press; 1990.
43. Sagawa S, Miki K, Tajima F, et al. Effect of dehydration on thirst and drinking during immersion in men. *J Appl Physiol.* 1992;72:128–134.
44. Denton D, Shade R, Zamarippa F, et al. Neuroimaging of genesis and satiation of thirst and an interoceptor-driven theory of origins of primary consciousness. *Proc Natl Acad Sci U S A.* 1999;96:5304–5309.
45. Figaro MK, Mack GM. Regulation of fluid intake in dehydrated humans: role of oropharyngeal stimulation. *Am J Physiol.* 1997;272:R1740–R1746.
46. Hubbard RW, Sandick BL, Matthew WT, et al. Voluntary dehydration and alliesthesia for water. *J Appl Physiol.* 1984;57:868–873.
47. Nose H, Mack GW, Shi XR, et al. Role of osmolality and plasma volume during rehydration in humans. *J Appl Physiol.* 1988;65:325–331.
48. Kenefick RW, Maresh CM, Armstrong LE, et al. Rehydration with fluid of varying tonicities: effects on fluid regulatory hormones and exercise performance in the heat. *J Appl Physiol.* 2007;102:1899–1905.

49. Merson SJ, Maughan RJ, Shirreffs SM. Rehydration with drinks differing in sodium concentration and recovery from moderate exercise-induced hypohydration in man. *Eur J Appl Physiol.* 2008;103:585–594.

50. Convertino VA, Brock PJ, Keil LC, et al. Exercise training-induced hypervolemia: role of plasma albumin, renin, and vasopressin. *J Appl Physiol.* 1980;48:665–669.

51. Gillen CM, Lee R, Mack GW, et al. Plasma volume expansion in humans after a single intense exercise protocol. *J Appl Physiol.* 1991;71:1914–1920.

52. Sawka MN, Convertino VA, Eichner ER, et al. Blood volume: importance and adaptations to exercise training, environmental stresses, and trauma/sickness. *Med Sci Sports Exerc.* 2000;32:332–348.

53. Gillen CM, Nishiyasu T, Langhans G, et al. Cardiovascular and renal function during exercise-induced blood volume expansion in men. *J Appl Physiol.* 1994;76:2602–2610.

54. Haskell A, Gillen CM, Mack GW, et al. Albumin infusion in humans does not model exercise-induced hypervolaemia after 24 hours. *Acta Physiol Scand.* 1998;164:277–284.

55. Haskell A, Nadel ER, Stachenfeld NS, et al. Transcapillary escape rate of albumin in humans during exercise-induced hypervolemia. *J Appl Physiol.* 1997;83:407–413.

56. Ray CA, Cureton KJ, Ouzts HG. Postural specificity of cardiovascular adaptations to exercise training. *J Appl Physiol.* 1990;69:2202–2208.

57. Nagashima K, Mack GW, Haskell A, et al. Mechanism for the posture-specific plasma volume increase after a single intense exercise protocol. *J Appl Physiol.* 1999;86:867–873.

58. Nagashima K, Cline GW, Mack GW, et al. Intense exercise stimulates albumin synthesis in the upright posture. *J Appl Physiol.* 2000;88:41–46.

59. Yang RC, Mack GW, Wolfe RR, et al. Albumin synthesis after intense intermittent exercise in human subjects. *J Appl Physiol.* 1998;84:584–592.

60. Mack GW, Bexfield N, Parcell A, et al. High intensity intermittent exercise training in rodents: impact on plasma volume and hepatic albumin mRNA expression. *Physiologist.* 2008;51:31.

61. Maw GJ, MacKenzie IL, Comer DA, et al. Whole-body hyperhydration in endurance-trained males determined using radionuclide dilution. *Med Sci Sports Exerc.* 1996;28:1038–1044.

62. Nagashima K, Wu J, Kavouras SA, et al. Increased renal tubular sodium reabsorption during exercise-induced hypervolemia in humans. *J Appl Physiol.* 2001;91:1229–1236.

63. Convertino VA, Mack GW, Nadel ER. Elevated central venous pressure: a consequence of exercise training-induced hypervolemia? *Am J Physiol.* 1991;260:R273–R277.

64. Kendall RG. Erythropoietin. *Clin Lab Haematol.* 2001;23:71–80.

65. Klausen T. The feed-back regulation of erythropoietin production in healthy humans. *Dan Med Bull.* 1998;45:345–353.

66. Connes P, Perrey S, Varray A, et al. Faster oxygen uptake kinetics at the onset of submaximal cycling exercise following 4 weeks recombinant human erythropoietin (r-HuEPO) treatment. *Pflugers Arch.* 2003;447:231–238.

67. Wilkerson DP, Rittweger J, Berger NJ, et al. Influence of recombinant human erythropoietin treatment on pulmonary O_2 uptake kinetics during exercise in humans. *J Physiol.* 2005;568:639–652.

68. Macdougall IC. Novel erythropoiesis-stimulating agents: a new era in anemia management. *Clin J Am Soc Nephrol.* 2008;3:200–207.

69. Fried W, Morley C. Effects of androgenic steroids on erythropoiesis. *Steroids.* 1985;46:799–826.

70. Christ ER, Cummings MH, Westwood NB, et al. The importance of growth hormone in the regulation of erythropoiesis, red cell mass, and plasma volume in adults with growth hormone deficiency. *J Clin Endocrinol Metab.* 1997;82:2985–2990.

71. Dardenne M, Mello-Coelho V, Gagnerault MC, et al. Growth hormone receptors and immunocompetent cells. *Ann N Y Acad Sci.* 1998;840:510–517.

72. Schmidt W, Eckardt KU, Hilgendorf A, et al. Effects of maximal and submaximal exercise under normoxic and hypoxic conditions on serum erythropoietin level. *Int J Sports Med.* 1991;12:457–461.

73. De Paoli Vitali E, Guglielmini C, et al. Serum erythropoietin in cross-country skiers. *Int J Sports Med.* 1988;9:99–101.

74. Chwalbinska-Moneta J, Krysztofiak F, Ziemba A, et al. Threshold increases in plasma growth hormone in relation to plasma catecholamine and blood lactate concentrations during progressive exercise in endurance-trained athletes. *Eur J Appl Physiol Occup Physiol.* 1996;73:117–120.

75. Christ F, Gamble J, Baschnegger H, et al. Relationship between venous pressure and tissue volume during venous congestion plethysmography in man. *J Physiol.* 1997;503:463–467.

76. Smith JA. Exercise, training and red blood cell turnover. *Sports Med.* 1995;19:9–31.

77. Schmidt W, Maassen N, Trost F, et al. Training induced effects on blood volume, erythrocyte turnover and haemoglobin oxygen binding properties. *Eur J Appl Physiol Occup Physiol.* 1988;57:490–498.

78. Weight LM, Alexander D, Elliot T, et al. Erythropoietic adaptations to endurance training. *Eur J Appl Physiol Occup Physiol.* 1992;64:444–448.

79. Telford RD, Sly GJ, Hahn AG, et al. Footstrike is the major cause of hemolysis during running. *J Appl Physiol.* 2003;94:38–42.

80. Gledhill N, Warburton D, Jamnik V. Haemoglobin, blood volume, cardiac function, and aerobic power. *Can J Appl Physiol.* 1999;24:54–65.

81. Buick FJ, Gledhill N, Froese AB, et al. Effect of induced erythrocythemia on aerobic work capacity. *J Appl Physiol.* 1980;48:636–642.

82. Mack GW, Thompson CA, Doerr DF, et al. Diminished baroreflex control of forearm vascular resistance following training. *Med Sci Sports Exerc.* 1991;23:1367–1374.

83. Sawka MN, Young AJ, Francesconi RP, et al. Thermoregulatory and blood responses during exercise at graded hypohydration levels. *J Appl Physiol.* 1985;59:1394–1401.

84. Takamata A, Mack GW, Gillen CM, et al. Osmoregulatory modulation of thermal sweating in humans: reflex effects of drinking. *Am J Physiol.* 1995;268:R414–R422.

85. Nose H, Yawata T, Morimoto T. Osmotic factors in restitution from thermal dehydration in rats. *Am J Physiol.* 1985;249:R166–R171.

86. Nose H, Mack GW, Shi XR, et al. Involvement of sodium retention hormones during rehydration in humans. *J Appl Physiol.* 1988;65:332–336.

87. Aloia JF, Vaswani A, Flaster E, et al. Relationship of body water compartments to age, race, and fat-free mass. *J Lab Clin Med.* 1998;132:483–490.

88. Davy KP, Seals DR. Total blood volume in healthy young and older men. *J Appl Physiol.* 1994;76:2059–2062.

89. Green HJ, Carter S, Grant S, et al. Vascular volumes and hematology in male and female runners and cyclists. *Eur J Appl Physiol Occup Physiol.* 1999;79:244–250.

CHAPTER 22

The Renal System

Edward J. Zambraski

Abbreviations

ACE	Angiotensin-converting enzyme	NO	Nitric oxide
ADH	Antidiuretic hormone	NSAID	Nonsteroidal anti-inflammatory drug
Ang II	Angiotensin II	PG	Prostaglandin
ARF	Acute renal failure	RBF	Renal blood flow
GFR	Glomerular filtration rate	RPF	Renal plasma flow
NE	Norepinephrine	RSNA	Renal sympathetic nerve activity

Introduction

The kidneys play an essential role in the maintenance of total body homeostasis. By varying the amount and chemical composition of the urine, the renal system can regulate total body water, extracellular volume and tonicity, plasma electrolyte levels, and plasma pH. The kidneys can also produce and release into the circulation a large number of compounds, such as angiotensin II (Ang II), prostaglandin (PG), norepinephrine (NE), erythropoietin, and nitric oxide (NO), that can affect circulatory function (blood pressure and flow), metabolism, thermoregulation, and red blood cell production. All of these responses are designed or intended to either maintain or restore homeostasis. The fact that acute exercise perturbs homeostasis therefore predicts that the renal response to exercise will be fundamental and essential in terms of our ability to do continued work. It follows that there should be a large amount of interest in and research on renal function and exercise, whereas, in fact, this has not always been the case. Historically, very few mechanistic studies have focused on the kidneys and exercise. The exercise studies of the 1930s and 1940s provided only a general description of the renal excretory and hemodynamic response to exercise. Interest in this topic increased during the 1970s to 1990s and more mechanistic

studies began to appear. Since then, there has been an increased interest in the renal response to exercise and to the factors that control this response. In this chapter, we describe the renal response to exercise, the mechanisms involved, and the relative importance of the renal response for acute and chronic exercise.

Extrinsic Control of Kidney Function during Exercise

To understand kidney function during exercise, one must be aware of the fundamental factors that control renal function. The three major controls are neural (autonomic nervous system), endocrine, and hemodynamic (blood pressure). During exercise, the kidneys are essentially targeted by these factors. The neural input to the kidney is largely sympathetic-adrenergic (i.e., NE-releasing), with essentially no functional parasympathetic innervation. Renal sympathetic nerve activity (RSNA) has the pote ntial to directly affect renal hemodynamics (renal blood flow [RBF] or glomerular filtration rate [GFR]), salt and water excretion, and the renal release of compounds such as renin, PG, and NE. The adrenoreceptors that are involved in the renal response include the α_1-receptor for renal vasoconstriction and augmented tubular sodium reabsorption, and the β_1-receptor for renin release. Endocrine and/or chemical control of renal function, via compounds such as antidiuretic hormone (ADH), aldosterone, atrial natriuretic peptide, and NO, influence GFR and RBF and the renal handling of sodium and water. Finally, because renal excretory function is totally dependent on filtration (i.e., adequate GFR), and GFR is directly dependent on blood pressure, changes in systemic blood pressure will markedly alter renal function. Even though renal autoregulation maintains RBF and GFR over a wide range of blood pressures, changes in blood pressure may alter the renal handling of sodium as well as the release of various renal endocrines. Consequently, the renal response to exercise is totally dependent on these three foci of control. Also, the greater the change in the control (e.g., increase in RSNA or endocrine level), the larger will be the magnitude of the renal response.

KEY POINT

The physiology of the kidneys is largely controlled by extrarenal factors. The degree to which these factors change during exercise will dictate the changes that occur in renal function.

TEST YOURSELF

The kidneys respond to various endocrines or hormones, such as aldosterone, ADH, atrial natriuretic peptide, and NE; however, they also release several endocrines or endocrine-like compounds that can have both renal and systemic effects. Identify these compounds.

Techniques to Assess Kidney Function with Exercise

To understand the renal response to exercise, one must understand the techniques and tools (and their inherent limitations) that are available to study renal function. Table 22.1 lists all of the techniques that have been used to assess renal function with exercise in animals and humans. Until the 1980s, the only techniques used in humans were urine collection and clearance methods. Only in the past two decades have more sophisticated techniques been used, in both humans and animals, to provide new, more mechanistic information.

TABLE 22.1	Techniques Used to Study Renal Function during Exercise in Conscious Humans and Animal Models
Humans	**Animals**
Single urine sample	Urine collection, clearance methods
Timed urine collection	Doppler, electromagnetic flow probes (RBF)
Clearance methodology (GFR, RPF)	Radioactive microspheres
Pharmacologic interventions	Pharmacologic interventions
Radiographic, NMR imaging	Surgical renal denervation
NE spillover estimates of RSNA	Renal vein cannulation, blood sampling
Radiowave renal denervation	Directly measured renal nerve activity

RBF, red blood flow; GFR, glomerular filtration rate; RPF, renal plasma flow; NMR, nuclear magnetic resonance; NE, norepinephrine; RSNA, renal sympathetic nerve activity.

Summary

The kidneys are excretory organs that play an important role in maintaining fluid and electrolyte homeostasis. This is especially essential during acute exercise, when large amounts of fluid and electrolytes may be lost through sweating. The kidney is also an important endocrine organ that releases renin, NE, and other compounds that can influence cardiovascular and metabolic functions during exercise. Kidney function is largely dictated by extrarenal control factors. One of the most important control factors is the RSNA (i.e., nerve activity that is increased during exercise) received by the kidneys.

Renal Hemodynamics and Exercise

Renal hemodynamics involve the RBF, GFR, intrarenal distribution of RBF (i.e., cortex vs. medulla), and the filtration fraction (the fraction of renal plasma flow [RPF] that is filtered). Table 22.2 illustrates the changes in renal hemodynamics that occur in response to progressive steady-state exercise at three different exercise intensities.

Renal Blood Flow

As measured by clearance techniques, RPF (both kidneys) is approximately 800 mL $\cdot$ min^{-1} at rest. When corrected for hematocrit, RBF is approximately 1300 mL $\cdot$ min^{-1}. With exercise at increasingly high intensities, RBF decreases in a linear fashion. The decline in RBF with exercise is somewhat greater if the subjects are exercising in the heat and/or

TABLE 22.2	Changes in Renal Hemodynamics and Excretory Function With Graded Exercise			
	Resting	25% $\dot{V}O_{2max}$	40% $\dot{V}O_{2max}$	>80% $\dot{V}O_{2max}$
RBF, mL · min$^{(-1)}$	1330.0	1250.0	1100.00	990
GFR, mL · min$^{(-1)}$	120.0	135.0	110.00	>80
UV, mL · min$^{(-1)}$	1.0	1.2	0.75	0.30–0.50
U Na V, % resting	100.0	125.0	60.00	20–50

Values represent workloads expressed as a percentage of $\dot{V}O_{2max}$.

UV, urine volume; U Na V, sodium excretion.

Data adapted from Freund BJ, Shizuru EM, Hashiro GM, et al. Hormonal, electrolyte, and renal responses to exercise are intensity dependent. *J Appl Physiol.* 1991;70:900–906.

dehydrated (1). At heavy or near-maximal exercise intensities, the absolute decrease in RBF is approximately 300 mL · min⁻¹. The decrease in RBF is due to active vasoconstriction of the renal blood vessels, and it is generally assumed that two strong renal vasoconstrictor mechanisms—increased RSNA and increased Ang II—are responsible for this reduction in RBF. Changes in directly measured RSNA in an exercising animal are shown in Figure 22.1. Indirect findings have suggested an important role for increased RSNA; however, no existing data support the concept that Ang II causes active renal vasoconstriction with dynamic exercise.

The change in RBF with exercise is almost exclusively described as a percentage of cardiac output rather than in an absolute fashion. At rest, RBF accounts for approximately 20% of cardiac output, whereas during maximal exercise this declines to 3% to 5% of cardiac output. This approach gives a false impression that the magnitude of change in RBF during exercise is large. What many fail to consider is that cardiac output goes from 5 to 25 to 30 L · min$^{(-1)}$ with heavy exercise; consequently, 3% of this larger amount is not very different from 20% of only 5 L · min$^{(-1)}$. The widely held belief that renal vasoconstriction during exercise is important because it redistributes a large quantity of blood from the kidneys to support active skeletal muscle is misleading (2). Relative to the cardiac output increase of 20 to 25 L · min$^{(-1)}$ seen with exercise, a 300-mL decline in RBF is negligible.

The importance of renal vasoconstriction during exercise relates to the change in total peripheral resistance. The intense renal vasoconstriction offsets the vasodilation seen in active skeletal muscle, and thus prevents total peripheral resistance from falling dramatically. Thus, this renal response helps maintain blood pressure (2).

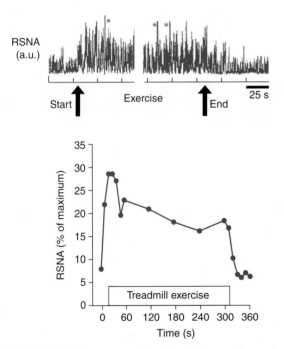

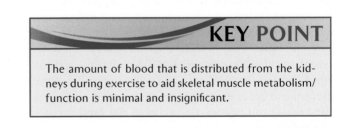

KEY POINT

The amount of blood that is distributed from the kidneys during exercise to aid skeletal muscle metabolism/function is minimal and insignificant.

FIGURE 22.1 With acute exercise, a rapid increase in renal sympathetic nerve activity (RSNA) occurs. *Top.* An actual renal nerve recording obtained from chronically instrumented rabbits at rest, during treadmill exercise, and during recovery. *Bottom.* The quantitative changes in RSNA expressed as a percentage of resting values. Note the rapidity with which the RSNA response turns on with exercise and diminishes with the end of exercise. (Data courtesy of Dr. K. O'Hagan, Department of Physiology, Midwestern University, Downers Grove, IL.)

Glomerular Filtration Rate

Glomerular filtration is essential for kidney function. Water and various chemical compounds must be filtered or translocated from the circulation to the renal tubule if they are to be excreted. The GFR is determined by the Starling forces at the glomerular capillary, as is the case for all capillaries. One unique factor in the kidney is that the glomerular capillary hydrostatic pressure, the major force favoring filtration, is usually high enough to ensure that filtration will always occur. This is in contrast to the situation in muscle capillaries, where filtration or absorption may occur. Filtration depends on two variables: the net filtration pressure and the permeability characteristics of the capillary membrane.

At rest, GFR is approximately 120 mL · min^{-1} (3). As shown in Table 22.2, GFR is either increased or maintained with light exercise, but it falls with moderate to heavy exercise (4). It has been hypothesized, but never proven, that the rise in GFR with light exercise may be due to increased atrial natriuretic peptide (4). With increased exercise intensity, there is more active renal preglomerular vasoconstriction, the effects of atrial natriuretic peptide are overridden, and GFR falls. The mechanisms responsible for the decline in GFR are the same as those described for the control of RBF. As noted above, GFR is also determined by the membrane permeability. Glomerular membrane permeability can differentially influence the movement of small molecules (*e.g.*, water and electrolytes) versus larger molecules (*e.g.*, plasma protein). Several compounds that increase during exercise may decrease glomerular capillary surface area and/or permeability to facilitate a decrease in GFR. These include ADH, Ang II, endothelin, thromboxane A2, and NE. A concomitant release of PGI$_2$, NO, and atrial natriuretic peptide, which increase glomerular capillary surface area and permeability, also occurs. Whether glomerular capillary surface area and/or permeability is actually altered during exercise, influencing water translocation across the glomerular capillary and contributing to the fall in GFR, is unknown. As discussed later in this chapter, glomerular permeability to larger molecules, such as albumin, is increased during acute dynamic exercise.

Site of Renal Vasoconstriction

The renal vasculature is densely innervated with sympathetic nerves. This innervation goes to both preglomerular and postglomerular vessels (5). Because these vessels are in series, constriction at either site will decrease RBF. In contrast, selective constriction of the preglomerular afferent arteriole will decrease glomerular capillary pressure and cause a fall in GFR, whereas constriction of the postglomerular efferent arteriole will have just the opposite effect. The fact that RBF and GFR decline in parallel during moderate to heavy exercise suggests that most renal vasoconstriction during exercise occurs at the preglomerular afferent arteriole.

Filtration Fraction and Exercise

The filtration fraction is the fraction of RPF that is filtered (*i.e.*, GFR/RPF). This value at rest is normally approximately 20%. With exercise, if GFR and RPF fall similarly, the filtration fraction will remain constant. The fact that GFR is unchanged or slightly increased with light exercise and decreases to a lesser extent with moderate to heavy exercise, as compared with RPF, means that the filtration fraction actually increases with the intensity and duration of exercise. The mechanism

may involve elevated postglomerular constriction. One possible mediator of this response is Ang II, which has been shown to act preferentially at the postglomerular vessels and to increase proportionally with exercise intensity (6). This possibility has not been confirmed or tested.

TEST YOURSELF

What is the difference between RBF and RPF? Why is the filtration fraction RPF/GFR and not RBF/GFR?

Distribution of RBF

It is known that >90% of the total RBF received by the kidneys perfuses the cortex, and the remaining 10% goes to the medulla through the special medullary circulation known as the vasa recta. In one study (7), small plastic spheres with radioactive labels were used to measure the distribution of blood flow within the kidney in various animal models. It was shown that the distribution of intrarenal blood flow does not change with exercise (*i.e.*, the decline in RBF) is proportional across the cortex and medulla. This finding, although negative, is important because if exercise increased medullary blood flow, it would have the potential to wash out the high concentrations of sodium and urea in the medullary interstitium. The resultant loss of the high medullary tonicity would dramatically impair the ability of ADH to produce concentrated urine (discussed further below).

Renal Handling of Sodium during Exercise

Sodium is one of the most important ions because it determines extracellular tonicity. The body must keep the extracellular tonicity constant; therefore, if the extracellular sodium content changes, more or less water will have to be added to that compartment to restore tonicity to normal. Thus, extracellular sodium content determines extracellular volume (including plasma volume). Under resting conditions, the amount of sodium in the body is determined by the amount of sodium ingested (dietary intake) versus sodium lost in the urine. At rest, various control factors regulate renal tubular sodium reabsorption to maintain sodium balance at zero (*i.e.*, intake equals loss). During exercise, especially when there is a thermal challenge, excessive sodium is lost via sweating. This can result in a net loss of total body sodium (*i.e.*, negative sodium balance). Conceptually, during exercise, the role of the kidney would be to decrease urinary sodium loss to offset sodium lost in the sweat and thereby maintain or restore sodium balance.

One of the primary controls over sodium excretion is GFR. If sodium (and/or water) is not filtered into the renal tubule, it cannot be excreted. The decrease in GFR with exercise is one of the fundamental responses to minimize urine sodium loss or to conserve sodium.

Absolute Changes in Sodium Excretion with Exercise

As shown in Table 22.2, sodium excretion declines with increases in exercise intensity. Studies have shown a very tight inverse linear relationship with sodium excretion and exercise intensity (percent $\dot{V}O_{2max}$) (4). With maximal exercise, sodium excretion can be as low as 10% to 20% of the resting value. Although the decline in GFR contributes to this antinatriuretic effect, it is also known that the magnitude of the reduction in sodium excretion with moderate to heavy exercise cannot be fully accounted for by the decrease in GFR or filtered sodium load (8). This means that an increase in renal tubular sodium reabsorption must be occurring.

Mechanisms of Control

The body has multiple redundant controls over renal tubular sodium reabsorption. Increased RSNA, Ang II, and aldosterone all directly stimulate tubular sodium reabsorption, and all of these factors increase with exercise. It is widely believed that during exercise an increase in aldosterone and/or Ang II is responsible for the renal conservation of sodium. Unfortunately, no data support this belief. In both animal and human studies, pharmacologic interventions to block Ang II or aldosterone have shown that these maneuvers do not alter the renal handling of sodium during exercise, and in fact, sodium ion conservation is unaffected (9,10). The control factor that is probably responsible for the augmented sodium reabsorption during exercise is the increase in RSNA (11). Definitive experiments to prove this assertion, even in animal models, are difficult to design and have not yet been undertaken.

Importance of Renal Sodium Conservation

The amount of sodium in the urine at rest is relatively small (approximately 130 mEq $\cdot$ L^{-1}). It has been shown in both laboratory and field experiments that sodium excretion decreases by approximately 50% to 75% with steady-state heavy exercise. Although this percent change appears impressive, when we calculate the absolute amount of sodium conserved (approximately 5 mEq $\cdot$ h^{-1}) and compare it with the amount lost in sweat (>30 mEq $\cdot$ h^{-1}), we can see that the kidneys are able to conserve only a small fraction of the total sodium that was lost. This demonstrates that the renal antinatriuretic response during exercise is inadequate, and large deficits in total body sodium will occur if dietary sodium intake is not supplemented. As indicated above, this will compromise extracellular and plasma volume.

An essential role of the kidneys in this regard is to restore normal body sodium content during the hours or days after long-term strenuous exercise. The control factors that operate in this setting are elevated aldosterone and Ang II (6).

TEST YOURSELF

If a person goes on a low-sodium diet or loses an excessive amount of sodium by sweating, what will be the renal response to these perturbations, and what mechanisms will be involved in the response?

KEY POINT

The amount of sodium the kidneys can conserve during exercise is minimal compared with the potential amount of sodium that can be lost by sweating.

Renal Handling of Water during Exercise

The excretion of water is necessary because it is the solvent that is required to remove dissolved electrolytes, acids, and metabolic wastes. Normal urine volume, or excretion of water, is approximately 1.0 mL $\cdot$ min^{-1} at rest. As shown in Table 22.2, urine volume goes down to 0.3 to 0.5 mL $\cdot$ min^{-1} with maximal exercise.

The renal handling of water, especially in the context of exercise stress, is largely misunderstood. Various factors should be clarified. First, the major control over the excretion of water is GFR. As was indicated above for sodium, if water is not filtered, it cannot be excreted. Second, 60% to 80% of the huge amount of water that is normally filtered (GFR 120 mL $\cdot$ min^{-1}) is reabsorbed or returned to the circulatory compartment via iso-osmotic reabsorption. This means that for every reabsorbed molecule of solute, such as sodium, chloride, or calcium, the resultant osmotic pressure is responsible for the reabsorption of a molecule of water. Because equal amounts of solute and solvent are being removed, the osmolarity of the fluid in the renal tubule does not change (hence the term *iso-osmotic*). This finding has two important implications. First, if mechanisms are activated to increase the reabsorption of sodium and other solutes, this will cause an increase in water reabsorption. Second, if all water reabsorption were accomplished solely by iso-osmotic reabsorption, the resultant osmolarity of urine would have to be similar to that of plasma (approximately 300 mOsm $\cdot$ L^{-1}). Because urine osmolarity varies from approximately 500 to 800 mOsm $\cdot$ L^{-1} in a well-hydrated person at rest to 1200 mOsm $\cdot$ L^{-1}

in someone who is exercising at maximum intensity and is likely dehydrated, another mechanism for water reabsorption must exist.

The ability to concentrate urine, or produce urine that is more concentrated than plasma, is derived from the effect of ADH. ADH increases the permeability of the collecting duct such that the high osmotic pressure of the medullary interstitium is allowed to extract water from the renal tubule. The higher the ADH, the greater will be the urine osmolarity and the lower the urine volume. If ADH is suppressed, a voluminous amount of urine with a low osmolarity will be excreted. Even if ADH is decreased, dilute urine can be produced only if an adequate amount of water is delivered to the distal tubule. With a decrease in GFR and augmented iso-osmotic reabsorption of water early in the renal tubule, minimal "free water" will be present in the collecting duct. In this situation, a decrease in ADH will not result in excretion of a high volume of dilute urine.

TEST YOURSELF

If a person has untreated diabetes and abnormally high blood glucose levels, why would this result in a large volume of urine?

Renal Excretion of Water during Exercise

As shown in Table 22.2, urine volume will decrease by 50% to 70% with moderate to heavy dynamic exercise. The primary mechanisms are a decrease in GFR and an increase in iso-osmotic reabsorption of water. All of the factors discussed with respect to increasing sodium reabsorption during exercise will also cause a proportional increase in water reabsorption. In addition, elevation of ADH will increase urine osmolarity and decrease volume.

Antidiuretic Hormone

ADH, also known as arginine vasopressin, is released from the posterior pituitary gland. One of the major factors that stimulate the release of ADH is increased tonicity sensed by osmoreceptors in the brain. If tonicity is elevated, ADH will be released, urine volume will be reduced, and the return of this water to the circulation will restore normal tonicity. ADH release is also stimulated by a wide variety of other factors, including stress, anesthesia, and exercise. With acute exercise, plasma levels of ADH do not increase appreciably until moderate to heavy exercise is performed (1). Resting ADH levels of 3 to 5 pg $\cdot$ mL^{-1} may increase 10-fold with exercise of maximum intensity (12).

ADH acts selectively on the cells of the renal tubule collecting duct. It promotes the formation of microtubules within the cytoplasm of these cells, which increases the ability of water to move through these cells. The driving force for this water movement is the high tonicity of the medullary interstitium.

Importance of Renal Water Conservation during Exercise

In similarity to beliefs regarding sodium (as discussed above), there is a widespread impression that the renal response to exercise is very important for conserving water to offset fluid lost by sweating. As shown in Table 22.2, urine flow rate is typically approximately 1.0 mL $\cdot$ min^{-1}. With heavy exercise, the excretion of water decreases to 0.3 to 0.5 mL $\cdot$ min^{-1}. If these values were to remain constant for one hour, the kidneys would be conserving only 30 to 42 mL $\cdot$ h^{-1}. These amounts are dwarfed by the amount of fluid that is lost in the sweat, which can be well above 1000 mL $\cdot$ h^{-1}. Because the kidneys do not excrete a large amount of water at rest, the antidiuretic effect seen with exercise is inconsequential. A key point, however, is that the renal conservation of water (and sodium) will persist for hours or days after exercise to restore total body water and electrolyte levels (6).

KEY POINT

Because the excretion of water at rest is only about 60 mL per hour, even if urine volume is reduced by 50% to 70% during exercise, the amount of water that can be conserved to prevent dehydration will be minimal.

Summary

The major renal responses to acute strenuous exercise are renal vasoconstriction, which decreases GFR and RBF, and decreased excretion of sodium and water. Although this conservation of sodium and water would appear to be advantageous, in order to offset losses due to sweating, the absolute amounts actually conserved during exercise must be minimal. The more important renal response is the longer term restoration of normal body water and electrolytes that may occur hours or even days after exercise.

Renal Acid Excretion and Metabolism during Exercise

At rest, the body excretes slightly acidic urine. With exercise, urine pH drops further to 4.0 to 5.0. This is the result of several mechanisms, including active secretion of hydrogen ions, excretion of fixed acids, and increased reabsorption of water resulting in concentrated urine.

The renal handling of lactic acid may vary with exercise. With exercise, lactic acid excretion increases. Lactic acid is freely filterable at the glomerular capillary, and it is also reabsorbed along the renal tubule. The excretion of lactic acid appears to involve a plasma threshold of 5 to 6 mmol $\cdot$ L^{-1} (13). Above this concentration, the maximal ability of the tubules to reabsorb lactic acid is exceeded and excretion increases. Nevertheless, the amount of lactic acid removed by excretion, relative to the total amount produced with heavy exercise, is estimated to be <2% (13).

It has been shown that the renal arterial-venous difference in lactic acid concentration is positive; that is, the kidneys remove lactic acid from the circulation during exercise, but the amount is not believed to be large. Lactic acid removed by the kidney could be used directly for energy or for gluconeogenesis. In one study, Krebs and Yoshida (14) observed that lactate-derived gluconeogenesis in the kidney increased by approximately 50% immediately after exercise.

TEST YOURSELF

During strenuous exercise, blood lactate levels increase. Does the decrease in GFR with acute exercise promote or reduce the ability of the kidneys to remove lactic acid from the plasma?

Water Intoxication

There are increasing reports of water intoxication in both competitive and recreational athletics. This occurs when an exercising individual consumes pure water in amounts that far exceed the amount of water lost by sweating (15). This causes a fluid imbalance (overhydration), expanded plasma volume, and lowered plasma electrolyte concentrations. Of particular concern is the lowering of plasma sodium (e.g., hyponatremia). Central nervous system and/or cardiac problems may ensue. It is unclear why the kidneys do not respond to this situation by excreting the excess water and thus preventing this condition. It has been suggested that this may reflect an abnormality in renal function (15). This is simply not correct; even when renal function is normal, certain control factors and conditions prevent excretion of the excess water in an exercising individual.

As indicated above, during exercise various control factors are activated to promote sodium and water reabsorption. When these controls are activated during acute exercise, they show a dramatic ability to minimize the excretion of sodium and water. For example, one study showed that if a subject drank 200 mL of water every 20 minutes and had resultant urine flow rates of 10 to 12 mL $\cdot$ min^{-1}, urine flow rates after exercise fell to 2 to 3 mL $\cdot$ min^{-1} even if the subject continued to drink the fluids (3). In individuals who are becoming water-intoxicated, ADH levels will be markedly suppressed. During exercise, if the free water that is being delivered to the distal tubule is limited, a reduction of ADH will have no effect because there will be a very limited volume of water to be excreted due to the decrease in ADH.

KEY POINT

During exercise, the kidneys are not able to prevent hyponatremia caused by excessive consumption of pure water.

Summary

The consumption of large amounts of pure water during prolonged exercise can cause water intoxication and hyponatremia (by definition, water intoxication means that symptomatic hyponatremia is present). During exercise, the kidneys will not excrete the excess water being consumed, because the GFR will be reduced and tubular reabsorption will be increased. This will result in a minimal amount of free water being delivered to the distal tubule and collecting duct, and limit the production of large volumes of urine.

TEST YOURSELF

For excretion of excess fluid due to the consumption of water during heavy exercise, which factor is more important or limiting: the decrease in free water at the collecting duct or the suppression of ADH?

Exercise Proteinuria

Exercise proteinuria is defined as an increase in urine protein concentration during or after exercise. Normally, because of the size and electrical charge of protein molecules, only a small amount of protein is filtered through the glomerular capillary membrane. A large percentage of this filtered protein (>90%) is reabsorbed by the renal tubule cells. Conceptually, exercise proteinuria could result from either an increase in the filtration of protein or decreased reabsorption, or both. In fact, studies have shown that both pathways are involved, with the major contributing mechanism being increased filtration due to an increase in glomerular membrane permeability (13). Acute exercise leads to an increase in membrane permeability to albumin as a result of the loss of the negative charge characteristics of the glomerular membrane (3). The anionic quality of the glomerular membrane normally prevents negatively charged plasma proteins from passing through it. In a diseased kidney, however, a damaged glomerular membrane will allow protein to pass through it, resulting in proteinuria. It is important to avoid confusing exercise proteinuria with disease-induced proteinuria. Exercise proteinuria is a benign, reversible process. Within 24 to 48 hours after exercise, the proteinuria will be resolved (3). Quantitatively, the amount of protein in the urine is proportional to both the intensity and the duration of exercise. Historically, it was commonly believed that the intense renal vasoconstriction associated with exercise was responsible for exercise proteinuria (3). Although this mechanism may contribute to the proteinuria, studies have shown that renal PGs are also involved. If exercising subjects are given a drug to block the renal production of PG, the exercise proteinuria will be markedly reduced in the absence of any renal hemodynamic changes (16). In addition, it is known that exercise-induced oxidative stress contributes to exercise proteinuria (17). NO production within the kidney during exercise may limit the amount of proteinuria; however, the mechanism of this effect is unknown (18).

TEST YOURSELF

Athletes may have their urine tested for the use of banned substances. Often these compounds are peptides. If a urine sample is obtained immediately after a race (*e.g.*, a marathon), why might there be a large number of false-positive results?

Summary

A large amount of protein in the urine is usually associated with renal disease. Exercise proteinuria, or the excretion of proteins after exercise, is a nonpathologic and benign process.

Renal Endocrine Release during Exercise

The importance of the kidney in the maintenance or restoration of fluid-electrolyte homeostasis is commonly accepted. Less well recognized is the fact that the kidneys also release into the circulation several endocrines, or compounds, with widespread effects that are important components of the integrated response to exercise. Several of these compounds are discussed next.

Renin and Angiotensin

Renin is released from the juxtaglomerular cells in the kidney. Renin release is proportional to exercise intensity. Resting plasma renin values of 1 to 3 $ng \cdot mL \cdot h^{-1}$ are significantly increased to levels of 10 to 12 $ng \cdot mL \cdot h^{-1}$, when exercise intensity exceeds 80% $\dot{V}_{O_{2max}}$ (12). Renin acts on angiotensinogen to form the decapeptide angiotensin I. Angiotensin I is converted to the octapeptide Ang II by an angiotensin-converting enzyme (ACE). Ang II is an extremely important biologically active compound. In brief, Ang II is a potent vasoconstrictor that affects systemic blood pressure, alters thirst, is a growth factor for various types of tissues, and promotes sodium reabsorption (5). In fact, there are at least two different converting enzymes (ACE and ACE2) that can result in chemically dissimilar angiotensin compounds with different physiologic actions (19). Numerous mechanisms are capable of causing an increase in renin release. The major mechanism for renin release during exercise is an increase in RSNA and stimulation of β_1-adrenoreceptors (20).

Renal Prostaglandins

The kidney has a very high capacity to produce PGs, a group of related compounds with diverse properties. The two major compounds, PGE_2 and PGI_2, are vasodilators that inhibit sodium transport (21).

PGs also serve a variety of other functions, such as mediating the inflammatory process (*e.g.*, in musculoskeletal injury). Nonsteroidal anti-inflammatory drugs (NSAIDs) are compounds that are designed to inhibit the synthesis of PG. Examples include widely used drugs such as ibuprofen (*e.g.*, Advil and Nuprin), indomethacin (Indocin), and meclofenamate (Meclofan). The major biochemical effect of aspirin is also to inhibit PG synthesis (21).

Exercise has the ability to increase renal PG synthesis and increase PGE_2 and PGI_2 in both urine and renal venous blood (22). Considering that these PGs are vasodilators and natriuretic, it is important to determine whether the use of NSAIDs during acute exercise, and the resultant reduction in renal PG, can alter the renal hemodynamic or excretory response, and even cause acute renal failure (ARF). Fortunately, studies examining the effects of renal PG synthesis inhibition, using NSAIDs or aspirin, have not shown deleterious changes in renal function during exercise in normal subjects tested under controlled laboratory conditions (16,22). It is known that PG control over renal function increases when a person is dehydrated, is in a negative sodium balance, and/or has very high levels of RSNA. The term *renal PG-dependent* has been used to describe the fact that under such conditions the use of an NSAID will predictably cause renal vasoconstriction and sodium retention (21). Such conditions would likely occur during a long-term endurance event, such as a marathon, especially with concomitant heat stress. There is anecdotal evidence that NSAIDs may cause kidney problems during such events. Investigators have replicated these combined conditions of sodium deprivation, dehydration, heat stress, and extended exercise in the laboratory to determine whether NSAIDs have a deleterious effect on kidney function under extreme physiologic circumstances. When ibuprofen was administered, an exaggerated renal vasoconstrictor response was observed; however, there were no reports of overt renal failure or salt and water retention (23). It has been suggested that during ultra-endurance events (*e.g.*, a triathlon), NSAID use is associated with hyponatremia (24,25). Although NSAIDs may decrease the kidneys' ability to excrete water during exercise, there is no direct proof that NSAIDs are directly responsible for hyponatremia.

TEST YOURSELF

Acetaminophen (*e.g.*, Tylenol) is a relatively weak inhibitor of PG synthesis compared with most NSAIDs. If I were a competitive athlete, and Tylenol and Advil gave me equal relief for my aches and pains, which compound would be better to use in terms of my kidney function? Why?

Norepinephrine

During exercise of various intensities in animals and humans, there is an increase in total body peripheral SNA. However, the sympathetic outflow is not uniform in all organs, as the kidneys receive a disproportionately elevated amount of SNA. Studies in animals have directly measured sympathetic nerve traffic over the renal nerves during exercise, as shown in Figure 22.1 (26,27).

In addition, investigations that measured NE spillover from the kidneys with exercise in humans confirmed that RSNA is markedly increased with exercise (28). The increase is proportional to the exercise intensity. This large increase in RSNA with exercise, together with the fact that the kidneys are densely innervated with sympathetic adrenergic nerves, has the effect that a large amount of NE will spill over from the synaptic spaces and enter the circulation through the renal vein. It has been estimated that at rest, renal spillover of NE accounts for about 20% of circulating NE in the plasma. In contrast, the adrenal gland's contribution to circulating NE at rest is <5% (29). With exercise, the marked increase in RSNA will increase the renal contribution to circulating NE, which, in turn, will have widespread systemic effects on cardiovascular function and metabolism.

Nitric Oxide

NO is produced in the endothelium by the NO synthase enzyme that acts on L-arginine. NO is a vasodilator that is believed to be responsible for setting the vascular tone and control of local blood flow. Acting as a vasodilator, NO contributes to muscle blood vessel dilation in response to dynamic exercise (30). Within the kidney, there is a potential for interaction among three control factors: RSNA, endothelin, and NO. Given that NO is a vasodilator, an increase in NO synthesis with acute dynamic exercise could attenuate the renal vasoconstrictor effects of increased RSNA and/or increased endothelin. Such an effect could assist in preventing renal failure during exercise (discussed further below). Alternatively, a decrease in NO synthesis during acute exercise could mediate the decrease in RBF.

In animal studies in which NO production was pharmacologically blocked, decreases in RBF with acute dynamic exercise were not changed (31). Other studies suggested that renal NO synthesis may be selectively reduced during exercise, perhaps as a result of an increase in endothelin (30). This reduction in NO could partially mediate the decrease in RBF (i.e., decreased vasodilatory NO may increase renal vascular resistance). One way to study the role of NO in various physiologic processes is to administer a false analog of L-arginine (e.g., L-NAME). This can be done in human subjects. One problem with trying to elucidate NO control of renal function during exercise using inhibitors such as L-NAME is that other systemic effects, such as an increase in blood pressure, will alter renal function. In one study, swine that were chronically treated with L-NAME for four weeks showed renal vasoconstrictor responses to submaximal and maximal exercise similar to those of controls (32). This suggests either the lack of a NO effect or the existence of other vasodilatory factors in the renal hemodynamic response to exercise.

Summary

When we think of the kidneys and endocrine function, we usually focus on the release of renin and the subsequent production of angiotensin. This is an important hormone system; however, the renal production and release of NE, PG, NO, and other compounds is an equally important process. PGs are major renal controls that can be easily modified (i.e., decreased) by aspirin or an NSAID. In certain situations, the inhibition of renal PG synthesis may induce renal failure or sodium retention, or increase the possibility of hyponatremia. New elements of the renin-angiotensin system (e.g., ACE and ACE2) are being discovered. The impact that exercise training has on these newly identified compounds is an important area of research.

KEY POINT

During exercise, the kidneys are an extremely important endocrine organ.

Injury or Acute Renal Failure Induced by Exercise

With exercise, the kidneys are stressed. Renal oxygen consumption, which is proportional to the amount of sodium being reabsorbed, is increased. At the same time, RBF, or oxygen delivery, is being compromised. At rest, the renal arteriovenous difference in oxygen is very small (i.e., oxygen extraction is minimal) compared with that of muscle. Oxygen extraction will increase with exercise to meet metabolic demands. It has never been shown that heavy exercise damages the kidney or the renal tubule cells in terms of an inadequate amount of oxygen. However, there are some concerns about individuals who exercise while they are also severely dehydrated, such as wrestlers attempting to lose weight. Studies have shown that the urine of wrestlers contains extremely high amounts of potassium and leucine amino peptidase (33). It has been suggested, but never proven, that the release of these compounds may be a response to renal tubule cell damage or death resulting from the combined effects of exercise and dehydration (11). To address this issue, we need to identify and validate novel biomarkers of renal damage that can be measured in the urine.

ARF is defined as a sudden decrease in renal function associated with a significant decline in GFR. Factors that result in a decrease in renal perfusion, or RBF, such as increased RSNA, increased Ang II, hypovolemia, and hypotension, can all contribute to ARF. Rhabdomyolysis (the breakdown of muscle tissue) can lead to ARF. Heavy exercise, especially when combined with dehydration, heat stress, and the sympathetic responses created by intense competition, can also cause ARF. Therefore, it is surprising that exercise-induced ARF is relatively rare (11). Although thousands of people participate in marathons and other long-term endurance events, only isolated cases of ARF have been reported. It has been hypothesized that some unidentified factor or factors vasodilate the kidney during exercise and thus protect against ARF (11). An additional protective mechanism may be the changes in RSNA observed with exercise training (discussed in the next section).

TEST YOURSELF

Rhabdomyolysis is a severe breakdown of muscle, resulting in the release of huge amounts of myoglobin into the plasma. Excessive myoglobin is filtered into the renal tubule. Could this also cause ARF? Why and how?

Changes in Kidney Function with Exercise Training

As indicated above, changes in kidney function are largely dictated by neural and endocrine controls activated by exercise. Therefore, changes in renal function with training would be anticipated if training altered the magnitude of change in a particular control factor.

In general, at rest there are no substantial measurable changes in either renal hemodynamics or excretory function as a consequence of training. This finding is consistent with the fact that training does not appear to change resting levels of ADH, atrial natriuretic peptide, aldosterone, or renin-Ang II (12). With exercise, the renal response (i.e., vasoconstriction and sodium reabsorption)

is proportional to the relative workload. Therefore, at the same absolute workload, some of the renal responses of the trained subject will be dampened compared with those of the untrained subject because the trained person is working at a lower relative workload.

Important recent findings suggest that exercise training may alter local tissue elements of the renin-angiotensin system (19). This may involve differential activation of ACE versus ACE2 converting enzymes and/or altered expression of AT1 and AT2 Ang-II receptors. The net effect may be less deleterious Ang-II-induced vasoconstriction, a very beneficial change for individuals with hypertension.

It is difficult to measure changes in kidney excretory function as a consequence of dynamic exercise training; however, another way to view or assess adaptations of the kidneys is to focus on sodium balance. If an individual's extracellular or plasma volume is undergoing a steady-state change, two things should be occurring. First, a person who is in a steady state must be in sodium balance. More importantly, if the plasma volume changes, the extracellular sodium content often changes as well. This is primarily caused by a change in sodium excretion. For example, an expansion of plasma volume can be achieved if the renal excretion of sodium initially decreases, allowing extracellular sodium to rise, with excretion subsequently finding a new steady state and reestablishing sodium balance. In other words, a maintained expansion of plasma volume often occurs with a change in the control of sodium excretion by the kidneys. It is well known that plasma volume is expanded with dynamic exercise training (2). This adaptation is often mediated or controlled by a change in sodium excretion; however, a redistribution of extracellular fluid to the plasma can also contribute via elevated circulating protein increasing the plasma oncotic pressure.

Changes in RSNA with Dynamic Exercise Training

One major change that occurs with training is an alteration in RSNA. In studies using NE spillover calculations and catheterization across the kidney in humans, investigators have been able to estimate RSNA both at rest and during exercise. In a landmark study in 1991, RSNA was measured in human subjects before and after a 4-week training program (34) (see *A Milestone of Discovery*). In these subjects, dynamic exercise training caused arterial NE levels to decrease by 21%. As shown in Figure 22.2, total body NE spillover also fell by 24%. The changes in RSNA were dramatic, in that the decreased RSNA accounted for 70% of the decrease in whole body NE spillover. In contrast, cardiac NE spillover, or sympathetic activity, was not altered by training, which suggests that exercise training has a selective effect on decreasing RSNA.

This decrease in RSNA with training suggests that certain renal parameters that are influenced by the renal nerves (e.g., RBF, GFR, sodium reabsorption, and renin release) are probably altered by training. These changes are undoubtedly very subtle, and they cannot be accurately measured with the techniques currently available.

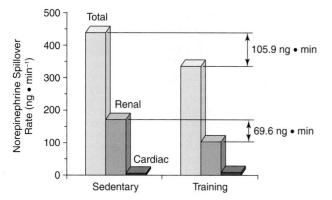

FIGURE 22.2 With exercise training, total peripheral sympathetic nerve activity (SNA) at rest decreases. This can be measured by means of the calculated total norepinephrine (NE) spillover. After 1 month of exercise training in humans, total NE spillover was decreased by approximately 25%. Renal SNA (RSNA) and renal NE spillover were also markedly decreased. The decrease in RSNA was responsible for approximately 70% of the change in total NE spillover. Cardiac sympathetic activity was unchanged with training. This shows that with training, a selective decrease in RSNA is responsible for most of the decrease in total sympathetic activity. This training adaptation may help protect the kidneys against acute renal failure. (Modified from Meredith IT, Friberg P, Jennings GL, et al. Exercise training lowers resting renal but not cardiac sympathetic activity in humans. *Hypertension.* 1991;18:579.)

As discussed in Chapter 7, in a trained individual the peripheral sympathetic response is reduced with a given exercise challenge, as reflected in notable decreases in plasma catecholamine concentrations. Animal studies in which renal neurograms were used to directly measure RSNA during exercise indicated that dynamic exercise training reduces RSNA in response to acute exercise (26,35).

The fact that exercise training results in a decreased RSNA at rest and during exercise has important ramifications because RSNA controls renal tubular sodium reabsorption (i.e., increased RSNA increases reabsorption or decreases excretion). Therefore, a decrease in RSNA could alter the total body sodium balance. With a decrease in RSNA, the resultant directional change would be a reduction in total body sodium and water. This response would be advantageous for an individual with hypertension, congestive heart failure, or other conditions in which sodium retention is problematic. Recent studies have confirmed that exercise training can normalize or reduce the exaggerated peripheral SNA and RSNA found in subjects with congestive heart failure (36).

A reduction in RSNA with exercise training can result in attenuation of renal vasoconstriction during exercise. This adaptation could be the most important protective mechanism responsible for the low incidence of exercise-induced ARF discussed above. It also means that an untrained person may be more likely to develop ARF after prolonged, strenuous exercise compared with a trained person who has this adaptation in RSNA response.

The mechanisms responsible for the decrease in RSNA with training have not been identified. Muscle tissue and organs such as the heart and kidneys have an extensive complex of afferent nerves that provide information to the central nervous system. In general, increases in renal or cardiac afferent activity have a tonic inhibitory effect on sympathetic outflow (5). Studies suggest that the increase in cardiac afferent nerve activity observed with exercise training is responsible for the measured reductions in RSNA seen with acute exercise (26). To date, the possible involvement of the renal afferent nerves in this response has not been examined.

Summary

Normally, when we consider the adaptations seen with chronic activity or physical training, we focus on specific biochemical, physiologic, and/or anatomical changes that occur within the tissue of interest (e.g., training can increase skeletal muscle oxidative capacity, endurance, and size). There do not appear to be any changes occurring within the various types of renal tissue as a result of exercise training. There are, however, significant and fundamental changes in the extrarenal control factors. As noted above, resting RSNA and the RSNA response to exercise are significantly decreased with exercise training. There also appear to be changes within the renin-angiotensin system. These adaptations can lead to subtle changes in innate renal function, as well as significant systemic changes, including prevention of ARF, decreased blood pressure in a hypertensive individual, and/or improved status of a person with congestive heart failure.

TEST YOURSELF

If RSNA and peripheral SNA are decreased at rest as a result of exercise training, by what mechanism would this decrease blood pressure in a hypertensive individual?

KEY POINT

The decrease in RSNA with exercise training is an adaptation that has extremely important clinical implications.

Aging, Exercise, and Renal Function

Age-related changes in renal function at rest have been well characterized and include a decrease in RBF and GFR, a decreased ability to excrete sodium, and a decline in renal

A MILESTONE OF DISCOVERY

Before the 1990s, it was well known that regular endurance exercise or training can lower circulating plasma norepinephrine (NE). This change reflects a general decrease in peripheral sympathetic nerve activity (SNA). It was also known that SNA is not uniform or global. The amount of SNA that is received by various sites or organs varies markedly, and the kidneys were believed to receive a disproportionately high amount of SNA. A research group from Australia headed by Murray D. Esler refined the technique of measuring NE spillover in human subjects to estimate SNA. In addition, by placing both arterial and venous catheters across different organs, such as the heart, kidneys, and liver, they were able to measure the amount of SNA going to each of these areas. This research group's influence on the exercise physiology research community began in 1991 when they examined the effects of exercise training on total body, renal, and cardiac NE spillover. Normal but sedentary men were exercise trained on a bicycle for 1 month. The program involved training only three times a week, 40 minutes per session, at an intensity of 60% to 70% of their maximal capacity.

With this minimal training regimen, plasma NE concentration and total body NE spillover fell by 20% to 24%. Of more importance, renal NE spillover, which reflects renal SNA (RSNA), fell by 41%. Two-thirds of this decrease in total body NE spillover was attributable to a selective decrease in RSNA. In contrast, as shown in Figure 22.2, cardiac NE spillover did not change. Blood pressure was also significantly reduced by training. This study showed that the decrease in total SNA seen with regular exercise is primarily due to a change in RSNA. Also, because RSNA is a major control factor in various aspects of renal function, the potential clinical implications of this decline in RSNA are extensive. In addition, the demonstration that this spillover technique could be used in conjunction with exercise and training led to several other studies that used this technique to assess RSNA in various exercise settings.

Meredith IT, Friberg P, Jennings GL, et al. Exercise training lowers resting renal but not cardiac sympathetic activity in humans. Hypertension. 1991;18:575–582.

concentrating ability. The most dramatic of these changes is the decrease in GFR, which is approximately 10% per decade starting at 30 years of age.

In contrast, the renal response to exercise in young subjects compared with older subjects has been assessed in only a limited number of studies. Experiments on exercise proteinuria suggest that the exercise proteinuric response to the same absolute workload is increased in older subjects [13]. It has been shown that the RBF response to exercise (i.e., vasoconstriction) is reduced in older subjects [37]. This change may be important for thermoregulation in that less blood will be available for heat transfer to the skin. In addition, there is good evidence that the decline in GFR with acute exercise is less pronounced in older subjects—a change that is beneficial in light of the noted decrease in resting GFR that accompanies aging [38]. At present, there is not enough information to determine whether any of these age-related changes in renal function with exercise are sex-specific.

Throughout this chapter, we have emphasized the importance of RSNA for controlling renal function. As people age, circulating plasma NE increases, and this increase in total-body peripheral sympathetic activity is believed to result from an increase in muscle SNA. RSNA does not appear to increase with aging [28]. In addition, it does not appear that the increase in RSNA stimulated by exercise is changed by aging [39]. One difference, however, is that the renal clearance of NE at rest is decreased in older subjects. This change contributes to higher levels of circulating NE. Whether the renal clearance of NE during exercise is also decreased with aging is unknown.

CHAPTER SUMMARY

The renal response to exercise is complex and involves hemodynamic changes, alterations in tubular function, and the release of a wide array of compounds into the circulation. The inaccessibility of the kidneys makes it extremely difficult to examine inherent kidney function in the exercise setting. The importance of the renal response to acute dynamic exercise is not, as most believe, conservation of sodium and water, but rather intense renal vasoconstriction to help maintain blood pressure and the release of large amounts of NE into the circulation. One of the fundamental changes that occur with exercise training is a decrease in RSNA, both at rest and during exercise. Changes in this control factor may be the crucial element in preventing exercise-associated ARF. Although the resultant changes in renal function with a training-induced decrease in RSNA have little effect on exercise performance, they may have widespread clinical benefits. With the newly discovered elements of the renin-angiotensin system, it will be important to assess the effects of physical activity and exercise training on this system, both within the kidney and the systemic vasculature.

REFERENCES

1. Radigan L, Robinson S. Effects of environmental heat stress and exercise on renal blood flow and filtration rate. *J Appl Physiol.* 1949;2:185–191.
2. Rowell LB. Human cardiovascular adjustments to exercise and thermal stress. *Physiol Rev.* 1974;54:75–159.

3. Poortmans JR. Exercise and renal function. *Sports Med.* 1984;1:25–53.
4. Freund BJ, Shizuru EM, Hashiro GM, et al. Hormonal, electrolyte, and renal responses to exercise are intensity dependent. *J Appl Physiol.* 1991;70:900–906.
5. Dibona GF, Kopp UC. Neural control of renal function. *Physiol Rev.* 1997;77:75–197.
6. Wade CE, Dressendorfer RH, O'Brien JC, et al. Renal function, aldosterone, and vasopressin excretion following repeated long-distance running. *J Appl Physiol.* 1981;50:709–712.
7. Sanders M, Rasmussen S, Cooper D, et al. Renal and intrarenal blood flow distribution in swine during severe exercise. *J Appl Physiol.* 1976;40:932–935.
8. Castenfors J. Renal function during prolonged exercise. *Ann NY Acad Sci.* 1977;301:151–159.
9. Wade C, Ramee S, Hunt M, et al. Hormonal and renal responses to converting enzyme inhibition during maximal exercise. *J Appl Physiol.* 1987;63:1796–1800.
10. Zambraski EJ. Renal regulation of fluid homeostasis during exercise. In: Gisolfi C, Lamb D, eds. *Fluid Homeostasis During Exercise.* Carmel, IN: Benchmark; 1990:247–280.
11. Zambraski EJ. The kidney and body fluid balance during exercise. In: Buskirk E, Puhl S, eds. *Body Fluid Balance, Exercise and Sports.* New York: CRC Press; 1996:75–95.
12. Wade C. Hormonal control of body fluid volume. In: Buskirk E, Puhl S, eds. *Body Fluid Balance, Exercise and Sports.* New York: CRC Press; 1996:53–73.
13. Poortmans JR, Vanderstraeten J. Kidney function during exercise in healthy and diseased humans: an update. *Sports Med.* 1994;18:419–437.
14. Krebs HA, Yoshida T. Muscular exercise and gluconeogenesis. *Biochem Z.* 1963;338:241–244.
15. Noakes TD, Goodman N, Rayner BL, et al. Water intoxication: a possible complication during endurance exercise. *Med Sci Sports Exerc.* 1985;17:370–375.
16. Mittleman KD, Zambraski EJ. Exercise-induced proteinuria is attenuated by indomethacin. *Med Sci Sports Exerc.* 1992;24:1069–1074.
17. Kocer G, Senturk UK, Kuru O, et al. Potential sources of oxidative stress that induce postexercise proteinuria in rats. *J Appl Physiol.* 2008;104:1063–1068.
18. Gunduz F, Kuru O, Senturk UK. Effect of nitric oxide on exercise-induced proteinuria in rats. *J Appl Physiol.* 2003;95:1867–1872.
19. Rush JWE, Aultman CD. Vascular biology of angiotensin and the impact of physical activity. *Appl Physiol Nutr Metab.* 2008;33:162–172.
20. Zambraski EJ, Tucker MS, Lakas CS, et al. Mechanisms of renin release in exercising dogs. *Am J Physiol.* 1984;246:E71–E78.
21. Vane JR, Bakhle YS, Botting RM. Cyclooxygenases 1 and 2. *Annu Rev Pharmacol Toxicol.* 1998;38:97–120.
22. Zambraski EJ, Dodelson R, Guidotti SM, et al. Renal prostaglandin E2 and F2 alpha synthesis during exercise: effects of indomethacin and sulindac. *Med Sci Sports Exerc.* 1986;18:678–684.
23. Farquhar WB, Morgan AL, Zambraski EJ, et al. Effects of acetaminophen and ibuprofen on renal function in the stressed kidney. *J Appl Physiol.* 1999;86:598–604.
24. Wharam PC, Speedy DB, Noakes TD, et al. NSAID use increases the risk of developing hyponatremia during an Ironman triathlon. *Med Sci Sports Exerc.* 2006;38:618–622.
25. Page AJ, Reid SA, Speedy BD, et al. Exercise-associated hyponatremia, renal function, and non-steroidal anti-inflammatory drug use in an ultraendurance mountain run. *Clin J Sports Med.* 2007;17:43–48.
26. DiCarlo SE, Stahl LK, Bishop VS. Daily exercise attenuates the sympathetic nerve response to exercise by enhancing cardiac afferents. *Am J Physiol.* 1997;273:H1606–H1610.
27. O'Hagan KP, Alberts JA. Uterine artery blood flow and renal sympathetic nerve activity during exercise in rabbit pregnancy. *Am J Physiol.* 2003;285:R1135–R1144.
28. Mazzeo RS, Rajkumar C, Jennings G, et al. Norepinephrine spillover at rest and during submaximal exercise in young and old subjects. *J Appl Physiol.* 1997;82:1869–1874.
29. Esler MG, Jennings P, Korner P, et al. Measurement of total and organ-specific norepinephrine kinetics in humans. *Am J Physiol.* 1984;247:E21–E28.
30. Miyauchi T, Maeda S, Iemitsu M, et al. Exercise causes a tissue specific change of NO production in kidney and lung. *J Appl Physiol.* 2003;94:60–68.
31. Shen W, Lundborg M, Wang J, et al. Role of EDRF in the regulation of regional blood flow and vascular resistance at rest and during exercise. *J Appl Physiol.* 1994;77:165–172.
32. McAllister RM, Newcomer SC, Pope ER, et al. Effects of chronic nitric oxide synthase inhibition on responses to acute exercise in swine. *J Appl Physiol.* 2008;104:186–197.
33. Zambraski EJ, Foster DT, Gross PM, et al. Iowa Wrestling Study: weight loss and urinary profiles of collegiate wrestlers. *Med Sci Sports.* 1976;8:105–108.
34. Meredith IT, Friberg P, Jennings GL, et al. Exercise training lowers resting renal but not cardiac sympathetic activity in humans. *Hypertension.* 1991;18:575–582.
35. Negrao CE, Irigoyen MC, Moreira ED, et al. Effect of exercise training on RSNA, baroreflex control, and blood pressure responsiveness. *Am J Physiol.* 1993;265:R365–R370.
36. Strickland MK, Miller JD. The best medicine: exercise training normalizes chemosensitivity and sympathoexcitation in heart failure. *J Appl Physiol.* 2008;105:779–781.
37. Kenney WL, Ho C. Age alters regional distribution of blood flow during moderate-intensity exercise. *J Appl Physiol.* 1995;79:1112–1119.
38. Poortmans JR, Ouchinsky M. Glomerular filtration rate and albumin excretion after maximal exercise in aging sedentary and active men. *J Gerontol.* 2006;61A:1181–1185.
39. Esler MD, Turner AG, Kaye DM, et al. Aging effects on human sympathetic neuronal function. *Am J Physiol.* 1995;268:R278–R285.

The Effects of Exercise in Altered Environments

CHAPTER 23

Physiologic Systems and Their Responses to Conditions of Heat and Cold

Michael N. Sawka, John W. Castellani, Samuel N. Cheuvront, and Andrew J. Young

Abbreviations

BAT	brown adipose tissue	NFCI	Nonfreezing cold injury
CHS	Compensated heat stress	PBMC	Peripheral blood mononuclear cell
CIVD	Cold-induced vasodilation	SkBF	Skin blood flow
CNS	Central nervous system	TBW	Total body water
EL	electrical stimulation	TNF	Tumor necrosis factor
HSP	Heat shock protein	UCHS	Uncompensated heat stress
IL	Interleukin	WBGT	Wet bulb globe temperature
MVC	Maximal voluntary contraction		

Introduction

Individuals exercise and work in a wide range of environmental conditions (*e.g.*, temperature, humidity, sun, wind, rain, and water). Depending on the environmental conditions and a person's metabolic rate and clothing, exercise can accentuate heat gain or heat loss, causing body temperature to rise or fall. Healthy humans normally regulate body (core) temperatures near 37°C at rest, and with environmental and/or exercise perturbations, body temperatures can fluctuate between 35°C and 41°C without adverse health consequences (1,2). Fluctuations outside that range can be associated with morbidity and mortality (3–5).

In this chapter, the term *exercise* refers to dynamic exercise, and *training* refers to repeated days of exercise in a specific modality leading to adaptations. The term *stress* refers to environmental and/or exercise conditions that tend to influence the body's heat content, and *strain* refers to the physiologic consequences of stress. The magnitude of stress and the resulting strain depend on a complex interaction among environmental factors (*e.g.*, ambient conditions and clothing) and the individual's biologic characteristics (*e.g.*, acclimatization status and body size) and activity level (*e.g.*, metabolic rate and duration). The term *acclimatization* refers to adaptations to both natural (acclimatization) and artificial (acclimation) environmental conditions.

In this chapter, we examine the effects of both heat stress and cold stress on physiologic responses and exercise capabilities. Human thermoregulation during exercise is addressed, but more detailed reviews on this process during environmental stress can be found elsewhere (6–8). This chapter includes information on the pathogenesis of exertional heat illness and hypothermia, since exercise can increase morbidity and mortality from thermal injury. Other chapters in this book emphasize acute and chronic (training) exercise, whereas in this chapter the focus is on acute and chronic (acclimatization) environmental exposure, although the effects of exercise training on physiologic responses during thermal (heat or cold) stress are discussed.

Thermal Balance and Control

Biophysics of Heat Exchange and Balance

Figure 23.1 schematically shows energy (heat) transfers in an exercising athlete. Muscular contraction produces metabolic heat that is transferred from the muscle to the blood and the body core. Because skeletal muscle contraction is about 20% efficient, about 80% of expended energy is released as heat that must be dissipated from the body to avoid heat storage and increased body temperature. Physiologic adjustments redirect blood flow from the body core to the periphery, thereby facilitating heat transfer from within the body to the skin, where it can be dissipated into the environment. Heat exchange between the skin and the environment is governed by biophysical mechanisms dictated by the surrounding air or water temperature; air humidity; air or water motion; solar, sky, and ground radiation; and clothing (9). The biophysical avenues of this heat exchange are conduction, convection, radiation, and evaporation. The nonevaporative avenues (conduction, convection, and radiation) are often collectively called dry heat exchange.

Conduction is the transfer of heat between two solid objects in direct contact, and convection is the exchange of heat between a surface and a moving fluid, including air or water. Heat exchange by conduction or convection occurs as long as there is a temperature gradient between the body surface and contacting object or surrounding fluid. When a person is standing, walking, or running and wearing shoes, heat exchange by conduction will be minimal because the thermal gradients between the body and contacted solids are usually small, as is the surface area for exchange. Convective heat exchange occurs when the surrounding fluid is moving (*e.g.*, wind and water circulation) relative to the body surface. In air environments, convective heat transfer can be significantly increased by wind if clothing does not create a barrier, and for swimmers convective heat loss can be very large, even when

the difference between the body surface and surrounding fluid temperature is small, because water has a much greater heat capacity than air (its conductive heat transfer coefficient is about 25 times that of air [7]). Heat loss by convection to air or water occurs when the air or water temperature is below body temperature; conversely, heat gain by convection from air or water occurs when the temperature exceeds that of the body.

Heat loss by radiation occurs when surrounding sun, sky, ground, or other large natural or manmade objects have lower surface temperatures than the body, and heat gain by radiation occurs when surrounding objects have higher surface temperatures than the body surface temperature. Radiative heat exchange is independent of air temperature or motion. Accordingly, temperature combinations of the sky, ground, and surrounding objects may result in body heat gain due to radiation even though the air temperature is below that of the body. For example, on a very sunny day, a mountaineer on a snowy surface may gain a significant amount of heat despite the low air temperature, and heat loss from exposed skin is greater under a clear night sky than in daylight due to radiative heat loss, even when ambient air temperatures are the same.

Evaporative heat loss occurs with the phase change when liquid turns to water vapor. In humans, evaporative heat loss is associated with breathing and perspiration. When water that is secreted onto the skin via sweat glands or is rained or splashed onto the skin evaporates, or water from respiratory passages evaporates, the kinetic energy of the motion of the water molecule (the latent heat of evaporation) will eliminate heat from the body. Evaporative cooling accounts for almost all heat loss during exercise at ambient temperatures equal to or above skin temperatures.

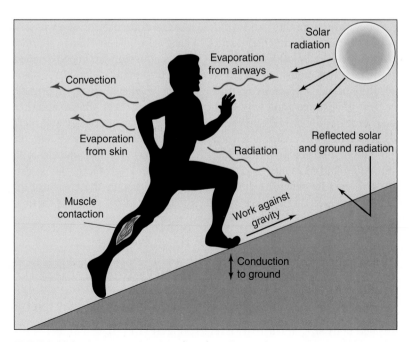

FIGURE 23.1   Avenues of energy (heat) exchange for an athlete performing exercise in air.

Body temperature reflects the balance between internal heat production and body heat transfer to the environment. The heat balance equation describes these relationships between the body and environment:

$$\pm S = M \pm \text{Work} \pm (R \pm C) \pm K \pm E \qquad [1]$$

where S = rate of body heat storage; M = rate of metabolic energy (heat) production; Work = mechanical work of either concentric (positive) or eccentric (negative) exercise; R ± C = rate of radiant and convective energy exchanges; K = rate of conduction (important only during direct contact with an object, such as clothing, or a substance, such as water); and E = rate of evaporative loss. The sum of these, heat storage, represents heat gain if positive or heat loss if negative. Body temperature increases when S is positive, decreases when S is negative, and remains constant when S equals zero (9).

Physiologic Thermoregulation

Humans regulate core temperature through two collaborative processes of temperature regulation: behavioral and physiologic (6). Behavioral temperature regulation operates through conscious alterations in behavior that can influence heat storage, such as modifying activity levels, changing clothes, and seeking shade or shelter. Physiologic temperature regulation operates through responses that are independent of conscious voluntary behavior, such as controlling the rate of metabolic heat production (*e.g.*, shivering), body heat distribution via the blood from the core to the skin (*e.g.*, cutaneous vasodilation and constriction), and

sweating. Persons often choose to ignore effective behavioral thermoregulation strategies because of their motivation to win or complete a task.

The function of the human thermoregulatory system is shown schematically in Figure 23.2 (6). This scheme presumes that thermal receptors in the core and skin send information about their temperature to some central integrator. Any deviation between the controlled variable (body temperature) and a reference variable (*e.g.*, set-point temperature) constitutes a load error that generates an efferent signal to control sweating, vasodilation, vasoconstriction, and shivering. The notion of such a thermal command signal is supported by two observations: (a) core temperature (70%–90%) and skin temperature (10%–30%) have similar influences on the control of both sweating and skin blood flow (SkBF) responses; and (b) the threshold temperatures for both sweating and SkBF are simultaneously shifted by similar magnitudes as a result of such factors as biologic rhythms, endogenous pyrogens, and heat acclimatization. It is useful to think of such similar and simultaneous shifts in various thermoregulatory thresholds as representing (or as being the result of) a shift in thermoregulatory set point (10). In contrast, dynamic exercise can increase the threshold temperature for SkBF but not alter the threshold for sweating, so this would not be interpreted as a change in the set-point temperature (11).

A disturbance in the regulated variable, core temperature, elicits graded heat loss or heat gain responses. Peripheral (skin) and central (brain, spinal column, and large vessels) thermal receptors provide afferent input into hypothalamic thermoregulatory centers (12), where this information is processed, producing a load error and

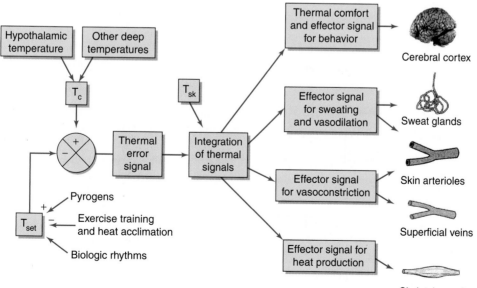

FIGURE 23.2 Human thermoregulation. (Adapted from Sawka MN, Wenger CB, Pandolf KB. *Thermoregulatory responses to acute exercise heat stress and heat acclimation.* In: Fregly MJ, Blatteis CM, eds. *Handbook of Physiology, Section 4. Environmental Physiology.* New York: Oxford University; 1996:160.)

proportionate thermoregulatory command signal to initiate responses to regain and maintain heat balance. In addition, very small changes in hypothalamus (anterior preoptic area) temperature elicit changes in the thermoregulatory effector responses, as this area contains many neurons that increase their firing rate in response either to warming or to cooling. The magnitudes of changes in heat loss (*e.g.*, sweating and SkBF), heat conservation (*e.g.*, vasoconstriction), or production (*e.g.*, shivering) are proportional to the displacement of the regulated variable (core temperature) from the thermoregulatory set-point temperature. The set-point temperature serves as a reference for the control of all thermoregulatory responses, somewhat similarly to a thermostat setting (13). There is controversy as to whether a set point truly exists, however, and there are alternative theories regarding this issue (14).

Exercise and fever both increase core temperature, but acute exercise does not alter the set point, whereas fever does (10). Figure 23.3 schematically shows the difference in thermoregulatory control between fever and exercise hyperthermia (15). Metabolic heat production increases immediately with the initiation of exercise, causing heat storage and thus a load error (−e) or difference between the set-point temperature and the elevated core temperature. The set-point temperature is unchanged, and therefore heat-dissipating responses are elicited as core temperature increases until heat loss responses sufficient to match heat production are achieved and a new thermal balance is established. When exercise stops, heat loss exceeds heat production, and thus the core temperature falls back toward the set point. This diminishes the signal (load error), eliciting the heat dissipation responses, and they decline to baseline levels as the thermal balance conditions prevailing before exercise are reestablished. Therefore, the primary event elevating core temperature during exercise is increased metabolic heat production.

In fever, the primary event is an elevation of the set-point temperature, which initially causes a negative load error (15). Heat-dissipating responses are inhibited and/or heat production is stimulated until core temperature increases enough to correct the load error and reestablish thermal balance at a new set-point temperature at which heat production and heat loss are near their values before the fever. The inhibition of heat dissipation and/or stimulation of heat production acts independently as a result of the person's thermal state and environmental temperature. When the fever abates (*i.e.*, the set point returns to normal), the heat-dissipating responses are increased and/or heat production is reduced until normal thermal balance is reestablished. If an individual exercises while having a fever, the exercise hyperthermia will be imposed above the fever temperature.

Summary

When changes in metabolic heat production or environmental temperature upset the thermal balance between heat dissipation and heat production, heat will be stored or lost from the body, and temperatures in the core or skin, or both, will change. Those temperature changes will be detected by the thermal receptors. In response to information from these receptors, the thermoregulatory controller in the central nervous system (CNS) will call for responses that alter heat loss and/or production. Unless the thermal stress exceeds the capacity of the thermoregulatory system, these responses will continue until they are sufficient to restore heat balance and prevent further change in body temperatures.

Core Temperature

The measurement of body core temperature is fundamental to the study of human temperature regulation. Core temperature is measured either to estimate the core temperature input to thermoregulatory control or to estimate average internal temperature to compute changes in heat storage in the core (6). Brain (*i.e.*, hypothalamic) temperature during exercise is generally accepted to be similar to blood temperature; however, recent evidence suggests that it could be slightly higher (16). There is no one true core temperature because temperature varies among sites deep inside the body. The temperature within a given deep body region depends on (a) the local metabolic rate of the surrounding tissues, (b) the source and magnitude of local blood flow, and (c) the temperature gradients between contiguous body regions. Considerable temperature gradients exist between and within orifices, body cavities, and blood vessels. For resting humans, internal organs and viscera within the body core produce about 70% of the metabolic heat. During dynamic exercise, however, skeletal muscles produce up to about 90% of the metabolic heat. Because metabolic heat sources change during exercise as compared with rest, the temperature

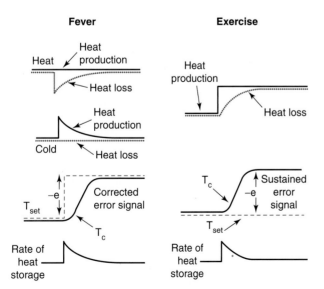

FIGURE 23.3   Differences between the elevation of core temperature in fever and during exercise. (Adapted from Stitt JT. Fever versus hyperthermia. *Fed Proc.* 1979;38:41–42.)

changes measured in one body region during exercise may be disproportionate to those measured in other body regions. These facts help explain the limitations of using two or even three compartment models for thermometric estimates of body heat storage (17). During rest in a comfortable environment, skeletal muscle temperature is lower than core temperature, but during exercise the temperature within active skeletal muscle often exceeds core temperature (temperature within inactive skeletal muscle usually does not increase) (18). Blood that is perfusing active skeletal muscles is warmed, and the blood then carries that heat to other body regions, resulting in an elevation in core temperature.

Core temperature during exercise is often measured at the esophagus, rectum, mouth, tympanum, or auditory meatus (6). The measurement methods employed for each of these locations, and the advantages and disadvantages of each, are summarized in Table 23.1. In brief, most thermal physiologists consider esophageal temperature to be the most accurate and reliable noninvasive index of core temperature for humans, followed in preference by rectal temperature and gastrointestinal tract temperature measured with the use of ingestible temperature sensor pills. Sensor pills are ideally suited for ambulatory monitoring outside of laboratories, but their values are variable and dependent on location within the gastrointestinal tract (19). Rectal and gastrointestinal tract temperatures are often slightly higher and slower to respond than esophageal temperature. Tympanic and auditory meatus temperatures are widely used to reflect core temperature, but are less reliable indices of core temperature than the other measures because they are influenced to some degree by head and face skin temperatures, ambient temperature, and positioning of the sensor.

Summary of Thermal Balance and Control

Thermal balance and control are affected by the biophysics of heat exchange and physiologic thermoregulation. Heat exchange between the skin and the environment is dictated by the surrounding air or water temperature; air humidity; air or water motion; solar, sky, and ground radiation; and clothing. Heat exchange occurs through conduction, convection, radiation, and evaporation. Humans regulate core temperature through behavioral and physiologic temperature regulation. Thermal receptors in the core and skin send information to a central integrator. A deviation between the body temperature and a set-point temperature generates

an efferent signal to control sweating, vasodilation, vasoconstriction, and shivering. Core temperature is measured either to estimate the core temperature input to thermoregulatory control or to estimate the average internal temperature to compute changes in heat storage in the core.

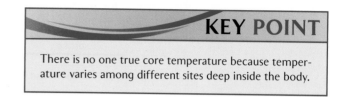

KEY POINT

There is no one true core temperature because temperature varies among different sites deep inside the body.

Heat Stress

Core Temperature Response to Exercise

Figure 23.4 illustrates core (rectal and esophageal) temperature responses to two exercise bouts separated by a brief rest period (20). During exercise and recovery, both measures of core temperature show similar patterns but with somewhat different kinetics and absolute values (rectal temperature is slower to respond and slightly higher). Heat production increases almost immediately at the onset of exercise; therefore, during the early stages of exercise, the rate of heat production exceeds the rate of dissipation, and the undissipated heat is stored, primarily in the core, causing the core temperature to rise. As the core temperature rises, heat-dissipating reflexes are elicited, the rate of heat storage decreases, and in turn the core temperature rises more slowly. As exercise continues, heat dissipation increases sufficiently to balance heat production, and steady-state values can be achieved. When exercise intensity or the combination of exercise intensity and environmental heat strain is high enough, a steady state may not be possible. When exercise is discontinued, the core temperature returns toward baseline levels, and with subsequent exercise the process is repeated.

The heat-exchange components that are necessary to achieve steady-state core temperature are dependent on the environmental conditions; however, exercise type (*e.g.*, arm vs. leg) can influence regional body heat exchange (21). Figure 23.5 illustrates the whole-body heat exchanges that might be expected during exercise (650-W metabolic rate) in a broad range of ambient temperatures (5°C–36°C, dry-bulb temperatures with low humidity) (22). The difference between metabolic rate and total heat loss represents

TABLE 23.1	Core Temperature Measurements	
Site	**Advantage**	**Disadvantage**
Esophageal	Accurate, rapid response	Uncomfortable, affected by swallowing
Rectal	Accurate, ease of measurement	Slow response, cultural objections
Auditory canal/ tympanic membrane	Ease of measurement	Inaccurate (biased by skin and ambient temperature; uncomfortable)
Oral	Ease of measurement	Inaccurate (affected by mouth breathing)
Pill	Accurate, ease of measurement	Pill movement from stomach and location influences measurement

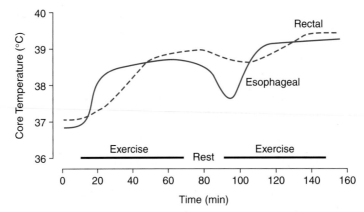

FIGURE 23.4   Core temperature (rectal and esophageal) responses to two exercise bouts separated by a brief rest period. (Reprinted from Sawka MN, Wenger CB. Physiologic responses to acute exercise heat stress. In: Pandolf KB, Sawka MN, Gonzalez RR, eds. *Human Performance Physiology and Environmental Medicine at Terrestrial Extremes*. Indianapolis, IN: Cooper; 1988:110.)

the energy used for mechanical work (and heat storage or heat debt, if there is no steady state). Total heat loss and therefore heat storage and elevation of core temperature are essentially the same in all environments. The relative contribution of dry and evaporative heat exchange to the total heat loss, however, varies with the environment. As the ambient temperature increases, the gradient for dry heat exchange diminishes and evaporative heat exchange becomes more important. When ambient temperature approaches or exceeds skin temperature, evaporative heat exchange will account for virtually all heat loss.

Heat stress can be classified as compensated heat stress (CHS) or uncompensated heat stress (UCHS) depending on biophysical factors (*e.g.*, environment, clothing, and metabolic rate) and biologic status (*e.g.*, heat acclimatization and hydration status). CHS exists when heat loss occurs at a rate in balance with heat production, so that a steady-state core

temperature can be achieved at a sustainable level for a requisite activity. UCHS occurs when the individual's evaporative cooling requirements exceed the environment's evaporative cooling capacity. During UCHS, an individual cannot achieve steady-state core temperature, and core temperature rises until exhaustion occurs at physiologic limits. A classic example of UCHS is that which occurs in people who work in a hot environment while wearing protective clothing, which adds thermal insulation and increases evaporative resistance (9).

During CHS and dynamic exercise, the magnitude of the steady-state core temperature elevation is largely independent of the environment and is proportional to the metabolic rate only within a specific range of CHS conditions, referred to as the prescriptive zone (23). Outside the prescriptive zone within CHS, steady-state core temperature will be achieved, but it will be elevated. Figure 23.6 provides an illustration of the steady-state core temperature elevation for a lightly

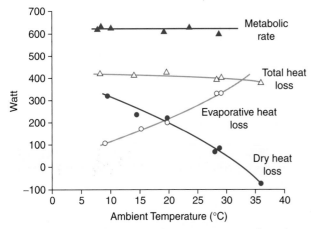

FIGURE 23.5   Heat exchange during exercise in a broad range of environmental temperatures with low humidity. (From Nielsen M. Die Regulation der Körpertemperatur bei Muskelarbeit. *Scand Arch Physiol* 1938;9:216.)

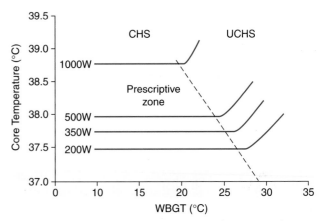

FIGURE 23.6   Possible core temperature (steady-state) responses during exercise at four metabolic rates during compensated heat stress (CHS) and uncompensated heat stress (UCHS) heat stress. (Adapted from Lind AR. A physiologic criterion for setting thermal environmental limits for everyday work. *J Appl Physiol*. 1963;18:53.)

clothed person that might be expected at several metabolic rates and wet bulb globe temperature (WBGT) conditions in low humidity (23). The 200-, 350-, and 500-W metabolic rates respectively approximate very light, moderate, and high-intensity dynamic exercise for occupational tasks. For many individuals, the upper limit for sustained exercise corresponds to a metabolic rate of about 1000 W. The prescriptive zone narrows as the metabolic rate increases.

During CHS, the core temperature increases in proportion to the metabolic rate during exercise (23,24). The greater the metabolic rate, the higher will be the steady-state core temperature during exercise. This relationship between metabolic rate and core temperature holds true for a given person but not always for comparisons between people. The use of relative intensity (percent of maximal oxygen uptake) rather than absolute metabolic rate (absolute intensity) reduces the variability between subjects for the core temperature elevation during exercise in CHS (25).

KEY POINT

Core temperature during exercise increases as a function of the metabolic rate.

Acute Exercise Heat Stress

Sweating and evaporative cooling

In humans, unlike most animals, respiratory evaporative cooling is much less efficient than total skin evaporative cooling. Human skin provides an advantage over the respiratory tract because it has a greater surface area that is directly exposed for evaporation. Thermoregulatory sweating can begin within a few minutes after the start of muscular exercise. The onset time of thermoregulatory sweating can vary and is influenced by skin temperature, acclimatization status, hydration status, and nonthermal stimuli (26), as well as reproductive hormones (27) and time of day (28). Although there is some evidence that sweat-gland output may be lower in women than in men (29), differences in sweat gland function with sex or age seem to be primarily linked to $\dot{V}O_{2max}$ (30,31).

The increase in thermoregulatory sweating closely parallels the increase in body temperature (26). As the sweating rate increases, sweat glands are recruited and the sweat secretion per gland increases. Therefore, the sweat secretion for a given region of skin reflects both the density of sweat glands and the secretion per gland (32). In addition, different body regions of skin have different sweating responses (threshold and/or sensitivity) for a given core temperature. The back and chest have the highest sweating rates, and the limbs have relatively high sweating rates only after a substantial elevation in core temperature (33).

The eccrine glands secrete sweat onto the skin, which allows evaporative cooling by conversion of sweat from liquid to water vapor. The evaporation rate is dependent on the gradient between the skin and water vapor pressure and the coefficient of evaporative heat transfer, and the wider the water vapor gradient, the greater will be the rate of evaporation for a given mass transfer coefficient (9). When 1 g of sweat is vaporized at 30°C, 2.43 kJ of heat energy becomes kinetic energy (latent heat of evaporation). The following calculations provide the minimal sweating requirements for a person performing exercise at a 600-W metabolic rate in severe heat in which only evaporative cooling is possible. If the activity is 20% efficient, the remaining 80% of metabolic energy produced is converted to heat in the body, such that 480 W (0.48 kJ $\cdot$ s^{-1}, or 28.8 kJ $\cdot$ min^{-1}) must be dissipated to avoid heat storage. The specific heat of body tissue (amount of energy required for 1 g of tissue to increase temperature by 1°C) approximates 3.5 kJ $\cdot$ °C^{-1}; thus, a 70-kg man would have a heat capacity of 245 kJ $\cdot$ °C^{-1}. If this person performed exercise in a hot environment that enabled only evaporative heat loss and he did not sweat, his body temperature would increase by approximately 1.0°C every 8.5 min (245 kJ per °C, 28.8 kJ $\cdot$ min^{-1}). Because the latent heat of evaporation is 2.43 kJ $\cdot$ g^{-1}, this person would need to evaporate approximately 12 g of sweat (28.8 kJ $\cdot$ min^{-1}/2.43 kJ $\cdot$ g^{-1}) per minute, or 0.72 L $\cdot$ h^{-1}. Sweating, however, is not 100% efficient, because some secreted sweat can drip from the body and not be evaporated. Therefore, higher sweat secretions than calculated may actually be needed to satisfy the demands for cooling.

Skin blood flow and dry heat loss

Blood transfers heat by convection from the deep-body tissues to the skin. When core and skin temperatures are low enough that sweating does not occur, raising SkBF will bring the skin temperature nearer to blood temperature, and lowering SkBF will bring the skin temperature nearer to ambient temperature. Thus, the body can control dry heat loss by varying SkBF and hence skin temperature. When sweating occurs, the tendency of SkBF to warm the skin is approximately balanced by the tendency of sweat evaporation to cool the skin. Therefore, after sweating has begun, SkBF serves primarily to deliver to the skin the heat that is being removed by sweat evaporation. SkBF and sweating thus work in tandem to dissipate heat.

Skin circulation is affected by temperature in two ways: local skin temperature affects the vascular smooth muscle directly, and temperatures of the core and the skin elsewhere on the body affect SkBF by reflexes operating through the sympathetic nervous system. Blood flow in much of the human skin is under dual vasomotor control (34). In the palm of the hand, sole of the foot, lips, ears, and nose, adrenergic vasoconstrictor fibers are probably the predominant source of vasomotor innervation, and the vasodilation that occurs in these regions during heat exposure is largely the result of withdrawing vasoconstrictor activity. Over most of the skin area, there is minimal vasoconstrictor activity at skin temperatures of about 39°C and above (35), and vasodilation during heat exposure depends on intact sympathetic innervation. This vasodilation depends on the action of neural signals and as such is sometimes referred to as active vasodilation. Both active vasoconstriction and active vasodilation play a major part in controlling SkBF on the arm, thigh, and calf. However, active vasodilation is primarily responsible for controlling SkBF on the torso. The mechanism or mechanisms responsible for active cutaneous vasodilation are not fully understood. It is known that active cutaneous vasodilation is usually closely associated with sweating. Whether this link is due to a cotransmitter or linkage to sudomotor neural activity is unresolved, but possible vasoactive substances include vasoactive intestinal peptide, calcitonin gene–related peptide, substance P, and nitric oxide (26,34,36).

The SkBF required to meet heat dissipation needs will change with skin conditions (*e.g.*, ambient conditions and sweat evaporation) and core temperatures. Table 23.2 provides calculations for minimal SkBF requirements at several core and skin temperature levels. These estimates assume that blood entering and leaving the cutaneous vasculature is equal to the core and skin temperatures, respectively (37). If the exercise-mediated heat production is 10 kcal · min^{-1} (about 698 W of heat production requires a metabolic rate of 872 W [about 2.5 L oxygen uptake] with 80% of energy converted to heat) and core temperature is 38°C, the minimal SkBF requirement will be about 5 L · min^{-1} if skin temperature is 36°C, but will decrease to 2.5 L · min^{-1} if skin temperature decreases to 34°C. This clearly demonstrates how evaporative cooling by a decrease in skin temperature reduces the cardiovascular strain associated with supporting SkBF.

When environmental conditions do not allow skin cooling, the body can employ a different approach to reduce SkBF requirements during exercise. Of importance, an additional elevation in core temperature may be tolerated. If skin temperature remains at 36°C, a core temperature elevation by 1°C will increase the core-to-skin temperature gradient and reduce the SkBF requirement from 5.0 to 3.3 L · min^{-1} (Table 23.2). Thus, an elevated core temperature is actually physiologically advantageous outside the prescriptive zone during CHS (Fig. 23.6) and reflects a strategy to reduce cardiovascular strain to sustain thermal balance and exercise performance.

Chronologic aging and menstrual cycle phase have been shown to alter nonacral SkBF during local and whole-body heating (30,31). However, with aging, SkBF is lower for any given increase in core temperature (38) and the response is independent of $\dot{V}O_{2max}$ (39). Age-related declines in SkBF are also associated with a smaller increase in cardiac output during passive heating and less redistribution of blood from the splanchnic and renal circulation to the skin (30,40).

Cardiovascular Effects

During exercise heat stress, the task of maintaining a high SkBF can impose a substantial burden on the cardiovascular system (37,41). SkBF can approach 8 L · min^{-1} for an average adult during heat stress. High SkBF can reduce right atrial pressure and filling (37) because the cutaneous venous bed is large and compliant, and dilates during heat stress. As the venous bed of the skin, especially below heart level, becomes engorged with blood, the central blood volume will decline as SkBF increases. Sweat secretion can result in a net loss of body water, reducing blood volume. Therefore, heat stress can reduce cardiac filling both through pooling of blood in the skin and reduced blood volume. To compensate for reduced cardiac filling during rest and exercise, cardiac contractility increases to maintain the stroke volume because of elevated sympathetic activity and parasympathetic withdrawal, and perhaps temperature effects on the cardiac pacemaker cells. In addition, whole body heating in resting subjects can reduce carotid baroreflex control of blood pressure and vagal baroreflex regulation of the heart rate, which may contribute to orthostatic intolerance during heat stress (42,43).

During exercise in the heat, the primary cardiovascular challenge is to increase cardiac output sufficiently to support both high SkBF for heat dissipation and high muscle blood flow for metabolism. Exercise heat stress increases SkBF and usually sustains muscle blood flow relative to temperate conditions; however, reduced muscle blood flow has been observed during maximal exercise with heat stress (44). Figure 23.7 provides an analysis of cardiac output and distribution during rest and dynamic exercise in temperate and hot climates (37). This figure depicts cardiac output as being elevated during mild and perhaps moderate exercise in the heat compared with similar exercise in temperate conditions. During high- and maximal-intensity exercise in the heat, cardiac output can be below levels observed during similar exercise in temperate conditions. The lower cardiac output during maximal exercise results largely from an inability of the heart rate to compensate for

TABLE 23.2	Skin Blood Flow Requirements for Several Core (T_c) and Skin (T_{sk}) Temperatures during Exercise Heat Stress				
Heat production (kcal/min)	Core temperature (°C)	Skin temperature (°C)	Core-to-skin gradient (°C)	SkBF (L/min)
10	38	36	2	5
10	38	34	4	2.5
10	39	36	3	3.3

SkBF = 1/SH × HP/T_c − T_{sk}.

SkBF, skin blood flow; SH, specific heat of blood (~1 kcal/°C/L blood); HP, heat production.

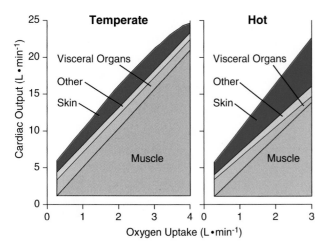

FIGURE 23.7 Comparison of cardiac output responses to exercise performed at various metabolic rates in temperate and heat stress conditions. (From Rowell LB. *Human circulation: regulation during physical stress.* New York: Oxford University Press; 1986:385.)

reductions in stroke volume associated with high SkBF and peripheral pooling of blood (45).

Coronary blood flow is believed to be unaffected by exercise heat stress. However, as a result of increased sympathetic activity and thermal receptor stimulation, visceral (splanchnic and renal) blood flow is reduced by both exercise and heat stress. The visceral blood flow reductions are graded with the intensity of exercise, and the effects of exercise and heat seem to be additive (37). The mechanisms that are responsible for changes in this splanchnic blood flow are probably quite complex (46). Reduced visceral blood flow allows a corresponding diversion of cardiac output to skin and exercising muscle, and helps support blood pressure (see Chapter 7). Also, secondary to reduced visceral blood flow, a substantial volume of blood can be mobilized from the compliant splanchnic beds to help maintain cardiac filling during exercise heat stress. If these compensatory responses are insufficient, skin, muscle, and even brain blood flow may be compromised. Although Figure 23.7 indicates that muscle blood flow decreases during severe exercise heat stress, this is controversial and probably occurs only with a combination of maximal exercise or severe heat strain and dehydration (44,47). Cerebral blood flow, however, can be reduced by 20% with only moderate-intensity exercise (50% $\dot{V}O_{2peak}$) during UCHS in which venous blood temperature increases from 38°C to 39.5°C (16). Similarly, heat stress and dehydration may mediate changes in cerebral vascular resistance that could contribute with reduced perfusion pressure to reduce cerebral blood flow (48,49).

Metabolism

The relationship between tissue temperature and metabolic processes is described by the temperature quotient (Q_{10}), which is the increase in a reaction that occurs as a function of a positive 10°C temperature change. Positive thermal dependence occurs when Q_{10} is greater than 1.0. Most mechanical (contraction velocity, power output) and chemical (enzymatic) reactions of skeletal muscle display thermal dependence on the order of 2.0 to 3.0 (50).

Acute heat stress increases the metabolic rate to perform submaximal exercise, possibly because the rate of adenosine triphosphate utilization to develop a given muscle tension is increased (i.e., increased cross-bridge cycling) as muscle temperature increases (51). Aerobic metabolism and muscle total adenine pool may decrease, whereas oxygen debt, blood and muscle lactate accumulation, skeletal muscle glycogen utilization, and inosine 5-monophosphate concentration may all increase during exercise with higher muscle temperatures (51,52). The increased glycogen utilization is probably mediated by elevated epinephrine and muscle hyperthermia. In addition, lactate uptake and oxidation by the liver and probably nonexercising muscle are impaired during exercise heat stress. Elevated muscle temperature does not appear to alter oxidative adaptations or mitochondrial biogenesis (53,54) (see Chapter 18).

Heat acclimatization usually lowers total metabolic rate during exercise because of reductions in aerobic and anaerobic components, but this effect is probably too small to reduce heat storage (51). On the other hand, changes in substrate metabolism induced by heat acclimatization may help improve endurance. Blood and muscle lactate accumulation and muscle glycogen depletion during exercise are often reduced after heat acclimatization. The fact that these metabolic effects of heat acclimatization are observed during exercise in both temperate and hot environments suggests that chronic heat exposure may result in metabolic adaptations that are independent of thermoregulatory and cardiovascular alterations (51,52).

Exercise Performance Limitations

Performance effects

Heat strain will degrade dynamic exercise performance and increase variability among athletes. High maximal aerobic power enables the performance of tasks that require sustained high metabolic rates; therefore, a lower maximal aerobic power often translates to reduced exercise performance. Most investigators find that maximal aerobic power is lower in hot climates than in temperate ones. For example, in one study, maximal aerobic power was 0.25 L · min⁻¹ (7%) lower at 49°C than at 21°C, and the state of heat acclimatization did not alter the magnitude of the maximal aerobic power decrement (55).

What physiologic mechanisms might be responsible for such a reduction in maximal aerobic power? Heat stress, by dilating the cutaneous vascular beds, may divert some cardiac output from skeletal muscle to skin, leaving less blood flow to support the metabolism of exercising skeletal muscle (44). In addition, dilation of the cutaneous vascular bed may increase cutaneous blood volume at the expense of central blood volume, reducing venous return and maximal cardiac output. For example, Rowell and associates

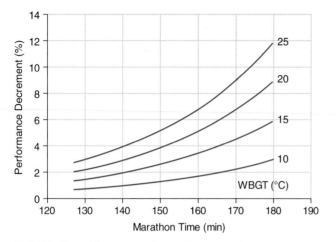

FIGURE 23.8 Nomogram for performance decrement (y-axis) based on projected marathon finishing time (x-axis) with increasing environmental heat stress (wet-bulb globe temperature [WBGT]). (From Ely MR, Cheuvront SN, Roberts WO, et al. Impact of weather on marathon-running performance. *Med Sci Sports Exer.* 2007;39:487.)

(45) reported that during intense exercise (73% of maximal aerobic power) in the heat, cardiac output can be reduced by 1.2 L · min^{-1} below control levels. Such a reduction in cardiac output during heat exposure could account for a 0.25 L · min^{-1} decrement in maximal aerobic power, assuming that each liter of blood delivers 0.2 L of oxygen (1.34 mL O$_2$ · g Hb^{-1} × 15 g Hb · 100 mL^{-1} of blood).

Submaximal exercise performance is also reduced by heat stress. It has been demonstrated that the performance of marathon runners becomes progressively slower with increased heat stress within a WBGT range of 5°C to 25°C (Fig. 23.8). The magnitude of slowing ranges from approximately 4 to 20 minutes, with the larger performance decrement observed in slower (3 hour) competitors (56). Figure 23.9 presents time-to-fatigue values

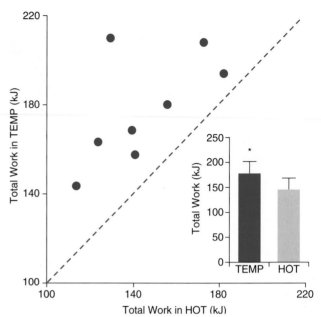

FIGURE 23.10 Exercise performance (15-min cycling time trial) in temperate (TEMP, 21°C) versus hot (HOT, 40°C) environments. The dotted line represents the line of identity (equal performances). *Inset*: Mean total work (mean, SD) in each environment; *denotes significant difference between conditions (*P* < 0.05). (Adapted from Ely BR, Cheuvront SN, Kenefick RW, et al. Aerobic performance is degraded, despite modest hyperthermia, in hot environments. *Med Sci Sports Exer.* 2010;42:135).

obtained during cycle ergometer exercise performed at four ambient temperatures (57). The subjects exercised 45% longer at an air temperature of 11°C compared with 31°C and had less cardiovascular strain. Core temperature at exhaustion was inversely related to air temperature but ranged narrowly from about 39°C to 40°C despite large differences in exercise duration. Likewise, time to fatigue in a cool (10°C) environment even after completion of a muscle-glycogen-reducing regimen was markedly longer (>30 min) than time to fatigue for glycogen-loaded subjects in a hot (30°C) environment (58). Muscle heating does not have a consistent effect on maximal voluntary contraction (MVC) and will generally reduce muscle endurance at a given percentage of MVC (50). However, in the absence of high core body temperatures, elevated skin temperatures alone can decrease $\dot{V}O_{2max}$ and reduce sustained submaximal exercise performance (59) (Fig. 23.10), likely by decreasing cardiovascular reserve (60).

Heat strain mechanisms of exhaustion

Table 23.3 presents physiologic mechanisms that can reduce exercise performance in the heat. These mechanisms include increased thermal and cardiovascular strain, diminished CNS drive for exercise, accelerated glycogen depletion with increased metabolite accumulation, and perhaps increased discomfort. The exact mechanism or mechanisms are unknown but probably depend on the

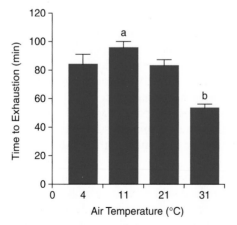

FIGURE 23.9 Exercise endurance time at a given metabolic rate in cold (4°C), cool (11°C), temperate (21°C), and warm (31°C) ambient temperatures. *P* < 0.05; a (>4, 21, 31°C); b (< 4, 11, 21°C). (Adapted from Galloway SD, Maughan RJ. Effects of ambient temperature on the capacity to perform prolonged cycle exercise in man. *Med Sci Sports Exer.* 1997;29:1242.)

TABLE 23.3	Physiologic Mechanisms that Contribute to Reduce Exercise Performance during Heat Stress	
Mechanism	**Cause**	**Consequence**
Cardiovascular strain	High skin blood flow	Inability to maintain required cardiac output and blood pressure
	Compliant skin	
	Dehydration	
Central fatigue	High brain temperature	Reduced neural drive to exercise
Thermal discomfort	Hot and wet skin	Insufficient carbohydrate substrate
	High heart rate	
Muscle glycogen depletion	High muscle temperature	Insufficient carbohydrate substrate
	High sympathetic activity	

specific heat stress, exercise task, and biomedical state of the individual. For example, increased glycogen depletion would be critical for reducing performance only if the individual could minimize the adverse consequences of elevated cardiovascular strain.

Core temperature provides the most reliable physiologic index to predict the incidence of exhaustion from heat strain during UCHS (61). However, as discussed above, the skin temperature associated with a given core temperature can greatly modify the physiologic strain. Figure 23.11 illustrates some relationships between core temperature and incidence of exhaustion from heat strain for heat-acclimated persons exercising during UCHS (most likely very hot skin) and CHS (most likely cool skin) (62). During UCHS, exhaustion is rarely associated with a core temperature below 38°C, and exhaustion will almost always occur before a core temperature of 40°C is attained (61). Remember, a skin temperature above 35°C,

as seen during UCHS, will be associated with greater cardiovascular strain for a given core temperature (60,63) and therefore result in earlier exhaustion. If skin is relatively cool, higher core temperatures can be better sustained during exercise. For example, some elite athletes can tolerate core temperatures above 41°C and continue to exercise as long as their skin temperature remains cool (64). Lower skin temperatures (and wider core-to-skin temperature gradients) decrease SkBF requirements (Table 23.2) and reduce cardiovascular strain. It is therefore intuitive to conclude that the larger cardiovascular reserve that accompanies training and is the hallmark of high fitness, confers an advantage. However, other factors may also contribute to a higher core temperature tolerance, such as extensive heat acclimatization, training practices, natural selection, or some combination thereof. For most people, the expected incidence of exhaustion will occur at core body temperatures somewhere along the continuum represented in Figure 23.11. However, higher skin temperatures and greater cardiovascular strain will generally produce exhaustion at modest core body temperatures (61).

The first convincing demonstration that the CNS can mediate reduced exercise performance in the heat was provided by Lars Nybo and Bodil Nielsen of Denmark (65) (see *A Milestone of Discovery* at the end of this chapter). Their experiments demonstrated that a core body temperature of 40°C markedly reduces voluntary force-generating capacity during a prolonged MVC in both active (leg) and inactive (forearm) muscles compared with that measured at a core temperature of 38°C. However, electrical stimulation (EL) of these hyperthermic muscles restored total force generation to that observed in a lower temperature trial. These data strongly suggest that the CNS contributes to the reduced exercise performance of individuals exercising under hyperthermic conditions. It is possible that CNS involvement is related to the reduction in brain blood flow (16) and reduced cerebral oxygen delivery. Strong evidence for a natural neurohumoral connection between heat stress and fatigue is lacking (66), and pharmacologic findings are mixed. However, drug manipulations of dopamine

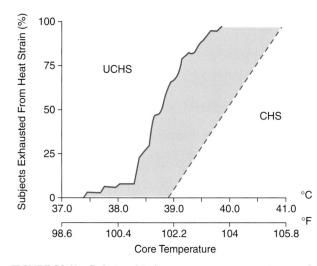

FIGURE 23.11   Relationship between core temperature and incidence of exhaustion from heat strain during exercise in compensated heat stress (CHS) and uncompensated heat stress (UCHS). (Adapted from Sawka MN, Young AJ. Physical exercise in hot and cold climates. In: Garrett WE, Kirkendall DT, eds. *Exercise and Sports Science.* Philadelphia: Lippincott Williams & Wilkins; 2000:389.)

(or the serotonin/dopamine ratio) show some promise for delaying heat stress fatigue (67). Indeed, exercise in the heat can induce changes in electroencephalographic activity from the frontal cortex (68) that are consistent with central fatigue based on changes in the concentrations of relevant monoamines (69,70).

It is not possible to say for certain whether measured losses of motor cortical output are the result of an unwilling or incapable participant, but psychological strain is probably an important factor in determining an individual's desire to continue exercise in the heat. Thermal discomfort is influenced by skin temperature and wetness (14), whereas rated perceived exertion is influenced by both of these factors as well as heart rate. Anticipatory models (71,72) that focus on the rate of body heat storage appear untenable (73,74). It is doubtful that high core temperature alone can be sensed, but high brain temperature may induce neurochemical changes that modify perception of strain. During exercise in the heat, skin temperature, wetness, and heart rate will increase. An athlete's tolerance to such perceptual cues will most likely influence his or her exercise capabilities. Thus, it appears that brain chemical manipulations that alter sensory perception may blunt the ill effects of heat stress on endurance performance by permitting greater tolerance (similar perception) to higher exercise intensities. Of importance, the remaining 19% performance decline from control (97) suggests a larger performance-limiting contribution by some other intact mechanism(s).

KEY POINT

The CNS contributes to reduced exercise performance in the heat.

Exercise Training and Heat Acclimatization

Exercise training

Exercise training in a temperate climate with emphasis on improved aerobic performance can reduce physiologic strain and improve exercise capabilities in the heat, but such exercise training programs alone cannot replace the benefits of heat acclimatization (75,76). Figure 23.11 depicts the effects of an exercise training program with heat acclimatization on reducing physiologic strain and improving endurance during exercise heat stress (77). After performing an initial (pretraining) exercise heat test (4 hours at about 35% maximal aerobic power under hot, dry conditions), the subjects completed the training program (1 hour a day, 4 times a week for 11 weeks in temperate conditions), then again underwent the exercise heat test. Finally, the subjects completed a heat acclimatization program (35% maximal aerobic power, 4 hours per day for 8 days) and again underwent the exercise heat test. The exercise training reduced physiologic strain and improved endurance,

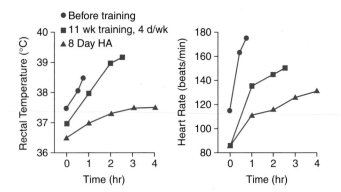

FIGURE 23.12 Core temperature and heart-rate responses during standardized exercise heat stress in an untrained subject not acclimatized to heat, after 11 weeks of physical training, and after 8 days of heat acclimatization. HA, heat acclimatization. (Adapted from Cohen JS, Gisolfi CV. Effects of interval training on work-heat tolerance of young women. *Med Sci Sports Exer.* 1982;14:46–52.)

but these improvements were modest compared with those obtained by heat acclimatization.

Dynamic exercise training in temperate climates can improve heat loss responses during exercise heat stress, but not to the same magnitude as achieved by heat acclimatization (75,76). Figure 23.12 illustrates the impact of training and heat acclimatization on improving sweating responses. Local sweating responses during exercise heat stress were measured on untrained and nonacclimatized subjects, after 10 days of exercise training (70%–80% maximal aerobic power in temperate conditions), and after 10 days of heat acclimatization (1 hour at 50% maximal aerobic power in hot, wet conditions) (78). Exercise training increased the slope of the sweating response, but heat acclimatization markedly reduced threshold temperature to initiate sweating as soon as core temperature started to rise. The net effect of heat acclimatization was a substantially increased sweating rate for a given core temperature during exercise. The SkBF responses changed in a manner similar to that observed for sweating after training and heat acclimatization.

To improve thermoregulation and exercise capabilities in the heat by training, the training sessions must produce a substantial elevation of core temperature and sweating rate (75). To achieve optimal improvement in thermoregulation with aerobic exercise training in temperate climates, the intensity should be at least 50% of maximal aerobic power for at least 1 week and perhaps as long as 8 weeks (45).

Heat Acclimatization

Heat acclimatization induces biologic adjustments that reduce the negative effects of heat stress. Heat acclimatization develops through repeated heat exposures that are sufficiently stressful to elevate both core and skin temperatures, and provoke profuse sweating. The biologic adjustments are mediated by integrated changes in thermoregulatory control, fluid balance, and cardiovascular responses. In addition to these systemic adaptations, research has shown that cellular adaptations may also occur (79).

The magnitude of biologic adaptations induced by heat acclimatization depends largely on the intensity, duration, frequency, and number of heat exposures. Exercising in the heat is the most effective method for developing heat acclimatization; however, even resting in the heat results in limited acclimatization. Usually, about 7 to 10 days of heat exposure are needed to induce heat acclimatization. Optimal heat acclimatization requires a minimum daily heat exposure of about 2 hours (or two 1-hour exposures) combined with dynamic exercise that requires cardiovascular endurance rather than resistance training for development of muscular strength (80). Shorter duration/higher intensity protocols are also effective for inducing heat acclimatization (81). Individuals should gradually increase the exercise intensity or duration each day of heat acclimatization.

During the initial exercise heat exposure, physiologic strain is high, as manifested by elevated core temperature and heart rate. The physiologic strain induced by the same exercise heat stress decreases each day of acclimatization. Most of the improvements in heart rate, skin and core temperatures, and sweat rate are achieved through daily exercise in a hot climate during the first week of exposure. The heart rate reduction develops most rapidly in 4 to 5 days. After 7 days, the reduction in heart rate is virtually complete. The thermoregulatory benefits from heat acclimatization are generally thought to be complete after 10 to 14 days of exposure (76). However, it may take longer to achieve improvements in physiologic tolerance (61).

Heat acclimatization is transient and gradually disappears if not maintained by continued repeated heat exposure (75,76). The benefits of heat acclimatization will be retained for about 1 week and then decay, with about 75% lost by about 3 weeks once heat exposure ends. A day or two of intervening cool weather will not interfere with acclimatization to hot weather. The heart rate improvement, which develops more rapidly during acclimatization, is also lost more rapidly than thermoregulatory responses.

Table 23.4 provides a brief description of the actions of heat acclimatization. Heat acclimatization improves thermal comfort and submaximal and maximal aerobic exercise capabilities (82). These benefits of heat acclimatization are achieved by improved sweating and SkBF responses, better fluid balance and cardiovascular stability, and a lowered metabolic rate (6). Heat acclimatization is specific to the climate (*e.g.*, desert or jungle) and physical activity level. However, heat acclimatization to one type of hot climate can markedly improve exercise capabilities in a different one.

TABLE 23.4	Actions of Heat Acclimatization
Thermal comfort improved	**Exercise performance improved**
Core temperature reduced	Cardiovascular stability improved
Sweating improved	Heart rate lowered
Earlier onset	Stroke volume increased
Higher rate	Blood pressure better defended
Redistribution (jungle)	Myocardial compliance improved
Hidromeiosis resistance (jungle)	Fluid balance improved
Skin blood flow improved	Thirst improved
Earlier onset	Electrolyte loss (sweat, urine) reduced
Higher rate	Total body water increased
Metabolic rate lowered	Plasma (blood) volume increased, better defended
	Acquired thermal tolerance improved

Heat acclimatization does not improve maximal exercise performance. For example, heat-stress–mediated reductions in maximal aerobic power are not abated by heat acclimatization (55). In addition, heat acclimatization probably does not alter the maximal core temperature a person can tolerate during exercise during CHS (83,84). There is some evidence, however, that persons who live and physically train over many weeks in the heat may be able to tolerate higher maximal core temperatures during UCHS (61).

The effects of heat acclimatization on submaximal exercise performance can be quite dramatic, and acclimatized subjects often find they can easily complete tasks in the heat that were previously difficult or impossible (Fig. 23.12). Heat acclimatization mediates improved submaximal exercise performance by reducing body temperature and physiologic strain (Fig. 23.12). The three classical signs of heat acclimatization are lower heart rate and core temperature, and higher sweat rate during exercise heat stress. Skin temperatures are often lower after heat acclimatization and thus dry heat loss is reduced (or, if the environment is warmer than the skin, dry heat gain is increased). To compensate for the changes in dry heat exchange, an increase in evaporative heat loss is necessary to achieve heat balance.

After acclimatization, sweating starts earlier and at a lower core temperature; that is, the core temperature threshold for sweating is decreased (Fig. 23.13). The sweat glands also become resistant to hidromeiosis and fatigue, so that higher sweat rates can be sustained. Sweating rate is often increased by the second day of heat acclimatization. Earlier and greater sweating improves evaporative cooling (if the climate allows evaporation) and reduces body heat storage

---

KEY POINT

Heat acclimatization reduces thermal and cardiovascular strain and improves thermal comfort and exercise performance.

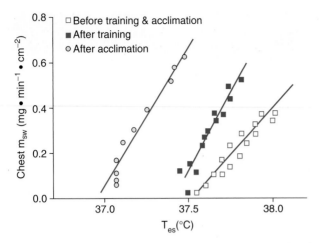

FIGURE 23.13 Local sweating responses during standardized exercise heat stress in an untrained subject unacclimatized to heat, after completion of a physical training program, and after completion of a heat acclimatization program. (From Roberts MF, Wenger CB, Stolwijk JAJ, et al. Skin blood flow and sweating changes following exercise training and heat acclimation. *J Appl Physiol.* 1977;43:135.)

and skin temperature. Lower skin temperatures decrease the cutaneous blood flow required for heat balance (because of the greater core-to-skin temperature gradient) and reduce cutaneous venous compliance so that blood volume can be redistributed from the peripheral to the central circulation. All of these factors reduce cardiovascular strain and enhance exercise performance in the heat.

The effects of heat acclimatization on cardiac output responses to exercise heat stress are not clear. Some studies have reported little change in cardiac output, but most have revealed an increase in cardiac output during submaximal exercise performed after heat acclimatization. Heart rate is much higher and stroke volume is lower during exercise heat stress, as compared with temperate conditions on the first day of heat acclimatization. Thereafter, heart rate begins to decrease as early as the second day. These changes are rapid at first but continue more slowly for about a week. It is likely that numerous mechanisms participate, and their relative contributions will vary both over the course of the program and among subjects (6). These mechanisms include (a) improved skin cooling and redistribution of blood volume, (b) plasma volume expansion, (c) increased venous tone from cutaneous and noncutaneous beds, and (d) reduced core temperature. In addition, heat acclimatization can increase compliance and reduce the myocardial energy cost (85).

Fluid balance improvements from heat acclimatization include better matching of thirst to body water needs, increased total body water, and increased blood volume (86,87). Most (but not all studies) have reported that heat acclimatization increases total body water (87). The magnitude of increase often approximates 2.0 liters, or about 5% of total body water. This increase is well within the measurement resolution for total body water, and thus appears to be a real physiologic phenomenon. The division of the total

body water increase between intracellular fluid and extracellular fluid varies: studies have reported that extracellular fluid accounts for greater, equal, or smaller amounts of the percentage increase compared with intracellular fluid after heat acclimatization (87). Because measures of extracellular fluid have a relatively high variability, it is difficult to interpret trends for such small changes. The extent to which intracellular fluid increases is unclear, because typically it is calculated as the difference between total body water and extracellular fluid, and thus measurement variability inherent in both these techniques is compounded in the calculation of intracellular fluid. If total body water and extracellular fluid increase after heat acclimatization, then expansion of plasma volume might be expected.

Plasma volume expansion is usually (but not always) present after repeated heat exposure and heat acclimatization (88). Erythrocyte volume does not appear to be altered by heat acclimatization. Heat-acclimatization studies have revealed that plasma volume expansion generally ranges from about 5% to about 30%, and the magnitude of increase somewhat depends on (a) whether the subject is at rest or performing exercise, (b) the day of heat acclimatization, and (c) the hydration state of the subject when measurements are made. Plasma volume expansion seems to be greatest during upright exercise on about the fifth day of heat acclimatization in fully hydrated persons who are living in the heat.

The mechanisms responsible for this hypervolemia are unclear, but they include an increase in extracellular fluid mediated by retention of crystalloids (primarily sodium chloride) and perhaps an increase in plasma volume selectively mediated by the oncotic effect of increased volume of intravascular protein (no change in content) (87). The increase in total body water can be explained in part by increased aldosterone secretion and/or renal sensitivity to a given plasma concentration. An unacclimatized person may secrete sweat with a sodium concentration of ≥ 60 mEq $\cdot$ L^{-1} and, if sweating profusely, can lose large amounts of sodium. With acclimatization, the sweat glands conserve sodium by secreting sweat with a sodium concentration as low as 10 mEq $\cdot$ L^{-1}. This salt-conserving effect of acclimatization depends on the hormone aldosterone, which is secreted in response to exercise and heat exposure, as well as to sodium depletion. The conservation of salt also helps to maintain the number of osmoles in the extracellular fluid and thus to maintain or increase extracellular fluid volume.

Acquired thermal tolerance and molecular adaptations

It has been shown that humans and animals repeatedly exposed to the hyperthermia of exercise can become more resistant to exertional heat injury and stroke. The repeated heating of body tissues results in acquired thermal tolerance, cellular changes resulting from severe, nonlethal heat exposure that allow the organism to survive a subsequent, otherwise lethal heat exposure (3,89). Acquired thermal tolerance and heat acclimatization are complementary processes, as acclimatization reduces heat strain and thermal tolerance increases survivability to a given heat load. For example, rodents with fully developed thermal tolerance can survive 60% more heat load compared with initially lethal levels (90).

Acquired thermal tolerance is associated with heat shock proteins (HSPs) that bind to denatured or nascent cellular polypeptides, providing protection against and accelerating repair from heat stress, ischemia, monocyte toxicity, and ultraviolet radiation in cultured cells and animals. These HSPs are grouped into families by molecular mass (89). They are found in a variety of cellular locations and their functions include processing stress-denatured proteins, managing protein fragments, maintaining structural proteins, and chaperoning proteins across cell membranes. For example, HSP-27 (sometimes referred to as sHSP) resides in the cytosol and nucleus and has anti-apoptotic and microfilament stabilization functions. The HSP-70 family resides in the cytosol (HSP-72, -73, -75, and -78), nucleus (HSP-72 and -73), endoplasmic reticulum (HSP-78), and mitochondria (HSP-75) and has molecular chaperone (HSP-73, -75, and -78), cytoprotection (HSP-72), and antiapoptotic (HSP-73) functions (89).

HSP responses increase within several hours after stress exposure and can last for several days. After the initial heat exposure, messenger ribonucleic acid levels peak within an hour, and subsequent HSP synthesis depends on both the severity of heat stress and cumulative heat stress (90). Both heat exposure and high-intensity dynamic exercise elicit HSP synthesis; however, the combination of dynamic exercise and heat exposure elicits a greater HSP response than does either stressor independently (91). HSPs respond to 10 days of heat acclimation in humans and may be important for conferring heat tolerance and reducing the risk of heat injury. Baseline HSP-72 levels in peripheral blood mononuclear cells (PBMCs) are increased after 6 to 10 days of heat acclimation (92,93), and HSP-90 concentrations in PBMCs are increased by 21% (93). Furthermore, cells taken from individuals who are heat-acclimated and then heat-shocked at 43°C exhibit a blunted HSP response that is related to the degree of physiologic heat acclimation (lower core temperature).

Heat acclimation may also confer protection in animals against novel stressors such as ischemia-reperfusion injury, hypoxia, and traumatic brain injury. This is known as acquired cross-tolerance (94). The mechanisms that mediate acquired cross-tolerance are believed to involve multiple pathways that confer cytoprotection and maintenance of DNA and chromatin integrity (94), as well as metabolic adaptations. Cytoprotection is mediated through increases in HSPs, and antiapoptotic and antioxidative pathways. Heat acclimation also induces hypoxic inducible factor 1α and its targeted metabolic pathways (glycolytic enzymes, glucose transporters, and erythropoietin), conferring protection against closed-head injury, hypoxia, and ischemia-reperfusion injury (94). Detailed gene and protein expression studies focusing on human heat acclimation are lacking; however, it has been shown that exercise and heat shock similarly affect stress response genes such as stress kinase (95), growth and transcription factors, and inflammatory and immune response genes (96), all of which may contribute to acquired thermal and cross-tolerance.

Fluid and Electrolyte Imbalances

Water balance represents the net difference between water intake and loss. During exercise in the heat, water is lost primarily by respiration and sweating. Renal water losses will be minimal and respiratory water losses will usually be approximately offset by metabolic water production (97). Therefore, sweat losses determine most of a person's water needs. Also, since sweat contains electrolytes (primarily sodium and chloride) and minerals (98), prolonged periods of high sweat losses can lead to electrolyte and possibly mineral deficits.

An individual's sweating rate depends on his or her exercise intensity, climatic conditions, and clothing. People who live in desert or tropical climates often have sweating rates of 0.3 to 1.0 L · h^{-1} while performing occupational activities. Competitive marathon runners' sweating rates average about 0.8 L · h^{-1} (range 0.7–1.4 L · h^{-1}) and about 1.2 L · h^{-1} (range 0.9–2.8 L · h^{-1}) in cool-to-temperate and warm-to-hot climates, respectively (99). For competitive athletes training in temperate and hot climates, daily fluid requirements may range from 3–5 L to 4–10 L, respectively (97).

Dehydration

People can become dehydrated (*i.e.*, sustain a body water deficit) during exercise if fluid is unavailable or there is a mismatch between thirst and body water requirements (100). In such instances, they may start an exercise task with normal total body water and then become dehydrated over time. This scenario is common for most athletic and occupational settings; however, sometimes a person will begin to exercise with a body water deficit. For example, in several sports (*e.g.*, boxing, power lifting, and wrestling), athletes purposefully dehydrate to compete in lower weight classes. Also, persons who have taken diuretics may be dehydrated prior to exercise. Dehydration from water deficit without excessive sodium chloride loss is the most common type of dehydration observed during relatively short-term exercise in the heat if the subject is consuming a normal diet. If the person has a large sodium chloride deficit, the extracellular fluid volume will contract and cause salt depletion dehydration. If the sodium chloride deficit is combined with excessive water consumption, it can result in hyponatremia, or water intoxication (101).

Regardless of the cause of dehydration, there is great similarity in the altered physiologic functions and performance consequences. Dehydration can decrease dynamic exercise performance, including maximal aerobic power (87). Dehydration by >2% of body weight degrades endurance exercise, especially in the heat (102). The magnitude of the performance decrement is variable and depends on the individual, the environment, and the exercise mode. Kenefick et al. (103) demonstrated that 4% dehydration degrades aerobic performance to a greater extent with increasing heat stress, and that when the skin temperature is >29°C, 4% dehydration degrades aerobic performance by 1.6% for each additional 1°C increase in skin temperature (Fig. 23.14). However, for a given person and event, the greater the dehydration level (after achieving the threshold for performance degradation), the greater will be the performance decrement. Dehydration seems to reduce muscle strength and power only minimally (1%–3%), but decreases muscular endurance by ~10% (104). In addition, dehydration of >2% often adversely influences cognitive function in the heat; however, this area requires more research (97). Of importance, a growing body of evidence indicates that the negative impact of dehydration on performance in laboratory settings also translates to team sports performance (105).

Physiologic factors that contribute to dehydration-mediated performance decrements include increased hyperthermia, increased cardiovascular strain, altered metabolic function, and perhaps altered CNS function (100). Although each factor is unique, evidence suggests that they interact to contribute in concert, rather than in isolation, to degrading exercise performance. The relative contribution of each factor may differ depending on the endurance event, environmental conditions, and athlete's prowess, but elevated hyperthermia probably acts to accentuate the performance decrement (102).

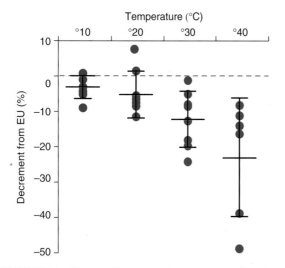

FIGURE 23.14 Percent decrement in exercise performance while 4% dehydrated relative to euhydration (EU) in 10°C, 20°C, 30°C, and 40°C. (From Kenefick RW, Cheuvront SN, Palombo LJ, et al. Skin temperature modifies the impact of hypohydration on aerobic performance. *J Appl Physiol.* 2010;109:79–86.)

Dehydration increases core temperature responses during exercise in temperate and hot climates (87). A body water deficit of as little as 2% of body weight can elevate core temperature during exercise. As the magnitude of water deficit increases, there is a concomitant graded elevation of core temperature during exercise in the heat (106). The magnitude of core temperature elevation approximates 0.2°C for every percent body weight lost and is influenced by the environment. The hotter the environment and greater the evaporative heat loss requirement, in general, the greater will be the core temperature elevation. Dehydration not only elevates core temperature, it also negates the core temperature advantages conferred by high aerobic fitness and heat acclimatization. In addition, dehydration lowers the core temperature that can be tolerated before exhaustion from heat strain during UCHS (107,108).

When a person is dehydrated, the elevated core temperature responses observed during exercise result from reduced heat dissipation. Both sweating and SkBF are reduced for a given core temperature during dehydration (87). For both of the thermoregulatory effector responses (sweat secretion and active cutaneous vasodilation), threshold temperature (body temperature at initiation of heat loss response) is increased and sensitivity (increase in heat loss for a given increase in body temperature) is reduced during dehydration. For thermoregulatory sweating, the increased threshold temperature and reduced sensitivity are proportional to the level of dehydration (106). Therefore, the degraded sweating response represents an attempt to conserve body water. Whole-body sweating is usually either reduced or unchanged during exercise at a given metabolic rate in the heat. However, even when dehydration is associated with no change in whole body sweating rate, core temperature is usually elevated, and thus the whole-body sweating rate for a given core temperature is lower when the subject is dehydrated.

Both the singular and combined effects of plasma hyperosmolality and hypovolemia mediate the reduced heat loss response seen during exercise heat stress (108). Plasma hyperosmolality with no change in blood volume can increase core temperature by reducing heat loss during rest or exercise in the heat through an increase in the core temperature threshold for vasodilation and sweating, and a reduction in the slope of the SkBF and sweating-temperature relationship (109). In addition, the reestablishment of blood volume that is still hyperosmotic does not alter the core temperature elevation compared with responses to dehydration during prolonged exercise in the heat. Plasma volume reductions with no change in osmolality can increase core temperature and impair heat loss during exercise in the heat (108).

Dehydration increases cardiovascular strain during dynamic exercise in temperate and hot climates (87). During submaximal dynamic exercise with little heat strain, dehydration elicits an increase in heart rate and decrease in stroke volume, but usually no change in cardiac output relative to euhydration levels (110,111). Heat stress and dehydration, however, have additive effects on cardiovascular strain (112). If evaporative cooling is reduced, the skin temperature will be elevated. This in turn increases compliance (superficial cutaneous veins) and acts to transfer blood from central to peripheral circulation. This transfer of blood volume, combined with the hypovolemia, acts to reduce cardiac filling and stroke volume, making it more difficult to sustain sufficient cardiac output to support muscle metabolism (47). The inability to sustain sufficient cardiac output provides a cardiovascular limitation to exercise in the heat (60). During submaximal dynamic exercise with moderate or severe heat strain, dehydration (3%–4% body weight) leads to a decrease in cardiac output. The dehydration-mediated cardiac output reduction (below euhydration levels) during heat stress is greater during high-intensity exercise (65% maximal aerobic power) than during low-intensity exercise (25% maximal aerobic power). In addition, severe water deficit (7% body weight) in the absence of heat strain can reduce cardiac output during submaximal exercise.

During severe exercise heat stress, when dehydration mediates a reduction in cardiac output, the skeletal muscle blood flow can also be decreased (47). Despite the decreased muscle blood flow, substrate delivery and lactate removal are not impaired by dehydration (113). However, dehydration can reduce free fatty acid uptake and increase muscle glycogen utilization and muscle lactate production during intense exercise (113). The dehydration-associated increase in muscle glycogen utilization during exercise is probably mediated by elevated catecholamine levels.

Dehydration may reduce exercise performance through mechanisms mediated by the CNS. As discussed above, dehydration elevates body temperature, and evidence suggests that hyperthermia can diminish the drive to exercise and reduce exercise tolerance time.

Hypervolemia and hyperhydration

Hypervolemia, or blood volume expansion, can improve thermoregulation and exercise performance in the heat if the erythrocyte volume alone or the erythrocyte volume and plasma volume together are expanded (87,114). Plasma volume expansion alone does not provide a thermoregulatory benefit, but it does reduce cardiovascular strain (87). Studies in which only erythrocyte volume was expanded showed small thermoregulatory benefits, but when both erythrocyte volume and plasma volume were expanded, more substantial benefits were observed. The former experiments were performed on unacclimatized subjects, and the latter experiments focused on heat-acclimatized subjects, so it is unclear whether the accentuated thermoregulatory benefits resulted from simultaneous expansion of both vascular volumes or the subjects' acclimatization state (114).

Hyperhydration, or above-normal amounts of body water, has been suggested to improve thermoregulation and exercise heat performance above euhydration levels (87). The concept that hyperhydration might be beneficial for exercise

performance arose from recognition of the adverse consequences of dehydration. It was theorized that an increase in body water might reduce cardiovascular and thermal strain of exercise by expanding blood volume and reducing blood tonicity, thereby improving exercise performance. In some studies that evaluated hyperhydration effects on thermoregulation in the heat, smaller core temperature elevations during exercise were observed with hyperhydration, but those studies generally had confounding factors in the experimental procedures used (e.g., if the control condition is hypohydration, this would change the heat acclimation status). Studies that were carefully controlled for these confounding factors did not observe any thermoregulatory advantages with either water hyperhydration or glycerol hyperhydration during exercise heat stress (87).

Hyponatremia

Symptomatic hyponatremia (serum sodium concentration of 125–130 mEq $\cdot$ L^{-1}) has been observed during prolonged marathon and ultramarathon competitions, military training, and recreational activities (101,115). Symptomatic hyponatremia is very rare, and hospitalizations occur at a rate of less than one per 100,000 person years for U.S. Army soldiers (116). The severity of symptoms is probably related to the serum sodium concentration and the rapidity with which it develops. If hyponatremia develops slowly over many hours, there may be less brain swelling and less adverse symptoms than when changes occur rapidly. Hyponatremia usually develops because a person drinks excessively large quantities of hypotonic fluids. However, other factors, such as excessive sodium losses, nausea (which increases vasopressin levels), and heat or exercise stress (which reduce renal blood flow and urine output), can contribute when excessively large volumes of fluids are consumed. For a person to become hyponatremic, total body water usually must be markedly increased, and excessive intake of hypotonic fluids and/or significant sodium loss must occur (101).

Table 23.5 presents a simplified prediction of the serum sodium response to prolonged exercise (90-km ultramarathon foot race) for two individuals of low and average body mass, respectively, with three different sweat sodium concentrations, who have replaced their sweat losses with sodium-free fluid (101). It is assumed that total body water is 63% of body mass, and that water distributes within the extracellular and intracellular fluids until osmotic equilibrium is reached. This analysis illustrates that sweat sodium losses are an important contributor to the reduction of serum sodium when water or a sodium-free solution is used to replace sweat lost during very prolonged exercise. In the example provided, if a 70-kg man had sweat sodium concentrations of 25, 50, and 75 mEq $\cdot$ L^{-1}, and drank sufficient sodium-free water to replace all of the 8.6 L of sweat loss, serum sodium would be expected to decline about 5, 10, and 15 mEq $\cdot$ L^{-1}, respectively. Sweat losses (8.6 L $\times$ sweat sodium) are divided by total body water (TBW) to

TABLE 23.5	Predicted Serum Sodium Values during Prolonged Exercise		
Body mass (kg)		50	70
Total body water (L)		31.5	44
ECF (L)		12.5	17.5
Serum [Na$^+$] (mEq/L)		140	140
ECF Na$^+$ (mEq)		1750	2450
Running velocity (km/h)		10	10
Sweat loss (L)		6.1	8.6
Calculations of serum sodium dilution when water intake = sweat loss			
Sweat [Na$^+$] (mEq/L)		25	25
		50	50
		75	75
Loss of Na$^+$ (mEq)		153	215
		305	430
		458	645
Δ TBW (osmol/L)		4.9	4.9
		9.7	9.8
		14.5	14.7
Serum [Na$^+$] (mEq/L)		135.1	135.1
		130.3	130.2
		125.5	125.3
Fluid excess to dilute serum		3.7	5.1
Na$^+$ to 121 mEq/L (L)		2.4	3.3
		1.2	1.6

Results are from a 90-km ultramarathon foot race, for two body masses when body mass was preserved by ingestion of sodium-free water. TBW, total body water.

determine the change in TBW (osmols · L^{-1}; *e.g.*, 8.6 × 50 mEq · L^{-1} sweat sodium = 430 mEq loss / 44 L TBW = 9.8 or ~10 osmol · L^{-1}). However, to lower the serum sodium to the average value reported for individuals with symptomatic hyponatremia (121 mEq · L^{-1}), the 70-kg man would still have to accrue a fluid excess of 5.1, 3.3, and 1.6 L at the low, moderate, and high sweat sodium concentrations, respectively. The calculation for a 70-kg person with 50 mEq · L^{-1} sweat sodium would be as follows:

$$x / 44 \text{ L TBW} \times 130 \text{ mEq} \cdot \text{L}^{-1} / 121 \text{ mEq} \cdot \text{L}^{-1} = 47.3 \text{ L}$$
$$47.3 - 44 = 3.3 \text{ L[2]} \qquad [2]$$

This analysis also illustrates that smaller individuals with similar sweat sodium concentrations will develop symptoms in the presence of less fluid excess to dilute serum sodium than larger persons. Therefore, if a group of people are drinking at the same rate (as might happen if they follow drinking schedules that are not adjusted for body mass), the individuals with smaller body mass will dilute their extracellular sodium levels more quickly and further than those with larger body mass. On the other hand, to

produce the magnitude of sodium dilution observed in symptomatic hyponatremia cases, persons who are larger than 70 kg would either have to substantially overdrink relative to sweating rate or have an abnormally high sweat sodium concentration. Although these mass balance equations are simplified, more quantitative accounting with standard equations (117) will produce the same results and agree well with careful quantitative experimental measurements (118,119).

TEST YOURSELF

The 70-kg man referenced above has a sweat sodium concentration of 35 mEq · L^{-1}. He completes a 42-km marathon in 4 hours on a cool day with a sweating rate equal to 0.5 L · h^{-1}. If we assume that he replaces 100% of sweat losses with water (0.5 L · h^{-1} drinking rate):

1. How much would his serum sodium drop from a starting value of 140 mEq · L^{-1}?
2. How much more water would be needed to reduce his serum sodium to 130 mEq · L^{-1}?
3. What is his new hourly drinking rate and how does it compare with his sweating rate? What does this suggest about the importance of overdrinking for hyponatremia risk in a marathon?
4. On a warmer day, a smaller runner (50 kg) has the same sweating rate, sweat sodium, serum sodium, %TBW, and finishing time. Perform the same calculations as above. What does this suggest about the importance of body size for hyponatremia risk? Manipulate other variables one at a time (sweat sodium, starting serum sodium, drinking rate, and finishing time) to better understand hyponatremia risk factors.

Environmental Heat Stress

Researchers in the fields of sports and occupational medicine commonly use the WBGT to quantify environmental heat stress and set limits on exercise in strategies designed to minimize the risk of serious exertional heat illness. The WBGT is an empirical index of climatic heat stress: outdoor WBGT = 0.7 natural wet bulb + 0.2 black globe + 0.1 dry bulb; and indoor WBGT = 0.7 natural wet bulb + 0.3 black globe. (The natural wet bulb is a stationary wet-bulb thermometer exposed to the sun and prevailing wind. The black globe thermometer consists of a 6-inch hollow copper sphere that is painted flat black on the outside and contains a thermometer with its bulb at the center of the sphere.) High WBGT values can be achieved through high air (dry bulb) temperature and solar load, as reflected in the black globe temperature, or through high humidity, as reflected in a high wet-bulb temperature. However, the WBGT underestimates heat stress risk for humid conditions, so different guidance tables should be used in low-, moderate-, and high-humidity climates. Table 23.6 shows the relative risks of excessive hyperthermia and possibly

TABLE 23.6	Risk of Hyperthermia and Possible Exertional Heat Illness for a Typical Marathon Runner			
Level of hyperthermia risk	Color code (flag)	WBGT, °C (°F) at RH of 100%	WBGT, °C (°F) at RH of 75%	WBGT, °C (°F) at RH of 50%
Excessive	Black	>28	>29	>33
High	Red	24–28 (73–82)	26–29 (77–85)	28–33 (82–92)
Moderate	Amber	18–23 (65–72)	20–25 (68–76)	24–27 (75–81)
Low	Green	<28 (<65)	<20 (<68)	<24 (<75)
Low (some risk of hypothermia)	White	<10 (<50)	<10 (<50)	<10 (<50)

Results based on wet bulb globe temperature (WBGT) and relative humidity (RH).

serious exertional heat illness for an individual exercising in the heat or an athlete competing in running events while lightly clothed and sustaining a high metabolic rate (120).

Exertional Heat Illness

Serious exertional heat illnesses occupy a continuum of increasing severity, ranging from heat exhaustion to heat injury and heat stroke (5). Heat exhaustion is defined as a mild to moderate illness that is characterized by an inability to sustain cardiac output with moderate (>38.5°C) to high (>40°C) body temperature resulting from strenuous exercise and environmental heat exposure and is frequently accompanied by hot skin and dehydration. Exertional heat injury is defined as a moderate to severe illness characterized by organ (e.g., liver and renal) or tissue (e.g., gut and muscle) injury with high body temperature resulting from strenuous exercise and environmental heat exposure, and body temperatures generally (but not always) >40°C. Exertional heat stroke is defined as a severe illness characterized by profound CNS dysfunction, organ (e.g., liver and renal) or tissue (e.g., gut and muscle) injury with high body temperatures resulting from strenuous exercise and environmental heat exposure. Heat stroke victims have profound neuropsychiatric impairments that develop early. Heat stroke can be complicated by liver damage, rhabdomyolysis, disseminated intravascular coagulation, water and electrolyte imbalances, and renal failure (5).

Risk factors for serious exertional heat illness include lack of heat acclimatization, low physical fitness, dehydration

and high body mass index, underlying health conditions, and certain medications (Table 23.7). However, serious exertional heat illness can occur in low-risk persons who are practicing sound heat mitigation procedures. Exertional heat injury and stroke often occur under conditions to which the victim has been exposed many times before, or while others are concurrently being exposed to the same condition without incident. This suggests that the victim was inherently more vulnerable that day and/or that some unique event triggered the heat injury.

It is suspected that some victims of exertional heat stroke were sick the previous day (121). Exertional heat stroke often occurs during the initial hours of exercise heat stress and does not always occur during the hottest part of the day (122). These facts suggest that on the day of the stroke, the victim began to exercise while already heat-stress compromised. Fever and inflammatory responses from muscle injury may adversely influence thermoregulation and may help mediate subsequent exertional heat injury or stroke (123). A plausible explanation is that increased circulating levels of interferon-γ may sensitize cells to a heat stress that is normally tolerated (96). Gastrointestinal problems will induce dehydration and increase the risk of serious exertional heat illness or may indicate previous heat injury (e.g., gut ischemia causing endotoxin leakage). Evidence suggests that some cases of exertional heat injury or stroke may be explained by an association between susceptibility to malignant hyperthermia and exertional heat stroke (122).

Recent research shows that exertional heat injury (unlike exercise or heat shock in vitro) produces a broad

TABLE 23.7	Factors that Predispose to Serious Heat Illness		
Individual factors	Health conditions	Medications	Environmental factors
Lack of acclimatization	Inflammation or fever	Anticholinergics	High temperature
Low fitness	Cardiovascular disease	Antihistamines	High humidity
Large body mass	Diabetes mellitus	Amphetamines	Little air motion
Dehydration	Gastroenteritis	Diuretics	Little shade
Age (old or young)	Sickle cell trait	Beta-blockers	Heat wave

Abbreviated list adapted from Winkenwerder W, Sawka MN. Disorders due to heat and cold. In: Goldman L, Ausiello D, eds. *Cecil Medicine.* 23rd ed. Philadelphia: Saunders Elsevier; 2008.

spectrum of gene expression changes (96). Of importance, the gene sequences that are upregulated with exertional heat injury but not by exercise consist of interferon-inducible genes. Elevated levels of circulating interferon-γ have been observed in victims of classic heat stroke, and this can increase cellular mortality by apoptosis after heat shock (96). A previous incident of cellular heat shock or some other unknown event may mediate expression of interferon genes, leading to elevated circulating interferon-γ or -α levels. Expression of this or another cytokine may contribute to the pathogenesis of exertional heat injury (124,125). Furthermore, exertional heat injury causes a downregulation in interferon-inducible gene sequences in T-cells and natural killer cells (96) that are not part of the normal response to exercise. These data suggest that the composition and distribution of circulating PBMCs, such as T- and natural killer cells, may change as a result of exertional heat injury. This difference in gene sequence downregulation for these immune cells may be a marker for exertional heat injury.

Figure 23.15 shows a diagram of the progression of heat strain to exertional heat injury and/or stroke (124). Hyperthermia and cardiovascular responses to exercise heat stress can result in reduced perfusion of the intestine and other body tissues, resulting in ischemia and excessively high tissue temperatures (heat shock, >42°C). The magnitude and duration of the heat shock will influence whether the cell responds by adaptation (acquired thermal tolerance), injury, or death (apoptotic or necrotic) (89,95). This can result in a variety of systemic coagulation and inflammatory responses (124). It is suspected that the inflammatory response is primed (e.g., by leukocytosis and expression of inflammatory cytokines) so that a subsequent exposure to severe exercise heat will induce an accentuated acute-phase response.

This exaggerated acute-phase response could mediate fever (in addition to exercise hyperthermia) and/or enhance the likelihood of tissue injury and cellular death. Cytokines are important mediators of the acute-phase response, and increased circulating levels have been observed in human heat-stroke patients and experimental animal models (125). Pro-inflammatory cytokines such as interleukin (IL)-6 and tumor necrosis factor (TNF) are thought to be important mediators of the thermoregulatory and tissue injury responses to heat stroke. Although enhanced mortality was observed in IL-6 and TNF receptor knockout mice, indicating that these cytokines have permissive (protective) effects, this process is not completely understood. It is likely that the role of cytokines in the heat-stroke syndrome has been misinterpreted as interaction(s) between these endogenous proteins and their soluble receptors, which may act as agonists (e.g., sIL-6R) or antagonists (e.g., sTNFR) of endogenous cytokine actions (125).

The severity of heat illness is often not apparent. An individual who is performing or competing in a strenuous activity in hot weather and exhibits symptoms of serious exertional heat illness (e.g., unsteady gait; sweaty, flushed skin; dizziness; headache; tachycardia; paresthesias; weakness; nausea; or cramps) should be immediately evaluated for mental status, core (rectal) temperature, and vital signs. Poor or worsening mental status (e.g., discoordination or confusion) is a true medical emergency, and this individual needs rapid intervention and evacuation to a medical treatment facility.

Regardless of the pathogenesis, serious exertional heat illness poses a risk to healthy persons who are active in warm weather. Guidelines for the prevention and treatment of serious exertional heat illness can be readily obtained

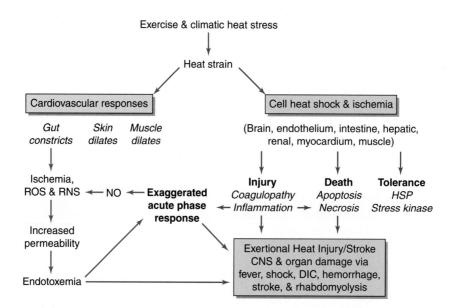

FIGURE 23.15   Possible pathogenesis of the progression of exercise heat strain to exertional heat injury and stroke. ROS, reactive oxygen species; RNS, reactive nitrogen species; HSP, heat shock protein; CNS, central nervous system, DIC, disseminated intravascular coagulation. (Adapted from Bouchama A, Knochel P. Heat stroke. *N Engl J Med.* 2002;346:1982.)

(http://www.usariem.army.mil/HeatInjury.htm and http://www.naspem.org/pos_stmts/) and should be followed.

Any person who is suspected of having exertional heat injury or stroke should be cooled as soon as possible. Delay in cooling is probably the single most important factor leading to death or residual serious disability. The patient should lie down, and as much clothing should be removed as is practical. Body cooling should be continued until the person's core temperature is <38.5°C. Immersion in cool or iced water with skin massage is the most rapid method, but ice sheets and ice packs can also be effective (126).

KEY POINT

The severity of heat illness ranges from heat exhaustion to heat injury and finally heat stroke.

Summary of Heat Stress

Heat stress can be classified as CHS or UCHS depending on biophysical factors (environment, clothing, and metabolic rate) and biologic status (heat acclimatization and hydration status). The increase in thermoregulatory sweating closely parallels the increase in body temperature (26). The back and chest have the highest sweating rates, whereas the limbs have relatively high sweating rates only after a substantial elevation in core temperature (33). During exercise in the heat, the primary cardiovascular challenge is to increase cardiac output sufficiently to support both high SkBF for heat dissipation and high muscle blood flow for metabolism. Heat strain will degrade dynamic exercise performance. Mechanisms include increased thermal and cardiovascular strain, increased discomfort and diminished CNS drive for exercise (neuro/psychological), and accelerated glycogen depletion with increased metabolite accumulation. Exercise training in a temperate climate with emphasis on improved aerobic performance can reduce physiologic strain and improve exercise capabilities in the heat, but such exercise training programs alone cannot replace the benefits of heat acclimatization. Usually, about 7 to 10 days of heat exposure are needed to induce heat acclimatization. Optimal heat acclimatization requires a minimum daily heat exposure of about 2 hours. Animals and humans who are repeatedly exposed to the hyperthermia of exercise can become more resistant to exertional heat injury and stroke. During exercise in the heat, water is lost primarily by respiration and sweating, and sweat losses determine most of a person's water needs. Because sweat contains electrolytes (primarily sodium and chloride) and minerals (98), prolonged periods of high sweat losses can lead to electrolyte and possibly mineral deficits. Serious exertional heat illnesses range in severity from heat exhaustion to heat injury and finally heat stroke (5).

Cold Stress

Environmental Cold Stress

The principal determinants of cold stress during outdoor events in cold weather are air temperature and wind speed. Most body heat loss during cold exposure occurs via conductive and convective mechanisms, so when ambient temperature is colder than body temperature, the thermal gradient favors body heat loss, and wind exacerbates heat loss by facilitating convection at the body (9). Windchill charts and tables have been constructed to depict, for every combination of air temperature and wind speed, a corresponding temperature in calm air (i.e., no wind) that is calculated to produce the same theoretical heat flow through bare skin, and this value is the equivalent chill temperature for the temperature and wind combination (127). The effect of increasing wind speed with decreasing air temperature on the equivalent chill temperature is illustrated in Figure 23.16. The windchill temperature index presents the relative risk of frostbite and the predicted times to freezing (Fig. 23.16) of exposed facial skin (128). Facial skin was chosen because this area of the body typically is not protected. Frostbite cannot occur if the air temperature is above 0°C (32°F). Wet skin exposed to the wind will cool even faster, and if the skin is wet and exposed to wind, the ambient temperature used for the windchill temperature table should be 10°C lower than the actual ambient temperature (129). One can greatly reduce windchill effects by wearing windproof clothing and/or engaging in strenuous exercise. Further, windchill provides no meaningful estimate of the risk of hypothermia. Thus, windchill tables probably somewhat exaggerate the risk of cold injury during endurance competition, and events in which participants are properly dressed and maintain high metabolic rates need not be canceled because of the windchill alone. Lacking a better tool, one can use the equivalent chill temperature as a factor in deciding whether to cancel outdoor activities; however, as with the WBGT, the limitations to this approach should be appreciated. Prudence does warrant increased safety surveillance of athletes when equivalent chill temperatures fall below −30°C, since injured or fatigued athletes may be unable to sustain high metabolic rates and skin temperatures that protect them from windchill.

As described at the beginning of this chapter, water has a much higher thermal capacity than air, and the heat transfer coefficient in water is 25 times greater than in air (7). Therefore, heat conduction away from the body is greater during exposure to a given cold air temperature when skin and clothing are wet (e.g., from rain) than when the skin is dry. With an air temperature of 5°C, heat loss in wet clothes may be double that in dry clothes (130). Even so, heat loss predictions (131) indicate that the core temperature of an average-sized individual performing high-intensity endurance exercise (metabolic rate of 600 W) in an air temperature of 5°C and continuous rain will not fall below 35°C for at least 7 hours, and experimental observations tend to

Wind Speed (mph)
↓

Air Temperature (°F)

	40	35	30	25	20	15	10	5	0	-5	-10	-15	-20	-25	-30	-35	-40	-45
5	36	31	25	19	13	7	1	-5	-11	-16	-22	-28	-34	-40	-46	-52	-57	-63
10	34	27	21	15	9	3	-4	-10	-16	-22	-28	-35	-41	-47	-53	-59	-66	-72
15	32	25	19	13	6	0	-7	-13	-19	-26	-32	-39	-45	-51	-58	-64	-71	-77
20	30	24	17	11	4	-2	-9	-15	-22	-29	-35	-42	-48	-55	-61	-68	-74	-81
25	29	23	16	9	3	-4	-11	-17	-24	-31	-37	-44	-51	-58	-64	-71	-78	-84
30	28	22	15	8	1	-5	-12	-19	-26	-33	-39	-46	-53	-60	-67	-73	-80	-87
35	28	21	14	7	0	-7	-14	-21	-27	-34	-41	-48	-55	-62	-69	-76	-82	-89
40	27	20	13	6	-1	-8	-15	-22	-29	-36	-43	-50	-57	-64	-71	-78	-84	-91
45	26	19	12	5	-2	-9	-16	-23	-30	-37	-44	-51	-58	-65	-72	-79	-86	-93
50	26	19	12	4	-3	-10	-17	-24	-31	-38	-45	-52	-60	-67	-74	-81	-88	-95
55	25	18	11	4	-3	-11	-18	-25	-32	-39	-46	-54	-61	-68	-75	-82	-89	-97
60	25	17	10	3	-4	-11	-19	-26	-33	-40	-48	-55	-62	-69	-76	-84	-91	-98

Frostbite Times

Frostbite could occur in 30 minutes
Frostbite could occur in 10 minutes
Frostbite could occur in 5 minutes

Air Temperature (°C)

Wind Speed (km/h)	5	0	-5	-10	-15	-20	-25	-30	-35	-40	-45	-50
5	4	-2	-7	-13	-19	-24	-30	-36	-41	-47	-53	-58
10	3	-3	-9	-15	-21	-27	-33	-39	-45	-51	-57	-63
15	2	-4	-11	-17	-23	-29	-35	-41	-48	-54	-60	-66
20	1	-5	-12	-18	-24	-30	-37	-43	-49	-56	-62	-68
25	1	-6	-12	-19	-25	-32	-38	-44	-51	-57	-64	-70
30	0	-6	-13	-20	-26	-33	-39	-46	-52	-59	-65	-72
35	0	-7	-14	-20	-27	-33	-40	-47	-53	-60	-66	-73
40	-1	-7	-14	-21	-27	-34	-41	-48	-54	-61	-68	-74
45	-1	-8	-15	-21	-28	-35	-42	-48	-55	-62	-69	-75
50	-1	-8	-15	-22	-29	-35	-42	-49	-56	-63	-69	-76
55	-2	-8	-15	-22	-29	-36	-43	-50	-57	-63	-70	-77
60	-2	-9	-16	-23	-30	-36	-43	-50	-57	-64	-71	-78
65	-2	-9	-16	-23	-30	-37	-44	-51	-58	-65	-72	-79
70	-2	-9	-16	-23	-30	-37	-44	-51	-58	-65	-72	-80
75	-3	-10	-17	-24	-31	-38	-45	-52	-59	-66	-73	-80
80	-3	-10	-17	-24	-31	-38	-45	-52	-60	-67	-74	-81

FROSTBITE GUIDE

Low risk of frostbite for most people
Increasing risk of frostbite for most people in 10 to 30 minutes of exposure
High risk for most people in 5 to 10 minutes of exposure
High risk for most people in 2 to 5 minutes of exposure
High risk for most people in 2 minutes of exposure or less

FIGURE 23.16 Windchill temperature index in Fahrenheit and Celsius. Frostbite times are for exposed facial skin (*Top*, from the U.S. National Weather Service; *bottom* from the Meteorological Society of Canada/Environment Canada).

confirm these predictions (132). The enhancement of conductive heat loss is much more pronounced during full or partial immersion. Skin heat conductance can be 70 times greater during exercise in water than during comparable exercise in air at the same temperature; thus, swimmers can lose considerable body heat even in relatively mild water temperatures. However, as will be explained later, anthropomorphic factors, exercise type and intensity, metabolic rate, aerobic capacity, and water temperature all interact in a complex manner to determine the net thermal balance during immersion in cold water. Therefore, individuals vary considerably with respect to the water temperature they can tolerate without incurring a dangerous decline in core temperature during exercise.

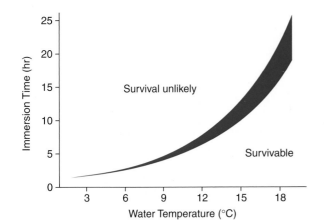

FIGURE 23.17 Approximate survival times during cold water immersion. (From Pandolf KB, Young AJ. Assessment of environmental extremes and competitive strategies. In: Shephard RJ, Astrand PO, eds. *Endurance in Sport.* Oxford: Blackwell Science; 2000:292.)

Safe limits for the duration of recreation involving immersion in water at different temperatures can be predicted with the use of thermoregulatory models (133–135) or estimated according to actual observations of survival times after accidental immersion (136), with the latter being the less conservative approach. Figure 23.17 illustrates both approaches for establishing water temperature safety limits for aquatic events (see Chapter 25). However, in both cases, the expected time to death due to hypothermia or drowning due to the inability to maintain consciousness or sustain useful physical activity is used to define the limits, and this approach may be too liberal for athletic competition. The American College of Sports Medicine Position Stand on the Prevention of Cold Injuries during Exercise (137) states that exercise can be safely performed in cold environments if the coaches, athletes, medical personnel, and officials follow a risk management strategy. Successful implementation of this strategy includes asking the following questions:

1. How cold is it?
2. What clothing protection is available?
3. Who is at risk for a cold weather injury?
4. What is the health condition of the exerciser?
5. What effective strategies are available to mitigate the cold stress and injury risk?
6. Is a contingency plan in place to deal with changing conditions?

Physiologic Responses to Cold

Acute cold exposure

Humans exhibit peripheral vasoconstriction upon exposure to cold. The resulting decrease in peripheral blood flow reduces convective heat transfer between the body's core and shell (skin, subcutaneous fat, and skeletal muscle), effectively increasing insulation by the body's shell. Because heat is lost from the exposed body surface faster than it is replaced, skin temperature declines. During whole body exposure to cold, the vasoconstrictor response extends beyond the fingers and spreads throughout the entire body's peripheral shell. Vasoconstriction begins when skin temperature falls below about 35°C and becomes maximal when skin temperature is about ≤31°C (138). Thus, the vasoconstrictor response to cold exposure helps retard heat loss and defend core temperature, but at the expense of a decline in the temperature of peripheral tissue.

Norepinephrine is a neurotransmitter that accounts for ~60% of the reflex cold-induced vasoconstriction in skin, and neuropeptide Y is responsible for ~20% to ~30% (139,140). In contrast, early in the local cooling response (with no reflex cooling occurring from other areas), vasoconstriction is mediated by norepinephrine and Rho kinase (141). However, as cooling continues, sympathetically mediated adrenergic vasoconstriction appears to be responsible for ~20% of cold-induced vasoconstriction, whereas nonadrenergic mechanisms (RhoA/rho kinase) mediates ~60% of the response (141,142). Local cooling enhances α_2 receptor sensitivity to norepinephrine by translocating α_{2C} receptors from the Golgi to the plasma membrane (142–144).

The reductions in vasoconstriction-induced blood flow and skin temperature probably contribute to the causation of peripheral cold injuries. Cold-induced vasoconstriction has pronounced effects in the hands and fingers, making them particularly susceptible to cold injury and loss of manual dexterity (145). In these areas, another vasomotor response, cold-induced vasodilation (CIVD), modulates the effects of vasoconstriction. Periodic fluctuations of skin temperature follow the initial decline during cold exposure resulting from transient increases in blood flow to the cooled finger. A similar CIVD in the forearm appears to reflect vasodilation of muscle as well as cutaneous vasculature (146). Although this was originally thought to just be a local cooling effect, evidence suggests that a CNS mechanism mediates CIVD (147) and the response is modulated by hypothermia (148).

Cold exposure also elicits increased metabolic heat production in humans, which can help offset heat loss. In humans, most cold-induced thermogenesis is attributable to skeletal muscle contractile activity. Humans initiate this thermogenesis by voluntarily modifying their behavior (*e.g.*, increasing physical activity such as exercise or fidgeting) or by shivering. It has been well established that rodents increase metabolic heat production by brown adipose tissue (BAT) in response to cold exposure, and it was thought for many years that adult humans lack this mechanism. However, a series of studies (149–151) using positron emission tomography and computed tomography scans along with the tracer 18F-fluorodeoxyglucose revealed that adult humans do indeed have active BAT that becomes active upon cold exposure. The highest BAT levels are found in the neck, supraclavicular tissue, and thoracic and abdominal paraspinal sites (152). BAT activation is negatively correlated with body mass index and %

body fat (149,151), and women appear to have more BAT than men (152). However, there is no evidence that BAT thermogenesis can increase high enough to defend core temperature during extended cold exposures.

Shivering consists of involuntary, repeated, rhythmic muscle contractions during which most of the metabolic energy expended is liberated as heat and little external work is performed. It may start immediately or after several minutes of cold exposure, and usually begins in torso muscles and then spreads to the limbs (153). The intensity and extent of shivering vary according to the severity of cold stress. As shivering intensity increases and more muscles are recruited to shiver, whole body metabolic rate increases, typically reaching about 200 to 250 W during resting exposure to cold air, but often exceeding 350 W during resting immersion in cold water. Maximal shivering is difficult to quantify, but the highest metabolic rate reported in the literature to date appears to be 763 W. This value was recorded while the test subject was immersed in 12°C water, and corresponded to 46% of the subject's maximal aerobic power (154).

Patterns of human cold acclimatization

People who are exposed to cold weather can acclimatize, but the specifics of the physiologic adjustments are modest, at best, and depend on the severity of the exposure. Cold acclimatization in persons who are repeatedly or chronically exposed to cold is manifested in three patterns of thermoregulatory adjustments: habituation, metabolic acclimatization, and insulative acclimatization. Figure 23.18 summarizes the characteristic features of each pattern (8).

The most commonly observed acclimatization pattern is habituation. With habituation, physiologic responses to

cold become less pronounced than before acclimatization. Blunting of both shivering and cold-induced vasoconstriction are the hallmarks of habituation (8). Sometimes (but not always) cold-habituated persons with blunted shivering and vasoconstrictor responses to cold also exhibit a more pronounced decline in core temperature during cold exposure than nonacclimatized persons, a pattern called hypothermic habituation. Taken together, findings from different cold acclimatization studies (see Young [8] for a detailed review) suggest that the distinction between studies that observed hypothermic habituation and those in which habituation of shivering and vasoconstriction occurred without effect on core temperature responses to cold probably reflect differences in experimental protocols rather than physiologic mechanisms.

The second distinct pattern of acclimatization induced by chronic cold exposure is characterized by a more pronounced thermogenic response to cold, and hence is termed *metabolic acclimatization* (8). In most studies in which subjects appeared to demonstrate an enhanced thermogenic response to cold exposure, the subjects were chronically exposed (for months to lifetime) to relatively mild whole-body cold that was tolerated without producing hypothermia (8). Enhanced thermogenic responses to cold could arise from an exaggerated shivering response or the development of nonshivering thermogenesis. Experimental evidence purporting to document the existence of both thermogenic adjustments has been reported (8), but a critical analysis of that evidence suggests little support for the development of a nonshivering thermogenic response in humans.

The third major pattern of cold acclimatization, referred to as insulative cold acclimatization, is characterized by enhanced heat conservation mechanisms (8). With insulative acclimatization, cold exposure elicits a more rapid and pronounced decline in skin temperature, and lower thermal conductance at the skin than in the unacclimatized state. The response is mediated by a pronounced vasoconstrictor response to cold, possibly due to enhanced sympathetic nervous response to cold. In addition, some data suggest that insulative cold acclimatization may also involve the development of enhanced circulatory countercurrent heat exchange mechanisms to limit convective heat loss. This notion is supported by the observation that before wet suits came into common use, Korean diving women immersed in cool water exhibited less forearm heat loss than control subjects, even though concomitant forearm blood flow remained higher in the diving women. After wet suit use became widespread, Korean diving women no longer exhibited any thermoregulatory adjustments compared with control subjects. This suggests that the previous differences truly reflected adjustments to frequent exposure to cold while diving (8).

The nature of the cold exposure may determine the pattern of acclimatization. In a suggested theoretical model, the key determinant for cold acclimatization is the

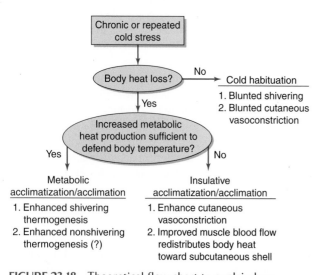

FIGURE 23.18 Theoretical flow chart to explain how humans develop different patterns of cold acclimatization. (From Young AJ. Homeostatic responses to prolonged cold exposure: human cold acclimatization. In: Fregly MJ, Blatteis CM, eds. *Handbook of Physiology, Section 4: Environmental Physiology*. New York: Oxford University; 1996:435.)

degree to which cold exposure results in body heat loss (8), and some recently reported experimental data support this concept (148). This model, illustrated in Figure 23.19, postulates that brief, intermittent cold exposures in which limited areas of the body surface are cooled and whole-body heat losses are negligible lead to habituation. By contrast, repeated cold exposures that are prolonged and/or severe enough to preclude increased metabolic heat production from balancing body heat loss (*i.e.*, deep body temperature declines) will induce insulative acclimatization. This model also postulates that an enhanced thermogenic capability will develop when repeated and prolonged cold exposures produce significant body heat loss, but increased body heat production can be sustained long enough to prevent significant decreases in core temperature. An alternative to that model's explanation for the development of different patterns of cold acclimatization is the notion that the metabolic, hypothermic, habituative, and insulative patterns do not represent different types of cold acclimatization but are actually different stages in the development of complete cold acclimatization. Thus, humans initially respond to whole-body cold exposure by shivering, which becomes more pronounced over time, and eventually the shivering disappears and is replaced by insulative adaptations to help limit body heat loss.

Compared with the effects of heat acclimatization, physiologic adjustments to chronic cold exposure are less pronounced, slower to develop, and less practical in terms of relieving thermal strain, defending normal body temperature, and preventing thermal injury. Therefore, researchers have directed less attention to these physiologic adjustments than to the effects of heat acclimatization. Nonetheless, physiologists need to appreciate these adjustments because they may be sufficient to influence the physiologic responses observed during exercise and/or exposure to environmental stress, particularly under controlled experimental conditions.

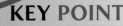

Individual Factors that Modify Responses to Cold

Anthropometric characteristics

Most of the variability observed among individuals in terms of their thermoregulatory responses and ability to maintain normal body temperature during cold exposure is attributable to anthropometric differences. Large individuals lose more body heat in the cold than smaller individuals because they have larger body surface areas. In general, persons with a large ratio of surface area to mass have greater declines in body temperature during cold exposure than those with a smaller ratio (7,9).

All body tissues provide thermal resistance to heat conduction (*i.e.*, insulation) from within the body. In resting individuals, unperfused muscle tissue provides a significant contribution to the body's total insulation. However, that contribution declines during exercise or other physical activity because increased blood flow through muscles facilitates convective heat transfer from the core to the body's shell. The thermal resistivity of fat is greater than that of other tissues (7), and as illustrated in Figure 23.19, subcutaneous fat provides significant insulation against heat loss in the cold. Consequently, fat persons have smaller body temperature changes and shiver less during cold exposure than lean persons (7).

Sex-associated differences in thermoregulatory responses and ability to maintain normal thermal balance during cold exposure appear to be almost entirely attributable to anthropometric characteristics (7). For example, men and women with equivalent total body masses have similar surface areas, but the women's greater fat content enhances insulation. However, in women and men with equivalent subcutaneous fat thickness, the women have a greater surface area but smaller total body mass (and lower total body heat content) than men. Thus, even though insulation is equivalent, total heat loss during resting cold exposure will be greater in women because they have a larger surface area for convective heat flux, and body temperature will tend to fall more rapidly for any given thermal gradient unless shivering thermogenesis is compensated for by a more pronounced increment than observed in men. This compensation may be possible when heat flux is low (mild cold conditions), but women's smaller lean body mass limits their maximal capacity for thermogenic response; therefore, under severely cold conditions, women might experience a more rapid core temperature decline compared with men of comparable body mass (155,156). However, during exercise in cold water, men and women with equivalent body fat percentages exhibit

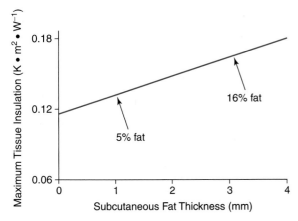

FIGURE 23.19 Tissue insulation during immersion in cold water as a function of subcutaneous fat thickness. (Adapted from Hong SK. Pattern of cold adaptation in women divers of Korea (Ama). *Fed Proc.* 1973;32:1618.)

similar thermoregulatory responses because women have a more favorable fat distribution over the exercising limbs compared with men (155).

Aging

As a result of reduced vasoconstriction and heat conservation, people who are older than 60 years may be less cold-tolerant than younger persons (157–160). Older people also experience a decline in physical fitness. Older persons who are exercising at the same absolute metabolic rates as younger individuals will be working at a higher $\%\dot{V}O_{2max}$, will fatigue sooner, and must decrease their absolute heat production if they fatigue, increasing the likelihood of a reduction in core temperature. Older individuals also appear to have a blunted thermal sensitivity to cold. For example, in studies in which subjects were able to control a thermostat as the ambient temperature fluctuated, older individuals allowed the air temperature to fall to lower levels before they adjusted the thermostat (161,162).

Aerobic Fitness and Training

Overall, exercise training and aerobic fitness appear to have only minor influences on thermoregulatory responses to cold. Most cross-sectional comparisons of aerobically fit and less-fit persons have revealed no relationship between maximal aerobic power and temperature regulation in the cold. In studies that purportedly demonstrated such a relationship, the differences in thermoregulation appear to be more attributable to anthropometric differences between the aerobically fit and less-fit subjects than to an effect of maximal aerobic power per se (163). Longitudinal studies showed that interval training had no measurable effects on thermoregulatory response to cold (164), and although endurance training was shown to improve cutaneous vasoconstrictor response during cold water immersion, that effect had little impact on core temperature changes during cold exposure (54). The effects of resistance training programs on thermoregulatory responses to cold have not been documented, but it seems likely that any such effects would be primarily attributable to training-related changes in body composition. The increased strength and aerobic power gained by exercise training provide a thermoregulatory advantage in that the fitter individual can sustain voluntary activity at higher intensity and thus higher rates of metabolic heat production for longer periods than less-fit persons during cold exposure.

TEST YOURSELF

In older individuals, is there a sex-specific effect on exercise thermoregulation in the cold? Keep in mind that differences in body composition and fitness between men and women are inherent biologic sex differences, and these characteristics change as a natural part of the aging process.

Clothing

A wide variety of athletic clothing is available to provide protection during exercise and recreational activity in cold conditions. A detailed consideration of the biophysics and heat transfer properties of cold weather athletic clothing can be found elsewhere (165) and is beyond the scope of this text. However, it should be intuitively obvious that the amount of clothing insulation required to maintain comfort and insulate against excessive body heat loss during cold-weather activity will depend on the combined effects of two opposing factors: the thermal gradient for heat loss (i.e., ambient temperature) and the rate of metabolic heat production (i.e., exercise intensity). Increasing clothing insulation will be required as the ambient temperature decreases, and decreasing clothing insulation will be required as the metabolic rate increases. Figure 23.20 depicts the insulation required to maintain thermal balance at different ambient temperatures and exercise intensities (165–168). Heat production during high-intensity exercise can be sufficient to prevent a fall in deep body temperature without the need for heavy clothing even when air temperature is extremely low. However, athletes who are dressed optimally for an event may be inadequately protected from the cold before the event starts or when exercise ceases because of fatigue, injury, or completion of the event. Therefore, modern cold-weather athletic clothes incorporate design features that provide for adjustable insulation, such as layers and ventilation. Further, since much of the insulation provided by cold-weather clothing is achieved by trapping stagnant air layers within the clothing or against the skin, the clothing must also provide a barrier against moisture and wind, which degrade insulation by disrupting the trapped air layers. Even during a high-intensity activity that produces enough metabolic heat to completely obviate the need for heavy cold-weather clothing to protect against hypothermia, any exposed skin of the fingers, nose, and ears may be susceptible to freezing injuries. Clothing to protect these regions from surface cooling should be worn when windchill conditions are extreme, although physical activity is an effective countermeasure to increase skin temperatures. For example, increasing the exercise intensity from 220 to 350 W (2.2–3.5 METS) can increase the nose temperature from 4.5°C to 8.9°C even in a 5 m · s^{-1} wind (129,169). Finally, because the insulation provided by cold-weather clothing adds to the insulation provided by body fat and other tissues, clothing requirements will vary among individuals depending on the anthropometric factors discussed above.

Exercise in the Cold

Oxygen uptake and systemic oxygen transport

As the noted environmental physiologist Dave Bass once observed, "A man in the cold is not necessarily a cold man" (170). Whether the physiologic responses to exercise are

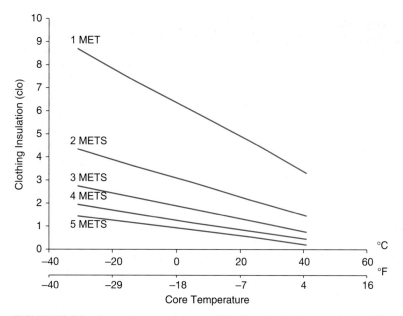

FIGURE 23.20 Approximate amount of clothing insulation needed at different air temperatures and physical activity levels. Wind speed is assumed to be <5 mph (2.2 m/s). 1 MET refers to energy expenditure at rest. One clo of insulation is the clothing necessary to allow a resting person to be comfortable when the air temperature is 21°C (70°F). MET, metabolic equivalent of task. (From Castellani JW, Young AJ, Ducharme MB, et al. American College of Sports Medicine position stand: prevention of cold injuries during exercise. *Med Sci Sports Exer.* 2006;38:2012.)

altered by a cold environment depends on whether the interactive effects of environment, clothing, anthropometric factors, and exercise intensity are such that cold stress elicits additional physiologic strain beyond that associated with the same exercise under temperate conditions.

If cold stress is severe enough to cause a significant decline in core or muscle temperature, maximal aerobic power can be reduced compared with that measured at normal core and muscle temperatures (171). The mechanism for this effect has not been definitively demonstrated, but it probably reflects an effect of low tissue temperature on contractile function of heart (171) and/or skeletal (172) muscle. An impairment of myocardial contractility could limit maximal cardiac output, thus accounting for the reduced maximal aerobic power. Further, impairment of the skeletal muscle contractile function associated with muscle cooling could reduce maximal aerobic power by impacting muscle oxygen use. However, there must be a threshold temperature for this effect, because it has been shown that exposure to cold conditions that lower core temperature ≤0.5°C has no significant effect on maximal aerobic power and associated responses (173).

Whether cold exposure influences oxygen uptake during steady-state submaximal exercise depends on whether exercise thermogenesis is sufficient to balance the rate of body heat loss to the ambient environment, and to keep core and skin temperatures warm enough to prevent shivering. During exercise at intensities too low for metabolic heat production to balance heat loss to the cold environ-

ment and prevent shivering, oxygen uptake will be higher than in warm conditions, with the increased oxygen uptake representing the added oxygen requirement for metabolism in the shivering muscles. With increasing exercise intensity, metabolic heat production rises, and core and skin temperatures are warmer. Therefore, the afferent stimulus for shivering declines along with the shivering-associated component of total oxygen uptake during exercise until exercise metabolism eventually becomes high enough to prevent shivering, and steady-state oxygen uptake at the same or higher intensity levels will be the same in cold and warm conditions.

Figure 23.21 illustrates conceptually the influence of exercise intensity on steady-state submaximal oxygen uptake during exercise (174). The precise effect of exercise intensity on the shivering component of total oxygen uptake during exercise, and the specific intensity at which metabolic heat production is sufficient to prevent shivering will depend on the severity of cold stress, clothing insulation, and anthropometric factors that influence body heat flux.

Cold exposure can also affect cardiovascular responses to submaximal exercise. When shivering occurs during exercise in the cold, cardiac output is elevated relative to the cardiac output elicited by that same exercise intensity in temperate conditions. However, the increment in cardiac output simply reflects the requirement for increased systemic oxygen transport to sustain shivering, so cardiac output for any given oxygen uptake level will remain

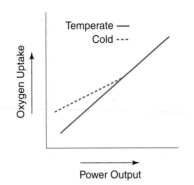

FIGURE 23.21   Steady-state oxygen uptake response during submaximal exercise at given power output in temperate and cold conditions. (From Young AJ, Sawka MN, Pandolf KB. Physiology of cold exposure. In: Marriott BM, Carlson SJ, eds. *Nutritional Needs in Cold and in High-Altitude Environments*. Washington: National Academy; 1996:137.)

unchanged (175,176). Nevertheless, shivering during exercise could somewhat increase cardiovascular strain for a given submaximal exercise bout in comparison with no shivering. Cold exposure can also alter the way in which a given cardiac output is achieved (175,176). During exercise in cold air or cold water, lower heart rates and increased stroke volume are observed for a given cardiac output and oxygen uptake level compared with exercise at the same oxygen uptake in temperate conditions (175,176). Increased central blood volume resulting from peripheral vasoconstriction (110,111) accounts partly for the lower heart rates and stroke volume increase seen during exercise during cold exposure, and other mechanisms (*e.g.*, baroreflex, a change in the inotropic state of the heart) await definitive experimental determination (175,176).

Muscle energy metabolism

Cold exposure may also affect muscle energy metabolism during exercise. If shivering occurs during exercise, higher blood lactate concentrations may be attained in cold than in temperate conditions, but when oxygen uptake is the same (*i.e.*, no shivering), blood lactate accumulation during exercise in cold and temperate conditions is the same (51). In one study, muscle glycogen depletion was observed to be more pronounced during low-intensity exercise (*e.g.*, below 25% maximal oxygen uptake) in the cold, when oxygen uptake levels were elevated compared with an exercise bout of similar intensity and duration performed under temperate conditions, but no differences were seen when bouts of higher intensity exercise were compared (51). These observations were interpreted as indicating that the added energy requirements of shivering increase glycogen breakdown during exercise, and that shivering preferentially metabolizes muscle glycogen as an energy source. However, recent findings show instead that shivering, like low-intensity exercise, relies on lipids as the predominant metabolic substrate, and blood glucose, muscle glycogen,

and even protein are metabolized as well (177). When glycogen reserves are low, the relative contributions from lipids, carbohydrates, and proteins change during cold exposure. When muscle glycogen levels are high, lipids, carbohydrates, and proteins respectively account for 25%, ~65%, and 10% of heat production. However, when muscle glycogen levels are low, the percent lipid contribution to heat production increases to ~60%, whereas carbohydrates and proteins account for only 20% and 25%, respectively (178). Furthermore, the type of shivering activity (*e.g.*, high-activity bursts versus continuous low-intensity shivering) will determine which metabolic fuel is used. Glycogen stores are primarily used during burst activity, and lipids are predominantly used during low-intensity shivering (178).

The accelerated muscle glycogen use observed during low-intensity exercise in cold conditions may result from increased motor unit recruitment to compensate for impaired force generation induced by muscle cooling. However, the cold exposure would probably have to be extreme or entail prolonged immersion in cold water to induce a sufficiently pronounced decline in muscle temperature to impair force generation during sustained dynamic exercise (172).

Body fluid balance

Cold exposure is thought to influence both physiologic and behavioral mechanisms that affect body fluid balance during exercise. For one thing, fluid intake can become inadequate during cold exposure. Thirst sensation may be blunted in cold persons (179), and cold environments often impose practical constraints against voluntary drinking (*e.g.*, because of frozen drinking supplies or the desire to avoid urinating outdoors in the cold). Cold exposure is also thought to exacerbate fluid losses, but the extent to which these effects are operational during exercise is unclear.

Perhaps the most widely recognized effect of exposure to cold air or immersion in cold water is an increased urine flow rate, or cold-induced diuresis; however, the precise mechanism behind this effect remains controversial. Experimental findings appear to rule out hormonal mechanisms and suggest that the increased systemic and renal blood pressure associated with cold-induced vasoconstriction may increase filtration and decrease reabsorption of water and solute by the kidney (180) (see Chapter 22). However, whatever mechanisms are involved, exercise can counteract or block them because cold-induced diuresis is prevented by even moderate exercise during cold exposure (180).

It has also been suggested that breathing cold air can exacerbate respiratory water loss during exercise, because cold air has a lower water content than warmer air, and it is assumed that each inspired breath warms to body temperature and becomes 100% saturated with water as it passes through the respiratory passages (180). However, this assumption may not be valid. Experimental observations (181) showed that cold inspired air ($-12°C$) did not warm to the same temperature as warmer air (23°C), and in fact, less rather than more water was lost in the exhaled cold air. The difference in temperature between ambient and inspired air temperature becomes even greater when ventilation rate increases, such as during exercise (181). Therefore, respiratory water losses are probably no more important for fluid balance during exercise in the cold than in warm conditions, and the most significant avenue of fluid loss during exercise in the cold—sweating—is the same as in warm conditions.

Even in cold environments, metabolic heat production can exceed heat loss, and the resulting heat storage can cause hyperthermia and initiate thermoregulatory sweating. The problem is that the clothing insulation needed for warmth and comfort in cold environments is much higher during rest and light activity than during strenuous activity (9). Therefore, if a person begins exercising vigorously while wearing clothes selected for sedentary activities in the cold, sweating and the resultant drinking requirements can increase substantially. If these increased drinking requirements go unmet, dehydration will ensue, just as with exercise in the heat, with possibly similar adverse physiologic and performance consequences (182) as discussed earlier in this chapter. However, moderate fluid loss may not be as important for exercise performance in the cold as it is for temperate and hot environments. Recent data show that if skin temperatures are very cool, 3% dehydration has no effect on aerobic cycling performance in the cold (183). Otherwise, there is little evidence that cold exposure has any unique impact on heat conservation, heat production, or cold CIVD responses (184,185), and thus does not appear to increase the likelihood of cold injuries.

Exercise Performance Limitations

As discussed above, cold exposure can reduce maximal aerobic power and increase metabolic and cardiovascular strain during submaximal exercise, both of which could be predicted to limit or impair exercise performance to some extent. However, both of those effects appear to be mediated by significant body heat loss and cooling of deep body and skeletal muscle. Thus, how exercise influences the ability to maintain thermal balance in the cold is probably the key factor in determining whether cold exposure is associated with performance decrements. In addition, certain pathophysiologic responses elicited by cold exposure can degrade performance by impairing an individual's ability to exercise.

Exercise and thermal balance

As described above, exercise elicits both thermogenesis and an increased peripheral blood flow (skin and muscles), which facilitates body heat loss by enhancing convective heat transfer from the central core to peripheral shell, and both responses increase concomitantly as exercise intensity increases. During exposure to cold air, the thermogenic

response during exercise is pronounced enough to ensure that the increased metabolic heat production will usually match or exceed any exercise-related facilitation of heat loss, and exercise performance will not be affected by the inability to maintain thermal balance (7). In contrast, because the higher conductive heat transfer coefficient is so much greater during water immersion than in air, the exercise-associated increase in heat loss during exercise in water can be so large that metabolic heat production during even intense exercise will be insufficient to maintain thermal balance (7).

Exercise affects thermal balance during cold exposure in two other ways. Arms have a greater ratio of surface area to mass, and thinner subcutaneous fat compared with legs, so exercise-induced increments in muscle and SkBF to the limb tend to increase convective heat transfer more during arm exercise than during leg exercise (21). As a result, metabolic heat production is less effective for sustaining thermal balance during arm than leg exercise at a similar intensity (7). In addition, limb movement disrupts the stationary boundary layer of air or water that develops at the skin surface in a still environment, and the loss of that insulation further favors increased convective heat loss from the body surface. Experimental observations confirm that these effects have a measurable influence on thermal balance during exercise in cold water (186). The practical implications of these effects for performance in the cold remain to be fully explored, but they may influence the design of cold-weather athletic clothing.

TEST YOURSELF

Galloway and Maughan (57) showed that exercise performance is optimal at an ambient temperature of 11°C, and a 13% decline in performance occurs at 4°C (Fig. 23.9). What factors might explain this decline in performance? Design a study to systematically determine the reason(s) for this decline in exercise performance as ambient temperature decreases.

Hiker's hypothermia: exertional fatigue and thermoregulation in the cold

Strenuous exercise can lead to exertional fatigue, and when strenuous exercise and high levels of energy expenditure are sustained for long periods, it can be difficult to maintain sufficiently high energy intakes to offset expenditures. It has been shown that fatigue due to exertion, sleep restriction, and underfeeding impairs an individual's ability to maintain thermal balance in the cold (187), and an anecdotal association between exertional fatigue and susceptibility to hypothermia has also been reported (188). This syndrome is sometimes referred to as hiker's hypothermia. The simplest explanation proposed is that prolonged exercise produces fatigue, so the exercise intensity and rate of metabolic heat production that can be sustained decline, and if ambient conditions are sufficiently cold, a negative thermal balance and declining core temperature will ensue. When underfeeding is a factor, effects probably result from the development of hypoglycemia, since acute hypoglycemia impairs shivering through a CNS-mediated effect. Also, declining peripheral carbohydrate stores probably contribute to the inability to sustain exercise or activity, and the associated exercise-induced thermogenesis in the cold. Recent studies also indicate that shivering and peripheral vasoconstriction may themselves be directly impaired after strenuous exercise (132,189), repeated or prolonged cold exposure (190), or both. Regardless of the mechanism(s) involved, when strenuous exercise produces fatigue (either acute or chronic), the ability to maintain thermal balance appears to be degraded, which in turn can further limit performance.

Cold-induced bronchospasm

For the most part, inhaling cold air during exercise has negligible effects. Upper airway temperatures, which normally remain unchanged during exercise under temperate conditions, can decrease substantially when extremely cold air is breathed during strenuous exercise; however, temperatures of the lower respiratory tract and deep body temperatures are unaffected (191). Pulmonary function during exercise in healthy athletes is usually unaffected by breathing cold air, but allergy-prone athletes frequently have bronchospasm (137,192). The triggering mechanism for bronchospasm in susceptible persons remains to be determined, but it may be related to thermally induced leakage in the lung's microcirculation with subsequent edema (181) or to airway drying caused by hyperventilation leading to the secretion of vasoconstrictor mediators (193,194). Persons who have bronchospasm when breathing cold air during heavy exercise exhibit a reduced forced expiratory volume (192), which can limit maximal ventilation and hence performance. Further, even healthy persons can experience an increase in respiratory passage secretions and decreased mucociliary clearance when breathing very cold air during exercise, and any associated airway congestion can impair pulmonary mechanics and ventilation during exercise, again impairing performance (137,195).

Cold Injury

Hypothermia

Clinically, hypothermia is defined as a core temperature below 35°C (95°F), which represents a ~2°C (3.5°F) decrease from normal body temperature (5,137). Physiologically, however, hypothermia is defined as a core temperature below the value observed typically observed during active phases (<36.8°C, 98°F). Hypothermia develops when heat losses exceed heat production, causing the body heat content to decrease. A drop in core temperature may eventually impact exercise performance.

Predisposing factors relevant to exercise include fatigue, wet clothing, hypoglycemia, and low physical fitness. For a complete list, see Winkenwerder and Sawka (5) and Castellani et al. (137).

Hypothermia is characterized as mild, moderate, or severe (5,137). Table 23.8 lists the core temperatures and physiologic changes associated with these low body core temperatures. The symptoms of hypothermia vary greatly from person to person, even at the same core temperature. Early symptoms of hypothermia include feeling cold, shivering, and exhibiting signs of apathy and social withdrawal. More pronounced hypothermia manifests as confusion or sleepiness, slurred speech, and a change in behavior or appearance. Severe hypothermia is associated with changes in cardiac rhythms that require immediate treatment to restore normal temperature. Resuscitation has been successful even with core temperatures as low as 13.7°C (56.7°F). At these temperatures, life signs are almost impossible to discern, and no one should be pronounced dead until he or she has been re-warmed (hence the adage, "a person is not dead until they are warm and dead").

Frostbite

Frostbite occurs when tissue temperatures fall below 0°C, 32°F. The freezing point of skin is slightly below the freezing point of water, due to the electrolyte content of the cells and extracellular fluid, with the skin surface reportedly freezing from −3.7°C to −4.8°C (25°F–23°F) (137). Wet skin will cool faster, reach a lower temperature, and freeze at a higher threshold (~−0.6°C, 31°F). Frostbite is most common in exposed skin (i.e., nose, ears, cheeks, and exposed wrists), but also occurs in the hands and feet because peripheral vasoconstriction significantly lowers tissue temperatures. Contact frostbite can occur by touching cold objects with bare skin (particularly highly conductive metal or stone), which causes rapid heat loss.

Usually, the first sign of frostbite is numbness. In the periphery, the initial sense of cooling begins at skin temperatures of 28°C, ~82°F, and pain appears at ~20°C, 68°F (137), but as skin temperature falls below 10°C, 50°F, these sensations are replaced by numbness (137). Individuals often report feeling a "wooden" sensation in the injured area. After the victim is re-warmed, the pain can be significant. The initial sensations are an uncomfortable sense of cold, which may include tingling, burning, aching, sharp pain, and decreased sensation. The skin color may initially appear red and then become waxy white. Note that peripheral temperatures (i.e., in hands and feet) may be indicative of a generalized whole-body cooling that may ultimately result in hypothermia.

Nonfreezing cold injuries

The most common nonfreezing cold injuries (NFCIs) are trenchfoot and chilblains. Trenchfoot typically occurs when deep tissues are exposed to temperatures between 0 and

TABLE 23.8	Core Temperature and Associated Physiologic Changes that Occur as Core Temperature Falls		

Stage	Core temperature		Physiologic changes
	°F	°C	
Normothermia	98.6	37.0	
Mild	95.0	35.0	Maximal shivering, increased blood pressure
	93.2	34.0	Amnesia, dysarthria, poor judgment, behavior change
	91.4	33.0	Ataxia, apathy
Moderate hypothermia	89.6	32.0	Stupor
	87.8	31.0	Shivering ceases, pupils dilate
	85.2	30.0	Cardiac arrhythmias, decreased cardiac output
	85.2	29.0	Unconsciousness
Severe hypothermia	82.4	28.0	Ventricular fibrillation likely, hypoventilation
	80.6	27.0	Loss of reflexes and voluntary motion
	78.8	26.0	Acid–base disturbances, no response to pain
	77.0	25.0	Reduced cerebral blood flow
	75.2	24.0	Hypotension, bradycardia, pulmonary edema
	73.4	23.0	No corneal reflexes, areflexia
	66.2	19.0	Electroencephalographic silence
	64.4	18.0	Asystole
	59.2	15.2	Lowest infant survival from accidental hypothermia
	56.7	13.7	Lowest adult survival from accidental hypothermia

Individuals respond differently at each level of core temperature (114).

15°C (32°F–60°F) for prolonged periods of time, whereas chilblains (defined as a more superficial NFCI) can occur after just a few hours of exposure to bare skin (137,196). These injuries may occur as a result of actual immersion or a damp environment inside boots caused by sweat-soaked socks. To diagnose NFCI, one must observe clinical symptoms over time as different, distinct stages emerge days to months after the initial injury.

Trenchfoot initially appears as a swollen, edematous foot with a feeling of numbness. The initial color is red but soon becomes pale and cyanotic if the injury is more severe. Peripheral pulses are hard to detect. Trenchfoot is accompanied by aches, increased pain sensitivity, and infection (137,196). The exposure time necessary to develop trenchfoot is quite variable, with estimates ranging from >12 hours to 3 to 4 days in cold, wet environments. Most commonly, trenchfoot develops when wet socks and shoes are worn continuously over many days. In most sporting activities, except for winter hiking, camping, and expeditions, the likelihood of developing trenchfoot is low.

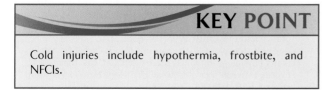

KEY POINT

Cold injuries include hypothermia, frostbite, and NFCIs.

CHAPTER SUMMARY

Body temperature is regulated by two distinct control systems: behavioral and physiologic. Behavioral thermoregulation involves the conscious, willed use of whatever means are available to minimize thermal discomfort. Physiologic thermoregulation employs unconscious responses that are controlled by the autonomic nervous system in proportion to the core and skin temperatures. The physiologic responses that modify body heat loss are increased SkBF and sweating, and those that modify heat conservation are vasoconstriction and shivering. Thermoregulatory responses are affected by an interaction among exercise duration, intensity, and mode, as well as environmental and individual characteristics.

Climatic heat stress and exercise interact synergistically and may push physiologic systems to their limits. Heat stress reduces an athlete's ability to exercise. Physiologic mechanisms that contribute to this reduced performance include cardiovascular, CNS, and metabolic perturbations. Heat acclimatization provides many physiologic adaptations to allow sustained exercise and protection from heat injury. Athletes routinely have high sweating rates during exercise heat stress that can lead to dehydration and adversely influence exercise performance.

In the cold, heat balance and requirements for shivering depend on the severity of the climatic cold stress, effectiveness of vasoconstriction, and intensity and mode

A MILESTONE OF DISCOVERY

Does central fatigue contribute to reduced exercise performance associated with hyperthermia? Human tissues retain their function and tolerate temperatures above 40°C without injury, but irrevocable damage can result beyond tissue temperatures >42°C (3,4). Therefore, an inability or unwillingness to exercise beyond destructive internal body temperatures may be a type of protection against catastrophic hyperthermia. Animal research has shown that exercise performance can sometimes decrease when hypothalamic temperature exceeds 42°C (independently of body temperature), suggesting that very high brain temperatures can mediate protective thermoregulatory behavior (197). However, such high brain temperatures would not normally be expected in exercising humans.

Before Nybo and Nielson (65) performed their study on hyperthermia and central fatigue, there was no conclusive evidence that central fatigue contributes to reduced performance for humans exercising in the heat. In that study, 14 subjects exercised at 60% of $\dot{V}o_{2max}$ for 1 hour in both a hot (40°C) and a temperate (18°C) climate. Immediately afterward, the subjects performed 2 minutes of sustained maximal voluntary contraction (MVC) of handgrip and knee extension with electrical stimulation (EL) periodically applied to the nervus femoralis. EL superimposed during the MVC generated the maximal total force (MVC + EL) and maximal voluntary activation percentage (MVC / MVC + EL). Core temperature increased to 40°C (exhaustion after 50 minutes of exercise) and 38°C (after 1 hour of exercise)

in the hot and temperate climates, respectively. Knee extension MVC force was initially unaffected by previous exercise, but after 5 seconds the decline in MVC force was greater after the hyperthermia than after the temperate trials. The total maximal forces were similar, and thus the voluntary activation percentage was lower after exercise in hot (54%) than in temperate (82%) conditions. Two subjects were passively heated to 39°C and demonstrated the same pattern of voluntary force decline during sustained maximal handgrip contractions. The experiments showed that hyperthermia significantly reduced force-generating capacity during a sustained MVC in both active (leg) and inactive (forearm) muscles compared with that measured at a lower core temperature. However, the capacity of the skeletal muscles was not altered by hyperthermia when EL was applied.

The results of this study provide strong support for the idea that central fatigue may contribute to reduced capabilities for dynamic exercise in hot weather. It is unclear whether the temperature of the brain or other tissues, or feedback inhibition from hot muscles, was influenced by the hyperthermia to send signals that affected motor activity. The precise mechanism for attenuated neuromuscular activity at a higher body temperature remains unresolved, but it may be linked to neurochemical alterations within the brain.

Nybo L, Nielsen B. Hyperthermia and central fatigue during prolonged exercise. J Appl Physiol. 2001;91:1055–1060.

of exercise. Cold-induced vasoconstriction decreases blood flow to peripheral tissues, which allows them to cool and makes them susceptible to cold injury. Cooling of peripheral tissues can degrade finger dexterity and impair skeletal muscle contractile function, whereas a reduced core temperature can degrade the body's ability to achieve maximal metabolic rates and submaximal endurance performance. Body composition is the most important physiologic determinant of thermoregulatory tolerance to cold exposure. The clothing requirement for warmth and comfort is much higher during rest and light activity than during strenuous activity, and overinsulation can cause heat stress that leads to sweating, wet clothing, and dehydration. Each of these factors can have undesirable affects on athletic performance and susceptibility to cold injury.

ACKNOWLEDGMENTS

The views, opinions, and findings in this report are those of the authors and should not be construed as an official Department of the Army position or decision unless so designated by other official documentation.

REFERENCES

1. Byrne C, Lee JK, Chew SA, et al. Continuous thermoregulatory responses to mass-participation distance running in heat. *Med Sci Sports Exer.* 2006;38:803–810.
2. Sonna LA, Kain JE, Hoyt RW, et al. Ambulatory physiological status monitoring during a mountaineering expedition. *Military Med.* 2000;165:860–866.
3. Katschinski DM. On heat cells and proteins. *News Physiol Sci.* 2004;19:11–15.
4. Bynum GD, Pandolf KB, Schuette WH, et al. Induced hyperthermia in sedated humans and the concept of critical thermal maximum. *Am J Physiol.* 1978;235:R228–R236.
5. Winkenwerder W, Sawka MN. Disorders due to heat and cold. In: Goldman L, Ausiello D, eds. *Cecil Medicine.* 23rd ed. Philadelphia: Saunders Elsevier; 2008.
6. Sawka MN, Wenger CB, Pandolf KB. Thermoregulatory responses to acute exercise heat stress and heat acclimation. In: Fregly MJ, Blatteis CM, eds. *Handbook of Physiology, Section 4: Environmental Physiology.* New York: Oxford University; 1996:157–185.
7. Toner MM. Human thermoregulatory responses to acute cold stress with special reference to water immersion. In: Fregly MJ, Blatteis CM, eds. *Handbook of Physiology, Section 4: Environmental Physiology.* New York: Oxford University; 1996:379–418.
8. Young AJ. Homeostatic responses to prolonged cold exposure: human cold acclimatization. In: Fregly MJ, Blatteis CM, eds. *Handbook of Physiology, Section 4: Environmental Physiology.* New York: Oxford University; 1996:419–438.
9. Gagge AP, Gonzalez RR. Mechanisms of heat exchange: biophysics and physiology. In: Fregly MJ, Blatteis CM, eds. *Handbook of Physiology, Section 4: Environmental Physiology.* New York: Oxford University; 1996:45–84.

10. Gisolfi CV, Wenger CB. Temperature regulation during exercise: old concepts, new ideas. *Exer Sport Sci Rev*. 1984;12:339–372.

11. Johnson JM, Park MK. Effect of upright exercise on threshold for cutaneous vasodilation and sweating. *J Appl Physiol*. 1981;50:814–818.

12. Boulant JA. Hypothalamic neurons regulating body temperature. In: Fregly MJ, Blatteis CM, eds. *Handbook of Physiology, Section 4: Environmental Physiology*. New York: Oxford University; 1996:105–125.

13. Cooper KE. Some historical perspectives on thermoregulation. *J Appl Physiol*. 2002;92:17–24.

14. Hensel HT. Neural processes in thermoregulation. *Phys Rev*. 1973;53:948–1017.

15. Stitt JT. Fever versus hyperthermia. *Fed Proc*. 1979;8:39–43.

16. Nybo L, Secher NH, Nielsen B. Inadequate heat release from the human brain during prolonged exercise with hyperthermia. *J Physiol*. 2002;545:697–704.

17. Jay O, Reardon FD, Webb P, et al. Estimating changes in mean body temperature for humans during exercise using core and skin temperatures is inaccurate even with a correction factor. *J Appl Physiol*. 2007;103:443–451.

18. Saltin B, Gagge AP, Stolwijk JAJ. Muscle temperature during submaximal exercise in man. *J Appl Physiol*. 1968;25:679–688.

19. Goodman DA, Kenefick RW, Cadarette BS, et al. Influence of sensor ingestion timing on consistency of temperature measures. *Med Sci Sports Exer*. 2009;41:597–602.

20. Sawka MN, Wenger CB. Physiological responses to acute exercise heat stress. In: Pandolf KB, Sawka MN, Gonzalez RR, eds. *Human Performance Physiology and Environmental Medicine at Terrestrial Extremes*. Indianapolis, IN: Cooper; 1988:97–151.

21. Sawka MN. Physiology of upper body exercise. *Exer Sport Sci Rev*. 1986;14:175–211.

22. Nielsen M. Die regulation der korpertemperatur bei muskelarbeit. *Skand Archiv Physiol*. 1938;9:193–230.

23. Lind AR. A physiological criterion for setting thermal environmental limits for everyday work. *J Appl Physiol*. 1963;18:51–56.

24. Nielsen B, Nielsen M. Body temperature during work at different environmental temperatures. *Acta Physiol Scand*. 1962;56:120–129.

25. Saltin B, Hermansen L. Esophageal, rectal, and muscle temperatures during exercise. *J Appl Physiol*. 1966;21:1757–1762.

26. Shibasaki M, Wilson TE, Crandall CG. Neural control and mechanisms of eccrine sweating during heat stress and exercise. *J Appl Physiol*. 2006;100:1692–1701.

27. Kolka MA, Stephenson LA. Control of sweating during the human menstrual cycle. *Eur J Appl Physiol*. 1989;58:890–895.

28. Stephenson LA, Wenger CB, O'Donovan BH, et al. Circadian rhythm in sweating and cutaneous blood flow. *Am J Physiol*. 1984;246:R321–R324.

29. Madeira LG, da Fonseca MA, Fonseca IA, et al. Sex-related differences in sweat gland cholinergic sensitivity exist irrespective of differences in aerobic capacity. *Eur J Appl Physiol*. 2010;109:93–100.

30. Kenney WL, Munce TA. Invited review: aging and human temperature regulation. *J Appl Physiol*. 2003;95:2598–2603.

31. Stephenson LA, Kolka MA. Thermoregulation in women. *Exer Sport Sci Rev*. 1993;21:231–262.

32. Sato K. The mechanism of eccrine sweat secretion. In: Gisolf CV, Lamb DR, Nadel ER, eds. *Exercise, Heat, and Thermoregulation*. Dubuque, IA: Brown & Benchmark; 1993:85–117.

33. Nadel ER, Mitchell JW, Saltin B, et al. Peripheral modifications to the central drive for sweating. *J Appl Physiol*. 1971;31:828–833.

34. Johnson JM, Proppe DW. Cardiovascular adjustments to heat stress. In: Fregly MJ, Blatteis CM, eds. *Handbook of Physiology, Section 4: Environmental Physiology*. New York: Oxford University; 1996:215–243.

35. Taylor WF, Johnson JM, O'Leary DS, et al. Modification of the cutaneous vascular response to exercise by local skin temperature. *J Appl Physiol*. 1984;7:18–84.

36. Holowatz LA, Thompson-Torgerson CS, Kenney WL. Altered mechanisms of vasodilation in aged human skin. *Exer Sport Sci Rev*. 2007;35:119–125.

37. Rowell LB. *Human Circulation: Regulation During Physical Stress*. New York: Oxford University; 1986.

38. Kenney WL, Morgan AL, Farquhar WB, et al. Decreased active vasodilator sensitivity in aged skin. *Am J Physiol Heart Circ Physiol*. 1997;272:H1609–H1614.

39. Armstrong CG, Kenney WL. Effects of age and acclimation on responses to passive heat exposure. *J Appl Physiol*. 2003;75:2162–2167.

40. Minson CT, Wladkowski SL, Cardell AF, et al. Age alters the cardiovascular response to direct passive heating. *J Appl Physiol*. 1998;84:1323–1332.

41. Gonzalez-Alonso J, Crandall CG, Johnson JM. The cardiovascular challenge of exercising in the heat. *J Physiol*. 2008;586:45–53.

42. Crandall CG. Carotid baroreflex responsiveness in heat-stressed humans. *Am J Physiol*. 2000;279:H1955–H1962.

43. Crandall CG, Zhang R, Levine BD. Effects of whole body heating on dynamic baroreflex regulation of heart rate in humans. *Am J Physiol*. 2000;279:H2486–H2492.

44. Gonzalez-Alonso J, Calbet JA. Reductions in systemic and skeletal muscle blood flow and oxygen delivery limit maximal aerobic capacity in humans. *Circulation*. 2003;107:824–830.

45. Rowell LB, Marx HJ, Bruce RA, et al. Reductions in cardiac output, central blood volume, and stroke volume with thermal stress in normal men during exercise. *J Clin Invest*. 1966;45:1801–1806.

46. Massett MP, Lewis SJ, Bates JN, et al. Effect of heating on vascular reactivity in rat mesenteric arteries. *J Appl Physiol*. 1998;85:701–708.

47. Gonzalez-Alonso J, Calbet JA, Nielsen B. Muscle blood flow is reduced with dehydration during prolonged exercise in humans. *J Physiol*. 1998;513:895–905.

48. Wilson TE, Cui J, Zhang R, et al. Heat stress reduces cerebral blood velocity and markedly impairs orthostatic tolerance in humans. *Am J Physiol*. 2006;291:R1443–R1448.

49. Carter R, Cheuvront SN, Vernieuw CR, et al. Hypohydration and prior heat stress exacerbates decreases in cerebral blood flow velocity during standing. *J Appl Physiol*. 2006;101:1744–1750.

50. Bennett A. Thermal dependence of muscle function. *Am J Physiol*. 1984;247:R217–R229.

51. Young AJ. Energy substrate utilization during exercise in extreme environments. *Exer Sport Sci Rev*. 1990;18:65–117.

52. Febbraio MA. Does muscle function and metabolism affect exercise performance in the heat? *Exer Sport Sci Rev*. 2000;28:171–176.

53. Mitchell CR, Harris MB, Cordaro AR, et al. Effect of body temperature during exercise on skeletal muscle cytochrome c oxidase content. *J Appl Physiol*. 2002;93:526–530.

54. Young AJ, Sawka MN, Levine L. Metabolic and thermal adaptations from endurance training in hot or cold water. *J Appl Physiol*. 1995;8:793–801.

55. Sawka MN, Young AJ, Cadarette BS, et al. Influence of heat stress and acclimation on maximal aerobic power. *Eur J Appl Physiol*. 1985;53:294–298.

56. Ely MR, Cheuvront SN, Robert WO, et al. Impact of weather on marathon-running performance. *Med Sci Sports Exer*. 2007;39:487–493.

57. Galloway SD, Maughan RJ. Effects of ambient temperature on the capacity to perform prolonged cycle exercise in man. *Med Sci Sports Exer*. 1997;29:1240–1249.

58. Pitsiladis SD, Maughan JR. The effects of exercise and diet manipulation on the capacity to perform prolonged exercise in the heat and in the cold in trained humans. *J Physiol*. 1999;517:919–930.

59. Ely BR, Cheuvront SN, Kenefick RW, et al. Aerobic performance is degraded. despite moderate hyperthermia, in hot environments. *Med Sci Sports Exer*. 2010;42:135–141.

60. Arngrimsson SA, Stewart DJ, Borrani F, et al. Relation of heart rate to percent $\dot{V}o_{2peak}$ during submaximal exercise in the heat. *J Appl Physiol*. 2003;94:1162–1168.

61. Sawka MN, Latzka WA, Montain SJ, et al. Physiological tolerance to uncompensable heat: intermittent exercise, field vs laboratory. *Med Sci Sports Exer*. 2001;33:422–430.

62. Sawka MN, Young AJ. Physical exercise in hot and cold climates. In: Garrett WE, Kirkendall DT, eds. *Exercise and Sport Science*. Philadelphia: Lippincott Williams & Wilkins; 2000:385–400.

63. Cheuvront SN, Kolka MA, Cadarette BS, et al. Efficacy of intermittent, regional microclimate cooling. *J Appl Physiol*. 2003;94:1841–1848.

64. Maron MB, Wagner JA, Horvath SM. Thermoregulatory responses during competitive marathon running. *J Appl Physiol*. 1977;42:909–914.

65. Nybo L, Nielsen B. Hyperthermia and central fatigue during prolonged exercise in humans. *J Appl Physiol*. 2001;91:1055–1060.

66. Nybo L, Nielsen B, Blomstrand E, et al. Neurohumoral responses during prolonged exercise in humans. *J Appl Physiol*. 2003;95:1125–1131.

67. Watson P, Hasegawa H, Roelands B, et al. Acute dopamine-noradrenaline reuptake inhibition enhances human exercise performance in warm, but not temperate conditions. *J Physiol.* 2005;565:873–883.

68. Nielsen B, Hyldig T, Bidstrup F, et al. Brain activity and fatigue during prolonged exercise in the heat. *Pflügers Arch Eur J Physiol.* 2001;442:41–48.

69. Davis JM, Bailey SP. Possible mechanisms of central nervous system fatigue during exercise. *Med Sci Sports Exer.* 1997;29:45–57.

70. Meeusen R, Watson P, Hasegawa H, et al. Central fatigue: the serotonin hypothesis and beyond. *Sports Med.* 2006;36:881–909.

71. Tucker R, Marle T, Lambert EV, et al. The rate of heat storage mediates an anticipatory reduction in exercise intensity during cycling at a fixed rating of perceived exertion. *J Physiol.* 2006;574:905–915.

72. Tucker R, Rauch L, Harley YX, et al. Impaired exercise performance in the heat is associated with an anticipatory reduction in skeletal muscle recruitment. *Pflügers Arch Eur J Physiol.* 2004;448:422–430.

73. Ely BR, Cheuvront SN, Kenefick RW, et al. Evidence against a 40 degrees C core temperature threshold for fatigue in humans. *J Appl Physiol.* 2009;107:1519–1525.

74. Jay O, Kenny GP. Current evidence does not support an anticipatory regulation of exercise intensity mediated by rate of body heat storage. *J Appl Physiol.* 2009;107:630–631.

75. Armstrong LE, Pandolf KB. Physical training, cardiorespiratory physical fitness and exercise heat tolerance. In: Pandolf KB, Sawka MN, Gonzalez RR, eds. *Human Performance Physiology and Environmental Medicine at Terrestrial Extremes.* Indianapolis: Benchmark; 1988:199–226.

76. Wenger CB. Human heat acclimatization. In: Pandolf KB, Sawka MN, Gonzalez RR, eds. *Human Performance Physiology and Environmental Medicine at Terrestrial Extremes.* Indianapolis: Benchmark; 1988:153–197.

77. Cohen JS, Gisolfi CV. Effects of interval training on work-heat tolerance of young women. *Med Sci Sports Exer.* 1982;14:46–52.

78. Roberts MF, Wenger CB, Stolwijk JAJ, et al. Skin blood flow and sweating changes following exercise training and heat acclimation. *J Appl Physiol.* 1977;43:133–137.

79. Horowitz M. Matching the heart to heat-induced circulatory load: heat acclimation responses. *News Physiol Sci.* 2003;18:215–221.

80. Lind AR, Bass DE. Optimal exposure time for development of acclimatization to heat. *Fed Proc.* 1963;22:704–708.

81. Houmard JA, Costill DL, Davis JA, et al. The influence of exercise intensity on heat acclimation in trained subjects. *Med Sci Sports Exer.* 1990;22:615–620.

82. Lorenzo S, Halliwill JR, Sawka MN, et al. Heat acclimation improves exercise performance. *J Appl Physiol.* 2010;109:1140–1147.

83. Nielsen B, Hales JRS, Strange S, et al. Human circulatory and thermoregulatory adaptations with heat acclimation and exercise in a hot, dry environment. *J Physiol.* 1993;460:467–485.

84. Nielsen B, Strange S, Christensen NJ, et al. Acute and adaptive responses in humans to exercise in a warm, humid environment. *Pflügers Arch Eur J Physiol.* 1997;434:49–56.

85. Horowitz M. Do cellular heat acclimation responses modulate central thermoregulatory activity? *News Physiol Sci.* 1998;13:218–225.

86. Mack GW, Nadel ER. Body fluid balance during heat stress in humans. In: Fregly MJ, Blatteis CM, eds. *Environmental Physiology.* New York: Oxford University; 1996:187–214.

87. Sawka MN, Coyle EF. Influence of body water and blood volume on thermoregulation and exercise performance in the heat. *Exer Sport Sci Rev.* 1999;27:167–218.

88. Sawka MN, Convertino VA, Eichner ER, et al. Blood volume: importance and adaptations to exercise training, environmental stresses, and trauma-sickness. *Med Sci Sports Exer.* 2000;32:332–348.

89. Kregel KC. Heat shock proteins: modifying factors in physiological stress responses and acquired thermotolerance. *J Appl Physiol.* 2002;92:1–10.

90. Maloyan A, Palmon A, Horowitz M. Heat acclimation increases the basal HSP72 level and alters its production dynamics during heat stress. *Am J Physiol.* 1999;276:R1506–R1515.

91. Skidmore R, Gutierrez JA, Guerriero V, et al. HSP70 induction during exercise and heat stress in rats: role of internal temperature. *Am J Physiol.* 1995;68:R92–R97.

92. Yamada PM, Amorim FT, Moseley P, et al. Effect of heat acclimation on heat shock protein 72 and interleukin-10 in humans. *J Appl Physiol.* 2007;103:1196–1204.

93. McClung JP, Hasday JD, He J, et al. Exercise-heat acclimation in humans alters baseline levels and ex vivo heat inducibility of HSP72 and HSP90 in peripheral blood mononuclear cells. *Am J Physiol.* 2008;294:R185–R191.

94. Horowitz M. Heat acclimation and cross-tolerance against novel stressors: genomic-physiological linkage. In: Sharma HS, ed. *Progress in Brain Research.* Amsterdam: Elsevier; 2007:373–392.

95. Gabai VL, Sherman MY. Interplay between molecular chaperones and signaling pathways in survival of heat shock. *J Appl Physiol.* 2002;92:1743–1748.

96. Sonna LA, Sawka MN, Lilly CM. Exertional heat illness and human gene expression. In: Sharma HS, ed. *Progress in Brain Research.* Philadelphia: Saunders Elsevier; 2007:321–346.

97. Institute of Medicine. Water. In: *Dietary Reference Intakes: Water, Potassium, Sodium, Chloride, and Sulfate.* Washington: National Academies; 2005:73–185.

98. Chinevere TD, Kenefick RW, Cheuvront SN, et al. Effect of heat acclimation on sweat minerals. *Med Sci Sports Exer.* 2008;40:886–891.

99. Cheuvront SN, Haymes EM. Thermoregulation and marathon running: biological and environmental influences. *Sports Med.* 2001;31:743–762.

100. Sawka MN, Burke LM, Eichner ER, et al. American College of Sports Medicine position stand: exercise and fluid replacement. *Med Sci Sports Exer.* 2007;39:377–390.

101. Montain SJ, Sawka MN, Wenger CB. Hyponatremia associated with exercise: risk factors and pathogenesis. *Exer Sport Sci Rev.* 2001;29:113–117.

102. Cheuvront SN, Carter R, Sawka MN. Fluid balance and endurance exercise performance. *Curr Sports Med Rep.* 2003;2:202–208.

103. Kenefick RW, Cheuvront SN, Palombo LJ, et al. Skin temperature modifies the impact of hypohydration on aerobic performance. *J Appl Physiol.* 2010;109:79–86.

104. Judelson DA, Maresh CM, Anderson JM, et al. Hydration and muscular performance: does fluid balance affect strength, power and high-intensity endurance. *Sports Med.* 2007;37:907–921.

105. Montain SJ. Hydration recommendations for sport 2008. *Curr Sports Med Rep.* 2008;7:187–192.

106. Montain SJ, Latzka WA, Sawka MN. Control of thermoregulatory sweating is altered by hydration level and exercise intensity. *J Appl Physiol.* 1995;79:1434–1439.

107. Sawka MN, Pandolf KB. Effects of body water loss on physiological function and exercise performance. In: Gisolfi CV, Lamb DR, eds. *Perspectives in Exercise Science and Sports Medicine, Volume 3: Fluid Homeostasis During Exercise.* Carmel, IN: Benchmark; 1990:1–38.

108. Sawka MN. Physiological consequences of hydration: exercise performance and thermoregulation. *Med Sci Sports Exer.* 1992;24:657–670.

109. Fortney SM, Wenger CB, Bove JR, et al. Effect of hyperosmolality on control of blood flow and sweating. *J Appl Physiol.* 1984;57:1688–1695.

110. Gonzalez-Alonso J, Mora-Rodriguez R, Coyle EF. Stroke volume during exercise: interaction of environment and hydration. *Am J Physiol.* 2000;278:H321–H330.

111. Kenefick RW, Mahood NV, Hazzard MP, et al. Hypohydration effects on thermoregulation during moderate exercise in the cold. *Eur J Appl Physiol.* 2004;92:565–570.

112. Gonzalez-Alonso J, Mora-Rodriguez R, Below PR, et al. Dehydration markedly impairs cardiovascular function in hyperthermic endurance athletes during exercise. *J Appl Physiol.* 1997;82:1229–1236.

113. Gonzalez-Alonso J, Calbet JA, Nielsen B. Metabolic and thermodynamic responses to dehydration-induced reductions in muscle blood flow in exercising humans. *J Physiol.* 1999;520:577–589.

114. Sawka MN, Young AJ. Acute polycythemia and human performance during exercise and exposure to extreme environments. *Exer Sport Sci Rev.* 1989;17:265–293.

115. Noakes TD, Goodwin N, Rayner BL, et al. Water intoxication: a possible complication during endurance exercise. *Med Sci Sports Exer.* 1985;17:370–375.

116. Carter R, Cheuvront SN, Williams JO, et al. Epidemiology of hospitalizations and deaths from heat illness in soldiers. *Med Sci Sports Exer.* 2005;37:1338–1344.

117. Montain SJ, Cheuvront SN, Sawka MN. Exercise associated hyponatraemia: quantitative analysis to understand the aetiology. *Brit J Sports Med.* 2006;40:98–105.

118. Baker LB, Lang JA, Kenney WL. Change in body mass accurately and reliably predicts change in body water after endurance exercise. *Eur J Appl Physiol.* 2009;105:959–967.

119. Baker LB, Lang JA, Kenney WL. Quantitative analysis of serum sodium concentration after prolonged running in the heat. *J Appl Physiol.* 2008;105:91–99.

120. Gonzalez RR. Biophysics of heat exchange and clothing: applications to sports physiology. *Med Exer Nutr Health.* 1995;4:290–305.

121. Kark JA, Burr PQ, Wenger CB, et al. Exertional heat illness in Marine Corps recruit training. *Aviat Space Environ Med.* 1996;67:354–360.

122. Gaffin SL, Hubbard RW. Pathophysiology of heatstroke. In: Office of the Surgeon General, ed. *Textbook of Military Medicine: Medical Aspects of Harsh Environments.* Washington, DC: Borden Institute; 2001:161–208.

123. Bouchama A, al-Sedairy S, Siddiqui S, et al. Elevated pyrogenic cytokines in heatstroke. *Chest.* 1993;104:1498–1502.

124. Bouchama A, Knochel P. Heat stroke. *N Engl J Med.* 2002;346:1978–1988.

125. Leon LR. Heat stroke and cytokines. In: Sharma HS, ed. *Progress in Brain Research.* Amsterdam: Elsevier; 2007:481–524.

126. Casa DJ, McDermott BP, Lee EC, et al. Cold water immersion: the gold standard for exertional heatstroke treatment. *Exer Sport Sci Rev.* 2007;35:141–149.

127. National Weather Service. Windchill temperature index. Washington: Office of Climate, Water, and Weather Services; 2001.

128. Ducharme MB, Brajkovic D. Guidelines on the risk and time to frostbite during exposure to cold wind. In: *Proceedings of the RTO NATO Factors and Medicine Panel Specialist Meeting on Prevention of Cold Injuries.* Amsterdam: NATO; 2005:21–29.

129. Brajkovic D, Ducharme MB. Facial cold-induced vasodilation and skin temperature during exposure to cold wind. *Eur J Appl Physiol.* 2006;96:711–721.

130. Kaufman WC, Bothe DJ. Wind chill reconsidered, Siple revisited. *Aviat Space Environ Med.* 1986;57:23–26.

131. Stolwijk JAJ, Hardy JD. Control of body temperature. In: Lee DHK, Falk HL, Murphy SD, et al., eds. *Handbook of Physiology, Section 9: Reactions to Environmental Agents.* Bethesda: American Physiological Society; 1977:45–68.

132. Castellani JW, Young AJ, Degroot DW, et al. Thermoregulation during cold exposure after several days of exhaustive exercise. *J Appl Physiol.* 2001;90:939–946.

133. Castellani JW, O'Brien C, Tikuisis P, et al. Evaluation of two cold thermoregulatory models for prediction of core temperature during exercise in cold water. *J Appl Physiol.* 2007;103:2034–2041.

134. Tikuisis P. Prediction of survival time at sea based on observed body cooling values. *Aviat Space Environ Med.* 1997;8:441–448.

135. Xu X, Tikuisis P, Gonzalez RR, et al. Thermoregulatory model for prediction of long-term cold exposure. *Comput Biol Med.* 2005;35:287–298.

136. Molnar GW. Survival of hypothermia by men immersed in the ocean. *JAMA.* 1946;131:1046–1050.

137. Castellani JW, Young AJ, Ducharme MB, et al. American College of Sports Medicine position stand: prevention of cold injuries during exercise. *Med Sci Sports Exer.* 2006;38:2012–2029.

138. Veicsteinas A, Ferretti G, Rennie DW. Superficial shell insulation in resting and exercising men in cold water. *J Appl Physiol.* 1982;2:1557–1564.

139. Stephens DP, Aoki K, Kosiba WA, et al. Nonnoradrenergic mechanism of reflex cutaneous vasoconstriction in men. *Am J Physiol.* 2001;280:H1496–H1504.

140. Stephens DP, Saad AR, Bennett LA, et al. Neuropeptide Y antagonism reduces reflex cutaneous vasoconstriction in humans. *Am J Physiol.* 2004;287:H1404–H1409.

141. Thompson-Torgerson CS, Holowatz LA, Flavahan NA, et al. Cold-induced cutaneous vasoconstriction is mediated by Rho kinase in vivo in human skin. *Am J Physiol.* 2007;292:H1700–H1705.

142. Johnson JM. Mechanisms of vasoconstriction with direct skin cooling in humans. *Am J Physiol.* 2007;292:H1690–H1691.

143. Chotani MA, Flavahan S, Mitra S, et al. Silent α_{2C}-adrenergic receptors enable cold-induced vasoconstriction in cutaneous arteries. *Am J Physiol.* 2000;278:H1075–H1083.

144. Chotani MA, Mitra S, Su BY, et al. Regulation of α_2-adrenoceptors in human vascular smooth muscle cells. *Am J Physiol.* 2004;286: H59–H67.

145. Brajkovic D, Ducharme MB, Frim J. Influence of localized auxiliary heating on hand comfort during cold exposure. *J Appl Physiol.* 1998;85:2054–2065.

146. Ducharme MB, Vanhelder WP, Radomski MW. Cyclic intramuscular temperature fluctuations in the human forearm during cold-water immersion. *Eur J Appl Physiol.* 1991;63:188–193.

147. Lindblad LE, Ekenvall L, Klingstedt C. Neural regulation of vascular tone and cold induced vasoconstriction in human finger skin. *J Auton Nerv Syst.* 1991;30:169–174.

148. O'Brien C, Young AJ, Lee DT, et al. Role of core temperature as a stimulus for cold acclimation during repeated immersion in 20°C water. *J Appl Physiol.* 2000;89:242–250.

149. van Marken Lichtenbelt WD, Vanhommerig JW, Smulders NM, et al. Cold-activated brown adipose tissue in healthy men. *N Engl J Med.* 2009;360:1500–1508.

150. Virtanen KA, Lidell ME, Orava J, et al. Functional brown adipose tissue in healthy adults. *N Engl J Med.* 2009;360:1518–1525.

151. Saito M, Okamatsu-Ogura Y, Matsushita M, et al. High incidence of metabolically active brown adipose tissue in healthy adult humans: effects of cold exposure and adiposity. *Diabetes.* 2009;58:1526–1531.

152. Cypess AM, Lehman S, Williams G, et al. Identification and importance of brown adipose tissue in adult humans. *N Engl J Med.* 2009;360:1509–1517.

153. Bell DG, Tikuisis P, Jacobs I. Relative intensity of muscular contraction during shivering. *J Appl Physiol.* 1992;72:2336–2342.

154. Golden FS, Hampton IF, Hervery GR, et al. Shivering intensity in humans during immersion in cold water. *J Physiol.* 1979;277:48.

155. McArdle WD, Magel JR, Spina RJ, et al. Thermal adjustment to cold-water exposure in exercising men and women. *J Appl Physiol.* 1984;56:1572–1577.

156. McArdle WD, Magel JR, Gergley TJ, et al. Thermal adjustment to cold-water exposure in resting men and women. *J Appl Physiol.* 1984;56:1565–1571.

157. Falk B, Bar-Or O, Smolander J, et al. Response to rest and exercise in the cold: effects of age and aerobic fitness. *J Appl Physiol.* 1994;76:72–78.

158. Kenney WL, Armstrong CG. Reflex peripheral vasoconstriction is diminished in older men. *J Appl Physiol.* 1996;80:512–515.

159. Smolander J. Effect of cold exposure on older humans. *Int J Sports Med.* 2002;23:86–92.

160. Young AJ, Lee DT. Aging and human cold tolerance. *Experimental Aging Research.* 1997;23:45–67.

161. Ohnaka T, Tochihara Y, Tsuzuki K, et al. Preferred temperature of the elderly after cold and heat exposures determined by individual self-selection of air temperature. *Journal of Thermal Biology.* 1993;18:349–353.

162. Taylor NA, Allsopp NK, Parkes DG. Preferred room temperature of young vs. aged males: the influence of thermal sensation, thermal comfort, and affect. *J Gerontol Biol Sci Med Sci.* 1995;50: 216–221.

163. Bittel JHM, Nonott-Varly C, Livecchi-Gonnot GH, et al. Physical fitness and thermoregulatory reactions in a cold environment in men. *J Appl Physiol.* 1988;65:1984–1989.

164. Savourey G, Bittel J. Thermoregulatory changes in the cold induced by physical training in humans. *Eur J Appl Physiol Occup Physiol.* 1998;78:379–384.

165. Gonzalez RR. Biophysical and physiological integration of proper clothing for exercise. *Exer Sport Sci Rev.* 1987;15:261–295.

166. Belding HS. Protection against dry cold. In: Newburgh LH, ed. *Physiology of Heat Regulation and the Science of Clothing.* Philadelphia: W.B. Saunders; 1949:351–366.

167. Holmer I. Assessment of cold stress in terms of required clothing insulation-IREQ. *Int J Indust Ergonom.* 1988;3:159–166.

168. ISO. Evaluation of cold environments—determination of required clothing insulation (IREQ). Geneva: International Organization for Standardization; 1993. Report No. 11079.

169. Gavhed D, Mäkinen T, Holmér I, et al. Face cooling by cold wind in walking subjects. *Int J Biometeorol*. 2003;47:148–155.

170. Bass DE. Metabolic and energy balances in men in a cold environment. In: Horvath SM, ed. *Cold Injury*. Montpelier, VT: Josiah Macy Foundation; 1960:317–338.

171. Bergh U, Ekblom B. Physical performance and peak aerobic power at different body temperatures. *J Appl Physiol*. 1979;46:885–889.

172. Bergh U, Ekblom B. Influence of muscle temperature on maximal muscle strength and power output in human skeletal muscles. *Acta Physiol Scand*. 1979;107:33–37.

173. Schmidt V, Brück K. Effect of a precooling maneuver on body temperature and exercise performance. *J Appl Physiol*. 1981;50:772–778.

174. Young AJ, Sawka MN, Pandolf KB. Physiology of cold exposure. In: Marriott BM, Carlson SJ, eds. *Nutritional Needs in Cold and in High-altitude Environments*. Washington: National Academy; 1996:127–147.

175. McArdle WD, Magel JR, Lesmes GR. Metabolic and cardiovascular adjustment to work in air and water at 18, 25, and 33. *J Appl Physiol*. 1976;40:85–90.

176. Pendergast DR. The effects of body cooling on oxygen transport during exercise. *Med Sci Sports Exer*. 1988;20:S171–S176.

177. Haman F, Peronnet F, Kenny GP, et al. Effect of cold exposure on fuel utilization in humans: plasma glucose, muscle glycogen, and lipids. *J Appl Physiol*. 2002;93:77–84.

178. Haman F. Shivering in the cold: from mechanisms of fuel selection to survival. *J Appl Physiol*. 2006;100:1702–1708.

179. Kenefick RW, Hazzard MP, Mahood NV, et al. Thirst sensations and AVP responses at rest and during exercise-cold exposure. *Med Sci Sports Exer*. 2004;36:1528–1534.

180. Freund BJ, Young AJ. Environmental influences on body fluid balance during exercise: cold exposure. In: Buskirk ER, Puhl SM, eds. *Body Fluid Balance: Exercise and Sport*. New York: CRC Press; 1996:159–181.

181. McFadden ER, Nelson JA, Skowronski ME, et al. Thermally induced asthma and airway drying. *Am J Resp Crit Care Med*. 1999;160:221–226.

182. Lennquist S, Granberg PO, Wedin B. Fluid balance and physical work capacity in humans exposed to cold. *Arch Environ Health*. 1974;29:241–249.

183. Cheuvront SN, Carter R, Castellani JW, et al. Hypohydration impairs endurance exercise performance in temperate but not cold air. *J Appl Physiol*. 2005;99:1972–1976.

184. O'Brien C, Young AJ, Sawka MN. Hypohydration and thermoregulation in cold air. *J Appl Physiol*. 1998;84:185–189.

185. O'Brien C, Montain SJ. Hypohydration effect on finger skin temperature and blood flow during cold-water finger immersion. *J Appl Physiol*. 2003;94:598–603.

186. Toner MM, Sawka MN, Pandolf KB. Thermal responses during arm and leg and combined arm-leg exercise in water. *J Appl Physiol*. 1984;6:1355–1360.

187. Young AJ, Castellani JW, O'Brien C, et al. Exertional fatigue, sleep loss, and negative energy balance increase susceptibility to hypothermia. *J Appl Physiol*. 1998;85:1210–1217.

188. Pugh LGCE. Cold stress and muscular exercise, with special reference to accidental hypothermia. *BMJ*. 1967;2:333–337.

189. Castellani JW, Young AJ, Kain JE, et al. Thermoregulation during cold exposure: effects of prior exercise. *J Appl Physiol*. 1999;87:247–252.

190. Castellani JW, Young AJ, Sawka MN, et al. Human thermoregulatory responses during serial cold-water immersions. *J Appl Physiol*. 1998;85:204–209.

191. Jaeger JJ, Deal EC, Roberts DE, et al. Cold air inhalation and esophageal temperature in exercising humans. *Med Sci Sports Exer*. 1980;12:365–369.

192. Helenius IJ, Tikkanen HO, Haahtela T. Exercise-induced bronchospasm at low temperatures in elite runners. *Thorax*. 1996;51:628–629.

193. Anderson SD, Daviskas E. Pathophysiology of exercise-induced asthma: the role of respiratory water loss. In: Weiler JM, ed. *Allergic and Respiratory Disease in Sports Medicine*. New York: Marcel Dekker; 1997:87–114.

194. Evans TM, Rundell KW, Beck KC, et al. Cold air inhalation does not affect the severity of EIB after exercise or eucapnic voluntary hyperventilation. *Med Sci Sports Exer*. 2005;37:544–549.

195. Giesbrecht GG. The respiratory system in a cold environment. *Aviat Space Environ Med*. 1995;66:890–902.

196. Lipman GS, Castellani JW. Nonfreezing cold-induced injuries. In: Auerbach PS, ed. *Wilderness Medicine*. 5th ed. Philadelphia: Mosby Elsevier; 2007:188–194.

197. Caputa M, Feistkorn G, Jessen C. Effect of brain and trunk temperatures on exercise performance in goats. *Pflügers Arch Eur J Physiol*. 2001;406:184–189.

CHAPTER 24

Physiologic Systems and Their Responses to Conditions of Hypoxia

Carsten Lundby

Abbreviations

A-aPO$_2$	Alveolar-arterial O$_2$ gradient	MSNA	Muscle sympathetic nervous activity
ATP	Adenosine Triphosphate	PAO$_2$	Alveolar partial pressure for oxygen
Cao$_2$	Arterial oxygen content	Pao$_2$	Arterial partial pressure for oxygen
C$_v$O$_2$	Venous oxygen content	P_{50}	Arterial oxygen partial pressure at which
EPO	Erythropoietin		oxygen saturation is 50%
F$_I$O$_2$	Inspired fraction of oxygen	P$_B$	Barometric pressure
[Hb]	Hemoglobin concentration	Q̇	Cardiac output
HIF-1	Hypoxia inducible factor 1	Sao$_2$	Arterial oxygen saturation
LHTH	Live high—train high	V̇A	Alveolar ventilation
LHTL	Live high—train low	V̇co$_2$	Pulmonary CO$_2$ output
LLTH	Live low—train high	V̇o$_{2max}$	Maximal pulmonary oxygen uptake

Introduction

On May 8, 1978, Reinhold Messner and Peter Habeler became the first humans to reach the summit of Mount Everest (8850 m) without the use of supplemental oxygen. This came as a surprise to many physiologists because sudden exposure to air at the oxygen concentrations found on the summit of Mount Everest usually results in unconsciousness within minutes and, if continued, death (1). Furthermore, the height of Mount Everest surpasses the level it has been predicted that humans can reach without using supplemental oxygen (2). However, Messner and Habeler had acclimatized themselves to the hypoxic environment by spending several weeks at altitudes above 5000 m, and this (besides factors involving technical and psychological aspects) was the main factor that made their historic feat possible. Subsequently, it was demonstrated that their V̇o$_{2max}$ on the summit must have been just sufficient to allow the necessary upward movements (2).

In this chapter, we focus on the physiologic responses and adaptations that occur when humans are exposed to hypoxia. We begin the chapter with a brief description of

cellular responses to hypoxia and then turn to O$_2$ transport using the O$_2$ cascade as a platform (i.e., starting with ventilation and then gradually moving toward the exercising skeletal muscles). This section is followed by a discussion on the effects of hypoxia on metabolism and fatigue. Subsequently, the effects of altitude exposure on sport performance and the use of altitude training are discussed. The physiologic response to exercise in high-altitude natives is discussed at the end of this chapter.

The Atmosphere

Barometric pressure (P$_B$) is a measure of the pressure exerted by the weight of the air above us. From sea level, the atmosphere is approximately 24 km wide, which equals a P$_B$ of 760 mm Hg. The air exerts much less pressure at the summit of Mount Everest than at sea level, and accordingly P$_B$ is reduced to ~250 mm Hg or ~⅓ of P$_B$ at sea level. At 5486 m, the pressure of a column of air at the earth's surface equals about one half of its pressure at sea level. At a given altitude, however, P$_B$ is not exactly the same everywhere. Because warm air weighs less than cool air, P$_B$ is dependent on air temperature. On the summit of Mount Everest, P_B has been measured to be 255 mm Hg in June, compared with 243 mm Hg in January. As we shall see later, this (in addition to low temperatures and high winds) makes the climb much more demanding during winter than summer. Moreover, the distribution of warm and cool air in the atmosphere is not uniform; for example, there is a slightly increased P_B along the equator compared with the North and South Pole regions for a given altitude.

Although an inverse relationship exists between P_B and altitude, the gas composition of the air is unaffected. The percentage distributions of O_2, CO_2, and N_2 in the air are always 20.93%, 0.03%, and 79.04%, respectively. Only the partial pressure (P) of the gasses changes, because it is a function of P_B (gas fraction $\times$ P_B). The partial pressure of inspired oxygen is moistened by the water vapor in the airways similarly at sea level and altitude. This reduces the oxygen pressure in the alveoli by about 47 mm Hg, which means relatively more the higher the altitude.

When it comes to the effect of altitude on the human body, the lower PO_2 causes the major difference between sea level and altitude. However, other factors, such as temperature, humidity, and radiation, are also affected by altitude. Air temperature is ~1°C lower for every 150 m of ascent. A temperature of 15°C at sea level thus corresponds to approximately −40°C at the summit of Mount Everest. The combination of low temperatures and high winds greatly increases the risks of hypothermia and frostbite at high altitudes. Because of the cold air, the absolute humidity is extremely low at high altitude. This promotes dehydration because the respiratory system needs to hydrate the less humid air, which can contribute to greater water loss. Much water is lost via the lungs due to increased ventilation. The atmosphere can absorb less of the ultraviolet light, and the reduced water content of the air further reduces the absorption of radiation from the sun. These two factors combined expose the individual to a higher solar radiation at altitude.

TEST YOURSELF

Explain why the partial pressure of a gas is decreased at altitude.

Oxygen Sensing

When the human body is exposed to either acute or chronic hypoxia, it attempts to maintain oxygen homeostasis by performing a complex series of adjustments. As discussed further below, all nucleated cells possess the protein hypoxia inducible factor 1 (HIF)-1, which is a transcription factor that is augmented in hypoxic conditions. This, in turn, facilitates the transcription of a variety of genes involved in oxygen transport (e.g., HO-1, I NOS, and Cox-2). At the cellular level, this is extremely important. At the systemic level, however, the hypoxic stimulation of the

carotid chemoreceptors (chemoreflex activation) is responsible for the important (and immediate) increase in sympathetic nervous activity and enhanced minute ventilation.

Hypoxia Inducible Factor 1 Pathway

All nucleated cells in the human body sense O_2 and respond to reduced O_2 availability (hypoxia), which can either be acute or chronic. The most important molecular responses to hypoxia are initiated by increases in the content of the transcription factor HIF-1. HIF-1 in turn augments the expression of a variety of genes that are primarily involved in oxygen delivery and glycolytic energy production in the cell. The expression of close to 200 genes is proposed to be activated at the transcriptional level by HIF-1, and although the list is extensive, it most likely underestimates the total number of genes induced by HIF-1. HIF-1 is the product of HIF-1α and HIF-1β. HIF-1β is constitutively expressed, whereas HIF-1α is stabilized under hypoxic conditions and therefore confers strictly to hypoxia. The specific DNA sequence to which HIF-1 binds on target genes is referred to as hypoxic response element. Hypoxic response element is located in the promoter or enhancer sequences of HIF-1 target genes, where HIF-1 binding may lead to increased transcription of the specific target gene (remember that activated genes need to be transformed to proteins in order to have functional significance). However, DNA binding to target genes alone is insufficient for gene upregulation, because coactivators must be present. HIF-1α contains two transactivation domains that mediate interactions with coactivators such as cAMP, response element-binding protein (CBP), and p300, which are crucial for the transcriptional activation of HIF-1 target genes. HIF-1α also consists of an oxygen-sensitive degradation domain that allows regulation of HIF-1α content by O_2 concentration. The most well-known physiologic consequence of HIF-1 activation is the increased synthesis of erythropoietin (EPO), which in turn increases the oxygen-carrying capacity of the blood. Other examples include glycolytic enzymes and factors involved in angiogenesis.

TEST YOURSELF

Explain how the expression of selected genes is augmented in the hypoxic environment.

Peripheral Chemoreceptors and the Autonomic Nervous System

The human body has two peripheral chemoreceptors, termed the aortic and carotid bodies. It is the carotid chemoreceptors that account for the main physiologic responses to hypoxia. The carotid chemoreceptors respond to a decrease in PaO_2 (Fig. 24.1), not arterial oxygen content (CaO_2). This is important because CaO_2 can be restored to

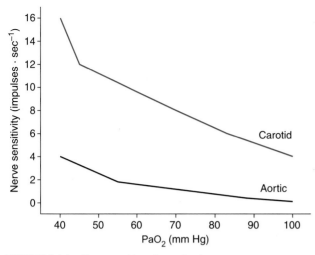

FIGURE 24.1   Cat carotid and aortic chemoreceptor sensitivity to a drop in Po_2. (Adapted from Fitzgerald RS, Lahiri S. Reflex responses to chemoreceptor stimulation. In: Cherniack NS, Widdicombe JG, eds. *The Respiratory System*. Bethesda: American Physiological Society; 1986:313–362.)

sea-level values with acclimatization (because of increased hemoglobin concentration [Hb]), whereas Pao_2 will increase only a little (because of hyperventilation). Carotid nerves project into several groups of neurons within the medulla that govern ventilation and sympathoexcitation. Parasympathetic stimulation may occur via nerve projections from the carotid body to the vagal nucleus and nucleus ambiguous. The ventilatory response to hypoxic carotid activation is described later in the sections on ventilation and the autonomic nervous system.

The sympathoadrenal response to hypoxia is characterized by an increase in adrenal medullary release of epinephrine, followed by a gradual increase in circulating norepinephrine. Circulating norepinephrine levels are the net result of synaptic norepinephrine release, reuptake, and clearance in the circulation. One study reported that in subjects who breathed an F_1O_2 of 0.10 for 30 minutes, plasma norepinephrine clearance increased by 20% compared with normoxia values (3). This means that a 46% increase in norepinephrine spillover was seen as a 20% increase in plasma norepinephrine levels. Today, investigators can access muscle sympathetic nervous activity (MSNA) by placing a thin needle in a nerve. Recordings obtained with this technique are shown in Figure 24.2 and reveal a gradual increase in sympathetic activity with increasing hypoxia. When the subjects were acutely exposed to a simulated height of 4000, 5000, and 6000 m in a hypobaric chamber, MSNA increased from sea level by 34%, 44%, and 48%, respectively (4). This initial increase in MSNA with acute hypoxic exposure was recently demonstrated to persist for several weeks in subjects exposed to high altitude (5). Sympathetic nervous activity is also increased during exercise in hypoxia. It is not possible to obtain MSNA recordings during full-body exercise;

therefore, the norepinephrine concentrations shown in Figure 24.3 were obtained during an incremental exercise test. It can be seen that (a) the norepinephrine and epinephrine responses to exercise in acute hypoxia are exacerbated compared with responses observed during the same exercise in normoxia; and (b) there is a marked further increase in arterial norepinephrine and epinephrine concentrations for any given work rate after 2 and 8 weeks, respectively, of continuous acclimatization to the same altitude (6,7). This is somewhat of a surprise because exercise heart rate is not changed from acute to chronic hypoxic exposure. This may be explained by an altitude-dependent decrease in β-adrenergic receptors in the right and left ventricles (8,9), resulting in a lowered change in heart rate at a given dosage of catecholamine. This interpretation is supported by the results found when isoproterenol is infused (10). However, this cannot explain the lowering of maximal heart rate with altitude exposure (see *Cardiac Output and Blood Flow, and O_2 Extraction by the Exercising Limbs*).

In contrast to our ability to directly quantify MSNA, we lack a direct technique to measure vagal nerve activity. However, there is plenty of evidence indicating that parasympathetic tone is increased at maximal exercise in hypoxia. For example, if parasympathetic nervous activity is blocked by glycopyrrolate, the altitude-dependent decrease in maximal heart rate will revert to sea-level values, suggesting an enhanced parasympathetic nervous activity at altitude (9). Noninvasive assessment of the variability of the R-R interval of the electrocardiogram allows examination of autonomic balance, and such a technique has been used to confirm the above-mentioned findings of increased MSNA and increased parasympathetic activity at

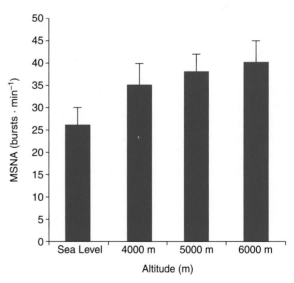

FIGURE 24.2   Dose-response stimulus of muscle sympathetic nervous activity (MSNA) by increasing levels of hypoxia in humans. (Adapted from Ashenden MJ, Gore CJ, Dobson GP, et al. "Live high, train low" does not change the total haemoglobin mass of male endurance athletes sleeping at a simulated altitude of 3000 m for 23 nights. *Eur J Appl Physiol*. 1999;80:479–484.)

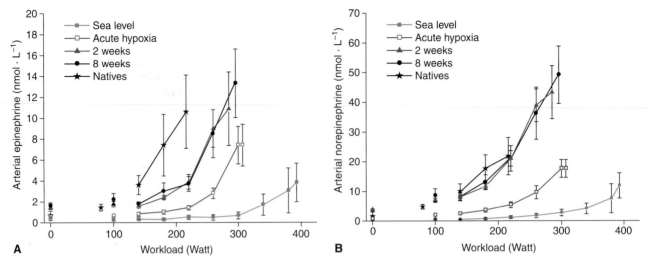

FIGURE 24.3 Arterial epinephrine and norepinephrine concentrations during incremental exercise at sea level, in acute hypoxia, and after 2 and 8 weeks of acclimatization. Values are also presented for high-altitude native Aymaras. (Adapted from Lundby C, Sander M, van Hall G, et al. Maximal exercise and muscle oxygen extraction in acclimatizing lowlanders and high altitude natives. *J Physiol.* 2006;573:535–547; and van Hall G, Lundby C, Araoz M, et al. The lactate paradox revisited in lowlanders during acclimatization to 4100 m and in high-altitude natives. *J Physiol.* 2009;587:1117–1129.)

altitude (11). Hence, at altitude there is a gradual increase in sympathetic nervous activity, and this is also true for parasympathetic activity during maximal exercise.

TEST YOURSELF

Explain why sympathetic activity remains elevated throughout exposure to high altitude even when arterial oxygen content is normalized.

Blood

Oxygen-sensing cells within the kidneys stabilize the transcription factor HIF-1, which in turn initiates the synthesis of EPO along with several other changes. EPO release stimulates the production of erythrocytes in the bone marrow. With exposure to high altitude, plasma EPO concentration peaks within the first 2 to 4 days and then gradually returns toward sea-level values (Fig. 24.4). However, although EPO concentration reaches a nadir early upon exposure to high altitude, it may take weeks for the new erythrocytes to mature and be released, and to eventually increase the total red cell mass (polycythemia). Despite this somewhat lengthy process, hematocrit is increased very rapidly with exposure to hypoxia, as a consequence of a reduction in plasma volume. This process is initiated within hours of exposure to hypoxia, and persists for several days. Plasma volume may decrease by as much as 20% over 12 days. This change appears to be an aspect of a generalized redistribution of fluids from the extracellular to the intracellular fluid compartment, with no net loss in total body water (12). The mechanisms

of this response are partially unknown, but volume-regulating hormones such as atrial natriuretic peptide, renin, and angiotensin could be involved, and at least atrial natriuretic peptide has been shown to be activated during acute hypoxia (13). As indicated above, true polycythemia develops when a person resides at high altitude for several weeks, and varies greatly among individuals. On average, the expansion of the red cell mass may require up to 1 month to become significant, and, in some individuals, the increased red cell mass may not prove sufficient to increase blood volume above sea-level values. Compared with lowlanders at sea level, natives living at high altitude have higher hematocrits as a result of an increased red cell

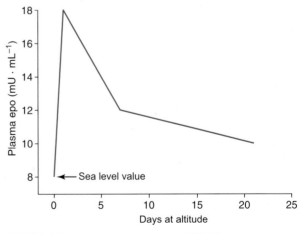

FIGURE 24.4 Plasma erythropoietin (EPO) concentration during 3 weeks of exposure to 2340 m altitude. (Adapted from Schuler B, Thomsen JJ, Gassmann M, et al. Timing the arrival at 2340 m altitude for aerobic performance. *Scand J Med Sci Sports.* 2007;17:588–594.)

mass. Because plasma volume is similar in lowlanders and highlanders, total blood volume is elevated in highlanders (14–16).

In sea-level residents, after a few weeks of exposure to high altitude, hematocrit and hemoglobin concentration may increase to levels found in high-altitude Andean indigenes. Indeed, with just 2 weeks of acclimatization to 4100 m, the hematocrit of lowlanders was increased from approximately 43% to 49%, compared with 50% observed in high-altitude natives. With such a hematocrit, arterial oxygen content at about 4000 m is approximately 200 mL $\cdot$ l^{-1} despite the lower saturations. This could explain why hematocrit does not increase to higher values even with further acclimatization (17).

TEST YOURSELF

Why is it advantageous to decrease plasma volume initially upon ascent to high altitude?

The sigmoid shape of the oxygen dissociation (equilibrium) curve facilitates blood oxygenation in the lung capillaries, because virtually all the hemoglobin is loaded (saturated) with oxygen, even at a relative low arterial oxygen tension. The ability of hemoglobin to bind with oxygen is expressed as the P_{50} value, which represents the arterial oxygen partial pressure at which oxygen saturation is 50%. The major determinant of the hemoglobin oxygen saturation is arterial oxygen pressure; however, the binding of oxygen to hemoglobin can be greatly influenced by many factors, including plasma pH; carbon dioxide tension; the concentration of 2,3-diphosphoglyceric acid, magnesium, adenosine triphosphate (ATP), and chloride; blood temperature; and the amount of hemoglobin bound to carbon monoxide. A leftward shift in the oxygen dissociation curve (i.e., a lowering of P_{50}) is advantageous for the uploading of oxygen in the pulmonary capillaries, whereas a rightward shift is supposed to facilitate oxygen unloading at the tissue level (18,19). Thus, in theory, if P_{50} is low, pulmonary oxygen uptake is enhanced and tissue oxygen unloading is impaired, and *vice versa* if P_{50} is high. With acclimatization to altitudes of 4000 to 5300 m, the blood-oxygen affinity of resting humans is decreased (rightward shift in the dissociation curve) and the standard P_{50} is increased by

0.3 to 0.7 mm Hg (17,20). This change is probably mediated by an increased blood content of 2,3-diphosphoglyceric acid, magnesium, ATP, or chloride (47,60). The result of these changes is a net decrease in blood-oxygen binding capacity. Although an increase in standard P_{50} with altitude exposure may seem paradoxical because the ability of hemoglobin to bind oxygen in the lung capillaries decreases, the effect of this change on oxygen unloading to the tissues may be beneficial.

TEST YOURSELF

Explain how a left or right shift in the oxygen dissociation curve affects O_2 loading in the lungs and O_2 unloading to the skeletal muscles. How could an increase or decrease in the standard P_{50} be beneficial for exercise at altitude?

Gas Exchange, Delivery, and Extraction

Ventilation

At altitude, ventilation is increased at rest and during exercise. The hypoxic ventilatory response results in an increase in the partial pressure for oxygen (P_AO_2) and hence in the arterial partial pressure for oxygen (P_aO_2), arterial oxygen saturation (S_aO_2), and ultimately C_aO_2. Thus, if no hypoxia-induced hyperventilation occurs, C_aO_2 for any given altitude will be lower.

At rest, the acute (seconds to minutes) ventilatory response to hypoxia results chiefly from hypoxic stimulation of the peripheral chemoreceptors, primarily those of the carotid bodies (see Chapter 8). Immediately after this increase, ventilation declines somewhat over the next 10 to 30 minutes above normoxic levels. This decline in ventilation is somewhat surprising, and the mechanisms behind it are the subject of considerable investigation. It has been concluded, however, that a decreased carotid body sensory output (reduced chemosensitivity) and hypocapnia are not involved, and that the response is most likely mediated within the central nervous system. After this initial decline, ventilation undergoes a progressive increase for a period of hours to days before reaching a plateau. Because ventilation is increased (or remains elevated) while at the same time arterial oxygen tension is increased and carbon dioxide tension is decreased, the elevated ventilation has often been ascribed to increased carotid body sensitivity (over time) to hypoxia. A considerable body of evidence indicates that the carotid bodies play a specific role in acclimatization. In this regard, increased gene expression in the carotid body, beginning on day 1 at high altitude, has been demonstrated to enhance cell number (23). This results in an increased number of hypoxic sensing cells

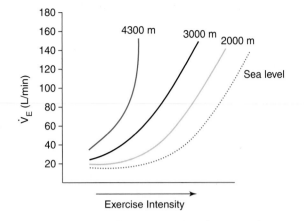

FIGURE 24.5 Effect of increasing altitude on ventilation during graded-intensity exercise. $\dot{V}_E$, minute ventilation.

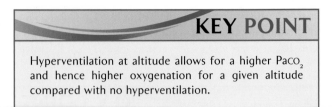

in the carotid body. Using the vascular isolated-perfused carotid body technique, Bisgard et al. (24) separated the circulation to the carotid body from the rest of the systemic circulation. When they rendered the carotid body hypoxic for several hours while maintaining the rest of the body normoxic, they observed essentially normal ventilatory acclimatization responses.

Exercise at altitude is accompanied by an increase in submaximal ventilation compared with that observed at sea level. The higher the altitude, the greater is the hypoxic ventilatory response at a given metabolic rate (Fig. 24.5), and in comparison with resting conditions, exercise ventilation is increased. The increased ventilation observed during exercise is not caused by the increase in relative exercise intensity (due to a reduction in $\dot{V}_{O_{2max}}$; discussed further below), but to chemoreceptor stimulation. In the case of elevated pH and lactate (see also *Metabolism and Energetics*), these chemicals will also be sensed by the chemoreceptors and ventilation will be adjusted accordingly. During exercise, the ventilatory response to acute hypoxia is sensitized by an unknown mechanism. At maximum effort, ventilation (in 1 minute) will be similar to that observed at sea level, even at extreme elevations. It should be noted, however, that the degree of hyperventilation ($\dot{V}_A/\dot{V}_{CO_2}$) is of much greater magnitude.

Alveolar-Arterial Oxygen Pressure Gradient and Arterial Oxygen Saturation

The pulmonary gradient between $P_{A}O_2$ and the partial pressure of O_2 in pulmonary capillary blood and the diffusion capacity of the lung for O_2 determine the rate of O_2 uptake by Hb during its transit through the lung capillaries. With altitude exposure, $P_{A}O_2$ and mixed venous PO_2 (and hence likely also pulmonary capillary PO_2) are reduced, whereas the diffusion capacity of the lung remains unchanged in acclimatizing lowlanders. However, the diffusion capacity of high-altitude natives is enhanced compared with lowlanders (see *High-Altitude Natives*).

Table 24.1 shows the typical response of $P_{A}O_2$ and $S_{a}O_2$ during acclimatization to 4300 m altitude. In this example, $P_{A}O_2$ initially decreases to 47 mm Hg, and with acclimatization there is a slight increase in $P_{A}O_2$ due to increased ventilation. Regardless of the acclimatization-induced slight enhancement in $P_{A}O_2$, $P_{a}O_2$ is reduced to its lower equilibrium, resulting in an $S_{a}O_2$ of approximately 80% during resting conditions at this altitude. Figure 24.6 illustrates the response of $S_{a}O_2$ at rest and during incremental exercise with acclimatization to 4100 m. The first thing that should be noticed is that at sea level, $S_{a}O_2$ is only slightly reduced with maximum exercise, whereas in hypoxia a substantial degree of arterial desaturation starts at submaximal exercise intensities. The exercise-induced desaturation in hypoxia obviously also decreases $C_{a}O_2$ during exercise (Fig. 24.6). During dynamic exercise, the increase in cardiac output reduces the transient time of the red blood cell through the pulmonary capillaries to a level that may be insufficient to allow equilibrium between $P_{A}O_2$ and capillary PO_2, resulting in a further reduction in $S_{a}O_2$. The resultant widening of the $P_{A}O_2$–$P_{a}O_2$ gradient (and reduced $S_{a}O_2$) at altitude may explain why $\dot{V}_{O_{2max}}$ is reduced at altitude in part due to diffusion limitations.

TABLE 24.1	Typical Resting Responses for P_{AO_2}, P_{ACO_2}, Ventilation, pH, and S_{aO_2} for a Sea-Level Resident Exposed to an Elevation of 4300 m for 2 Weeks			
	Sea level	Day 1	Day 7	Day 14
P_{AO_2}	100	47	52	56
P_{ACO_2}	39	35	31	28
Ventilation (L · min⁻¹)	8	9	11	12
pH	7.40	7.46	7.50	7.45
S_{aO_2} (%)	97	80	86	88

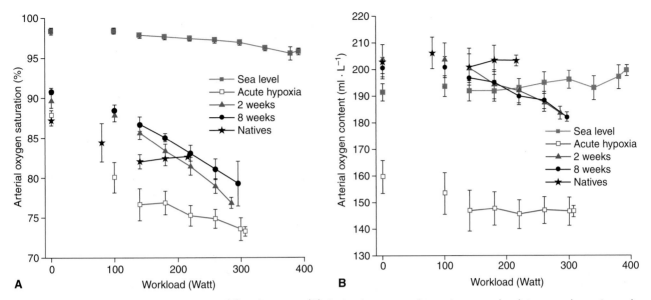

FIGURE 24.6 Arterial oxygen saturation **(A)** and content **(B)** during incremental exercise at sea level, in acute hypoxia, and after 2 and 8 weeks of acclimatization. Values are also presented for high-altitude native Aymaras. (Adapted from Lundby C, Sander M, van Hall G, et al. Maximal exercise and muscle oxygen extraction in acclimatizing lowlanders and high altitude natives. *J Physiol*. 2006;573:535–547.)

Gas exchange across the lung also depends on the ratio of alveolar ventilation to blood perfusion ($\dot{V}_A/\dot{Q}$) throughout the lung. At rest, the upper lobes are ventilated more but the lower lobes have a higher perfusion, and hence the $\dot{V}_A/\dot{Q}$ is not distributed uniformly. With altitudes above approximately 2500 m, an increase in blood flow to poorly perfused areas is ensured by hypoxia-induced vasoconstriction, and the concomitant increase in $\dot{V}_A$ increases the surface for gas exchange. Hence, both a diffusion limitation and a $\dot{V}_A/\dot{Q}$ mismatch contribute to the desaturation, but the contribution of diffusion limitation becomes proportionally greater with increasing exercise intensity and altitude (25).

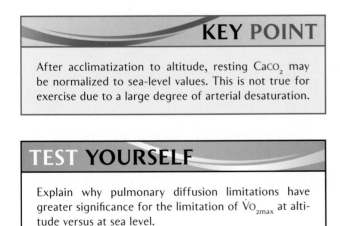

KEY POINT

After acclimatization to altitude, resting C_aCO_2 may be normalized to sea-level values. This is not true for exercise due to a large degree of arterial desaturation.

TEST YOURSELF

Explain why pulmonary diffusion limitations have greater significance for the limitation of $\dot{V}_{O_{2max}}$ at altitude versus at sea level.

Cardiac Output and Blood Flow, and O₂ Extraction by the Exercising Limbs

Systemic O_2 transport is the product of C_aO_2 and cardiac output ($\dot{Q}$). With acute hypoxic exposure when C_aO_2 is reduced, systemic oxygen transport is maintained at rest and during submaximal exercise by a higher cardiac output. Thus, cardiac output increases to ensure that oxygen delivery matches metabolic demand. At maximal exercise, $\dot{Q}$ is reduced as compared with sea-level values, and consequently, maximal blood flow to the exercising legs is reduced. Ultimately, the decrease in O_2 delivery to the exercising muscles is the main factor in reduced $\dot{V}_{O_{2max}}$.

The initial increase in resting cardiac output with an acute exposure to hypoxia is, for the most part, a function of an increased heart rate (chronotropic response). This change is sustained directly by hypoxia-dependent sympathetic activation and vagal withdrawal and stimulation of the peripheral chemoreceptors, and indirectly by an increase in ventilation. With acclimatization to altitudes >3000 m (which corresponds to the commencement of the relatively flat part of the oxygen dissociation curve), the elevation in resting heart rate persists, slightly decreasing toward sea level after 2 to 3 weeks. With acute hypoxic exposure, β-receptor blockade can diminish most of the initial increase in resting heart rate. However, this is not the case with acclimatization. During the course of this adaptation, heart rate remains somewhat elevated, even after administration of supplemental oxygen or beta blockers. At altitudes above approximately 3000 m, maximum heart rate is reduced (26). This is the effect of an elevated parasympathetic nervous activity, and maximum heart rate can be restored to sea-level values by blocking the parasympathetic activity (27). Of interest, when maximum heart rate is restored (by blocking parasympathetic activity), maximum stroke volume is reduced, thus leaving maximum $\dot{Q}$ unaltered. Therefore, it would seem that the regulated variable is $\dot{Q}$ (27). The reduced $\dot{Q}$ at maximum effort at altitude could serve to decrease the transit time of the red blood cell in the pulmonary capillaries to prevent further arterial desaturation.

As mentioned above, the initial increase in resting cardiac output is usually not a function of an augmented stroke volume. However, changes in stroke volume become important with acclimatization. Because heart rate is consistently elevated at altitude, the reduction in cardiac output noted above must be a consequence of a decreased stroke volume, and this has been confirmed in various studies. This reduction is caused mainly by a decrease in plasma volume. Because the stroke volume is the difference between the end-diastolic and end-systolic volumes, the stroke volume can only be reduced if the end-systolic volume is increased due to impaired contractile function or if end-diastolic volume is reduced due to impaired left-ventricular filling. Laboratory studies conducted as part of Operation Everest II showed that myocardial contractility is well preserved even at extreme altitudes (28), and stroke volume is therefore reduced in parallel with changes in left-ventricular end-diastolic volume. Such changes are secondary to a hypoxia-induced plasma (blood) volume reduction (29).

The reduced maximum cardiac output at high altitude ultimately reduces maximal blood flow to the exercising legs during whole body exercise (6). With acclimatization to high altitude, there is a gradual decrease in maximal leg blood flow, but with a concomitant gradual increase in C_aO_2, O_2 delivery to the exercising legs during exercise is similar throughout acclimatization (at least up to 8 weeks). Because arterial O_2 extraction at maximal exercise is similar at altitude and sea level (usually between 80% and 93%), also $\dot{V}O_{2max}$ does not change from acute to chronic exposure at altitudes above approximately 4000 m. At lower altitude, $\dot{V}O_{2max}$ may increase over time, as discussed below.

KEY POINT

Maximal cardiac output and leg blood flow are reduced with acclimatization to high altitudes.

TEST YOURSELF

By what mechanism is maximal cardiac output reduced at altitude, and what could be the rationale for such a reduction?

Maximal Aerobic Exercise

Maximal oxygen uptake ($\dot{V}O_{2max}$) is the product of the total quantity of blood transported to the tissue by the heart (*i.e.*, cardiac output, $\dot{Q}$) and the difference in systemic

arterial and venous O_2 content. This is referred to as the Fick equation:

$$\dot{V}O_{2max} = \dot{Q} \times (C_aO_2 - C_vO_2)$$

C_aO_2 can be accessed from any artery, but for quantification of systemic differences, C_vO_2 is obtained by sampling from the right atrium or the inferior vena cava. Altitude-related adjustments in any of these parameters will affect $\dot{V}O_{2max}$, and, as described above, both $\dot{Q}$ and C_aO_2 are reduced at maximal exercise in hypoxia, whereas oxygen extraction is maintained.

During the transition from rest to maximal dynamic exercise, such as running or cycling, $\dot{Q}$ is redistributed. In resting conditions, the skeletal muscles receive approximately 20% of $\dot{Q}$, whereas at maximal effort this is increased to around 85%. Accordingly, the distribution of $\dot{Q}$ to the liver and kidney is reduced from approximately 50% in resting conditions to <5% at maximal exercise. Of interest, recent studies described a redistribution of $\dot{Q}$ at maximal exercise in humans exposed to high altitude when compared with data obtained at sea level, such that the percent of $\dot{Q}$ going to the exercising legs was decreased with acclimatization. Therefore, blood flow must be increased to other, nonexercising areas because $\dot{Q}$ was unchanged at the same time (6).

The solid line in Figure 24.7 illustrates the curvilinear relationship of the measured decrease (%) in $\dot{V}O_{2max}$ with

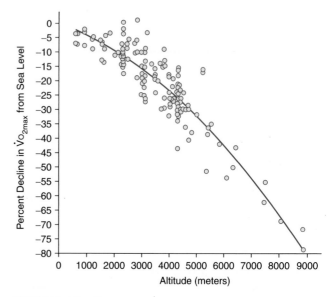

FIGURE 24.7 Changes in $\dot{V}O_{2max}$ with changes in altitude. Each of the 146 points represents the average $\dot{V}O_{2max}$ decrement of a group of test subjects participating in one of 67 research studies conducted at actual or simulated altitudes from 580 to 8848 m. Because each data point is a mean value of many intrastudy individual determinations of $\dot{V}O_{2max}$, the drawn regression line represents thousands of $\dot{V}O_{2max}$ test values. (Reprinted with permission from Fulco CS, Rock PB, Cymerman A. Maximal and submaximal exercise performance at altitude. *Aviat Space Environ Med.* 1998;69:794.)

increasing degree of altitude. The data were obtained from 67 research studies carried out in acute hypoxia (in the laboratory or at altitude) or after exposure to hypoxia (in the laboratory or at altitude) of varying duration. In general, a decrease in $\dot{V}_{O_{2max}}$ is observed from approximately 1500-m altitude, and thereafter by a 1% reduction for every 100 m of altitude gained (100). For example, on average, $\dot{V}_{O_{2max}}$ declines by about 9%, 14%, 24%, and 32% at 2000, 3000, 4000, and 5000 m, respectively. At the summit of Mount Everest, at 8850 m, the reduction in $\dot{V}_{O_{2max}}$ is approximately 80% and leaves very little exercise capacity left for climbing. When men and women are matched to the sea-level aerobic fitness level, there is generally no difference in the altitude-induced decline in $\dot{V}_{O_{2max}}$. In elite athletes, however, a decrease in $\dot{V}_{O_{2max}}$ has been observed at altitudes as low as 580 m (30). As mentioned above, this is normally not the case for the majority of human beings, and one of the biggest contributors to the variation in the decline in $\dot{V}_{O_{2max}}$ at altitude is the aerobic fitness level before exposure. Figure. 24.8 illustrates the difference in the decline of $\dot{V}_{O_{2max}}$ in trained versus untrained subjects. This difference may become substantial; for example, at 4000 m, a trained individual's $\dot{V}_{O_{2max}}$ may be decreased by 22%, whereas an untrained individual's $\dot{V}_{O_{2max}}$ may only be decreased by 13%. Wehrlin and Hallen (31) analyzed studies that included male, unacclimatized, endurance-trained athletes with a mean $\dot{V}_{O_{2max}}$ >60 mL · min^{-1} · kg^{-1}. In this population, $\dot{V}_{O_{2max}}$ was reduced by 7.7% per 1000 m of altitude. Furthermore, in an attempt to find a threshold altitude for reduced $\dot{V}_{O_{2max}}$ in individual athletes, the authors observed a uniform and highly linear decline in $\dot{V}_{O_{2max}}$ at altitude, beginning as low as 800 m altitude and extending through 2800 m with a decline of 6.3% per 1000 m altitude. The greater decrease in $\dot{V}_{O_{2max}}$ of trained versus untrained humans seems to be dependent on a higher degree of arterial desaturation occurring in the more trained male and female subjects (30,32,33) and is the consequence of either a greater capillary diffusion limitation or a greater ventilation-perfusion mismatch (25).

The issue of whether $\dot{V}_{O_{2max}}$ is increased significantly with acclimatization has been debated for decades. Confounding factors such as the degree of altitude-independent muscle atrophy and an individual's ability to maintain training certainly do not make the picture any clearer. The different fatigue patterns observed at different altitudes also add to the controversy. Recent studies have revealed that from a certain altitude threshold, the origin of fatigue during whole-body exercise changes from being predominantly peripheral to predominantly central (34) (discussed further below). In degrees of hypoxia where the O_2 transport system may not be the limiting factor for $\dot{V}_{O_{2max}}$, it makes sense that restoring, or even surpassing, sea-level C_aO_2 does not increase $\dot{V}_{O_{2max}}$ as much as expected. In an attempt to reduce the potential negative influence of altitude acclimatization on $\dot{V}_{O_{2max}}$, investigators performed studies with acute hypoxic exposure before and after 1 to 2 months of EPO treatment (36). After EPO treatment, C_aO_2 was significantly increased

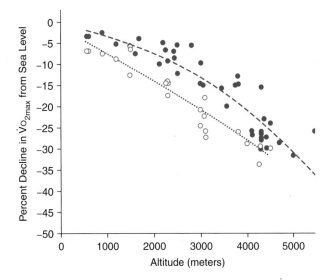

FIGURE 24.8 Effect of sea-level physical fitness on $\dot{V}_{O_{2max}}$ decrements at high altitude. *Closed circles* represent untrained subjects and *open circles* represent trained subjects. (Reprinted with permission from Fulco CS, Rock PB, Cymerman A. Maximal and submaximal exercise performance at altitude. *Aviat Space Environ Med.* 1998;69:794.)

during maximum exercise at sea level and at 1500, 2500, 3500, 4100, and 4500 m, but $\dot{V}_{O_{2max}}$ was only increased from sea level and up to 3500 m. These experimental laboratory data support the notion that $\dot{V}_{O_{2max}}$ increases with acclimatization to altitudes below 3500 to 4000 m (37), but not above (6,38,39).

TEST YOURSELF

Explain why the $\dot{V}_{O_{2max}}$ at altitude is usually reduced more in trained individuals than in nontrained individuals.

Submaximal Aerobic Exercise Performance

As described above, $\dot{V}_{O_{2max}}$ does not increase with acclimatization to high altitudes above approximately 4000 m. Does this mean that athletes should not acclimatize to altitude before competing at altitude? The answer is that, unlike $\dot{V}_{O_{2max}}$, submaximal exercise capacity is increased with acclimatization, and therefore athletes should indeed reach the altitude of competition at least 14 days before an event (Fig. 24.9).

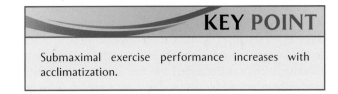

KEY POINT

Submaximal exercise performance increases with acclimatization.

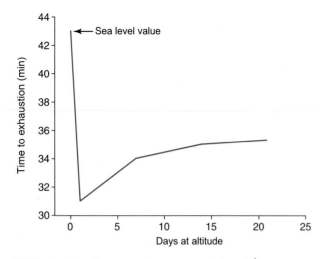

FIGURE 24.9 Time to exhaustion at 80% of $\dot{V}_{O_{2max}}$ at sea level, and after 1, 7, 14, and 21 days of exposure to 2340 m altitude. (Adapted from Schuler B, Thomsen JJ, Gassmann M, et al. Timing the arrival at 2340 m altitude for aerobic performance. *Scand J Med Sci Sports.* 2007;17:588–594.)

The metabolic cost for a particular exercise task performed in a steady state at a specified absolute power output is similar at sea level and at altitude. Therefore, leg $\dot{V}_{O_2}$ remains unchanged at a given submaximal exercise intensity. It should be remembered, however, that due to the increase in ventilation and heart rate at any given work rate, the whole body energy turnover must also be increased, (*i.e.*, there must be a higher pulmonary $\dot{V}_{O_2}$ for any given work rate). However, because the extra O_2 requirements are only of small magnitude, increases in submaximal pulmonary $\dot{V}_{O_2}$ are generally not observed at altitude (40).

Because of the progressive decrease in $\dot{V}_{O_{2max}}$ with increasing elevation, a fixed power output represents progressively greater relative exercise intensity (*i.e.*, a higher percentage of $\dot{V}_{O_{2max}}$) as the elevation increases. The greater relative stress during exercise at a fixed power output requiring an identical $\dot{V}_{O_2}$ can shorten the time to exhaustion at altitude. Similarly, for activities in which a fixed distance or amount of work must be performed, competition times will be extended (Fig. 24.9). Hence, it is clear that submaximal exercise performance, as is the case with $\dot{V}_{O_{2max}}$, is decreased at altitude. However, whereas $\dot{V}_{O_{2max}}$ only seems to increase with acclimatization to altitudes below approximately 4000 m, submaximal exercise performance increases at all altitudes with acclimatization, provided that the individual is not affected by confounding factors such as acute mountain sickness or lack of familiarity with the altitude environment. In one study performed at 2340 m altitude, a group of elite cyclists (average sea level $\dot{V}_{O_{2max}}$ ~80 mL $\cdot$ min^{-1} $\cdot$ kg^{-1}) were investigated on days 1, 7, 14, and 21 for time to exhaustion at 80% of sea level $\dot{V}_{O_{2max}}$. Compared with sea level, the average time to exhaustion was decreased by 26% on day 1, but then gradually increased by 6% on day 7, by a further 5.7% on

day 14, and a further 1.4% on day 21 (37) (Fig. 24.9). This clearly indicates that athletes competing at this altitude should arrive at least 14 days before the start of competition to optimize their performance (37). The 2340-m altitude is relevant for disciplines such as bicycling and cross-country skiing because competitions may be held at this altitude. At 4300 m altitude, which is relevant for alpine climbers (and a few more extreme events), submaximal exercise performance is also improved with acclimatization. Endurance time to exhaustion at a given power output while residing at 4300 m improved by 45% on day 10 (59) and by 59% on day 16 (41) compared with day 2 for individuals with $\dot{V}_{O_{2max}}$ of approximately 49 mL $\cdot$ min^{-1} $\cdot$ kg^{-1} at sea level. At 2340 m altitude, the acclimatization-induced increase in submaximal exercise performance could be related to an acclimatization-induced increase in $\dot{V}_{O_{2max}}$, and hence a gradual reduction in the relative exercise intensity. At 4300 m, however, $\dot{V}_{O_{2max}}$ is usually not increased with acclimatization and other factors must be involved. At present, such factors are speculative, but one possibility is that at submaximal exercise, the increase in CaO_2 allows a given $\dot{V}_{O_2}$ to be achieved with a lower $\dot{Q}$, thus reducing cardiac work. It is clear, however, that endurance performance at 4300 m improves with residence for a few weeks at altitude independently of changes in $\dot{V}_{O_{2max}}$ or training volume.

TEST YOURSELF

If an athlete plans to compete at around 2500 m altitude, how long of an acclimatization period would you recommend? Also discuss muscle versus whole-body $\dot{V}_{O_2}$ during submaximal exercise in an individual exposed to hypoxia.

Metabolism and Energetics

Resting metabolism is increased slightly with exposure to altitude (as shown in Fig. 24.10) and is most likely the consequence of an elevated energy expenditure caused by an elevated heart rate or ventilation. Whether the initial spike in basal O_2 consumption with acute exposure to hypoxia represents increased energy requirements that are only present in this phase is unknown, but it is clear that resting metabolism is increased at altitude. If this is not compensated for by an increase in caloric intake, loss of body mass will be unavoidable (42).

In a variety of experimental models, hypoxia has been shown to cause a shift in substrate use to favor increased dependence on glucose. One explanation for this phenomenon could be a selective advantage derived from the increased metabolic economy (*i.e.*, more ATP derived per unit oxygen consumed) that results when glucose is oxidized rather than lipid. In support of this hypothesis, it was observed that when subjects acclimatized to

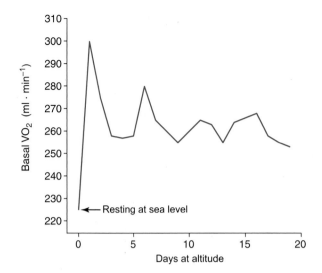

FIGURE 24.10 Basal oxygen uptake at sea level and during acclimatization to 4300 m altitude. (Adapted from Butterfield GE, Gates J, Fleming S, et al. Increased energy intake minimizes weight loss in men at high altitude. *J Appl Physiol.* 1992;72:1741–1748.)

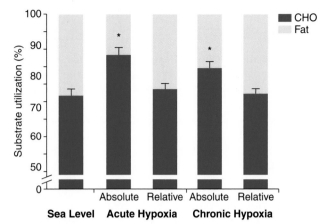

FIGURE 24.11 Substrate utilization during submaximal exercise at sea level, and again at the same relative and absolute intensities in acute and chronic hypoxia. CHO, carbohydrate. (Adapted from Lundby C, van Hall G. Substrate utilization in sea level residents during exercise in acute hypoxia and after 4 weeks of acclimatization to 4100 m. *Acta Physiol Scand.* 2002;176:195–201.)

hypoxia exercised at the same absolute exercise intensity as at sea level, and hence at a higher relative exercise intensity given the altitude-dependent reduction in $\dot{V}O_{2max}$, an elevated dependence on blood glucose as a substrate was observed (43). However, because exercise intensity is of major importance for substrate preference during exercise, the enhanced glucose oxidation during exercise at altitude could be associated with relative higher exercise intensity. To isolate the potential intensity-dependent increase in glucose oxidation at altitude, investigators studied lowlanders during 60 minutes of cycle exercise at 50% of sea level $\dot{V}O_{2max}$. The protocol was repeated in acute hypoxia and also after 4 weeks of acclimatization to 4100 m. In the hypoxic conditions, the 60-minute exercise trial was performed at the same absolute exercise intensity as at sea level (now corresponding to approximately 65% of hypoxic $\dot{V}O_{2max}$) and at the same relative exercise intensity (*i.e.*, 50% of the hypoxic $\dot{V}O_{2max}$). The results obtained from this study confirmed the previous studies (*i.e.*, increased glucose oxidation at the same absolute exercise intensities), but when the intensity was reduced to elicit the same relative intensity found at sea level, no differences in substrate utilization as compared with sea level were observed (Fig. 24.11) (44). This suggests that, at least during exercise, the previously observed increase in glucose oxidation seems to be caused by the increased exercise relative intensity, and not directly by hypoxia.

Since the 1930s, the issue of lactate metabolism at submaximal and maximal exercise intensities with acclimatization has been the subject of a lively debate. For years, the predominant view was that in spite of the hypoxemia, less lactate accumulates in blood during exercise after prolonged exposure to altitude. This phenomenon is referred to as the lactate paradox. Recent studies, however, have questioned this concept. After 2 and 8 weeks of acclimatization in lowland Danes, no differences as compared with acute exposure were found in arterial lactate concentrations (Fig. 24.12). Also, muscle biopsy specimens obtained in the same experiments showed no signs of "paradoxical" lactate levels.

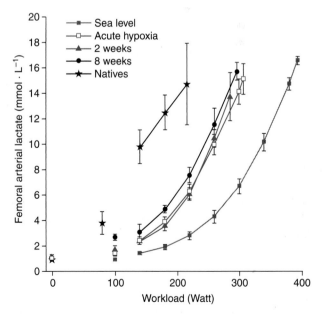

FIGURE 24.12 Arterial lactate concentrations during incremental exercise at sea level, in acute hypoxia, and after 2 and 8 weeks of acclimatization. Values are also presented for high-altitude native Aymaras. (Adapted from van Hall G, Lundby C, Araoz M, et al. The lactate paradox revisited in lowlanders during acclimatization to 4100 m and in high-altitude natives. *J Physiol.* 2009;587:1117–1129.)

KEY POINT

Most of the metabolic effects seen at altitude during exercise can be explained by changes in exercise intensities (*i.e.*, absolute vs. relative intensities) rather than by hypoxia.

Summary

Upon altitude exposure, the lactate curve is shifted to the left with acute exposure, and thereafter remains left-shifted with acclimatization. The left shift seems to be related to changes in relative exercise intensity, because when lactate concentration/release is expressed relative to exercise intensities, no changes in these parameters are observed compared with sea-level values. At maximal intensities, lactate values similar to those found at sea level may be observed.

TEST YOURSELF

Does altitude exposure affect substrate metabolism during submaximal exercise?

Fatigue

An increasing number of studies are now examining the mechanisms of fatigue in acute hypoxia. To a lesser extent, important information has also emerged concerning the effects of chronic hypoxia. The main question addressed in the experiments performed in acute hypoxia is whether the fatigue is of peripheral or central origin. In brief, peripheral fatigue refers to fatigue originating at or distal to the neuromuscular junction, whereas central fatigue includes the failure of the central nervous system to adequately excite motor neurons. Blunted O_2 delivery exaggerates the rate of fatigue, whereas an augmentation in O_2 delivery attenuates the rate of fatigue development. Alterations in O_2 delivery to the working muscle affect the development of peripheral fatigue during whole-body exercise via its effects on relative exercise intensity and changes in intracellular metabolism. Both of these factors alter the rate of accumulation of metabolites known to cause failure of excitation-contraction coupling within the muscle fiber, which has been identified as the main factor in evoking loss of tension development during the fatigue process under conditions of high-intensity exercise. Central fatigue may be elicited by low brain oxygenation, which may cause a mismatch between brain O_2 demand and supply, leading to reduced interstitial and cellular PO_2. Near-infrared spectroscopy measurements of prefrontal, premotor, and motor cortex deoxygenation during exercise with acute hypoxic exposure (45) revealed that,

as compared with normoxic controls, deoxygenation was more profound in hypoxia. It was concluded that this could contribute to an individual's decision to stop exercising sooner than he or she would otherwise. The critical interstitial PO_2 levels that lead to central fatigue are unknown, but an "altitude threshold" has been shown to exist. Amann et al. (34) assessed neuromuscular function (quadriceps twitch force by supramaximal magnetic femoral nerve stimulation) before and immediately after constant-load exercise to exhaustion with various fractions of inspired O_2 (F_IO_2 = 0.21, 0.15, and 0.10). The quadriceps twitch force was reduced from preexercise baseline after exercise in all settings, but the reduction in force became less with an increase in hypoxia, indicating that the muscle was not as fatigued as in normoxia and mild hypoxia. They concluded that the major determinant of central motor output and exercise performance switches from a predominantly peripheral origin of fatigue to a hypoxia-sensitive central component of fatigue, probably involving brain hypoxic effects on effort perception. An interesting issue to be addressed is whether altitude acclimatization increases brain oxygenation enough to revert to the normoxic fatigue pattern.

A study by van Hall et al. (7) clearly showed that peripheral signs of fatigue were unchanged throughout the process of acclimatization to 4100 m. In muscle biopsies obtained a few seconds after the termination of an incremental exercise test until exhaustion, metabolites normally associated with fatigue were not altered after 2 and 8 weeks of acclimatization as compared with acute exposure or values obtained in normoxia. Analyses of ATP, adenosine diphosphate, adenosine monophosphate, inosine monophosphate, creatine phosphate, creatine content, inorganic phosphate, lactate, and glycogen content showed no signs of a change in the peripheral fatigue pattern. As mentioned above, it has been shown that from a certain threshold altitude, the origin of fatigue during exercise changes from being of predominantly peripheral to being a predominantly central (34). When central fatigue becomes prevailing, one might expect peripheral signs of fatigue to be reduced. However, this does not seem to be the case, because plasma lactate is equally high in both situations, and hence it seems unlikely that this could explain the low lactate concentrations observed at extreme altitudes in some studies.

TEST YOURSELF

Explain how changes in fatigue pattern could explain why $\dot{V}O_{2max}$ is not increased with acclimatization despite increases in arterial oxygen content.

Athletic Performance

The term *athletic performance* refers to the integrated response of some of the physiologic systems described above. The effect of altitude on athletic performance became very clear during the 1968 Olympic Games in Mexico City, which is located at an altitude of 2240 m. Two main factors are responsible for the effects of altitude on athletic performance: (a) the decrease in air density, which parallels the reduction in P_B and hence reduces air resistance (this is especially important for disciplines that require the athlete to overcome air resistance, such as throwing events and events performed at high speeds, since air resistance quadruples when speed is doubled); and (b) the progressive decrease in $\dot{V}O_{2max}$ with increasing altitude.

Sports that involve mainly anaerobic capacity, such as weight lifting, are unaffected by altitude exposure, whereas throwing events will show increased performance because of the decrease in air density. At 2300 m, the 24% reduction in air density will increase shot put-, hammer-, javelin-, and discus-throwing distances by 6, 53, 69, and 162 cm, respectively (46). Sprint-running (60, 100, 200, and 400 m) times may be decreased with increasing altitude because of a reduced air resistance and reliance on anaerobic metabolism (which is mostly unaffected) (47). However, the recovery from anaerobic sprints seems to be affected. Analyses of ATP regeneration after fatiguing exercise have demonstrated that resynthesis of ATP may be slowed in hypoxia (48–50). Therefore, although a single sprint may be faster at altitude than at sea level, repetitive sprints (such as in soccer) may be more fatiguing. The magnitude of this effect depends on the work duration and the work/rest ratio. In 15-second sprints performed over the course of six sprints between low altitude (585 m) and moderate altitude (2100 m), no decrease in peak power was observed as long as the work/rest ratio was 1:3 (51). At 2320 m altitude, repetitive 400-m sprints could be performed 10% to 15% farther at sea level if a 1- or 2-minute rest was allowed between sprints. The difference was eliminated when a 5-minute interval between sprints was allowed (52).

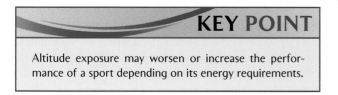

KEY POINT

Altitude exposure may worsen or increase the performance of a sport depending on its energy requirements.

In sport disciplines that rely on aerobic energy utilization, such as distance running and cross-country skiing, performance is reduced because of an altitude-induced decrease in $\dot{V}O_{2max}$. Figure 24.13 demonstrates decrements in physical performance as a function of event duration and elevation up to 4300 m. In general, for events lasting more than 2 minutes at sea level, the longer the event, the greater is the impairment at a given altitude, and the higher the elevation, the greater is the impairment for long events. The figure can also be used to predict the approximate elevation at which measurable performance impairments might consistently be detected.

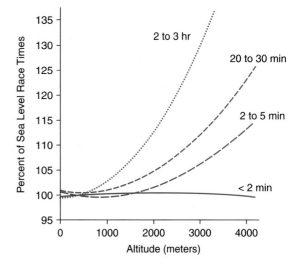

FIGURE 24.13 Physical performance decrements as a function of event duration and elevations up to 4300 m. Each regression line illustrates how performance changes at altitude for sea level events that lasted less than 2 minutes, 2 to 5 minutes, 20 to 30 minutes, and 2 to 3 hours. (Reprinted with permission from Fulco CS, Rock PB, Cymerman A. Maximal and submaximal exercise performance at altitude. *Aviat Space Environ Med.* 1998;69:793–801.)

For example, impaired performance during events lasting 2 to 5 minutes at sea level might not be detected until the elevation exceeds approximately 1600 m, whereas for an event lasting 20 to 30 minutes at sea level, the impairment might occur at a somewhat lower altitude (about 800 m). In sports such as speed skating and track cycling, in which velocities are much higher than in running, the reduced air density allows a greatly increased performance compared with sea level, even though $\dot{V}O_{2max}$ may be significantly reduced. In fact, a theoretical model suggests that 4000 m would be the optimal elevation for breaking the 1-hour unaccompanied cycle record (53) despite an approximately 25% decline in $\dot{V}O_{2max}$. At higher elevations, cycling performance would be impaired by the further reduction in $\dot{V}O_{2max}$ that would more than offset the improving aerodynamic benefit.

TEST YOURSELF

Explain why some sports are negatively impacted by acute altitude exposure and some are positively affected.

Improving Athletic Performance at Sea Level by Altitude Training

Athletes and coaches use various types of altitude training regimens to increase performance at sea level. Here, we discuss the advantages and disadvantages of these different regimens.

Live high—train high

The overall rationale for living and training at altitude (usually 1500–3000 m) is to increase red cell mass and impose an additional training stimulus. There are numerous anecdotal reports about world class athletes who incorporate this type of altitude training into their preparations, but well-controlled studies investigating the effects of a live high—train high (LHTH) regimen on sea-level performance are scarce. In one such study by Levine and Stray-Gundersen (54), 39 college runners were subjected to 2 weeks of lead-in training, followed by 4 weeks of supervised sea-level training. The subjects were then randomly assigned to 4 weeks of either living at 2500 m and training at 2500 to 2700 m (LHTH), living and training at sea level (control), or living at 2500 m and training at 1200 to 1400 m (live high—train low [LHTL]). After the various training periods, $\dot{V}O_{2max}$ was increased in LHTH and LHTL, but 5000-m running performance was increased only in the LHTL group. The authors speculated that running performance was not increased with LHTH because running speeds during training could not be maintained at altitude due to the reduction in $\dot{V}O_{2max}$. However, other investigators have not found an increase in sea-level $\dot{V}O_{2max}$ after 4 weeks at altitudes between 1500 and 2000 m (55), or in $\dot{V}O_{2max}$ and 3.2-km running performance after 4 weeks at 1740 m (56). It may be that these altitudes were too low to elicit the desired increase in Hb mass. Indeed (albeit in less controlled studies), no increases in performance were reported in recent studies lasting 13 days to 1 month at altitudes below 1900 m (57–59), whereas sea-level time trials have been reported to be increased after approximately 3 weeks at altitudes between 2100 and 2650 m (60,61).

Summary

From the current literature, it is difficult to draw any clear-cut conclusions regarding the effects of LHTH on athletic performance at sea level. However, it seems that LHTH may increase sea-level performance for some (but not all) individuals. It must be assumed that this is especially true for individuals who can maintain their daily training regimen despite being exposed to altitude. Current evidence indicates that living at altitudes of at least 2000 m and not exceeding 3000 m can improve performance. The duration of exposure should not be less than 3 to 4 weeks, and the training intensity should be carefully monitored to avoid overtraining or undertraining.

Live high—train low

The general idea behind the LHTL regimen is to increase performance at sea level through an altitude-induced augmentation of red cell mass. Training at sea level (and not at the residing altitude) can be effective because training intensity cannot be maintained at altitude, and a reduction in training intensity may affect performance negatively. Levine and Stray-Gundersen (54) showed that LHTL was effective at increasing sea-level performance in college runners. As mentioned above, in their study $\dot{V}O_{2max}$ was increased after LHTH and LHTL, but running performance was increased only in the LHTL group (54). Subsequently, Stray-Gundersen et al. (62) confirmed that LHTL was effective for both elite male and female athletes. In the latter study, subjects were enrolled in training camps immediately after they performed in national championship competitions, and thus would be expected to be in peak physical condition. This suggests that LHTL may improve sea-level performance in elite athletes even if they are at their limit for training-induced adaptations. Before going into detail with the results from more recent LHTL studies, we should note that the studies undertaken by Levine and Stray-Gundersen (54) seem far more controlled and carefully conducted than other studies in this area. In addition to reducing the confounding factors typically associated with training studies, they also applied an impressive battery of tests. Of the tested variables, the only factor that was associated with improved sea-level performance was an improvement in red cell mass when coupled with the maintenance of training velocities and O_2 flux (63). In confirmation of these studies, it was recently demonstrated that red cell mass was increased in subjects who lived at 2500 m with concomitant training at lower altitudes for 24 days, and at the same time $\dot{V}O_{2max}$ was increased (64). From the above studies, it seems clear that (a) living at 2100 to 2800 m for approximately 3 weeks can increase red cell mass, and (b) if at the same time training intensity can be maintained by descending to lower altitudes for training, then sea-level endurance performance can be increased. It should be noted, however, that the term "train low" in these studies does not refer to training at sea level (this is also the case for the French studies described below). Although the training altitudes were low (i.e., 1200–1800 m), it should be remembered that $\dot{V}O_{2max}$ (and hence also training intensity) may be reduced in athletes at altitudes as low as 580 m (30). If the training had been conducted at sea level, it is possible that more pronounced effects on subsequent sea-level performance would have been observed. Finally, although performance was increased in these studies, the magnitude of this increase most likely does not justify recommending amateur athletes to engage in this type of activity; rather, they should be advised to add an additional training session.

For practical reasons, it may not be convenient for athletes to spend time at altitude. To overcome this potential problem, investigators have tried simulating altitude exposure with the use of nitrogen housing (i.e., indoor living areas are flushed with N_2 to decrease F_IO_2). From the many studies that have examined the so-called "sleep high–train low" regimen, it has become clear that a certain cumulative hypoxia threshold has to be surpassed. For example, several studies from Australia found no increase in red cell mass or $\dot{V}O_{2max}$ after 8 to 10 hours/day sleeping in hypoxia up to

3000 m stimulated altitude for 3 weeks (65–67), except for one study (approximately 46 nights at 2860 m, 8–9 hours/night) in which an increase of 4.9% was observed in Hb mass but no changes in $\dot{V}O_{2max}$ were observed (68). A series of experiments in France (69) demonstrated that red cell volume and performance were unaffected in cross-country skiers who spent 11 hours/day in hypoxia for a total of 18 nights (6 days 2500 m + 6 days at 3000 m + 6 days at 3500 m). Among swimmers who spent 16 hours/day in hypoxia for a total of 13 days (5 days at 2500 m + 8 days at 3000 m), red cell volume was increased by 8.5% and $\dot{V}O_{2max}$ by 4.5% (70). Among runners who spent 14 hours/day in hypoxia for 18 days (6 days at 2500 m + 12 days at 3000 m), both red cell volume and $\dot{V}O_{2max}$ were increased (71). Neya and co-workers (72) studied long- and middle-distance runners before and after 29 nights (11 hours/night) at 3000 m and reported no change in total Hb mass or $\dot{V}O_{2max}$. Summarizing these sleep high–train low studies, it seems that Hb mass is increased if (a) the altitude exceeds 2100 m; (b) the duration of exposure is approximately 3 weeks; and (c) daily time in hypoxia exceeds 14 hours. The factors seem to depend on each other (*i.e.*, inducing more severe hypoxia) (*e.g.*, 3000 m) does not allow a concomitant reduction in daily exposure time. It may be advantageous to supplement with daily iron intake because ferritin levels of >35 ng $\cdot$ mL^{-1} are necessary to obtain the optimal effect of hypoxia on erythropoiesis. It should also be remembered that approximately 3 weeks after termination of the hypoxic stimulus, Hb mass is usually reduced by 50%, and the time from altitude training to competition should not exceed this period. It should also be mentioned that two research groups (68,72,73) support the idea that LHTL increases sea-level performance by increasing exercise economy rather than by increasing $\dot{V}O_{2max}$. The underlying mechanism could be associated with changes in muscle buffer capacity. Lundby et al. (40) analyzed the results of three independent studies and found no changes in exercise economy after acclimatization to moderate or high altitude. In the light of the overwhelming number of LHTL studies that reported no changes in economy, it seems doubtful that this is a major variable contributing to enhancements in sea-level performance.

Live low—train high

The rationale for performing LLTH, according to Lundby et al. (40), is that during exercise at sea level, tissue hypoxia is a major stimulus for training-induced adaptations. When training sessions are performed in hypoxic conditions, the oxygen partial pressure is lower (74), and thus training adaptations may be of greater magnitude. Indeed, the transcription factor HIF-1, which is augmented in hypoxia, is known to induce the expression of a variety of genes (75), many of which may also contribute to enhancements in performance and increased protein levels. LLTH-induced adaptations at the muscular level seem to be the main consequence of this type of training, as Hb

concentration generally remains unaffected. Two studies have reported changes in hematocrit and Hb concentration likely related to uncontrolled changes in plasma volume (76,77). A further argument (78) in support of LLTH over LHTL is that permanent exposure to severe hypoxia (5000 m and higher) leads to a considerable deterioration of skeletal muscle tissue. However, this argument is somewhat misleading because (a) LHTL is not recommended for altitudes above 3000 m; (b) even at 4559 m, altitude muscle protein synthesis is not decreased (79); and (c) if nutritional intake and physical activity are maintained, deterioration of skeletal muscles may deteriorate at 5250 m (80) but not at 4100 m (81).

Since the year 2000, more than 15 studies have reported on the effects of LLTH. However, it is difficult to establish clear guidelines from the results of these investigations. The studies are confounded by variations in exposure duration (10 days to 8 weeks), degree of hypoxic exposure (2300–5700 m), and the subjects examined (ranging from untrained to athletic). The discrepancies among these studies could also be related to the great variation in exercise intensity (50%–80% of $\dot{V}O_{2max}$). Because $\dot{V}O_{2max}$ is reduced at altitude, the intensity that can be sustained during training is also reduced. This is the main criticism of LLTH studies. It should also be noted that almost all of these studies were conducted unblinded (*i.e.*, both the experimenter and the subjects are aware of the treatment). As with the LHTL studies, the Levine group seems to have conducted the most thoroughly controlled studies in this area. In the studies by Truijens et al. (82,83), both subjects and investigators were blinded, and no gains in performance in comparison with normoxic training were observed. Other research groups reported no effect on performance (84,85), whereas still others observed an increase (86).

Summary

It seems that no clear conclusion can be drawn as to whether LLTH improves sea-level performance, but the hypothesis that a distinct functional phenotype is associated with LLTH must be rejected.

Intermittent Hypoxia

The term *intermittent hypoxic exposure* can refer to (a) repeated switching between breathing hypoxic and normoxic air during a period of usually 60 to 90 minutes (because the hypoxic exposures are brief [five minutes in some cases], the severity of hypoxia can be high [4500–6000 m]); or (b) one session of daily hypoxic exposure of rather severe hypoxic magnitude (4000–5500 m). The precise mechanisms behind this increase in sea-level performance are less clear than in LHTL and LLTH, and at present the mechanisms remain obscure. In recent years, a large number of well-controlled studies, all including a double-blind design, have been performed, and again the Levine group has published extensively in this area. In one of their studies, 14 national-class distance runners completed a 4-week regimen (5:5-minute hypoxia/normoxia ratio for 70 minutes, five times a week) of intermittent normobaric hypoxia or placebo control at rest. After the experimental period, no significant differences in $\dot{V}O_{2max}$ or 3000-m time-trial performance were observed (87). Subsequently, the group performed a double-blind, randomized, placebo-controlled trial to examine the effects of 4 weeks of resting exposure to intermittent hypobaric hypoxia (3 hours/day, 5 days/week at 4000–5500 m). No differences in $\dot{V}O_{2max}$, performance (88) or exercise economy were reported (83). Tadibi et al. (89) reported similar results after addressing the question with a similar setup. For 15 consecutive days, 20 endurance-trained men were exposed each day to breathing either a gas mixture or compressed air, six times for 6 minutes, followed by 4 minutes of breathing room air for a total of six consecutive cycles. The results of this study demonstrated that 1 hour of intermittent hypoxic exposure for 15 consecutive days had no effect on aerobic or anaerobic performance (89). Therefore, it appears that the use of intermittent hypoxic exposure does not increase sea-level performance.

> ### KEY POINT
>
> The LHTL regimen seems to be the only justifiable altitude-training approach to increase performance at sea level.

> ### TEST YOURSELF
>
> Explain the main principle behind LLTH, and give recommendations regarding optimal degrees and durations of exposure.

High-Altitude Natives

High-altitude natives, such as the Sherpas from the Himalayas and the Aymaras from the Andes, have been exposed to chronic hypoxia for generations. One clear advantage of high-altitude natives is that their increased pulmonary diffusion capacity keeps the alveolar-arterial O_2 gradient (A-aPO_2) small. At maximum exercise, however, high-altitude native skeletal muscle extracts less arterial O_2, reducing some of the advantage of a high pulmonary diffusion capacity at maximal aerobic exercise.

The likely basis of the low A-aPO_2 gradient observed in Aymaras is the higher diffusion capacity associated with larger lung volumes (20,90,91). The larger lung volumes may be the result of multiple factors, and from animal

studies it is known that hypoxic exposure is associated with larger alveolar septal tissue volume and surface areas (92), which are further augmented by a smaller alveolar duct volume and smaller mean harmonic diffusion-barrier thickness. In these animal studies, structural changes induced a higher oxygen diffusing capacity during exercise (93). For lung adaptations to occur in animals, high-altitude exposure has to be initiated during lung maturation, and altitude exposure in adult animals does not induce structural or volume changes (94). Once such adaptations are made, however, even 2 years of reexposure to normoxia does not reverse them (93). Together, these studies suggest that increases in gas-exchange efficiency arise largely from developmental exposure to hypoxia, and this notion is further supported by the similar diffusion capacities of natives from Colorado, the Andes, and Tibet. It seems unlikely that the superior diffusion capacities of high-altitude natives, which depend on structural adaptations in the lungs, can become available to acclimatizing individuals. Due to the differences in A-aPO_2 between acclimatizing lowlanders and highlanders, the response of SaO_2 to graded exercise also differs between groups (Fig. 24.6). Quite remarkably, in one study (95), the exercise-induced desaturation was only 4.6%, as compared with approximately 12% in acclimatizing lowlanders. This has major effects on the arterial oxygen content (CaO_2), which is kept almost constant throughout exercise in high-altitude natives (Fig. 24.6). Hence, one clear advantage the Aymara have is that exercise at altitude is not associated with the same degree of arterial desaturation that is known to occur in lowlanders. In the above-mentioned experiment, however, at maximal exercise intensity the lowlanders extracted 90% to 91% of arterial O_2, whereas the Aymaras extracted 83%. The decreased fractional extraction of arterial O_2 at maximal exercise in high-altitude Aymara offsets the advantage of a high pulmonary diffusion capacity.

Although they have a hypothetical advantage, high-altitude natives do not possess a higher fraction of oxidative skeletal muscle fibers, and also capillarization is not increased compared with that in lowlanders. In one study (81), lowlanders had 4.0 ± 0.6 capillaries fiber^{-1}, and this ratio was not significantly changed with acclimatization. By comparison, the high-altitude natives had 2.4 ± 0.3 capillaries fiber^{-1}. However, due to a smaller cross-sectional area of the individual fibers in the high-altitude natives, the actual capillary count per muscle fiber was identical in lowland and high-altitude natives (81). This is in agreement with other published data from a similar experimental population (96), and similar muscle fiber areas have been observed in high-altitude Sherpas (97).

> ### TEST YOURSELF
>
> Explain the main physiologic and anatomical differences between high-altitude and sea-level natives.

CHAPTER SUMMARY

From the above text, it should be clear that most humans tolerate exposure to altitude well. It should also be clear that this depends on a number of very important physiologic responses. Among the first important responses to hypoxia is an increased ventilatory drive, which increases the arterial oxygen saturation beyond what could be expected for a given altitude. This in turn increases arterial oxygen content. Another important immediate response is an increase in cardiac output, which occurs secondary to stimulation of the peripheral chemoreceptors and vagal withdrawal, and ensures a match between O_2 delivery and demand. After a few hours of hypoxic stimulation, the concentration of plasma EPO is increased transiently (peaking on day 2–4). However, it may take weeks for the new erythrocytes to mature and be released, and to eventually increase the total red cell mass. The hematocrit increases

A MILESTONE OF DISCOVERY

In the fall of 1985, a team of investigators began what is now known as Operation Everest II. This multifaceted project, which had been in preparation for approximately 5 years, was conducted in a hypobaric chamber in Natick, Massachusetts, under the direction of the U.S. Army Research Institute of Environmental Medicine. This investigation resulted in more than 40 published works that have significantly added to our understanding of the adaptations made by the human body in response to extremely high altitude. The study by John Sutton and his associates specifically examined the role of oxygen transport during exercise under such conditions. Because ambient oxygen pressure decreases with increasing altitude, their goal in this study was to examine how well oxygen transport is maintained under such extreme conditions, particularly when the added demands of exercise are placed upon the body. They also assessed the extent to which the various links in the oxygen transport chain or cascade can respond and function. Nine subjects began the investigations, and six of these subjects completed all phases of the experiment. A simulated ascent to the summit of Mount Everest (8848 m) was accomplished by gradual decompression over time, with the subjects spending a total of 40 days inside the chamber. The subjects were studied at rest and while cycling on a bicycle ergometer to maximal capacity, with each workload lasting 5 to 8 minutes. The main finding was that oxygen transport at extreme altitude was defended primarily by the first (pulmonary ventilation) and last (diffusion from capillary and mitochondrial utilization) links in the oxygen transport chain.

Table 24.2 shows data for the highest exercise power output achieved, which was common to all altitudes (PIo_2)

studied. The observation of a progressive increase in both resting and exercise ventilation indicated that the hypoxic ventilatory control was maintained at these extreme altitudes. Further, the results suggested that despite severe hypoxemia, there was no depression of ventilatory drive or respiratory muscle fatigue.

Although the next link in the chain, diffusion of oxygen from the alveoli to capillary blood, was diffusion limited at altitude, it was found to contribute only marginally to the reduction in Pao_2. The finding that at high altitude cardiac output for a given workload was similar to that observed at sea level led the authors to conclude that cardiac output defends oxygen transport only at the higher exercise workloads. This was further supported by the observation that tissue oxygen extraction, indicated by decrements in mixed venous Po_2, during the initial workloads was significantly greater at altitude than at sea level. Thus, at a given submaximal power output at high altitude, muscle $\dot{V}o_2$ is defended by increasing tissue oxygen extraction in preference to increasing cardiac output. Only at higher workloads, when oxygen extraction becomes limited, are adjustments made in cardiac output. The time and effort required for such a multifaceted study, the number of subjects and investigators involved, and the voluminous amount of data collected and analyzed under such finely controlled conditions makes Operation Everest II truly a remarkable achievement in high-altitude physiology.

Sutton JR, Reeves JT, Wagner PD, et al. Operation Everest II: oxygen transport during exercise at extreme simulated altitude. J Appl Physiol. 1988;64:1309–1321.

TABLE 24.2	Data Collected at Power Output of 120 W during Operation Everest II				
Elevation (m)	PIo_2	$\dot{V}_E$ (L · min^{-1})	Pao_2 (Torr)	$\dot{Q}$ (L · min^{-1})	Pvo_2 (Torr)
Sea level	150	47.7 ± 3.5	99.7 ± 5.8	16.5 ± 2.4	26.0 ± 2.0
4527	80	71.8 ± 6.8	42.2 ± 2.7		
6100	63	92.4 ± 12.7	33.8 ± 2.9	14.6 ± 1.7	15.4 ± 1.7
7620	49	161.8 ± 18.0	33.1 ± 1.2	15.9 ± 0.6	14.4 ± 1.4
8848	43	183.5 ± 34.0	27.6 ± 0.6	16.1 ± 0.1	13.8 ± 0.6

PIo_2, inspired Po_2; $\dot{V}_E$, minute ventilation (BTPS); Pao_2, arterial Po_2; $\dot{Q}$, cardiac output; Pvo_2, mixed venous Po_2; Values are means ± SD. For sea level and 4572 m, $n = 8$; for 6100 m, $n = 6$; for 7620 and 8848 m, $n = 3$.

during the first days of altitude exposure due to reductions in plasma volume. Exercise physiologists may think of this as a maladaptation, because a reduction in blood volume can decrease $\dot{V}O_{2max}$. However, the increase in hematocrit caused by a reduction in plasma volume should be seen as a survival/defense mechanism against hypoxia.

Because resting ventilation and cardiac output are increased, the basal metabolic rate is increased at altitude, and if this is not compensated for by increased caloric intake, weight loss will occur. During submaximal exercise, increases in ventilation, cardiac output, blood flow, and oxygen extraction by the exercising skeletal muscles ensure that O_2 demand for a given work rate will be maintained. Although all of these processes require higher O_2 consumption, this is usually not reflected by a measurably higher pulmonary $\dot{V}O_2$. At maximal exercise, diffusion limitations and reductions in blood flow to the exercising muscles reduce $\dot{V}O_{2max}$. In general, the reduction in $\dot{V}O_{2max}$ is greater in athletes than in nonathletes. Although acclimatization to high altitude increases arterial oxygen content, $\dot{V}O_{2max}$ is not increased with acclimatization at altitudes above approximately 4000 m. However, this does not mean that athletes who are planning to compete at high altitude should not arrive at the site of competition in advance because submaximal exercise capacity is increased tremendously with acclimatization. Athletes who wish to increase their performance at sea level could make use of the LHTL approach. Most humans can achieve performance gains by living at 2100–3000 m altitude for 3 weeks and ensuring that daily altitude exposure exceeds 14 hours.

REFERENCES

1. West JB, Wagner PD. Predicted gas exchange on the summit of Mt. Everest. *Resp Physiol.* 1980;42:1–16.
2. Buskirk ER, Kollias J, Akers RF, et al. Maximal performance at altitude and on return from altitude in conditioned runners. *J Appl Physiol.* 1967;23:259–266.
3. Leuenberger U, Gleeson K, Wroblewski K, et al. Norepinephrine clearance is increased during acute hypoxemia in humans. *Am J Physiol Heart Circ Physiol.* 1991;261:H1659–H1664.
4. Saito M, Mano T, Iwase S, et al. Responses in muscle sympathetic activity to acute hypoxia in humans. *J Appl Physiol.* 1988;65:1548–1552.
5. Hansen J, Sander M. Sympathetic neural overactivity in healthy humans after prolonged exposure to hypobaric hypoxia. *J Physiol.* 2003;546:921–929.
6. Lundby C, Sander M, van Hall G, et al. Maximal exercise and muscle oxygen extraction in acclimatizing lowlanders and high altitude natives. *J Physiol.* 2006;573:535–547.
7. van Hall G, Lundby C, Araoz M, et al. The lactate paradox revisited in lowlanders during acclimatization to 4100 m and in high-altitude natives. *J Physiol.* 2009;587:1117–1129.
8. Kacimi R, Richalet JP, Corsin A, et al. Hypoxia-induced down-regulation of beta-adrenergic receptors in rat heart. *J Appl Physiol.* 1992;73:1377–1382.
9. Voelkel NF, Hegstrand L, Reeves JT, et al. Effects of hypoxia on density of beta-adrenergic receptors. *J Appl Physiol.* 1981;50:363–366.
10. Richalet JP, Larmignat P, Rathat C, et al. Decreased cardiac response to isoproterenol infusion in acute and chronic hypoxia. *J Appl Physiol.* 1988;65:1957–1961.
11. Hughson RL, Yamamoto Y, McCullough RE, et al. Sympathetic and parasympathetic indicators of heart rate control at altitude studied by spectral analysis. *J Appl Physiol.* 1994;77:2537–2542.
12. Hannon JP, Shields JL, Harris CW. Effects of altitude acclimatization on blood composition of women. *J Appl Physiol.* 1969;26:540–547.
13. Albert TS, Tucker VL, Renkin EM. Atrial natriuretic peptide levels and plasma volume contraction in acute alveolar hypoxia. *J Appl Physiol.* 1997;82:102–110.
14. Claydon VE, Norcliffe LJ, Moore JP, et al. Orthostatic tolerance and blood volumes in Andean high-altitude dwellers. *Exp Physiol.* 2004;89:565–571.
15. Gamboa A, Gamboa JL, Holmes C, et al. Plasma catecholamines and blood volume in native Andeans during hypoxia and normoxia. *Clin Auton Res.* 2006;16:40–45.
16. Sanchez C, Merino C, Figallo M. Simultaneous measurement of plasma volume and cell mass in polycythemia of high altitude. *J Appl Physiol.* 1970;28:775–778.
17. Lundby C, Calbet JAL, van Hall G, et al. Pulmonary gas exchange at maximal exercise in Danish lowlanders during 8 wk of acclimatization to 4,100 m and in high-altitude Aymara natives. *Am J Physiol Regul Integr Comp Physiol.* 2004;287:R1202–R1208.
18. Bencowitz HZ, Wagner PD, West JB. Effect of change in P50 on exercise tolerance at high altitude: a theoretical study. *J Appl Physiol.* 1982;53:1487–1495.
19. Winslow RM. Red cell properties and optimal oxygen transport. *Adv Exp Med Biol.* 1988;227:117–136.
20. Wagner PD, Araoz M, Boushel R, et al. Pulmonary gas exchange and acid-base state at 5,260 m in high-altitude Bolivians and acclimatized lowlanders. *J Appl Physiol.* 2002;92:1393–1400.
21. Lenfant C, Torrance JD, Reynafarje C. Shift of the O2-Hb dissociation curve at altitude: mechanism and effect. *J Appl Physiol.* 1971;30:625–631.
22. Mairbaurl H, Oelz O, Bartsch P. Interactions between Hb, Mg, DPG, ATP, and Cl determine the change in Hb-O2 affinity at high altitude. *J Appl Physiol.* 1993;74:40–48.
23. Wang ZY, Olson EB Jr, Bjorling DE, et al. Sustained hypoxia-induced proliferation of carotid body type I cells in rats. *J Appl Physiol.* 2008;104:803–808.
24. Bisgard GE, Busch MA, Forster HV. Ventilatory acclimatization to hypoxia is not dependent on cerebral hypocapnic alkalosis. *J Appl Physiol.* 1986;60:1011–1015.
25. Wagner PD, Sutton JR, Reeves JT, et al. Operation Everest II: pulmonary gas exchange during a simulated ascent of Mt. Everest. *J Appl Physiol.* 1987;63:2348–2359.
26. Lundby C, Araoz M, van Hall G. Peak heart rate decreases with increasing severity of acute hypoxia. *High Alt Med Biol.* 2001;2:369–376.
27. Boushel R, Calbet JA, Radegran G, et al. Parasympathetic neural activity accounts for the lowering of exercise heart rate at high altitude. *Circulation.* 2001;104:1785–1791.
28. Reeves JT, Groves BM, Sutton JR, et al. Operation Everest II: preservation of cardiac function at extreme altitude. *J Appl Physiol.* 1987;63:531–539.
29. Grover RF, Lufschanowski R, Alexander JK. Alterations in the coronary circulation of man following ascent to 3,100 m altitude. *J Appl Physiol.* 1976;41:832–838.
30. Gore CJ, Hahn AG, Scroop GC, et al. Increased arterial desaturation in trained cyclists during maximal exercise at 580 m altitude. *J Appl Physiol.* 1996;80:2204–2210.
31. Wehrlin JP, Hallen J. Linear decrease in $\dot{V}O_{2max}$ and performance with increasing altitude in endurance athletes. *Eur J Appl Physiol.* 2006;96:404–412.
32. Mollard P, Woorons X, Letournel M, et al. Role of maximal heart rate and arterial O2 saturation on the decrement of $\dot{V}O_{2max}$ in moderate acute hypoxia in trained and untrained men. *Int J Sports Med.* 2007;28:186–192.
33. Woorons X, Mollard P, Lamberto C, et al. Effect of acute hypoxia on maximal exercise in trained and sedentary women. *Med Sci Sports Exerc.* 2005;37:147–154.
34. Amann M, Romer LM, Subudhi AW, et al. Severity of arterial hypoxaemia affects the relative contributions of peripheral muscle fatigue to exercise performance in healthy humans. *J Physiol.* 2007;581:389–403.

35. Lundby C, Damsgaard R. Exercise performance in hypoxia after novel erythropoiesis stimulating protein treatment. *Scand J Med Sci Sports.* 2006;16:35–40.

36. Robach P, Calbet JAL, Thomsen JJ, et al. The ergogenic effect of recombinant human erythropoietin on O_2max depends on the severity of arterial hypoxemia. *PLos ONE.* 2008;3:e2996.

37. Schuler B, Thomsen JJ, Gassmann M, et al. Timing the arrival at 2,340 m altitude for aerobic performance. *Scand J Med Sci Sports.* 2007;17:588–594.

38. Calbet JAL, Boushel R, Radegran G, et al. Why is $\dot{V}o_{2max}$ after altitude acclimatization still reduced despite normalization of arterial O_2 content? *Am J Physiol Regul Integr Comp Physiol.* 2003;284:R304–R316.

39. Lundby C, Møller P, Kanstrup IL, et al. Heart rate response to hypoxic exercise: role of dopamine D2-receptors and effect of oxygen supplementation. *Clin Sci (Lond).* 2001;101:377–383.

40. Lundby C, Calbet JAL, Sander M, et al. Exercise economy does not change after acclimatization to moderate to very high altitude. *Scand J Med Sci Sports.* 2007;17:281–291.

41. Horstman D, Weiskopf R, Jackson RE. Work capacity during 3-wk sojourn at 4,300 m: effects of relative polycythemia. *J Appl Physiol.* 1980;49:311–318.

42. Butterfield GE, Gates J, Fleming S, et al. Increased energy intake minimizes weight loss in men at high altitude. *J Appl Physiol.* 1992;72:1741–1748.

43. Brooks GA, Butterfield GE, Wolfe RR, et al. Increased dependence on blood glucose after acclimatization to 4,300 m. *J Appl Physiol.* 1991;70:919–927.

44. Lundby C, van Hall G. Substrate utilization in sea level residents during exercise in acute hypoxia and after 4 weeks of acclimatization to 4,100 m. *Acta Physiol Scand.* 2002;176:195–201.

45. Subudhi AW, Miramon BR, Granger ME, et al. Frontal and motor cortex oxygenation during maximal exercise in normoxia and hypoxia. *J Appl Physiol.* 2009;91:475.

46. Dickinson ER, Piddington MJ, Brain T. Project Olympics. *Schweitz Zeit Sportmed.* 1966;14:305–308.

47. Peronnet F, Thibault G, Cousineau DL. A theoretical analysis of the effect of altitude on running performance. *J Appl Physiol.* 1991;70:404.

48. Haseler LJ, Hogan MC, Richardson RS. Skeletal muscle phosphocreatine recovery in exercise-trained humans is dependent on O_2 availability. *J Appl Physiol.* 1999;86:2013–2018.

49. Haseler LJ, Lin A, Hoff J, et al. Oxygen availability and PCr recovery rate in untrained human calf muscle: evidence of metabolic limitation in normoxia. *Am J Physiol Regul Integr Comp Physiol.* 2007;293:R2046–R2051.

50. Haseler LJ, Lin AP, Richardson RS. Skeletal muscle oxidative metabolism in sedentary humans: 31P-MRS assessment of O_2 supply and demand limitations. *J Appl Physiol.* 2004;97:1077–1081.

51. Brosnan MJ, Martin DT, Hahn AG, et al. Impaired interval exercise responses in elite female cyclists at moderate simulated altitude. *J Appl Physiol.* 2000;89:1819–1824.

52. Feriche B, Delgado M, Calderon C, et al. The effect of acute moderate hypoxia on accumulated oxygen deficit during intermittent exercise in nonacclimatized men. *J Strength Cond Res.* 2007;21:413–418.

53. Capelli C, Di Prampero PE. Effects of altitude on top speeds during 1 h unaccompanied cycling. *Eur J Appl Physiol.* 1995;71:469–471.

54. Levine BD, Stray-Gundersen J. "Living high-training low": effect of moderate-altitude acclimatization with low-altitude training on performance. *J Appl Physiol.* 1997;83:102–112.

55. Bailey DM, Davis B, Romer L, et al. Implications of moderate altitude training for sea-level endurance in elite distance runners. *Eur J Appl Physiol.* 1998;78:360–368.

56. Gore CJ, Hahn AG, Burge CM, et al. $\dot{V}o_{2max}$ and haemoglobin mass of trained athletes during high-intensity training. *Int J Sports Med.* 1997;18:477–482.

57. Friedmann B, Jost J, Rating TWE, et al. Effects of iron repletion on blood volume and performance capacity in young athletes. *Int J Sports Med.* 1999;20:78–85.

58. Roels B, Hellard P, Schmitt L, et al. Is it more effective for highly trained swimmers to live and train at 1,200 m than at 1,850 m in terms of performance and haematological benefits? *Br J Sports Med.* 2006;40:e4.

59. Svendenhag J, Piehl-Aulin K, Skog C, et al. Increased left ventricular muscle mass after long-term altitude training in athletes. *Acta Physiol Scand.* 1997;161:63–70.

60. Friedmann B, Frese F, Menold E, Bärtsch P. Individual variation in the reduction of heart rate and performance at lactate thresholds in acute normobaric hypoxia. *Br J Sports Med.* 2005;39:148–153.

61. Gore CJ, Craig NP, Hahn AG, et al. Altitude training at 2690m does not increase total haemoglobin mass or sea level $\dot{V}o_{2max}$ in world champion track cyclists. *J Sci Med Sport.* 1998;1:156–170.

62. Stray-Gundersen J, Chapman RF, Levine BD. "Living high-training low" altitude training improves sea level performance in male and female elite runners. *J Appl Physiol.* 2001;91:1113–1120.

63. Stray-Gundersen J, Levine BD. Live high, train low at natural altitude. *Scand J Med Sci Sports.* 2008;18:21–28.

64. Wehrlin JP, Zuest P, Hallen J, et al. Live high–train low for 24 days increases hemoglobin mass and red cell volume in elite endurance athletes. *J Appl Physiol.* 2006;100:1938–1945.

65. Ashenden MJ, Gore CJ, Dobson GP, et al. "Live high, train low" does not change the total haemoglobin mass of male endurance athletes sleeping at a simulated altitude of 3,000 m for 23 nights. *Eur J Appl Physiol.* 1999;80:479–484.

66. Ashenden MJ, Gore CJ, Martin DT, et al. Effects of a 12-day "live high, train low" camp on reticulocyte production and haemoglobin mass in elite female road cyclists. *Eur J Appl Physiol.* 1999;80:472–478.

67. Roberts AD, Clark SA Townsend NE, et al. Changes in performance, maximal oxygen uptake and maximal accumulated oxygen deficit after 5, 10, and 15 days of live high:train low altitude exposure. *Eur J Appl Physiol.* 2003;88:390–395.

68. Saunders PU, Telford RD, Pyne DB, et al. Improved running economy and increased hemoglobin mass in elite runners after extended moderate altitude exposure. *J Sci Med Sport.* 2009;12:67–72.

69. Robach P, Schmitt L, Brugniaux JV, et al. Living high-training low: effect on erythropoiesis and maximal aerobic performance in elite Nordic skiers. *Eur J Appl Physiol.* 2006;97:695–705.

70. Robach P, Schmitt L, Brugniaux JV, et al. Living high-training low: effect on erythropoiesis and aerobic performance in highly trained swimmers. *Eur J Appl Physiol.* 2006;96:423–433.

71. Brugniaux JV, Schmitt L, Robach P, et al. Eighteen days of "living high, training low" stimulate erythropoiesis and enhance aerobic performance in elite midwe-distance runners. *J Appl Physiol.* 2006;100:203–211.

72. Neya M, Enoki T, Kumai Y, et al. The effects of nightly normobaric hypoxia and high-intensity training under intermittent normobaric hypoxia on running economy and hemoglobin mass. *J Appl Physiol.* 2007;103:828–834.

73. Gore CJ, Hahn AG, Aughey RJ, et al. Live high: train low increases muscle buffer capacity and submaximal cycling efficiency. *Acta Physiol Scand.* 2001;173:275–286.

74. Richardson RS, Duteil S, Wary C, et al. Human skeletal muscle intracellular oxygenation: the impact of ambient oxygen availability. *J Physiol.* 2006;571:415–424.

75. Semenza GL, Shimoda LA, Prabhakar NR. Regulation of gene expression by HIF-1. *Novartis Found Symp.* 2006;272:2–8.

76. Hendriksen IJ, Meeuwsen T. The effect of intermittent training in hypobaric hypoxia on sea-level exercise: a cross-over study in humans. *Eur J Appl Physiol.* 2003;88:396–403.

77. Meeuwsen T, Hendriksen IJ, Holewijn M. Training-induced increases in sea-level performance are enhanced by acute intermittent hypobaric hypoxia. *Eur J Appl Physiol.* 2001;84:283–290.

78. Hoppeler H, Klossner S, Vogt M. Training in hypoxia and its effects on skeletal muscle tissue. *Scand J Med Sci Sports.* 2008;18:38–49.

79. Imoberdorf R, Garlick PJ, McNurlan MA, et al. Skeletal muscle protein synthesis after active or passive ascent to high altitude. *Med Sci Sports Exerc.* 2006;38:1082–1087.

80. Mizuno M, Savard GK, Areskog NH, et al. Skeletal muscle adaptations to prolonged exposure to extreme altitude: a role of physical activity? *High Alt Med Biol.* 2008;9:311–317.

81. Lundby C, Pilegaard H, Andersen JL, et al. Acclimatization to 4,100 m does not change capillary density or mRNA expression of potential angiogenesis regulatory factors in human skeletal muscle. *J Exp Biol.* 2004;207:3865–3871.

82. Truijens MJ, Toussaint HM, Dow J, et al. Effect of high-intensity hypoxic training on sea-level swimming performances. *J Appl Physiol.* 2003;94:733–743.

83. Truijens MJ, Rodriguez FA, Townsend NE, et al. The effect of intermittent hypobaric hypoxic exposure and sea level training on submaximal economy in well-trained swimmers and runners. *J Appl Physiol.* 2008;104:328–337.

84. Geiser J, Vogt M, Billeter R, et al. Training high-living low: changes of aerobic performance and muscle structure with training at simulated altitude. *Int J Sports Med.* 2001;22:579–585.

85. Ventura N, Hoppeler H, Seiler R, et al. The response of trained athletes to six weeks of endurance training in hypoxia or normoxia. *Int J Sports Med.* 2003;24:166–172.

86. Dufour SP, Ponsot E, Zoll J, et al. Exercise training in normobaric hypoxia in endurance runners, I: Improvement in aerobic performance capacity. *J Appl Physiol.* 2006;100:1238–1248.

87. Julian CG, Gore CJ, Wilber RL, et al. Intermittent normobaric hypoxia does not alter performance or erythropoietic markers in highly trained distance runners. *J Appl Physiol.* 2004;96:1800–1807.

88. Rodriguez FA, Truijens MJ, Townsend NE, et al. Performance of runners and swimmers after four weeks of intermittent hypobaric hypoxic exposure plus sea level training. *J Appl Physiol.* 2007;103:1523–1535.

89. Tadibi V, Dehnert C, Menold E, et al. Unchanged anaerobic and aerobic performance after short-term intermittent hypoxia. *Med Sci Sports Exerc.* 2007;39:585–564.

90. Schoene RB. Limits of human lung function at high altitude. *J Exp Biol.* 2001;204:3121–3127.

91. Zhuang J, Droma T, Sutton JR, et al. Smaller alveolar-arterial O2 gradients in Tibetan than Han residents of Lhasa (3,658 m). *Resp Physiol.* 1996;103:75–82.

92. Hsia CCW, Carbayo JJ, Yan X, et al. Enhanced alveolar growth and remodeling in Guinea pigs raised at high altitude. *Resp Physiol Neurobiol.* 2005;147:105–115.

93. McDonough P, Dane DM, Hsia CCW, et al. Long-term enhancement of pulmonary gas exchange after high-altitude residence during maturation. *J Appl Physiol.* 2006,100:474–481.

94. Johnson RL Jr, Cassidy SS, Grover RF, et al. Functional capacities of lungs and thorax in beagles after prolonged residence at 3,100 m. *J Appl Physiol.* 1985;59:1773–1782.

95. Lundby C, Calbet JAL. Why are high altitude natives so strong at altitude? Maximal oxygen transport to the muscle cell in altitude natives. *Adv Exp Med Biol.* Accepted for publication: 2011.

96. Desplanches D, Hoppeler H, Tuscher L, et al. Muscle tissue adaptations of high-altitude natives to training in chronic hypoxia or acute normoxia. *J Appl Physiol.* 1996;81:1946–1951.

97. Kayser B, Hoppeler H, Claassen H, et al. Muscle structure and performance capacity of Himalayan Sherpas. *J Appl Physiol.* 1991;70:1938–1942.

98. Sutton JR, Reeves JT, Wagner PD, et al. Operation Everest II: oxygen transport during exercise at extreme simulated altitude. *J Appl Physiol.* 1988;64:1309–1321.

99. Fitzgerald RS, Lahiri S. Reflex responses to chemoreceptor stimulation. In: Cherniack NS, Widdicombe JG, eds. *The Respiratory System.* Bethesda: American Physiological Society; 1986:313–362.

100. Fulco CS, Rock PB, Cymerman A. Maximal and submaximal exercise performance at altitude. *Aviat Space Environ Med.* 1998;69:794–801.

CHAPTER 25

Physiologic Systems and Their Responses To Conditions of Hyperbaria

John R. Claybaugh, Keizo Shiraki, Robert Elsner, and Yu-Chong Lin

Abbreviations

atm	Atmosphere	P_{ACO_2}	Alveolar carbon dioxide partial pressure
atm abs	Atmospheres absolute—a measure of underwater pressure	P_{O_2}	Partial pressure of oxygen
		psi	pounds per square inch
AVP	Arginine vasopressin	SCUBA	Self-contained underwater breathing apparatus
BH	Breath hold		
FSW	Feet sea water	torr	Torricell unit (mm Hg)
kPa	kilopascals	$\dot{V}_E$	Ventilatory volume
MET	Metabolic equivalents		

Introduction

When humans enter a hyperbaric environment, their purpose is typically to exercise or work. Such work includes the age-old occupations of breath-hold (BH) diving and helmet diving, as well as diving with self-contained underwater breathing apparatus (SCUBA). In addition, underwater tunnel construction and deep-saturation diving are often done in dry pressurized-gas environments. The work force in these occupations is relatively small. For instance, there are approximately 20,000 commercial BH divers currently. The Association of Diving Contractors International estimates that there are 4200 commercial divers in the United States. Most of these divers are helmet divers, some use SCUBA, and approximately 600 are engaged in saturation diving. It has been estimated that there are 13,000 to 15,000 commercial divers worldwide. These figures do not include workers whose job may occasionally involve diving, such as policemen, firemen, military workers, commercial fishermen, and scientists. In addition, the Professional Association of Diving Instructors certified 932,486 SCUBA divers worldwide in 2008, and approximately 15 million over the past 20 years. Thus, a labor force and a large recreational population are exposed to hyperbaric work and exercise,

justifying consideration of the unique problems associated with this environment.

Unfortunately, the units of pressure used to describe high-pressure environments are not consistent. Pressures are given in units of pounds per square inch (psi), bar, atmospheres (atm), atmospheres absolute (atm abs), torr, and pascals (Table 25.1), and the depth is usually given in feet sea water (FSW) or meters sea water (MSW). In this text, pressure is expressed in atm abs (sometimes abbreviated ATA in the older literature). The term *absolute* indicates that the atmospheric pressure at sea level is included in the value. For instance, for every 33-FSW increase in depth, there is an additional 1 atm of pressure in the environment. Thus, at a depth of 66 FSW, the absolute pressure is 2 atm plus 1 atm at the surface if the surface is assumed to be sea level.

The hyperbaric environment poses many obstacles that must be overcome before human habitation is possible. The most elementary obstacle is that the underwater environment lacks gaseous oxygen, and therefore lung-breathing animals must hold their breath. If long stays under water are required, oxygen from compressed gas must be used. At depths of approximately 180 FSW (55 MSW), the partial pressure of nitrogen is more than

TABLE 25.1	Pressure Unit Equivalents of 1 atm
1.01325 bar	760 torr
101.325 kPa	33.08 FSW
14.6959 psi	10.13 MSW

The unit of pressure defined by the International System of Unit is the pascal (Pa = N · m⁻²), which is often the preferred unit of pressure in current publications. atm, atmosphere; kPa, kilopascal; psi, pounds per square inch; torr, Torricelli unit (mm Hg); FSW, feet sea water; MSW, meters sea water.

six times higher than that at sea level, which can lead to a narcotic effect. At greater depths, helium is used instead of nitrogen in the compressed-gas mixture. In addition, the high partial pressures of oxygen (Po_2) become poisonous because of the induction of free radicals at depths of only 33 FSW. Therefore, at depths of several atmospheres, a reduced percentage of oxygen is used in the gas mixture, but it is usually maintained at about twice the sea-level Po_2 (0.4–0.5 atm abs). Thus, the mixture of gas is a factor to be considered.

Other factors to be considered when a human body is under water include the state of weightlessness, which causes blood to be displaced from the legs to the thorax (see Chapter 26 for a discussion of the physiologic consequences of this fluid shift). This in turn causes an increase in preload to the heart and affects certain exercise responses. The partial pressures of all gases become higher in the body tissues at high pressure, and the risk of bubbles forming upon decompression, similar to opening a bottle of champagne, can be influenced by exercise. Therefore, divers must practice slow decompression to ensure that the gases are exhaled from the body without forming bubbles in the tissues.

When divers descend to greater and greater depths, the amount of time they can spend at depth becomes shorter relative to the amount of time that is required for safe decompression. Therefore, during dives of several hundred feet, the body is allowed to come to equilibrium with gases in the environment. In this way, extended bottom times can be achieved with a constant amount of decompression time necessary for safe decompression. Such dives are called saturation dives, and human performance has been studied at great pressures equivalent to >2000 FSW (1) (see *A Milestone of Discovery* at the end of this chapter). The advantage of saturation dives is that they allow divers to work at depth for several days. The divers can remain at pressure in a dry chamber on a surface vessel for sleep and rest. Complications resulting from the dry high-pressure environment, including changes in insensible water loss and hormonal control of water balance, also become a factor affected by exercise.

Therefore, the definition of a hyperbaric environment that is compatible with human habitation changes with increasing depth and with the state of immersion or dry-

ness. This means that the response to exercise is likely to change as a function of depth or immersion not only because of the depth per se, but also because of changes in other characteristics of the environment that are necessary to support human life, such as gas mixture and density.

TEST YOURSELF

At sea level, we breathe air that is 20% O_2. How can humans comfortably satisfy oxygen requirements at a depth of 660 FSW by breathing gas mixtures of only 1% O_2?

Exercise During Submersion

Three important physiologic disturbances occur with exercise during submersion. First, humans must hold their breath or breathe from a pressurized source, since there is no gaseous source of oxygen. These two modes of underwater diving cause distinct differences in the physiologic responses to dynamic exercise and are considered separately here. Second, the hydrostatic gradient in air causes a certain proportion of blood to be sequestered in the legs, but submersion removes the gradient. This shifts blood from the legs to the thorax. The third disturbance involves the physiologic adjustments that must take place for a person to tolerate the challenges to thermal regulation. Exercise or work in water usually takes place in a cooler setting than thermal neutral, and the impact of heat loss and its interaction with exercise are important factors.

Exercise During Breath Holding

Cessation of respiration by breath holding fundamentally contradicts what seems natural and supports life. It deprives an organism of oxygen and the ability to dump carbon dioxide. It is the first step toward asphyxia (i.e., the threatening combination of tissue hypoxia, hypercapnia, and acidosis). This triad disrupts physiologic integrations and ultimately leads to the reversal of life-sustaining functions. Human breath-holding performance appears trivial when compared with that of aquatic mammals. We do not hold our breath comfortably, as seals and whales routinely do in their underwater excursions. Nevertheless, BH skin diving is the most immediate and simplest means of diving for work or pleasure.

Marine mammals: a model of breath-hold diving

Whereas asphyxia refers to the cessation of respiration by an organism, ischemia refers to the reduction or occlusion of blood flow within an organ or tissue. Resistance to asphyxia varies among species, and tolerance of ischemia varies from tissue to tissue. Although some seal and whale species can tolerate breath-holding apnea for more than an hour; most humans struggle to hold their breath for 1 minute. We lose consciousness when our brain is deprived of blood circulation for longer than a few seconds, but we can tolerate limb ischemia by a tourniquet for 30 minutes or more.

The superior breath-holding capacities of seals, especially the phocid or "true" seals, depend on several physiologic characteristics that support their diving habits. Strictly speaking, seals' adaptive mechanisms are not unique to them; rather, these animals exploit fundamental mammalian functions and regulations, and expand them quantitatively. Their combined adaptations result in some impressive dive depths and durations. Harbor seals (*Phoca vitulina*), which are common on both U.S. coasts, can dive to 200 m and remain submerged for 25 minutes. Antarctic Weddell seals (*Leptonychotes weddelli*) can stay at 700 m for more than 1 hour, and northern elephant seals (*Mirounga angustirostris*) can dive to 1500 m.

Marine mammals derive their advantages for underwater living from several specializations, including enhanced oxygen supply in high blood volume and enriched hemoglobin concentration, and physical features such as collapsible lungs, which may prevent inert gas bubble formation upon decompression (*i.e.*, the bends) in these species. However, seals display other mechanisms of oxygen conservation during a dive, such as a reduction and redistribution of circulation heralded by bradycardia, the marked slowing of heart rate that is characteristic of most dives but is less noticeable in breath-holding terrestrial animals. The redirected circulation favors continued blood flow to the most vulnerable and obligatory aerobic organs—the brain and heart—at the expense of organs with greater anaerobic facilities, such as the kidney, gut, and skin. Another advantage that seals have for underwater excursions is a high tolerance for low oxygen and pH levels, well beyond human limits (2). For instance, harbor seals and Weddell seals can reach arterial Po_2 levels of 10 torr and pH values of 6.8 and can recover without incident.

Muscle perfusion in seals is partially reduced during dives, and this tissue depends on richly oxygenated myoglobin content. As a consequence of these various reductions in circulatory perfusion, overall metabolism declines, and body temperature falls slightly during long dives. Ultimately, the metabolic resources are exhausted; however, the seal's superior mechanisms for dealing with problems of acid–base balance and cerebral tolerance of hypoxia can further extend the diving time (2,3). The responses are variable in timing and intensity; brief dives, for example, sometimes show relatively little effect, whereas longer submersions are supported by more profound reactions. The result is metabolic conservation and lowering of energetic demands during apneic dives in support of extending the underwater episode. Therefore, this metabolic conservation can be adjusted to some extent by behavioral alterations of swimming activity.

Summary

Marine mammals have several physiologic characteristics that allow them to remain underwater for significant periods of time. This is achieved for the most part by a metabolic conservation brought about by the redistribution of blood supply away from tissues that are not critical for short-term survival, such as the kidney, gut and skin, and maintenance of an adequate blood supply to the muscles. Despite greatly reduced heart rates, the enriched hemoglobin concentration and richly oxygenated myoglobin content in the muscle provide enough oxygen to maintain neurologic and muscular function well beyond what is possible in humans.

Human breath-hold diving

Many people tend to think of BH diving as a recreational sport. Throughout human history, however, this type of diving has been important for occupations such as harvesting food, gathering pearls, and performing various underwater operations. These activities continue today in several locations, including Japan, Korea, Indonesia, Oceania, and to a lesser extent other coastal regions of the world. Currently, approximately 16,000 men and women in Japan and 3000 women in Korea are employed in such occupations. The Japanese ama divers are active during the summer, and Korean divers work throughout the year. Diving activity patterns vary depending on local customs and harvesting conditions. Invertebrates such as abalone and sea snails are an important part of the products foraged from the sea floor.

Japanese and Korean BH divers traditionally worked in very cold conditions, but modern divers are better protected by wet suits. This relief from severe cold exposure permits the full expression of diving capabilities without the need for frequent interruptions for rewarming. Dives typically last for 5 to 20 minutes, and seldom exceed 1 minute. Some divers average 100 dives during a 5-hour workday (4).

HUMAN DIVE RESPONSES   Human breath-holding capabilities pale by comparison with those of the marine diving specialists, seals and whales. Still, some traces of their responses can be seen in humans. Most human subjects show bradycardia and reductions of peripheral circulation during submersion, even when only the face is immersed. For example, immediately upon immersion, a seal's heart rate will drop to 5% to 30% of its rate before the dive, but the human diver usually undergoes a slow decline in heart rate over 30 seconds to about 70% of the value before the dive. These effects are consistently more responsive to water immersion than to breath holding in air, whether the immersion involves the whole body or the face alone. Over the past half century, roughly 1000 subjects have been studied in various apneic diving experiments under different conditions (2,5). Of these, nearly all exhibited a slowing of the heart rate, usually of considerably less magnitude than that of diving seals. However, a few human subjects have shown remarkably slow cardiac rates: less than 20 beats per minute. Limb blood flow was reduced in subjects in whom it was measured (6). Despite these reactions suggesting physiologic possibilities that might extend the usable dive duration, the overall savings in oxygen demand for humans is small. Still, an oxygen-saving response to face immersion can be demonstrated in human subjects during dynamic exercise. For example, Andersson and associates (7) reported that the reduction in arterial oxygen saturation resulting from a BH for 30 seconds in air while exercising at 100 W was 6.8%, but with a BH during face immersion and exercising at a similar rate, the decrement in oxygen saturation was only 5.2%. Accompanying these responses were corresponding reductions in heart rate of 21% to 33%, and the blood pressure increases were augmented by 34% to 42%.

TEST YOURSELF

What physiologic alterations occur during a breath-hold dive that would tend to reduce O_2 consumption compared with those observed in an individual performing similar work and breathing at the surface?

Contradictions of breath holding and exercise

Apneic diving is usually accompanied by swimming. In several respects, the reactions to breath holding are antithetical to those of exercise and work in direct opposition to each other. The demands for increased oxygen consumption during exercise and oxygen conservation during apneic diving are in fundamental conflict. Increased cardiovascular responses of exercise (*i.e.*, tachycardia and elevated muscle blood flow) act directly against the requirements of sustained apneic dives. It is the resolution of this conflict that defines the practical range of underwater activities for seals and skin divers alike. Seal dive times are shortened when accompanied by vigorous swimming, and humans are similarly affected by underwater exercise. Several investigations have been undertaken for the specific purpose of examining this issue.

The results of studies that combined BH dives and dynamic exercise showed, somewhat surprisingly, that reduced heart rate is the prevailing cardiac response and usually overrides the tachycardia of exercise. Some examples of profound human bradycardia have been observed in apneic diving or simple face immersion by inexperienced subjects while performing moderate exercise (2,8,9). Jung and Stolle (10) demonstrated that a swimmer's heart rate levels off at 55 beats/minute during a 50-m underwater swim. Such activity requires 5 to 10 times the resting oxygen consumption rate. In fact, abundant examples show

that exercise potentiates rather than attenuates apneic bradycardia. As shown in Figure 25.1, the heart rates of two individuals were decreased by 90% during exercise with face immersion compared with preapneic levels (11). The lowest heart rate of 5.6 beats/minute was recorded in a resting subject during face immersion in cold water (12). This point and two other points fit on a line corresponding to a 90% reduction in the pre-BH heart rate. A potent bradycardia is observed when humans exercise in cold water while holding their breath. Vagus nerves mediate apneic bradycardia in diving mammals and nondiving vertebrates alike. Exercise reduces or abolishes the vagus activity to the heart, which accounts in part for the exercise tachycardia. Cessation of respiratory movement promptly activates the vagus nerves, and an accentuated bradycardia occurs against the sympathetic activity.

KEY POINT

In most cases, the bradycardia caused by breath holding has a greater effect on reducing heart rate during exercise than during rest. Notice in Figure 25.1 that the triangles, representing conditions of work, are dominant among the reductions in heart rate of 30% or more.

A variety of factors can modify the duration of breath holding. From a simple supply-and-demand relationship, we can roughly estimate the length of a BH as follows:

$$\text{BH time with air (in min)} \propto \text{TLC} \times F_IO_2 / \dot{V}O_2$$

where TLC represents the total lung capacity in liters, F_IO_2 is the fraction of O_2 in the inspired air, and $\dot{V}O_2$ is the O_2 consumption rate in liters/minute. Therefore, elevation of F_IO_2 or lowering of $\dot{V}O_2$ prolongs the BH time. In practical terms, hyperventilation is the most effective way of prolonging the BH time because it blows off CO_2 and elevates O_2 concentration in the lung. As shown in Table 25.2, the estimates match well with published records of BH time (5). A lung full of air should allow apnea for about 4 minutes (20% of 6 L of air divided by the O_2 consumption rate at 0.25 L/min). Likewise, when a BH is performed with 100% O_2, the available amount of O_2 is 6 L minus the residual volume and divided by 0.25, which should last for ≥15 minutes according to this simple estimate, a value that also aligns with those in Table 25.2. In a study by Elsner et al. (6), a BH of 5 minutes after hyperventilation with 100% O_2 was achieved with only moderate discomfort by all five subjects in the study, demonstrating the general effectiveness of this procedure for extending a BH. Nevertheless, as effective as hyperventilation may be, its use prior to underwater activities should be discouraged. The low P_{CO_2} due to hyperventilation at the onset of an apnea dive keeps the alveolar P_{CO_2} from reaching a level that normally induces the urge to resume breathing. Meanwhile, O_2 concentration falls continuously while

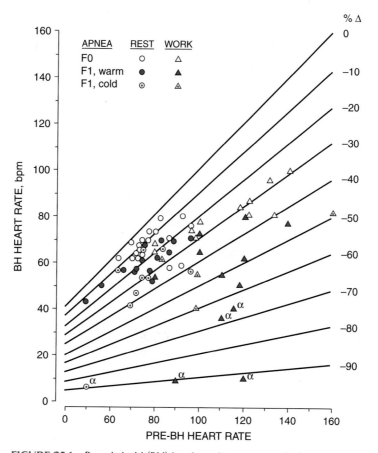

FIGURE 25.1 Breath-hold (BH) bradycardiac response in humans at rest and during exercise. FI and FO stand for BH with and without facial immersion, respectively, in cold or warm water. The symbol α denotes two individuals who decreased their heart rates by 90% during exercise with face immersion. (Reproduced with permission from Lin YC. Physiologic limitations of humans as breath-hold divers. In: Lin YC, Shida KK, eds. *Man in the Sea, vol 2.* San Pedro, CA: Best Publishing Co; 1990: 33–56.)

TABLE 25.2 Published Records for Breath-Hold Time

Conditions	BH time min:sec	Subject	Reference
Air	4:30	Subject SKH	13
	4:00	Student	14
Air, hyperventilation	4:11	Subject PM	15
	5:04	Subject EM	15
	5.09	Subject RM	15
Oxygen	6.29	Pouliquen	GBWR 1984
Oxygen, hyperventilation	13:00	Subject SKH	16
	13:48	Subject MT	16
	14:00	Subject HR	16
	15.13	Student	17
	20:05	Frechette	18
Oxygen, hyperventilation, total immersion in water	13:34	Foster	GBWR 1981

GBWR, Guinness Book of World Records.

Reproduced with permission from Lin YC, Hong SK. Hyperbaria: breath-hold diving. In: Fregly MJ, Blatteis CM, eds. *Handbook of Physiology, Section 4: Environmental Physiology, Vol 2.* New York: Oxford University; 1996:979–995; and Lin YC. Physiological limitations of humans as breath-hold divers. In: Lin YC, Shida KK, eds. *Man in the Sea, Vol 2.* San Pedro, CA: Best Publishing Co; 1990. p. 33–56.

at depth but P_{O_2} remains high. During ascent, P_{O_2} falls with the decreasing ambient pressure, and loss of consciousness often occurs before the diver reaches the surface. The Centers for Disease Control reported 3381 deaths from drowning in the United States in 2007, and drowning remains a leading cause of accidental death, ranked number 3 in all people up to 40 years of age. Approximately 1400 deaths from drowning occur during the active, adolescent, and young adult ages of 10 to 40 years, but accurate estimates of the incidence of shallow-water blackout in these cases are not available (www.cdc.gov). The danger of hyperventilating before engaging in underwater activity should be taught in all swimming and diving programs.

KEY POINT

After hyperventilation and BH diving, as a diver uses up O_2 at depth, and the delayed rise in alveolar carbon dioxide partial pressure (P_{ACO_2}) finally reaches a breathing stimulus level, the diver ascends. However, as the diver ascends, the P_{O_2} in the alveoli and arterial blood is reduced as a consequence of the reduced atmospheric pressure (shallower water), and the diver may simply lose consciousness before reaching the surface.

An exception to the general reactions of untrained human BH divers has been observed in highly experienced professional Japanese and Korean ama divers. In contrast to the responses of relatively untrained human subjects, further activation of diving bradycardia in ama divers is suppressed by exercise, and they have moderately higher heart rates during underwater exercise than during resting immersion (19). The explanation for these diverse results is not readily discernible. The ama divers may, through long underwater experience with apneic exercise, have become readapted for sustained circulatory support of exercising muscle, thus maintaining higher cardiovascular integrity compared with untrained divers.

TEST YOURSELF

The term *shallow-water blackout* correctly implies that the risk of blacking out during a prolonged breath-hold dive increases as the depth of the dive becomes shallower during ascent. Aside from the fact that usually this part of a dive occurs later in the BH, what other factor in the shallow water exacerbates the problem compared with deeper water?

Effects of Submersion on Cardiorespiratory Responses to Exercise

Whether a diver is performing a BH dive or using SCUBA, his or her body will become weightless in the water. This results in a shift of the blood from the legs into the thoracic cavity. Intuitively, this suggests that an increased preload probably exists and therefore results in alterations of exercise-induced cardiorespiratory responses (see also *Effects of Immersion* in Chapter 27). For instance, in a study by Christie et al. (20), when measured with the subject in the resting seated position during water immersion to the suprasternal notch, right atrial pressure increased 10.7 mm Hg, pulmonary arterial pressure increased 9.9 mm Hg, and the cardiac index and stroke index both increased >70% compared with similar measurements taken in the dry environment. Mean arterial pressure was not affected by immersion.

Christie and colleagues (20) performed these measurements in the same subjects at similar percentages of $\dot{V}_{O_{2max}}$ in both dry and immersed conditions, and noted that these determinations remained at a similar absolute difference despite increasing during exercise. For instance, the mean differences in pulmonary arterial pressure at rest between immersion and dry land were approximately 10 mm Hg, and this difference remained 10 mm Hg during exercise at 41%, 60%, 83%, and 100% of $\dot{V}_{O_{2max}}$, even though the exercise in both conditions caused increases in pulmonary arterial pressure. In this study, heart rates were similar at lower workloads performed during immersion compared with air, but at higher workloads and maximal exercise, heart rates were lower during immersion. Despite the reduced maximal heart rate during immersion, a similar $\dot{V}_{O_{2max}}$ was achieved in the two conditions of exercise. Similar results were reported more than 20 years earlier for subjects performing cycling exercise while completely submerged and breathing with a SCUBA. These results indicate that bradycardia occurs only at heavy workloads, but is accompanied by modest or no differences in $\dot{V}_{O_2}$ at heavy or maximal workloads. Despite reductions in maximal heart rate by approximately 10 beats per minute and ventilatory volume ($\dot{V}_E$) by 15 L $\cdot$ min^{-1} compared with the air environment, $\dot{V}_{O_{2max}}$ remains similar during exercise while the subject is submerged and breathing by SCUBA or during exercise performed during head-out immersion as tested by cycle exercise (21). The ability to deliver adequate supplies of oxygen to reach $\dot{V}_{O_{2max}}$ despite reduced heart rate and reduced $\dot{V}_E$ is apparently achieved by the increased cardiac output owing to the increased stoke volume. However, this reduction in heart rate during immersed exercise occurs only at high workloads, in contrast to BH diving, in which the relative heart rate is reduced by ≥30 beats per minute even at lower workloads (8).

KEY POINT

The state of immersion causes a reduction in heart rate relative to dry-land conditions at higher workloads (not at rest or low workloads). However, despite a reduced exercise-induced maximum heart rate, maximum oxygen consumption is not impaired, because of the increased stroke volume.

At greater depths, equivalent to 1600 FSW (22), $\dot{V}_E$ is greatly reduced in subjects exercising on a bicycle ergometer while breathing through a mouthpiece to about 50% relative to sea-level control values under similar conditions, and sensations of breathlessness seem to limit the performance of work at high oxygen consumption levels. For instance, three divers able to work with a $\dot{V}_{O_2}$ of >3 L · min^{-1} on a bicycle while submersed at 1 atm abs were able to work only at a $\dot{V}_{O_2}$ of 1.9 L · min^{-1} at 1600 FSW (22). This inability to perform work at high $\dot{V}_{O_2}$ requirements is apparently a consequence of the state of submersion and breathing through a mouthpiece, because similar exercise performed in the dry gas environment at similar pressures does not cause great reductions in $\dot{V}_{O_{2max}}$ (1).

Interactions of Water Submersion and Exercise, and their Effects on Thermal Balance

Heat is conducted from the human body about 25 times faster in water than in air, and the heat capacity of water (the product of density and specific heat) is about 3500 times greater than that of air. Because of these physical characteristics, human thermoregulatory mechanisms are incapable of preventing a decrease in internal body heat during prolonged cold-water exposure without additional insulation.

Divers can protect themselves against the cold by wearing thick underwear covered by a drysuit or a closed-cell foam-rubber wet suit. Drysuits usually provide satisfactory thermal protection for most cold-water diving, but they often limit the diver's mobility. Most contemporary divers who are engaged in BH or SCUBA diving protect themselves from cold-water stress by wearing a wet suit. However, as the closed-cell foam is compressed when hydrostatic pressure increases, it loses thickness, resulting in a loss of protection (23).

Effects of Water Submersion on Thermal Balance

Body temperature represents a balance between rates of metabolic heat production and heat dissipation. Heat loss in humans occurs mainly through the skin and partly through the respiratory tract. The range of ambient temperature in air between 28°C and 31°C is considered as the zone of vasomotor regulation of body temperature in an unclothed human; this is known as the thermoneutral zone. In water, the range of the thermoneutral zone is approximately 33°C to 35°C, which is much narrower than the range in air. *Tissue conductance* is a term used to describe the delivery of heat from the core to surface, and the reciprocal of conductance is defined as tissue insulation. The lowest value of the zone of vasomotor regulation is called the *critical temperature*, and in water is termed

the *critical water temperature*. Below these values, core temperature cannot be maintained in the normal range without an increase in metabolic heat production by shivering. However, the shivering markedly increases the convective heat loss in water because of body movements, leading to increases in conductance and total heat loss. The faster body heat loss in water is the dominant thermal problem for divers, and in fact it determines the duration of dive exposure.

The primary pathways of heat transfer from the body surface to the surrounding water are convection and conduction. The combined heat transfer coefficient for convection and conduction varies from 38 kcal · (m^2 · h · °C)$^{-1}$ in still water to an average of 55 kcal · (m^2 · h · °C)$^{-1}$ in stirred water. Shivering in still water raises the heat transfer coefficient considerably. According to Rapp (24), the conductive heat transfer coefficient is about 9 kcal · (m^2 · h · °C)$^{-1}$ regardless of the degree of stirring, whereas the convective heat transfer coefficient increases from 81 kcal · (m^2 · h · °C)$^{-1}$ in still water to 344 kcal · (m^2 · h · °C)$^{-1}$ at a swimming speed of 0.5 m · s^{-1}. These values are 100 to 200 times greater than those found in air (1–2 kcal · [m^2 · h · °C]$^{-1}$). Despite such marked differences in the convective heat transfer coefficient between air and water, the heat loss in water has been estimated to be only about two to five times greater than that in air at the same temperature. This indicates that heat loss in water is largely determined by core-to-skin tissue insulation.

The range of neutral water temperature for a resting, unprotected human is 33°C to 35°C, and it varies inversely with the thickness of the subcutaneous fat (25). The critical water temperature for humans is 29°C to 33°C, which is also inversely dependent on the thickness of subcutaneous fat (26). Because the water temperature in typical dives is lower than this neutral temperature range, divers are often exposed to cold-water stress.

Effects of Dynamic Exercise on Thermal Balance During Submersion

When the cold-water stress is moderate (water temperature 25°C–32°C), humans can maintain reasonable thermal equilibrium by increasing heat production with exercise. For instance, humans can maintain their normal body temperature in water of 32°C when they are engaged in continuous underwater work that doubles their resting oxygen consumption (2-MET exercise), and a 3-MET exercise keeps body temperature normal in water temperature at 26°C (27). However, when the water temperature falls below 24°C, heat loss becomes so great that it is virtually impossible to maintain thermal balance by an increased metabolic rate without the use of protective clothing. Thus, the core temperature of humans immersed in water is determined by several physical and physiologic factors, including the water temperature, intensity and type of exercise, subcutaneous fat thickness, ratio of surface area to mass, and duration of immersion (28).

TEST YOURSELF

Immersion in the upright position causes a redistribution of blood from the legs to the thorax. Theoretically, how might this response to immersion influence heat loss?

Effects of Exercise Intensity on Maintenance of Body Temperature during Cold-Water Submersion

Exercise accelerates the rate of heat loss from the body compared with that seen during rest in cold water. However, this does not necessarily reduce the core temperature. The intensity of exercise influences the core temperature's response to cold water immersion; in fact, the performance of heavy exercise during immersion in water of 17°C to 24°C can lessen the rate of decline of the core temperature as compared with that observed during static immersion. The type of exercise also plays a role in determining the core temperature's response to cold-water immersion. For instance, leg exercise is more effective than whole body exercise at maintaining the core body temperature in water of 18°C (29).

The exercise intensity required to keep the core body temperature within the physiologic range in water has been investigated over a range of exercise intensities and water temperatures. In a group of male subjects, Sagawa and associates (27) conducted experiments in which a 30-minute rest in water of various temperatures was followed by a series of graded leg exercises of 2 to 4 MET for 30 minutes. Four water temperatures were used: (a) 2°C below critical water temperature (29°C), (b) critical water temperature (31°C), (c) thermoneutrality (34°C), and (d) 2°C above thermoneutrality (36°C). Figure 25.2A illustrates the typical effects of leg exercise on the esophageal temperature at critical water temperature (31°C). During rest in water, esophageal temperature gradually decreased. During 30 minutes of exercise, however, esophageal temperature increased to a higher level than recorded after 30 minutes of rest in water, and the rise in core temperature depended on the exercise intensity.

The time course of cumulative heat storage is shown in Figure 25.2B, which reveals changes in body heat content during rest and exercise at different intensities in water of various temperatures. During 30 minutes of rest in thermoneutral water, cumulative heat storage remained near zero, whereas it increased in water above thermoneutrality and decreased in water below thermoneutrality. Leg exercise increased cumulative heat storage in proportion to the intensity at all water temperatures, indicating that heat production during underwater exercise exceeded heat loss into the water at these temperatures. After a 30-minute rest in water at critical temperature (31°C), negative heat storage occurred, but 30 minutes of work intensity at 4 MET returned the heat storage to the initial level. In contrast, heat storage did not return to the initial level (zero heat storage) even during the 4-MET exercise at 2°C below critical water temperature. Thus, leg exercise is effective at maintaining core temperature during cold-water exposure, and the effectiveness increases with increasing intensity of exercise. In practice, an exercise intensity of >200 kcal · m^2 · h^{-1} (about 4 MET) cannot last long in water, but this level of exercise intensity, as determined from several related exercise studies (27), can maintain body temperature in water at a temperature of about 25°C. Therefore, 25°C approaches the lowest water temperature in which an average unprotected person can continue to perform dynamic exercise without lowering the core temperature, and this water temperature can be defined as the crucial water temperature. Below this value, the body temperature continues to decrease even with continued exercise at an intensity of approximately 4 MET.

Summary

The increased heat production caused by exercise can maintain the core temperature in 25°C water at a maximal sustainable exercise intensity of 4 MET. Beyond this exercise level, the work cannot be sustained, and at lower water temperatures the heat production from the exercise cannot keep up with heat losses.

Tissue Insulation and Muscle Mass

Classically, a close inverse relationship has been observed between the fall in core temperature and the skinfold thickness of subjects during immersion (28). However, Veicsteinas and associates (30) suggested that during rest in cold water, the muscle acts in series with fat and skin to provide tissue insulation. Furthermore, the vasoconstricted muscle provides the major tissue insulation in the resting state. During swimming or severe shivering, the variable insulation of muscle will be lost because of increased blood perfusion through exercising muscle, leaving only the fixed insulation of the subcutaneous fat and skin. It thus seems that during static cold-water immersion one might expect the fall in core temperature to be more closely related to body weight (or muscle mass) than to subcutaneous fat thickness. On the other hand, during dynamic cold-water immersion, the variable insulation of muscle is reduced and the role of

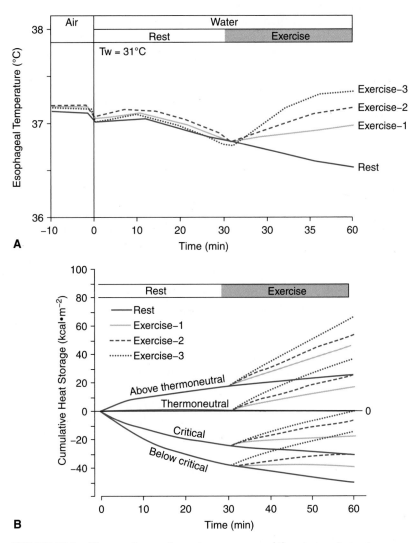

FIGURE 25.2 Changes in esophageal temperature (**A**) and cumulative heat storage (**B**) during underwater exercise at various work intensities. **A.** Typical time changes in core (esophageal) temperature at different work levels during immersion in water of critical temperature (31°C). Exercise 1, 2, and 3 refer to exercise intensity at 2, 3, and 4 MET, respectively. (Adapted from Shiraki K, Claybaugh JR. Effect of diving and hyperbaria on response to exercise. *Exerc Sport Sci Rev.* 1995;23:464, with permission of Lippincott Williams and Wilkins.) **B.** Average time course of cumulative heat storage during rest and the three different exercises in water of above thermoneutral (36°C), thermoneutral (34°C), critical (31°C), and below critical (29°C) temperatures. (Adapted with permission from Sagawa S, Shiraki K, Yousef MK, et al. Water temperature and intensity of exercise in maintenance of thermal equilibrium. *J Appl Physiol.* 1988;65:2416.)

subcutaneous fat becomes a more important factor in tissue insulation (30).

The results of limb exercise studies suggest that the arms are a significant source of heat loss during whole body exercise in cold water (27,29), and most swimming strokes require a high level of energy expenditure by the arms. Even at similar work levels, the arms, because of their smaller muscle mass, will receive higher blood flows per unit of weight than the legs. This will result in more circulatory delivery of heat to the arms. In other words, the arms have less ability than the legs to retain heat because the arms have approximately twice the ratio of surface area to mass of the legs, and the conductive pathway from the core to the surface of the limbs is shorter in the arms than in the legs.

Regional Heat Loss During Dynamic Exercise in Water

There are regional differences in tissue insulation during underwater exercise (27). Specifically, the trunk has less insulation than the limbs in water of cooler than critical temperature (29°C). This is probably because of a longer conduction pathway in the limbs, an enhanced counter-current heat exchange in the limbs, and/or the predominance of shivering in the trunk. On the other hand, during immersion in water of neutral (34°C) or warmer (36°C) temperature, limb insulation decreases more than that of the trunk, probably because of an attenuated counter-current heat exchange in the limbs. The results indicate that when water temperature is lower than thermoneutral (<34°C) but above critical temperature, leg exercise facilitates heat loss from the limbs by releasing vasoconstrictor tone in skin vessels. By contrast, dynamic exercise in water warmer than thermoneutral (36°C) causes trunk vasodilation and facilitates heat loss to the water. Exercise in water cooler than thermoneutral does not increase heat loss from the trunk as exercise intensity increases. If this observation applies to other dynamic immersions, one might expect exercise-generated heat to be preserved more efficiently in the trunk than in the limbs, and the trunk to maintain its maximum insulation during muscular exertion as well as at rest in cold water. Tissue insulation in the limbs, on the other hand, is high during rest but decreases as the intensity of leg exercise increases.

Summary

Several factors determine whether exercise during cold water immersion will accelerate or retard a decrease in core temperature. These factors include the water temperature, water agitation, the fitness (muscle mass) and fatness (subcutaneous fat thickness) of the individual, the type of clothing worn, and the intensity and type of dynamic exercise.

TEST YOURSELF

Given the preceding discussion, would a diver performing work underwater derive the most benefit from thermal protection of the torso or the limbs?

Thermal Balance in Wet-suited Divers and Effects of Pressure

The insulation of neoprene wet suits is provided by trapped air. Therefore, the volume of the trapped air, and thus the suit insulation, will be inversely proportional to the depth of immersion (hydrostatic pressure). The apparent suit insulation is reduced by approximately 45% at 2 atm abs (10 m sea water) and 52% at 2.5 atm abs (15 m) compared with the 1 atm abs (sea level) value (23). When the reciprocal relation of depth to insulation is extended to high pressure, suit insulation at 31 atm abs (300 m) during a saturation dive, for instance, would be almost negligible. Fortunately, however, this is not the case in a prolonged

helium–oxygen saturation dive, because the wet suit regains its original thickness in 24 hours by diffusion of environmental gas into the neoprene. During a typical SCUBA dive, suit insulation decreases curvilinearly as the diving depth increases, and the diver loses heat even in moderately cold water (23).

Park and associates (23) observed changes in the critical water temperature in subjects wearing wet suits at 2 and 2.5 atm abs in comparison with 1 atm abs, with the average critical water temperature of wet-suited subjects being 22°C, 26°C, and 28°C at 1, 2, and 2.5 atm abs, respectively. The reduction in wet suit insulation at pressure is exactly compensated for by an increase in the critical water temperature, such that the suit heat loss remains similar at different pressures, resulting in a similar degree of skin cooling when measured at critical water temperature. Consequently, the vasomotor control for transfer of internal heat loss at critical water temperature is identical at all pressures. These data indicate that the increase in the critical water temperature of wet-suited subjects at high pressure is most likely a simple consequence of changes in suit insulation, rather than alterations in the physiologic mechanisms that control body heat conservation. The available data on critical water temperature at depth are limited to a maximum pressure of 2.5 atm abs.

Another potentially critical problem associated with dives is related to heat loss from the respiratory tract. A diver who is engaged in heavy exercise and breathing cold gas (7°C) at 3 atm abs loses heat through the respiratory system, which represents 65% of metabolic heat production (31). The respiratory heat loss of a diver in cold water at depth can lead to a severe negative heat balance unless the breathing gas is heated.

TEST YOURSELF

If a saturation diver leaves a pressurized chamber and enters the water at 100 FSW, and another diver, equipped with the same wet suit for thermal protection, dives from the surface to a depth of 100 FSW, which diver will suffer the greatest loss of body heat?

Decompression Sickness

Work in the hyperbaric environment is not restricted to activities during immersion. Early applications of hyperbaric work began with the development of the first caisson in 1788 (32). The caisson was originally devised as a bell, open at the bottom, with air supplied to the top. This design allowed workers to remove silt and clay from river bottoms until bedrock could be located for the positioning of bridge piers. The first major caisson project in the United States was the Eads Bridge over the Mississippi River in St. Louis, Missouri, which was completed in 1874. The caisson builders worked at a depth of 112 feet, and decompression sickness had not yet been defined. Of the 352 workers employed, 13 died and 30 others were seriously injured. Similar incidences during the construction of the Brooklyn Bridge led to the use of the words "bends" and "bent," reflecting the bent-over posture that caisson workers developed from the effects of decompression sickness. With the advent of more sophisticated underwater breathing support for free swimming workers, fewer cases of decompression sickness in hyperbaric conditions have been reported. The neurologic damage caused by decompression likely results from the formation of gas bubbles in the brain and spinal tissues.

General Concepts Regarding Bubble Formation upon Decompression

The formation of gas bubbles during decompression depends on two major factors (33). The first is a requirement for supersaturation of a gas in a fluid, such that the pressure of the gas in the fluid plus the vapor pressure of the gas exceeds the atmospheric pressure. It is possible for supersaturation to occur without bubble formation. Other factors, therefore, contribute to the process of bubble formation, and the second major factor is the presence of pre-existing gas nuclei in solution because of surface tension. As decompression proceeds and supersaturation becomes greater, bubbles from the gas nuclei form. Thus, theoretical approaches to prevent bubble formation include limiting the supersaturation by slow decompression rates and reducing the number of gas nuclei. For example, several *in vitro* and animal experiments (33) have demonstrated that prior compression can remove gas nuclei and hence reduce bubble formation upon decompression.

KEY POINT

Approaches to prevent decompression sickness, or the bends, focus on limiting supersaturation by slow decompression rates and reducing the number of gas nuclei.

Caisson work, which is also used in tunnel construction, continues today with improvements in safety owing to scheduled decompressions that allow more time for gas elimination from the body and the use of oxygen during decompression. Sometimes oxygen is substituted for nitrogen because it can be eliminated from the body by metabolism to carbon dioxide. This metabolism converts the relatively insoluble oxygen into carbon dioxide that is 21 times more soluble and therefore less likely to come out of solution to form bubbles. The inert nitrogen can be eliminated only by diffusion down a concentration gradient, and therefore it is a slower process than the elimination of oxygen (33). With these added precautions in more recent projects, the reported rate of decompression illness is about 1.5%, based on the number of workers affected seriously enough to report for treatment. The greatest practical

pressure that is used in compressed air work is about 4.4 atm abs (445 kPa), about the depth of the Eads Bridge piers, because slightly beyond this pressure, mixed gases become necessary and the cost becomes prohibitive.

TEST YOURSELF

The previous discussion dealt with the logic of increasing O_2 partial pressure during ascent from saturation dives to reduce the incidence of bubble formation and the bends. By what mechanism is this procedure proposed to work?

Exercise and Decompression Sickness

Generally held concepts regarding exercise and bubble formation resulting from decompression involve the understanding that exercise at depth will increase blood flow and consequently nitrogen uptake. With more nitrogen in the body, the time required to unload the additional nitrogen will be greater. Studies have shown, for instance, that more nitrogen is eliminated from a person at sea level after a dive in which exercise was performed at depth compared with a dive without exercise (34). This observation is in agreement with the finding that more bubbles are detected when subjects exercise during or immediately after decompression, and the intravascular bubbles impede the elimination of inert gases. An analysis of previous reports led to the conclusion that dynamic exercise performed either before or during exposure to pressure increases the risk of decompression sickness (33).

Such impressions led to conclusions that otherwise unexplainable cases of decompression sickness may have been due to heavy exercise performed before an incident. On the other hand, more recent reports indicated that when moderate arm or leg exercise was performed during decompression, Doppler-detected gas emboli were reduced by >50% at all body sites monitored (35). Doppler-detected gas emboli in the venous circulation (*i.e.*, venous gas emboli) can be detected in subjects lacking symptoms of decompression sickness. Furthermore, these circulating gas emboli are not believed to cause decompression sickness, which is most likely caused by the formation of bubbles in the tissues. Thus, there is no direct correlation between the detection of venous gas emboli and decompression sickness, but high incidence rates of venous gas emboli are associated with a significant probability of developing decompression sickness (35). The potential beneficial effects of dynamic exercise during decompression are similarly thought to be a result of increased blood flow, but in this case cause increased gas elimination. Therefore, the timing of exercise performed at depth and the intensity of the exercise become critical factors in determining whether the effects are harmful or beneficial.

Recently, a new theory regarding exercise and decompression sickness was proposed by a research group in Norway (36,37). Studies conducted in rats showed that bubble formation and death from decompression could be prevented by exercise 20 hours before a dive to 7 atm abs. This beneficial effect did not occur if the exercise was performed too close to the dive time (*e.g.*, within 10 h) or too much in advance of the dive time (*e.g.*, 48 h before) (37). The authors proposed a mechanism whereby exercise-induced suppression of bubble formation is related to nitric oxide production, which may reduce the number of gas nuclei. In an earlier study, they showed that nitric oxide inhibition exacerbated the occurrence of decompression sickness in this animal model (38). They then demonstrated that administration of a nitric oxide–releasing agent reduced bubble formation (37). However, this could be demonstrated when the nitric oxide was given just 30 minutes before hyperbaric exposure. Thus, the timing of the responses between exercise and nitric oxide administration were quite different, suggesting that the mechanism of the exercise response may not be resolved.

Perhaps most interesting is their subsequent report that dynamic exercise performed in human subjects 24 hours before a dive to 2.8 atm abs reduced venous gas emboli by 78% (36). The exercise involved treadmill running at 90% of maximum heart rate for 3 minutes followed by running at 50% of maximum heart rate for 2 minutes. This series was repeated eight times. It is not clear why dynamic exercise, performed only within a window of time near 24 hours before a dive, can produce the effect if the mechanism is linked to a nitric oxide–dependent reduction in bubble nuclei. Whether the exercise-dependent reduction of bubble formation operates through the formation of nitric oxide, as the authors hypothesized, or through another mechanism, these studies provide new avenues for ameliorating the formation of bubbles upon decompression in humans. Further standardization and study of the contribution of this effect is necessary before it can be widely used as a predictable safeguard against decompression sickness.

Summary

The incidence of decompression illness has decreased dramatically since it was first discovered. This is primarily due to our understanding that this illness is caused by a state of supersaturation of nitrogen in the body tissues that develops when a person breathes air in a high atmospheric pressure and then subsequently moves to a lesser pressure. The dissolved nitrogen will form bubbles around preexisting nuclei if the decompression occurs too rapidly, similar to a carbonated beverage. Thus, slow decompression in proportion to the time spent at pressure and the magnitude of pressure has been the key factor in reducing the incidence of decompression illness. In addition, substituting O_2 for N_2 will reduce the N_2 concentration and the likelihood of bubble formation because O_2 is cleared more rapidly than N_2. Lastly, a reduction in the number of preexisting bubble nuclei, through specific regimens of exercise or other maneuvers, may further reduce the incidence of bubble formation.

Breath-Hold Divers and Decompression Sickness

There is a persistent question about whether BH divers may under some circumstances be susceptible to the bends. Little information about this issue is available, and the most direct evidence comes from an experiment conducted by a Danish submarine officer to test the potential for inert gas accumulation precipitated by an enforced severe bout of frequent and deep BH diving. In this experiment, the officer performed 60 20-minute apneic dives over a period of 5 hours, with only brief intervals at the surface. At the conclusion of the diving bout, he had incipient decompression symptoms. He promptly recovered after being placed in a recompression chamber, which verified that he had indeed experienced decompression sickness (39). The extreme circumstances of this experiment are noteworthy, and it seems clear that ordinarily benign apneic diving is unlikely to impose a hazard of inert gas sequestration.

Exercise in a Dry Hyperbaric Environment

When humans encounter increased atmospheric pressure in the air (approximately 80% nitrogen and 20% oxygen), several factors with a bearing on exercise performance immediately change. First, the density of the air increases. At 33 FSW (2 atm abs), the gas is twice as dense as at sea level. With increasing gas density, the resistance to breathing increases and the work involved in breathing increases. Second, the P_{O_2} increases. Studies conducted nearly eight decades ago by Hill and associates (40) demonstrated that breathing 50% oxygen could increase $\dot{V}_{O_{2max}}$. One might expect, therefore, that the increased P_{O_2} at hyperbaria could also result in an increased $\dot{V}_{O_{2max}}$. Third, the heart rate decreases (41,42).

Effects of Compressed Gas Environments on Cardiorespiratory Responses to Exercise

Many studies have shown that an increase in environmental gas pressure greatly reduces the maximum voluntary ventilation. This is evident even at pressures of 3 atm abs (approximately 66 FSW). Of particular importance is the demonstration by Maio and Fahri (43) that altering the density of the gas could duplicate the changes in maximum voluntary ventilation observed at high pressure. The authors were able to demonstrate sequentially greater decrements in maximum voluntary ventilation with increasing gas density by replacing the nitrogen in air with helium or sulfur hexafluoride to achieve breathing gas densities that were approximately one-third and four times the density of air, respectively.

The increase in breathing resistance caused by the increased gas density also contributes to a predictable decrease in maximum $\dot{V}E$. Fagraeus (44) studied maximal exercise in subjects in compressed-air environments ranging from 1 to 6 atm abs (Fig. 25.3).

With increasing pressures, $\dot{V}O_{2max}$ decreased but $\dot{V}O_{2max}$ was not greatly affected. It can be seen in the figure that $\dot{V}O_{2max}$ was actually enhanced at 1.4 atm abs compared with 1 atm abs in the air. This confirms the observation that at least in some instances, a small increase in $\dot{V}O_{2max}$ can be achieved by breathing higher concentrations of oxygen (Table 25.3). At higher pressures of air, however, these workers and others reported no increase in $\dot{V}O_{2max}$. Thus, it can be seen from Figure 26.3 that reductions in $\dot{V}E_{max}$ by >40% can still be accompanied by only modestly reduced $\dot{V}O_{2max}$ values. Also, it can be seen that the reduction in ventilation is accompanied by a significant increase in P_{ACO_2}. This decrease in $\dot{V}E$ associated with exercise is not only evident during maximum efforts (Table 25.3); it is also uniformly reported at submaximal workloads and at pressures ranging from 2 atm abs to 66 atm abs.

The reduction in $\dot{V}E$ is a consequence of both increased airway resistance caused by the increased gas density, and a reduced ventilatory drive caused by increased pressure and gas density in response to carbon dioxide (45,46). For instance, Lambertsen and associates (45) demonstrated a slowing of the incremental increase in respiration in response to increased carbon dioxide produced by rebreathing expired carbon dioxide while maintaining inspired oxygen constant. They tested rebreathing at increasing gas densities up to the equivalent of 5000 FSW in the helium–oxygen environment, 25 times the density at sea level. This was accomplished by substituting neon as the inert gas in a chamber pressurized to 1200 FSW. Through these experiments it was observed that maximum voluntary ventilation decreased rather steeply up to gas densities equivalent to about 2000 FSW in a helium–oxygen environment and then leveled off at a decrement of about 60%. On the other hand, the $\dot{V}E$ at about 80% $\dot{V}O_{2max}$ steadily decreased, reaching an 80% decrement at the gas

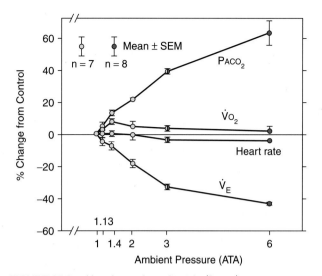

FIGURE 25.3 Alveolar carbon dioxide (P_{ACO_2}), oxygen consumption ($\dot{V}O_2$), heart rate, and expiratory volume ($\dot{V}E$) responses to maximal exercise at different pressures in a dry compressed-air environment. SEM, standard error of the mean; ATA, atmosphere absolute. (Modified with permission from Fagraeus L. Cardiorespiratory and metabolic functions during exercise in the hyperbaric environment. *Acta Physiol Scand Suppl.* 1974;414:20.)

densities equivalent to 5000 FSW in the helium–oxygen environment. Thus, they constructed a "predicted work load maximum" at which maximum voluntary ventilation equals $\dot{V}E$ at maximum $\dot{V}O_2$. In their experiments on two subjects, this point would be reached at 5000 FSW in the helium–oxygen environment. These two subjects were able to exercise for 4 minutes of a scheduled 6-minute bout before voluntarily stopping. The P_{ACO_2} was approximately 60 mm Hg and was not considered limiting; instead, it was believed that $\dot{V}E$ had been reduced to maximum voluntary ventilation and the oxygen demand could not be met.

TABLE 25.3	Exercise-Induced Changes in Heart Rate, Expiratory Volume, and Oxygen Consumption at Maximal Exercise					
Total pressure ATA	P_{O_2} (ATA)	Density (g · L^{-1})	ΔHR_{max} (%)	$\Delta \dot{V}E_{max}$ (%)	$\Delta \dot{V}O_{2max}$ (%)	Reference
1.4 (air)	0.28	1.5	$\times$	↓7	↑11	44
3 (air)	0.60	3.3	↓3	↓33	$\times$	44
3 (He-O$_2$)	0.60	1.08	↓<3	↓14	↑13	44
6 (air)	1.20	7.2	↓5	↓46	$\times$	44
18.6 (He-O$_2$)	0.30	3.8	↓4	↓26	↑3	50
18.6 (He-O$_2$)	0.21	2.8	↓4	↓21	$\times$	50
31 (He-O$_2$)	0.40	7.3	↓9	↓45	↓13	46
37 (He-N$_2$-O$_2$)	0.50	9.2	↓7	↓41	↓10	47
47–66 (He-N$_2$-O$_2$)	0.50	12.3–17.1	↓4	↓16	↓13	1

Intensities in dry pressurized environments of various gas mixtures and densities.

ΔHR_{max}, change in maximal heart rate; $\Delta \dot{V}E_{max}$, change in maximal expiratory volume; $\Delta \dot{V}O_{2max}$, change in maximal oxygen consumption.

Summary

Increased atmospheric pressure causes an increase in gas density, which has been shown to cause a reduction in $\dot{V}E$. Most deep-saturation divers use helium as the inert gas because of its low density and non-narcotic effects. In these predictive studies, neon was used as the inert gas in a simulated dive to 1200 FSW, mimicking the gas density that a helium–oxygen environment would have at 5000 FSW. At this density, the maximum ventilation accompanying maximum exercise is similar to maximum voluntary ventilation and is therefore a limiting factor in the achievement of maximum oxygen consumption.

Surprisingly, even at these extreme environmental gas densities, the subjects were able to exercise at 80% of their sea-level maximums with no reports of dyspnea. Although no studies have been performed at such extreme depths, in one study, maximum exercise was performed at 37.5 atm abs (equivalent to slightly greater than 1200 FSW) with no evidence of dyspnea despite a 30% reduction in $\dot{V}E$, and nearly sea-level values for $\dot{V}O_{2max}$ were achieved (46). Similarly, Salzano and associates (1) reported dyspnea as a "rare occurrence" at nearly maximum workloads performed by subjects at >2000 FSW. Thus, predictive experiments and direct observations indicate that relatively similar levels of exertion can be performed at hyperbaria with negligible respiratory consequences. However, this interpretation must be considered with caution because, as mentioned earlier in this chapter, at moderate workloads at 1600 FSW, other investigators observed dyspnea that severely limited exercise performance in upright subjects breathing through a mouthpiece during submersion (22). These and similar reports suggest an effect of submersion and/or a need to optimize the equilibration pressure of the breathing apparatus; however, this issue remains unresolved.

TEST YOURSELF

In the studies by Fagraeus (44), men performed maximal exercise in compressed air environments at pressures ranging from 1 to 6 atm abs. The maximal ventilation decreased by approximately 40% at 6 atm abs compared with the values at 1 atm abs. How were the responses of P_{ACO_2} and $\dot{V}O_{2max}$ affected by the environmental pressure of 6 atm abs?

Effects of Compressed Gas Environments on Water Balance and Hormonal Responses to Dynamic Exercise

The increased gas density at hyperbaria also decreases insensible water loss that is not accompanied by a decrease in water intake. Thus, the accumulation of free water must be voided in the urine. This seems to be accomplished by a chronic reduction in circulating arginine vasopressin (AVP), which is accompanied by the production of about an additional 200 to 500 mL of relatively dilute urine per day (41). This new setpoint for the homeostatic regulation of fluid and electrolytes would be expected to alter the hormonal and renal responses to exercise. To date, this possibility has been investigated in only one study (47). At sea level, maximal dynamic exercise is invariably accompanied by severalfold increases in levels of AVP, atrial natriuretic peptide, renin, and aldosterone (48). In addition, for reasons that are unclear, urine osmolality decreases during exercise despite the increase in plasma AVP concentration and plasma osmolality. In contrast, the AVP and atrial natriuretic peptide responses to maximal dynamic exercise are greatly blunted, whereas the renin and aldosterone responses are unaffected in the hyperbaric environment at 37 atm abs (47). Despite the greatly reduced rise in plasma AVP, maximal and submaximal exercise was associated with increases in urine osmolality and a decrease in urine flow in hyperbaria. An explanation for the blunted AVP response is not readily apparent. It seems likely that the decreased insensible water loss associated with the hyperbaric environment may result in a slight state of hyperhydration. This could lead to small reductions in plasma osmolality that may contribute to the significant decrease in the resting plasma AVP. However, a state of hyperhydration would not be expected to blunt the atrial naturetic factor response. Such a response is more expected with dehydration, which is in better agreement with the increased hematocrit and decreased plasma volume observed in other studies (41). Thus, the blunted AVP response to dynamic exercise at hyperbaria is probably a result of other factors in addition to plasma osmolality.

TEST YOURSELF

The classic "chicken and egg" dilemma is at the core of the AVP and drinking response to hyperbaria (i.e., is the increased drinking relative to the state of hydration causal or in response to the reduced AVP observed in hyperbaria?) Given complete freedom and money to design an experiment, how might you resolve this issue?

Hyperbaric Bradycardia

As mentioned above, heart rate is reduced during exercise associated with breath holding, face immersion, and head-out immersion. The dry hyperbaric environment is also accompanied by a slight decrease in heart rate but apparently driven by different mechanisms (31,42). Consequently, when exercise is performed at hyperbaria, the heart rate at any given workload and at all pressures studied is reduced relative to 1 atm abs values (Fig. 25.4).

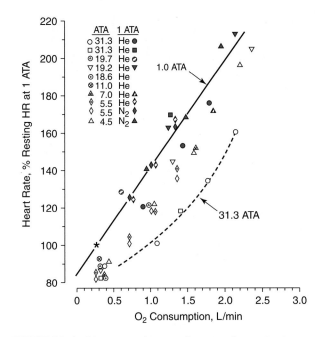

FIGURE 25.4 Heart rate during submaximal exercise in hyperbaric environments. ATA, atmospheres absolute; HR, heart rate. (The data for this figure are based on multiple sources cited in the original publication. Redrawn with permission from Lin YC, Shida KK. Brief review: mechanisms of hyperbaric bradycardia. *Chinese J Physiol.* 1988;31:5.)

However, as noted earlier, the effects on oxygen consumption and the ability to perform work do not appear to be greatly affected. There appear to be several reasons for this so-called hyperbaric bradycardia, the most obvious of which is the increase in oxygen concentration. Breathing increased concentrations of oxygen will reduce the heart rate by a combination of vasoconstriction, increased vagal tone, and decreased sympathetic activity via baroreceptor and chemoreceptor input (41,42). Experimental data support such responses in hyperbaria. For instance, significantly reduced basal plasma norepinephrine (15%) and muscle sympathetic nerve activity (60%) were shown in a study comparing human subjects at 3 atm abs in compressed air with subjects at 1 atm abs. In addition, the baroreceptor stimulation of

these measurements, as assessed by lower body negative pressure applications, were blunted in the hyperbaric environment (49). However, when oxygen concentration was held constant by breathing 100% oxygen at 1 atm abs and breathing normal air at 4.5 atm abs, Fagraeus (44) observed greater bradycardia at pressure. Also, if normoxia was maintained between 1 atm abs and 18.6 atm abs, maximal exercise at hyperbaria was accompanied by 4% bradycardia (50). Thus, hyperoxia is not the only factor that causes bradycardia. Another factor that can be shown to reduce the heart rate response to exercise, independently of oxygen, is an increase in the partial pressure of nitrogen. However, hyperbaric bradycardia is also observed in a helium–oxygen hyperbaric environment with nitrogen essentially absent. Therefore, factors other than hyperoxia and increased nitrogen reduce heart rate in the hyperbaric environment; however, these factors remain to be identified.

CHAPTER SUMMARY

Exercise in the hyperbaric environment is never a unifactorial effect of high pressure on the human physiologic response to dynamic exercise. In fact, that single effect (if it exists) is difficult to identify and perhaps meaningless, since it is invariably commingled with other, more profound factors such as breath holding, immersion, cold exposure, and gas density. For the most part, these effects on exercise have been shown to be unaffected by different ambient pressures. For instance, we have discussed evidence for increasing ambient pressure up to 2.5 atm abs with no effects on critical temperature and duplication of ventilatory effects of hyperbaria by changing gas density with no changes in atmospheric pressure. Finally, when physical barriers are minimized, humans can perform at near-maximal intensities even at pressures of 66 atm abs or depths greater than 2000 FSW. This performance most likely does not represent a limit of pressure tolerance, but rather a limit due to practical considerations as well as to a lack of need for humans at these great depths because robots and highly manageable submarines have been developed for these purposes.

A MILESTONE OF DISCOVERY

In the late 1970s, it was not clear whether humans could safely perform strenuous work at extreme pressures. Predictive studies had shown that moderate work up to 80% of $\dot{V}_{O_{2max}}$ at sea level could be performed with no severe dyspnea in dry hyperbaric environments at gas densities equivalent to 5000 FSW in a helium–oxygen environment. Thus, it was concluded that breathing limitations pose no significant barrier to the performance of fairly intense exercise at gas densities 22 times greater than those found at sea level. However, when moderate

work was performed during submersion at 1600 FSW, severe dyspnea was encountered. This raised the question of whether gas density is the single limiting feature in breathing during exercise at extreme hyperbaria or if high pressure has an effect in addition to gas density. Alternatively, the disparate results could be attributable to the submersed state.

At the same time, others explored the utility of adding some nitrogen (5%–10% of total gases) to the helium–oxygen gas mixture, a mixture called trimix, as a means of reducing high-pressure nervous syndrome associated with compression to depths of >1000 FSW. Trimix provided a means of safely placing divers at a greater depth, up to 2250 FSW, but at the same time increased gas density and therefore raised additional questions regarding the effect of trimix on exercise performance at high pressure.

As shown in Figure 25.5, through a series of dry-saturation dives, Salzano and associates [1] studied exercise-induced changes in cardiorespiratory measurements at rest and work rates of 360, 720, 1080, and 1440 kpm · min⁻¹, at gas densities of 1.1 g · L⁻¹ (air with 50% oxygen), 10.1 g · L⁻¹ (trimix with 5% nitrogen at 47 atm abs), 12.3 g · L⁻¹ (trimix with 10% nitrogen at 47 atm abs), and 17.1 g · L⁻¹ (trimix with 10% nitrogen at 66 atm abs).

A work rate of 1080 kpm · min⁻¹ produced oxygen consumption of 75% to 92% of sea-level maximum for four individuals. The fifth subject was able to perform work at 1440 kpm · min⁻¹ at approximately 80% of sea level $\dot{V}O_{2max}$ at 66 atm abs.

Two decades later, these experiments represent the most extreme environmental pressures under which exercise responses have been studied in humans. They demonstrated that work performed at 360 kpm · min⁻¹ at approximately three to four times resting $\dot{V}O_2$ results in essentially the same physiologic responses found at sea level. Also, greater workloads could be achieved, with most individuals able to perform work at about 80% of their sea-level $\dot{V}O_{2max}$ at pressures of 47 atm abs, and one subject able to do so at 66 atm abs.

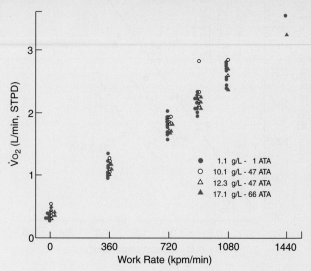

FIGURE 25.5 Cardiorespiratory responses to exercise at 47 and 66 ATA (atmospheres absolute) by five subjects at different work rates and gas densities. Each symbol represents one exercise session among five subjects. STPD, standard temperature and pressure, dry. (Redrawn with permission from Salzano JV, Comporesi EM, Stolp BW, et al. Physiological responses to exercise at 47 and 66 ATA. *J Appl Physiol.* 1984;57:1060.)

Salzano JV, Camporesi EM, Stolp BW, et al. Physiological responses to exercise at 47 and 66 ATA. J Appl Physiol. 1984;57:1055–1068.

ACKNOWLEDGMENT

The views expressed in this chapter are those of the authors and do not reflect the official policy or position of the Department of the Army, Department of Defense, or the United States government.

REFERENCES

1. Salzano JV, Comporesi EM, Stolp BW, et al. Physiological responses to exercise at 47 and 66 ATA. *J Appl Physiol.* 1984;57:1055–1068.
2. Elsner R, Gooden B. Diving and asphyxia: a comparative study of animals and man. Monographs of the Physiological Society, No. 40. Cambridge: Cambridge University; 1983:168–189.
3. Elsner R. Living in water: solutions to physiological problems. In: Reynolds JE, Rommel SA, eds. *Biology of Marine Mammals.* Washington, DC: Smithsonian Institution; 1999:73–116.
4. Mohri M, Torii R, Nagaya K, et al. Diving patterns of Ama divers of Hegura Island, Japan. *Undersea Biomed Res.* 1995;22:137–143.
5. Lin YC, Hong SK. Hyperbaria: breath-hold diving. In: Fregly MJ, Blatteis CM, eds. *Handbook of Physiology, Section 4: Environmental Physiology, Vol 2.* New York: Oxford University; 1996:979–995.
6. Elsner R, Gooden BA, Robinson SM. Arterial blood gas changes and the diving response in man. *Aust J Exp Biol Med Sci.* 1971:435–444.
7. Andersson JP, Linér MH, Runow E, et al. Diving response and arterial oxygen saturation during apnea and exercise in breath-hold divers. *J Appl Physiol.* 2002;93:882–886.
8. Butler PJ, Woakes AJ. Heart rate of humans during underwater swimming with and without breath-hold. *Resp Physiol.* 1987;69:387–399.
9. Strømme SB, Kerem D, Elsner R. Diving bradycardia during rest and exercise and its relation to physical fitness. *J Appl Physiol.* 1970;28:614–621.
10. Jung K, Stolle W. Behavior of heart rate and incidence of arrhythmia in swimming and diving. *Biotelem Pat Monit.* 1981;8:228–239.
11. Lin YC. Physiological limitations of humans as breath-hold divers. In: Lin YC, Shida KK, eds. *Man in the Sea, vol 2.* San Pedro, CA: Best Publishing Co; 1990:33–56.
12. Arnold RW. Extremes in human breath hold, facial immersion bradycardia. *Undersea Biomed Res.* 1985;12:183–190.
13. Hong SK, Rahn H. The diving women of Korea and Japan. *Sci Am.* 1967;216:34–43.
14. Hong SK, Rahn H, Kang DH, et al. Diving pattern, lung volumes, and alveolar gas of the Korean diving women (ama). *J Appl Physiol.* 1963;18:457–465.
15. Ferrigno M, Grassi B, Ferretti G, et al. Electrocardiogram during deep breath-hold dives by elite divers. *Undersea Biomed Sci.* 1991; 18:81–91.
16. Klocke FJ, Rahn H. Breath-holding after breathing of oxygen. *J Appl Physiol.* 1959;14:689–693.

17. Schneider EC. Respiration at high altitude. *Yale J Biol Med.* 1932;4:537–550.

18. Mithoefer JC. The breaking point of breath holding. In: Rahn H, Yokoyama T, eds. *Physiology of Breath-Hold Diving and the Ama of Japan.* Washington, DC: NAS-NRC Publication; 1965:195–205.

19. Shiraki K, Elsner R, Sagawa S, et al. Heart rate of Japanese male ama divers during breath-hold dives: diving bradycardia or exercise tachycardia? *Undersea Hyperbaric Med.* 2002;29:59–62.

20. Christie JL, Sheldahl LM, Tristani FE, et al. Cardiovascular regulation during head-out water immersion exercise. *J Appl Physiol.* 1990;69:657–664.

21. Dressendorfer RH, Morlock JF, Baker DG, et al. Effects of head-out water immersion on cardiorespiratory responses to maximal cycling exercise. *Undersea Biomed Res.* 1976;3:177–87.

22. Spaur WH, Raymond LW, Knott MM, et al. Dyspnea in divers at 49.5 Atm Abs; mechanical, not chemical in origin. *Undersea Biomed Res.* 1977;4:183–198.

23. Park YH, Iwamoto J, Tajima F, et al. Effect of pressure on thermal insulation in humans wearing wet suits. *J Appl Physiol.* 1988;64:1916–1922.

24. Rapp GM. Convection coefficients of man in a forensic area of thermal physiology: heat transfer in underwater exercise. *J Physiol (Paris).* 1971;63:392–396.

25. Craig Jr AB, Dvorak M. Thermal regulation during water immersion. *J Appl Physiol.* 1966;21:1577–1585.

26. Rennie DW. Thermal insulation of Korean diving women and non-divers in water. In: Rahn H, Yokoyama T, eds. *Physiology of Breath-Hold Diving and the Ama of Japan.* Washington, DC: National Academy of Science National Research Council; 1965. p. 315–24.

27. Sagawa S, Shiraki K, Yousef MK, et al. Water temperature and intensity of exercise in maintenance of thermal equilibrium. *J Appl Physiol.* 1988;65:2413–2429.

28. Craig AB Jr, Dvorak M. Thermal regulation of man exercising during water immersion. *J Appl Physiol.* 1968;25:28–35.

29. Toner MM, Sawka MN, Pandolf KB. Thermal responses during arm and leg and combined arm-leg exercise in water. *J Appl Physiol.* 1984;56:1355–60.

30. Veicsteinas A, Ferretti G, Rennie DW. Superficial shell insulation in resting and exercising men in cold water. *J Appl Physiol.* 1982;52:1557–1564.

31. Shiraki K, Claybaugh JR. Effects of diving and hyperbaria on responses to exercise. *Exerc Sport Sci Rev.* 1995;23:459–485.

32. Kindwall EP. Compressed air work. In: Bennett PB, Elliott DH, eds. *The Physiology and Medicine of Diving.* 4th ed. Philadelphia: Saunders; 1993:1–18.

33. Vann RD, Thalmann ED. Decompression physiology and practice. In: Bennett PB, Elliott DH, eds. *The Physiology and Medicine of Diving.* 4th ed. Philadelphia: Saunders; 1993:376–432.

34. Dick APK, Vann RD, Mebane GY, et al. Decompression induced nitrogen elimination. *Undersea Biomed Res.* 1984;11:369–380.

35. Jankowski LW, Nishi RY, Eaton DJ, et al. Exercise during decompression reduces the amount of venous gas emboli. *Undersea Hyperbaric Med.* 1997;24:59–65.

36. Dujic' Z, Duplanc˘ic' D, Marinovic'-Terzic' I, et al. Aerobic exercise before diving reduces venous gas bubble formation in humans. *J Physiol (Lond).* 2004;555:637–642.

37. Wisløff U, Richardson RS, Brubakk AO. NOS inhibition increases bubble formation and reduces survival in sedentary but not exercised rats. *J Physiol (Lond).* 2003;546:577–582.

38. Wisløff U, Richardson RS, Brubakk AO. Exercise and nitric oxide prevent bubble formation: a novel approach to the prevention of decompression sickness? *J Physiol (Lond).* 2004;555:825–829.

39. Paulev P. Decompression sickness following repeated breath-hold dives. *J Appl Physiol.* 1965;20:1028–1031.

40. Hill AV, Long CNH, Lupton H. Muscular exercise, lactic acid, and the supply and utilization of oxygen. Parts VII and VIII. *Proc R Soc Edinb B Biol.* 1924;97:155–176.

41. Hong SK, Bennett PB, Shiraki K, et al. Mixed-gas saturation diving, part V: the hyperbaric environment. In: Blatteis CM, Fregley MJ, eds. *Handbook of Physiology, Section 4: Adaptation to the Environment.* New York: Oxford University; 1995:1023–1045.

42. Lin YC, Shida KK. Brief review: mechanisms of hyperbaric bradycardia. *Chinese J Physiol.* 1988;31:1–22.

43. Maio DA, Fahri LE. Effect of gas density on mechanics of breathing. *J Appl Physiol.* 1967;23:687–693.

44. Fagraeus L. Cardiorespiratory and metabolic functions during exercise in the hyperbaric environment. *Acta Physiol Scand Suppl.* 1974;414:5–40.

45. Lambertsen CJ, Gelfand R, Peterson R, et al. Human tolerance to He, Ne, and N2 at respiratory gas densities equivalent to He-O$_2$ breathing at 1200, 2000, 3000, 4000 and 5000 feet of sea water (predictive studies III). *Aviat Space Environ Med.* 1977;48:843–855.

46. Ohta Y, Arita H, Nakayama H, et al. Cardiopulmonary functions and maximal aerobic power during a 14-day saturation dive at 31 ATA (Seadragon IV). In: Bachrach AJ, Matzen MM, eds. *Underwater Physiology VII: Proceedings of the VII Symposium on Underwater Physiology.* Bethesda, MD: Undersea Medical Society; 1981:209–221.

47. Claybaugh JR, Freund BJ, Luther G, et al. Renal and hormonal responses to exercise in man at 46 and 37 atmospheres absolute pressure. *Aviat Space Environ Med.* 1997;68:1038–1045.

48. Freund BJ, Shizuru EM, Hashiro GM, et al. The hormonal, electrolyte, and renal responses to exercise are intensity dependent. *J Appl Physiol.* 1991;70:900–906.

49. Yamauchi K, Tsutsui Y, Endo Y, et al. Sympathetic nervous and hemodynamic responses to lower body negative pressure in hyperbaria in men. *Am J Physiol.* 2002;282:R38–R45.

50. Dressendorfer RH, Hong SK, Morlock JF, et al. Hana Kai II: a 17-day dry saturation dive at 18.6 ATA. V. Maximal oxygen uptake. *Undersea Biomed Res.* 1977;4:283–296.

CHAPTER 26

Physiologic Systems and Their Responses to Conditions of Microgravity and Bed Rest

Suzanne M. Schneider and Victor A. Convertino

Abbreviations

$a\text{-}vO_{2diff}$	The difference in oxygen content between arterial and venous blood	ISS	International Space Station
BMD	Bone mineral density	SLS-1, SLS-2	Space Life Sciences missions 1 and 2
BR	Bed rest	$\dot{V}A/\dot{Q}$	Ventilation-perfusion matching
EVA	Extravehicular activity	$\dot{V}O_2$	Oxygen uptake
HR_{max}	Maximal heart rate	$\dot{V}O_{2max}$	Maximal oxygen uptake
		$\dot{V}O_2pk$	Peak oxygen consumption

Introduction

When Columbus set sail for the New World, skeptics predicted that his ships would sink, his men would die of scurvy or some other disease, and they would be unable to find their way home. Prior to April 12, 1961, similar catastrophes were predicted for human space travel: the rocket would explode on takeoff, the astronauts would die of weightlessness, or they would burn up during reentry. Happily for Yuri Gagarin, the first human to fly in space, the skeptics were wrong. We now know that the human body can adapt and function quite well during extended spaceflight (the longest flight to date was made by Valeri Polykov, who returned safely after 437.7 days onboard the Mir Space Station in 1995). However, we must wait for further data to understand the consequences of very long exposures to flight (e.g., during interplanetary travel) on the physiologic functions of crew members who have resumed normal terrestrial activities. In the process of unraveling the mechanisms by which physiologic systems respond to changes in gravity, we are obtaining new insights into how the human body adapts to environmental and disease stressors. The techniques and procedures (countermeasures) that have been developed to ease the transition between spaceflight and normal gravity may prove useful for ameliorating the adverse consequences of aging or chronic illness. For example, the decrease in bone mass that occurs during spaceflight is similar in many ways to the osteoporosis of aging, and the loss of muscle mass is similar to that observed in immobilized patients. As examined in this chapter, one of the most effective countermeasures for preventing spaceflight-induced deconditioning is exercise.

Microgravity and Weightlessness

The term *microgravity* describes a condition in which gravitational forces acting on the long axis of the body are minimized. This is a technical (physics) definition that applies to the low gravitational forces in space. Humans can experience brief periods of microgravity on Earth during free fall, such as occurs on some amusement park rides. There are several ways to simulate microgravity. For example, during bed rest (BR), subjects are confined to a horizontal or head-down tilt position, which minimizes the effects of gravity on the body. These subjects are in a condition of simulated microgravity.

Astronauts are often said to be weightless during spaceflight, but that is not technically correct. According to Newton's law of gravitation, every particle in the universe attracts every other particle with a force that is directly proportional to the product of their masses and inversely proportional to the square of the distance between them (1). For a human being standing on Earth, gravity therefore depends on the product of that person's mass, the Earth's mass, and the distance from the center of the Earth. During orbital spaceflight, the distance between the astronaut and the center of the Earth is about 5% greater than when the astronaut is standing on the Earth, and the mass of the Earth and the astronaut are relatively constant. Thus, orbital spaceflight is associated with only a minor decrease in gravity (2). Instead, weightlessness during orbital spaceflight results from the fact that the spacecraft is in free fall. The spacecraft circles the Earth at a rate such that the craft's centrifugal force counterbalances the force of gravity, and thus the scale used for weighing and the mass to be measured (the astronaut) are accelerating at the same rate. The crew member therefore seems weightless, even in the presence of gravity.

Weightlessness is therefore a term that refers to what the crew perceives during spaceflight, and it is one of the major factors that contribute to the total syndrome of spaceflight deconditioning. During BR, simulated microgravity is a major factor in the total syndrome of BR deconditioning. These two types of deconditioning have many similar physiologic adaptations, but one must also consider other unique stressors associated with spaceflight (*e.g.,* altered day/night cycles) or BR (*e.g.,* confinement) when comparing data from these two conditions.

Spaceflight

During spaceflight, an astronaut is exposed to a variety of environmental and psychological stressors (3). A potent environmental stressor felt immediately upon insertion into orbit is microgravity, which unloads body tissues and redistributes body fluids. Also, during orbital flight, external light and dark cycles occur every 90 minutes, disrupting normal pituitary-hypothalamic regulation. Ultraviolet radiation is nearly abolished, which decreases vitamin D production. Ionizing radiation exposure is elevated, posing potential health hazards. Microflora in the air and water proliferate in the enclosed spacecraft, and immune responses may become compromised. Carbon dioxide levels inside the craft are chronically elevated to about 0.4% during nominal crew activity, with peaks of 1% to 3% observed during intense exercise and when other crews are visiting. Stress levels may be high in the diverse crew members exposed to relatively confined quarters, high noise levels, and altered sleeping and eating patterns. The crew members are required to exercise vigorously during long flights, often more intensely than they did before flight. Therefore, it is a misconception to view spaceflight as a condition of reduced activity (hypodynamia). The physiologic changes that occur in response to all of these stressors are collectively referred to as spaceflight deconditioning. Astronauts are deconditioned in relation to how they could perform upon return to a 1-g environment, but during spaceflight, they adapt appropriately and can function normally.

Free Fall and Parabolic Flight

Free fall occurs when a person plunges downward at the rate of acceleration due to gravity ($980 \text{ cm} \cdot \text{s}^{-2}$). This can happen in a falling elevator, after release from a drop tower, on some amusement park rides, or in a diving aircraft. Astronauts first experience weightlessness while training in a special plane that flies parabolic arcs (3). During this maneuver, the airplane dives to gain speed and then pulls up at a 45-degree angle into the first arm of the parabolic arc, producing hypergravity (1.8 g). The pilot then powers back the engines, allowing the plane to glide over the top of the arc and begin a controlled, 45-degree nose-down dive. The passengers inside the plane immediately go into free fall (weightlessness). As the plane reaches the bottom of its parabola, the passengers again are subjected to 1.8 g. The average duration of weightlessness during this maneuver is 20 to 25 seconds. If you watch the movie "Apollo 13" closely, you can see that the actors actually are weightless; scenes from this movie were filmed during parabolic flight. During parabolic flight, the brief exposures to microgravity interspersed with exposures to hypergravity make interpretation of physiologic responses challenging and often unique to the parabolic flight condition.

Simulated Microgravity

Microgravity can be simulated by changing the angle of the person relative to the gravitational vector or by unweighting all or portions of the body. Unweighting can be achieved by immersion in water, by suspension, or by immobilization of limbs.

Bed rest

The most common model used to simulate the physiologic effects of microgravity in humans is prolonged BR. Subjects are placed in a slightly head-down tilt position (to simulate microgravity during spaceflight) or a 10-degree head-up tilt position (to simulate a Lunar 1/6-g environment) for the duration of a study that can last for hours or longer than a year. The physiologic responses to BR depend on the duration of the study and the angle of tilt. The earliest BR studies were performed with subjects in a horizontal position. Then, in the mid-1970s, Kakurin and coworkers demonstrated that an antiorthostatic head-down tilt position of 4 to 16 degrees induces body fluid and cardiovascular responses to tilting or exercise similar to those that accompany spaceflight (4). Since then, because responses to a 6-degree head-down tilt most closely approximate those observed during spaceflight deconditioning, this angle is used most frequently to study cardiovascular responses to microgravity (3).

Physiologic systems respond to BR with different rates of deconditioning. A decrease in muscle mass and loss of strength become apparent after approximately 2 weeks of BR (5), whereas it takes about 12 weeks to detect a decrease in bone mineral density (BMD) by standard dual-energy absorptiometry imaging (6), although changes in bone biochemical markers appear within days (7,8). A decrease in cardiac mass is measurable after approximately 6 weeks of BR without exercise (9). Impairment in exercise responses is evident after only a few days of BR, but maximal exercise capacity may not decline for a few weeks, and it will depend on the initial fitness level of the subject (5). Thus, it is important to consider the most appropriate BR protocol when designing a study to simulate a particular effect of spaceflight.

KEY POINT

The most frequently used simulation for spaceflight is BR; however, one must use caution when extrapolating BR results to flight conditions, because BR does not replicate many of the stressors of living and working in space.

Immersion

Immersion is another model that is used to simulate microgravity. American astronauts prepare to perform extravehicular activity (EVA) by training in the Neutral Buoyancy Laboratory at the Johnson Space Center. This laboratory has a 6.2-million-gallon pool that contains a mockup of the Space Station at the bottom. The astronauts don their EVA suits and are slowly lowered into the pool. As they stand completely submerged on a platform, weights are added to their suits until they reach neutral buoyancy. Astronauts report that the sensations of working underwater are similar to those of working in space. This model of microgravity has obvious limitations for performing experimental investigations.

Unconfined water immersion (without a spacesuit) has also been used to simulate microgravity. Subjects are usually immersed in a small pool of thermoneutral (34.5°C) water either with their head just above water or submerged while breathing through a snorkel. A major difficulty of such studies is the high rate of heat transfer between the subject and the surrounding water, which necessitates close monitoring of the subject's body temperature. This model is used to simulate responses of body fluids and electrolytes during the first few days of microgravity. During immersion, the water pressure against the surface of the body causes a central fluid redistribution from legs to thorax, resulting in slightly more pronounced body fluid and cardiovascular responses than those observed during spaceflight or with other microgravity simulation models (3).

To avoid problems during immersion associated with heat exchange and from prolonged exposure of the skin to the immersion fluid, some investigators enclose the subjects in a waterproof material. This "dry immersion method"

was first used during the 1960s and is still used occasionally by Russian investigators (3). Physiologic responses are similar to those during wet water immersion, and study duration can be weeks.

Suspension and immobilization

Musculoskeletal unloading can be produced by suspending subjects above the ground with springs or by supporting them from below with air jets (air-bearing floors). Such methods create regions of tissue compression that can be tolerated for only short periods. Limb immobilization or casting has been used to study regional changes in muscle. A limb is casted at a fixed angle, and the reported changes in muscle generally are greater and occur more rapidly than those observed during BR or spaceflight. However, fixing the limb may not replicate the conditions of spaceflight, since astronauts can move their limbs freely during such flights (10).

Two methods of unilateral lower limb suspension can be used to unweight a limb to simulate microgravity. In one method, a support strap is used to suspend one limb while the other limb is used for mobilization via crutches. In the other method, a high platform shoe is fitted on one foot while the subject walks with crutches, allowing the unloaded leg to hang freely. The strap method produces muscle changes similar to those obtained with casting, possibly because of the limited movement of the limb. The platform-shoe method produces muscle responses similar to those reported in astronauts during flight and in subjects during BR (10).

Summary
Spaceflight exposes astronauts to extreme environmental conditions imposed by a variety of stressors that result in pronounced deconditioning upon their return to Earth. Microgravity simulations often are used to study the mechanisms of the physiologic responses to spaceflight and to develop countermeasures against deconditioning. The most frequently used simulation is BR; however, one must use caution when extrapolating BR results to flight because BR does not replicate many of the stressors of living and working in space.

TEST YOURSELF

How would you design a ground-based model to mimic an actual spaceflight mission? What factors would you need to control besides gravitational loading? If you plan to exercise using this model, how might you have to modify the exercise equipment or protocols? List the positives and negatives of each microgravity model you develop.

Effects of Microgravity on Human Physiologic Systems

Exposure to microgravity can affect human tissues through several mechanisms. First, the reduction in apparent body mass unloads the postural or supportive tissues, resulting in atrophy of these tissues. Second, microgravity causes body fluids to redistribute caudally, such that hydrostatic forces equilibrate throughout the body, increasing perfusion in upper body regions and decreasing perfusion in lower body regions. A result of the increased upper body fluid volume is the activation of intravascular pressure receptors, such as carotid and aortic baroreceptors, resulting in a reduction in total blood volume. The concomitant changes in regional intravascular pressures must be counterbalanced by modifications in vascular permeability and tissue oncotic pressures to reestablish homeostatic body fluid exchange. Microgravity engenders much smaller fluctuations in vascular pressures than would naturally occur during a change in posture in terrestrial gravity. Without such pressure fluctuations, the baroreceptors and other reflexes that regulate blood pressure become less responsive and less able to maintain blood pressure upon return to 1 g or during positive acceleration (11). Third, the effects of increased stress and altered light and dark cycles may result in alterations of the hypothalamic-pituitary-adrenal axis or the sympathetic-adrenal medullary axis, resulting in marked changes in hormonal, neural, and immune functions. As we will see later in this chapter, exercise may be an important countermeasure for many of these physiologic changes.

Cardiovascular System

Exposure to microgravity initiates alterations in the body's homeostasis that can lead to profound effects on the capacity of the body to maintain orthostatic (fainting) tolerance and perform physical exercise. Data from both spaceflight and BR experiments demonstrate an early reduction in blood volume due to contraction of the plasma, followed by a more gradual stabilization between 30 and 60 days of exposure (Fig. 26.1). Results from BR experiments indicate that plasma volume decreases within 24 to 72 hours as a result of diuresis and natriuresis induced by the headward fluid shifts. A gradual decrease in red cell mass also occurs and becomes evident after about 2 weeks. Loss of circulating blood volume probably contributes directly to a limitation of cardiac filling, as evidenced by a reduction in echocardiographic end-diastolic and stroke volumes (5,12–16). The reduction in blood volume observed during flight and BR may involve different mechanisms. An early diuresis has not been observed during flight. It has been hypothesized that dehydration or fluid movements associated with the prelaunch position (lying supine with the feet above heart level) may attenuate the body fluid

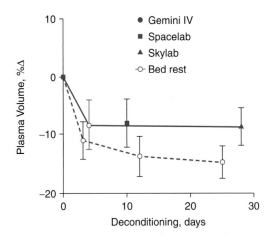

FIGURE 26.1 Time courses of percent change (%Δ) in plasma volume during spaceflights (*closed symbols, solid line*) and BR (*open circles, broken line*). (Adapted from Convertino VA. Exercise and adaptation to microgravity environments. In: Fregly MJ, Blatteis CM, eds. *Handbook of Physiology. Section 4: Environmental Physiology, Vol 3. The Gravitational Environment.* New York: Oxford University; 1996:824.)

redistribution upon insertion into microgravity (17). Alternately, microgravity during spaceflight may reduce intrathoracic pressure, allowing blood to move into the pulmonary circulation and prevent the rise in central venous pressure and diuresis that occurs during BR (see *Pulmonary System*).

In addition to a reduced circulating blood volume, cardiovascular structures adapt to microgravity and its simulations. Magnetic resonance imaging measurements of the heart before and after exposure to spaceflight and BR reveal a smaller myocardial mass afterward (9,14,18). Cardiac atrophy may contribute to the reduced cardiac filling and stroke volume observed after adaptation to microgravity. Contrary to human data on myocardial atrophy in space and BR, evidence from ground-based and flight experiments on animals suggests that cardiac atrophy may not occur in microgravity, and that reports of atrophic effects on the myocardium may simply reflect the negative caloric balance routinely observed in astronauts during spaceflight (19). Measures of myocardial function curves, ejection fraction, and arterial pulse wave velocities all suggest that short exposures to microgravity have little effect on cardiac contractility (5,13–15).

Alterations in cardiac mechanical factors have been associated with exposure to microgravity. The observation that stroke volume remained higher at any given filling pressure during confinement to BR for less than 2 weeks (13) suggests that cardiac compliance is increased in the early stage of exposure. Elevated cardiac compliance (the change in intraventricular pressure for a given change in cardiac filling) may be a mechanism to defend stroke volume in the presence of hypovolemia and reduced cardiac filling pressure. However, when the duration of BR or flight exceeds about 2 weeks, ventricular remodeling occurs and myocardial compliance and cardiac filling are reduced (20).

Increased venous compliance in the lower body has also been observed during exposure to spaceflight and BR (5,13,14,21). Greater compliance and impaired constriction of capacitance vessels (22) would compound the effect of hypovolemia and impair venous return and stroke volume by providing a greater capacity to pool blood at the same hydrostatic pressure. A positive correlation between the magnitudes of reduction in leg muscle mass and elevated calf compliance has been observed in BR subjects. This relationship supports the premise that increased venous compliance may be influenced by a loss of tissue mass that normally provides structural support for the veins. When the muscle compartment is reduced, compliance increases (5); when the muscle compartment loss is attenuated by exercise during BR, the compliance changes are eliminated (5).

> ## KEY POINT
>
> Both short-term and prolonged spaceflight result in significant orthostatic intolerance in the post-flight period.

Exposure to spaceflight or BR is also associated with impaired baroreflex mechanisms that control cardiovascular functions. Data from spaceflight and BR have provided evidence for reduced cardiac vagal nerve activity, increased heart rate response with aortic baroreceptor stimulation, elevated sympathetic nerve activity and circulating catecholamines, and greater cardiac β-adrenergic receptor reactivity (14). These alterations in autonomic function alone or in combination could explain, at least in part, the tachycardia and compromised orthostatic response observed after exposure to spaceflight or BR.

Exposure to microgravity causes alterations in the structure and function of vascular smooth muscle. Elevated peripheral vascular resistance (14) after exposure to spaceflight or BR reflects a reflex compensatory response to the reduction in stroke volume and cardiac output. Because maximal vasoconstriction is finite, an elevated resting vasoconstriction reflects a reduction in vasoconstrictive reserve and lowers the capacity to buffer alterations in blood pressure. Increased vascular β-adrenoreceptor (vasodilatory) sensitivity after BR has been reported (14). In the presence of elevated sympathetic nerve traffic, increased vasodilatory adrenergic receptor reactivity could limit vasoconstrictive capacity. Another explanation for attenuated vasoconstriction after BR or flight is that the vasoconstrictor response is impaired due to reduced release or end-organ sensitivity to norepinephrine (23,24). Furthermore, consistent and compelling evidence from animal experiments indicates that vascular smooth muscle contraction is reduced during exposure to low gravity and is associated with altered morphology, atrophy, and lower vasoreactivity (25).

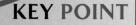

> ## KEY POINT
>
> Exposure to spaceflight or BR is associated with impaired baroreflex mechanisms that control several cardiovascular functions.

Summary

Gravity is crucial for the regulation of cardiovascular function. In microgravity, body fluids redistribute centrally, blood volume is reduced, and remodeling occurs in both cardiac and vascular tissues. Cardiovascular reflexes may be accentuated at rest but impaired in response to a sudden fall in blood pressure. Decreased cardiac filling and systemic resistance may induce an initial cardiac atrophy, although contractile function is maintained at least during short-duration flights. These cardiovascular adaptations are appropriate for a microgravity environment but reduce orthostatic tolerance and exercise capacity upon a sudden transition back to 1 g.

Pulmonary System

Gravity profoundly influences the lung. In a 1-g environment, gravity helps determine the shape of the lungs, distribution of ventilation and blood flow, alveolar size, intrapleural pressure, chest mechanics, and gas exchange. Therefore, it is predicted that pulmonary function will be altered greatly during microgravity, although the direction of change is uncertain because some alterations may impair pulmonary function while others may be beneficial. Prisk and coworkers (26,27) argued that the effects of "true microgravity," such as spaceflight or parabolic flight, differ from the effects caused by simulated microgravity, such as BR. For this reason, we will discuss spaceflight and BR responses separately.

Lung function during spaceflight

Prisk (26) extensively reviewed the effects of spaceflight on pulmonary function, and many of his findings are summarized in Table 26.1. He reported that lung volumes decreased upon entry to microgravity in part because of the headward fluid shifts. Both vital capacity and forced vital capacity decreased during the first 24 hours as compared with a preflight standing control, and then returned to preflight levels by 72 hours and remained there for the remainder of the 9-day flight. The initial decrease in lung volumes was attributed to the rapid increase in intrathoracic blood volume and the later recovery to a gradual reduction in thoracic blood volume as plasma volume decreased. A 10% decrease in functional residual capacity also occurred immediately as a result of an upward movement of the diaphragm and abdominal contents, and an outward movement of the rib cage with gravitational unloading. Residual volume decreased compared with preflight standing and

TABLE 26.1	Respiratory Changes during 1–17 Days of Spaceflight	
Physiologic Response	**Flights**	**Changes**
Pulmonary blood flow		
Total pulmonary blood flow (cardiac output)	SLS1, SLS2, D2	Initial 35% increase, then reduction to about 25% above preflight upright
Diffusing capacity (carbon monoxide)	SLS1	25% increase
Pulmonary capillary blood volume		25% increase
Diffusing capacity of alveolar membrane	SLS1	25% increase
Pulmonary tissue volume		No change at 24 h, 20%–25% decrease after 9 d
Pulmonary blood flow distribution	SLS1	More uniform but some inequality remained
Pulmonary ventilation		
Respiration frequency	SLS1, SLS2	9% increase
Tidal volume	SLS1, SLS2	15% decrease
Alveolar ventilation	SLS1, SLS2	Unchanged
Total ventilation	SLS1, SLS2	7% decrease
Ventilatory distribution	SLS1, SLS2, D2	More uniform but some inequality remained
Maximal peak expiratory flow	SLS1	Decreased $\leq 12.5\%$ early in flight then returned to normal by fourth day
Gas Exchange		
Oxygen uptake	SLS1, SLS2	Unchanged
CO_2 output	SLS1, SLS2	Unchanged
End-tidal P_{O_2}	SLS1	Unchanged
End-tidal P_{CO_2}	SLS1	Small increase when CO_2 concentration in spacecraft increased
$\dot{V}_A/\dot{Q}$ matching	SLS1, SLS2	Increase but still some mismatching remains
Lung Volumes		
Vital capacity	SLS1	5% decrease at 24 h, return to control values by 72 h
Functional residual capacity	SLS1	15% decrease
Residual lung volume	SLS1	18% decrease
Closing volume (argon bolus)	SLS1	Unchanged
Control of Breathing		
Hypoxic response	Neurolab, LMS	50% reduction
Hypercapnic response	Neurolab, LMS	No change

Flight durations: Space Life Sciences mission 1 (SLS1), 9 days; SLS2, 14 days; D2, 10 days; Neurolab, 16 days; and Life and Microgravity Spacelab (LMS), 17 days. Data are summarized from Prisk GK. Microgravity and the lung. *J Appl Physiol.* 2000;89:385–396.

was attributed to a more uniform closure of airways in dependent lung regions such that less air was trapped in the bottom of the lungs during expiration. Airway resistance, assessed by measurement of peak expiratory flow, decreased early in flight but recovered after 9 days. Prisk (26) suggested that this airway response was due to measurement difficulties and requires further verification.

The most surprising finding from the Space Life Sciences mission 1 (SLS-1) and mission 2 (SLS-2; 9 and 14 days, respectively) was that the normal ventilation ($\dot{V}_A$) and perfusion ($\dot{Q}$) gradients in the lung, although improved, still persisted during weightlessness. This remaining nongravitational inhomogeneity in ventilation and perfusion was unexpected, and the cause remains unclear. An improvement in the $\dot{V}_A/\dot{Q}$ matching would be expected to enhance gas exchange and possibly increase arterial P_{O_2}

and lower arterial P_{CO_2}. Instead, arterial oxygen pressure fell, as estimated from arterialized capillary blood samples obtained during long-duration Soviet Mir missions. Arterial desaturation has yet to be confirmed with direct arterial measurements.

An unexpected finding from the 16-day Neurolab mission (26) was that the ventilatory response to hypoxia was reduced during spaceflight. This altered hypoxic drive was attributed to an increase in arterial pressure at the carotid bodies, which may decrease the sensitivity of these chemoreceptor organs. In contrast, the ventilatory response to hypercapnia was unchanged during the flight (26).

Resting oxygen consumption and carbon dioxide production were unchanged during the SLS-1 and SLS-2 missions (26). Tidal volume was smaller and breathing frequency was faster, but not fast enough to compensate totally because ventilation was reduced by about 7% compared with pre-flight values. However, alveolar ventilation was maintained because of a reduction in physiologic dead space.

A particular concern during spaceflight is that aerosol deposition (*i.e.*, the trapping of small particles in the airways) will be impaired. Gravity plays an important role in causing potentially toxic inhaled particles to be deposited and cleared in the airways before reaching the alveoli. There have been no studies of aerosol deposition during spaceflight; however, during parabolic flight there is an almost linear positive relationship between the gravity level and the amount of particle deposition (26).

Lung function during bed rest

During spaceflight, the changes in mechanical forces on the lungs—caused by removal of gravity from the surface of the lungs, chest, and abdominal walls—are greater than those observed during BR. True microgravity causes the ribcage to expand slightly, creating more negative intrapleural pressure. A decrease in central venous pressure at the heart has been measured during spaceflight despite an increase in intrathoracic blood volume (26). These mechanical influences are not replicated during BR, where the body tissues continue to be compressed by gravity, and the central venous pressure increases transiently upon assumption of a supine or head-down position (11). Although the changes in lung volumes, pulmonary blood flow, $\dot{V}_A/\dot{Q}$ matching, gas diffusion, and physiologic dead space occur in the same direction as during spaceflight (11), they are not as pronounced. In agreement with spaceflight data, pulmonary tissue volume does not increase during exposure to BR despite the increase in thoracic blood volume and central venous pressure. This resistance to formation of pulmonary edema is explained by the ample compliance of the pulmonary circulation (26).

As BR continues and the central blood volume returns toward pre-BR levels, lung volumes also return to pre-BR values (11). BR differs from spaceflight in this respect. During BR, the lung volumes and diffusing capacity recover toward the pre-BR supine value, whereas during spaceflight these values return toward the preflight standing value. Prisk and associates (27) attributed this difference to the different mechanical influences on the lung, chest, and abdominal wall. Peak expiratory flow rate is unaffected even during prolonged BR, which has been interpreted as evidence against respiratory muscle deconditioning during microgravity (28). In agreement with spaceflight data, some authors have reported arterial desaturation during prolonged BR, which they attributed to pulmonary circulatory stasis or to a reduced threshold for airway closure (11). In contrast to spaceflight, carbon dioxide sensitivity was reduced after 120 days of BR (11). Changes in breathing mechanics during BR were similar to those observed during spaceflight (*i.e.*, an increase in breathing frequency and a decrease in tidal volume), although ventilation was unchanged (11).

Summary

Changes in pulmonary function during exposure to microgravity for as long as 4 to 6 months have been reported to be minimal (29). Much of the inhomogeneity of perfusion that was originally thought to be the result of gravity is now known to relate to the morphologic structure of the lungs, which has evolved in a gravity environment. The large vascular compliance allows fluid redistribution without large changes in pulmonary pressures. Changes in control of breathing during flight may be influenced by blood flow changes around the carotid bodies during flight, and by exposure to a mildly elevated carbon dioxide in the environment.

Muscular System

Exposure to spaceflight and BR causes unloading and relative disuse atrophy of skeletal muscles, especially those of the lower extremities. The magnitude of the resulting decrease in limb size is similar in individuals exposed to flight and BR and has been used as an indication of muscle atrophy (Fig. 26.2). Muscle biopsies taken from thigh or calf muscles before and after exposure to flight or BR reveal significant muscle-fiber atrophy afterward, as evidenced by a reduction in cross-sectional areas of slow-twitch (type I) and fast-twitch (type II) muscle fibers of the vastus lateralis (30,31), and the gastrocnemius and soleus muscles (32). Muscle atrophy was accompanied by a reduced ratio of capillaries to fiber in both slow- and fast-twitch fibers after exposure to BR and flight (30,31). Various ultrastructural abnormalities (*e.g.*, disorganized myofibrils, cellular edema, irregular Z-bodies, and fiber necrosis [disrupted fiber membranes], as indicated by disrupted sarcolemma,

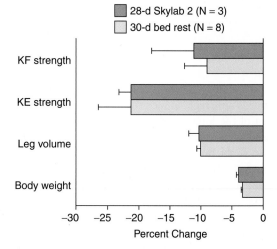

FIGURE 26.2 Percent change in strength of knee flexors (KF), knee extensors (KE), leg volume, and body weight after 30 days of BR compared with 28 days of spaceflight (*Skylab 2*). Values are mean ± SE. (Adapted from Convertino VA. Neuromuscular aspects in development of exercise countermeasures. *Physiologist*. 1991;34(suppl):S125–S128.)

abnormal mitochondria, disrupted striation patterns, and mitochondria in the intercellular spaces) were observed from electron microscopic analyses of muscle biopsy samples obtained from humans confined to BR (30). The molecular pathways by which gravitational unloading initiates muscle atrophy and remodeling are only partially understood (see Chapter 5). The net result is a decrease in muscle protein synthesis, perhaps mediated by changes in the protein kinase B–mammalian target of rapamycin signaling pathway. But even more important is an up regulation of protein degradation pathways, such as the ATP-dependent ubiquitin-proteosome pathway.

In addition to changes in muscle mass, exposure to microgravity has been associated with histochemical alterations. In studies by Convertino (30) and Edgerton et al. (31), although there were no significant changes in activities of glycolytic enzymes (e.g., adenosine triphosphatase, α-glycerophosphate dehydrogenase, lactate dehydrogenase, and phosphofructokinase) in soleus and/or vastus lateralis muscles following BR or flight, the activities of enzymes associated with aerobic metabolic pathways (succinate dehydrogenase, citrate synthase, β-hydroxyacyl-coenzyme A dehydrogenase) were reduced in both slow- and fast-twitch muscle fibers. After 6 months of spaceflight, there was a 12% to 17% shift in myosin heavy chain phenotype (a slow to fast fiber-type transition) in the gastrocnemius and soleus muscles of nine crew members on the International Space Station (ISS), despite their participation in exercise countermeasures (33). These data indicate that in addition to a compromised ability to generate force, the effects of prolonged muscle unloading and the reduced energy requirements associated with microgravity may reduce the capacity for oxygen delivery and utilization by muscle fiber cells.

KEY POINT

Skeletal muscle atrophy and biochemical adaptations occur during BR and spaceflight, resulting in reduced force production and endurance capacity.

Skeletal System

Bone mass and mineral density decrease during exposure to microgravity, and this loss of bone tissue is one of the critical issues that must be resolved before planetary exploration can be pursued. Factors that influence bone remodeling include gravitational forces, dynamic mechanical forces during movement, nutrition, hormonal changes, and biochemical effects produced during mineral and acid–base imbalances. Age, sex, and ethnicity also have important effects on bone homeostasis. Bone loss begins immediately upon unloading and is evidenced by a rapid and sustained increase in calcium excretion. The increased blood and urinary calcium concentrations increase the risk of cardiac arrhythmias and kidney stones (3).

Similar qualitative changes are observed in the bones of subjects after BR and flight, as well as patients with disuse osteoporosis (34). For this reason, gravitational unloading and reduced dynamic mechanical forces are believed to be the primary stimuli for bone changes in microgravity. One study reported that during spaceflights lasting 4 to 14 months, whole-body BMD decreased at approximately 0.6% per month (6), faster than during BR, despite the fact that the crew members were exercising 1 to 2 h $\cdot$ day^{-1} and the BR subjects were not exercising. It is unclear from these results whether the spaceflight subjects would have lost bone at an even greater rate without the exercise countermeasures, or whether the in-flight exercise was totally ineffective at preventing bone loss.

Decreases in BMD during BR and flight are not uniform; 95% of the changes occur from weight-bearing regions of the body, including the hip, spine, and legs (6). Smith and coworkers (35) predict that the rate of bone loss during flight and recovery is linear, but it takes approximately 2.5 times longer to regain bone than to lose it. However, the rate of recovery varies greatly among individuals and among different regions of the body (36). A regression model developed from data from 45 crew members who served on flights of 4 to 6 months predicts a 50% restoration of BMD for all bone sites within 9 months of normal reambulation (37). However, in 16 crew members after 4- to 6-month flights, bone stiffness estimated by quantitative computed tomography measurements of the proximal femur made 1 year after flight indicated that bone strength in this site still had not recovered despite full recovery of BMD (38).

The decline in bone mass and strength with BR and flight is attributed primarily to mechanical factors, such as gravitational unloading, and a lack of dynamic forces on bones during walking. However, nongravitational effects may account for the faster rate of bone loss that occurs during spaceflight as compared with BR. Changes in secretion of calcium-regulating hormones, such as parathyroid hormone, vitamin D, and calcitonin, during flight have been reported (39), whereas other hormonal changes, such as reduced growth hormone and increased cortisol, may contribute to the bone loss but are not observed consistently during spaceflight (3). Nutritional factors, including reduced energy and calcium intake, impaired absorption of calcium from the gastrointestinal tract, and possible effects related to a high-sodium diet, also may contribute to bone loss (39).

Bone calcium (Table 26.2) is lost at rates of up to 140 mg $\cdot$ day^{-1} during flight (35), and countermeasures such as exercise, increased calcium intake, reduced sodium intake, vitamin D supplementation, and exposure to ultraviolet light have proved ineffective for preventing these bone losses (34). Bisphosphonate administration (alendronate) appears to be a promising countermeasure to reduce bone loss (36). However, data from BR experiments showed that pharmacologic treatment alone does not prevent all bone loss, and treatment with two of the early bisphosphonates

| TABLE 26.2 | Calcium and Bone during Bed Rest and Spaceflight | | | | |

Bed Rest			Spaceflight		
Time	Change	Reference[a]	Time	Change	Reference[b]
2 d	Urinary calcium increased Resorption markers increased	Baecker et al., 2003	21 d	Ionized calcium increased Serum 1,25 vitamin D decreased Formation markers decreased Resorption markers increased	Turner, 2000
7 d	Resorption markers increased Formation markers increased or no change	Lueken et al., 1993	28–48 d	BMD decrease in flight and no return in 5 yr	Turner, 2000
10 d	Hydroxyproline increased Urinary calcium increased Serum calcium, phosphate increased Vitamin D decreased	Van der Wiel, 1991	28–84 d	Urinary calcium increased during flight	Turner, 2000
20 d	Formation markers no change Resorption markers increased Cytokines transiently increased	Fukuoka et al., 1994	28–84 d	Urinary collagen breakdown markers increased	Turner, 2000
			51 d	Resorption markers increased Formation markers no change	Turner, 2000
			60 d	Urinary calcium increased during flight	Turner, 2000
3 mo	BMD in spine and hip decreased Urinary, serum calcium increased Serum calcium increased PTH, vitamin D decreased Formation markers no change Resorption markers increased	Zerwekh et al., 1998	1, 6 mo	Formation markers decreased Resorption markers no change	Collet et al., 1997
4 mo	BMD decreased in lower body BMD no change in upper body Resorption markers increased Formation markers no change PTH, vitamin D decreased	LeBlanc et al., 2002	4–14.5 mo	BMD decreased in lower body BMD no change in upper body	LeBlanc et al., 2000
			3 mo	Calcium intake and absorption decreased Urinary calcium increased Resorption markers increased Formation markers increased	Smith et al., 1999
			180 d	Serum PTH decrease Formation markers decreased Resorption markers increased	Turner, 2000

(continued)

TABLE 26.2	Calcium and Bone during Bed Rest and Spaceflight *(continued)*					
Bed Rest				**Spaceflight**		
Time	Change	Reference[a]		Time	Change	Reference[b]
210 to 252 d	Urinary calcium, sustained increase Fecal calcium increased Sweat calcium not increased Whole body calcium loss 4.2% Phosphorus balance similar to calcium Os Calcis, 25%–45% loss in mass in central region	Donaldson et al., 1970		30–438 d	Serum calcium increased PTH increased Calcitonin decreased	Turner, 2000
				115 d	Intestinal calcium absorption decreased GI and kidney calcium excretion increased	Turner, 2000

BMD, bone mineral density; PTH, parathyroid hormone; GI, gastrointestinal.

[a]BR references

Baecker N, Tomic A, Mika C, et al. Bone resorption is induced on the second day of bed rest: results of a controlled crossover trial. *J Appl Physiol.* 2003;95:977–982; Lueken SA, Arnaud SB, Taylor AK, et al. Changes in markers of bone formation and resorption in a bed rest model of weightlessness. *J Bone Miner Res.* 1993;8(12):1433–1438; Van der Wiel HE. Biochemical parameters of bone turnover during ten days of bed rest and subsequent mobilization. *Bone Miner.* 1991;13:123–129; Fukuoka H, Kiriyama M, Nishimura Y, et al. Metabolic turnover of bone and peripheral monocyte release of cytokines during short-term bed rest. *Acta Physiol Scand Suppl.* 1994;616:37–41; Zerwekh JE, Ruml LA, Gottschalk F, et al. The effects of twelve weeks of bed rest on bone histology, biochemical markers of bone turnover, and calcium homeostasis in eleven normal subjects. *J Bone Miner Res.* 1998;13(10):1594–1601; LeBlanc AD, Driscol TB, Shackelford LC, et al. Alendronate as an effective countermeasure to disuse induced bone loss. *J Musculoskelet Neuronal Interact.* 2002;2(4):335–343; and Donaldson CL, Hulley SB, Vogel JM, et al. Effect of prolonged bed rest on bone mineral. *Metabolism.* 1970;19(12):1071–1084.

[b]Spaceflight references

Turner RT. Physiology of a microgravity environment invited review: what do we know about the effects of space flight on bone? *J Appl Physiol.* 2000;89:840–847; Collet PH, Uebelhart D, Vico L, et al. Effects of 1- and 6-month spaceflight and bone mass and biochemistry in two humans. Bone. 1997;20:547–551; LeBlanc A, Schneider V, Shackelford L, et al. Bone mineral and lean tissue loss after long duration space flight. *J Musculoskelet Neuronal Interact.* 2000;1(2):157–160; and Smith SM, Wastney ME, Morukov BV, et al. Calcium metabolism before, during, and after a 3-mo space flight: kinetic and biochemical changes. *Am J Physiol.* 1999;277:R1–R10.

(etidronate and clodronate) was most effective when combined with exercise (36). In an ongoing collaboration, U.S. and Japanese scientists are currently evaluating the effectiveness of alendronate tablets before and during flight, and zolendronic acid (another bisphosphonate) injections before flight to reduce bone loss in ISS crew members.

Intensive research is being conducted to discover the mechanisms by which unloading (deconditioning) causes bone loss. Bone mass turnover is determined by the net balance between resorption and formation. Bone resorption, as indicated by the urinary markers hydroxyproline and urinary collagen crosslinks, increase within the first few days of BR and flight (2,35). Kinetic tracer data indicate a 50% increase in bone resorption during long flights (35). On the other hand, findings regarding the changes in bone formation conflict. Biochemical markers, including osteocalcin and bone-specific alkaline phosphatase, are unchanged or slightly decreased during BR (36) and flight (35,39). After both flight and BR, bone formation markers increase promptly to well above the preflight values (35). Thus, it seems that bone

loss in microgravity is due to increased bone resorption compounded by a slowly developing decrease in bone formation. Animal data suggest that decreased bone blood perfusion during microgravity simulations may alter nutrient delivery and vascular wall shear forces to stimulate endothelial cytokine activity that results in regional bone loss (40).

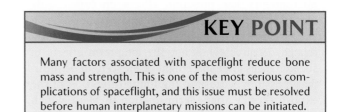

KEY POINT

Many factors associated with spaceflight reduce bone mass and strength. This is one of the most serious complications of spaceflight, and this issue must be resolved before human interplanetary missions can be initiated.

Immune Function

Humans who travel in space have compromised immune function (see Sonnenfeld [41] for a recent overview of results from human and animal studies during flight). During the Apollo missions, 15 of 29 astronauts reported bacterial or viral infections either during flight or within the first week after landing. During the infamous *Apollo 13* mission, the travails of one of the crew members were compounded by a severe urinary tract infection. Most human spaceflight studies have examined the effects of flight on cell-mediated immunity. Blood samples drawn from astronauts and cosmonauts after the *Apollo-Soyuz* test project, Skylab, and space shuttle flights revealed inhibition of mitogen-induced formation of leukocytes. After a joint Soviet and Hungarian flight, it was found that the cosmonauts' leucocytes had a decreased ability to produce interferon-α and interferon-β. Crew members immediately after flight have an increased leukocyte count, including neutrophils, monocytes, $CD3^+CD4^+$ T-helper cells, $CD19^+$ B-cells, and reduced natural killer cell activity (42). Delayed hypersensitivity responses to skin tests are inhibited after short- and long-term spaceflights, and reactivation of latent viruses (*e.g.,* Epstein-Barr) may occur, possibly in response to the elevated catecholamine levels.

The causes of these changes in immune function are uncertain. Changes that occur during spaceflight could be a direct effect of microgravity or they could be related to the confined environment, increased stress, exercise countermeasures (see Chapter 20), exposure to radiation, altered nutrition, sleep deprivation, or other as-yet-undefined factors. The concern is that changes in immune function may make the crew more susceptible to bacterial or viral infections, tissue radiation damage, and future development of tumors and cancers.

Alterations in immune responses after BR have also been reported (43). Many of these responses are similar to those observed during flight, such as decreased interleukin-2 production and increased interleukin-1 production by monocytes, which may be involved in promoting bone mineral loss. Other changes that occur during flight, such as alterations in leukocyte subsets, have not been consistently observed in humans during BR (44).

Summary

Microgravity has profound effects on human tissues that can result in physiologic responses such as those observed in aging, detraining, or inactivity-related diseases. Thus far, the long-term effects of such changes after spaceflight or BR seem to be minimal, possibly because of the limited duration of the exposures. For a long-term mission to Mars, which is estimated to require at least 3 years in continuous microgravity, the most significant concerns involve the health consequences of bone loss and the effects of radiation. As discussed later in this chapter, it is hoped that exercise countermeasures can help prevent bone loss, improve immune function, and minimize radiation effects.

TEST YOURSELF

Compare and contrast the physiologic changes associated with spaceflight and aging. Explain how the responses are similar and how they are different. Which changes are most likely to be improved by a combined aerobic and resistive exercise program?

Changes in Aerobic and Anaerobic Exercise Responses during and after Spaceflight or Bed Rest

Many of the adaptive responses to microgravity discussed above can have a significant impact on aerobic and anaerobic exercise responses when astronauts return to 1 g. For example, a loss of aerobic capacity during spaceflight could impair an astronaut's ability to perform appropriately during an emergency landing. Deconditioning in a bedridden patient could compound the effects of illness; for example, the hypovolemia and increased blood calcium associated with BR (11) could complicate the management of arrhythmias in a cardiac patient.

Cardiorespiratory Responses

After exposure to microgravity, the circulatory and respiratory responses to exertion will be impaired before a significant change in maximal exercise capacity occurs. For example, one study revealed that after only 5 days of BR, the heart rate and respiratory exchange ratio were elevated during submaximal cycle exercise, yet the peak oxygen uptake ($\dot{V}O_{2pk}$) was maintained (45). This finding raises questions about results from BR or flight, when a change in aerobic capacity is assumed because of changes observed in submaximal exercise responses.

Cardiorespiratory responses during exposure to microgravity

A consistent cardiorespiratory response to exercise during BR and spaceflight is impaired cardiac filling (46). Investigators measured cardiac output (using the single-breath carbon dioxide rebreathing method) several times during the 9- and 15-day SLS-1 and SLS-2 shuttle missions. At rest, the cardiac output was similar to preflight supine levels, with slightly larger stroke volume and slightly lower heart rate. During exercise at 30% and 60% of preflight $\dot{V}O_{2pk}$, the in-flight heart rate increased more rapidly than before the flight, whereas stroke volume decreased with increased exercise intensity. As a result of this unusual decrease in stroke volume, the increase in cardiac output was attenuated significantly from preflight levels, such that the slope of the cardiac output (L · min^{-1}) to oxygen uptake ($\dot{V}O_2$) (L · min^{-1}) relationship was only 3.5 compared with the normal value of 6.0. Blood pressure responses at rest and during exercise were similar to those observed in the supine subject before the flight. The reason for the attenuated cardiac output response to exercise in microgravity is unclear. Shykoff and coworkers (46) suggested that it may be due to lower cardiac output requirements in flight, as the peripheral muscle tissues may have better perfusion and hence a better ability to extract oxygen from the circulating blood. Given the reduced red cell mass and generally attenuated perfusion found in the lower extremities during flight, this explanation seems unlikely. Alternatively, a reduction in circulating blood volume due to sequestration of blood in the pulmonary circulation could limit the body's ability to increase cardiac output.

During a 237-day Russian spaceflight, cosmonauts exercising at 125 and 175 W also had lower stroke volume, cardiac output, and end-diastolic volume than before the flight (5). Also, end-systolic volumes were smaller and ejection fractions were larger than before the flight, suggesting that a reduced cardiac contractility could not account for the reduced cardiac output. Perhonen and associates (9) evaluated cardiac function before and after flight, and after 2, 6, and 12 weeks of BR, and noted significant cardiac muscle atrophy after 2 to 6 weeks of BR and a 12% reduction in cardiac mass after only 10 days of flight. The authors cautioned that a reduction in cardiac mass does not necessarily indicate impairment in cardiac contractile function, as patients with spinal cord injury have a much smaller heart but normal systolic function. Instead, an important clinical outcome of cardiac atrophy is a decline in diastolic function caused by a leftward shift in the ventricular diastolic pressure-volume curve for any given filling pressure. This would result in reduced cardiac filling and thus contribute to the reduced stroke volume during exercise and orthostatic stress (9).

Cardiorespiratory responses after exposure to microgravity

Cardiorespiratory responses are further compromised after flight, even in crew members whose aerobic capacity was maintained or increased during flight (3,47). Sitting submaximal cycle exercise was performed during Skylab flights at 25%, 50%, and 75% of preflight $\dot{V}_{O_{2}pk}$. When this test was performed on landing day, cardiac output was 30% lower and stroke volume was 50% lower than before the flight. Heart rate and total peripheral resistance were elevated, whereas arterial blood pressure was similar to those before the flight. A profound reduction in cardiac output and stroke volume during exercise postflight was also reported after Russian flights of 30, 63, and 96 days (5), whereas the accompanying systolic blood pressure was elevated and diastolic blood pressure was similar to that observed before the flight (unchanged during exercise).

Interpretation of exercise responses postflight depends on the position of the subject during testing. Cardiorespiratory changes that occur during exercise postflight are more pronounced when the exercise is performed in a sitting position compared with a supine position. For example, on landing day after the *Skylab* 4 mission, three crew members exercised at approximately 25% of their preflight $\dot{V}_{O_{2}pk}$

while sitting or in a supine position. During supine exercise, the cardiac output was maintained despite a decrease in stroke volume. However, during sitting exercise, the cardiac output fell and was accompanied by an accentuated increase in heart rate and a decrease in stroke volume (48). Similar changes in cardiorespiratory responses to exercise and effects of posture after BR have also been reported (5).

Oxygen uptake and mechanical efficiency

$\dot{V}_{O_{2}}$ at the same absolute power output on a cycle ergometer is consistently lower during flight and BR than baseline $\dot{V}_{O_{2}}$ values measured before such exposures (5,13,49) and is greater with dynamic exercise during recovery from flight and BR (5). Thus, the lower submaximal $\dot{V}_{O_{2}}$ at equal power outputs may be explained by increased mechanical efficiency in flight. Alternatively, the lower in-flight $\dot{V}_{O_{2}}$ may involve a change in the time constant for the $\dot{V}_{O_{2}}$ to reach a steady state. If the rate change of $\dot{V}_{O_{2}}$ during the transient phase of exercise were lengthened during flight or BR, the $\dot{V}_{O_{2}}$ measured after 3 to 5 minutes of exercise might not have reached steady state, and it would be lower than preexposure levels without a change in mechanical efficiency. This idea is supported by the measurement of a slower $\dot{V}_{O_{2}}$ kinetics during the transient phase of exercise after BR with a slower recovery of oxygen uptake after exercise (Fig. 26.3). These attenuated changes in $\dot{V}_{O_{2}}$ kinetics during the transient periods at the beginning and end of exercise after deconditioning may reflect a greater requirement for anaerobic metabolism to provide for adequate energy demand, and these findings are further supported by higher blood lactate and ventilation and respiratory exchange ratios after BR (5).

When exercise metabolism reaches steady state during post-BR cycle ergometry, the energy requirement is equal

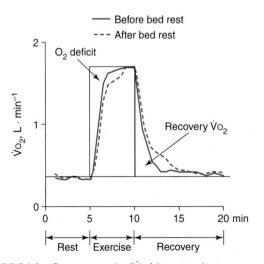

FIGURE 26.3 Oxygen uptake ($\dot{V}_{O_{2}}$) kinetics during constant-load exercise (115 W) before (*solid line*) and after (*broken line*) bed rest. (Modified from Convertino VA. Exercise and adaptation to microgravity environments. In: Fregly MJ, Blatteis CM, eds. *Handbook of Physiology. Section 4: Environmental Physiology, vol 3. The Gravitational Environment.* New York: Oxford University; 1996:818.)

to the pre-BR level (5), which suggests that mechanical efficiency does not change. These BR results have been verified during flight, in that a predicted $\dot{V}O_2$ of 2.25 L · min^{-1} during in-flight exercise at 160 W on a cycle ergometer was virtually equal to the measured $\dot{V}O_2$ of 2.31 L · min^{-1} (approximately 20% mechanical efficiency, the same as that generally observed on the ground). Because the basal metabolic rate is similar before and during exposure to BR or flight, the gross efficiency of performing exercise on a mechanically stabilized device (cycle ergometer) seems to be unaltered during flight.

> ## KEY POINT
>
> The energy cost of performing work in space is not similar to that required for doing the same tasks on earth.

The energy cost of locomotion in flight may be much higher when the body cannot be stabilized by postural muscles as it is in terrestrial gravity. This hypothesis is supported by comparisons of the average power output and metabolic cost of exercise on a cycle ergometer with those on a treadmill during flight. The energy expenditure during treadmill exercise, with a system of bungee cords used to stabilize the subject, was 7.4 kcal · min^{-1} during flight versus 5.7 kcal · min^{-1} when the same treadmill exercise was performed on Earth (5). Thus, the predicted mechanical efficiency of 20% on Earth was reduced to 15% in flight. These findings demonstrate the importance of taking gravity stabilization of the body into account when measuring mechanical efficiency during in-flight exercise in microgravity.

Maximal oxygen uptake

Maximum aerobic capacity, whether expressed as maximal oxygen uptake ($\dot{V}O_{2max}$) or $\dot{V}O_{2pk}$ (*i.e.*, subjects exercise to voluntary exhaustion without attaining a plateau of the oxygen consumption–work level curve), is reduced by 5% to 35% in individuals exposed to BR or flight, and the magnitude of this loss is dependent upon the duration of the exposure (Fig. 26.4). Because $\dot{V}O_{2max}$ is regarded as a very good single indicator of maximal endurance and aerobic physical fitness, measurement of the reduction in $\dot{V}O_{2max}$ during BR or flight should provide a good assessment of the magnitude of the deconditioning process on the cardiorespiratory and other physiologic systems. The Fick equation expresses the relationship between oxygen uptake (oxygen utilized by the total body), a-vO_{2diff} (the difference between arterial and venous oxygen concentrations resulting from the amount of oxygen extracted by working muscles), and cardiac output (heart rate × stroke volume):

$$\dot{V}O_2 = \text{heart rate} \times \text{stroke volume} \times \text{a-}vO_{2diff}$$

Thus, one can assess the mechanisms that underlie reduction in $\dot{V}O_{2max}$ during adaptation to deconditioning by eval-

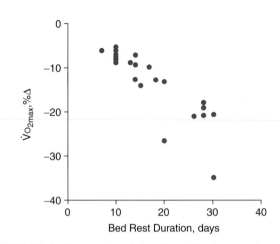

FIGURE 26.4 Regression of duration of bed rest and percent change (%Δ) in maximal oxygen uptake ($\dot{V}O_{2max}$). Compilation of data from 19 independent investigations. The linear regression of best fit is %Δ$\dot{V}O_{2max}$ = −0.85 [days] + 1.4; r = .73. (Modified from Convertino VA. Exercise and adaptation to microgravity environments. In: Fregly MJ, Blatteis CM, eds. *Handbook of Physiology. Section 4: Environmental Physiology, vol 3. The Gravitational Environment.* New York: Oxford University; 1996:819.)

uating changes in factors that influence the control of heart rate, stroke volume, and oxygen delivery.

After BR or spaceflight, the heart rate is increased at each level of oxygen uptake, including that at $\dot{V}O_{2max}$ (Fig. 26.5). The mechanisms of elevated exercise heart rate after BR or flight represent a combination of several probable factors, including increased sympathetic nerve activity at maximal levels, as evidenced by higher plasma norepinephrine concentrations (13). In addition, the heart rate response to a 0.02 µg · kg · min^{-1} steady-state dose of isoproterenol is increased significantly

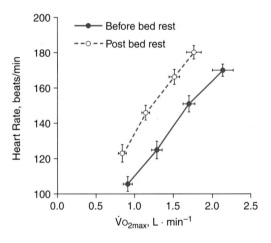

FIGURE 26.5 Mean (±SE) relationship between oxygen uptake and heart rate before (*closed circles, solid line*) and after (*open circles, broken line*) 10 days of bed rest in 12 healthy middle-aged men. (Modified from Hung J, Goldwater D, Convertino VA, et al. Mechanisms for decreased exercise capacity following bed rest in normal middle-aged men. *Am J Cardiol.* 1983;51:344–348.)

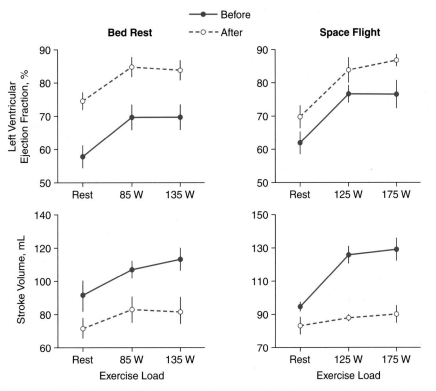

FIGURE 26.6   Mean (± SE) left-ventricular ejection fraction (*top*) and stroke volume (*bottom*) during rest and graded exercise before and after bed rest (*left*) and spaceflight (*right*). (Bed rest data adapted from Hung J, Goldwater D, Convertino VA, et al. Mechanisms for decreased exercise capacity following bed rest in normal middle-aged men. *Am J Cardiol.* 1983;51:344–348. Spaceflight data adapted from Convertino VA. Exercise and adaptation to microgravity environments. In: Fregly MJ, Blatteis CM, eds. *Handbook of Physiology. Section 4: Environmental Physiology, vol 3. The Gravitational Environment.* New York: Oxford University; 1996:827–828.)

after BR (13), which suggests that cardiac β-adrenergic receptor sensitivity may be increased. Therefore, increased sympathetic nerve activity and sensitivity of cardiac adrenergic receptors may partly explain an elevated maximal heart rate (HR_{max}) after microgravity deconditioning.

Despite a normal or increased HR_{max}, cardiac output during maximal exercise is decreased after exposure to BR and flight deconditioning (5,13,15,49). Thus, the reduction in maximal cardiac output is mostly due to a reduced stroke volume. The absence of change in a-vo_{2diff} suggests that the primary mechanism for the reduction in $\dot{V}O_{2max}$ after deconditioning is a severely compromised stroke volume.

The lower resting heart volume (measured echocardiographically) after deconditioning suggests that reduced stroke volume during exercise reflects a decreased ventricular performance resulting from myocardial atrophy (9,16). To test this hypothesis, Hung et al. (15) measured cardiac output and stroke volume in exercising subjects before and after BR using radionuclide imaging. They reported that the 17% reduction in $\dot{V}O_{2max}$ was due solely to a 23% reduction in cardiac output and 28% decrease in stroke volume, with little change in the a-vo_{2diff}. Despite a significant reduction in the exercise stroke volume after BR, the ejection fraction actually increased at rest and during exercise (Fig. 26.6, left panels).

This reduction in stroke volume and an increased ejection fraction at baseline rest and during exercise have been substantiated during flight (Fig. 26.6, right panels). The reduced stroke volume in the presence of a higher ejection fraction suggests that ventricular performance is maintained, and functional myocardial deterioration is not significant after exposure to microgravity.

In the absence of any evidence of significant loss of myocardial function, the reduced cardiac output with increased ejection fraction and heart rate during exercise after deconditioning points to reductions in venous return and cardiac filling, which probably constitute the primary mechanism by which maximal stroke volume is decreased. Reduced myocardial compliance and increased peripheral venous pooling (compliance) could limit cardiac filling. However, a rapid decrease in maximal stroke volume and $\dot{V}O_{2max}$ occurs during the initial period of microgravity (Fig. 26.7), when cardiac compliance may be unchanged or even increased (13).

Because limited cardiac filling cannot be explained by compromised myocardial mechanics during the first few weeks of BR (13), a primary factor associated with reduced stroke volume during maximal exercise is lower circulating blood (plasma) volume. This hypothesis is supported by the close relationship between the magnitude of changes in

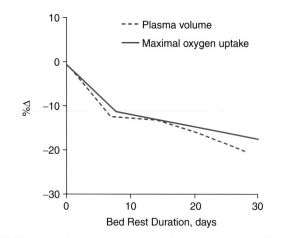

FIGURE 26.7 Average time course of percent change (%Δ) in plasma volume and maximal oxygen uptake from five male subjects during bed rest. (Modified from Greenleaf JE, Bernauer EM, Ertl AC, et al. Work capacity during 30 days of bed rest with isotonic and isokinetic exercise training. *J Appl Physiol.* 1989:1820–1826.)

blood volume and in $\dot{V}O_{2max}$ (5,13). The time course of the relative reduction in $\dot{V}O_{2max}$ shows a steep decline within the first few days of BR, followed by a more gradual reduction thereafter, which is similar to the time course of hypovolemia (Fig. 26.7). Cross-sectional comparison of data from 12 independent investigations demonstrated a high correlation ($r = .85$) between the percent change in plasma volume and $\dot{V}O_{2max}$ (Fig. 26.8). This relationship suggests that reduction in plasma volume contributes significantly (approximately 70% of the variability) to the limitation of maximal stroke volume, cardiac output, and $\dot{V}O_2$ following flight deconditioning. The effect of lower circulating blood volume on venous return and cardiac filling may be com-

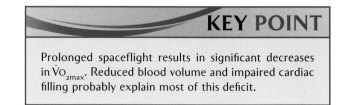

KEY POINT

Prolonged spaceflight results in significant decreases in $\dot{V}O_{2max}$. Reduced blood volume and impaired cardiac filling probably explain most of this deficit.

pounded by the increased venous pooling (compliance) in the lower extremities, which is supported by observations that the reductions in maximal stroke volume and $\dot{V}O_{2max}$ after BR are greater during exercise in the sitting position than in the supine position (5,13,15).

Peripheral mechanisms of oxygen delivery and utilization may also contribute to lower $\dot{V}O_{2max}$ during extended spaceflight. Oxygen utilization by exercising muscle appears to be lower during BR, as evidenced by a greater accumulation of blood lactate at the same work rate as before BR (5,16). Lower muscle oxygen utilization is consistent with reduced oxidative enzyme activities and compromised capacity for oxygen delivery because of less capillary density, lower maximal conductance, and decreased red blood cell volume. Although changes in the peripheral mechanisms associated with restricted delivery to and utilization of oxygen by skeletal muscle could contribute to lower $\dot{V}O_{2max}$ after BR, this mechanism is not apparent from a calculation of maximal a-vO_{2diff} (15,16). It is probable that the reduction of cardiac output is such an overwhelming limiting factor that the input from peripheral mechanisms is relatively insignificant. However, if blood volume and cardiac filling are not fully limiting, or the duration of deconditioning is prolonged, the influence of peripheral mechanisms for limiting $\dot{V}O_{2max}$ may become more important.

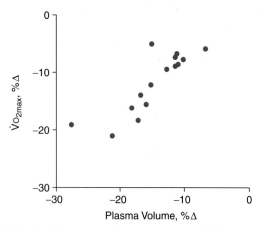

FIGURE 26.8 Regression of percent change (%Δ) in maximal oxygen uptake ($\dot{V}O_{2max}$) on %Δ in plasma volume after bed rest. Data were obtained from 12 investigations. The linear regression equation is $\%\Delta\dot{V}O_{2max} = + 0.82 [\%\Delta PV] + 0.3$; $r = .84$. (Modified from Convertino VA. Cardiovascular consequences of bed rest: effects on maximal oxygen uptake. *Med Sci Sports Exerc.* 1997;29:191–196.)

Summary

The deconditioning effects of BR or spaceflight on $\dot{V}O_{2max}$ can be accounted for initially by alterations in central (cardiac) and later by peripheral mechanisms (Fig. 26.9). An increased sympathetic activity (norepinephrine release) and cardiac β-adrenergic reactivity initially maintain cardiac contractility. However, stroke volume and maximal cardiac output still are compromised due to reduced cardiac filling associated with the lower blood volume, altered cardiac pressure-volume relationship, and peripheral blood pooling. Although a-vO_{2diff} initially is unaltered after BR and flight, reductions in oxidative enzymes, capillary density, and maximal blood flow to skeletal muscle limit oxygen delivery and utilization as the duration of microgravity exposure increases. The ultimate consequence of these alterations in cardiovascular and muscle properties is a marked reduction in aerobic power.

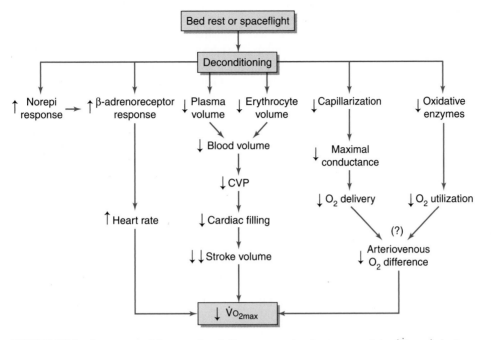

FIGURE 26.9 Summary of factors that influence maximal oxygen uptake ($\dot{V}O_{2max}$) during bed rest and spaceflight. CVP, central venous pressure.

Exercise endurance

Results from both spaceflight and BR experiments designed to determine the effects of microgravity exposure on exercise endurance are limited. However, in one study (5), increased heart rate and reduced stroke volume were associated with decreased endurance in two crew members, as evidenced by their inability to complete a 5-minute standardized exercise test at relatively low work intensity on the 24th day of a 96-day flight aboard the Soviet *Salyut 6* space station. Results from numerous BR investigations have provided quantitative evidence of reduced endurance after BR by demonstrating that less time was required to reach volitional exhaustion during graded exercise tests (5). However, information about the ability of a crew to complete prolonged submaximal work tasks after flight is limited because all experiments on this subject to date employed exercise durations of no more than 5 to 10 minutes.

Thermoregulation

Both resting and exercise body temperatures are altered during BR and spaceflight. In one study (11), basal temperatures were unchanged after 14- and 30-day BR but were decreased by 0.05° to 0.07° C after 56 days of horizontal BR. Body temperature circadian rhythm was blunted during BR and flight, with increases in the minimum night temperature (0.22°C) and decreases in the maximal daily temperature (0.20°C). Thermal sensations were altered, and the subjects felt cooler than normal, especially in the legs.

During dynamic exercise after BR or flight, the ability to dissipate body heat is impaired, resulting in a faster rise in core temperature for a given absolute level of work. Skin blood flow is reduced at rest, possibly because of enhanced sympathetic vasoconstriction, and during exercise the sensitivity of the active vasodilatory response is reduced. Crandall and associates (50) postulated that the reduced skin blood flow observed during exercise may be due not only to enhanced sympathetic vasoconstriction but also to vascular remodeling, which limits maximal blood flow, and a reduced vascular responsiveness or release of nitric oxide. The sweating response is also impaired after BR or flight. Although 14 days of BR did not alter the sensitivity of the sweat glands to exogenously applied acetylcholine, and did not affect the number of active sweat glands, the maximal sweat output per gland was reduced, possibly because of sweat gland atrophy (50). Dynamic exercise training (90 min · day^{-1} at 75% of pre-BR HR$_{max}$) during 14 days of BR prevented these exercise-induced changes in skin blood flow and sweating (51).

Age and sex

Female astronauts account for approximately 30% of active U.S. astronauts. Thus, they constitute a small sample size and a relatively homogeneous age group, which makes it difficult to evaluate the effects of age and sex factors on exercise responses in women after spaceflight. To date, the longest single flight by a woman was made by Sunita Williams in 2007 and lasted for 195 days. The oldest astronaut studied so far is John Glenn, at 77 years in 1988, and the youngest was Gherman Titov, at 25 years in 1961. In BR studies, despite differences in baseline $\dot{V}O_{2max}$ between men and women and young and middle-aged subjects, the relative (percent) changes in $\dot{V}O_{2max}$ after similar durations of BR were similar. $\dot{V}O_{2max}$, measured during supine cycle ergometry, decreased by 9% in young men, 10% in young women, 8% in middle-aged men, and 8% in middle-aged women (5). The corresponding changes in maximal work rate and exercise duration, both indices of functional work capacity, were also similar for the age and sex comparisons. However, the slope of the regression line between initial $\dot{V}O_{2max}$ and post-BR change in $\dot{V}O_{2max}$ was significantly steeper in the younger subjects than in the older subjects (52), suggesting that the rate of absolute reduction in aerobic power is greater in younger subjects. The attenuated reduction in absolute $\dot{V}O_{2max}$ for older subjects is most likely explained by their lower pre-BR fitness.

Level of physical fitness

An active (fit) individual with a large $\dot{V}O_{2max}$ reserve has a greater potential to lose that reserve during spaceflight or BR than does a more sedentary individual with a smaller $\dot{V}O_{2max}$ reserve (16). This idea is supported by early descriptive reports of a 22% reduction in $\dot{V}O_{2max}$ following BR in a subject with an initial $\dot{V}O_{2max}$ of 4.15 L · min^{-1} compared with a 13% reduction observed in a subject with initial $\dot{V}O_{2max}$ of 3.54 L · min^{-1} (5). Also, two subjects with greater aerobic capacity showed greater relative loss of their $\dot{V}O_{2max}$ than three less-fit subjects after 20 days of BR (16). In a more systematic approach, changes in $\dot{V}O_{2max}$ before and after BR in 10 moderately fit subjects ($\dot{V}O_{2max}$ = 48.5 ± 1.9 mL · kg^{-1} · min^{-1}) compared with those in 10 less-fit subjects ($\dot{V}O_{2max}$ = 38 ± 1.8 mL · kg^{-1} · min^{-1}) revealed that the percent reduction in blood volume and $\dot{V}O_{2max}$ was nearly threefold greater in the moderately fit subjects than in the less-fit group (5). Although some analyses have not supported this relationship, general findings are consistent with the hypothesis that the relative magnitude of reduction in aerobic capacity during microgravity is associated with the initial $\dot{V}O_{2max}$ reserve, and that levels of physical conditioning may influence the results.

Changes in Muscle Strength and Endurance after BR and Spaceflight

As discussed previously, microgravity results in changes not only in muscle mass but also in the biochemical properties of skeletal muscles. Lean body mass, muscle volume, and postural muscle cross-sectional areas decrease after approximately 2 weeks of BR or after a few days of flight (5). Both type 1 and type 2 muscle fibers become smaller, capillarity density decreases, and enzymatic properties and myosin isoforms adapt, resulting in a smaller, faster, more anaerobic phenotype (10,32,33).

Muscular strength

Investigators have used standard clinical methods to assess muscle strength after spaceflight. The most frequently used methods were isokinetic because of perceived greater

safety for the crew (Table 26.3). However, strength tests during flight have been performed rarely and only when special hardware was flown. Changes in strength occur during two phases during flight: an initial rapid decline in which the decrease after flight is much greater than predicted by the change in muscle volume, and a later, slower decline in strength. In BR and flight studies, this initial decrease in strength (attributed to neuromotor changes) is followed by a more gradual decrease in strength that is more closely related to the decreased muscle mass. However, the changes in strength after flight are highly variable among crew members and do not correlate positively with flight length. This variability may be related to a protective effect provided by in-flight exercise countermeasures. For example, in a recent study of nine ISS crew members, those who performed more than 200 hours per week of treadmill exercise had a partial preservation of preflight calf muscle properties, including less muscle volume and single-fiber atrophy than crew members who exercised on a treadmill less than 100 hours per week (32,33). In general, strength changes are greater in lower body muscle groups than in upper body groups, and in extensor than in flexor muscles (Table 27.3). Few flight follow-up data are available to describe changes in the force or torque-velocity relationship of muscles. From the biochemical changes in muscle favoring a greater expression of fast-twitch myosin isoforms and increased glycolytic enzymes, one might predict that strength would be better maintained at faster contraction velocities. However, this hypothesis has not been supported by spaceflight findings. After 6 months of flight, greater losses in ankle plantar flexor strength occurred at faster angular velocities (180°/s) compared with slower ones (60°/s) (10,33). Thus, changes in muscle morphology with prolonged microgravity exposure (32) or changes in neural drive may alter torque-velocity curves after flight.

Results generated from BR experiments have consistently substantiated that the strength in both small-muscle (e.g., arm, forearm, and hand) and large-muscle (e.g., trunk, thigh, and leg) groups is decreased. An analysis of cross-sectional data reveals that the relative reduction in the strength of muscle groups does not substantially decrease until after 7 to 14 days of BR and is dependent on the specific muscle group and duration of BR (Fig. 26.10). A linear regression of cross-sectional changes in maximal muscle force development over 120 days of BR suggests average decreases in strength in all muscle groups at a rate of 0.4% per day. However, the mean reductions in handgrip (−8%) and arm (−6%) strengths are only about one-third as great as the strength losses in the trunk (−22%) and leg (−20%) muscle groups during periods of 1 to 120 days. The fact that arms are used more frequently than legs during flight may explain in part why upper body muscles decondition more slowly. Another reason may be that arm muscles normally generate smaller forces during terrestrial movement than do the antigravity muscles of the lower extremities. This difference in preflight use could account for smaller strength losses in the upper body after BR or flight.

TABLE 26.3	Muscle Changes after Spaceflight		
Variable	**Flight Length**	**Changes**	**Reference[a]**
Muscle volume (MRI)	17 d	Largest changes in calf, back muscles, 12% and 10%	LeBlanc et al., 2000
Muscle volume (MRI)	112–196 d	Largest changes in calf, back muscles, 24% and 20%	LeBlanc et al., 2000
Muscle volume (MRI)	6 months on ISS	Soleus decreased 13%, gastroc. decreased 10%	Trappe et al., 2009
Muscle volume (MRI)	6 months on ISS	Calf decreased 10%, thigh decreased 7%	Gopalakrishnan et al., 2010
Isokinetic strength 5 d postflight	Skylab 2, 28 d, 30-min cycle exercise	10% decrease in arm flexor extensor isokinetic strength 25% decrease in leg extensors, 5% decrease in leg flexors	Rummel et al., 1975
Isokinetic strength 5 d postflight	Skylab 3, 56 d, 60-min cycle, some resistive arm exercise	Minimal change in arm strength 18% decrease in leg flexors, 25% decrease in leg extensors	Rummel et al., 1975
Isokinetic strength 5 d postflight	Skylab 4, 84 d, 90-min cycle, some resistive arm exercise, passive treadmill plate	No change in arm flexors; 15% decrease in arm extensors 5% decreases in leg flexors, extensors	Rummel et al., 1975
Isokinetic strength, landing day	Shuttle 5–13-d flights, minimal in-flight aerobic exercise	No change biceps, triceps, deltoids, tibialis anterior, gastrocnemius, soleus	Greenisen et al., 1999
		Back, 23% concentric, 14% eccentric	
		Abdomen, 10% concentric, 8% eccentric	
		Quads, 12% concentric, 7% eccentric	
		Hamstrings, no change	
Isokinetic strength, 5–7 d postflight	ISS missions, 129–145 d	Knee extension, 26% decrease	Lee et al., 2003
	2 h · d⁻¹ in-flight countermeasures	Knee flexion, 29% decrease	
Isokinetic endurance, 5–7 d postflight	ISS missions, 129–145d	Knee extension, 19% decrease	Lee et al., 2003
	2 h · d⁻¹ in-flight countermeasures	Knee flexion, 24% decrease	
Isometric strength	17-d LSM mission, frequent strength measurements	No change in calf muscle strength	Trappe et al., 2001
Isometric strength	Mir missions, 180 d	Triceps surae group, 42% decrease	Koryak, 2001
Isometric force, endurance	180 d	Plantar flexor force decreased 20%–48% Force decrease not correlated with decreases in muscle volume Shortened endurance due to reduced metabolic efficiency	Zange et al., 1996
Peak tetanic force	Mir missions, 180 d	Triceps surae group, 25% decrease	Koryak, 2001
Maximal explosive power	30 d	Reduced 30%	Di Prampero and Antonutto, 1997

(continued)

TABLE 26.3 Muscle Changes after Spaceflight (continued)

Variable	Flight Length	Changes	Reference[a]
Maximal explosive power	180 d	Reduced 55%	Antonutto et al., 1999
Myosin isoforms	11 d	Reduced proportion of vastus lateralis fibers expressing only slow myosin heavy chain	Zhou et al., 1995
Fiber size, capillarity, ATPase, GPD	5 and 11 d	6%–8% fewer slow fibers; 16%–32% decrease fiber cross-sectional area; ATPase activity increased in type 2 (fast) fibers; GPD activity in type 1 fibers increased 80%; 24% decrease capillarity	Edgerton et al., 1995
Skinned myofiber velocity of shortening	17 d	Increased force and velocity of shortening of slow fibers	Widrick et al., 1999
Fiber size	6 mo	Soleus Type 1 decreased > soleus Type II > gastroc. Type I > gastroc. Type II	Fitts et al., 2010
Thin filament density	6 mo	Increased in proportion to reduced fiber velocity of shortening	Fitts et al., 2010

MRI, magnetic resonance imaging; ISS, International Space Station; ATPase, adenosine triphosphatase; GPD, glycoprotein D.

[a]References for tables

LeBlanc A, Lin C, Shackelford L, et al. Muscle volume, MRI relaxation times (T2), and body composition after spaceflight. *J Appl Physiol.* 2000;89:2158–2164; Trappe S, Costill D, Gallagher P, et al. Exercise in space: human skeletal muscle after 6 months aboard the International Space Station. *J Appl Physiol.* 2009;106:1159–1168; Gopalakrishnan R, Genc KO, Rice AJ, et al. Muscle volume, strength, endurance, and exercise loads during 6-month missions in space. *Aviat Space Environ Med.* 2010;81:91–102; Rummel JA, Sawin CF, Michel EL, et al. Exercise and long duration space flight through 84 days. *J Am Med Womens Assoc.* 1975;30:175–187; Greenisen MC, Hays JC, Siconolfi SF, et al. Functional performance evaluation. In: NASA/SP-199-534. 1999;3-1–3-8; Lee SMC, Loehr JA, Guilliams ME, et al. Isokinetic strength and endurance after international space station (ISS) missions. *Med Sci Sport Exerc.* 2003;35:S262; Trappe SW, Trappe TA, Lee GA, et al. Comparison of a space shuttle flight (STS-78) and bed rest on human muscle function. *J Appl Physiol.* 2001;91:57–64; Koryak YU. Electrically evoked and voluntary properties of the human triceps surae muscle: effects of long-term spaceflights. *Acta Physiol Pharmacol Bulg.* 2001;26(1–2):21–27; Zange J, et al. Changes in calf muscle performance energy metabolism, and muscle volume caused by long-term stay on space station MIR. *Proc 6th Eur Symp Life Sci Res Space.* ESA SP-390; 1996:287–290; di Prampero PE, Antonutto G. Cycling in space to simulate gravity. *Int J Sports Med.* 1997;18(suppl 4): S324–S326; Antonutto G, Capelli C, Girardis M, et al. Effects of microgravity on maximal power of lower limbs during very short efforts in humans. *J Appl Physiol.* 1999;86:85–92; Zhou MY, Klitgaard H, Saltin B, et al. Myosin heavy chain isoforms of human muscle after short-term spaceflight. *J Appl Physiol.* 1995;78:1740–1744; Edgerton VR, Zhou MY, Ohira Y, et al. Effect of a 17-day spaceflight on contractile properties of human soleus muscle fibres. *J Physiol.* 1999;516(pt 3):915–930; Fitts RH, Trappe SW, Costill DL, et al. Prolonged spaceflight-induced alterations in the structure and function of human skeletal muscle fibres. *J Physiol.* 2010;588(pt 18):3567–3592.

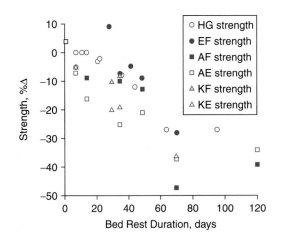

FIGURE 26.10   Regression of percent change (%Δ) in strength of handgrip (HG), elbow flexors (EF), ankle flexors (AF), ankle extensors (AE), knee flexors (KF), and knee extensors (KE) on duration of bed rest. Compilation of data from 17 independent investigations. (Adapted from Convertino VA. Exercise and adaptation to microgravity environments. In: Fregly MJ, Blatteis CM, eds. *Handbook of Physiology. Section 4: Environmental Physiology, vol 3. The Gravitational Environment.* New York: Oxford University; 1996:823.)

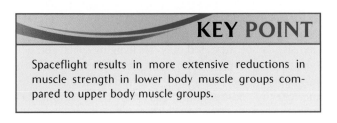

KEY POINT

Spaceflight results in more extensive reductions in muscle strength in lower body muscle groups compared to upper body muscle groups.

After 2 to 4 weeks of BR, the average decrease in angle-specific peak torque across multiple speeds of concentric muscle action is approximately 20% for knee extensors and 10% for knee flexors of the dominant leg (Fig. 26.2). These decreases in muscle strength are associated with average body weight losses of about 3% and average leg volume reduction of about 10%. These changes in body weight, leg volume, and muscle function after BR compare favorably with similar changes in the same muscle groups after flights of similar duration (Fig. 26.2). The general conclusion is that microgravity reduces strength approximately twice as much in extensor muscles as in flexor muscles (30).

A change in the torque-velocity relationship of BR subjects demonstrated a reduction in force development across all speeds of limb movement during concentric muscle contractions. Strength loss occurred with eccentric as well as concentric muscle actions, and the reduction of angle-specific peak torque was not significantly influenced by the type or speed of muscle action.

Muscle endurance

Investigators have assessed muscle endurance after short and long spaceflights by measuring the total isokinetic work performed during multiple contractions. After short shuttle flights, the total work during knee flexion and extension was reduced on landing day, but returned to baseline within 7 days (53). After 129- to 145-day space-station missions, knee extensor and flexor endurance (21 contractions at $180° \cdot s^{-1}$) were reduced by 19% (extension) and 24% (flexion) 7 days after landing and had not recovered to preflight levels by 20 days of recovery (54).

Data regarding the fatigability characteristics of muscle groups in humans after BR are limited. Right-leg plantar flexor exercise (60 contractions per minute with a target force of 588 N) was performed by seven supine men before and after 16 days of BR during which the lower limb was made ischemic by inflation of a pneumatic cuff just above the knee. After BR, the time to fatigue (inability to maintain cadence and/or force for >5 seconds) during ischemic plantar flexion exercise was decreased by 18% (55). Upper body muscular strength and endurance are especially important for crew members who perform EVAs. During an EVA, the crew member must move against the pressurized spacesuit to move and perform work. Such activities involve mostly upper body exertions at approximately 26% to 32% of the crew member's upper body $\dot{V}O_{2max}$ (56). Normally this would not be a problem, except that this work must be continued for 5 to 8 hours, during which time the crew member has limited access to fluids and may become dehydrated by up to 2.6% of body weight. During BR simulations without exercise countermeasures, arm strength decreased by 10% to 20% (56). This decrease in strength also would reduce upper body endurance and thus compromise the EVA timeline and possibly even the success of the EVA.

Neuromotor function

The decrease in strength observed after flight is often much greater than would be expected from the corresponding decreases in muscle mass. For example, in one study (10), the peak isometric force of the legs was reduced by 17%, whereas the corresponding muscle mass was reduced by only 11% in 14 cosmonauts after 90 to 180 days of flight. Electromyographic activity from the contracting muscles was reduced by 39%. The authors concluded that the results were due to impairment of neuromotor function from either an effect on the intrinsic characteristics of the motor units or a change in their recruitment pattern.

Maximal explosive power

In a spaceflight emergency, maximal explosive power may be critical for survival. Antonutto and coworkers (57) measured maximal explosive power (single maximal contractions with both legs) with a dynamometer after as long as 180 days of flight. The maximal explosive power was reduced by 30% after 1 month and by 45% after 6 months of flight. Because these reductions in maximal explosive power were much larger than the concomitant decrease in muscle mass of 9% to 13%, these results support the hypothesis that both motor control and coordination deteriorate after flight.

Summary

Loss of muscle mass, strength, and endurance are frequently observed after microgravity exposure, although the changes are not a simple function of the duration of exposure. The greatest changes occur in muscle groups involved in postural control or locomotion. The initial rapid decline in strength is most likely caused by changes in neuromotor function. The continuing decline in strength and changes in endurance are related to muscle atrophy and biochemical changes (a more glycolytic, fast-twitch phenotype). Although microgravity is the primary stimulus for deconditioning, changes in nutrition and endocrine and immune functions may compound the unloading effects.

TEST YOURSELF

Draw a diagram of all the factors that determine $\dot{V}O_{2max}$. Now consider how a prolonged spaceflight might influence each of these factors. Make a case for which of these factors is most important and why.

Exercise Countermeasures

A prescription containing both dynamic (aerobic) and resistive exercise would be expected to prevent most of the deconditioning effects of microgravity described above. Dynamic exercise should be effective in preventing cardiorespiratory changes, and resistive exercise should help to maintain muscle function. In addition, high-impact dynamic exercise and high-intensity resistive exercises may prevent decreases in bone mass and BMD.

Exercise to Maintain Exercise Tolerance after Flight

After BR or flight, deconditioning of the cardiorespiratory system is evident from the reductions in orthostatic tolerance and exercise capacity (*i.e.,* decreased $\dot{V}O_{2max}$). Specific exercises performed during flight or BR may provide a therapeutic benefit by helping to preserve cardiac function, cardiovascular reflexes, skeletal muscle mass, oxidative capacity of muscle fibers, neuromotor coordination, and body fluid homeostasis (5). Few studies have been performed during spaceflight to determine the most

effective exercise prescription. In the Skylab program, as the duration of each mission increased from 28 to 56 to 84 days, in-flight exercise was increased from 30 to 60 to 90 min $\cdot$ day^{-1}, respectively. Submaximal cycle exercise tests were performed before flight, every 5 to 6 days during flight, and 2 days after flight. When the in-flight exercise responses were maintained, exercise responses after flight (including decreased cardiac output, stroke volume, and oxygen pulse, and elevated heart rate and ventilation) significantly decreased. The decrement after flight did not worsen with increasing flight duration, which led the investigators to conclude that the in-flight exercise was useful for shortening the recovery period after flight (3,48).

The effects of in-flight dynamic exercise during shuttle missions to improve exercise responses aferflight was evaluated in 30 shuttle crew members who performed various levels of in-flight exercise (53). The investigators evaluated exercise responses after flight by measuring the change in heart rate during a graded cycle exercise test. Even moderate volumes of in-flight dynamic exercise (cycle or treadmill exercise performed three times per week for >20 minutes per session) reduced the exercise heart rate response after flight.

On the ISS, crew members perform moderate-intensity dynamic treadmill or cycle exercise for approximately 5 hours per week (32,33). Treadmill exertion in microgravity is typically less than that in 1 g, for two reasons. First, intensity can be increased only by changing speed and not by increasing grade. Second, most crew members run with only approximately 50% of 1 g footward loading due to the microgravity and discomfort caused by the treadmill harness system (58) (Fig. 26.11). Cycle exercise may provide similar cardiorespiratory loading as in a 1-g environment, but is less favored by most crew members and activates a smaller muscle mass across a limited range of motion compared with treadmill running. Cycle exercise also does not provide high-impact loading to help preserve bone.

BR findings strongly support the notion that dynamic exercise can help prevent the deconditioning effects of simulated microgravity. Numerous studies have demonstrated that various modes of dynamic exercise performed daily with intensities from 50% to 100% of $\dot{V}O_{2max}$ for 15 to 60 minutes minimize the reduction in $\dot{V}O_{2max}$ in comparison with no exercise training (5,59). These observations indicate the importance of regular physical exercise for maintenance of $\dot{V}O_{2max}$ during prolonged exposure to BR.

Exercise to Prevent Orthostatic Intolerance

Although dynamic exercise training with a high aerobic component has proved successful in maintaining $\dot{V}O_{2max}$ when performed during BR (5,59,60), exercise training alone has failed to protect against orthostatic intolerance (5,14,61,62). Few studies have been performed during flight to determine the most effective exercise prescription for orthostatic intolerance postflight. However, there is evidence that a single bout of maximal dynamic exercise

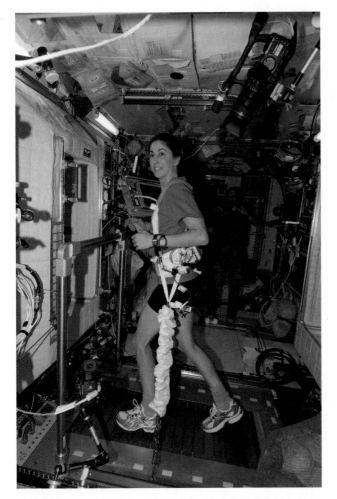

FIGURE 26.11 Astronaut Nicole Scott performing treadmill exercise during Expedition 20 on the International Space Station. (Photo courtesy of Stuart Lee, Johnson Space Center.)

within 24 hours of the end of BR can increase or restore blood volume, stroke volume, sympathetic nerve activity, vascular α-receptor reactivity, and various baroreflex functions associated with control of heart rate and vascular peripheral resistance (14). Orthostatic hypotension and intolerance also were ameliorated by a single bout of maximal dynamic exercise in individuals restrained for extended periods to wheelchairs or to BR (5,14,63). To test the hypothesis that a single bout of maximal exercise would improve orthostatic function after spaceflight, four shuttle crew members performed maximal cycle exercise within 24 to 48 hours of landing, and cardiovascular responses to the operational 10-minute stand test were examined before and after flight. Four control crew members from the same flights did not perform the exercise countermeasure. Although the postflight heart rate and blood pressure responses to standing were similar for both groups, cardiac stroke volume (by echocardiography) was better maintained in the exercisers (64). In the BR studies, a smaller reduction in stroke volume was found in the subjects who had the smallest decrement in orthostatic tolerance (5,14). However, to validate the effectiveness of this maximal exer-

cise countermeasure and evaluate improvements in orthostatic tolerance, a more provocative orthostatic test and results from longer flights are needed.

Submaximal dynamic exercise performed frequently during short flights may improve orthostatic responses after flight (65). Heart rate and blood pressure responses to standing were evaluated for the same 30 shuttle crew members described above, who were categorized as high-, medium-, or low-volume exercisers. The medium- and high-volume exercisers had significantly smaller increases in heart rate and decreases in pulse pressure during the stand test. These results suggest that even moderate amounts of in-flight dynamic exercise may reduce orthostatic stress after short flights. Again, however, more provocative tests must be performed to validate an effect to protect orthostatic tolerance.

To totally ameliorate orthostatic intolerance, however, a combination of aerobic exercise and extensive volume loading may be required. Shibata and coworkers (62) attributed postflight deconditioning to two factors: cardiac atrophy (which results in a stiffer ventricle with impaired diastolic function) and hypovolemia. These researchers were able to completely prevent orthostatic intolerance in subjects after 2 weeks of BR by a combination of moderate supine cycling exercise for 90 minutes per day (to maintain cardiac function) and a dextran infusion (to restore both plasma volume and left-ventricular filling pressure) performed 30 minutes before post-BR orthostatic testing.

Exercise to Prevent Muscle Deconditioning

During the 17-day Life and Microgravity Spacelab (LMS) mission, a torque velocity dynamometer was flown to assess changes in muscle function during flight in four crew members. However, since strength tests were performed frequently during the mission, no significant changes in isometric or isokinetic calf strength, force–velocity characteristics, or muscle fiber composition or size were found after flight (66). Thus, infrequent maximal contractions may be sufficient to preserve muscle function in microgravity.

An elastomer-based interim resistive exercise device was used on the ISS from 2001 until 2009. It consisted of two canisters that were capable of producing a peak resistance of up to 136 kg (300 lb). A serious deficiency of this exercise device was that resistance during eccentric phase of each exercise was only approximately 70% of the concentric phase due to the elastic property of the resistance mechanism. Nine crew members performed squats, heel raises, and dead lifts 3 to 6 d · wk^{-1} using this device during approximately 6-month-long missions. After these missions, their calf muscle volume was reduced by 13% ± 2%, peak power was reduced by 32%, and microgravity-induced changes in muscle-fiber structure and function were evident (32). The failure of this device to prevent muscle deconditioning most likely was due to its failure to provide sufficient resistance and eccentric loading.

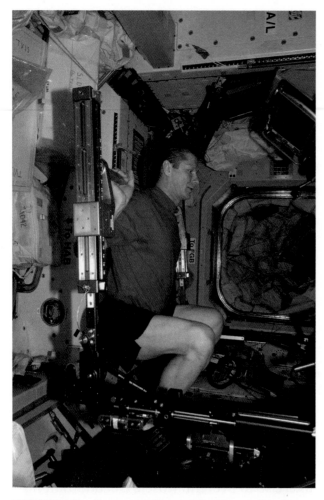

FIGURE 26.12   Cosmonaut Gennady Padalka performing a squat exercise using the advanced resistance exercise device during Expedition 19 on the International Space Station. (Photo courtesy of Stuart Lee, Johnson Space Center.)

In November 2009, an advanced resistive exercise device was deployed on the ISS (Fig. 26.12). This exercise device uses vacuum cylinders to provide up to 272 kg (600 lb) of resistance. It has a more constant force curve through the range of motion during exercise, and provides an eccentric/concentric ratio of >90%. Anecdotal reports from the first few crew members to use this exercise device suggest that the advanced resistive exercise device may attenuate or even prevent postflight reductions in lower body muscle mass and strength.

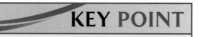

KEY POINT

Resistance exercise has been proven to be an effective countermeasure for reducing muscle atrophy in space.

Results from muscle strength tests and biopsies obtained from subjects before and after BR also argue that resistive exercise can counteract the muscle atrophy and dysfunction that occurs during exposure and adaptation to

extended microgravity (67,68). The application of regular axial-loaded resistance to the musculoskeletal system of the arms, legs, and torso by means of various resistance-exercise devices can ameliorate many of the expected changes in muscle size, strength, and morphology associated with BR (5,66,67).

Promising results from spaceflight and BR experiments suggest that preservation or restoration of muscle structure and function during microgravity can be obtained by means of appropriately designed exercise protocols and adequate nutrition. Nearly all muscle actions in flight or BR require fiber shortening (concentric actions), whereas fiber lengthening (eccentric actions) is virtually eliminated in both environments because of the negation of effects of gravity. An efficient exercise countermeasure designed to ameliorate muscle atrophy during flight and BR should include intense eccentric contractions in addition to concentric contractions.

Exercise to Prevent Bone Deconditioning

Bone loss during spaceflight was first suspected from radiographic changes observed in Gemini and Apollo crewmen postflight. Bone loss was observed (by photon absorptiometry) after Skylab flights despite the progressive increase in dynamic exercise volume during the three missions (3). During Mir missions, cosmonauts and astronauts performed approximately 2 h · day^{-1} of treadmill (footward loading of approximately 50% body weight), cycle, and expander-resistive exercises. Yet all crew members had decreases in BMD in their lower extremities that directly correlated with flight length (6). This continuing loss of bone mass during spaceflight, even with the various exercise training regimens being used, will persist until more effective countermeasures (*e.g.*, exercise, drugs, and hormones) are developed.

In early BR studies of 5 to 36 weeks' duration, investigators evaluated the effectiveness of various exercise training programs for preventing increases in calcium excretion (69). The countermeasures included a resistance pulley system (Exer-Genie) used for 80 min · day^{-1}, a static body longitudinal compression device applied for 4 h · day^{-1} at a force of 80% body weight, and impact loading with longitudinal compression of 80% body weight. However, these countermeasures failed to attenuate the negative calcium balance after 12 or 17 weeks of BR. During 120 days of BR (70), 1 hour of heavy exercise (with isokinetic cycle and isokinetic devices and bungee expanders) performed during 3 out of every 4 BR days maintained bone formation but did not prevent resorption. Ingested diphosphonates reduced bone resorption and bone formation. Exercise plus diphosphonates also decreased resorption, but exercise alone did not prevent the reduction in bone formation. In a subsequent 360-day BR study (71), 1 h · day^{-1} of dynamic exercise (horizontal treadmill, cycling) during the first 120 days of BR did not prevent the negative calcium balance, which was similar to that observed in controls who did not exercise. During the second 120 days, when the dynamic exercise training regimen was increased to two 60-minute exercise sessions per day, bone resorption was reduced, which improved the calcium balance significantly (by 52%). When exercise was combined with bisphosphonate administration (900 mg daily), the calcium balance was normalized throughout BR. Thus, from these early Russian BR studies, it seemed that very vigorous and prolonged exercise training could reduce but not prevent bone loss. In a recent 30-day BR study, 30 min · day^{-1} of treadmill exercise (6 days per week) within a lower body negative pressure chamber (which provides a ground reaction force of 1–1.2 times body weight) significantly reduced the increase in bone resorption markers observed in the subjects who did not exercise (72). Thus, high-impact dynamic exercise or heavy-intensity resistive exercise may help to maintain bone integrity during simulated microgravity.

Summary

Exercise countermeasures are used extensively (approximately 1–2 h · day^{-1}) during ISS missions. Dynamic (aerobic) exercises are intended to preserve cardiorespiratory function, as assessed by responses to exercise and orthostatic challenges postflight. Continuing decrements in these responses suggest that further improvements in these countermeasures are necessary. The implementation of a new, more effective resistive exercise device may ameliorate at least some of the muscle deconditioning that occurs after spaceflight. Further studies are required to verify this muscle effect and to determine whether intense resistance exercise might also prevent flight-induced changes in bone.

TEST YOURSELF

Considering flight limitations in terms of space, power, noise, vibration of the station during exercise, and crew time, what exercise prescription would you design to prevent changes in aerobic capacity and endurance? Considering the same limitations, can you describe the requirements for a resistive exercise device that might prove effective in a microgravity environment? What type of resistive exercise program (in terms of intensity, duration, frequency, and progression) would you prescribe to prevent the changes in muscle associated with spaceflight?

Exercise to Prevent Decompression Sickness during Extravehicular Activity

A lesser-known role for exercise during spaceflight is to prevent decompression sickness. Decompression sickness is a risk during EVA because the pressure surrounding the astronaut decreases from 14.7 psi (normal ambient pressure in the spacecraft) to 4.3 psi (the pressure in the U.S. EVA suit). With a sudden reduction in ambient pressure, nitrogen in the tissues forms bubbles that move into the circulation and block blood flow. To prevent decompression sickness during spaceflight, the shuttle is decompressed to 10.2 psi for 12 hours before an EVA. The EVA crew members then breathe 100% oxygen for 1 hour to reduce their tissue nitrogen before donning their EVA suits. Without the 10.2-psi cabin decompression, crew members would have to breathe oxygen for 4 hours before an EVA. On the ISS, however, it is impractical to decompress the entire space station, so the crew members use exercise to accelerate nitrogen elimination (73). The ISS crew members perform 10 minutes of moderate arm and leg exercise during a 2-hour oxygen-breathing period before each EVA to increase tissue perfusion and retard nitrogen bubble formation during the EVA.

Repeated Exposures to Bed Rest and Space Flight

Although more than 100 crew members have flown more than once in space, no systematic evaluation has been conducted to compare the physiologic effects of repeated spaceflights. Do repeated spaceflights result in adaptations that can attenuate the physiologic changes, or do the detrimental effects accumulate with repeated spaceflights? Is the interval (recovery) between flights important? Cardiorespiratory responses to exercise seem to recover within 30 days and have no lasting effect. Cosmonaut V. V. Ryumin performed a 185-day flight only 6 months after landing from a 175-day flight. His preflight aerobic capacity was nearly identical before both missions, suggesting full recovery (5). Bone decrements, on the other hand, may be additive, since full recovery often takes several years. LeBlanc and coworkers (6) found that the rate of bone loss in three cosmonauts who flew twice was similar, suggesting no protective effect on their second flight. The best protection against bone loss may be to select crew members who have the greatest BMD, or to screen for those who show resistance to bone loss during flight. A possible countermeasure for long space missions would be to perform DNA screening to select candidates with genetic profiles that indicate resistance to bone demineralization.

CHAPTER SUMMARY

Astronauts during spaceflight and BR subjects both undergo profound physiologic changes. Some immediate effects of spaceflight and BR occur in the cardiovascular system in response to the headward redistribution of body fluids. Within hours of assuming a horizontal or head-down position, a person will experience a reduction in plasma volume and impaired orthostatic and exercise responses. With continued exposure to spaceflight or BR, changes in baroreceptor function, cardiac function, venous tone, and vascular reactivity will further impair blood pressure regulation and the ability to maintain stroke volume and cardiac output during subsequent orthostatic or exercise stresses.

Pulmonary function is also susceptible to the effects of gravity. During spaceflight and BR, the lung volume decreases in relation to changes in thoracic blood volume, the residual volume decreases in response to upward movement of the abdominal contents, and the ventilation-perfusion nonhomogeneity is improved but still persists. Pulmonary responses to spaceflight are generally in the same direction but larger than responses to BR.

Muscle mass is reduced during spaceflight and BR. Initially, muscle strength declines more rapidly than muscle mass. Maximal explosive power also is reduced to a greater extent than the decline in muscle mass, suggesting an impairment in neuromotor function. Morphologic and biochemical changes include smaller muscle fibers with faster velocity of shortening and greater reliance on glycolytic metabolism. These changes reduce strength and endurance.

A MILESTONE OF DISCOVERY

Although the debilitating effects of bed rest (BR) confinement on physical performance have been well recognized and described for decades in the clinical literature, the physiology underlying the reduction in $\dot{V}O_{2max}$ and working capacity was not well understood until 1968. In a landmark investigation of the effects of BR and training on responses to exercise, Saltin and coworkers (16) demonstrated an average reduction in treadmill $\dot{V}O_{2max}$ of 26% in five young male subjects (19–21 years old) after they were confined in bed for 21 days. Specific hemodynamic and pulmonary function measurements performed during baseline rest and exercise provided the first evidence for the mechanisms behind the reduction in $\dot{V}O_{2max}$ after exposure to BR. The magnitude of the decrease in $\dot{V}O_{2max}$ was equal to the average 26% reduction in maximal cardiac output from 20.0 L · min^{-1} before to 14.8 L · min^{-1} after BR. A slight compensatory elevation in HR_{max} after BR failed to compensate for the average reduction in stroke volume from 104 to 74 mL. The absence of a significant change in pulmonary function or arterial-venous oxygen difference indicated that the primary cause for the reduction in $\dot{V}O_{2max}$ during BR was a severely compromised stroke volume (a central cardiac effect) rather than decrements in gas exchange or in peripheral oxygen delivery or utilization. The authors gained new insights into the adaptation process during exposure to microgravity by comparing responses during upright and supine exercise, as well as measurements of heart volume, blood volume, and various blood biochemical parameters at rest and during exercise. It is clear that this study has stimulated numerous investigations designed to test new hypotheses regarding the effects of deconditioning on structural and functional relationships of cardiac and skeletal muscles, blood pressure regulation, and metabolic and hemodynamic responses during exercise and their clinical implications.

Although their subject sample was small, Saltin and associates introduced the premise that persons with a large $\dot{V}O_{2max}$ (physiologic) reserve incur a greater absolute loss of that reserve during deconditioning than do more sedentary individuals with a smaller $\dot{V}O_{2max}$ reserve. They found that the two subjects with the highest $\dot{V}O_{2max}$ before BR (average = 4.48 L · min^{-1}) showed a greater absolute loss of their $\dot{V}O_{2max}$ (average = −1.01 L · min^{-1}) than three less-fit subjects (average $\dot{V}O_{2max}$ = 2.52 L · min^{-1} before BR) with an average absolute reduction of $\dot{V}O_{2max}$ of 0.75 L · min^{-1}. Subsequent data from several different physiologic systems have provided support for this hypothesis.

Data from this study are often cited as evidence in favor of the use of exercise training to enhance recovery from the deleterious effects of deconditioning on exercise performance after BR. In the three sedentary subjects, $\dot{V}O_{2max}$ was restored within 10 to 14 days of recovery from BR and continued to increase by 36% above baseline levels at 60 days of recovery. However, the two habitually active subjects required 30 to 40 days of physical activity to restore $\dot{V}O_{2max}$ to baseline levels. These results emphasize the importance of regular exercise in the rehabilitation of BR patients, particularly in relatively fit individuals.

In an interesting 30-year follow-up investigation, McGuire and associates (74) studied these same five subjects to assess their maximal aerobic capacity. On average, their $\dot{V}O_{2max}$ had decreased by 11%. Their body weight had increased 25%, entirely because of a 100% change in body fat with little change in fat-free mass. Their HR_{max} had declined by 6% and maximal stroke volume had increased by 16%, resulting in no change in maximal cardiac output. Their entire decline in $\dot{V}O_{2max}$ could be accounted for by a 15% decrease in the maximal arterial-venous oxygen difference. Thus, 3 weeks of BR when these men were 20 years old had a more profound effect on their physical work capacity than did 30 years of aging.

In 2009, McGavock et al. (75) performed a 40-year follow-up study in these same five men. During the most recent 10 years of aging, there was a fourfold increase in the rate of decline in $\dot{V}O_{2max}$ (compared with the first 30 years), caused by decreases in both maximal cardiac output and peripheral oxygen extraction. Thus, advanced aging effects on the heart are similar to the BR effects seen in young men.

Saltin B, Blomqvist G, Mitchell JH, et al. Response to exercise after bed rest and after training. Circulation. 1968;38(suppl 7):1–78.

Bone mineral content and density decrease gradually during spaceflight and BR as a result of a rapid increase in bone resorption and a more gradual decrease in bone formation. The recovery of bone mass and density varies for different body regions and often takes several months or even years.

Aerobic capacity decreases during spaceflight and BR, primarily because of the body's inability to maintain stroke volume and hence maximal cardiac output. Reduced muscle capillarity and decreased activity of muscle oxidative enzymes also impair cardiorespiratory endurance. Previous in-flight exercise countermeasures, consisting primarily of treadmill and cycle dynamic exercises and low-intensity resistive exercise, were shown to be capable of attenuating the decline of aerobic capacity during flight. However, after flight, especially during upright exercise, cardiac filling was impaired and aerobic capacity was reduced for several weeks. High-intensity resistance-exercise training performed only two to three times per week during BR is effective at preventing muscle deconditioning. The use of resistive exercise during flight to improve muscle or bone responses has not been systematically tested.

Exercise-training treatments and procedures developed to prevent spaceflight- or BR-induced deconditioning have been used to treat many Earth-based conditions, such as disuse osteoporosis, orthostatic intolerance, muscle diseases associated with sarcopenia, sedentary disease syndrome, and aging. Finally, there is no evidence of additional detrimental effects from repeated spaceflights or BR exposures.

REFERENCES

1. McArdle WD, Katch KI, Katch VL. Microgravity: the last frontier. In: *Exercise Physiology*. Baltimore: Lippincott Williams & Wilkins; 2001:678–748.
2. Turner RT. Physiology of a microgravity environment invited review: what do we know about the effects of spaceflight on bone? *J Appl Physiol*. 2000;89:840–847.
3. Nicogossian AE, Huntoon CL, Pool SL. *Space Physiology and Medicine*. Philadelphia: Lea & Febiger; 1994.
4. Kakurin LI, Lobachik I, Mikhailov VM, et al. Antiorthostatic hypokinesia as a method of weightlessness simulation. *Aviat Space Environ Med*. 1976;47:1083–1086.
5. Convertino VA. Exercise and adaptation to microgravity environments. In: Fregly MJ, Blatteis CM, eds. *Handbook of Physiology: Section 4. Environmental Physiology, vol 3. The Gravitational Environment*. New York: Oxford University; 1996:815–843.
6. LeBlanc A, Schneider V, Shackelford L, et al. Bone mineral and lean tissue loss after long duration spaceflight. *J Musculoskelet Neuron Interact*. 2000;1:157–60.
7. Lueken SA, Arnaud SB, Taylor AK, et al. Changes in markers of bone formation and resorption in a bed rest model of weightlessness. *J Bone Miner Res*. 1993;8:1433–1438.
8. Baecker N, Tomic A, Mika C, et al. Bone resorption is induced on the second day of bed rest: results of a controlled cross-over trial. *J Appl Physiol*. 2003;95:977–982.
9. Perhonen MA, Franco F, Lane LD, et al. Cardiac atrophy after bed rest and spaceflight. *J Appl Physiol*. 2001;91:645–653.
10. Adams GR, Caiozzo VJ, Baldwin KM. Invited review: skeletal muscle unweighting: spaceflight and ground-based models. *J Appl Physiol*. 2003;95:2185–2201.
11. Fortney SM, Schneider VS, Greenleaf JE. The physiology of bed rest. In: Fregly MJ, Blatteis CM, eds. *Handbook of Physiology. Section 4: Environmental Physiology, vol 3. The Gravitational Environment*. New York: Oxford University; 1996:889–939.
12. Bungo MW, Johnson PC Jr. Cardiovascular examinations and observations of deconditioning during the space shuttle orbital flight test program. *Aviat Space Environ Med*. 1983;54:1001–1004.
13. Convertino VA. Cardiovascular consequences of bed rest: effects on maximal oxygen uptake. *Med Sci Sports Exerc*. 1997;29:191–196.
14. Convertino VA. Mechanisms of microgravity-induced orthostatic intolerance and implications of effective countermeasures: overview and future directions. *J Grav Physiol*. 2002;9:1–12.
15. Hung J, Goldwater D, Convertino VA, et al. Mechanisms for decreased exercise capacity following bed rest in normal middle-aged men. *Am J Cardiol*. 1983;51:344–348.
16. Saltin B, Blomqvist G, Mitchell JH, et al. Response to exercise after bed rest and after training. *Circulation*. 1968;38(suppl 7):1–78.
17. Linnarsson D, Tedner B, Lindborg B. Lower leg fluid displacement during a simulated space shuttle launch. *Eur J Appl Physiol*. 1998;78:65–68.
18. Dorfman TA, Levine BD, Tillery T, et al. Cardiac atrophy in women following bed rest. *J Appl Physiol*. 2007;103:8–16.
19. Ray CA, Vasques M, Miller TA, et al. Effect of short-term and long-term hindlimb unloading on rat cardiac mass and function. *J Appl Physiol*. 2001;91:1207–1213.
20. Levine BD, Zuckerman JH, Pawelczyk JA. Cardiac atrophy after bed-rest deconditioning: a nonneural mechanism for orthostatic intolerance. *Circulation*. 1997; 96:517–525.
21. Arbeille P, Kerbeci P, Mattar L, et al. WISE-2005: tibial and gastrocnemius vein and calf tissue response to LBNP after a 60-day bed rest with and without countermeasures. *J Appl Physiol*. 2008;104:938–943.
22. Arbeille P, Kerbeci P, Mattar L, et al. Insufficient flow reduction during LBNP in both splanchnic and lower limb areas is associated with orthostatic intolerance after bedrest. *Am J Physiol. Heart Circ Physiol*. 2008;295:H1846–H1854.
23. Buckley JC, Lane LD, Levine BD, et al. Orthostatic intolerance after spaceflight. *J Appl Physiol*. 1996;81:7–18.
24. Fritsch-Yelle JM, Whitson PA, Bondar RL, et al. Subnormal norephinephrine release relates to presyncope in astronauts after spaceflight. *J Appl Physiol*. 1996;81:2134–2141.
25. Delp MD, Colleran PN, Wilkerson MK, et al. Structural and functional remodeling of skeletal muscle microvasculature is induced by simulated microgravity. *Am J Physiol*. 2000;H1866–H1873.
26. Prisk GK. Physiology of a microgravity environment invited review: microgravity and the lung. *J Appl Physiol*. 2000;89:385–396.
27. Prisk GK, Fine JM, Elliott AR, et al. Effect of 6° head-down tilt on cardiopulmonary function: comparison with microgravity. *Aviat Space Environ Med*. 2002;73:8–16.
28. Montmerle S, Spaak J, Linnarsson D. Lung function during and after prolonged head-down bed rest. *J Appl Physiol*. 2002;92:75–83.
29. Prisk GK, Fine JM, Cooper TK, et al. Lung function is unchanged in the 1 G environment following 6-months exposure to microgravity. *Eur J Appl Physiol*. 2008; 103:617–623.
30. Convertino VA. Neuromuscular aspects in development of exercise countermeasures. *Physiologist*. 1991;34(suppl):S125–S128.
31. Edgerton VR, Zhou MY, Ohira Y, et al. Human fiber size and enzymatic properties after 5 and 11 days of spaceflight. *J Appl Physiol*. 1995;78:1733–1739.
32. Fitts RH, Trappe SW, Costill DL, et al. Prolonged spaceflight-induced alterations in the structure and function of human skeletal muscle fibres. *J Physiol*. 2010;588(Pt 18):3567–3592.
33. Trappe S, Costill D, Gallagher P, et al. Exercise in space: human skeletal muscle after 6 months aboard the International Space Station. *J Appl Physiol*. 2009;106:1159–1168.
34. Vico L, Collet P, Guignandon A, et al. Effects of long-term microgravity exposure on cancellous and cortical weight-bearing bones of cosmonauts. *Lancet*. 2000;355:1607–1611.
35. Smith SM, Wastney ME, Morukov BV, et al. Calcium metabolism before, during, and after a 3-mo spaceflight: kinetic and biochemical changes. *Am J Physiol*. 1999;277:R1–R10.
36. LeBlanc AD, Driscol TB, Shackelford LC, et al. Alendronate as an effective countermeasure to disuse induced bone loss. *J Musculoskel Neuron Interact*. 2002;2:335–343.

37. Sibonga JD, Evans HJ, Sung HG, et al. Recovery of spaceflight-induced bone loss: bone mineral density after long-duration missions as fitted with an exponential function. *Bone.* 2007;41:973–978.

38. Lang TF, LeBlanc AD, Evans HJ, et al. Adaptation of the proximal femur to skeletal reloading after long-duration spaceflight. *J Bone Miner Res.* 2006;21:1224–1230.

39. Smith SM, Heer M. Calcium and bone metabolism during space-flight. *Nutrition.* 2002;18:849–852.

40. Colleran PN, Wilkerson MK, Bloomfield SA, et al. Alterations in skeletal muscle perfusion with simulated microgravity: a possible mechanism for bone remodeling. *J Appl Physiol.* 2000;89:1046–1054.

41. Sonnenfeld G. The immune system in space and microgravity. *Med Sci Sports Exerc.* 2002;34:2021–2027.

42. Mills PJ, Meck JV, Waters WW, et al. Peripheral leukocyte sub-populations and catecholamine levels in astronauts as a function of mission duration. *Psychosom Med.* 2001;63:886–890.

43. Sonnenfeld G. Spaceflight, microgravity, stress, and immune responses. *Adv Space Res.* 1999;23:1945–1953.

44. Schmitt DA, Schaffar L, Taylor GR, et al. Use of bed rest and head-down tilt to simulate spaceflight-induced immune system changes. *J Interferon Cytokine Res.* 1996;16:151–157.

45. Lee SMC, Bennett BS, Hargens AR, et al. Upright exercise or supine lower body negative pressure exercise maintains exercise responses after bed rest. *Med Sci Sport Exerc.* 1997;29:892–900.

46. Shykoff BE, Farhi LE, Olszowka AJ, et al. Cardiovascular response to submaximal exercise in sustained microgravity. *J Appl Physiol.* 1996;81:26–32.

47. Sawin CF, Rummel JA, Michel EL. Instrumented personal exercise during long-duration spaceflights. *Aviat Space Environ Med.* 1975;46:394–400.

48. Michel EL, Rummel JA, Sawin CF, et al. Results of medical experiment M171—metabolic activity. In: Biomedical Results from Skylab, NASA SP-377. Washington, DC: 1977:372–387.

49. Levine BD, Lane LD, Watenpaugh DE, et al. Maximal exercise performance after adaptation to microgravity. *J Appl Physiol.* 1996;81:686–694.

50. Crandall CG, Shibasaki M, Wilson TE, et al. Prolonged head-down tilt exposure reduces maximal cutaneous vasodilator and sweating capacity in humans. *J Appl Physiol.* 2003;94:2330–2336.

51. Shibasaki M, Wilson TE, Cui J, et al. Exercise throughout 6 degrees head-down tilt bed rest preserves thermoregulatory responses. *J Appl Physiol.* 2003;95:1817–1823.

52. Convertino VA, Goldwater DJ, Sandler H. Bedrest-induced peak Vo₂ reduction associated with age, gender and aerobic capacity. *Aviat Space Environ Med.* 1986;57:17–22.

53. Greenisen MC, Hayes JC, Siconolfi SF, et al. Functional performance evaluation. In: Extended duration orbiter medical project final report. NASA SP-1999–534. Houston: 1999:3-1–3-17.

54. Lee SMC, Loehr JA, Guilliams ME, et al. Isokinetic strength and endurance after international space station (ISS) missions (Abstract). *Med Sci Sport Exerc.* 2003;35:S262.

55. Engelke KA, Convertino VA. Restoration of peak vascular conductance after simulated microgravity by maximal exercise. *Clin Physiol.* 1998;18:544–553.

56. Cowell SA, Stocks JM, Evans DG, et al. The exercise and environmental physiology of extravehicular activity. *Aviat Space Environ Med.* 2002;73:54–67.

57. Antonutto G, Capelli C, Girardis M, et al. Effects of microgravity on maximal power of lower limbs during very short efforts in humans. *J Appl Physiol.* 1999;86:85–92.

58. Gopalakrishnan R, Genc KO, Rice AJ, et al. Muscle volume, strength, endurance, and exercise loads during 6-month missions in space. *Aviat Space Environ Med.* 2010;81:91–102.

59. Schneider SM, Lee SM, Macias BR, et al. WISE-2005: exercise and nutrition countermeasures for upright Vo₂ₚₖ during bed rest. *Med Sci Sport Exerc.* 2009;41:2165–2176.

60. Greenleaf JE, Bernauer EM, Ertl AC, et al. Work capacity during 30-days of bed rest with isotonic and isokinetic exercise training. *J Appl Physiol.* 1989;67:1820–1826.

61. Greenleaf JE, Wade CE, Leftheriotis G. Orthostatic responses following 30-day bed rest deconditioning with isotonic and isokinetic exercise training. *Aviat Space Environ Med.* 1989; 60:537–542.

62. Shibata, S, Perhonen M, Levine BD. Supine cycling plus volume loading prevent cardiovascular deconditioning during bed rest. *J Appl Physiol.* 2010;108:1177–1186.

63. Engelke KA, Doerr DF, Crandall CG, et al. Application of acute maximal exercise to protect orthostatic tolerance after simulated microgravity. *Am J Physiol.* 1996;271:R837–R847.

64. Moore AD, Lee SMC, Charles JB, et al. Maximal exercise as a countermeasure to orthostatic intolerance after spaceflight. *Med Sci Sport Exerc.* 2001;33:75–80.

65. Lee SMC, Moore AD, Fritsch-Yelle JM, et al. Inflight exercise affects stand test responses after spaceflight. *Med Sci Sport Exerc.* 1999;31:1755–1762.

66. Trappe SW, Trappe TA, Lee GA, et al. Comparison of a space shuttle flight (STS-78) and bed rest on human muscle function. *J Appl Physiol.* 2001:57–64.

67. Trappe S, Trappe T, Gallagher P, et al. Human single muscle fiber function with 84 day bed-rest and resistance exercise. *J Physiol.* 2004;557(pt 2):501–503.

68. Trappe TA, Burd NA, Louis ES, et al. Influence of concurrent exercise or nutrition countermeasures on thigh and calf muscle size and function during 60 days of bed rest in women. *Acta Physiol.* 2007;19:147–159.

69. Schneider VS, McDonald J. Skeletal calcium homeostasis and countermeasures to prevent disuse osteoporosis. *Calcif Tissue Int.* 1984;36:S151–S154.

70. Vico L, Chappard D, Alexandre C, et al. Effects of a 120-day period of bed rest on bone mass and bone cell activities in man: attempts at countermeasure. *Bone Miner.* 1987;2:383–394.

71. Grigoriev AI, Morukov BV, Oganov VS, et al. Effect of exercise and bisphosphonate on mineral balance and bone density during 360-day antiorthostatic hypokinesia. *J Bone Miner Res.* 1992;7(suppl 2):S449–S455.

72. Smith SM, Davis-Street JE, Fesperman JV, et al. Evaluation of treadmill exercise in a lower body negative pressure chamber as a countermeasure for weightlessness-induced bone loss: a bed rest study with identical twins. *J Bone Miner Res.* 2003;18: 2223–2230.

73. Webb JT, Fischer MD, Heaps CL, et al. Exercise-enhanced preoxygenation increases protection from decompression sickness. *Aviat Space Environ Med.* 1996;67:618–624.

74. McGuire DK, Levine BL, Williamson JW, et al. A 30-year follow-up of the Dallas Bedrest and Training study: II. Effect of age on cardiovascular adaptation to exercise training. *Circulation.* 2001;104:1358–1366.

75. McGavock JM, Hastings JL, Snell PG, et al. A forty-year follow-up of the Dallas Bed Rest and Training Study: the effect of age on the cardiovascular response to exercise in men. *J Gerontol Ser A Biol Sci Med Sci.* 2009;64:293–299.

Genomics in the Future of Exercise Physiology

CHAPTER 27

Exercise Genomics and Proteomics

Frank W. Booth and P. Darrell Neufer

Abbreviations

AAV	Adeno-associated virus	mg	Milligram
AMPK	adenosine monophosphate-activated protein kinase	MHC	Myosin heavy chain
		miRNA	MicroRNAs
Ca^{++}	Calcium ion	mm Hg	Millimeters of mercury
cDNA	Complementary DNA	mRNA	Messenger RNA
ChIP	Chromatin immunoprecipitation	MS	Mass spectrometry
ChIP-seq	DNA sequencing of DNA regions immunoprecipitated with an antibody	NMDA	N-methyl D-aspartate
		PCR	Polymerase chain reaction
FRT	Flp recognition target	PDH	Pyruvate dehydrogenase
GLUT$_4$	Glucose transporter 4	PDK$_4$	Pyruvate dehydrogenase kinase 4
GO	Gene ontology	P$_{O_2}$	Partial pressure of oxygen
IL-6	Interleukin-6	P$_{CO_2}$	Partial pressure of carbon dioxide
MEF2	Myocyte enhancer factor 2	SNP	Single-nucleotide polymorphism

Introduction

The concept of a gene as a functional unit of hereditary information was first proposed in the mid-nineteenth century by Gregor Mendel. In the early 1900s, scientists surmised that genes were located in chromosomes. However, despite the detailed information about inheritance and development that was being provided by the field of genetics, the prevailing wisdom for several decades was that genes are simple substances that serve to support the structure of cells, and only proteins are structurally complex enough to carry genetic information. The discovery of the double-helix structure of DNA by James Watson and Francis Crick in 1953 definitively transformed this way of thinking by providing a new concept of how genetic information can be encoded in the structure of nucleic acids and transmitted from one generation to the next. Soon it became evident that each protein within a cell is encoded for by a single gene, and that variations in the sequence of a gene can alter the amino acid sequence of the resulting protein, sometimes with profound physiologic and clinical consequences.

In this chapter we introduce genomics, proteomics, and bioinformatics and discuss their applications to exercise physiology. Genomics is a rapidly evolving discipline, and therefore much of this chapter offers perspectives for future research for the aspiring student. To serve as a foundation, we first provide a comprehensive discussion of the principles of homeostasis (the driving force that leads all cells to respond and adapt) in the context of physical activity or inactivity (i.e., exercise or lack of exercise). Particular emphasis is placed on the potential application of genomic and proteomic approaches and technologies to decipher the mechanisms that are responsible for diseases linked to chronic physical inactivity, as well as the cellular and molecular basis for preventing or treating such diseases by means of increased physical activity. Next, methods and concepts to form hypotheses regarding the functions of genes altered by physical activity or inactivity and how they might be integrated to orchestrate a new phenotype are discussed. Finally, methods of genomics research are briefly introduced. Because this is the final chapter in this text, we have made a particular effort to provide insights into what the future may hold for research in physical activity or inactivity and exercise physiology. The tides of technology will undoubtedly shift the research sands in ways we cannot foresee; however, it is the unknown that we look forward to the most.

Genomics: Terms and Definitions

Genomics is traditionally defined as the study of the genetic material (genome) of an organism, that is, all of the DNA in the chromosomes of an organism. The year 2000 is an approximate demarcation in genomics research between the twentieth century, when genomics was largely confined to geneticists working to identify and sequence one or a few genes at a time, and the twenty-first century, when scientists from nearly every discipline have the opportunity to examine the function and interaction of all genes within cells, tissues, and organ systems. This transition can be attributed in large part to the recent sequencing of the entire genome (all of the nucleotide sequences, including structural genes, regulatory sequences, and noncoding DNA segments) for several species (*e.g.,* human, mouse, *Caenorhabditis elegans*, and yeast) and to the tremendous advances that have been made in biotechnology, that is, the methods of science.

Functional, Physiologic, and Environmental Genomics

This transition has also spawned a number of new terms, such as *functional genomics*, *physiologic genomics*, and *environmental genomics*, to name a few. Genomics is obviously common to all three terms, reflecting an evolution in its connotation. In other words, the field of genomics now addresses questions such as, What proteins are encoded for by every gene in the genome, and what is the function of these proteins? How do variations in the gene sequence (polymorphisms) affect gene expression and function? What is the genetic basis for diversity in physical performance of everyday life and in sports? What genes are expressed in specific cell types, and how does gene expression in those cell types change under different conditions, such as physical activity? Although it is still evolving, the discipline of functional genomics generally refers to the study of the function of all gene products within a cell. Physiologic genomics addresses the functional interaction among gene products within a larger setting (tissue, organ, or whole body) to maintain homeostasis. Environmental genomics focuses on how factors outside of the cell, tissue, organ, or whole body (*e.g.,* physical activity or inactivity, diet, oxygen content, and toxins) can affect the regulation of gene expression. It also addresses how such regulation is influenced by polymorphisms among individuals (*e.g.,* susceptibility to obesity because of variations in specific genes in the environmental context of sedentary behavior or a high-fat diet, or elite vs. nonelite performance).

> ## KEY POINT
>
> Genomics is a tool to explain the molecular basis for differences in physical ability that affect performance and health.

Application of Genomics to Exercise: Exercise Genomics

How does exercise physiology fit into the genomics era? It is now recognized that athleticism is at least in part inherited. However, it also became appreciated in the latter half of the twentieth century that exercise training improves physical performance through changes in gene expression. Thus, it is now clear that elite athletes must also train to optimize the expression of an undefined subpopulation of genes that predispose to superior physical performance (application of exercise to genomics). Indeed, numerous investigators have shown that training can change protein levels within cells by altering both their concentration (milligrams per unit of cell) and content (milligrams of tissue) in a manner that improves the functional capacity of muscle as well as the whole body (6). The challenge for exercise physiologists in the twenty-first century is not only to identify all of the genes that are responsive to exercise but to decipher the mechanisms by which those genes are regulated, the functional impact of the proteins that are encoded by those genes, how such protein interactions form the basis for the cellular adaptations generated by exercise training, and how such adaptations among all affected organs integrate to improve whole-body function and health. Exercise biochemistry is thus a basic science that can be used not only to enhance athletic performance but also to improve the health of children, adults, and the elderly.

Application of Genomics to Sedentary Diseases

In the last decade of the twentieth century, it was firmly established that a lack of daily dynamic exercise in otherwise healthy individuals significantly increases their risk of developing chronic health disorders. The application of genomics research to study diseases caused by sedentary living represents a clear challenge for twenty-first-century exercise scientists. For example, the ability of an individual to perform increased maximal aerobic work is linked to a reduced prevalence of chronic disease. This raises an obvious and important question: What genes play a role in both maximal aerobic performance and the prevention of chronic health disorders? Since the twentieth century, exercise genomics has grown from the study of a small number of elite athletes to a science that can be used to address the health needs of sedentary individuals. An additional challenge for the exercise physiologist in the twenty-first century will be to decipher the mechanisms by which physical inactivity alters the expression of disease susceptibility genes until ultimately a biologic threshold is passed, resulting in overt clinical disease.

Principles of Homeostasis: The Foundation for Exercise Genomics and Proteomics

An understanding of the principles of homeostasis provides a foundation for future genomics- and proteomics-based research efforts to identify the essential mechanisms that mediate the effects of physical inactivity on the etiology of chronic disease, as well as the ability of regular physical activity to prevent disease.

KEY POINT

Most exercise adaptations are initiated as an effort by cells, organs, and systems to stay within limits that are consistent with maintaining life by changing levels of proteins.

Definitions of Homeostasis: The Pregenomic Era

Homeostasis is classically defined as the ability to maintain relative constancy or uniformity in the internal environment in the face of significant changes in the external environment. This definition can be applied in many contexts. For example, cells are surrounded by membranes that allow nutrients, ions, gases, and so forth to move in and out passively or selectively while maintaining their own internal consistency or milieu, a property known as cell homeostasis. Physiologists also define homeostasis as the ability of the whole body or organism to maintain constancy under varying environmental conditions outside of the body. In this context, various organs contribute to maintaining whole body homeostasis. For example, the lungs facilitate the exchange of carbon dioxide for oxygen in the blood to maintain arterial blood partial pressure of carbon dioxide (P_{CO_2}) within a narrow range of 40 mm Hg in a resting, healthy individual. The cardiovascular system delivers oxygen to the peripheral tissues to keep skeletal muscle partial pressure of oxygen (P_{O_2}) within a range of 6 to 10 mm Hg at rest. The gastrointestinal system assists in maintaining blood Ca^{++} within a narrow range by absorbing Ca^{++} under the control of the parathyroid glands, and the kidneys remove metabolic byproducts and help maintain ion and fluid balance. All of the above are perturbed by exercise.

Definition of Homeostasis: The Era of the Genome

With the genome sequencing of an ever-growing list of species, basic science is evolving rapidly in terms of the complexity level at which researchers view cellular, organ, and whole-body physiology. By recognizing that every gene contains information required for the product of that gene (protein) to function (e.g., localization, enzymatic activity, and binding properties), we can begin to get a sense of how the baseline or genetic set point of each cell is determined by the collective functions and interactions of all proteins that are expressed within that cell type, and how the expression of these proteins can contribute to homeostasis. Of course, cells are not isolated entities but reside within an aqueous environment of extracellular fluid and blood, and neighboring cells that may secrete autocrine or paracrine factors. In other words, two cells of the same type (e.g., two hepatocytes) may differ slightly in their gene expression profile depending on their surrounding environment (i.e., fluid milieu, proximity to other cell types). It is the context of this surrounding environment that establishes the homeostatic set point of a given cell, that is, the adjustment of the genetic set point according to the surrounding environment. Other environmental influences, such as exercise, can challenge the maintenance of cellular homeostasis, as described in the next section.

Homeostasis in skeletal muscle

The external environment for cells in skeletal muscle is a composite derived from the various cell types that occupy the tissue, including skeletal myofibers, satellite cells, neurons, vascular endothelial and smooth muscle cells, fibroblasts, and various cells of the immune system. Homeostasis within a resting myofiber is a balance among competing systems, such as substrate flux through the various metabolic pathways, ion distribution across the plasma membrane, calcium sequestration in the sarcoplasmic reticulum, and contractile protein cycling (to name but a few). An analogy to homeostasis is the set point of the body's thermostat, which defends against changes in core body temperature (the set point) in response to both internal and external environmental challenges. Collectively, the relative set points of all of the dynamic systems of a cell define the resting homeostatic state of the myofiber. In the face of changes to the environment outside and inside the cell (*e.g.,* oxygen concentration, ion concentration, and substrate delivery), cellular systems react to ensure that homeostasis, be it metabolic, electrochemical, or physical, is maintained during the initial perturbation.

Not all myofibers are defined by the same homeostatic set point. Skeletal muscle fibers are broadly divided into two categories—slow and fast—based on their speed of contraction, although a continuum exists between the two extremes (1). The homeostatic level of high-energy phosphates (*e.g.,* adenosine triphosphate) is almost twice as high in fast fibers as in slow fibers. Muscle fiber types also differ in their calcium-handling properties, glycolytic and oxidative capacities, mitochondrial content, and capillary density. For example, the homeostatic level of resting free Ca^{++} is twice as high in slow fibers versus fast fibers. The variation in homeostatic regulation among fiber types is relevant because each muscle fiber (and likely each myonuclear domain) has to provide slightly different global gene expression patterns to maintain different (local) homeostatic levels at rest. Future research will likely reveal that the molecular mechanisms that defend against disruptions of homeostasis in exercising muscle also vary among myonuclei within a single fiber and among different muscle fiber types.

Contribution of other organ systems to homeostasis in skeletal muscle

At rest, most of the body's energy is used to support organs such as the heart, lung, liver, kidney, gastrointestinal system, adipose tissue, and brain. The cardiovascular and gastrointestinal systems, lung, and liver all contribute to maintaining homeostasis in skeletal muscle by facilitating the exchange of oxygen and metabolic substrates for carbon dioxide and metabolic byproducts. In fact, one could argue that skeletal muscle is a rather selfish tissue, relying on other organs to maintain its own homeostasis while offering little in return. During exercise, muscle's reliance on other organ systems obviously intensifies. Under most conditions of exercise, the priority of other organ systems is to provide the support necessary for skeletal muscle to maintain contractile activity (*e.g.,* increased cardiac output to allow increased muscle blood flow, and enhanced respiratory minute volume to permit maintenance of a constant arterial P_{O_2}). However, as the exercise continues, particularly under adverse conditions such as a hot environment, the needs of these other organ systems begin to increase in priority, limiting their support to skeletal muscle and therefore the ability to continue exercise. Competition for blood volume between exercising muscle and skin to dispose of the metabolic byproduct heat, particularly in a hot environment, and the competing need for glucose between exercising muscle and the brain are two prime examples of times when the requirements of contracting muscle may be overridden in favor of homeostatic needs elsewhere in the body. This topic is discussed in detail in Chapter 19.

Contribution of skeletal muscle to other organs and whole-body homeostasis

Does muscle contribute to whole-body homeostasis and, if so, how? Cardiac muscle makes an obvious contribution by pumping blood to other organs. The contribution by skeletal muscle, however, is less obvious. Skeletal muscle plays a major role in blood glucose homeostasis. It can also communicate with other organs during exercise by (a) type III (mechanoreceptors) and IV (metabolically sensitive) sensory nerves from skeletal muscle to stimulate the exercise pressor effect, which increases heart rate and blood pressure; and (b) myokines, such as interleukin-6 (IL-6), that are released by skeletal muscle and are thought to help coordinate organ function (see Chapter 20).

Simply put, skeletal muscle is a major consumer of energy. It constitutes about 40% of total body weight and 20% to 25% of basal metabolic rate. When carbohydrate intake is insufficient (*e.g.,* as a result of prolonged physical activity, fasting, malnutrition, or cachexia), defending blood glucose concentration, the major source of energy for the brain, becomes the metabolic priority for the body. Under such conditions, glucose utilization must be conserved by peripheral tissues. Skeletal muscle, which normally relies heavily on blood glucose, shifts to alternative fuel sources (*i.e.,* free fatty acids and proteins). This conservation of glucose, coupled with the activation of glucose production by the liver in response to numerous counterregulatory hormones (*e.g.,* glucagon, epinephrine, and cortisol), ensures that the brain can continue to be supplied with a sufficient amount of glucose. As these conditions persist, skeletal muscle also becomes the major source of amino acids (released via protein breakdown), many of which serve as gluconeogenic precursors for the liver.

Skeletal muscle can also communicate with other organs via nerves and the bloodstream. Muscle generates an exercise pressor reflex (a peripheral neural reflex originating in skeletal muscle) whose afferent arm originates by activation of mechanically (muscle mechanoreflex) and chemically sensitive (muscle metaboreflex) skeletal muscle receptors during skeletal muscle contraction. Contracting skeletal muscle can also communicate with other organs via the release of signals into the blood. These signals are cytokines and other peptides that are produced, expressed, and released by muscle fibers (termed *myokines*) that exert either paracrine or endocrine effects. IL-6 meets the definition of a myokine because it is expressed by and released from contracting human skeletal muscle. IL-6 also has metabolic effects in humans in vivo. The effect of IL-6 on insulin-stimulated glucose disposal and fatty acid oxidation in skeletal muscle and adipose tissue of humans in vivo appears to be mediated by activation of adenosine monophosphate-activated protein kinase (AMPK) (see Chapter 14).

This example serves to illustrate a future challenge in genomic and proteomic profiling: to integrate multiple changing gene expression profiles in various organs to determine organ integration in whole body stresses such as physical exercise. A future research endeavor will thus be to put together the changes in global gene expression that communicate signals among individual organs to integrate a reduction in homeostatic disruptions.

In times of plenty, skeletal muscle's contribution to metabolic homeostasis can go awry with devastating consequences. In healthy, physically fit individuals, skeletal muscle is responsible for about 80% of the clearance of both glucose and lipids from the blood after a meal. However, when a chronic positive caloric imbalance exists in the body (particularly associated with high-fat diets), skeletal muscle can begin to lose its ability to clear glucose from the circulation, resulting in a condition known as insulin resistance. If insulin resistance persists for years, the pancreas in some individuals may no longer be able to produce enough insulin to maintain hyperinsulinemia to compensate for the insulin resistance in skeletal muscle. Consequently, blood glucose concentration remains elevated both after and between meals—the clinical transition to type 2 diabetes.

Although the mechanism of insulin resistance in skeletal muscle is not fully understood, it is clear that a chronic disturbance to metabolic homeostasis in the form of a chronic positive caloric balance generated by excess intake and/or inadequate expenditure is a major underlying factor. This should make it readily apparent that the level of daily physical activity and thus the level of energy that is consumed by skeletal muscle to support that activity are major determinants of energy balance (*i.e.*, metabolic homeostasis) on a day-to-day basis. When considered in the context of obesity and type 2 diabetes (two disease states classified as epidemics in the United States), the contribution of skeletal muscle to glucose homeostasis and overall energy balance is profound and yet often underappreciated. Therefore, a major goal of future research will be to elucidate the mechanisms underlying physical-inactivity–induced chronic health disorders. Information gained from genomics, proteomics, and bioinformatics will be needed to identify which genes in skeletal muscle orchestrate the pathologies of insulin resistance, and which of those genes serve as metabolic signals among all involved organs or tissues when insufficient physical activity produces metabolic dysfunctions from a chronic positive caloric imbalance.

TEST YOURSELF

How does skeletal muscle contribute to whole-body homeostasis during aerobic exercise?

Principles of Cellular Homeostasis

The maintenance of cellular homeostasis is a dynamic process. To optimize survival, a cell must retain the ability to adapt to changes in its external environment, and thus the proteins that control these adjustments must be able to

increase or decrease, which means they have to be continuously turning over, replacing the old with the new. (If a protein had no turnover, it would likely have no synthesis or degradation processes to call upon when an adaptive change in protein level was required to adjust to a new external environment.) The concentration of any protein at any given time thus reflects the balance between its rate of synthesis and rate of degradation. As long as these rates remain equal, the concentration of the protein will remain the same. This is known as the steady-state concentration. In the following sections, we provide a series of examples to illustrate how specific changes in protein synthesis and degradation lead to a change in the steady-state level of proteins. Because the proteome represents the future of research in exercise physiology as well as all biomedical research, an understanding of the principles that govern protein turnover in all cells is required.

KEY POINT

For a protein to adapt from one level to a new level, the balance between the rate of synthesis and degradation must change via a process termed *protein turnover*.

Protein turnover: kinetics of normal cellular life

To be able to appropriately design and interpret research studies, the exercise scientist must understand the principles that govern protein turnover. The same principles apply to any change in regular physical activity, whether it involves a sedentary person who is beginning a training program, an elite athlete who is detraining due to injury, or an elite athlete who is retraining to regain peak condition. In this section, we discuss the principles upon which all adaptations to a habitual change in activity level are based.

Imagine that you can turn off the synthesis of a particular protein in a cell. By following the decrease in concentration of that protein in the cell over time, you can determine its rate of degradation or turnover rate. By plotting time on the X axis and protein concentration on the Y axis, you will discover that the rate of change in protein concentration per unit of time (*i.e.*, the turnover rate) is not linear; rather, it is a curvilinear or exponential decay (Fig. 27.1A). This is known as a first-order relationship and is given by the following equation:

$$\textbf{Turnover Rate} = \frac{d[\text{protein}]}{dt} = k \cdot [\text{protein}] \qquad [1]$$

where k = the fractional degradation rate constant expressed as reciprocal units of time (*i.e.*, fraction or percentage degraded per minute or per day). This is called a first-order reaction because the degradation or turnover rate depends on k (which is unique for every protein) and the concentration of

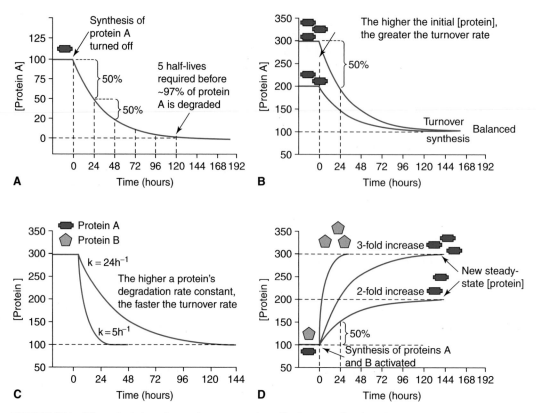

FIGURE 27.1 The principles of protein turnover in cells. See text for details.

the protein. In other words, the turnover rate is a certain percentage of the concentration of the protein at any given time. This means that as the protein concentration decreases over time, less and less protein will be available to be degraded. This accounts for the exponential decrease in protein concentration shown in Figure 27.1A. This also means that the absolute turnover rate (i.e., the absolute amount of protein degraded per unit of time) will decrease exponentially.

The integrated form of Eq. 27.1, which is more useful for making calculations, is

$$\log \frac{[A_o]}{[A_t]} = \frac{kt}{2.303}$$

where $[A_o]$ is the initial concentration of protein A at time zero, and $[A_t]$ is the concentration at any time t. To allow for comparison among proteins when synthesis is artificially set to zero, the loss of protein can be set to 50% ($[A_o]/[A_t] = 2$). Solving for t gives the half-life ($t_{1/2} = 0.693 \cdot k^{-1}$) of the protein (i.e., the time required for half of the protein concentration to be degraded). Under these conditions, the fractional turnover rate is synonymous with the half-life. In the example shown in Figure 27.1A, protein A has a half-life of 24 hours; thus 50% of the decrease in protein A concentration occurs during the first 24 hours, another 50% loss (of the remaining protein concentration) occurs during the next 24 hours, and so on, such that a total of five half-lives, or 5 days, are required before about 97% of the initial protein is degraded.

Now we move our example to the context of the cell. As mentioned above, the concentration of a particular protein at any given time reflects the balance between its rate of synthesis and rate of degradation. When homeostasis is disturbed within a cell, the rate of synthesis and/or degradation of a target protein may be adjusted to allow for an adaptive change in the protein level to minimize either acute or chronic disruptions in homeostasis. For the purpose of discussion, we will assume that the fractional degradation rate constant remains unchanged and that control for change in the protein level is exerted only by changing the rate of synthesis. In the example shown in Figure 27.1B, the stimulus to the cell requires the concentration of protein A to be lowered from 200 to 100 (milligrams per muscle weight). The protein synthesis rate will be reduced to the level required to generate the new desired concentration (in this case halved), resulting in a loss in the concentration of protein A that follows a pattern identical to that shown in Figure 27.1A, requiring about 5 days (five half-lives) before the degradation rate of protein A equals the synthesis rate and the new steady-state concentration of protein A is established. What if the initial concentration of protein A is 300 instead of 200 mg per muscle weight? How long will it take to reduce protein A to the same baseline concentration of 100 mg per muscle weight, again assuming that the fractional degradation rate constant (k) is unchanged? As depicted in Figure 27.1B, the answer is the same: about 5 days. The protein synthesis rate will again be reduced to the level required to generate a concentration of 100 mg per muscle weight. Because the fractional turnover rate of any protein is directly proportional to the concentration of that protein (see Eq. 27.1), the higher initial concentration will result in a greater absolute amount (milligrams) of protein being degraded per day. Thus, when the synthesis of a given protein is abruptly changed to a new rate, the time required to achieve the new steady-state concentration will be independent of the initial protein concentration and solely a function of the fractional degradation rate constant, or half-life of the protein.

Thus far, we have considered protein A with a characteristic half-life of 24 hours. The fractional turnover rate, as you might imagine, varies considerably among proteins and is typically given as percent per day (*e.g.,* 50% per day for a protein with a half-life of 24 hours). For proteins with a much shorter half-life, the time required to reach a new steady-state concentration will be much less. Figure 27.1C compares the fractional turnover rate of protein A, with a half-life of 24 hours, and protein B, with a half-life of 5 hours. Adjusting the concentration of both proteins from an initial concentration of 300 to a new steady-state concentration of 100 mg protein per muscle weight will require a total of 25 hours (five half-lives) for protein B compared with 5 days (five half-lives) for protein A. This example illustrates the concept that the time required to achieve a new steady-state concentration is solely a function of the fractional degradation rate constant, or half-life of each individual protein.

This section has three take-home points. First, the absolute turnover rate of a protein is a product of the fractional degradation rate constant (percent per given time period) for that specific protein and the concentration (milligrams of protein per whole muscle or other tissue) of the protein at any given time. Second, regardless of the initial concentration of a particular protein, a change in the synthesis rate (with no change in the fractional degradation rate constant) will require five half-lives before the concentration of that protein reaches about 97% of its new steady-state concentration. The new concentration simply represents the balance between the new rate of synthesis (expressed as milligrams of protein synthesized per day per whole muscle) and the absolute rate of degradation (milligrams of protein degraded per day per whole muscle). Third, the higher the fractional degradation rate constant (*i.e.,* the shorter the half-life), the less total time will be required for the protein to assume its new steady-state concentration (five half-lives).

TEST YOURSELF

The swim coach at your university wants to know how fast his swimmers will lose their trained state after the last meet of the season. You decide to take biopsies of the deltoid muscle on the day of the final meet and 1, 7, and 14 days later to measure the concentrations of proteins X, Y, and Z. You know that proteins X, Y, and Z have half-lives of 10 hours, 3 days, and 7 days, respectively. What percent change in protein do you expect to measure for proteins X, Y, and Z at each time point?

The rate of adaptive increase in protein concentration is also a function of protein turnover

Up to this point, we have considered only the dynamics governing a decrease in protein concentration. What if the disturbance to cell homeostasis requires an increase in protein concentration? It turns out the same principles apply. Remember that with any increase in protein concentration, more protein will be available for degradation. In this example, let us assume that the stimulus doubles the protein concentration by doubling the protein synthesis rate (milligrams of protein synthesized per day) while keeping the protein degradation rate unchanged (percent per day). Thus, the doubling in protein synthesis is partially offset by an increase in the milligrams of protein degraded per day (determined by constant percent degraded per day multiplied by progressively increasing protein concentration in milligrams of protein per whole muscle). Returning to protein A, with a half-life of 24 hours, a plot of the concentration of protein A versus time in response to an inducing stimulus shows that 50% of the adaptive change in protein concentration occurs during the first half-life, 50% of the remaining adaptive increase occurs in the second half-life, and so on, resulting in a nonlinear or exponential rate of increase in protein concentration (Fig. 27.1D). As with protein degradation, the overall time required for protein A to adjust from its initial concentration to the new steady-state concentration is about five half-lives, or 5 days, irrespective of the level of increase in protein synthesis rate or magnitude of the final increase in protein concentration (twofold vs. threefold in Fig. 27.1D). Again, the new steady-state concentration simply reflects the point at which the elevated amount of protein synthesized per day is balanced by the increased amount of protein degraded per day. In effect, the set point for homeostasis within the cell, at least with respect to protein A, has been reset in the context of the new environmental conditions. As long as these conditions persist, the concentration of protein A will remain stable at its new higher level.

It should also be clear from Figure 27.1D that the time required to reach the new steady-state concentration depends entirely on the half-life of the protein. For example, protein B, with a half-life of only 5 hours, will reach its new steady-state level in 25 hours. This is because the fractional turnover rate is much faster, effectively allowing adjustments in concentration to occur at a much greater rate. At this point, you may be thinking that if protein A and protein B have the same initial concentration (*e.g.,* 100 mg per muscle weight), how can the concentration of protein B, with the higher fractional turnover rate constant, increase faster than the concentration of protein A, with the lower fractional turnover rate constant? The key to thinking about this question is to recognize that even though protein A and protein B have the same initial concentrations, the basal synthesis rate of protein B is five times that of protein A because the half-life of protein B (5 hours) is about one-fifth of the half-life of protein A (24 hours). Thus, to triple the concentration of both protein A and protein B, the absolute increase in synthesis (milligrams of protein synthesized per day) of protein B will have to be five times greater than for protein A; that is, the relative rates of protein synthesis will have to be tripled for both A and B. Under these conditions, protein B will reach its new steady-state concentration much sooner than protein A (Fig. 27.1D).

What if the intensity of the stimulus to increase protein A is far greater, and sufficient to induce a 10-fold increase in protein A concentration? How long will it take to generate the full response? The answer should be evident from the discussion about protein B: the half-life of protein A has not changed, so it will still require about 5 days to achieve the new steady-state concentration. The concentration (milligrams of protein A per whole muscle) will be 10 times greater, but the total time required for the adaptive response will remain the same.

Points of cellular control regulating protein expression

During resistance training, skeletal muscle increases in size, so more protein must appear. In contrast, during aerobic training, mitochondrial proteins increase in skeletal muscle, but muscle mass may not increase. Exactly how do muscle cells adjust the concentration of specific proteins? In response to a stimulus, components of both protein synthesis (e.g., messenger RNA [mRNA] concentration, translation initiation, processing, and assembly), and protein degradation (e.g., ubiquitination) are subject to regulation, usually in a coordinated manner. Of course, genetic information ultimately flows from DNA (via transcription) to mRNA (via translation) to protein. The steady-state level of expression of a given gene product (protein) therefore reflects a series of synthetic and degradative processes and is ultimately determined by the kinetics of the rate-limiting step. Although it is difficult to determine in living animals, the rate-limiting step likely varies considerably among proteins and may shift from one step to another in response to a given stimulus. For example, proteins that are constitutively expressed in skeletal muscle (e.g., contractile proteins and many metabolic enzymes) tend to be fairly stable (i.e., with long half-lives) and are backed by relatively steady rates of transcription, such that adjustments in protein concentration may be fine-tuned by altering protein translation or stability and altered on a larger scale by changes in mRNA.

In contrast, for proteins that fluctuate or are expressed as needed (e.g., stress proteins and certain transcription factors), the rate of synthesis for the final product (protein) is often primarily a function of the concentration of the corresponding mRNA. In similarity to proteins, the concentration of a given mRNA in a cell is a function of its rate of synthesis (transcription) and fractional degradation rate (mRNA turnover). In addition, all mRNAs have a characteristic turnover rate, or half-life. Thus, the principles that govern protein turnover also apply to the control of mRNA turnover. In fact, the half-life of most mRNAs is typically much shorter than the half-life of the corresponding

proteins, which means that adjustments in mRNA concentration in response to a given stimulus occur much more rapidly. This also implies that although regulation may be exerted at multiple steps, the rate-limiting step for altering the expression of many acutely regulated proteins likely resides at the level of transcription of the corresponding gene. Knowledge of the degree and time course of change in protein level can be used as one criterion to form hypotheses regarding the functions of gene expression altered by physical activity or inactivity, as discussed further below.

Principles Governing the Adaptive Response to Altered Physical Activity

The principles of protein turnover discussed in the preceding sections are based on the responses of a cell in the face of a constant change in the environment that evokes a challenge to homeostasis. In other words, the stimulus to a cell will be the same throughout the adaptive period. But what if the disturbance to homeostasis in a cell is not constant? Exercise training, for example, is an intermittent stimulus that induces only temporary disruptions to homeostasis; yet, when such exercise is performed daily for several weeks, it is a stimulus that evokes clear adaptations. In the next section, we discuss the kinetic principles that govern cellular responses to intermittent stimuli, such as repeated exercise bouts.

Dynamic exercise transiently activates transcription of select metabolic genes

The use of molecular biology approaches in the late 1980s revealed that dynamic training-induced increases in mitochondrial proteins (such as the cytochromes of electron transport and Krebs cycle enzymes) are preceded by increases in their corresponding mRNAs (see A Milestone of Discovery at the end of this chapter). This suggests that at least a portion of the adaptive response to training is mediated at the pretranslational level (i.e., transcription and/or mRNA stability). Indeed, over the past two decades, a number of studies have provided direct evidence that contractile activity activates transcription of select metabolic genes. Of importance, these regulatory events were found to be acute and transient, occurring primarily over several hours during the recovery period after exercise. The implication from these studies is that the training adaptations generated by exercise training likely stem from the cumulative effects of the acute transient responses to each individual exercise bout. As illustrated in the next section, whether a particular exercise-responsive protein will accumulate during the course of a training program is determined solely by the half-life of that protein.

Kinetics of the acute adaptive response to exercise

In Figures 27.2 to 27.4, we employ an analogy to conceptualize how the dynamics that govern changes in gene expression in response to an acute bout of exercise ultimately

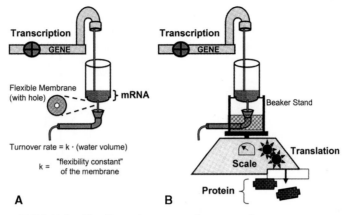

FIGURE 27.2 The flow of genetic information from a gene to messenger RNA (mRNA) (**A**) to protein (**B**). See text for details.

provide the underlying basis for the adaptations to endurance training. In this analogy (Fig. 27.2A), the transcriptional activity of a gene is represented by the rate of water flowing out of a faucet, regulated by an on/off valve.

The water collects in a glass beaker, the volume of which represents the concentration of mRNA at any given time. To account for the turnover of mRNA, the bottom of the beaker is constructed from a flexible rubber membrane with a small hole in the middle, allowing water to drain

from the beaker. Because the membrane is flexible, the hole in the membrane expands in direct proportion to the volume of water in the beaker. This increases the volume of water lost as a constant fraction of the total water volume (representing the fractional degradation rate constant). Different beakers possess membranes with different flexibility constants, representing the different degradation rate constants among mRNAs. Thus, the fractional turnover rate of the water (mRNA) is a function of the membrane flexibility

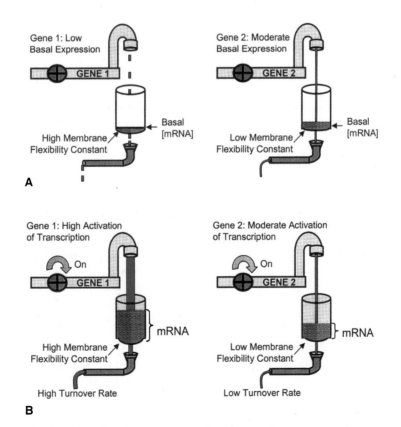

FIGURE 27.3 The dynamics governing changes in gene expression for two different genes in response to an acute bout of exercise.
A. Regulation at rest. **B.** The 2-hour period immediately after exercise. See text for details.

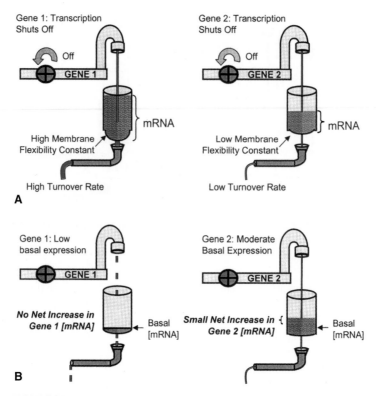

FIGURE 27.4 The dynamics governing changes in gene expression for two different genes in response to an acute bout of exercise. **A.** Regulation at 2 to 6 hours. **B.** Regulation 24 hours after exercise. See text for details.

constant (mRNA fractional degradation rate constant) and the amount of water in the beaker (mRNA concentration) similar to Eq. 27.1, which describes protein turnover.

To complete the analogy, the beaker is placed on a balance. The balance is mechanically linked to a machine that makes building blocks representing new proteins. The balance is designed to activate the building block machine (protein synthesis) in direct portion to the weight of the beaker. For the sake of simplicity, mRNA stability, translation, and protein turnover are not subject to regulation in this analogy. Thus, the level of water (mRNA) in the beaker will determine the rate of building-block production (protein synthesis).

Let us consider the response to exercise of two genes (Fig. 27.3A). Gene 1 encodes for a specialized protein (*e.g.,* a transcription factor) that is needed by the cell only under certain conditions. Expression of gene 1 in the basal state is very low. The basal water flow from this faucet (transcriptional activity) is low, the membrane flexibility constant (mRNA fractional degradation rate constant) is high, and as a result the basal level of water in the beaker (mRNA concentration) is low. Gene 2 encodes for a protein that is required for normal day-to-day function in the cell (*e.g.,* a mitochondrial enzyme). It possesses a modest level of basal water flow from the faucet, a moderate membrane flexibility constant, and consequently a modest basal level of water in the beaker.

This stable level of water in the beaker produces a constant rate of building block synthesis (gene 2 encoded protein).

In response to a single bout of exercise, the faucet valve (transcription) for gene 1 is fully turned on (Fig. 27.3B). During the initial 2 hours or so of recovery, water accumulates quickly in the beaker, followed by a rapid rise in the rate of gene 1 building block (protein). (Note: For the sake of simplicity, this example assumes a constant proportion between the concentration of a given mRNA and its translation into protein, which often is not maintained upon the transition from rest to exercise.) The valve for gene 2 is also turned on, but not nearly to the same extent, producing a relatively small increase in water flow from the faucet and a small rise in the water level in the beaker. The inherently high membrane flexibility constant of gene 1 also results in a much greater rate of water loss (mRNA fractional turnover) from the beaker.

Nevertheless, as the flow of water from each faucet (transcription) slows during the next several hours of recovery (about 2–6 h), the total accumulation of water in the beaker (mRNA concentration) for gene 1 will still far exceed that of gene 2 (Fig. 27.4A). However, within 24 hours after exercise, the level of water in the beaker for gene 1 will return to its initial low basal level, whereas the level of water in the beaker for gene 2, because of the much slower rate of water loss for gene 2, will remain slightly higher than basal (Fig. 27.4B). Thus, for gene 2, there will be a small net accumulation of water in the beaker (mRNA concentration) 1 day after exercise. When this scenario is repeated day after day, the water for gene 2 will gradually accumulate with each transient response to exercise, eventually producing a net two- to threefold increase in water (mRNA) level, or training adaptation. Presumably, the gradual or net cumulative increase in the water level (mRNA concentration) of gene 2 will translate into a corresponding overall increase in the rate of synthesis for its protein and accumulation of building block 2 (protein). In contrast, despite the dramatic transient activation of water flow for gene 1 occurring in response to each exercise bout, the rate of water loss from the gene 1 beaker postexercise will prevent any net mRNA accumulation from 1 day to the next. Assuming that the turnover rate for gene 1 protein is also rapid, protein 1 concentration will spike in response to each exercise bout but will return to baseline before the next bout. Thus, for gene 1 mRNA and protein, no cumulative training adaptation will occur.

What are the two key points to take away from this analogy? First, the magnitude of increase in a specific mRNA or protein to an acute stimulus, such as exercise, depends largely on the degree of activation of the rate-limiting process (i.e., activation of transcription in the analogy), whereas the duration of increase depends primarily on the fractional degradation rate constants (half-lives) of the specific mRNAs and proteins involved. Second, for an mRNA or protein to undergo a cumulative increase in concentration in response to repeated bouts of exercise, as with exercise training, the half-life of the mRNA or protein must be long enough to result in a net increase between each exercise bout. Although it is not depicted specifically, the rate-limiting step in the synthetic process for a given gene may involve something other than transcription (e.g., posttranscriptional processing, mRNA stability, translation, and assembly), may vary with the type of stimulus, and/or may shift during the course of the adaptive period. Regardless of the site of control, however, the disturbance to homeostasis during any training program is intermittent and therefore governed by standard kinetic principles.

TEST YOURSELF

From your last study with the swimmers, you have become particularly interested in protein X because other studies have shown that it is a key transcription factor for activating the genes that encode for proteins Y and Z. You want to do a study on the swimmers at the beginning of the new season to measure proteins X, Y, and Z in the deltoid muscle before and after 8 weeks of training (the same proteins you studied at the end of the last swim season; see page 675). Your mentor instructs you to take a biopsy before training and 48 hours after the last training bout at the end of the 8 weeks to avoid any potential acute effects from the last training bout. You do not agree with this design. Why? How would you design the study?

Implications regarding the kinetic principles governing exercise and exercise training

EXERCISE: A TRANSIENT DISTURBANCE TO HOMEOSTASIS Although the concept is predominantly theoretical, it seems reasonable to assume that the acute molecular responses to exercise that occur in muscle are triggered by the relative stress imparted on the cell (i.e., the disturbance to homeostasis and the cell's effort to reestablish homeostasis). The time required for the various systems in myofibrils to recover and to return can vary on the order of minutes (ion balance) to several days or more (protein synthesis for damage repair). Thus, it is apparent that the cellular and molecular responses to exercise can extend well beyond the period of contractile activity. This implies that the signaling mechanisms within muscle may not simply reflect the residual effects of the exercise bout; rather, they may be sensitive to specific disturbances in homeostasis regardless of how they are evoked. In other words, until that disturbance is resolved, the specific regulatory mechanism will remain activated in an attempt to restore that portion of cell homeostasis.

KEY POINT

Muscle senses changes in homeostasis evoked by the level of daily exercise and sends signals for the changes in protein levels to minimize the disturbance. The net result is less disruption to homeostasis upon exercise the next day.

A perfect example of this concept is the regulation of glucose uptake during recovery from exercise. Despite the absence of contractile activity or insulin (two known activators of glucose uptake), glucose uptake remains elevated in muscle during the initial 30-minute recovery period after exercise (42). Moreover, insulin sensitivity (the amount of glucose taken up for a given amount of insulin) is also enhanced and remains elevated in a previously exercising muscle until muscle glycogen content is fully restored. Although the mechanisms are not well understood, it is reasonable to suggest that signaling mechanisms that are sensitive to muscle glycogen content, rather than the contractile activity itself, may remain activated to ensure that glucose continues to enter the cell until substrate reserves are replenished.

ACUTE RESPONSES TO EXERCISE LIKELY DEPEND ON THE RELATIVE INTENSITY, DURATION, AND MODE OF EXERCISE   The magnitude of increase in the mitochondrial protein cytochrome c in response to a 12-week endurance training program is directly related to the intensity and duration of exercise (7,48). Although data at the molecular level are limited, we can conjecture that the acute activation of gene expression is also directly related to the intensity, duration, and mode of exercise (27). Clearly, the impact of a given exercise bout will depend on the relative stress perceived by a particular cellular system. For example, one might expect genes that help conserve whole body glucose reserves to be induced in response to a long bout of endurance exercise. Likewise, growth-promoting resistance exercise would be expected to elicit a much different set of genes compared with those induced by endurance exercise. Identifying the full complement of genes that respond under different intensities, durations, and modes of exercise is a challenge for future research in exercise physiology. Furthermore, identifying the polymorphisms that account for the wide variation in adaptive response to the same exercise stimulus among humans and animals also represents a particularly challenging but important area for future research.

CHRONIC EXERCISE (TRAINING) PRODUCES A RELATIVELY STEADY-STATE CHANGE IN PROTEIN CONCENTRATION

As exercise training continues over the course of several weeks, the products of genes with a sufficiently long half-life (*e.g.*, cytochrome *c*) will continue to gradually accumulate (5). If a progressive training program is used (*i.e.*, low intensity gradually increasing to high intensity), and protein concentration is measured at the same time each week, the change in protein concentration may appear to be linear and fairly slow. However, if the daily exercise stimulus follows the pattern of a square wave (*i.e.*, high intensity every day), the change in protein concentration will be exponential. After several weeks of training, the acute increase in synthesis in response to each exercise bout will be balanced by an increased absolute degradation rate. In addition, as the adaptations to training continue, a progressive resetting of the homeostatic set point will occur such that the disruption to homeostasis in response to each exercise bout will be lessened. If the training intensity is not increased, no further net increase in protein concentration will occur, and the protein will level off at a new, higher relative steady state. However, maintenance of the trained state is dependent on regular intervals of exercise. Thus, in a sense, the concentration of proteins adapting to an intermittent stimulus is in a constant state of flux.

CUMULATIVE INCREASES IN GENE EXPRESSION LIKELY DEPEND ON THE FREQUENCY OF TRAINING

In addition to the intensity and duration of exercise, it is well established that the frequency of exercise during a training program directly influences the rate at which mitochondrial protein concentration increases. Again, although information at the molecular level is limited, it is reasonable to assume that the level of an acute increase in protein or mRNA is inversely related to the time between exercise bouts. In other words, the shorter the period between exercise bouts, the more protein or mRNA will remain from the adaptive response to the previous bout and the faster the accumulation will be during training. In one study (26), for example, 2 hours of dynamic exercise for 2 or 6 days

a week increased cytochrome *c* protein concentration 30% and 85%, respectively, after 14 weeks. Furthermore, it is also likely that with shorter intervals between exercise bouts, the expression of a greater number of genes will be elevated and thus they will accumulate with successive bouts of exercise. However, if a minimal rest period is not obtained, some components, such as contractile proteins, will decrease in quantity, as in the continuous chronic stimulation of skeletal muscle.

SOME TRAINING ADAPTATIONS ARE RAPIDLY LOST WITH THE CESSATION OF TRAINING

It is painfully obvious to anyone who has undergone a period of detraining that training adaptations disappear rapidly, and recovery to the trained state requires a disproportionately longer time than detraining. This, of course, is due to the first-order nature of protein turnover as discussed above; that is, 50% of the loss of a protein occurs in one half-life (which for this example was the duration of the detraining), and five half-lives are required to regain the total protein lost once training resumes. In many studies, the effects of an endurance training program were assessed 48 to 96 hours after the last training session to avoid the acute effects of the last exercise bout and ascertain the "true training" effect. Although this strategy may be fine for proteins with relatively long half-lives (>1 wk; *e.g.*, citrate synthase and succinate dehydrogenase have an estimated half-life of 12 d), it will significantly underestimate the training effect for proteins with shorter half-lives (<2–3 d). Moreover, some regulatory proteins with half-lives on the order of less than 1 day (*e.g.*, transcription factors) may return to their resting concentration less than 24 to 48 hours after exercise.

Although it is difficult to directly measure the degradation rates of specific proteins in living animals, indirect estimates suggest that protein degradation rates increase as a result of enhancements in skeletal muscle usage. The higher the protein degradation rate, the shorter will be the protein's half-life (*i.e.*, the more rapid will be the turnover rate). Thus, it is likely that protein turnover occurs more rapidly in exercise-trained muscle.

Summary

Thus far, we have focused on the molecular and cellular basis of adaptations made in response to changes in the level and type of physical activity. We will now describe some of the wondrous genomics and proteomics tools that are available to dissect exercise mechanisms.

Methods of Genomics and Proteomics Research

Thanks to recent advances in technology, many important hypotheses regarding the scientific basis of physical activity can now be tested and applied to exercise research.

Here we describe various approaches to decipher the functions of the thousands of changes in gene expression that occur with physical activity, and discuss some potential applications of genomics in physical activity research. This will be followed by a section on proteomics. It is assumed that the reader is familiar with basic molecular biology techniques (*e.g.,* DNA sequencing, Northern blotting, and reverse transcriptase polymerase chain reaction [PCR]). In the following section, we present newly developed techniques for global analyses.

KEY POINT

A variety of molecular techniques can be employed to investigate the multiple, sequential steps (from gene to protein) that contribute to the final level of a protein.

Human Research

DNA and genes

The amino acid sequence of every protein in the body largely determines the location, three-dimensional structure, and function of that protein. Because the amino acid sequence is derived from the gene that encodes for that protein, it is not hard to imagine that specific variations in DNA sequence (*e.g.,* insertions, deletions, or single-nucleotide polymorphisms [SNPs, pronounced *snips*]) may alter the amino acid sequence in a way that affects the function of the protein. In fact, it is this natural variation in gene sequence that accounts for the uniqueness of each human being. As one might expect, the frequency of SNPs varies considerably across all genes depending on the functional impact of the particular variation and the evolutionary pressure to conserve critical sequences.

SINGLE-NUCLEOTIDE POLYMORPHISMS Although some diseases result from a single gene defect (*e.g.,* cystic fibrosis), most complex diseases do not (*e.g.,* cancer and diabetes); rather, they are caused by a host of environmental factors interacting with multiple genes over the course of many years. Each individual's susceptibility to such a disease is thought to stem from his or her polymorphic profile. One strategy being employed by geneticists is to identify the frequency and locations of all SNPs, under the assumption that specific SNPs will be associated with specific diseases. Of particular interest and importance is to determine which of these polymorphisms double as SNPs that are responsive to physical activity or inactivity.

However, the hunt for genetic markers of disease susceptibility thus far has been an extremely daunting task. SNPs occur as frequently as one in every 1000 bases, which means that huge numbers of SNPs must be analyzed in large populations before links between DNA and disease can be truly correlated. An alternative to a genome-wide search is to employ a selective strategy in which the search for disease-associated SNPs is restricted to previously suspected regions of a chromosome associated with a disease. For example, such a strategy was used to identify, in a 66,000-nucleotide stretch of chromosome 2, three SNPs associated with a heightened susceptibility to diabetes in a population of Mexican Americans (24). It is anticipated that restricting searches to the promoter regions, protein coding segments (exons), and 3′ untranslated regions of candidate genes, thereby eliminating the intron sequence from the analysis, may prove to be a more efficient and fruitful strategy for identifying meaningful SNPs.

By identifying disease and activity SNPs, we may be able to more accurately predict predisposition to disease on an individual basis and establish primary preventive treatments (individualized medicine). However, the task will be challenging because (a) the data are initially associative, not causal; (b) very large populations must be studied to attain statistical confidence; and (c) multiple SNPs can contribute to the risk for a single disease, and thus the contribution of each individual SNP may be too low to detect.

EPIGENETIC MODIFICATIONS THAT ALTER TRANSCRIPTIONAL ACTIVITY Whereas genetic information is encoded by DNA sequences, epigenetic information is encoded by differential methylation of DNA on cytosines (primarily in CpG dinucleotides), by proteins that associate with DNA and their covalent modifications, and by the chromatin structures that form within the nucleus. DNA-associated proteins include histones (which may be modified covalently by acetylation, methylation, phosphorylation, and/or ubiquitination) and methyl-CpG–binding proteins (19). For example, activation of muscle-specific genes by members of the myocyte enhancer factor 2 and MyoD families of transcription factors is coupled to histone acetylation and inhibited by class II histone deacetylases 4 and 5, which interact with myocyte enhancer factor 2 (55).

DNA–PROTEIN INTERACTIONS Chromatin immunoprecipitation (ChIP) permits global analysis of the interaction of a particular protein (*e.g.,* transcription factor) with DNA. In a ChIP assay, protein and DNA interactions are first cross-linked in a muscle or nuclear homogenate (33). The specific protein is then immunoprecipitated by antibody, and the DNA fragments are amplified by PCR and sequenced to determine whether proteins bind to the specific DNA region of interest. An advantage of this method is that it can be used to determine chromatin regulation at both local and global levels. Local effects refer to regulation of single genes, and ChIP can be used to determine whether a specific transcription factor is binding to a specific gene regulatory region. The ChIP-seq method combines ChIP with sequencing, which allows all sequences/genes associated with a given transcription factor or histone modification to be identified. Thus, ChIP assays can also be used to determine global effects on gene expression.

RNA

To analyze changes in pretranslational regulation produced by exercise, one can obtain mRNA from skeletal muscle or adipose tissue biopsies, myonuclei isolated from the biopsies, and tissue sections. As opposed to DNA, which is the same in different cell types, mRNA expression varies by cell type and experimental treatment.

MICRORNAs MicroRNAs (miRNAs) are noncoding or nonmessenger, single-stranded RNAs, 19 to 25 nucleotides in length, that are processed from longer endogenous hairpin-shaped transcripts originating mainly from noncoding regions of the genome (45). They regulate target mRNAs by binding to complementary sequences in 3′-UTRs base pairing, which can lead to translational repression, decapping, deadenylation, and/or cleavage of the target mRNA. A single miRNA can regulate many mRNA targets, and several miRNAs can regulate a single mRNA. In one study (34), after 7 days of functional overload-induced hypertrophy of the plantaris muscle, miRNAs miR-1 and miR-133a expression levels decreased 50%, whereas miR-206 expression was unchanged.

MICROARRAY ANALYSIS It is now possible to simultaneously analyze all mRNAs in a given cell type or tissue. Complementary DNA (cDNA) or oligonucleotide microarrays can be used to measure the expression patterns of thousands of genes in parallel, generating clues to gene function. The cDNA microarray technique uses discrete DNA sequences that have been arrayed onto a glass slide and then interrogated with fluorescently labeled cDNA probes reverse transcribed from an mRNA population. Each oligonucleotide is paired with its identical cDNA sequence, which has a single base mismatch to serve as a control. Both techniques can result in false-positive differences in gene expression between two experimental groups if the sample sizes are small and/or improper (or no) statistics are employed. Although oligonucleotide microarrays allow the simultaneous analysis of thousands of mRNAs, they require larger sample sizes to maximize the ability to detect significant differences while minimizing the percentage of false positives.

Microarray analysis offers a comprehensive snapshot of mRNA expression under a given experimental condition; however, there is not always a direct relationship between the concentration of an mRNA and its encoded protein. Differential rates of mRNA translation into protein, protein assembly, and variations in specific rates of protein degradation influence the predictive power of mRNA expression to protein expression profiles. The correlation coefficients between changes in mRNA and protein in yeast are not high. Microarrays have been applied to isolated polysomes to determine the differential expression of mRNAs attached to ribosomes. Although microarrays are not quantitative, they provide an unbiased global database from which unique insights and new hypotheses can be generated based on the identification of specific genes of interest that would otherwise remain unknown. As such, microarrays should be viewed as an initiator of new information for novel hypotheses (14).

REAL-TIME PCR Because many microarray analyses involve a small sample size and/or do not employ rigorous statistical evaluations, differentially expressed mRNAs identified for further study require confirmation with an independent measurement, which is usually real-time PCR. Real-time PCR technology combines rapid thermocycling with real-time fluorescent probe detection of amplified target mRNAs or nucleic acids with high sensitivity. Once the analysis of a given mRNA is established for real-time PCR, a high-throughput analysis may be feasible. However, each mRNA quantified by PCR must be normalized to account for potential differences in total RNA content in each sample. This is done by normalizing to the total amount of template in reaction (total RNA-single-stranded DNA generated by the reverse transcriptase reaction) or to an mRNA that is unaffected by the experimental treatment. This accounts for potential differences in the initial total mRNA concentration across samples. It can be very difficult to find an mRNA or ribosomal RNA for real-time PCR analysis that is not changed in a comparison of two physical activity levels because exercise often produces global changes in mRNA expression. For example, a recent study (38) reported that the quantity of almost every housekeeping gene and ribosomal RNA in the soleus muscle of rats was altered by 10 days of hindlimb immobilization. Even mRNAs that were not statistically significant according to the microarray analysis became statistically different when they were reanalyzed by the more sensitive real-time PCR method. Thus, the normalization of mRNA expression data continues to present a challenge for experimental researchers.

Proteomics

Proteins are at the end point of gene expression, and a protein's activity will determine its function. The study of all proteins in a cell, tissue, or organism is called proteomics.

It has been estimated that humans possess approximately 23,000 genes. All proteins encoded by the human genome are subject to modification by phosphorylation, acetylation, acylation, glycosylation, and/or myristoylation and an unknown percentage of these modifications can change the bioactivity of the modified protein. Thus, the number of proteins with different bioreactivities exceeds 23,000 and is likely greater than 200,000 because each protein has multiple bioreactivities. An advantage of proteomics in gene function over determination of adaptations by mRNAs with microarrays is that its methodology can determine the cellular response to any perturbation at the level of protein activation, such as phosphorylation (phosphoproteome), and it can determine the downstream consequences in terms of gene expression changes. Because different levels of daily physical activity are associated with adaptive alterations in protein levels, information about the tens of thousands of proteins and their modified forms will be required to decipher the precise mode by which the human body functions in daily life.

TWO-DIMENSIONAL FLUORESCENCE DIFFERENCE GEL ELEC-TROPHORESIS The two-dimensional fluorescence difference in-gel electrophoresis method uses two different protein samples labeled with one of two different charge-matched fluorescent dyes (Cy3 or Cy5) to resolve and separate proteins initially by charge (*i.e.,* the isoelectric point) and then by molecular weight in the second dimension. After electrophoresis is performed, the gel is scanned for the fluorescence of each dye and images are then overlaid to identify differentially expressed proteins in the control and experimental samples. Changes in protein content from as little as 1.3-fold to >100-fold between control and experimental samples may be detected. Spots of interest may then be excised for further analysis (*e.g.,* trypsin digestion followed by mass spectrometry [MS]) and possible identification by comparison with existing peptide databases.

MASS SPECTROMETRY MS-based proteomics can be used to analyze complex protein samples. The advantages of MS include sensitivity, resolution, speed, and high throughput, which enable investigators to analyze huge data sets using advanced bioinformatics. In standard MS, molecules are ionized and accelerated through a vacuum by an electric field. The particles are then separated according to their ratio of mass to charge by either deflection in a magnetic field or by measurement of their time of flight to the detector. The multiple types of MS available today allow identification of a protein as well as modifications to that protein, such as glycosylation and phosphorylation.

ADVANTAGES AND LIMITATIONS An overriding advantage of proteomics is that proteins are the unit of biologic action in a cell. Because physical activity likely alters the expression of thousands of proteins, categorization of these changes is necessary to decipher the signals that react to and counterbalance disturbances to homeostasis during exercise and the signals that lead to long-term adaptations with training to improve function during physical activity. Proteomics will continue to progress to the forefront of biomedical research, as existing techniques are improved and new techniques are developed.

KEY POINT

Understanding the complex process involved in regulating hundreds of genes to produce new cellular architecture in proteins during exercise requires software, computers, and human interpretation.

Bioinformatics

Genomics- and proteomics-based research presents an enormous challenge in terms of the sheer volume of raw data that must be managed. Thousands and thousands of data points (each corresponding to a single SNP, mRNA, or protein) are obtained with each sample. Each experiment, in turn, requires multiple samples or subjects to obtain sufficient statistical power to determine with some confidence that a given finding is truly relevant. Adding to the complexity is the fact that the locations, functions, and activities of proteins are continually subject to allosteric interactions, covalent modifications, and binding to other proteins. Thus, deciphering all of the molecular, cellular, and physiologic events responsible for the improvements in physical performance and health that accompany exercise, or the decrements associated with the development of overt clinical disorders in response to physical inactivity, is a daunting task. It is not unreasonable to estimate that up to 200,000 individual gene expression or protein changes will occur in all tissues with physical activity or inactivity, and all of these changes must be cataloged, interpreted, and integrated to explain the normal and pathologic functions of the human body. To categorize findings and make predictions, one must employ specific software (*in silico* science).

Bioinformatics is a discipline that applies computationally intensive techniques to analyze molecular biology approaches. The Gene Ontology (GO) project is a collaborative effort to address the need for consistent descriptions of gene products in different databases (1). The GO project has developed three structured controlled vocabularies (ontologies) that describe gene products in terms of their associated biologic processes, cellular components, and molecular functions in a species-independent manner. GO enrichment analysis categorizes identified mRNAs/miRNAs into families with similar functions, and into signaling pathways/networks/causal cascades (21). A GO analysis of mRNAs altered with human endurance training demonstrated a significant biologic overlap with mRNAs found in cancer biology (30), which is reminiscent of an observation made in 2002 using mRNA microarrays of altered regulation of growth regulatory genes in a single bout of resistance exercise by rats (11).

The necessity for bioinformatics was reinforced by a recent review article in which the authors noted that the biggest challenge for exercise physiologists in the forthcoming years will be to link signaling cascades to defined metabolic responses and specific changes in gene expression that occur during and after exercise (25). Computers will allow investigators to store and sort a vast amount of information about the cross-talk, feedback regulation, and transient activation that occur during and after exercise.

Animal Research

This section is subdivided into two parts: techniques and physical activity interpretations of genetically modified animals.

Historical perspective

As early as the 1930s, investigators had learned to identify new hormones by removing a tissue (*e.g.,* the thyroid gland) from an animal, observing the phenotype, grinding up the gland, and injecting it into the animal to see if the initial phenotype could be rescued. If the phenotype was rescued, the proteins were isolated from the ground-up gland, and then each individual isolated protein was injected alone until a specific biochemical (*e.g.,* thyroxine) restored the original phenotype. The rescue identified the chemical (hormone) responsible for the phenotype. These same principles can be applied to understand current gene manipulation methods that are used to identify the genes responsible for phenotypical adaptations in response to physical activity.

> **KEY POINT**
>
> Techniques to modify the level of a gene allow researchers to make an educated guess as to the normal function of genes during exercise if both sedentary and trained populations are studied.

Transgenic animals

Transgenic technologies originated in the early 1980s with the development of pronuclear microinjection in which the gene of interest is directly injected into the pronuclei of fertilized eggs and the functional outcome is observed. In the late 1980s to early 1990s, Mario Capecchi, Martin Evans, and Oliver Smithies achieved a major breakthrough in altering gene expression, for which they were awarded the Nobel Prize in Physiology and Medicine in 2007. With the use of homologous recombination, it was discovered that DNA could be exchanged between the host genome and a transgene (a new gene transferred into the host genome), that is, a transgene could be inserted into a precise location in the mouse genome (49).

This finding gave investigators the ability to knock out a specific endogenous gene and replace it with a DNA sequence of their design (Fig. 27.5). It also enabled researchers to insert extra copies of a gene or insert genes with special promoters to cause overexpression of a gene. With these transgenic technologies, genetically modified animals can be created and studied to reveal the functions of individual genes and gene-related diseases (53). In this section, we explain the many advantages of genetic modification technologies in living animals and their great potential for advancing our understanding of exercise science. We also discuss the potential limitations of using genetically modified animals to study exercise adaptations.

THE KNOCKOUT ANIMAL The term *knockout* refers to a mutant animal in which the function of a particular gene has been eliminated by the insertion of a replacement DNA

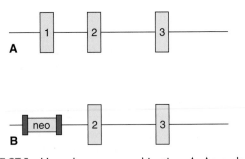

FIGURE 27.5 Homologous recombination. **A.** An endogenous gene with three exons (*rectangles 1–3*) that can make protein A. The line between the rectangles represents introns. **B.** A new gene constructed from gene A such that a neomycin (*neo*) coding sequence replaces a part of the promoter A and exon 1, inactivating the coding sequence of gene A; thus, no protein A would be made if gene B were to replace gene A in an egg by homologous recombination.

sequence. Normally, the replacement sequence causes a portion of the original gene to be lost, and thus the original gene fails to function normally. Phenotypes of the knockout mice are compared with those of wild-type mice (with intact genes), allowing researchers to deduce the function of the knocked-out gene. This method is analogous to a loss-of-function study in which removal of a gland is used to prove that the gland produces the missing hormone. For example, if a gene that is necessary for muscle hypertrophy is knocked out, the knockout animal may no longer exhibit muscle growth with training. One advantage of a knockout model is that it can show a loss-of-function phenotype, that is, the animal loses a function or ability to adapt. Another advantage is that the gene disruption is made in the germ line, and thus subsequent generations will carry the same genetic composition. Because some gene knockout models faithfully mimic the phenotype of human diseases, they can be used as model systems for the study of human diseases. For example, apoprotein E knockouts develop cardiovascular disease and are being used to study the development of atherosclerosis and potential treatments for cardiovascular disease (18). Knockout mice can also be used to test specific hypotheses about exercise. For example, one study (13) reported that hippocampal neurogenesis increased within 3 weeks when mice were housed in cages with running wheels. Activation of N-methyl D-aspartate (NMDA) receptors is thought to be involved in neurogenesis; therefore, it was hypothesized that NMDA receptor signals may be involved in exercise-induced neurogenesis. To test this hypothesis, knockout mice lacking the NMDA receptor-ε_1 subunit gene were housed in cages with running wheels. No increases in hippocampal neurogenesis and brain-derived neurotrophic factor occurred in the knockout mice, whereas wild-type mice with the intact NMDA receptor gene showed marked increases in brain-derived neurotrophic factor production and neurogenesis. These findings led to the suggestion that hippocampal neurogenesis in mice induced by voluntary running is likely mediated, at least in part, by NMDA receptor signaling (31).

A disadvantage of knockout animals is that they sometimes show surprisingly little phenotypic change, often because they have alternative or redundant genes or mechanisms that compensate for the deficient gene during development and maturation. Sometimes it takes a bout of exercise to elicit an abnormal phenotype in a knockout animal, which means that the knocked-out gene likely was selected during evolution to function during physical activity for survival. Another disadvantage of traditional knockout models is that some genes are necessary for normal development, and animals lacking these genes may die in utero or shortly after birth as a result of developmental defects. Even if the animals survive, some genetically modified models have somewhat different phenotypes from their human counterparts, limiting their utility as models of human disease. Another limitation is that it may be impossible to delineate whether the observed phenotype is the result of a deficiency that occurred during development, adolescence, or adulthood. The latter shortcoming with the traditional knockouts can be overcome with a new technology known as conditional knockout or tissue-specific gene targeting (reviewed later in the chapter). Another disadvantage of knockout animals could be the unintended removal of an intron-located sequence for an miRNA, which disrupts the normal mechanisms that regulate expression of the protein.

THE OVEREXPRESSION ANIMAL   Transgenic animals are often designed to overexpress a gene so that its protein product is overproduced, yielding a gain-of-function phenotype. This technique is also employed to misexpress a mutated nonfunctional copy (also known as a negative copy, because the overexpression of a catalytically inactive protein overwhelms the amount of endogenous protein) in animals. In some instances, it is desirable to restrict expression of the target gene to a specific tissue. For example, selection of a skeletal-muscle–specific promoter restricts expression to skeletal muscle myofibers as opposed to other tissues or cell types in skeletal muscle, such as fibroblasts and smooth muscle cells. This strategy was employed to generate transgenic mice overexpressing hexokinase II by using a construct consisting of the muscle creatine kinase promoter fused to the human hexokinase II cDNA (10,23). These mice were generated to examine whether hexokinase II, which catalyzes the first step (phosphorylation) in the metabolism of glucose once it enters the cell, plays a role in determining the rate of glucose uptake in muscle. Under basal conditions, glucose uptake into muscle did not differ between wild-type mice and mice overexpressing hexokinase II. However, in response to both hyperinsulinemia and exercise, mice overexpressing hexokinase II had a significantly greater rate of glucose uptake into muscle than their wild-type littermates, providing evidence that hexokinase II–mediated phosphorylation of glucose may be an important determinant of the overall rate of glucose uptake in skeletal muscle during exercise.

Another potentially useful strategy is to select a promoter that contains one or more binding sites for a specific transcription factor of interest, and place it in front of a reporter gene. When the transcription factor is present and active, the reporter gene will be expressed. This strategy was used to examine the molecular pathways involved in the control of exercise-responsive genes.

A disadvantage of gene overexpression is that the transgenic technique can result in the transgene randomly inserting into the genome at an unknown integration site, which may affect the expression of a second, unknown gene. Another limitation inherent to this technique is that the copy number of inserted genes is variable (1–100 copies of the transgene can be inserted). The variable copy number can lead to inconsistent phenotypic characteristics (e.g., expression pattern and level of expression). Thus, to verify the phenotype in transgenic animals, the development of several independent transgenic lines is required. A final limitation to overexpression technology is that the gene may be expressed at a supraphysiologic level, producing an abnormal phenotype.

CONDITIONAL KNOCKOUTS   The purpose of conditional knockouts, in contrast to traditional knockouts, is to delete a gene in a specific organ, tissue type, or cell type at a specific time determined by the investigator. This technique can be used to knock out portions of genes, entire genes, or even promoter regions of genes. The creation of a conditional knockout is typically executed through a mechanism of site-specific recombination. The most widely used method is the Cre-loxP recombinase system. The second most popular system is the Flp-Flp recognition target (FRT) system. Both Cre and Flp are site-specific recombinases, that is, the enzymes act to trade DNA segments by recognizing specific DNA sequences. Recombinases act like molecular scissors (targeting their actions to the specific DNA recognition sites of loxP or FRT) to cut out designated regions of DNA flanked on both sides by loxP or FRT and replace the region with a new DNA fragment. These systems are referred to as binary systems because they require the interaction of two components: the recombinase and the splice site.

In practice, a researcher can design a transgenic mouse with a tissue-specific promoter that drives the Cre recombinase gene. The investigator can then create a second transgenic animal that contains loxP sites around the region of DNA (typically in introns [noncoding sequences surrounding a regulatory exon]) to be spliced out. These two transgenic animals are mated to produce progeny with tissue-specific knockout of a specific gene. Because Cre will be expressed only in the tissue or cells where the promoter is activated to transcribe Cre, the targeted gene will be knocked out only in the specified tissue or cells. Thus, the mouse will express its wild-type phenotype until the tissue-specific promoter is induced, at which time the Cre protein will be expressed and its recombinase activity will delete the gene segment between its recombinase recognition sites. This approach makes it possible to circumvent the problem of embryonic lethality, if an appropriate promoter is chosen to be activated only in the adult animal, not during embryogenesis. Both recombination systems offer exquisite specificity for testing gene function. Thus, the advantage of a tissue-specific conditional knockout is that it allows the scientist to study a gene's mechanism of action in a specific tissue (without the complications of observing the side effects of the gene deficiency in other surrounding tissues) and by choice of promoter. Tissue-specific conditional knockouts also give a higher level of specificity and control over whole body knockouts, but they do not allow the investigator to turn the gene on again once the gene has been excised from the genome. In one effective conditional knockout experiment, inactivation of the myostatin gene in striated muscle by the Cre-lox system was shown to result in generalized muscular hypertrophy (20). Although these findings were similar to that observed with constitutive myostatin knockout mice, the conditional knockout system eliminated the possibility of mitigating developmental influences in the general knockout mice by using a muscle-specific promoter expressed only in differentiated skeletal muscle, leading the researchers to suggest the hypothesis that a myostatin antagonist could be used to treat muscle wasting and to promote muscle growth in humans and animals.

INDUCIBLE TRANSGENIC SYSTEMS   In an ideal research design, an exercise investigator would have control over a genetic switch that could be flipped to activate or to silence a transgene. In addition, the transgene would have a high level of gene expression when on, and no expression when off. The switch would be a chemical that would be foreign to the animals and would not interfere with or be affected by other cellular components. Most of the qualities of the ideal genetic switch have been achieved through the use of conditional (tissue specific) or inducible transgenic systems (44). Conditional or inducible systems allow gene manipulation not only in a specific organ, tissue type, or cell type, as with the conditional knockout, but also at a stage of development or life selected by the investigator. The tetracycline system allows for the control of target gene expression in eukaryotic systems via the application of the antibiotic tetracycline or a tetracycline analogue, such as doxycycline, to study gain of function or loss of function for any given gene. The use of this kind of technology allows tissue-specific gene expression to be turned on or off by a drug (tetracycline) that is not normally present in the body. Additionally, because these systems are inducible, genes that are critical for development can express normally through development, and then later in adolescence or adulthood be manipulated by the addition or subtraction of the drug. Because the amount of transgene expression is roughly proportional to the amount of drug administered, the investigator may be able to titrate the levels of target gene expression. The biggest advantage of these techniques

is that they can overcome the limitation of a gene alteration being present throughout the life of the animal. Thus, the gene can be turned on in a mature animal just before or during exercise training and compared with an animal whose gene is kept off during the exercise training. This temporal control of gene expression gives the researcher exquisite control for analyzing the functional significance of a gene with exercise. When tetracycline systems were first introduced, they were leaky and it was nearly impossible to completely silence the expression of the transgene. Since then, however, researchers have redesigned the promoters to achieve nearly complete silencing. Although in general gene expression is barely detectable or undetectable in the noninduced state, transcription is usually stimulated to levels $>10^5$-fold above background in the induced state. Finally, tissue-specific expression of inducible transgenes is now possible.

FUTURE GENETICALLY MODIFIED ANIMAL MODELS   Current transgenic technologies permit the generation of double knockouts (i.e., a single mouse with two genes functionally eliminated). It is anticipated that future technologic developments will permit researchers to selectively activate or deactivate the expression of multiple genes in a given tissue or animal to allow for a more comprehensive study of signaling pathways and regulatory mechanisms. Because exercise alters multiple signaling pathways simultaneously, an ideal future model would be to block multiple signaling events instantaneously at the start of an exercise bout.

Gene transfer techniques

NAKED DNA INJECTIONS   Gene transfer into skeletal muscle by the direct injection of naked plasmid DNA results in sustained gene expression in a small percentage of muscle fibers. Detection of the exogenous gene product is facilitated by incorporation of a reporter gene that encodes for a fluorescent or otherwise easily detected protein (e.g., luciferase). This strategy was used to characterize the effects of mutations of the skeletal α-actin promoter (driving a reporter gene) in a plasmid injected into a mechanically overloaded muscle (8). Deletional mutations identified a hypertrophy-responsive region, which was later confirmed by site-specific mutations of suspected promoter elements within the responsive region. The hypertrophy response was blocked by a plasmid expressing a mutated serum response element 1 DNA regulatory region, suggesting that in this overload model, serum response element 1 is a hypertrophy-responsive element on the skeletal α-actin promoter. A limitation of gene transfer of plasmids is the highly variable level of promoter expression among animals. Although this limitation can be lessened by coinjection with and normalization to a second, non–exercise-sensitive promoter driving a second reporter gene, exercise can often alter the expression of the putative non–exercise-responsive promoter. Naked plasmid gene transfer has not been shown to be very successful in tissues other than skeletal muscle.

ELECTROPORATION The temporary application of an electric field to skeletal muscle can increase the uptake of injected DNA by 100-fold or more, enhancing both the quantity and consistency of expression from the exogenous gene. Although the mechanism of electroporation is not entirely clear, the electric field is thought to cause temporary formation of pores across the sarcolemma, allowing the normally impermeable DNA to gain access to the cytoplasm (17). Although almost 99% of the injected DNA is lost or degraded within 24 hours, a portion of it winds up in the nucleus, where it remains viable and expresses for up to 2 to 3 months. A certain degree of muscle damage and the presence of an inflammatory infiltrate have also been reported with the electroporation technique, and the altered gene expression of the damage and inflammation must be separated from the exercise-induced change in gene expression. Electroporation can also be used in adipose tissue or cell culture.

VIRAL INJECTIONS Vectors for the adeno-associated virus (AAV) used for gene transfer into skeletal muscle have minimal or no immune response; however, if genes engineered into these vectors express proteins that are novel to the animal receiving the vector, an immune reaction to the novel protein can occur in the host. Adenovirus infection of adult

skeletal muscle has been shown to be unsuccessful because the virus fails to diffuse through sheets of connective tissue in muscle formed during maturation. However, the use of replication-defective AAV vectors has been shown to successfully transfer genes into adult muscle. This strategy has been used to rescue aged mouse skeletal muscle from sarcopenia with a single injection of an AAV expressing insulin-like growth factor 1 into skeletal muscle (4). The advantage of injection into skeletal muscle with AAV over plasmids is that 80% of the muscle fibers may be infected with AAV, whereas only 1% to 2% may take up and express a plasmid. A lentivirus vector was recently reported as a tool for gene transfer and expression in mature muscle fibers (17).

Interpretation of chronic exercise responses in genetically modified animals

As challenging as (or more challenging than) the production of a transgenic animal is the need to interpret results from the perspective of the exercise literature while integrating vast amounts of information from multiple organs and disciplines. A definitive cause-and-effect relationship for the function of a gene altered by physical activity or inactivity will normally require a sequence of gene modification experiments that may be published in separate venues (Fig. 27.6). The next example illustrates this approach. In 1998, it was reported that overexpression of calcineurin in the mouse heart induced cardiac hypertrophy, providing

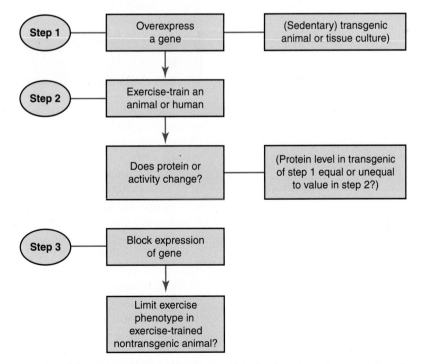

FIGURE 27.6 Experimental steps to establish the function of a gene altered by physical activity or inactivity. This shows a suggested protocol for determining a more definitive cause-and-effect function for a protein in exercise experiments.

evidence that calcineurin participates in signal transduction leading to cardiac hypertrophy (36). In Figure 27.6, overexpression of a gene to obtain an exercise phenotype is designated as step 1 in a process of determining cause and effect for exercise.

However, little was known about whether calcineurin actually participates in the signaling of exercise-induced hypertrophy, as most studies on this issue used animals with pathologic hypertrophy to study calcineurin signaling. The breakthrough came in 2000, when it was found that calcineurin was activated by 150% in the enlarged hearts of rats that ran 2.4 km each night for 10 weeks as compared with caged controls (16). This is shown in step 2 of Figure 27.6, in which it is determined that physiologic exercise increases the protein concentration or activity to a similar degree as found in the transgenic animal in step 1. Although treatment with the calcineurin antagonist drug cyclosporin A completely inhibited the development of left-ventricular hypertrophy in a subgroup of the voluntarily running rats, a controversy arose over whether cyclosporin could block pathologic hypertrophic responses in the hearts of animal models of pressure overload or genetic cardiomyopathy. A different experimental approach would be necessary to resolve this controversy. In 2001, the forced overexpression of the calcineurin-inhibitory protein myocyte-enriched calcineurin-interacting protein-1 (hMCIP1) in hearts of transgenic mice was found to attenuate 57% of the hypertrophic response from voluntary running (step 3 in Fig. 27.6) (43). Thus, only after step 3 does it become possible to claim a cause-and-effect role for calcineurin in the hypertrophic response of the myocardium triggered by exercise as performed by mice in voluntary running wheels.

KEY POINT

Animal models of changes in daily levels of physical activity allow the study of mechanisms controlling adaptations in levels of proteins setting limits to performance and health.

Use of the Concept of Physiologic Exercise and Models to Show the Limits of Adaptation with Nonphysiologic Models

Although electrical stimulation of skeletal muscle $24 \text{ h} \cdot \text{d}^{-1}$ induces a number of adaptive responses similar to those achieved by dynamic exercise training (39), it is clear that the changes evoked by chronic stimulation exceed those induced by any other form of increased contractile activity. In effect, the chronic stimulation model provides information as to the limits of muscle adaptation. Unfortunately, results from this model are often translated as occurring in humans at exercise levels that are lower than chronic stimulation. For example, many contend that sedentary humans switch

from type II to I fibers with dynamic training, as in the nonphysiologic model of chronic stimulation of muscle for $24 \text{ h} \cdot \text{d}^{-1}$. Unfortunately, the published literature does not support this contention. Sedentary humans and animals do not increase their type I percentage with endurance exercise training. On the other hand, humans and animals do switch from type I to II fibers when sedentary populations undergo hindlimb unloading, hindlimb immobilization, or spinal isolation, and upon retraining, they switch back toward the percentage level found in sedentary populations (22). Thus, a future challenge will be to differentiate between physiologic exercise and models that provide information about the limits of muscle adaptation when interpreting results from transgenic animals.

Summary

In this section, we describe multiple approaches for manipulating gene expression in animals prior to exercise testing. The challenge will be to interpret the exercise results. A best-guess interpretation regarding the functional outcome of a single modified gene in a sea of at least 200,000 other exercise-induced changes in multiple tissues of genetically modified animals will require a strong working knowledge of the literature.

Application of Theoretical Concepts to Predict Functions of Proteins Whose Activities Are Altered by Exercise

The application of transcript profiling techniques will undoubtedly lead to the identification of novel proteins that change with physical activity or inactivity. One enlightening way to approach the interpretation of changes in gene expression with alterations in physical activity or inactivity is to question the existence of a gene. For example, do activity-induced changes in the levels of some proteins reflect evolutionary selection of those genes for a particular survival function? Should the assignment of function for genes whose expression changes during physical training be based on the concept that the gene usurped an exercise function from a gene selected by evolution to perform a function other than exercise? Or is it possible that exercise research in the new millennium is unmasking, in an otherwise sedentary population, the function of genes that evolved to support physical activity as a means of survival? With the advent of genomics, proteomics, and bioinformatics, some of the concepts listed in Table 27.1 may be used to form hypotheses regarding the functions of identified changes in protein levels with physical activity or inactivity.

TABLE 27.1 Concepts Allowing Generation of Potential Functions of Proteins or mRNAs Changing as a Result of Physical Activity or Inactivity

Pattern of change with physical activity or inactivity
Homeostasis
Phenotype of elite physical performer
Environment–gene interaction
    Physical activity–gene interaction
    Thrifty genotype or gene hypothesis
Chronic diseases
Bioinformatics
    Search through multiple databases containing
        protein functions
    Chromosomal position

Application of Various Time Courses or Patterns of Changes in Gene Expression to Identify Potential Functions for Genes Altered by Physical Activity

The pattern of change in the expression of a gene can provide clues to the function of that gene. If the response pattern shows an abrupt spike or repression, it will be designated as an acute response as described in the next two examples. In example 1, the IL-6 gene is markedly activated in muscle during the latter stages of long-term exercise (3–4 h) but then shuts off immediately upon cessation of exercise (29). Such a pattern suggests a potential function downstream in an exercise sensor pathway communicating that exercise is ongoing. A second transient pattern is exemplified by the uncoupling protein 3 gene, which encodes for a mitochondrial protein whose expression increases dramatically during the first several hours after exercise but then returns to resting levels within 24 hours after exercise (27,41). Recent findings suggest that uncoupling protein 3 is induced to prevent excessive reactive oxygen species production during recovery from exercise, a metabolic state characterized by a sudden reduction in energy demand with elevated substrate supply (2). Abrupt changes in mRNA per protein are possible only for gene products with very short half-lives. Because many regulatory proteins and rate-limiting enzymes have short half-lives to allow for speedy adjustments in control mechanisms, it is reasonable to hypothesize that proteins with similar transient expression patterns may perform similar functions. Many of these types of proteins are also normally not expressed at appreciable levels under resting conditions, as they may fulfill a specific need of the cell that under normal conditions is not required or even potentially detrimental.

However, if the pattern is a gradual change over days to weeks, different potential functions may be proposed. The protein may serve to reduce an exercise-induced disruption in homeostasis rather than to regulate other protein expression. The level of the mRNA or protein is often relatively high in sedentary subjects and requires multiple exercise bouts to generate a measurable increase in the mRNA or protein level. Proteins in this category have a relatively long half-life (days). One substance that falls into this category is cytochrome *c*. The half-life of cytochrome *c* protein is 7 days in rat skeletal muscle undergoing training or detraining, and it thus takes several days of daily exercise before a significant increase in its concentration can be detected.

Application of the Concept of Homeostasis to Identify Potential Functions for Genes Altered by Physical Activity

If at least one function of a gene and its pattern of change in response to a change in physical activity are known, an educated guess can be made as to whether the protein plays a role in homeostasis. If the directional change that occurs in the protein with exercise training is sufficient to predict that the exercise-induced disruption of homeostasis would be attenuated, it is feasible to hypothesize that the adaptive change in protein level might minimize the disturbance to homeostasis in response to exercise. An example of an adaptation that was eventually shown to minimize homeostatic disruption is the doubling of mitochondrial density, using cytochrome *c* protein concentration as an index, with endurance training. Investigators hypothesized that muscle with twice as many mitochondria but consuming the same oxygen as other muscle would have only half the flux through each electron transport chain, implying that adenosine diphosphate concentration would increase only half as much. The hypothesis was later proved, that is, the disruption of the homeostatic level of adenosine diphosphate is less in the muscle with twice as much mitochondrial density at the same workload (15).

Homeostasis is classically defined as the maintenance of a constant level of a chemical. However, some functions of the body involve cycling and are considered normal. For example, the cycling of biochemical and hormonal events associated with the menstrual cycle can be considered as homeostatic cycling (see Chapter 19). Another example of homeostatic cycling is the hormonal response to ingestion of food, which includes a transient pulse in blood insulin and subsequent effects of insulin receptor signaling, all of which are a normal response to the ingestion of food (with ingestion being periodical, not constant). Therefore, homeostatic cycling includes the physiologic cycling of various biochemicals, such as insulin and glucose, in normal human functions. Consequently, it is reasonable to propose that biochemical cycling associated with the exercise–recovery cycle is a normal function. During the last few thousands of years, the final selection of the current 23,000 human genes was made. Because the survival of a gene pool involves the cycling of fundamental life processes such as reproduction, food consumption, physical labor related to food gathering, and defense against the environment, these may be designated as homeostatic cycling processes. The absence of cycling (*e.g.,* amenorrhea, starvation, or immobility) are surmised to be associated with selection for extinction. Therefore, it is speculated that the proper fluctuation of biochemicals supporting the exercise–recovery cycle was likely selected during evolution and still occurs today when exercise is performed. Thus, exercise–recovery cycles are an example of homeostatic cycling. In the presence of chronic physical inactivity, however, the normal homeostatic cycling of biochemicals stalls, leading to chronic metabolic dysfunctions that underlie chronic health conditions. Thus, if proteins that cycle in tandem with exercise and recovery do not cycle in physical inactivity, we can hypothesize that they may play some role in metabolic diseases. A protein whose concentration cycles in accordance with exercise and rest in healthy subjects but not in a disease state may be a candidate for affecting health. For example, glucose transporter protein glucose transporter 4 (GLUT4) cycles from intracellular vesicles to the sarcolemma in response to both insulin and exercise, returning to its intracellular location 12 hours after the last meal or bout of physical activity. Exercising diabetic patients have increased sarcolemmal GLUT4 concentrations, which leads to the hypothesis that GLUT4 protein has dual exercise functions, that is, a role after exercise to replenish muscle glycogen and prevent type 2 diabetes.

Summary

A key concept is that physical activity is a natural cycle that is integrated into most other cycles in humans and animals. A disruption in the expected daily cycle of physical activity elicits disruptions in other cycles, leading to abnormal gene expression and systemic dysfunctions.

Application of Elite Physical Performance to Identify Potential Functions for Genes Altered by Physical Activity

In the 1960s, most applications of exercise physiology were directed toward improving the physical performance of world-class athletes. In studies involving the use of muscle biopsies, cyclists were shown to have an 80% higher mitochondrial density in their legs than in their arms, whereas canoeists had 36% higher mitochondrial density in their arms (12). Distance runners had a very high percentage of type I fibers compared with the average population, and sprinters had a high percentage of type II fibers. Costill (12) noted that although the percentages of type 1 fibers can distinguish between good and elite distance runners of both sexes, fiber composition alone is a poor predictor of distance running success. Thus, by associating world-class performance with phenotype differences investigators were able to deduce functions (*e.g.,* higher mitochondrial density and type I fiber percentage related to endurance athletic events). The identification of the functions of novel genes is allowing new experiments to determine whether these genes have a role in elite performance. One example is the myostatin gene, which was identified in 1997. Knockout of

the myostatin gene in mice doubled skeletal muscle mass and created excited speculation that variations in sequence or expression might explain differences in human muscle mass (35). Although two common polymorphisms were subsequently identified in the myostatin gene, neither was found to be related to the change in muscle mass in response to strength training in either whites or African Americans (35). In addition, no significant correlations were observed between myostatin expression and any muscle strength or volume measure.

Application of the Concept of Environmental Gene Interaction to Identify Potential Functions for Genes Altered by Physical Activity or Inactivity

Gene expression (defined by the concentration of specific proteins) is not constant throughout an individual's lifespan. Although some genes have programmed changes in expression (development) and others are regulated by biologic clocks (menstrual cycle or sleep), the environment also plays a major role in eliciting altered gene expression. Here, the term *environment* refers to the milieu within and surrounding a cell. The environment can alter the periodicity of the menstrual cycle. For example, the menstrual cycle can be overridden by chronic excessive physical exercise due to a negative caloric balance producing an alteration in the hypothalamic-pituitary-gonadal axis, which is responsible for menstrual disorders (see Chapter 19). Another example of an environmental factor is resistance training, which increases skeletal muscle size and strength. Thus, physical activity or inactivity is an environmental perturbation of gene expression.

KEY POINT

From a purely biologic perspective, two factors determine physical ability: genes inherited from parents and the interaction of physical activity levels with genes predisposing to high or low levels of physical performance.

Application of the Physical Activity–Gene Interaction to Understand Protein Function

The concept of interaction between physical activity and genes received strong support at the biochemical level in 1967, when John Holloszy (28) reported increases in mitochondrial protein and enzyme activities in the skeletal muscles of rats that had been forced to run on treadmills while their cage mates remained sedentary. As detailed in Chapter 18, Holloszy showed that the expression of mitochondrial proteins can be modified by the level of habitual physical activity. Thus, he applied known information about exercise to explain an observed interaction between physical activity and a gene.

Another example of interaction between physical activity and genes comes from recent research on the effects of exercise on cognitive ability. As discussed earlier in the chapter, providing mice with voluntary running wheels is associated with improved hippocampal neurogenesis and cognitive function (13). Epidemiologic data show that women who are 65 years or older will have a 50% reduction in cognitive impairment, Alzheimer disease, and dementia of any type if they engage three or more times per week in exercise at an intensity greater than walking (32). Therefore, a future research endeavor will be to further define the interactions between removal of running activity and changed gene expression that allow a biologically significant threshold to be passed, leading to overt clinical cognitive dysfunction.

Application of the Thrifty Genotype Hypothesis to Identify Potential Functions for Genes Altered by Physical Activity or Inactivity

Thrifty gene hypothesis

In 1962, Neel (37) hypothesized that a "thrifty" genotype would be exceptionally efficient for the intake and/or utilization of food. Most published interpretations of Neel's hypothesis emphasized that humans who could most efficiently store foods as fat were more likely to survive a famine than those without thrifty fat storage, since the former would start out with a store of fat. More recently, it was proposed that individuals whose gene pools contain polymorphisms that allow for more efficient storage of fat were more likely to survive via natural selection than those who could not store fat as efficiently. Less often mentioned in current interpretations of the original thrifty genotype hypothesis is the other part of Neel's original definition, that is, the role of exceptional efficiency in the utilization of stored fat during a famine.

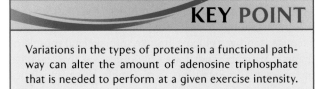

KEY POINT

Variations in the types of proteins in a functional pathway can alter the amount of adenosine triphosphate that is needed to perform at a given exercise intensity.

Simply stated, individuals with polymorphisms that can conserve the limited body stores of carbohydrate and triglycerides longer during physical activity will have a survival advantage. In 1986, Åstrand and Rodahl (3) concluded that because food was not continuously available for 99% of human existence, physical activity must have been obligatory for survival. Both humans and animals had to endure periods when food was not available (famine). Thus, the selection of polymorphisms is surmised to have

occurred during thousands of years of feast-and-famine cycles when the environmental component of physical activity was required for food procurement during starvation (9). Humans without an ability to undertake physical activity or without polymorphisms that relatively efficiently conserve glycogen in the search for food were likely to be selected for extinction because during evolution, food was not acquired from grocery stores or restaurants. Such logic, if valid, supports the hypothesis that a subpopulation of the human genotype was selected to support physical activity during food shortage. Interaction between the environment and genes was likely a fundamental determinant in the conjectured selection of the thrifty genotype that was more efficient in the usage of carbohydrate and fat during physical activity. Therefore, the thrifty genotype is an example of a hypothesis that can be addressed by future exercise physiologists studying the functions of polymorphisms identified by genomic scans.

Extension of the thrifty genotype hypothesis to protein functions during exercise

It is interesting to consider that during evolution, specific genes, in addition to polymorphisms, were selected to maximize the efficiency of physical activity required for survival, particularly during periods of starvation, and the efficiency of energy restoration during feeding. To address this concept further, the next sections provide examples of candidate thrifty genes in the context of the regulation of fuel metabolism during physical activity.

GLUCOSE HOMEOSTASIS DURING PHYSICAL ACTIVITY AS AN EVOLUTIONARY FORCE FOR THE SELECTION OF THRIFTY GENES   The energy required to support life is derived from the metabolism of carbohydrate, fat, and proteins. In the absence of food intake, existing stores of fat and protein can supply the needed energy for several weeks. Carbohydrate reserves (i.e., muscle and liver glycogen), however, are extremely limited and will be depleted within about 24 hours. This presents a serious challenge to intermediary metabolism because the brain relies almost exclusively on blood glucose to support its energy needs; free fatty acids bound to albumin cannot cross the blood–brain barrier. Fortunately, metabolic catastrophe is avoided under such conditions because of the liver's ability to activate endogenous synthesis of both glucose (gluconeogenesis) and ketone bodies, an alternative fuel that can cross into and be metabolized by the brain. In fact, most hormonal control exerted over intermediary metabolism is targeted to the regulation of blood glucose to ensure that hypoglycemia does not occur during prolonged periods with limited or no carbohydrate intake.

Prolonged physical activity also represents a significant challenge to intermediary metabolism and specifically to glucose homeostasis. Although skeletal muscle, unlike the brain, can utilize carbohydrate, fatty acids, and amino acids to meet the energy demands of contractile activity, it is well established that when muscle glycogen concentration approaches zero during exercise, work cannot be continued at the same intensity. That is, fatigue occurs if the same exercise power is continued. Obviously, the challenge to both glucose homeostasis and exercise endurance is exacerbated if physical activity is performed under conditions of limited fuel intake. The thrifty gene hypothesis postulates that genes (and polymorphisms within, *i.e.,* the original thrifty genotype hypothesis) that could most efficiently conserve muscle glycogen during work would be more likely to be conserved during evolution. In other words, being unable to perform the level of physical activity necessary for survival (hunting, gathering) because of an unfavorable metabolic gene profile would be incompatible with survival.

Here, we use the "exercise-responsive" gene known as pyruvate dehydrogenase kinase 4 (PDK4) to illustrate how insight into functions for genes identified as being altered by physical activity may be gained when viewed in the context of both cellular homeostasis and evolutionary selection (*e.g.,* thrifty gene hypothesis). The PDK4 enzyme is discussed in detail in Chapter 16. PDK4 is expressed primarily in skeletal and cardiac muscle, where it catalyzes the phosphorylation of the E1 component of pyruvate dehydrogenase enzyme complex, inhibiting the conversion of pyruvate to acetyl-coenzyme A and thus preventing the entry of glycolytic products into the mitochondria for oxidation (47). The pyruvate dehydrogenase complex is a pivotal step in metabolism because (a) the decarboxylation of pyruvate represents the irreversible loss of a major three-carbon gluconeogenic precursor; and (b) skeletal muscle, which comprises a large percentage of total body mass, accounts for nearly 20% to 25% of the resting energy expenditure in young adults. PDK4 mRNA is nearly undetectable in muscle under normal resting conditions when carbohydrate reserves are plentiful. However, transcription of the PDK4 gene to PDK4 mRNA increases dramatically during the late stages of prolonged low-intensity exercise (27,41). This induction of PDK4 mRNA is consistent with the steady decline in oxidation of carbohydrates that occurs in muscle during such exercise. Thus, PDK4 induction may be an important mechanism for reducing the rate of both glucose and muscle glycogen utilization during prolonged activity as a means of delaying hypoglycemia, glycogen depletion, and therefore fatigue.

If PDK4 is to qualify as a candidate thrifty gene, regulation of this gene must be consistent in response to other metabolic challenges (*e.g.,* prolonged exercise, fasting, diabetes). Indeed, both starvation and streptozotocin-induced diabetes also elicit marked increases in PDK4 expression in skeletal muscle (54). In each of these metabolic states, there is a real or at least a perceived deficit in carbohydrate availability in the form of either low blood glucose or low muscle glycogen concentration. Consistent with this view is the finding that activation of the PDK4 gene is significantly enhanced when exercise is initiated with low muscle glycogen concentration (40), presumably reflecting the need to conserve glucose and/or glycogen utilization much earlier during exercise than in the fed state. In the big picture, these findings collectively raise

the possibility that PDK4 may have been selected as a gene for induction in skeletal muscle during feast-and-famine cycles to minimize carbohydrate utilization during periods of starvation when physical activity was required to maintain survival. In other words, fatigue precipitated by an inability to conserve adequate carbohydrates when reserves are limited would be incompatible with survival.

ENERGY HOMEOSTASIS DURING PHYSICAL ACTIVITY AS AN EVOLUTIONARY FORCE FOR THE SELECTION OF THRIFTY GENES   Another candidate for a thrifty gene that would more efficiently utilize stored energy for physical activity is myosin heavy chain (MHC) I protein. More than two decades ago, it was found that muscles with a preponderance of MHC type I fibers use less than half the energy to perform the same contractile work as expended by muscles with a preponderance of MHC type II fibers. Thus, MHC I uses fuels more efficiently, fitting Neel's definition of thrifty.

Summary

The preceding examples show how expanding the context in which exercise research findings regarding the regulation of a particular gene can provide further insight into the function of that gene product. One of the primary adaptations to dynamic exercise training is a reduced utilization of carbohydrate stores by the working muscle at a given absolute exercise intensity. A future research interrogation using genomics or proteomics could include a search for genes selected to permit a more efficient usage of substrate; that is, conservation of muscle glycogen and body glucose during exercise after endurance training. The conjecture is that genes involved in conserving muscle glycogen during physical activity can be called thrifty genes.

Application of Chronic Disease to Identify Potential Functions for Genes Altered by Physical Activity or Inactivity

Type 2 diabetes is associated with defective postreceptor insulin signaling. It has been known for a century that exercise improves glucose uptake into skeletal muscle of diabetic patients, and it was hypothesized that exercise increases insulin signaling. Surprisingly, however, studies testing this hypothesis revealed that contractile activity did not increase proximal insulin signaling. As a result, investigators were forced to look for candidates other than insulin-signaling proteins to determine which proteins were involved in the exercise-induced increase in glucose uptake by skeletal muscle. Attention was soon focused on an energy-sensing protein known as AMPK. It was found that (a) exercise increased AMPK activity; (b) increasing AMPK activity by administering a drug also activated glucose transport in muscle of resting animals; and (c) expression of a dysfunctional form of AMPK in transgenic mice at least partially attenuated the activation of glucose transport in muscle. Thus, these studies proved that AMPK is at least one of the signaling proteins required for the exercise-induced increase in glucose uptake by skeletal muscle.

> ## KEY POINT
>
> Low physical ability levels are associated with a greater prevalence of chronic diseases. The genomics of a lack of exercise provides insights into the primary causes of most chronic diseases.

A study (56) published in the early 1950s reported an apparent association between increased physical activity levels and decreased coronary heart disease. Later investigations showed that exercise training increased coronary blood flow transport capacity, but not as a result of an enhanced structural capacity of blood vessels. Rather, they showed that blood vessels in trained animals and humans had better vasodilation than those in sedentary subjects, allowing more blood flow. Building on earlier findings that nitric oxide produces vasodilation, investigators were able to support the hypothesis that exercise training increases endothelial nitric oxide synthase mRNA and protein in vascular endothelial cells in the heart (see Chapter 11).

Summary

Hypotheses in genomics research must be stated with a clear understanding of the principles that guide not only the immediate homeostasis of the cells, tissues, and whole organism but also the factors that allow for the selection and reinforcement of the genes in the human genome during evolution. A future genomic research endeavor in exercise physiology will be to prove the postulate that some of the molecular adaptations to physical training consist of genes that are permitted to invoke their ancient functions during physical activity or training by sedentary humans or animals. Thousands of genes change expression during physical activity or inactivity. Exercise-induced genes can be used to determine why some of the 23,000 genes in the human genome survived selection and are still present. The inclusion of the concept of thrifty genes in physical activity adaptations may provide an additional approach to delineate the true function for genes whose expression is altered by physical activity or inactivity. If the truth is that some genes that comprise the human genome were selected for their survival functions to support physical activity, then basic science demands that the original role of this subset of genes must be determined to fully elucidate the human genome. After all, discerning the correct function of a gene will lead to a true understanding of the essence of life.

The Role of Exercise in Future Genomic Research

Individualized Medicine for the Prediction of Disease

Grand Challenge II-3 of the Human Genome Project is to develop genome-based approaches to predict disease susceptibility. The discovery of variants that affect risk of disease could be used in individualized preventive medicine, including diet, exercise, lifestyle, and pharmaceutical interventions, to maximize the likelihood of staying well. Individualization of an exercise prescription for prevention of disease (primary, secondary, and tertiary) must include the recognition that individuals exhibit heterogeneity in terms of the threshold that must be passed to induce a significant change in an exercise adaptation. One example of heterogeneity among individuals is the variation in minimal work volume required to induce a significant increase in maximal O_2 uptake. This concept is illustrated in a study in which work volumes in three groups of subjects were 4, 8, and 12 kcal/kg/wk (46). Tripling of work volume decreased the percentage of nonresponders from 41% to 15%. Another study revealed variation in responsiveness to different training regimens (50). Some of the highest responders to increasing maximal O_2 uptake with aerobic training were the lowest responders for an increased performance time in an exercise test, whereas other high responders to maximal O_2 uptake were high responders for performance time (50).

> ## KEY POINT
>
> The use of genomics to investigate inherited genes will allow predictions on an individual basis regarding the types, durations, and intensities of physical training that will optimize health.

Therefore, variability in responsiveness exists both within a single adaptive change to exercise and among multiple adaptations to aerobic exercise within the same individual. A more accurate term than nonresponsiveness to exercise is heterogeneity in exercise-induced adaptations. Further compounding the complexity of individualized exercise prescription is the necessity to include such factors as exercise type variance (endurance versus strength); gene variance (at least 1000 genes predispose to chronic diseases; the metabolic syndrome includes multiple chronic diseases, so it would contain more predisposing genes than a single chronic condition); subject variance (age, sex, starting fitness level, and special conditions such as pregnancy); cultural variance (*e.g.,* religious practices); environmental variance (*e.g.,* air quality and weather conditions); and societal variance (*e.g.,* neighborhood safety, accessibility of exercise facilities, and work schedules). Furthermore, an exercise prescription must include compliance as well as the heterogeneity of the responsiveness of exercise genes. All the above will make it challenging to determine the optimum exercise prescription for each human being.

It is also clear that inheritance plays a major role in predisposing an individual to a specific disease and that physical inactivity determines whether the expression of inherited genes surpasses a biologic threshold for the overt occurrence of this disease (*i.e.*, gene–environmental interaction). Figure 27.7 illustrates the role of gene–physical inactivity interaction in determining the risk of type 2 diabetes.

In "population medicine," the same amount of physical activity is prescribed for everyone. For example, the current prescription is a minimum of 30 minutes of moderate physical activity per day to provide a minimal health benefit (U.S. Surgeon General) or 60 minutes of physical activity per day to prevent weight gain based on the average U.S. caloric intake (U.S. Institute of Medicine). However, as discussed above, a shortcoming of population medicine for physical activity is that not all individuals respond identically to physical training. Thus, individualized medicine ideally must take into account the gene polymorphisms for a given individual and formulate exercise prescriptions based on the identified cocktail of disease-susceptible and physical inactivity polymorphisms present in the individual's genome.

Population studies are ongoing in the United States with the goal of locating polymorphisms related to physical inactivity and chronic health conditions. In the HERITAGE Family Study, the aim is to use genome-wide scans, including targeted dense SNP mapping and skeletal muscle gene expression studies with serial analysis of gene expression, to search for genes and mutations. The investigators hope to document the contribution of cardiovascular and metabolic responses to endurance training, and of genetic factors to the concomitant risk of cardiovascular disease and type 2 diabetes risk factors among nearly 1000 individuals. A second population study aims to characterize environmental effects on 87 biologic and positional candidate genes for genotyping in a population-based sample of 11,000 subjects. The study addresses dietary measures, obesity, measures of physical activity, smoking, and (in women) menopause status and hormone use. The outcome of these studies could provide a foundation of polymorphisms for future personalized physical activity prescriptions by physicians to primarily prevent chronic health conditions (individualized medicine for physical activity). The success of such studies will depend on large populations of subjects. Within 100 years, it is possible that healthy patients will have access to gene chips that can predict susceptibility to future diseases based on the polymorphisms in their genome, including genes that are susceptible to physical inactivity. The goal will be to provide a personalized, preventive lifestyle prescription to prevent the interaction of physical inactivity

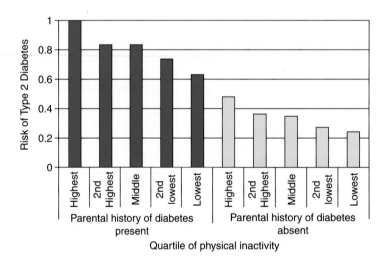

FIGURE 27.7 Predisposition to risk of type 2 diabetes depends on inherited genes (deduced from a greater prevalence with parental history of type 2 diabetes) and on environmental interaction with genes predisposing to type 2 diabetes. This figure shows the quartile of physical inactivity instead of physical activity on the X axis as the cause of type 2 because exercise does not cause type 2 diabetes, whereas physical inactivity does. The risk of type 2 diabetes respectively increases 59% and 100% from the lowest to the highest quartile of physical inactivity in siblings with and without a parental history of type 2 diabetes. The subjects were 70,102 women (46–72 years old) who had no diagnosed diabetes, cardiovascular disease, or cancer at the start of the 6-year study. (Modified with permission from Hu F, Sigal RJ, Rich-Edwards JW, et al. Walking compared with vigorous physical activity and risk of type 2 diabetes in women: a prospective study. *JAMA.* 1999;282:1433–1439.)

genes (by including a personalized physical activity plan) with existing disease susceptibility genes, and avoid crossing the threshold for development of overt clinical disease. Although the hypothesis is as yet unproved, it is anticipated that an individualized, genomics-based preventive approach to medicine will result in an improved, more cost-effective health care system.

Designation of Control Group Based on Genomics

If it is true that hunter-gatherers were more physically active in acquiring food than members of sedentary cultures, and some genes exist in the human genome because they were selected to support physical activity, then the control group based on the human genome must be the physically active group. It is speculated that the gene pool of most sedentary humans in hunter-gatherer societies would have been selected for the human genome (the lack of physical activity would not permit food gathering, and thus an early death is presumed). Thus, physical activity was the norm for nearly all of the population during nearly all of human existence on earth. It is presumed that the control group would have consisted of physically active individuals throughout evolution until sometime in the 1900s. Sedentary individuals, by virtue of their rareness (<1% of the population), could not be considered a representative control group for most of the population during more than 99% of human existence on earth. Thus, a future challenge is to designate physically active individuals as the control group for genomic studies seeking to elucidate the function of genes.

KEY POINT

Inherited genes were optimized to support physical activity for survival. In the absence of historical physical activity levels, inherited genes "misfire" and function incorrectly.

In the early 1900s, the average person included in the control group was more physically active in his or her daily routine than the average person in the late 1900s. The exercise group in the early 1900s consisted of the same cohort and was called the treatment group. The initial terminology has been retained; that is, the less physically active group is still designated as the control group. However, as of 2000, the control group has changed from including physically active individuals (*e.g.*, those who walk for transportation or perform manual labor) in 1900 to individuals who are physically inactive or sedentary. The levels of physical activity in experimental groups can be described as follows: A trained group of physically active individuals in the early 1900s was more active than in the physically active control group in the 1900s. Controls in the 1900s were about as active as

the exercise-trained group of physically active individuals in 2000, who are more active than the sedentary control group in 2000. Between 1900 and 2000, the control group designation has been retained for the group not undergoing the experimental exercise treatment, but the control group went from being physically active in 1900 to sedentary in 2000. Thus, in the future, physically active individuals should be designated as the control group because their activity levels are closer to those of the control group in the early 1900s and to the hunter-gatherer than are the sedentary majority in the United States in 2009.

Jeremy N. Morris and Ralph S. Paffenbarger, Jr., were awarded the 1996 Olympic Prize for their pioneering studies that showed that exercise protects against heart disease (56). Their research findings changed the practice of medicine, inspired the fitness revolution, and stimulated additional studies that have provided insight into the relationship between physical activity and the incidence of coronary heart disease. Morris's early studies showed that bus drivers, who of course are sedentary on the job, had more clinical heart disease than conductors, who continuously walked around a double-decker London bus. It is now well established that sedentary women have a 40% higher prevalence of coronary heart disease and stroke than middle-aged women who walk a minimum of 30 min · d^{-1}. It is a tenet in research medicine that healthy individuals are the control group and the sick patients are the treatment group. The exercise literature calls healthier, physically active individuals the treatment group and the sicker, sedentary subjects the controls. Thus, exercise physiologists are one of a few (if not the only) medical groups that designate the sicker population as the controls for experimental purposes. This assignment has led to the perception by some scientists in disciplines other than exercise that exercise as the treatment group is not normal and that sedentary is physiologically the norm. Thus, in the future, physically active individuals should be designated as the control group.

A negative byproduct of the misdesignation of the proper physical activity level for the control group is the misconception by some that the cellular and molecular mechanisms underlying exercise adaptations explain with 100% fidelity the cause of inactivity-related diseases. However, this experimental approach is flawed because exercise does not cause obesity or type 2 diabetes. To understand the mechanistic etiology of inactivity-related diseases, we must make physical inactivity the research focus. A similar tenet of medicine is that understanding the molecular mechanisms of diseases will provide the scientific basis for therapy and prevention. Again, the only way to decipher the mechanisms of disease prevention is to study the process itself as it is evoked by increased physical activity, diet, and so forth. It is therefore anticipated that future research will investigate the molecular mechanisms of the sicker, physically inactive population because physical inactivity, not activity, causes genes to misexpress proteins, producing the metabolic dysfunctions that can result in overt clinical disease if continued long enough.

Drug Development

Remarkable development of pharmaceutical agents is predicted to occur with the sequencing of the human genome. Multiple references to an exercise pill have appeared in news reports. However, attractive this idea may be, the term *exercise pill* is a misnomer because a true full-exercise pill would produce at least some of the following effects:

- Physiologic cardiac hypertrophy
- Bradycardia
- Enhanced nitric oxide synthase in vascular endothelial cells
- Lower systolic blood pressure
- Decreased arterial stiffness
- Less prevalence of stroke
- Cardioprotective effect
- Higher blood levels of high-density lipoprotein
- Improved cognitive function
- Lower incidence of depression
- Better immune function
- Less C-reactive protein
- Skeletal muscle hypertrophy and prevention of physical frailty
- Increased skeletal muscle mitochondria and capacity to oxidize fatty acids
- Increased whole body insulin sensitivity
- Reduction in colon and breast cancers
- Increased bone density
- Normal body mass index

Any single pill that could incorporate one or two of the aforementioned benefits would accurately be termed a *small-part exercise pill*. People would miss out on the many health benefits that can be gained from exercise if they were induced to give up physical activity. Nonetheless, such a pill would be of great benefit to those who are unable to exercise. However, the developers of such a drug would have a responsibility to ensure its proper usage.

Future Research Questions That Can Be Addressed with Genomics and Proteomic Methods

KEY POINT

In this chapter, we have provided a look into the future. As such, the answers to the following questions are not answered here. They remain to be addressed in future studies.

- What are the mechanisms by which mechanical loading hypertrophies human skeletal muscle?
- Why is mechanical loading in microgravity less effective for stimulating hypertrophy of skeletal muscle than loading in full gravity?
- What are the differential gene expressions between exercise-induced physiologic cardiac hypertrophy and cardiac pathophysiology?
- Should exercise-induced hypertrophic hearts rather than atrophied sedentary hearts be the norm for clinical medicine?
- What are the mechanisms by which bone loading during physical activity reduces the risk of osteoporosis?
- What are the underlying mechanisms for loss of muscle fibers and motor units with aging? Which is lost first? Do muscle fibers cause the loss of nerves, or does motor neuron loss initiate the loss of muscle fibers?
- What are the mechanisms that cause aged skeletal muscle to exhibit defective muscle regrowth after atrophy?
- By what mechanisms does physical inactivity increase the risk of most site-specific cancers, including breast, colon, lung, rectal, and pancreatic cancer?
- By what mechanisms does physical activity maintain somatic cells in a nonimmortalized condition?
- How is blood flow regulated through the microcirculation during exercise?
- By what mechanisms does moderate exercise enhance the immune system?
- What mechanisms are involved in moderate exercise that can suppress local inflammation, such as in the walls of arterial blood vessels?
- How does muscle inactivity cause insulin resistance?
- By what mechanisms does muscle inactivity initiate prediabetes?
- What additional signaling mechanisms to AMPK activate glucose transport in response to contractile activity?
- What is the connection among physical inactivity, mitochondrial dysfunction, and insulin resistance?
- How many ways does skeletal muscle communicate with other organs and tissues?
- Is skeletal muscle an endocrine organ?
- How is the metabolic state of the working skeletal muscle communicated to the brain? Does it use type III or IV sensory neurons?
- What are the mechanisms by which physical activity improves learning, memory, and cognitive function?
- By what mechanisms does physical activity reduce the risk of disorders of cognitive dysfunction?
- What are the physical activity mechanisms by which satellite cells are activated, proliferate, and fuse into muscle fibers?
- Are there genes whose expression produces sedentary behavior?
- What are the connecting pathways by which the lack of food drives increased physical activity?

A MILESTONE OF DISCOVERY

In July of 1984, Watson and colleagues (51) published what appears to be the earliest study in which changes in a specific messenger RNA (mRNA) in response to altered contractile activity were measured. Their study was preceded by numerous works that reported changes in specific mRNAs during myoblast differentiation in culture. However, the study by Watson et al. differed in that it reported the relative content of α-actin-mRNA in gastrocnemius muscle of living rats. They found that α-actin mRNA significantly decreased after 7 days of rat hindlimb immobilization, but was not changed after 6 or 72 hours of immobilization. In contrast, actin protein synthesis decreased at the sixth hour of immobilization, which led them to conclude that a change in the content of alpha-actin mRNA did not contribute significantly to the rapid onset of the decreased actin protein synthesis rate observed after 6 hours of immobilization. In 1986, Williams et al. (52) reported that after 21 days of electrical stimulation of a motor nerve, aldolase mRNA fell to one-fourth of control levels, whereas cytochrome *b* mRNA increased fivefold. These two studies inaugurated the era of exercise molecular biology.

Watson PA, Stein JP, Booth FW. Changes in actin synthesis and alpha-actin-mRNA content in rat muscle during immobilization. Am J Physiol. 1984;247:C39–C44.

ACKNOWLEDGMENTS

J. Scott Pattison and Matthew J. Laye assisted in writing the section on genomic methodology. The chapter was written while the authors were supported by National Institutes of Health grants AR19393 (FWB) and AR45372 (PDN), and the chapter was revised while the authors were supported by grants AG18780 (FWB) and DK073488 (PDN) and DK074825 (PDN).

REFERENCES

1. Ashburner M, Ball CA, Blake JA. Gene Ontology: tool for the unification of biology. The Gene Ontology Consortium. *Nat Genet.* 2000;25:25–29.
2. Anderson EJ, Yamazaki H, Neufer PD. Induction of endogenous uncoupling protein 3 suppresses mitochondrial oxidant emission during fatty acid-supported respiration. *J Biol Chem.* 2007;282:31257–31266.
3. Astrand PO, Rodahl K. *Textbook of Work Physiology.* New York: McGraw-Hill; 1986.
4. Barton-Davis ER, Shoturma DI, Musaro A, et al. Viral-mediated expression of insulin-like growth factor I blocks the aging-related loss of skeletal muscle function. *Proc Natl Acad Sci USA.* 1998;95:15603–15607.
5. Booth FW. Effects of endurance exercise on cytochrome *c* turnover in skeletal muscle. *Ann N Y Acad Sci.* 1977;301:431–439.
6. Booth FW, Baldwin KM. Muscle plasticity: energy demand and supply processes. In: Rowell LB, Shepherd JT, eds. *The Handbook of Physiology. Exercise: Regulation and Integration of Multiple Systems.* New York: Oxford University; 1996:1075–1023.
7. Booth FW, Thomason DB. Molecular and cellular adaptation of muscle in response to exercise: perspectives of various models. *Physiol Rev.* 1991;71:541–585.
8. Carson JA, Schwartz RJ, Booth FW. SRF and TEF-1 control of chicken skeletal alpha-actin gene during slow-muscle hypertrophy. *Am J Physiol.* 1996;270:C1624–C1633.
9. Chakravarthy MV, Booth FW. Eating, exercise, and "thrifty" genotypes: connecting the dots toward an evolutionary understanding of modern chronic diseases. *J Appl Physiol.* 2004;96:3–10.
10. Chang PY, Jensen J, Printz RL, et al. Overexpression of hexokinase II in transgenic mice: evidence that increased phosphorylation augments muscle glucose uptake. *J Biol Chem.* 1996;271:14834–14839.
11. Chen YW, Nader GA, Baar KR, et al. Response of rat muscle to acute resistance exercise defined by transcriptional and translational profiling. *J Physiol.* 2002;545:27–41.
12. Costill D. *A Scientific Approach to Distance Running.* Los Altos: Track and Field News; 1979.
13. Cotman CW, Berchtold NC. Exercise: a behavioral intervention to enhance brain health and plasticity. *Trends Neurosci.* 2002;25:295–301.
14. Curtis RK, Brand MD. Control analysis of DNA microarray expression data. *Mol Biol Rep.* 2002;29:67–71.
15. Dudley GA, Tullson PC, Terjung RL. Influence of mitochondrial content on the sensitivity of respiratory control. *J Biol Chem.* 1987;262:9109–9114.
16. Eto Y, Yonekura K, Sonoda M, et al. Calcineurin is activated in rat hearts with physiological left ventricular hypertrophy induced by voluntary exercise training. *Circulation.* 2000;101:2134–2137.
17. Fattori E, La Monica N, Ciliberto G, et al. Electro-gene-transfer: a new approach for muscle gene delivery. *Somat Cell Mol Genet.* 2002;27:75–83.
18. Fazio S, Linton MF. Mouse models of hyperlipidemia and atherosclerosis. *Front Biosci.* 2001;6:D515–D525.
19. Fitzpatrick DR, Wilson CB. Methylation and demethylation in the regulation of genes, cells, and responses in the immune system. *Clin Immunol.* 2003;109:37–45.
20. Grobet L, Pirottin D, Farnir F, et al. Modulating skeletal muscle mass by postnatal, muscle-specific inactivation of the myostatin gene. *Genesis.* 2003;35:227–238.
21. Gusev Y. Computational methods for analysis of cellular functions and pathways collectively targeted by differentially expressed microRNA. *Methods.* 2008;44:61–72.
22. Haggmark T, Eriksson E, Jansson E. Muscle fiber type changes in human skeletal muscle after injuries and immobilization. *Orthopedics.* 1986;9:181–185.
23. Halseth AE, Bracy DP, Wasserman DH. Overexpression of hexokinase II increases insulin and exercise-stimulated muscle glucose uptake in vivo. *Am J Physiol.* 1999;276:E70–E77.
24. Hanis CL, Boerwinkle E, Chakraborty R, et al. A genome-wide search for human non-insulin-dependent (type 2) diabetes genes reveals a major susceptibility locus on chromosome 2. *Nat Genet.* 1996;13:161–166.
25. Hawley JA, Zierath JR. Integration of metabolic and mitogenic signal transduction in skeletal muscle. *Exerc Sport Sci Rev.* 2004;32:4–8.
26. Hickson RC. Skeletal muscle cytochrome *c* and myoglobin, endurance, and frequency of training. *J Appl Physiol.* 1981;51:746–749.
27. Hildebrandt AL, Pilegaard H, Neufer PD. Differential transcriptional activation of select metabolic genes in response to variations in exercise intensity and duration. *Am J Physiol Endocrinol Metab.* 2003;285:E1021–E1027.

28. Holloszy JO. Biochemical adaptations in muscle: effects of exercise on mitochondrial oxygen uptake and respiratory enzyme activity in skeletal muscle. *J Biol Chem.* 1967;242:2278–2282.

29. Keller C, Steensberg A, Pilegaard H, et al. Transcriptional activation of the IL-6 gene in human contracting skeletal muscle: influence of muscle glycogen content. *FASEB J.* 2001;15:2748–2750.

30. Keller P, Vollaard N, Babraj J, et al. Using systems biology to define the essential biological networks responsible for adaptation to endurance exercise training. *Biochem Soc Trans.* 2007;35:1306–1309.

31. Kitamura T, Mishina M, Sugiyama H. Enhancement of neurogenesis by running wheel exercises is suppressed in mice lacking NMDA receptor epsilon 1 subunit. *Neurosci Res.* 2003;47: 55–63.

32. Laurin D, Verreault R, Lindsay J, et al. Physical activity and risk of cognitive impairment and dementia in elderly persons. *Arch Neurol.* 2001;58:498–504.

33. Massie CE, Mills IG. ChIPping away at gene regulation. *EMBO Rep* 2008;9:337–343.

34. McCarthy JJ, Esser KA. MicroRNA-1 and microRNA-133a expression are decreased during skeletal muscle hypertrophy. *J Appl Physiol.* 2007;102:306–313.

35. McPherron AC, Lawler AM, Lee SJ. Regulation of skeletal muscle mass in mice by a new TGF-beta superfamily member. *Nature.* 1997;387:83–90.

36. Molkentin JD, Lu JR, Antos CL, et al. A calcineurin-dependent transcriptional pathway for cardiac hypertrophy. *Cell.* 1998; 93:215–228.

37. Neel JV. Diabetes mellitus: a "thrifty" genotype rendered detrimental by "progress"? *Am J Hum Genet.* 1962;14:353–362.

38. Pattison JS, Folk LC, Madsen RW, et al. Expression profiling identifies dysregulation of myosin heavy chains IIb and IIx during limb immobilization in the soleus muscles of old rats. *J Physiol.* 2003;553:357–368.

39. Pette D, Vrbova G. Adaptation of mammalian skeletal muscle fibers to chronic electrical stimulation. *Rev Physiol Biochem Pharmacol.* 1992;120:115–202.

40. Pilegaard H, Keller C, Steensberg A, et al. Influence of pre-exercise muscle glycogen content on exercise-induced transcriptional regulation of metabolic genes. *J Physiol.* 2002;541:261–271.

41. Pilegaard H, Ordway GA, Saltin B, et al. Transcriptional regulation of gene expression in human skeletal muscle during recovery from exercise. *Am J Physiol Endocrinol Metab.* 2000;279:E806–E814.

42. Richter EA, Derave W, Wojtaszewski JF. Glucose, exercise and insulin: emerging concepts. *J Physiol.* 2001;535:313–322.

43. Rothermel BA, McKinsey TA, Vega RB, et al. Myocyte-enriched calcineurin-interacting protein, MCIP1, inhibits cardiac hypertrophy in vivo. *Proc Natl Acad Sci USA.* 2001;98:3328–3333.

44. Ryding AD, Sharp MG, Mullins JJ. Conditional transgenic technologies. *J Endocrinol.* 2001;171:1–14.

45. Singh SK, Pal Bhadra M, Girschick HJ, et al. MicroRNAs—micro in size but macro in function. *FEBS J.* 2008;275:4929–4944.

46. Sisson SB, Katzmarzyk PT, Earnest CP, et al. Volume of exercise and fitness nonresponse in sedentary, postmenopausal women. *Med Sci Sports Exerc.* 2009;41:539–545.

47. Sugden MC, Holness MJ. Recent advances in mechanisms regulating glucose oxidation at the level of the pyruvate dehydrogenase complex by PDKs. *Am J Physiol Endocrinol Metab.* 2003;284:E855–E862.

48. Terjung RL, Hood DA. Biochemical adaptations in skeletal muscle induced by exercise training. In: Washington LD, ed. *Nutrition and Aerobic Exercise.* Washington, DC: American Chemical Society; 1986:8–27.

49. van der Neut R. Targeted gene disruption: applications in neurobiology. *J Neurosci Methods.* 1997;71(1):19–27.

50. Vollaard NB, Constantin-Teodosiu D, Fredriksson K, et al. Systematic analysis of adaptations in aerobic capacity and submaximal energy metabolism provides a unique insight into determinants of human aerobic performance. *J Appl Physiol.* 2009;106:1479–1486.

51. Watson PA, Stein JP, Booth FW. Changes in actin synthesis and alpha-actin-mRNA content in rat muscle during immobilization. *Am J Physiol.* 1984;247:C39–C44.

52. Williams RS, Salmons S, Newsholme EA, et al. Regulation of nuclear and mitochondrial gene expression by contractile activity in skeletal muscle. *J Biol Chem.* 1986;261:376–380.

53. Williams RS, Wagner PD. Transgenic animals in integrative biology: approaches and interpretations of outcome. *J Appl Physiol.* 2000;88:1119–1126.

54. Wu P, Sato J, Zhao Y, et al. Starvation and diabetes increase the amount of pyruvate dehydrogenase kinase isoenzyme 4 in rat heart. *Biochem J.* 1998;329(pt 1):197–201.

55. Zhang CL, McKinsey TA, Olson EN. Association of class II histone deacetylases with heterochromatin protein 1: potential role for histone methylation in control of muscle differentiation. *Mol Cell Biol.* 2002;22:7302–7312.

56. Morris JN, Heady JA, Raffle PAB, et al. Coronary heart disease and physical activity of work. *Lancet.* 1953;2:1053–1057.

INDEX

Note: Page numbers in *italics* refer to illustrations; page numbers followed by "t" refer to tables.

699